Lauri Matey, MSN, RN, CHPN
Clinical Services Director
Hospice of Southern Maine
Scarborough, Maine
Chapter 4. Overview of Cancer and Cancer Treatment

Haleigh E. Mistry, MS, PA-C
Physician Assistant
Department of Lymphoma and Myeloma
University of Texas MD Anderson Cancer Center
Houston, Texas
Chapter 15. Gastrointestinal and Mucosal Toxicities

Sandra A. Mitchell, PhD, CRNP, AOCN®
Research Scientist
Outcomes Research Branch
Division of Cancer Control and Population Sciences
National Cancer Institute
Bethesda, Maryland
Chapter 23. Fatigue

Kathy Mooney, MSN, RN, ACNS-BC, BMTCN®, OCN®
Clinical Nurse Specialist
Sidney Kimmel Comprehensive Cancer Center at Johns Hopkins Hospital
Baltimore, Maryland
Chapter 21. Cutaneous Toxicities and Alopecia

Ryan W. Naseman, PharmD, MS, BCPS
Assistant Director of Pharmacy
James Cancer Hospital
The Ohio State University Wexner Medical Center
Columbus, Ohio
Chapter 6. Chemotherapy

Elizabeth Ness, MS, BSN, RN
Director, Office of Education and Compliance
Center for Cancer Research
National Cancer Institute
National Institutes of Health
Bethesda, Maryland
Chapter 5. Clinical Trials and Drug Development

Martha Polovich, PhD, RN, AOCN®
Assistant Professor
Byrdine F. Lewis College of Nursing and Health Professions
Georgia State University
Atlanta, Georgia
Chapter 12. Safe Handling of Hazardous Drugs

Zandra R. Rivera, DNP, RN, ANP-BC, BMTCN®
Advanced Practice Registered Nurse
University of Texas MD Anderson Cancer Center
Houston, Texas
Chapter 18. Hepatic Toxicities

Lisa Schulmeister, MN, RN, FAAN
Oncology Nursing Consultant
New Orleans, Louisiana
Chapter 13. Infusion-Related Complications

Brenda K. Shelton, DNP, RN, APRN-CNS, CCRN, AOCN®
Clinical Nurse Specialist
Sidney Kimmel Comprehensive Cancer Center at Johns Hopkins Hospital
Baltimore, Maryland
Chapter 17. Pulmonary Toxicities

Lisa Hartkopf Smith, MS, RN, AOCN®, CHPN
Oncology Clinical Nurse Specialist
OhioHealth Riverside Methodist Hospital
Columbus, Ohio
Chapter 1. Professional Practice Considerations; Chapter 11. Administration Considerations

Darryl Somayaji, PhD, RN, CCRC
Assistant Professor
School of Nursing, University at Buffalo
Buffalo, New York
Chapter 26. Post-Treatment and Survivorship Care

Kelli Thoele, MSN, RN, ACNS-BC, BMTCN®, OCN®
Robert Wood Johnson Foundation Future of Nursing Scholar
PhD Student, Indiana University
Clinical Nurse Specialist
Indiana University Health
Indianapolis, Indiana
Chapter 15. Gastrointestinal and Mucosal Toxicities

Barbara J. Wilson, MS, RN, AOCN®, ACNS-BC
Director, Oncology Professional Practice
WellStar Health System
Marietta, Georgia
Chapter 14. Myelosuppression

Disclosure

Editors and authors of books and guidelines provided by the Oncology Nursing Society are expected to disclose to the readers any significant financial interest or other relationships with the manufacturer(s) of any commercial products.

A vested interest may be considered to exist if a contributor is affiliated with or has a financial interest in commercial organizations that may have a direct or indirect interest in the subject matter. A "financial interest" may include, but is not limited to, being a shareholder in the organization; being an employee of the commercial organization; serving on an organization's speakers bureau; or receiving research funding from the organization. An "affiliation" may be holding a position on an advisory board or some other role of benefit to the commercial organization. Vested interest statements appear in the front matter for each publication.

Contributors are expected to disclose any unlabeled or investigational use of products discussed in their content. This information is acknowledged solely for the information of the readers.

The contributors provided the following disclosure and vested interest information:

MiKaela M. Olsen, APRN-CNS, MS, AOCNS®, FAAN: Becton, Dickinson and Company, honoraria

Kristine B. LeFebvre, MSN, RN, AOCN®: American Nurses Credentialing Center, other remuneration

Kelly J. Brassil, PhD, RN, AOCNS®: Genentech, Inc., Premier, Inc., consultant or advisory role; Oncology Nursing Society, honoraria; Genentech, Inc., research funding

Kristine D. Abueg, RN, MSN, OCN®, CBCN®: Greater Sacramento Chapter Oncology Nursing Society, honoraria

Mary K. Anderson, BSN, RN, OCN®: Rigel Pharmaceuticals, Inc., Taiho Oncology, Inc., consultant or advisory role

Fedricker D. Barber, PhD, ANP-BC, AOCNP®: Oncology Nursing Society, employment or leadership position

Virginia Rose Bayer, BSN, RN, CCRP: University of Texas MD Anderson Cancer Center, expert testimony

Lanell M. Bellury, PhD, RN, AOCNS®, OCN®: Georgia Center for Oncology Research and Education, consultant or advisory role

Veronica Joyce Brady, PhD, MSN, FNP-BC, BC-ADM, CDE: Diabetes Improvement Through Management and Education Study, consultant or advisory role; Nevada Health Information Management Association, Nevada Primary Care Association, honoraria

Victoria Tkacz Brown, PharmD, BCOP: Hematology/Oncology Pharmacy Association, honoraria

Bradley Burton, PharmD, BCOP: Oncology Reimbursement Management, consultant or advisory role

Nancy Corbitt, BSN, RN, OCN®, CRNI: Bristol-Myers Squibb, consultant or advisory role

Sheryl G. Forbes, PhD, MEd, RN, CCRP: International Association of Clinical Research Nurses, employment or leadership position

RuthAnn Gordon, MSN, FNP-BC, OCN®: Creative Educational Concepts, consultant or advisory role

Natalie Jackson, MSN, FNP-C: Oncology Nursing Society, honoraria

Patricia Jakel, RN, MN, AOCN®: Genentech, Inc., Merck and Co., Inc., consultant or advisory role; Genentech, Inc., ONS Foundation, honoraria

Alice S. Kerber, MN, APRN, ACNS-BC, AOCN®, AGN-BC: Pfizer Inc., honoraria

Martha Polovich, PhD, RN, AOCN®: Becton, Dickinson and Company, honoraria, other remuneration

Lisa Hartkopf Smith, MS, RN, AOCN®, CHPN: Genentech, Inc., honoraria

Barbara J. Wilson, MS, RN, AOCN®, ACNS-BC: Amgen Inc., Genentech, Inc., honoraria

Contents

Abbreviations Used

ABC—adenosine triphosphate–binding cassette
AC—anthracycline plus cyclophosphamide
ACCC—Association of Community Cancer Centers
ACE—angiotensin-converting enzyme
ACoS CoC—American College of Surgeons Commission on Cancer
ACS—American Cancer Society
ACVBP—doxorubicin, cyclophosphamide, vindesine, bleomycin, prednisone
ADL—activities of daily living
AE—adverse event
AHRQ—Agency for Healthcare Research and Quality
AI—aromatase inhibitor
AIDS—acquired immunodeficiency syndrome
AJCC—American Joint Committee on Cancer
AKI—acute kidney injury
ALK—anaplastic lymphoma kinase
ALL—acute lymphoblastic leukemia
ALP—alkaline phosphatase
ALT—alanine aminotransferase
AML—acute myeloid leukemia
ANA—American Nurses Association
ANC—absolute neutrophil count
ANLL—acute nonlymphocytic leukemia
anti-HBc—hepatitis B core antibody
APL—acute promyelocytic leukemia
APOE—apolipoprotein E
ara-C—cytarabine
ARDS—acute respiratory distress syndrome
ASCO—American Society of Clinical Oncology
ASHP—American Society of Health-System Pharmacists
ASM—aggressive systemic mastocytosis
AST—aspartate aminotransferase
ATRA—all-trans-retinoic acid
AUC—area under the plasma concentration versus time curve
BCG—bacillus Calmette-Guérin
BCRP—breast cancer resistance protein
BDNF—brain-derived neurotrophic factor
BID—twice daily
BMD—bone mineral density
BMI—body mass index
BNP—B-type (brain) natriuretic peptide
bpm—beats per minute
BRCA—breast cancer gene
BSA—body surface area
BSC—biosafety cabinet
BTK—Bruton tyrosine kinase
BUN—blood urea nitrogen
CAB—combined androgen blockade
CACI—compounding aseptic containment isolator
CAR—chimeric antigen receptor
CBC—complete blood count
CBT—cognitive behavioral therapy
CBT-I—cognitive behavioral therapy for insomnia
CD—cluster of differentiation
CDK—cyclin-dependent kinase
CHF—congestive heart failure
CHOP—cyclophosphamide, doxorubicin, vincristine, prednisone
CI—confidence interval
CIN—chemotherapy-induced neutropenia
CINV—chemotherapy-induced nausea and vomiting
CIPN—chemotherapy-induced peripheral neuropathy
CLL—chronic lymphocytic leukemia
CML—chronic myeloid leukemia
CNS—central nervous system
COPD—chronic obstructive pulmonary disease
C-PEC—containment primary engineering control
CPK—creatine phosphokinase
CR—complete response
CrCl—creatinine clearance
CRF—cancer-related fatigue
CRS—cytokine release syndrome
CSTD—closed-system drug-transfer device
CT—computed tomography
CTCAE—Common Terminology Criteria for Adverse Events
CTEP—Cancer Therapy Evaluation Program
CTLA-4—cytotoxic T-lymphocyte antigen 4
CTZ—chemoreceptor trigger zone
CVD—cardiovascular disease
CYP—cytochrome P450
D5W—5% dextrose in water
DBP—diastolic blood pressure
DEHP—di(2-ethylhexyl) phthalate
DHEA—dehydroepiandrosterone
DLBCL—diffuse large B-cell lymphoma
DLCO—diffusing capacity of the lung for carbon monoxide
DNA—deoxyribonucleic acid
DTR—deep tendon reflexes
EBMT—European Society for Blood and Marrow Transplantation
ECG—electrocardiogram
echo—echocardiography
ECOG—Eastern Cooperative Oncology Group
EEG—electroencephalogram
EGFR—epidermal growth factor receptor
EGFRI—epidermal growth factor receptor inhibitor
EML4—echinoderm microtubule-associated protein-like 4
EPO—erythropoietin
ESA—erythropoiesis-stimulating agent
estCrCl—estimated creatinine clearance
FAACT—Functional Assessment of Anorexia/Cachexia Therapy
FDA—U.S. Food and Drug Administration
FDG—fluorodeoxyglucose
^{18}F-FDG—fluorine-18 fluorodeoxyglucose
FiO_2—fraction of inspired oxygen
5-FU—5-fluorouracil
$5\text{-}HT_3$—5-hydroxytryptamine-3
FLT3—FMS-like tyrosine kinase 3
FLT3-ITD—FLT3–internal tandem duplication
FSH—follicle-stimulating hormone
G_0—gap 0
G_1—gap 1
G_2—gap 2
G-CSF—granulocyte–colony-stimulating factor
GD2—ganglioside
GFR—glomerular filtration rate
GGT—gamma glutamyl transferase
GI—gastrointestinal
GIST—gastrointestinal stromal tumor
GM-CSF—granulocyte macrophage–colony-stimulating factor
GVHD—graft-versus-host disease
Gy—gray
H—histamine
HAMAs—human anti-mouse antibodies
HBsAg—hepatitis B surface antigen
HBV—hepatitis B virus
HCl—hydrochloride
HCV—hepatitis C virus

HCW—healthcare worker
HD—hazardous drug
HDAC—histone deacetylase
HEPA—high-efficiency particulate air
HER—human epidermal growth factor receptor
Hgb—hemoglobin
HGFR—hepatocyte growth factor receptor
HIF-1—hypoxia-inducible factor-1
HIPEC—heated intraperitoneal chemotherapy
HIV—human immunodeficiency virus
HL—Hodgkin lymphoma
HNC—head and neck cancer
HNSCC—head and neck squamous cell carcinoma
HPV—human papillomavirus
HR—hormone receptor
HSC—hematopoietic stem cell
HSCT—hematopoietic stem cell transplantation
HTN—hypertension
IAP/APA—International Association of Pancreatology/American Pancreatic Association
IC—informed consent
IDH2—isocitrate dehydrogenase
IFN—interferon
IFRT—involved-field radiation therapy
Ig—immunoglobulin
IgE—immunoglobulin E
IGF-1R—insulin-like growth factor 1 receptor
IL—interleukin
ILD—interstitial lung disease
IM—intramuscular
IND—investigational new drug
INR—international normalized ratio
INSR—insulin receptor
irAE—immune-related adverse event
IRB—institutional review board
ISMP—Institute for Safe Medication Practices
ISONG—International Society of Nurses in Genetics
ISOO—International Society of Oral Oncology
IT—intrathecal
IV—intravenous
IVP—intravenous push
IVPB— intravenous piggyback
JAK2—Janus kinase-2
LDH—lactate dehydrogenase
LFT—liver function test
LH—luteinizing hormone
LHRH—luteinizing hormone–releasing hormone
LLN—lower limit of normal
LV—leucovorin
LVEF—left ventricular ejection fraction
M—mitosis
mAb—monoclonal antibody
MAP—mitogen-activated protein
MASCC—Multinational Association of Supportive Care in Cancer
MCV—mean corpuscular volume
MDR1—multidrug resistance protein 1
MDS—myelodysplastic syndrome
MHC—major histocompatibility complex
MI—myocardial infarction
MIU—million international units
MOPP—mechlorethamine, vincristine, procarbazine, prednisone
MRI—magnetic resonance imaging
mRNA—messenger RNA
MRSA—methicillin-resistant *Staphylococcus aureus*
ms—millisecond
MTD—maximum tolerated dose
mTOR—mammalian target of rapamycin
MUGA—multigated acquisition
NaCl—sodium chloride
NCCN—National Comprehensive Cancer Network
NCI—National Cancer Institute
NDA—new drug application
NET—neuroendocrine tumor
NHL—non-Hodgkin lymphoma
NIDDK—National Institute of Diabetes and Digestive and Kidney Diseases
NIOSH—National Institute for Occupational Safety and Health
NK_1—neurokinin-1
NK—natural killer
NKT—natural killer T
NLM—National Library of Medicine
NPH—neutral protamine Hagedorn
NS—normal saline
NSAID—nonsteroidal anti-inflammatory drug
NSCLC—non-small cell lung cancer
n/v—nausea and vomiting
NYHA—New York Heart Association
O_2—oxygen
OAC—oral agent for cancer
OBI—on-body injector
ONS—Oncology Nursing Society
OSHA—Occupational Safety and Health Administration
PAP—prostatic acid phosphatase
PARP—poly(ADP-ribose) polymerase
PCR—polymerase chain reaction
PD-1—programmed cell death protein 1
PDE5—phosphodiesterase type 5
PDGF—platelet-derived growth factor
PDGFR—platelet-derived growth factor receptor
PD-L1—programmed cell death-ligand 1
PD-L2—programmed cell death-ligand 2
PE—pulmonary embolism
PEB—cisplatin, etoposide, bleomycin
PEG-G-CSF—pegylated granulocyte–colony-stimulating factor
PEP—Putting Evidence Into Practice
PERCIST—Positron Emission Tomography Response Criteria in Solid Tumors
PET—positron-emission tomography
PET-CT—positron-emission tomography–computed tomography
PFT—pulmonary function test
PFU—plaque-forming units
P-gp—P-glycoprotein
Ph—Philadelphia chromosome
PI3K—phosphoinositide 3-kinase
PJP—*Pneumocystis jiroveci* pneumonia
PML—progressive multifocal leukoencephalopathy
PMN/poly—polymorphonuclear neutrophil
pNET—pancreatic neuroendocrine tumor
PO—by mouth
PPE—personal protective equipment
PPI—proton pump inhibitor
PR—partial response; progesterone receptor
PRES—posterior reversible encephalopathy syndrome
PRN—as needed
PRO—patient-reported outcomes
PROMIS SexFS—Patient-Reported Outcomes Measurement Information System Sexual Function and Satisfaction Measure
PT—prothrombin time
PVC—polyvinyl chloride
Q5M—every 5 minutes
Q10M—every 10 minutes
Q15M—every 15 minutes
QID—four times daily
QOL—quality of life
QTc—QT interval corrected
QTcF—corrected QT interval using Fridericia's calculation
RANK—receptor activator of nuclear factor kappa-B
RANKL—receptor activator of nuclear factor kappa-B ligand
RBC—red blood cell
RCC—renal cell carcinoma
RECIST—Response Evaluation Criteria in Solid Tumors
rHu—recombinant human
RIT—radioimmunotherapy
RNA—ribonucleic acid
RPLS—reversible posterior leukoencephalopathy syndrome
RR—relative risk
RSO—radiation safety officer
RT—radiation therapy
S—synthesis
SBP—systolic blood pressure
SC—subcutaneous
SCF—stem cell factor
SCLC—small cell lung cancer
SCP—survivorship care plan
SCr—serum creatinine
SDS—safety data sheet
segs—segmented neutrophils
SERM—selective estrogen receptor modulator
SIADH—syndrome of inappropriate antidiuretic hormone secretion
SIR—standardized incidence ratio
6-MP—6-mercaptopurine
SLAMF7—signaling lymphocytic activation molecule family member 7
SLL—small lymphocytic lymphoma
SMN—second malignant neoplasm

SOS—sinusoidal obstruction syndrome
SPF—sun protection factor
SpO_2—blood oxygen saturation level
SSRI—selective serotonin reuptake inhibitor
TBI—total body irradiation
T-DM1—ado-trastuzumab emtansine
TdP—torsades de pointes
TEC—toxic erythema of chemotherapy
T4—thyroxine
TH1, TH2—helper T cells
TID—three times daily
TKI—tyrosine kinase inhibitor
TLS—tumor lysis syndrome
TPO—thrombopoietin
Tregs—regulatory T cells
TSH—thyroid-stimulating hormone
UA—urinalysis
ULN—upper limit of normal
USP—U.S. Pharmacopeial Convention
UV—ultraviolet
VAD—venous access device
VC—vomiting center
VEGF—vascular endothelial growth factor
VEGFR—vascular endothelial growth factor receptor
VOD—veno-occlusive disease
VSP—vascular signaling pathway
VTE—venous thromboembolism
WBC—white blood cell
WHO—World Health Organization

Preface

It is with great pride that we introduce the first edition of the Oncology Nursing Society's *Chemotherapy and Immunotherapy Guidelines and Recommendations for Practice.* This book is an update of the classic foundational volume, *Chemotherapy and Biotherapy Guidelines and Recommendations for Practice,* which had four editions published. The new title emphasizes the existence of many new categories of drugs that use the immune system to support or treat patients with cancer.

In fact, the book has been completely reorganized to include a new chapter on immunotherapy. This chapter details six categories of immunotherapeutic approaches: checkpoint inhibitors, chimeric antigen receptor T-cell therapy, cytokines, monoclonal antibodies (including radioimmunotherapy), immunomodulators, and oncolytic viral therapies. Other chapters that have been added or expanded include those on chemotherapy agents, molecularly targeted antineoplastic agents, and hormone therapy. Drug tables in each chapter include detailed information to guide nurses during administration of antineoplastic therapy and supportive care medications. New figures, tables, and algorithms are included to provide quick access to content.

The pathophysiology and management of toxicities related to antineoplastic treatment are extensively detailed within individual chapters, with evidence-based guidelines to direct nursing practice. The timely addition of the unique side effects of immunotherapy agents and their management is important, as nurses gain knowledge to expertly recognize and manage these serious and potentially life-threatening toxicities. Safe administration of cancer therapies, including a chapter to guide oncology nurses in the prevention and management of infusion-related reactions (e.g., hypersensitivity, cytokine release syndrome, infiltration and extravasation), is included, with current evidence-based strategies.

The new volume provides content on professional considerations such as scope and standards, professional education, policies and procedures, antineoplastic medication safety, ethical and legal issues, and patient education. Adhering to national, state, and institutional standards is a fundamental responsibility of all nurses. The guidelines explain and reference standards that oncology nurses should be aware of and follow. Each section details the requirements of these standards for nurses.

The editors want to thank all the contributors who came forward to make this publication a reality. This work builds upon the knowledge of many generations of oncology nurses and has been used both nationally and internationally to inform oncology nursing practice. We are proud to continue to serve oncology nurses throughout the world with an essential resource to guide their practice.

MiKaela M. Olsen, APRN-CNS, MS, AOCNS®, FAAN
Kristine B. LeFebvre, MSN, RN, AOCN®
Kelly J. Brassil, PhD, RN, AOCNS®

SECTION I

Professional Practice Considerations

CHAPTER 1

Professional Practice Considerations

A. Scope and standards

1. Administration of chemotherapy, targeted therapy, and immunotherapy in a variety of settings is within the oncology nurse's scope of practice (Brant & Wickham, 2013).
2. Professional nursing practice is defined and regulated at four levels (American Nurses Association, 2015).
   a) Practice is defined nationally through the scopes and standards of practice, codes of ethics, and specialty certifications.
   b) States regulate practice through boards of nursing and nurse practice acts.
   c) Institutions outline policies and procedures.
   d) Nurses are individually licensed and consequently are responsible for their individual decisions and actions.
3. In 2008, the American Society of Clinical Oncology (ASCO) and the Oncology Nursing Society (ONS) began an ongoing collaboration to define and later revise safety standards for chemotherapy and other antineoplastic agents. The ASCO/ONS Chemotherapy Administration Safety Standards (Neuss et al., 2016) address staffing-related issues, antineoplastic therapy planning, documentation, orders, preparation, patient education, administration, and monitoring, with application to all settings and patient populations.

B. Professional education

1. To promote a safe level of care for individuals receiving chemotherapy, targeted therapy, and immunotherapy, each institution or supporting agency should provide specialized education and preparation consisting of didactic learning followed by successful completion of a clinical practicum (ONS, 2017).
2. Didactic content is comprehensive, current, and evidence based. At the conclusion of the didactic course, the nurse demonstrates an understanding of the following, as identified in the ONS (2017) position statement on the education of the nurse who administers chemotherapy, targeted therapy, and immunotherapy:
   a) Types, classifications, and routes of administration
   b) Pharmacology of agents, regardless of indications for use
   c) Pertinent molecular biomarkers
   d) Chemotherapy and radiation therapy protectants
   e) Principles of safe preparation, storage, labeling, transportation, and disposal of agents
   f) Administration procedures
   g) Appropriate use and disposal of personal protective equipment (PPE)
   h) Assessment, monitoring, and management of patients receiving therapy in the care setting
   i) Patient and family education for these agents, specific to side effects and related symptom management, and process for urgent and ongoing follow-up
   j) Assessment of, education on, and management of post-treatment care, including follow-up care procedures, late or long-term side effects, and physical and psychosocial aspects of survivorship
3. The clinical practicum allows the nurse to apply the knowledge gained in the didactic component to direct patient care situations. Emphasis is placed on the clinical skills that a nurse must demonstrate prior to being deemed competent to administer chemotherapy, targeted therapy, and immunotherapy (see Appendices A and B). At the completion of the clinical practicum, the nurse will be able to perform the following:
   a) Demonstrate proficiency regarding the safe preparation (when applicable), storage, transport, handling, spill management, adminis-

tration, and disposal of antineoplastic drugs and equipment.

b) Identify appropriate physical and laboratory assessments for specific agents.

c) Demonstrate skill in venipuncture, including vein selection and maintenance of the site during and after drug administration.

d) Demonstrate skill in the care and use of various vascular access devices.

e) Identify patient and family education needs in relation to agents.

f) Identify acute local or systemic reactions (including extravasation and anaphylaxis) in association with antineoplastic drugs, and identify appropriate interventions.

g) Demonstrate proficiency in the safe administration of hazardous drugs (HDs) and disposal of contaminated waste and equipment.

h) Demonstrate knowledge of institutional policies and procedures regarding antineoplastic administration.

i) Document pertinent information in the medical record.

4. Clinical activities

a) Pair nurses who are new to antineoplastic drug administration with an experienced nurse who can serve as preceptor, providing clinical supervision and instruction (Lockhart, 2016).

b) The preceptor and the nurse establish specific objectives at the beginning of the clinical practicum. Ideally, the nurse and preceptor select an assignment of patients, and the nurse assumes responsibility for planning and providing care for these patients under the guidance and supervision of the preceptor.

c) The length of time spent in the clinical practicum should be individualized depending on the nurse's ability and skill in meeting the specific objectives and institutional requirements.

d) The nurse should become proficient and independent in administering nonvesicants before progressing to vesicant administration.

e) Various clinical settings can be used for the nurse to demonstrate competence in antineoplastic drug administration. It may not be realistic for all settings or agencies to provide on-site education and training. Alternative methods can be used, such as the following:

(1) Contracting with larger institutions for didactic education or clinical experience, including experience for specific needs (e.g., vesicant, nonvesicant, IV push, short infusion, continuous infusion)

(2) Creating or using a simulated laboratory to substitute for the clinical component

5. Evaluation: An evaluation tool based on the desired outcomes should be used to document the nurse's knowledge of and competency in the following:

a) Agents and the associated nursing implications

b) Technical skills required for the administration of agents (e.g., dose calculation, venipuncture, access device management)

c) Patient and family education about the treatment regimen

d) Steps to take in the event of an untoward response following drug administration (e.g., anaphylaxis, hypersensitivity reaction, extravasation)

6. Competency may be verified in a simulated setting (e.g., skills laboratory) or as a precepted experience in the clinical setting. Individualize the evaluation/documentation tool to meet the needs of the new nurse and the practice setting, including a minimum number of observed and documented antineoplastic drug administrations. Observed administration of at least three different agents, types, and routes (i.e., nonvesicant and vesicant; IV push and short-term infusion) is recommended.

7. Annual continuing education and ongoing competency assessment are required of staff who order, prepare, and administer antineoplastic agents (Neuss et al., 2016).

a) Educational content should be designed to meet the needs of staff in the healthcare setting and emphasize new information available.

(1) Methods that may be used to identify needs include but are not limited to clinical observation, literature review, staff or patient survey, chart audits, and quality improvement studies.

(2) Potential topics include new drugs or drug delivery, reinforcement or training on policies and procedures, and prevention and management of treatment toxicities.

b) Competency assessment is ongoing, may be done by peers or supervisory staff, and is measured in several ways (Lockhart, 2016). Examples include the following:

(1) Testing: Provide a packet of articles for the staff to read or a live educational program followed by an open-book

test to measure knowledge. Consider a pre- and post-test to measure individual knowledge gains.

(2) Return demonstration: Competency checklists can be used to document performance of a technical skill, such as the donning and doffing of PPE used during drug administration. Staff can also be observed and evaluated using a scoring rubric with a checklist of criteria detailing the steps to take in practice. Examples include monitoring a nurse administering a vesicant or completing dose verification. Actions can be observed in practice or a simulated environment and later debriefed.

(3) Simulation: Simulation provides a safe environment for staff to practice clinical and critical-thinking skills. Staff can face a clinical challenge and problem-solve the steps to be followed, such as a patient experiencing an infusion reaction or extravasation. Asking nurses, "What would you do if . . ." challenges them to consider the implications of their actions. When a simulation lab is not available, it can be done through role-playing and mock scenarios in nearly any location.

8. Antineoplastic medications administered outside designated oncology areas: The ONS (2017) position statement on the education of the nurse administering and providing care to patients receiving chemotherapy, targeted therapy, and immunotherapy applies to antineoplastic drugs regardless of route, indication, patient population, or setting.
   a) All nurses should be knowledgeable about the drugs they administer: the mode of action, side effects, and toxicity; dosage range, rate of administration, and route of excretion; potential responses; and interactions with other medications and foods.
   b) The format, length, and specific focus of educational initiatives, both didactic education and the clinical experience, may vary according to the needs of the staff and setting. Select staff may require drug- or disease-specific education, whereas others will require comprehensive education for all antineoplastic medications.
   c) Address the educational plan for all individuals working with chemotherapy, targeted therapy, and immunotherapy within institutional policy.

C. Policies and procedures

1. Policies should be developed using a systematic, evidence-based approach to promote standardization of practice within an institution. They identify and communicate expectations of practice (Dols et al., 2017).
2. Once a policy has been implemented, it is imperative that it be enforced and followed by staff. Individuals can be held liable if patient harm results from failure to follow a policy. Institutions can have liability if a policy is not clear, contrasts with another policy, or could be interpreted in different ways.
3. Collaboration between departments and professionals is recommended when creating antineoplastic policies and procedures. Input from pharmacy, medicine, nursing, environmental services, occupational health, and other departments will result in a more comprehensive policy.
4. Policies related to antineoplastic drug therapy address processes designed to promote the safe and efficient care of patients receiving these medications, regardless of setting or department. Topics include the following (Neuss et al., 2016):
   a) Qualifications, including initial educational and ongoing competency requirements, credentialing process, and documentation of staff who order, prepare, and administer chemotherapy, targeted therapy, and immunotherapy
   b) HD management, including safe drug receipt, storage, compounding, transport, PPE, equipment used to administer HDs, administration, post-treatment care, spill management, disposal of HDs, alternative duty, and medical surveillance (U.S. Pharmacopeial Convention, 2016)
   c) Order writing and dose verification, including process, standard regimens, rounding, cumulative dose, order format, and communication of modifications
   d) Informed consent process
   e) Toxicity monitoring, including standardized documentation and communication of toxicities
   f) Procedures for care in medical emergencies
   g) Communication of status during transitions of care
   h) Reporting of adverse events and near misses

D. Antineoplastic medication safety

1. Prevalence of medication errors: Medication errors cause nearly one death daily and 1.3 million injuries annually (U.S. Food and Drug Administration [FDA], 2017b).

2. Chemotherapy and other antineoplastic drugs are classified as high-alert medications by the Institute for Safe Medication Practices (ISMP, 2014). These medications have narrow therapeutic indices and multiple potential toxicities and often are administered in complex regimens, protocols, and schedules (Griffin, Gilbert, Broadfield, Easty, & Trbovich, 2016; Kullberg, Larsen, & Sharp, 2013).
3. Errors may occur at any point during the drug delivery process (Kullberg et al., 2013; Schwappach & Wernli, 2010; White, Cassano-Piché, Fields, Cheng, & Easty, 2014).
   a) Ordering/prescribing: unclear or erroneous orders, drug calculation errors, omission of antineoplastic or supportive drugs or hydration, input and transcription errors, errors in cycle or day, cumulative dose documentation or tracking
   b) Drug preparation: staging/loading the biosafety cabinet with incorrect equipment and supplies, rounding doses, reconstitution, compounding, label application, dispensing
   c) Drug administration: incorrect drug or dose, schedule or timing errors, patient identification errors, infusion rate errors, route errors
4. Contributing factors to medication errors (Fyhr, Ternov, & Ek, 2017; Keers, Williams, Cooke, & Ashcroft, 2013; Shulman, Miller, Ambinder, Yu, & Cox, 2008; World Health Organization, n.d.)
   a) Poor communication among healthcare professionals or with patients
   b) Look-alike, sound-alike medications
   c) "Batching" or preparing more than one agent at a time
   d) Distractions/interruptions
   e) Heavy workload, fatigue, stress
   f) Lack of systematic processes
   g) Medication supply and storage issues (e.g., drugs of similar names or dosage strengths stored in close proximity)
   h) Equipment failures
   i) Inadequate knowledge or experience of those ordering, preparing, or administering agents
   j) Patient factors: literacy, language barriers, complexity of care
5. System safeguards: The following strategies have been used to reduce the risk of medication errors in antineoplastic administration (Goldspiel et al., 2015; ISMP, 2014; Neuss et al., 2016; ONS, 2017).
   a) Develop policies and procedures using interprofessional collaboration, and include strategies to promote adherence.
   b) Establish a process of educational preparation and competency of those administering, preparing, or ordering chemotherapy, targeted therapy, or immunotherapy. Nurses administering antineoplastic agents are RNs qualified by education and training.
   c) Ensure current drug information and resources for drug dosing, administration, and side effects are readily available.
   d) Follow standards regarding chemotherapy, targeted therapy, and immunotherapy orders.
      (1) Orders are signed manually or by electronic approval by credentialed prescribers (ISMP, 2017; Neuss et al., 2016).
      (2) Verbal orders for chemotherapy, targeted therapy, and immunotherapy medications are not permitted, except to hold or stop drugs (ISMP, 2017; Neuss et al., 2016).
      (3) Text messaging of patient care orders is not permitted (Joint Commission, 2016).
      (4) Standardized electronic or preprinted orders should be used for chemotherapy, targeted therapy, and immunotherapy (ISMP, 2010; Neuss et al., 2016).
         (a) Orders should be regimen based and include the elements outlined by current safety standards.
         (b) Use of standardized, regimen-based preprinted or electronic orders has been shown to increase evidence-based oncology care and decrease errors (Meisenberg, Wright, & Brady-Copertino, 2014). The National Comprehensive Cancer Network® (www.nccn.org) has disease-specific guidelines and chemotherapy order templates that include suggested patient monitoring for cancer type and stage (e.g., type and timing of imaging) and treatment regimen (e.g., toxicity monitoring). See Appendix C for an example of a chemotherapy order template.
         (c) Avoid the use of abbreviations, acronyms, and other ambiguous methods of communicating drug information.
      (5) Safety advantages reported with the use of electronic prescribing over preprinted orders include the removal of interpretation or transcription errors, availability of information about drug doses and schedules, automatic calcu-

lation of medication doses, and alert and error-checking functions (Aita et al., 2013). However, some errors specific for oncology include "cut and paste" errors—propagation of errors from cutting and pasting, and errors resulting from dose reduction or medication changes not being propagated into future cycles.

(6) A policy should be in place for prescribing chemotherapy, targeted therapy, and immunotherapy regimens that vary from standard regimens. For example, the prescriber may be required to document supporting references for the variance.

e) Use safety measures provided in electronic health record systems, such as drug interaction alerts, cumulative dose calculation (when applicable), and override restrictions (Weingart, Zhu, Young-Hong, Vermilya, & Hassett, 2014).

f) Require at least two practitioners approved by the healthcare setting to administer or prepare antineoplastic agents to perform dose and drug verification for all routes of delivery before preparation, upon preparation, and prior to the administration of chemotherapy, targeted therapy, and immunotherapy (Neuss et al., 2016).

(1) Independent dual verification (i.e., independent double checks): A process in which a second person conducts a verification of the accuracy of the prescribed therapy, without revealing findings to the other verifier until both have completed the process (ISMP Canada, 2005).

(2) Numerous studies have demonstrated the ability of independent double checks to detect up to 95% of errors (Grasha, Reilley, Schell, Tranum, & Filburn, 2001; White et al., 2010).

(3) Checklists may help promote a consistent process (White et al., 2010; see Appendix D).

(4) Prior to administering antineoplastic agents, review the treatment plan and verify orders, the medication, the patient, and the pump programming (Neuss et al., 2016). See Chapter 11 for greater detail on dose verification.

(5) Conducting a comprehensive review of the medication orders rather than simply comparing the product to the order is invaluable in catching prescribing errors (ISMP, 2013).

(6) Perform drug and dose verification in a distraction-free setting.

g) Establish procedures for emergency preparedness.

(1) Provide 24/7 triage to a provider—for example, on-call practitioners or emergency departments (Neuss et al., 2016).

(2) At least one clinical staff member certified in basic life support must be present during chemotherapy administration. Staff certified in advanced cardiac life support or pediatric advanced life support may be indicated depending on the setting and types of treatments delivered (Neuss et al., 2016).

(3) Policies, procedures, and standardized orders should be in place for the management of medical emergencies (Schiavone, 2009). Procedures include the process for monitoring/tracking the availability and readiness of emergency equipment and expiration date on medications, including antidotes and rescue agents.

(4) Educate staff regarding who to call and the process for contacting the provider/team (e.g., outpatient nurses need to be clear as to whether they should contact 911 or the institution's code team).

(5) Orders for the treatment of infusion emergencies should be available to enable immediate intervention without waiting for the provider's order. Indications for each medication should be clearly defined (e.g., indications for epinephrine, diphenhydramine, steroids).

(6) All team members should understand their role and responsibilities in an emergency situation.

(7) Verify that emergency equipment and supplies, including oxygen, are available and working and that staff are aware of their location. Infusion chairs should be functional to change position if needed.

(8) Extravasation: Establish policies, procedures, and standardized orders and have antidotes in place for the management of vesicant extravasation (ISMP, 2016; Neuss et al., 2016; see Chapter 13).

(*a*) Staff must be knowledgeable regarding the management of extravasation, the location of orders, and the process for obtaining antidotes.

(*b*) Coupled order sets (e.g., inclusion of an order on the antineoplastic therapy order set, such as "Initiate extravasation orders for suspected extravasation") permit the prompt and evidence-based management of emergencies such as extravasation (ISMP, 2016).

(9) Ensure that antidotes or rescue agents (where applicable) and directions for use are readily available (ISMP, 2016; Nelson, Moore, Grasso, Barbarotta, & Fischer, 2014).

(10) Conduct process improvement projects and educational programs designed to provide patients with prompt, evidence-based interventions.

(*a*) Evaluate previous emergent situations to determine what worked and areas for improvement.

(*b*) Consider running mock codes and mock infusion reactions. Numerous studies have shown that these drills increase practitioner proficiency and confidence and decrease anxiety (Dorney, 2011; Ruesseler et al., 2012; Scaramuzzo, Wong, Voitle, & Gordils-Perez, 2014).

h) Communication and handoffs: Implement a standardized process to promote effective handoffs between nurses and between care sites (as applicable to role) for patients receiving antineoplastic therapy (Neuss et al., 2016).

(1) Nursing bedside rounds and interprofessional rounds have been found to increase communication and decrease errors (Garcia-Alonso, 2011; Taylor, 2015).

(2) Document any missed patient appointments or treatments, and follow up with the patient and other members of the healthcare team (Neuss et al., 2016).

(3) Document an accurate treatment summary, including history, previous cancer treatments, and current treatment when a patient is transferred to a different healthcare setting. The ASCO Institute for Quality has example templates on its website (www.instituteforquality.org/cancer-treatment-plan-and-summary-templates).

i) Provide ongoing patient education, including information, motivation, and encouragement to patients to become "vigilant partners" in safety measures (Bruce, 2013; Schwappach & Wernli, 2010).

6. Drug shortages

a) Drug shortages can have significant clinical effects (Becker et al., 2013; Fox, Sweet, & Jensen, 2014; McBride et al., 2013).

(1) Treatment outcomes can be affected by omitted or reduced doses from delays or changes in treatment regimens.

(2) Medication errors

(*a*) Healthcare providers are not knowledgeable about substitute medications when the preferred drug is unavailable, potentially resulting in errors in dosing, adverse effects, and drug interactions.

(*b*) A different concentration or brand is purchased, potentially affecting how the dose is prepared, dispensed, and administered.

(*c*) Look-alike/sound-alike medications are purchased from a different manufacturer.

(3) Increased costs

(*a*) Cost of replacement medications may be significant. Becker et al. (2013) noted a 1,704% cost increase when paclitaxel was replaced by docetaxel for a single treatment.

(*b*) Labor costs are associated with seeking sources for replacement supplies, managing inventory, updating computer systems for replacement medications, and educating staff.

b) The Food and Drug Administration Safety and Innovation Act, which became law in 2012, requires pharmaceutical companies to notify FDA when a product may be affected by production changes or manufacturing interruptions (U.S. FDA, 2014).

c) FDA (2017a) works with manufacturers to minimize the impact of drug shortages. A list of drugs in short supply is maintained on the FDA website (www.fda.gov/Drugs/DrugSafety/DrugShortages/default.htm).

References

Aita, M., Belvedere, O., De Carlo, E., Deroma, L., De Pauli, F., Gurrieri, L., ... Fasola, G. (2013). Chemotherapy prescribing errors: An observational study on the role of information technology and computerized physician order entry systems. *BMC Health Services Research, 13,* 522. https://doi.org/10.1186/1472-6963-13-522

American Nurses Association. (2015). *Nursing: Scope and standards of practice* (3rd ed.). Silver Spring, MD: Author.

Becker, D.J., Talwar, S., Levy, B.P., Thorn, M., Roitman, J., Blum, R.H., ... Grossbard, M.L. (2013). Impact of oncology drug shortages on patient therapy: Unplanned treatment changes. *Journal of Oncology Practice, 9,* e122–e128. https://doi.org/10.1200/JOP.2012.000799

Brant, J.M., & Wickham, R. (Eds.). (2013). *Statement on the scope and standards of oncology nursing practice: Generalist and advanced practice.* Pittsburgh, PA: Oncology Nursing Society.

Bruce, S.D. (2013). Before you press that button: A look at chemotherapy errors. *Clinical Journal of Oncology Nursing, 17,* 31–32. https://doi.org/10.1188/13.CJON.31-32

Dols, J.D., Muñoz, L.R., Martinez, S.S., Mathers, N., Miller, P.S., Pomerleau, T.A., ... White, S. (2017). Developing policies and protocols in the age of evidence-based practice. *Journal of Continuing Education in Nursing, 48,* 87–92. https://doi.org/10.3928/00220124-20170119-10

Dorney, P. (2011). Code blue: Chaos or control, an educational initiative. *Journal for Nurses in Staff Development, 27,* 242–244. https://doi.org/10.1097/NND.0b013e31822d6ee4

Fox, E.R., Sweet, B.V., & Jensen, V. (2014). Drug shortages: A complex health care crisis. *Mayo Clinic Proceedings, 89,* 361–373. https://doi.org/10.1016/j.mayocp.2013.11.014

Fyhr, A., Ternov, S., & Ek, A. (2017). From a reactive to a proactive safety approach. Analysis of medication errors in chemotherapy using general failure types. *European Journal of Cancer Care, 26,* e12348. https://doi.org/10.1111/ecc.12348

Garcia-Alonso, A. (2011). Improving the chemotherapy process and service to cancer patients. *Risk Management and Healthcare Policy, 4,* 41–45. https://doi.org/10.2147/RMHP.S16059

Goldspiel, B., Hoffman, J.M., Griffith, N.I., Goodin, S., DeChristoforo, R., Montello, M., ... Patel, J.T. (2015). ASHP guidelines on preventing medication errors with chemotherapy and biotherapy. *American Journal of Health-System Pharmacy, 72,* e6–e35. https://doi.org/10.2146/sp150001

Grasha, T., Reilley, S., Schell, K., Tranum, D., & Filburn, J. (2001). *Process and delayed verification errors in community pharmacy: Implications for improving accuracy and patient safety* (Cognitive Systems Performance Laboratory Technical Report No. 112101). Retrieved from http://www.ibrarian.net/navon/paper/Process_and_Delayed_Verification_Errors_In_Commun.pdf?paperid=3382578

Griffin, M.C., Gilbert, R.E., Broadfield, L.H., Easty, A.E., & Trbovich, P.L. (2016). ReCAP: Comparison of independent error checks for oral versus intravenous chemotherapy. *Journal of Oncology Practice, 12,* 168–169, e180–e187. https://doi.org/10.1200/JOP.2015.005892

Institute for Safe Medication Practices. (2010). *ISMP's guidelines for standard order sets.* Retrieved from http://www.ismp.org/tools/guidelines/standardordersets.pdf

Institute for Safe Medication Practices. (2013, June 13). Independent double checks: Undervalued and misused: Selective use of this strategy can play an important role in medication safety. Retrieved from http://www.ismp.org/newsletters/acutecare/showarticle.aspx?id=51

Institute for Safe Medication Practices. (2014). High-alert medications in acute care settings. Retrieved from https://www.ismp.org/Tools/institutionalhighAlert.asp

Institute for Safe Medication Practices. (2016). *ISMP guidelines for safe preparation of compounded sterile preparations.* Retrieved from https://www.ismp.org/Tools/guidelines/IVSummit/IVCGuidelines.pdf

Institute for Safe Medication Practices. (2017, May 18). Despite technology, verbal orders persist, read back is not widespread, and errors continue. Retrieved from https://www.ismp.org/newsletters/acutecare/showarticle.aspx?id=1167

Institute for Safe Medication Practices Canada. (2005). Lowering risks of medication errors: Independent double checks. *ISMP Canada Safety Bulletin, 5,* 1–2. Retrieved from http://www.ismp-canada.org/download/safetyBulletins/ISMPCSB2005-01.pdf

Joint Commission. (2016, December 22). Clarification: Use of secure text messaging for patient care orders is not acceptable. Retrieved from https://www.jointcommission.org/clarification_use_of_secure_text_messaging

Keers, R.N., Williams, S.D., Cooke, J., & Ashcroft, D.M. (2013). Causes of medication administration errors in hospitals: A systematic review of quantitative and qualitative evidence. *Drug Safety, 36,* 1045–1067. https://doi.org/10.1007/s40264-013-0090-2

Kullberg, A., Larsen, J., & Sharp, L. (2013). 'Why is there another person's name on my infusion bag?' Patient safety in chemotherapy care—A review of the literature. *European Journal of Oncology Nursing, 17,* 228–235. https://doi.org/10.1016/j.ejon.2012.07.005

Lockhart, J.S. (2016). *Nursing professional development for clinical educators.* Pittsburgh, PA: Oncology Nursing Society.

McBride, A., Holle, L.M., Westendorf, C., Sidebottom, M., Griffith, N., Muller, R.J., & Hoffman, J.M. (2013). National survey on the effect of oncology drug shortages on cancer care. *American Journal of Health-System Pharmacy, 70,* 609–617. https://doi.org/10.2146/ajhp120563

Meisenberg, B.R., Wright, R.R., & Brady-Copertino, C.J. (2014). Reduction in chemotherapy order errors with computerized physician order entry. *Journal of Oncology Practice, 10,* e5–e9. https://doi.org/10.1200/JOP.2013.000903

Nelson, W.K., Moore, J., Grasso, J.A., Barbarotta, L., & Fischer, D.S. (2014). Development of a policy and procedure for accidental chemotherapy overdose. *Clinical Journal of Oncology Nursing, 18,* 414–420. https://doi.org/10.1188/14.CJON.18-04AP

Neuss, M.N., Gilmore, T.R., Belderson, K.M., Billett, A.L., Conti-Kalchik, T., Harvey, B.E., ... Polovich, M. (2016). 2016 updated American Society of Clinical Oncology/Oncology Nursing Society chemotherapy administration safety standards, including standards for pediatric oncology. *Journal of Oncology Practice, 12,* 1262–1271. https://doi.org/10.1200/JOP.2016.017905

Oncology Nursing Society. (2017, October). *Education of the nurse who administers and cares for the individual receiving chemotherapy, targeted therapy, and immunotherapy* [Position statement]. Retrieved from https://www.ons.org/advocacy-policy/positions/education/chemotherapy-biotherapy

Ruesseler, M., Weinlich, M., Müller, M.P., Byhahn, C., Marzi, I., & Walcher, F. (2012). Republished: Simulation training improves ability to manage medical emergencies. *Postgraduate Medical Journal, 88,* 312–316. https://doi.org/10.1136/pgmj-2009-074518rep

Scaramuzzo, L.A., Wong, Y., Voitle, K.L., & Gordils-Perez, J. (2014). Cardiopulmonary arrest in the outpatient setting: Enhancing patient safety through rapid response algorithms and simulation teaching. *Clinical Journal of Oncology Nursing, 18,* 61–64. https://doi.org/10.1188/14.CJON.61-64

Schiavone, R. (2009). Emergency response in outpatient oncology care: Improving patient safety. *Clinical Journal of Oncology Nursing, 13,* 440–442. https://doi.org/10.1188/09.CJON.440-442

Schwappach, D.L.B., & Wernli, M. (2010). Medication errors in chemotherapy: Incidence, types and involvement of patients in prevention. A review of the literature. *European Journal of Cancer Care, 19,* 285–292. https://doi.org/10.1111/j.1365-2354.2009.01127.x

Shulman, L.N., Miller, R.S., Ambinder, E.P., Yu, P.P., & Cox, J.V. (2008). Principles of safe practice using an oncology EHR system for chemotherapy ordering, preparation, and administration, part 1 of 2. *Journal of Oncology Practice, 4,* 203–206. https://doi.org/10.1200/JOP.0847501

Taylor, J.S. (2015). Improving patient safety and satisfaction with standardized bedside handoff and walking rounds. *Clinical Journal of Oncology Nursing, 19,* 414–416. https://doi.org/10.1188/15.CJON.414-416

U.S. Food and Drug Administration. (2014). Center for Drug Evaluation and Research manual of policies and procedures: Drug shortage management. Retrieved from https://www.fda.gov/downloads/AboutFDA/CentersOffices/OfficeofMedicalProductsandTobacco/CDER/ManualofPoliciesProcedures/UCM079936.pdf

U.S. Food and Drug Administration. (2017a, November 30). Drug shortages. Retrieved from https://www.fda.gov/Drugs/DrugSafety/DrugShortages/default.htm

U.S. Food and Drug Administration. (2017b, August 2). Medication error reports. Retrieved from https://www.fda.gov/Drugs/DrugSafety/MedicationErrors/ucm080629.htm

U.S. Pharmacopeial Convention. (2016). General chapter 800: Hazardous drugs—Handling in healthcare settings. In *The United States Pharmacopeia–National Formulary* (USP 39–NF 34). Rockville, MD: Author.

Weingart, S.N., Zhu, J., Young-Hong, J., Vermilya, H.B., & Hassett, M. (2014). Do drug interaction alerts between a chemotherapy order-entry system and an electronic medical record affect clinician behavior? *Journal of Oncology Pharmacy Practice, 20,* 163–171. https://doi.org/10.1177/1078155213487395

White, R.E., Cassano-Piché, A., Fields, A., Cheng, R., & Easty, A.C. (2014). Intravenous chemotherapy preparation errors: Patient safety risks identified in a pan-Canadian exploratory study. *Journal of Oncology Pharmacy Practice, 20,* 40–46. https://doi.org/10.1177/1078155212473000

White, R.E., Trbovich, P.L., Easty, A.C., Savage, P., Trip, K., & Hyland, S. (2010). Checking it twice: An evaluation of checklists for detecting medication errors at the bedside using a chemotherapy model. *Quality and Safety in Health Care, 19,* 562–567. https://doi.org/10.1136/qshc.2009.032862

World Health Organization. (n.d.). Patient safety: Medication without harm. Retrieved from http://www.who.int/patientsafety/medication-safety/en

CHAPTER 2

Ethical and Legal Issues

A. Ethical issues related to cancer therapy

1. The healthcare environment necessitates that nurses be sensitive to ethical and legal issues. Concerns arise in the care of all patients, but the intensity is often greater in the cancer population, as patients, families, and healthcare professionals face frequent and potentially difficult moral choices.
2. Ethical issues related to cancer therapy
   a) Healthcare realities that present potential ethical issues
      (1) Major advances with increased availability and access to medical technology, heightened expectations, and changing moral attitudes combine to generate complex ethical and legal problems related to cancer and palliative care (Bressler, Hanna, & Smith, 2017; Butts & Rich, 2016). In particular, the use of life-sustaining measures may raise ethical questions when healthcare professionals do the following:
         (a) Fail to discuss patient requests before a crisis develops
         (b) Are reluctant or fail to communicate medical treatment options with a stressed and grief-stricken family
         (c) Fail to consider supportive care measures
         (d) Experience moral distress related to personal values or biases (Kates, 2017; Sirilla, Thompson, Yamokoski, Risser, & Chipps, 2017; Sisk, Frankel, Kodish, & Isaacson, 2016; Sullivan & Dickerson, 2016)
      (2) Changing healthcare environment: Staffing shortages, reallocation of resources, consolidation, and corporatization have resulted in growing administrative dominance over clinical practice (Agency for Healthcare Research and Quality, 2017; Centers for Medicare and Medicaid Services, n.d.; Page, 2004).
   b) Large numbers of underinsured and undocumented individuals: Even for people with health insurance, copayments or deductibles can lead to substantial debt.
      (1) *Financial toxicity* has been described as the devastating impact of out-of-pocket costs to individuals in their efforts to balance payments for cancer care with other life expenses, such as food, family, home, and transportation.
      (2) Children and the working poor are most affected by limited coverage and higher deductibles. Other protected groups include prisoners and the homeless, whose payment for care must also be addressed (Lyckholm & Glancey, 2016; Zafar, 2016).
      (3) Some people with insurance are unable to obtain reimbursement for certain treatments, such as bone marrow transplantation, clinical trials, or off-label use of medications (Brown, Markus, & Bales, 2016; Centers for Medicare and Medicaid Services, n.d.; Shaw, Asomugha, Conway, & Rein, 2014).
   c) Expanding awareness and appreciation of cultural diversity
      (1) Cultural diversity includes factors such as social status, culture, religion, personality, race/ethnicity, age, gender, sexual orientation, and decision-making ability.
      (2) Cultural and communication differences and protections present a range of challenges, from discussion of surveillance, diagnosis, and prognosis to decisions about who will provide long-term care (Agency for Healthcare Research and Quality, 2017; Bressler et al., 2017; Butts & Rich, 2016).

d) Use of alternative therapies
(1) Evidence-based complementary and alternative medicine, in conjunction with or as a substitute for conventional treatment, is affected by variations in individual response to cancer and its treatment, the need for a sense of control, belief in individual rights and determination, and cultural and spiritual beliefs. The use of such therapies is often limited by caregiver beliefs.
(2) In the search for cancer care with minimal side effects, survivors and families often embark on unproven therapies, which can cause adverse outcomes and insurmountable cost (Johnson, Park, Gross, & Yu, 2017).
(3) Oncology nurses must be educated about alternative methods to provide education about reliable options (American College of Surgeons Commission on Cancer, 2015; Butts & Rich, 2016; Cox et al., 2017; Fouladbakhsh, 2013).

e) Heightened use of targeted therapies, growth of management guidance for those with genetic mutations, and molecular testing: As personalized therapies become more common, healthcare professionals are expected to apply this knowledge to practice and be aware of the molecular targets. Awareness of types of testing and impact on care are a daily process. Reimbursement for testing and services, extensive family history collection, and costs of targeted and biologic therapies offer more challenges to patients, the healthcare system, and professionals (American Nurses Association [ANA] & International Society of Nurses in Genetics [ISONG], 2016; Mohammed, Peter, Gastaldo, & Howell, 2016; Roeland, Dullea, Hagmann, & Madlensky, 2017).

3. Ethical issues that oncology nurses face in daily practice (de Groot et al., 2017; Fiore & Goodman, 2016; Sisk et al., 2016; Sullivan & Dickerson, 2016)
a) Autonomy
(1) Patient autonomy and decision-making capacity
(2) Informed consent
(3) Cancer risk reduction (e.g., prophylactic surgeries)
(4) Treatment during pregnancy
(5) The right to refuse treatment

b) The healthcare environment and reform
(1) Undertreatment of pain, particularly in light of opioid crisis
(2) Inequities in cancer care
(3) Access to care, clinical trials
(4) Access to high-cost cancer drugs, drug shortages
(5) Cultural diversity and potential bias
(6) Balance and justice in cancer care

c) End-of-life/prolongation of life decisions
(1) Assisted dying (legal in several states)
(2) Treatment futility versus continuing experimental treatment
(3) Prognosis-related discussions

d) Confidentiality
(1) Genomic testing and disclosure of results
(2) Scientific integrity
(3) Big data collection and warehousing

e) Conflict resolution/critical conversations
(1) Intrafamily conflicts
(2) Nurse–family conflicts
(3) Nurse–physician conflicts
(4) Physician–family conflicts
(5) Clarity in communications

f) Professional boundaries
(1) Giving or receiving gifts
(2) Social media (e.g., friend requests from patients)

4. The Joint Commission (2016) requires accredited institutions to provide access to an ethics consultation to assist in evaluating the decision-making capacity of an individual as well as to assist with problem resolution.
5. The ethical principles guiding decision making are summarized in Table 2-1.
6. The ANA (2015a) Code of Ethics serves as an ethical framework for practice, providing direction regarding ethical relationships, nursing responsibilities, appropriate behaviors, and decision making. Components of the framework include the following:
a) Respect for the inherent dignity, worth, and unique attributes of every person
b) Primary commitment to the patient
c) Protection of the rights, health, and safety of the patient
d) Authority, accountability, and responsibility for nursing practice
e) Same duties owed to self as to others
f) Establishment, maintenance, and improvement of the ethical environment of work setting and conditions of employment
g) Advancement of the profession through research and scholarly inquiry
h) Protection of human rights, promotion of health diplomacy, and reduction of health disparities

Table 2-1. Ethical Principles

Principle	Description	Clinical Examples
Autonomy	Independent decision making by an individual in accordance with his or her own best interest	Respecting an individual's choice even when different from one's own Providing supportive services
Nonmaleficence	The duty to do no harm	Providing complete information Providing survivorship services Recognizing professional limitations and seeking consultation/collaboration Adhering to professional standards of care
Beneficence	The duty to act in the best interest of the involved person	Personalizing care based on individual desires, culture, disease, and other factors Providing evidence-based care
Justice	Equitable distribution of available resources	Offering/providing treatment regardless of ability to pay, culture, or socioeconomic status Assisting with or referring for financial support
Veracity	Truth telling	Explaining treatment in understandable terms before it is initiated Providing accurate information and educational materials
Fidelity	Faithfulness to promises made	Following up as promised Providing survivorship care planning Fostering collegiality

Note. Based on information from Beauchamp & Childress, 2013.

i) Articulation of nursing values, maintenance of integrity of the profession, and integration of the principle of social justice

B. Legal issues related to cancer therapy
1. Adhering to national, state, and institutional standards is a fundamental responsibility of all nurses (ANA, 2015a; Brown et al., 2016; Centers for Medicare and Medicaid Services, n.d.).
2. Acts and standards guiding oncology nursing practice (not all-inclusive, as the changing environment requires knowledge of specialty competencies depending on practice setting)
   a) Nurse practice acts are state laws that define nursing performance in fundamental terms for each state (ANA, 2015b).
   b) The Oncology Nursing Society's (ONS's) *Statement on the Scope and Standards of Oncology Nursing Practice: Generalist and Advanced Practice* (Brant & Wickham, 2013) describes the minimum standard of care to which a patient with cancer is entitled.
   c) The American Society of Clinical Oncology/ONS Chemotherapy Administration Safety Standards (Neuss et al., 2016) describe the safety standards for chemotherapy prescription, preparation, and administration, with the recent addition of pediatric and oral chemotherapy standards.
   d) *Genetics/Genomics Nursing: Scope and Standards of Practice* (ANA & ISONG, 2016) describes standards and scope of practice for general and advanced practice nurses addressing genetic/genomic issues with examples from a variety of practice settings.
   e) ONS's *Access Device Standards of Practice for Oncology Nursing* (Camp-Sorrell & Matey, 2017) describes the current standards for use of venous access devices in cancer care.
   f) *Infusion Therapy Standards of Practice* (Infusion Nurses Society, 2016) describes the current standards of nursing practice for IV therapy.
   g) American College of Surgeons Commission on Cancer's *Cancer Program Standards: Ensuring Patient-Centered Care* encompasses the requirements that cancer programs must meet to earn and maintain Commission on Cancer accreditation (American College of Surgeons Commission on Cancer, 2015).
   h) Institution-specific standards may be set forth in the following:
      (1) Standards of practice
      (2) Nursing policy and procedure manuals
      (3) Job descriptions
      (4) Institutional review board decisions and guidance
3. Common legal issues
   a) Medication errors (see Chapter 1)

b) Documentation issues: The duty to keep accurate records is a fundamental nursing responsibility. The medical record is scrutinized in the event of litigious action and is believed to reflect the care rendered (American Society of Health-System Pharmacists, 2011; Neuss et al., 2016; Scott, 2016).

(1) Common documentation errors

(a) Omitting significant observations

(b) Failing to document response to an intervention

(c) Failing to document patient teaching and understanding

(d) Failing to document what was taught and to whom

(2) Nursing actions to include in documentation

(a) Telephone, text, or other digital communications or conversations, particularly those in which the nurse gives the patient instructions or advice

(b) Fax and email communications, particularly those in which the nurse gives the patient instructions or advice

(c) Virtual face-to-face communications, particularly those in which the nurse gives the patient instructions or advice, including the type of communication, who was included, and the location (such as online meetings, forums, email distribution lists, telemedicine, etc.)

(d) Pertinent conversations with the patient, family, or other caregivers

(e) Interagency referrals, including telephone conversations with provider(s)

(f) Antineoplastic drug administration (see Appendices A and B)

(g) Treatment-related documentation including the following, when applicable:

i. Completion of independent verification of drug and dose

ii. Two unique patient identifiers (such as name, medical record number, or date of birth)

iii. Patient-specific measurements used to calculate doses (e.g., body surface area)

iv. Pertinent laboratory and diagnostic test results

v. Date and time of therapy

vi. Drug name, dose, route, and location of administration, and infusion duration

vii. Volume and type of IV fluids administered

viii. Assessment of the IV site before, during, and after infusion

ix. Information about the infusion device (e.g., vein selection, needle size, type of device, infusion pump)

x. Verification of venous access device patency, including presence of a blood return before, during, and after IV therapy (also any issues with venous access)

(h) Patient assessment and evaluation of the patient response to and tolerance of treatment

(i) Patient and family education related to the drugs received, toxicities, toxicity management, and follow-up care (especially when and who to call with specific resource numbers and times)

(j) Post-treatment or discharge instructions

c) Informed consent

(1) Process: Patients must give informed consent for treatment, enrollment in a clinical trial, or participation in nursing research (Beauchamp & Childress, 2013; Butts & Rich, 2016; Klimaszewski, 2016). With the exception of research, each institution determines its own practice related to how and if a patient must provide written informed consent before receiving cancer treatment such as antineoplastic agents, targeted therapies, or immunotherapies (Neuss et al., 2016). It is important to maintain consistency between policy and practice throughout the institution. Regardless of the method used to document informed consent, all needed elements of the informed decision-making process must be included. The following approaches have been used:

(a) The patient signs a designated antineoplastic therapy consent form designed specifically for the administration of chemother-

apy, targeted therapy, or immunotherapy. This document reflects patient education, remains part of the medical record, and may be preferred by risk management. A sample template for chemotherapy consent is provided in Appendix E.

(b) The general hospital "consent to treat" document serves as the signed permission to provide antineoplastic medications.

(c) Some centers use a general procedure consent form for cancer treatment.

(d) A specific form is not signed, but consent is documented within the medical record.

(2) Elements of consent (Elements of Informed Consent, 2017)

(a) Disclosure: The patient is informed of his or her diagnosis of cancer, including the type, location, and stage.

(b) Nature of the proposed treatment: The patient is informed of the prognosis and goal of proposed treatment (cure, control, palliation).

(c) Possible benefits of the treatment are discussed.

(d) Possible risks and adverse effects, including short- and long-term side effects, are discussed.

(e) Alternatives to treatment and associated risks are covered. Palliative care should be offered as an option, when appropriate.

(f) Children younger than age 18 may be legally able to give informed consent if they are emancipated minors. *Assent* is willingness to participate in a treatment by people who are, by definition, too young to give informed consent but are old enough to understand the diagnosis and proposed treatment (Neuss et al., 2016).

i. If assent is given, informed consent must still be obtained from the patient's parents or guardian.

ii. The main goal of child assent is to provide protection for children involved in clinical trials (Tait & Geisser, 2017).

(3) Requirements

(a) The informed consent document must state the right of the patient to refuse or discontinue treatment at any time.

(b) The informed consent document and, subsequently, healthcare providers assure patients that ongoing support and care will be provided if they decline or discontinue treatment connected with the trial or research.

(c) Nurses and physicians have different but complementary roles in the informed consent process.

(d) See Chapter 5 for additional information on the informed consent process related to clinical trials and the nurse's role.

References

Agency for Healthcare Research and Quality. (2017, July). *2016 national healthcare quality and disparities report* (AHRQ Pub. No. 17-0001). Retrieved from https://www.ahrq.gov/research/findings/nhqrdr/nhqdr16/index.html

American College of Surgeons Commission on Cancer. (2015). *Cancer program standards: Ensuring patient-centered care* (2016 ed.). Chicago, IL: Author.

American Nurses Association. (2015a). *Code of ethics for nurses with interpretive statements.* Silver Spring, MD: Author.

American Nurses Association. (2015b). *Nursing: Scope and standards of practice* (3rd ed.). Silver Spring, MD: Author.

American Nurses Association & International Society of Nurses in Genetics. (2016). *Genetics/genomics nursing: Scope and standards of practice* (2nd ed.). Silver Spring, MD: American Nurses Association.

American Society of Health-System Pharmacists. (2011). ASHP statement on bar-code verification during inventory, preparation, and dispensing of medications. *American Journal of Health-System Pharmacy, 68,* 442–445. https://doi.org/10.2146/sp100012

Beauchamp, T.L., & Childress, J.F. (2013). *Principles of biomedical ethics* (7th ed.). New York, NY: Oxford University Press.

Brant, J.M., & Wickham, R. (Eds.). (2013). *Statement on the scope and standards of oncology nursing practice: Generalist and advanced practice.* Pittsburgh, PA: Oncology Nursing Society.

Bressler, T., Hanna, D.R., & Smith, E. (2017). Making sense of moral distress within cultural complexity. *Journal of Hospice and Palliative Nursing, 19,* 7–14. https://doi.org/10.1097/NJH.0000000000000308

Brown, S., Markus, S., & Bales, C.A. (2016). Legal, regulatory, and legislative issues. In A.D. Klimaszewski, M. Bacon, J.A. Eggert, E. Ness, J.G. Westendorp, & K. Willenberg (Eds.), *Manual for clinical trials nursing* (3rd ed., pp. 51–65). Pittsburgh, PA: Oncology Nursing Society.

Butts, J.B., & Rich, K.L. (2016). *Nursing ethics: Across the curriculum and into practice* (4th ed.). Burlington, MA: Jones & Bartlett Learning.

Camp-Sorrell, D., & Matey, L. (Eds.). (2017). *Access device standards of practice for oncology nursing.* Pittsburgh, PA: Oncology Nursing Society.

Centers for Medicare and Medicaid Services. (n.d.). Regulations and guidance. Retrieved from https://www.cms.gov/regulations-and-guidance/regulations-and-guidance.html

Cox, A., Lucas, G., Marcu, A., Piano, M., Grosvenor, W., Mold, F., ... Ream, E. (2017). Cancer survivors' experience with telehealth: A systematic review and thematic synthesis. *Journal of Medical Internet Research, 19,* e11. https://doi.org/10.2196/jmir.6575

de Groot, F., Capri, S., Castanier, J.-C., Cunningham, D., Flamion, B., Flume, M., ... Wong, O. (2017). Ethical hurdles in the prioritization of oncology care. *Applied Health Economics and Health Policy, 15,* 119–126. https://doi.org/10.1007/s40258-016-0288-4

Elements of Informed Consent, 21 C.F.R. § 50.25 (2017).

Fiore, R.N., & Goodman, K.W. (2016). Precision medicine ethics: Selected issues and developments in next-generation sequencing, clinical oncology, and ethics. *Current Opinion in Oncology, 28,* 83–87. https://doi.org/10.1097/CCO.0000000000000247

Fouladbakhsh, J. (2013, June 26). *Integrative therapies in oncology* [Webinar]. Retrieved from http://event.on24.com

Infusion Nurses Society. (2016). *Infusion therapy standards of practice.* Norwood, MA: Author.

Johnson, S.B., Park, H.S.M., Gross, C.P., & Yu, J.B. (2017). Use of alternative medicine for cancer and its impact on survival. *International Journal of Radiation Oncology, Biology, Physics, 99,* E401. https://doi.org/10.1016/j.ijrobp.2017.06.1562

Joint Commission. (2016). *2016 hospital accreditation standards.* Oakbrook Terrace, IL: Author.

Kates, J. (2017). Advance care planning conversations. *Journal for Nurse Practitioners, 13,* e321–e323. https://doi.org/10.1016/j.nurpra.2017.05.011

Klimaszewski, A.D. (2016). Informed consent. In A.D. Klimaszewski, M. Bacon, J.A. Eggert, E. Ness, J.G. Westendorp, & K. Willenberg (Eds.), *Manual for clinical trials nursing* (3rd ed., pp. 113–125). Pittsburgh, PA: Oncology Nursing Society.

Lyckholm, L.J., & Glancey, C.L. (2016). Ethical issues in caring for prison inmates with advanced cancer. *Journal of Hospice and Palliative Nursing, 18,* 7–12. https://doi.org/10.1097/NJH.0000000000000216

Mohammed, S., Peter, E., Gastaldo, D., & Howell, D. (2016). The "conflicted dying": The active search for life extension in advanced cancer through biomedical treatment. *Qualitative Health Research, 26,* 555–567. https://doi.org/10.1177/1049732315572772

Neuss, M.N., Gilmore, T.R., Belderson, K.M., Billett, A.L., Conti-Kalchik, T., Harvey, B.E., ... Polovich, M. (2016). 2016 updated American Society of Clinical Oncology/Oncology Nursing Society chemotherapy administration safety standards, including standards for pediatric oncology. *Journal of Oncology Practice, 12,* 1262–1271. https://doi.org/10.1200/JOP.2016.017905

Page, A. (Ed.). (2004). *Keeping patients safe: Transforming the work environment of nurses.* Retrieved from http://www.nationalacademies.org/hmd/Reports/2003/Keeping-Patients-Safe-Transforming-the-Work-Environment-of-Nurses.aspx

Roeland, E.J., Dullea, A.D., Hagmann, C.H., & Madlensky, L. (2017). Addressing hereditary cancer risk at the end of life. *Journal of Oncology Practice, 13,* e851–e856. https://doi.org/10.1200/JOP.2017.021980

Scott, L. (2016). Medication errors. *Nursing Standard, 30*(35), 61–62. https://doi.org/10.7748/ns.30.35.61.s49

Shaw, F.E., Asomugha, C.N., Conway, P.H., & Rein, A.S. (2014). The Patient Protection and Affordable Care Act: Opportunities for prevention and public health. *Lancet, 384,* 75–82. https://doi.org/10.1016/S0140-6736(14)60259-2

Sirilla, J., Thompson, K., Yamokoski, T., Risser, M.D., & Chipps, E. (2017). Moral distress in nurses providing direct patient care at an academic medical center. *Worldviews on Evidence-Based Nursing, 14,* 128–135. https://doi.org/10.1111/wvn.12213

Sisk, B., Frankel, R., Kodish, E., & Isaacson, J.H. (2016). The truth about truth-telling in American medicine: A brief history. *Permanente Journal, 20*(3), 74–77. https://doi.org/10.7812/TPP/15-219

Sullivan, S.S., & Dickerson, S.S. (2016). Facing death: A critical analysis of advance care planning in the United States. *Advances in Nursing Science, 39,* 320–332. https://doi.org/10.1097/ANS.0000000000000138

Tait, A.R., & Geisser, M.E. (2017). Development of a consensus operational definition of child assent for research. *BMC Medical Ethics, 18,* 41. https://doi.org/10.1186/s12910-017-0199-4

Zafar, S.Y. (2016). Financial toxicity of cancer care: It's time to intervene. *Journal of the National Cancer Institute, 108,* jv370. https://doi.org/10.1093/jnci/djv370

CHAPTER 3

Patient Education

A. Patient education
   1. Patient education is a combination of learning experiences that empower individuals or a community with health information and instruction used to understand the risk of illness, prevent illness, care for themselves throughout the treatment trajectory, and know when to obtain help in their care.
   2. Patient education is a continuous process throughout the cancer experience (Gidron, 2016; Vaartio-Rajalin et al., 2015; World Health Organization, n.d.).
      a) Health teaching and health promotion are key aspects of the role of nurses and oncology nurses at all levels of practice, in all care settings, and are a necessity for patients, their significant others, and the public. Using the models of patient engagement and shared decision making, all practitioners are to be involved in health teaching and promotion, requiring collaboration and open communication, both interprofessionally and across healthcare settings (American Nurses Association, 2015; Blecher, Ireland, & Watson, 2016; Brant & Wickham, 2013; Tariman et al., 2016; Vaartio-Rajalin et al., 2015).
      b) The Agency for Healthcare Research and Quality (AHRQ, 2015a) has identified universal precautions for health literacy; steps are aimed at improving communication of healthcare information, leading to improved comprehension and access; improving patients' ability to navigate the healthcare system; and supporting patients in their self-care.

B. Short-term outcomes of patient education (Blecher et al., 2016; Neuss et al., 2016)
   1. Empowering active participation in care
   2. Understanding of diagnosis and treatment options
   3. Ability to communicate understanding of the goals and duration of treatment
   4. Identification of short- and long-term side effects, including those that need to be reported
   5. Demonstration of the ability to perform self-care or adapt to potential limitations
   6. Promotion of adaptive skills in a life-threatening situation
   7. Autonomous decision making regarding treatment options or a decision of no treatment
   8. Identification and use of community resources

C. Long-term outcomes of patient education (Joint Commission, 2017)
   1. Improvement in self-care behaviors
   2. Improvement in health-related quality of life
   3. Decreased healthcare costs
   4. Increased customer satisfaction
   5. Improved ability to make informed healthcare decisions

D. Barriers to patient education
   1. Barriers should be assessed on an individual basis, and an individualized learning needs assessment should be performed and documented (Gumusay et al., 2016; Joint Commission, 2017; Neuss et al., 2016).
   2. Barriers to learning
      a) The individual's cognitive resources, including potential for problems with attention, working memory, or information processing ability related either to the disease or treatment (Jewitt et al., 2016; Vaartio-Rajalin et al., 2015)
      b) Lack of knowledge or understanding of the diagnosis and treatment plan, as well as differences in professional and patient knowledge expectations (Jewitt et al., 2016; Vaartio-Rajalin et al., 2015)
      c) Differing expectations or understanding of the purpose of treatment among the patient, caregiver, and healthcare team
      d) Concerns or misconceptions regarding therapy due to prior experience or the experience of a friend or relative, which may deter the patient from undergoing treatment

e) Patient or provider language barriers and lack of access to effective translator resources

f) Educational barriers

(1) Seventeen percent of young people in the United States do not graduate from high school. Graduation rates are lower among minorities, with graduation rates of 78% or lower for Hispanic, Black, and Native American students (National Center for Education Statistics, 2017).

(2) Older individuals may not have the same levels of education, as the rate of high school graduation improved dramatically from 6.4% in 1900 to 77% in 1969 (Education Week, n.d.).

g) Health literacy barriers (AHRQ, 2015b; Centers for Disease Control and Prevention, 2015, 2016; Joint Commission, 2017; Katz, 2017; Nielsen-Bohlman, Panzer, & Kindig, 2004)

(1) Inability to complete health forms

(2) Lack of knowledge regarding medical history and management of chronic conditions

(3) Nonadherence to preventive medicine guidelines

(4) Lack of knowledge regarding the connection between risky behaviors and health

(5) Inability to understand directions on medication containers

(6) Nonadherence to medication instructions

(7) Person is unable to name medications and explain their purpose or dosing.

h) Physical barriers, including pain, visual disturbances, auditory or cognitive impairments, and inability to speak, can interfere with comprehension (Joint Commission, 2017).

i) Geographic barriers may include distance traveled to the treatment facility, as well as availability of transportation to the facility.

j) Psychosocial or emotional issues may create barriers to learning and may need to be addressed before learning can take place (Joint Commission, 2017).

k) Interprofessional care coordination and communication barriers (Joint Commission, 2017; Tariman et al., 2016; Vaartio-Rajalin et al., 2015)

(1) Ineffective communication among healthcare team members

(2) Ineffective communication among healthcare facilities

(3) Differences among healthcare professionals in their perceptions of the patient education process

l) Methods of overcoming barriers

(1) Allow patients time to express their concerns and attempt to manage their anxiety.

(2) Assess cognitive resources and knowledge expectations of the individuals being educated, keeping in mind that educational level alone does not always give the complete picture of an individual's abilities.

(3) Include the patient's support system (family, friends, significant others) in the patient education process, providing support to the patient and help with learning.

(4) Manage physical barriers, such as pain, and ensure that learners have all necessary assistive devices (glasses, hearing aids) available.

(5) Provide access to translators, either in person or through telecommunications (Joint Commission, 2017).

(a) Hospitals are required to ensure the competency of interpreters and translators.

(b) Use of significant others as translators is not recommended, because of role conflicts or inability to communicate complex medical terminology.

(c) Cancer-related Spanish-language literature is available through the National Cancer Institute at www.cancer.gov and the American Cancer Society at www.cancer.org.

(6) Offer explanations for any misconceptions concerning diagnosis, treatment, and follow-up care using teach-back techniques (AHRQ, 2015b).

(7) Perform and document a learning needs assessment that addresses cultural/religious beliefs and preferences and desire and motivation to learn, as well as the previously listed items, and share with all individuals involved in the care of the patient (Joint Commission, 2017).

(8) Assess patients individually and tailor teaching to their level of understanding using short simple words, chunking (short sections of information), active voice, and concrete examples (AHRQ, 2014; Cancer Patient Edu-

cation Network, 2013; Joint Commission, 2017; U.S. Department of Health and Human Services Office of Disease Prevention and Health Promotion, n.d.). Cancer-related literature for low-literacy patients is available through the National Cancer Institute at www.cancer.gov and the American Cancer Society at www.cancer.org.

(9) Engage patients in the learning process through the use of patient portals, interactive activities, and patient-reported outcome measurement.

(10) Effective care coordination/transition may be facilitated through the use of handoff tools to improve continuity of care and collaboration between professionals. Patient navigators can provide an effective link for both patient and healthcare provider communication and satisfaction.

3. Barriers to educator effectiveness (AHRQ, 2015b; Blecher et al., 2016)
   a) The educator's expertise regarding information provided
   b) The educator's understanding of teaching-learning principles
   c) The educator's understanding of differences in learning styles
   d) The methods available to the educator for patient education
   e) The educator's ability to match the appropriate teaching methods and language to specific content and learning styles. Language must be adapted to individuals' learning abilities and healthcare-related literacy, as well as their ability to speak, read, and understand English.
   f) The educator's ability to involve individuals in the learning process
   g) The educator's ability to communicate with other members of the healthcare team to provide continuity of care between the various points of care, hospital, physician practice, home, or extended care facilities

E. Methods of patient education (Blecher et al., 2016; Hopmans et al., 2014; Laszewski et al., 2016; LeFebvre & Felice, 2016; Neuss et al., 2016; Şahin & Ergüney, 2016; Sullivan et al., 2016)

1. Educational methods should be selected based on preferences and abilities. They may include any combination of the following:
   a) Auditory, such as audiotapes or face-to-face live presentations
   b) Printed/visual materials, including videotaped education, booklets, chemotherapy cards, infographics, and printed instructions regarding procedures or self-care measures
   c) Computer-based learning using CDs, flash drives, or preloaded devices
   d) Web-based learning, including patient portals, learning management systems, and reliable external websites
      (1) National Cancer Institute: www.cancer.gov
      (2) American Cancer Society: www.cancer.org
      (3) American Society of Clinical Oncology: www.cancer.net
   e) Demonstration
2. Patient education in any format includes teach-back techniques to reinforce learning along with documentation of the strategies used and an evaluation of current learning.
3. Patient education is the responsibility of all nurses and continues as an ongoing process throughout the cancer care continuum (American Nurses Association, 2015).

F. Scope of information

1. Provide verbal, video, audio, written, or web-based information that is easily understandable. If printed material is used, ensure that the sentences and paragraphs are short. Bullet points are helpful. Always encourage patients and significant others to ask questions, provide feedback, and participate actively (AHRQ, 2015b; Frentsos, 2015; Narwani, Nalamada, Lee, Kothari, & Lakhani, 2016; Truccolo, 2016; UnityPoint Health, Picker Institute, Des Moines University, & Health Literacy Iowa, 2017).
2. Include patients and significant others, and provide education on the following topics (Gumusay et al., 2016; LeFebvre & Felice, 2016; Neuss et al., 2016; Şahin & Ergüney, 2016; Sullivan et al., 2016):
   a) Disease and treatment plan
   b) Goals of treatment
   c) Duration and schedule of treatment
      (1) Cancer medication names, including generic and brand names; the dose and frequency of the treatment and number of cycles (length of therapy); and the implications and plan for missed or delayed doses, especially with the use of oral anticancer medications
      (2) Supportive care medications, including generic and brand names, as well as their doses and frequency

(3) Drug–drug and drug–food interactions based on the most current medication list
(4) Potential short- and long-term adverse effects along with a variety of management strategies

d) When and how to contact the healthcare team
e) Symptoms that require immediate discontinuation of self-administered medications/treatments
f) Procedure for handling medications in the home, including safe storage, handling, and management of unused medication
g) Procedures for handling body secretions and waste in the home
h) Follow-up schedules, including laboratory and healthcare provider visits
i) Contact information for healthcare team members and directions regarding communicating with healthcare team members
j) A list of credible resources where more information can be obtained if desired
k) Encourage patients to write down questions they think of between visits and bring them to follow-up appointments. At each visit, healthcare providers should address patient and caregiver questions.

G. Documentation

1. Nurses assess and document patients' understanding of the content presented after education takes place to meet regulatory (e.g., Joint Commission) standards, manage risk, and enhance staff communication (Joint Commission, 2017).
2. Documentation of understanding includes the patients' ability to verbalize or demonstrate learning and needs for reinforcement of information. If patients cannot comprehend the information or they refuse education, this also must be documented, along with alternative plans.
3. Methods of assessing patient understanding (Joint Commission, 2017; UnityPoint Health et al., 2017)

a) Patient/significant other communicates an understanding of the information presented, including medication names and the purpose of the therapy.
b) Patient/significant other identifies crucial instructions for self-care.
c) Patient/significant other identifies symptoms/side effects to report and how to contact the providers if needed.
d) Patient brings new prescriptions to a follow-up visit and correctly states the instructions for use.
e) Patient performs a return demonstration of procedures such as temperature monitoring and handwashing.
f) Patient/significant other accurately identifies the date and time of the next follow-up visit.
g) For oral agents, the patient/significant other can verbalize the name of the medication, the correct procedure for administration (e.g., with or without food), and appropriate safe handling and disposal procedures. See Chapter 4 for discussion of adherence to oral antineoplastics.
h) Patient/significant other shares where or how to obtain additional information if desired.
i) Patient/significant other communicates the need for additional teaching sessions if issues are identified or if complex or multimodal treatments are planned.

References

Agency for Healthcare Research and Quality. (2014). *The SHARE approach—Using the teach-back technique: A reference guide for health care providers* (Workshop curriculum: Tool 6). Retrieved from https://www.ahrq.gov/professionals/education/curriculum-tools/shareddecisionmaking/tools/tool-6/index.html

Agency for Healthcare Research and Quality. (2015a). *AHRQ health literacy universal precautions toolkit* (2nd ed.). Retrieved from https://www.ahrq.gov/professionals/quality-patient-safety/quality-resources/tools/literacy-toolkit/index.html

Agency for Healthcare Research and Quality. (2015b). Health literacy: Hidden barriers and practical strategies [Slide presentation]. Retrieved from https://www.ahrq.gov/professionals/quality-patient-safety/quality-resources/tools/literacy-toolkit/tool3a/index.html

American Nurses Association. (2015). *Nursing: Scope and standards of practice* (3rd ed.). Silver Spring, MD: Author.

Blecher, C.S., Ireland, A.M., & Watson, J.L. (2016). *Standards of oncology education: Patient/significant other and public* (4th ed.). Pittsburgh, PA: Oncology Nursing Society.

Brant, J.M., & Wickham, R. (Eds.). (2013). *Statement on the scope and standards of oncology nursing practice: Generalist and advanced practice.* Pittsburgh, PA: Oncology Nursing Society.

Cancer Patient Education Network. (2013). *Establishing comprehensive cancer patient education programs: Standards of practice.* Retrieved from http://www.cancerpatienteducation.org/docs/CPEN/Educator%20Resources/CPENStandardsofPractice.Nov14.pdf

Centers for Disease Control and Prevention. (2015). Healthy People 2010. Retrieved from https://www.cdc.gov/nchs/healthy_people/hp2010.htm

Centers for Disease Control and Prevention. (2016). What is health literacy? Retrieved from https://www.cdc.gov/healthliteracy/learn/index.html

Education Week. (n.d.). The nation's long and winding path to graduation. Retrieved from https://www.edweek.org/media/34gradrate-c1.pdf

Frentsos, J.M. (2015). Use of videos as supplemental education tools across the cancer trajectory [Online exclusive]. *Clinical Journal of Oncology Nursing, 19,* E126–E130. https://doi.org/10.1188/15.CJON.E126-E130

Gidron, Y. (2016). Education, patient. In M. Gellman & J.R. Turner (Eds.), *Encyclopedia of behavioral medicine.* https://doi.org/10.1007/978-1-4614-6439-6_105-2

Gumusay, O., Cetin, B., Benekli, M., Gurcan, G., Ilhan, M.N., Bostankolu, B., … Buyukberber, S. (2016). Factors influencing chemotherapy goal perception in newly diagnosed cancer patients. *Journal of Cancer Education, 31,* 308–313. https://doi.org/10.1007/s13187-015-0827-y

Hopmans, W., Damman, O.C., Timmermans, D.R.M., Haasbeek, C.J.A., Slotman, B.J., & Senan, S. (2014). Communicating cancer treatment information using the Web: Utilizing the patient's perspective in website development. *BMC Medical Informatics and Decision Making, 14,* 116. https://doi.org/10.1186/s12911-014-0116-4

Jewitt, N., Hope, A.J., Milne, R., Le, L.W., Papadakos, J., Abdelmutti, N., … Giuliani, M.E. (2016). Development and evaluation of patient education materials for elderly lung cancer patients. *Journal of Cancer Education, 31,* 70–74. https://doi.org/10.1007/s13187-014-0780-1

Joint Commission. (2017). *Standards of patient education.* Oakbrook Terrace, IL: Author.

Katz, A. (2017). Health literacy: What do you know? *Oncology Nursing Forum, 44,* 521–522. https://doi.org/10.1188/17.ONF.521-522

Laszewski, P., Zelko, C., Andriths, L.A., Cruz, E.V., Bauer, C., & Magnan, M.A. (2016). Patient preference for instructional reinforcement regarding prevention of radiation dermatitis. *Clinical Journal of Oncology Nursing, 20,* 187–191. https://doi.org/10.1188/16.CJON.187-191

LeFebvre, K.B., & Felice, T.L. (2016). Nursing application of oral chemotherapy safety standards: An informal survey. *Clinical Journal of Oncology Nursing, 20,* 258–262. https://doi.org/10.1188/16.CJON.258-262

Narwani, V., Nalamada, K., Lee, M., Kothari, P., & Lakhani, R. (2016). Readability and quality assessment of internet-based patient education materials related to laryngeal cancer. *Head and Neck, 38,* 601–605. https://doi.org/10.1002/hed.23939

National Center for Education Statistics. (2017, April). The condition of education: Public high school graduation rates. Retrieved from https://nces.ed.gov/programs/coe/indicator_coi.asp

Neuss, M.N., Gilmore, T.R., Belderson, K.M., Billett, A.L., Conti-Kalchik, T., Harvey, B.E., … Polovich, M. (2016). 2016 updated American Society of Clinical Oncology/Oncology Nursing Society chemotherapy administration safety standards, including standards for pediatric oncology. *Journal of Oncology Practice, 12,* 1262–1271. https://doi.org/10.1200/JOP.2016.017905

Nielsen-Bohlman, L., Panzer, A.M., & Kindig, D.A. (Eds.). (2004). *Health literacy: A prescription to end confusion.* Retrieved from http://www.nationalacademies.org/hmd/Reports/2004/Health-Literacy-A-Prescription-to-End-Confusion.aspx

Şahin, Z.A., & Ergüney, S. (2016). Effect on symptom management education receiving patients of chemotherapy. *Journal of Cancer Education, 31,* 101–107. https://doi.org/10.1007/s13187-015-0801-8

Sullivan, C.M., Dalby, C., Gross, A.H., Chesnulevich, K., Lilienfeld, C.W., Hooper, C., … Kochanek, T. (2016). Oral chemotherapy education: Using innovation to ensure broad access. *Clinical Journal of Oncology Nursing, 20,* 126–128. https://doi.org/10.1188/16.CJON.126-128

Tariman, J.D., Mehmeti, E., Spawn, N., McCarter, S.P., Bishop-Royse, J., Garcia, I., … Szubski, K. (2016). Oncology nursing and shared decision making for cancer treatment. *Clinical Journal of Oncology Nursing, 20,* 560–563. https://doi.org/10.1188/16.CJON.560-563

Truccolo, I. (2016). Providing patient information and education in practice: The role of the health librarian. *Health Information and Libraries Journal, 33,* 161–166. https://doi.org/10.1111/hir.12142

UnityPoint Health, Picker Institute, Des Moines University, & Health Literacy Iowa. (2017). *10 elements of competence for using teach-back effectively.* Retrieved from http://www.teachbacktraining.org/assets/files/PDFS/Teach%20Back%20-%2010%20Elements%20of%20Competence.pdf

U.S. Department of Health and Human Services Office of Disease Prevention and Health Promotion. (n.d.). *Quick guide to health literacy.* Retrieved from https://health.gov/communication/literacy/quickguide/default.htm

Vaartio-Rajalin, H., Huumonen, T., Iire, L., Jekunen, A., Leino-Kilpi, H., Minn, H., & Paloniemi, J. (2015). Patient education process in oncologic context: What, why, and by whom? *Nursing Research, 64,* 381–390. https://doi.org/10.1097/NNR.0000000000000114

World Health Organization. (n.d.). Health education. Retrieved from http://www.who.int/topics/health_education/en

SECTION II

Cancer and Cancer Treatment

CHAPTER 4

Overview of Cancer and Cancer Treatment

A. Definition of cancer

1. Cancer is a large group of diseases with the following traits (American Cancer Society [ACS], 2018; Block et al., 2015; Eggert, 2018):
   a) Sustained proliferation of abnormal cells and the ability to replicate indefinitely
   b) Uncontrolled growth and cell division, and deregulation of repair of defective DNA
   c) Ability to grow new blood vessels (angiogenesis)
   d) Ability to spread to distant sites (metastasize)
   e) Evasion of normal protective mechanisms of growth suppression, immunologic suppression, and programmed cell death (apoptosis)
   f) Genetic instability, inflammation, and fibrosis that enable malignant cell transformation
2. Models of cancer evolution (Eggert, 2018; see Figure 4-1)
   a) Clonal: Initial DNA changes result in benign growth, from which cloned cells accumulate multiple genetic mutations over time, resulting in a malignancy.
   b) Cancer stem cell: Cancer cells arise from cancer stem cells, which may have limited proliferative capability, but from which at least one cell line becomes tumorigenic.
   c) Plasticity model: This model builds on the cancer stem cell model, suggesting that noncancer stem cell versions of cells have the ability to change throughout their life cycle and are converted to cancer stem cells.
   d) Inflammation theory: Infectious agents and interaction with inflammatory cells induce chronic inflammation, causing cancer.
3. Genetic mutations and other genetic errors that drive oncogenesis (Hassen, Eggert, & Loud, 2018)
   a) Normal genes involved in cell growth are called *proto-oncogenes. Tumor suppressor genes* direct the programmed suppression of normal cell growth. Normal cells with some mutations can typically be restored to premutation function through normal DNA repair processes.
   b) Genetic mutations in proto-oncogenes and tumor suppressor genes disrupt normal cell processes—inhibiting apoptosis, disrupting DNA repair processes, and inducing immortality. Replication of the mutated genes allows development of malignancy. Mutated proto-oncogenes can be activated into oncogenes, which then exhibit uncontrolled cell proliferation.
   c) Driver mutations, such as those associated with the *TP53* gene (associated with about 50% of sporadic [acquired] cancers), are associated with oncogenesis and can often be targeted specifically for treatment (Block et al., 2015; Eggert, 2018).
   d) Epigenetic changes (changes in genetic expression rather than a genetic mutation) can affect the efficacy of DNA repair genes, altering specific gene expression and disrupting normal expression of proto-oncogenes and tumor suppressor genes.
   e) Other genetic errors such as deletions, translocations, or mismatched nucleotide pairs can initiate ongoing mutations that result in malignancy.
   f) Transcription errors of DNA when transcribed into messenger RNA (mRNA) can result in mutations.
      (1) A small percentage of cancers are caused by mutations of inherited DNA between generations in the germ line (sperm and ova).
      (2) Most cancers are sporadic and caused by a series of acquired mutations in somatic DNA over time (Eggert, 2018).
   g) Many microRNAs regulate genetic mechanisms and are deregulated in multiple tumor

Figure 4-1. Theories of Cancer Evolution

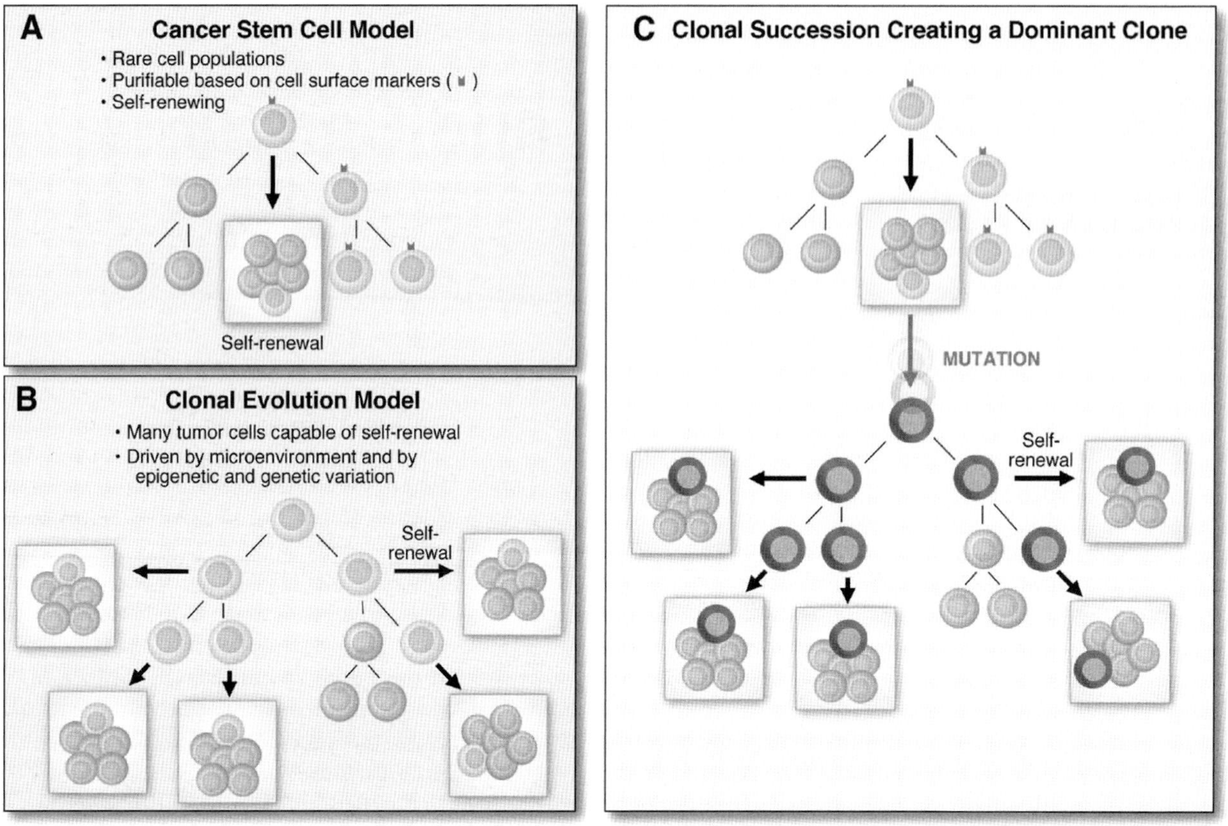

Note. From "Immunologic Targeting of the Cancer Stem Cell," by C.J. Wu in L. Girard (Ed.), *StemBook* [Internet], 2008, Cambridge, MA: Harvard Stem Cell Institute. Retrieved from https://www.ncbi.nlm.nih.gov/books/NBK27075. Copyright 2008 by Catherine J. Wu; distributed under CC BY 3.0 (https://creativecommons.org/licenses/by/3.0), which permits unrestricted use, distribution, and reproduction, provided the original work is properly cited.

types, making them a target for future therapies (Eggert, 2018).

4. Multiple factors often interact, leading to the development of cancer. Normal cells may undergo changes because of the following:
   a) Spontaneous transformation: No causative agent is identified, but cellular characteristics are typical of cancer cells.
   b) Chronic or occupational exposure to substances such as asbestos, benzene, radiation, tobacco, arsenic, nickel, and some chemotherapy agents is implicated in cancer development. The International Agency for Research on Cancer (2017) has identified 120 substances as carcinogens and another 375 substances as possibly or probably carcinogenic, while the National Toxicology Program (2016) has estimated the number of known carcinogens to be over 200.
   c) Changes in the microenvironment, such as cancer cell plasticity, immune cell and signaling molecule involvement, and even metabolic changes brought about by changes in oncogenes and tumor suppressor genes all contribute to the progression of cancer growth (Eggert, 2018).
   d) Exposure to viruses: Genetic changes can occur to cells through viral infections (e.g., human papillomavirus [HPV] is the primary cause of cervical cancer) (Inan et al., 2017).

B. Cancer staging and grading (American Joint Committee on Cancer [AJCC], 2017a, 2017b; Vogel, 2018)
   1. Staging: Verifies the extent of the disease by assessing the location and size of the primary tumor and determining if it has spread to other tissues or organs. Staging informs prognosis, treatment planning, identification of suitable clinical trials, and treatment response. Staging conventions provide a common language with which the healthcare team can communicate about a patient's case. Staging criteria are unique for many types of cancer (AJCC, 2017b; National Cancer Institute [NCI], 2015a).

a) Four types of staging (AJCC, 2017b)
   (1) Clinical: Based on physical examination, imaging, and biopsy
   (2) Pathologic: Based on tissue, fluids, or exploration during surgery; is combined with clinical staging
   (3) Post-therapy/postneoadjuvant therapy: Used for confirming cancer remaining after systemic chemotherapy or hormone therapy, or radiation therapy prior to surgery, or when no surgery is done
   (4) Restaging: Used for determining the extent of recurrence

b) The tumor-node-metastasis staging system is maintained jointly by AJCC and the Union for International Cancer Control. It is the most commonly used anatomic staging system and is based on specific criteria. It is then combined with a staging number (0–IV) and sometimes with substage designations (such as IIa or IIb). In general, stage I cancer confers a more favorable prognosis than stage IV (AJCC, 2017b; NCI, 2015a; Vogel, 2018).
   (1) Tumor (local involvement, invasion): Describes the original tumor (primary) and ranges from TX (cannot be evaluated) to T0–T4 (measurement of size/extent)
   (2) Node (lymph node involvement): Ranges from NX (cannot be evaluated) to N0–N3 (number of nodes involved and extent of spread)
   (3) Metastasis: Ranges from M0 (no distant metastasis) to M1 (presence of metastasis)

c) Hematologic malignancies, malignant melanoma, brain cancers, and some other cancers are staged according to other systems. For example, the Ann Arbor staging system is used to stage Hodgkin lymphoma, the Rai staging system is used to stage chronic lymphocytic leukemia, and the International Staging System is used for multiple myeloma (American Brain Tumor Association, n.d.; Leukemia and Lymphoma Society, n.d.-a, n.d.-b; Multiple Myeloma Research Foundation, n.d.; Vogel, 2018).

d) The American College of Surgeons Commission on Cancer requires that childhood cancers are staged either by AJCC criteria or pediatric clinical trial staging systems, the most common being the Children's Oncology Group staging system (NCI, n.d.-c, 2015a).

e) Prognostic information is provided by an increasing number of nonanatomic factors that may predict the effectiveness of specific therapies. Gender, overall health status, and genetic variants or specific biologic properties of tumor cells are characteristics that may affect patient outcomes and have been incorporated into some staging algorithms (AJCC, 2017b).

2. Grading: Cellular differentiation is based on how closely tumor cells resemble normal cells in their structure and maturity.
   a) Differentiation is graded from GX (cannot be assessed) to G4 (undifferentiated, where the parent cell is impossible to distinguish).
   b) Cells are obtained by biopsy or surgical removal for microscopic examination by a pathologist. Cancer cell differentiation can vary over time, and cells with several grades of differentiation can exist within a single tumor.
   c) Tumor grade is a prognostic indicator. The higher the grade, the more aggressive the tumor (NCI, 2013; Vogel, 2018).

C. Cancer treatment modalities

1. Table 4-1 summarizes the history of cancer therapy. A variety of modalities are used to treat cancer.
2. Surgery (Lester, 2018)
   a) Precise local treatment, which may be robotic-assisted (Doyle-Lindrud, 2015b)
   b) May remove all or a portion of the primary tumor, lymph nodes, and adjacent tissues
   c) Can be used to obtain specimens for cytopathology
   d) May be the only treatment a patient requires
   e) May be preceded or followed by other modalities
   f) May be used in the palliative setting to alleviate or lessen intolerable symptoms
3. Radiation therapy (Behrend, 2018; Doyle-Lindrud, 2015a; Gosselin, 2018)
   a) Local treatment in which energy is precisely directed at a specific target
   b) May be given before surgery to decrease tumor burden or after surgery to prevent recurrence of the primary tumor
   c) More effective for some diseases than others
   d) Multiple methods of treatment delivery, including various external beam treatments, stereotactic radiosurgery, image-guided CyberKnife® radiosurgery, brachytherapy, and sealed and unsealed radionuclide therapy

e) Often given in combination with chemotherapy (chemoradiation) or as radioimmunotherapy

4. Chemotherapy (Bender et al., 2014; Dowling, McDonagh, & Meade, 2017)
   a) Most commonly administered as a systemic treatment
   b) May be used locally for instillations (e.g., bladder, peritoneum) and topical therapy
   c) May be used as single agents or, more commonly, in combination
   d) Limited by nonspecific cytotoxic effects on normal tissues
   e) Generally affect the cell cycle and cell kinetics

Table 4-1. History of Cancer Treatments

Period	Events
Pre-20th century	1500s: Heavy metals are used systemically to treat cancers; however, their effectiveness is limited, and their toxicity is great (Burchenal, 1977). 1890s: William Coley, MD, develops and explores the use of Coley toxins, the first nonspecific immunostimulants used to treat cancer.
World War I	Sulfur-mustard gas is used for chemical warfare; servicemen who are exposed to nitrogen mustard experience bone marrow and lymphoid suppression (Gilman, 1963; Gilman & Philips, 1946).
World War II	Congress passes National Cancer Act in 1937, establishing the National Cancer Institute (NCI). Alkylating agents are recognized for their antineoplastic effect (Gilman & Philips, 1946). Thioguanine and mercaptopurine are developed (Guy & Ingram, 1996). 1946: NCI-identified cancer research areas include biology, chemotherapy, epidemiology, and pathology. 1948: Divisions within NCI and external institutions are identified to conduct research (Zubrod, 1984). Folic acid antagonists are found to be effective against childhood acute leukemia (Farber et al., 1948). Antitumor antibiotics are discovered.
1950s	1955: The National Chemotherapy Program, developed with Congressional funding, is founded to develop and test new chemotherapy drugs. 1957: Interferon is discovered. The Children's Cancer Group, the first cooperative group dedicated to finding effective treatments for pediatric cancer, is formed.
1960s–1970s	Development of platinum compounds begins. Multidrug therapy improves remission rates without severe toxicity; mechlorethamine, vincristine, procarbazine, and prednisone (MOPP), the first combination chemotherapy, is used and found to be curative against Hodgkin lymphoma (Noonan, 2007). Clinical trials of bacillus Calmette-Guérin and *Corynebacterium parvum*, nonspecific immunostimulants, begin. Chemotherapy is used with surgery and radiation as cancer treatment. Development of hybridoma technology begins. NCI starts its Biological Response Modifiers Program. Tamoxifen is synthesized in 1962 and first used in 1969.
1970s	The National Cancer Act of 1971 provides funding for cancer research; NCI director is appointed by and reports to the president of the United States. Doxorubicin phase 1 trials begin. Adjuvant chemotherapy begins to be a common cancer treatment (Bonadonna et al., 1995; Fisher et al., 1986). Discovery of human leukocyte antigen histocompatibility system expands the use of and survival from bone marrow transplantation (Perry & Linch, 1996).
1980s	Community Clinical Oncology Programs are developed in 1983 to contribute to NCI chemotherapy clinical trials. Use of multimodal therapies increases (Eilber et al., 1984; Marcial et al., 1988). Focus turns to symptom management to alleviate dose-limiting toxicities related to neutropenia, nausea and vomiting, and cardiotoxicity. Clinical trials for dexrazoxane (ICRF-187) as a cardioprotectant begin (Speyer et al., 1988). New chemotherapy agents are available. Scientists begin to investigate recombinant DNA technology. Trials of monoclonal antibodies and cytokines begin. Effector cells (lymphokine-activated killer cells and tumor-infiltrating lymphocytes) are grown ex vivo. 1986: U.S. Food and Drug Administration (FDA) approves interferon alfa. 1989: FDA approves erythropoietin. High-dose chemotherapy is used for myeloablation prior to bone marrow and stem cell transplantation (Perry & Linch, 1996).

(Continued on next page)

Table 4-1. History of Cancer Treatments *(Continued)*

Period	Events
1990s	New classifications of drugs (e.g., taxanes) are developed. In clinical trials, paclitaxel is found to be effective against ovarian and breast cancers (Rowinsky et al., 1992). FDA approves granulocyte–colony-stimulating factor and granulocyte macrophage–colony-stimulating factor, interleukin-2, interleukin-11, rituximab, trastuzumab, and denileukin diftitox. Clinical trials of gene therapy and antiangiogenic agents begin. FDA approves filgrastim for use in bone marrow transplantation and chemotherapy-induced neutropenia, severe chronic neutropenia, and peripheral blood stem cell transplantation. FDA approves ondansetron for prevention of chemotherapy-induced nausea and vomiting; other 5-hydroxytryptamine-3 receptor antagonists are in clinical trials (Perez, 1995). Because of improved symptom management, dose intensity becomes a focus. FDA approves new analogs (e.g., vinorelbine) (Abeloff, 1995). Scientists focus on the sequencing of agents (Bonadonna et al., 1995). The genetic basis of cancers becomes an important factor in cancer risk research (e.g., *BRCA1* for breast cancer, renal cell cancer) (Gnarra et al., 1995; Hoskins et al., 1995; Miki et al., 1994). Aromatase inhibitors are approved for breast cancer treatment. This marks a step forward for hormone therapy.
2000–2009	The Children's Oncology Group (www.childrensoncologygroup.org), a cooperative group combining the efforts of several groups, is formed to further the advancement of cancer treatment for children. Scientists complete a working draft of the human genome (American Society of Clinical Oncology [ASCO], n.d.). Theory of immune surveillance continues to develop, and biotherapy is used to target and mount a defense against certain antigens on malignant cells (e.g., gemtuzumab ozogamicin binds to CD33 on leukemic cells, rituximab binds to CD20-positive non-Hodgkin lymphoma cells). Radioimmunotherapy is used to deliver radioactivity directly to select tumor cells, avoiding damage to healthy tissue (e.g., ibritumomab tiuxetan, tositumomab and iodine-131). FDA approves targeted therapies attacking epidermal growth factor receptor for lung cancer (gefitinib and erlotinib) and colon cancer (cetuximab and panitumumab) (ASCO, n.d.). FDA approves antiangiogenic agents (bevacizumab was the first) (ASCO, n.d.). A neurokinin-1 antagonist (aprepitant) is used in combination with other antiemetic drugs to prevent chemotherapy-induced nausea and vomiting. Therapeutic vaccine trials begin for existing cancers (e.g., OncoVAX®, an autologous tumor cell vaccine, is in phase 3 studies for stage II colon cancer). FDA approves a prophylactic vaccine (Gardasil®) for the prevention of human papillomavirus infections that cause cervical cancer (ASCO, n.d.).
2010–present	2010: Patient Protection and Affordable Care Act is signed into law. American cancer survivors number 13.7 million, the highest number to date (ASCO, n.d.). FDA approves the first cancer treatment vaccine (sipuleucel-T), utilizing the patient's dendritic cells in the immune system to attack cancer cells (Anassi & Ndefo, 2011). 2011: FDA approves ipilimumab for unresectable or metastatic melanoma. Its mechanism of action is to stimulate the body's immune system to attack cancer cells (Bristol-Myers Squibb Co., 2011; NCI, 2015b). 2013: FDA approves ado-trastuzumab emtansine (T-DM1), an antibody–drug conjugate, linking trastuzumab (the monoclonal antibody) and mertansine (the cytotoxic drug) to block microtubule formation in cancer cells (Amiri-Kordestani et al., 2014). 2014: FDA grants accelerated approval for checkpoint inhibitor pembrolizumab for advanced melanoma for patients whose disease progressed following ipilimumab and/or a BRAF inhibitor (if BRAF positive) (Raedler, 2015). 2016: FDA approves atezolizumab, the first programmed cell death-ligand 1 (PD-L1) checkpoint inhibitor for treatment of advanced bladder cancer (ASCO, 2017). Pembrolizumab becomes a new standard option for previously treated patients with advanced non-small cell lung cancer (NSCLC); later the same year, it is FDA approved for use as first-line treatment for PD-L1–positive NSCLC. National debate begins about the importance to test select patients to determine those who may benefit from immune checkpoint inhibitors (ASCO, 2017). 2017: FDA approves avelumab for the treatment of Merkel cell carcinoma; this is the first FDA-approved product for this disease (U.S. FDA, 2017d). FDA approves a chimeric antigen receptor T-cell therapy for select patients with B-cell acute lymphoblastic leukemia, the first gene therapy that uses technology to reprogram the patient's own immune system to destroy cancer cells (Novartis Pharmaceuticals Corp., 2017). FDA approves Mvasi™ (bevacizumab-awwb, Amgen Inc.), the first biosimilar approved in the United States for the treatment of cancer (U.S. FDA, 2017c).

f) Includes alkylating agents, antimetabolites, antitumor antibiotics, nitrosoureas, and plant alkaloids (e.g., taxanes, vinca alkaloids, camptothecins)

5. Hormone therapy (Tortorice, 2018)
   a) Systemic treatment, often combined with other antineoplastic agents to treat cancer
   b) Have various mechanisms of action and unique side effect profiles
   c) Includes corticosteroids, androgens, antiandrogens, selective estrogen receptor modulators, estrogen receptor antagonists, aromatase inhibitors, and luteinizing hormone–releasing hormone antagonists and agonists (see Chapter 7)
6. Immunotherapies and gene therapies (Bayer et al., 2017; Lea, 2018; Martin, 2017; Muehlbauer, Callahan, Zlott, & Dahl, 2018; Vioral, 2018; see Chapter 10)
   a) Systemic treatments that use the patient's own immune system through various pathophysiologic mechanisms
   b) May be synthetic (such as chimeric antigen receptor [CAR] T cells), biologically derived (such as monoclonal antibodies), or nonpathogenic or pathogenic (requiring modification for use) viruses
   c) Includes CAR T-cell therapies, checkpoint inhibitors, monoclonal antibodies, cancer vaccines, immunomodulators, cytokines, and oncolytic viruses
   d) May cause significant cytokine release syndrome or hypersensitivity reactions, as well as unique side effect profiles due to immune response to drug
   e) Rapidly evolving class of treatment options
   f) Gene therapies correct defective genes typically by inserting a normal gene into the nuclei of a gene to repair, replace, or alter the function of an abnormal gene by use of viral vectors.
7. Targeted therapies (McIntyre, 2015; Wujcik, 2018)
   a) Systemic therapies (see Chapter 8)
   b) Targeted therapies may be so specific as to target a single molecular feature on the surface of tumor cells or an enzyme within the cell; they block or turn off signals causing cell growth, initiate apoptosis, or kill cancer cells directly (Kreamer & Riordan, 2015).
   c) Toxicities are primarily nonhematologic and have unique side effect profiles (Kreamer & Riordan, 2015).
   d) Includes tyrosine kinase inhibitors (TKIs), anaplastic lymphoma kinase inhibitors, cyclin-dependent kinase inhibitors, and epidermal growth factor receptor (EGFR) inhibitors
8. High-dose chemotherapy with hematopoietic stem cell support: Administration of high doses of chemotherapy with the intention of ablation of the bone marrow, with subsequent rescue using peripheral, bone marrow, or umbilical stem cells. Transplants can be autologous, allogeneic, syngeneic, or haploidentical. The use of high-dose chemotherapy with hematopoietic stem cell rescue is standard of care for many hematologic malignancies (Tortorice, 2018).
9. Emerging therapies
   a) Tumor treatment fields generate alternative electromagnetic fields that disrupt cell division for patients newly diagnosed with glioblastoma multiforme (Chang, 2017; Saria & Kesari, 2016).
   b) Nano/microbubbles delivered via ultrasound to specific genes, followed by drug introduction, has demonstrated significant tumor reduction in tumors in mice and may be a new method for gene delivery for cancer gene therapy (Mitra et al., 2015; Wujcik, 2018).
   c) Biosimilars are biologic products that are similar to, but not exactly the same as, the reference drug that they mimic (U.S. Food and Drug Administration [FDA], 2017a). They are not generic forms of a reference drug (which are chemically identical to the reference drug) but instead are chemically similar, and structural and chemical changes should not affect efficacy (Griffith, McBride, Stevenson, & Green, 2014). Biosimilars are produced through an abbreviated manufacturing process and are therefore expected to be an affordable alternative to some therapeutic agents.

D. Treatment approaches

1. Chemoprevention: Use of selected pharmacologic agents to prevent cancer in high-risk individuals (e.g., tamoxifen for women whose personal health history indicates they are at a statistically increased risk for developing breast cancer) (Smith, Richmond, & Dunn, 2018).
2. Neoadjuvant therapy: Use of one or more treatment modalities prior to the primary therapy (e.g., chemotherapy before surgery). Goal is to debulk the primary tumor prior to surgery or to address micrometastases (Tajima et al., 2017; Tortorice, 2018).
3. Adjuvant therapy: Therapy following the primary treatment modality (e.g., chemotherapy or radi-

ation after surgery). Goal is to target minimal disease or micrometastases for patients at high risk for recurrence (Tortorice, 2018).

4. Conditioning or preparative therapy: Administration of chemotherapy, sometimes with total body irradiation, to eliminate residual disease or ablate the marrow space prior to receiving a hematopoietic stem cell transplant (also referred to as *myeloablation*).
   a) Myeloablative: Obliteration of bone marrow with chemotherapy agents typically administered in high doses in preparation for hematopoietic stem cell transplantation. Myeloablative therapy does not allow for spontaneous marrow recovery because of the lethal doses of agents used; therefore, it must be followed by transplantation to prevent death (Gyurkocza & Sandmaier, 2014; Zack, 2018).
   b) Nonmyeloablative: Reduced-intensity conditioning using doses that are not lethal to bone marrow (Epperla et al., 2017; Gyurkocza & Sandmaier, 2014). This type of transplant is dependent on the graft-versus-tumor effect. Use of nonmyeloablative regimens has expanded options and transplant eligibility for older adult patients or those with comorbidities (Gyurkocza & Sandmaier, 2014).
5. Immunosuppression: Administration of antineoplastic agents at doses sufficient to blunt a patient's immune response. Agents such as methotrexate are given post-transplantation to prevent graft-versus-host disease. Select agents are used to treat noncancerous conditions, such as autoimmune diseases.

E. Treatment strategies

1. Combination versus single therapies: Combinations of drugs or combination of therapies (e.g., drug alone vs. drug plus radiation therapy) generally provides superior efficacy and a survival advantage over monotherapy in many tumor types and combination regimens, although the mechanism by which this occurs is not fully understood in some cases (Haque, Verma, Butler, & Teh, 2017; Jin, Fan, Pan, & Jin, 2017; Mokhtari et al., 2017; Pritchard et al., 2013; Tortorice, 2018; Zhang et al., 2017). Hypotheses include that one agent may potentiate the effect of another, or that the combined agent or therapies create effects that together are distinctly unique.
   a) Tumor cell populations are heterogeneous; therefore, a combination of agents or therapies with different mechanisms of action is able to increase the proportion of cells killed at any one time.
   b) Combination agents or therapies with different mechanisms of action also reduce the possibility of drug resistance, as researcher consensus concludes that many mechanisms of resistance are likely to be occurring within a single tumor (Mokhtari et al., 2017; NCI, 2016).
   c) Combinations of drugs can be used synergistically to access sanctuary sites, as one drug's solubility or affinity for specific tissues may be different than, but complementary to, another particular drug's characteristics (Mokhtari et al., 2017).
   d) Drugs with similar toxicities generally are avoided, although this is not always possible. Therapy combinations may potentiate the toxic effects of either or both therapies or may be lessened because of different targeted mechanisms of action (Mokhtari et al., 2017).
2. Dosing of cytotoxic chemotherapy
   a) Treatment cycles are designed to permit recovery from damage to normal tissues and organs and are based on the known pharmacokinetics of agents. Because the average white blood cell nadir is 10–14 days, many regimens are based on this time frame (Drooger, van Pelt-Sprangers, Leunis, Jager, & de Jongh, 2016; Tortorice, 2018).
   b) *Dose density* refers to the drug dose per unit of time. Higher dose density is achieved by shortening the intervals between treatments (Lambertini et al., 2017). Reducing the time between chemotherapy cycles may diminish tumor regrowth.
   c) *Dose intensity* is the amount of drug that is delivered over time. Dose reduction or delay resulting from chemotherapy side effects, scheduling conflicts, or any other reason reduces dose intensity and may negatively affect patient survival (Matikas, Foukakis, & Bergh, 2017). The prophylactic use of the myeloid growth factor pegfilgrastim has allowed for administration of dose-dense and dose-intense chemotherapy regimens that would otherwise result in unacceptable neutropenia (Kourlaba et al., 2015).
   d) Relative dose intensity is calculated by comparing the received dose to the referenced (standard) dose of the standard regimen. Proactively managing symptoms and educating patients on the importance of maintaining the prescribed dosing schedule are paramount to optimal outcomes (Havrilesky, Reiner, Morrow, Watson, & Crawford, 2015).

e) Dose density and intensity and relative dose intensity concepts may not apply to targeted therapies, immunotherapies, and hormone therapies because of their different toxicity profiles.

F. Goals of cancer therapy
1. Treatment planning includes shared decision making that integrates the patient's personal goals, needs, and values as part of care planning (Cranley, Curbow, George, & Christie, 2017; Lilley, Bader, & Cooper, 2015).
2. Prevention (Mahon, 2018)
a) Primary cancer prevention: Measures taken to avoid carcinogen exposure and promote health or to prevent disease development (e.g., avoidance of tobacco products, immunization against HPV)
(1) Chemoprevention (e.g., tamoxifen for women at risk for breast cancer; HPV vaccine to protect against HPV infection, which can cause cancers of the cervix, vagina, penis, anus, and oropharynx)
(2) Lifestyle and behavioral modification of risk factors (e.g., dietary choices, obesity, smoking) associated with the development of some cancers (Smith et al., 2018)
b) Secondary cancer prevention: Early detection and treatment of cancer (e.g., mammogram and colonoscopy screening)
c) Tertiary cancer prevention: Monitoring for or preventing recurrence of the original cancer or secondary malignancies (e.g., rehabilitation and exercise programs, nutritional changes, psychosocial support) (Smith et al., 2018)
3. Curative intent: Defined as treatment that has the potential to eliminate disease (ACS, 2016b)
4. Control: When cure is not possible, the goal may be to administer treatment to slow the growth or spread of cancer and allow patients to live longer than if therapy had not been given (ACS, 2016a).
5. Palliation: An interprofessional team-based approach that improves the quality of life for patients and families through expert assessment and treatment of physical, spiritual, psychological, and social problems associated with serious illness (World Health Organization [WHO], n.d.)
a) Both the Oncology Nursing Society (ONS, 2014) and the American Society of Clinical Oncology (ASCO; Peppercorn et al., 2011) maintain position statements associated with integration of personalized palliative care that includes recognition of the patient's goals, needs, and values as key to effective cancer care.
b) Integration of palliative care early in the cancer care experience is key to effective patient management (Hui & Bruera, 2016; Salins et al., 2016). It may include surgery, radiation therapy, complementary and integrative therapies, chemotherapy, targeted therapies, or immunotherapies, individually or in combination (WHO, n.d.).
c) Palliative care can be offered at any point in the cancer care continuum and can be provided in inpatient, ambulatory, primary care, and community settings.

G. Measuring response
1. Objective tumor response
a) Quantitative measurement: Objective tumor response is assessed through a quantitative measurement such as surgical examination, imaging studies, or serum tumor markers. Baseline measurements recorded at the time of diagnosis are compared to those recorded after treatment completion.
(1) The earliest measures of determining response date back to 1976 when oncologists treating patients with lymphoma developed a system by measuring simulated tumor masses with rulers and calipers. The developers recommended that to avoid error when measuring, a 50% decrease in tumor diameter be used as the criteria for determining the efficacy of treatment. Thus, the decision to use reduction of tumor size by 50% was chosen to reduce error, not because it indicated a clinical benefit (Fojo & Bates, 2015).
(2) WHO Tumor Response Criteria were developed in 1981 as a standardized approach to reporting response to treatment and marked the advent of using a common language to describe response criteria (Fojo & Bates, 2015).
(a) Tumor measurements are obtained by using the cross product, which is determined by multiplying the longest diameters of the axial and perpendicular planes.
(b) Although used for several decades, the limitations and deficiencies of these response criteria became obvious over time. For example, there

were no guidelines for what type of imaging may be used, and the bidimensional measuring technique was cumbersome. Several modifications were attempted, but none of these methods was uniformly accepted (Sandrasegaran, 2015).

(3) The Response Evaluation Criteria in Solid Tumors (RECIST) guidelines were published in 2000 by a task force that included members of the European Organisation for Research and Treatment of Cancer, NCI, and the National Cancer Institute of Canada. These guidelines addressed most but not all of the deficiencies in the WHO criteria.

(*a*) RECIST guidelines recommended the use of one-dimensional tumor measurements (the longest diameter) rather than the cross product (Sandrasegaran, 2015).

i. Complete response (CR): Complete disappearance of all disease

ii. Partial response (PR): At least 30% reduction in the sum of the longest diameter of the target lesion

iii. Stable disease: Change not meeting criteria for response or progression

iv. Progression: 20% or more increase in the sum of the longest diameter of target lesions

(*b*) RECIST 1.1 was developed in 2009 as technology and medicine advanced. Using the same criteria for response from 1.0, it also identified and addressed problems with RECIST 1.0. For example, the criteria were updated to include nodal disease (Fojo & Bates, 2015). RECIST 1.1 has also been known to have limitations.

i. The criteria depend solely on anatomic measurements and do not consider tumor vascularity or the parameters of functional imaging.

ii. Traditional cytotoxic chemotherapy often results in the reduction of tumor size, but newer targeted agents that interfere or inhibit cell growth and division by inhibiting molecular pathways are considered *cytostatic*, meaning they block tumor cell proliferation, whereas standard chemotherapy agents are cytotoxic, meaning they kill tumor cells.

(*c*) Studies of several cancer types such as prostate cancer, mesothelioma, soft tissue sarcoma, and neuroendocrine tumors have also shown that RECIST 1.1 criteria are inaccurate in reporting response to therapy (Sandrasegaran, 2015).

2. Clinical benefit response: The concept of clinical benefit response was developed when patients did not have measurable tumor shrinkage but experienced a reduction in symptoms (e.g., pancreatic cancer). *Clinical benefit* is defined as a combination of reduction or improvement in pain, performance status, and weight (Fojo & Bates, 2015).
3. The severity-weighted assessment tool was designed to assign a factor to cutaneous T-cell lymphoma where skin lesions can vary widely in severity rather than size, ranging from individual skin lesions to involving the entire epidermis (Fojo & Bates, 2015).
4. Pathologic complete response in breast cancer is the endpoint used to evaluate response after neoadjuvant treatment. After the standard neoadjuvant chemotherapy regimen, the breast is resected and evaluated for remaining breast cancer cells. The absence of cancer cells in the resected breast is referred to as *pathologic complete response* (Fojo & Bates, 2015).
5. Computed tomography–based tumor density is frequently used with diseases that have response to treatment but have minimal tumor shrinkage such as gastrointestinal stromal tumor, renal cell cancer, or hepatocellular cancer (Fojo & Bates, 2015).
6. Glucose analog tracer, fluorine-18 fluorodeoxyglucose positron-emission tomography (^{18}F-FDG PET)

a) In 2007, the International Working Group incorporated guidelines using PET assessments in metabolically active lymph nodes. Although widely used in clinical trials as part of the standardized response criteria for lymphoma, PET imaging in solid tumors is used for detection of new or recurrent sites of disease and can be used as an adjunct for evaluating disease progression when using RECIST criteria (Fojo & Bates, 2015).

b) The most recent effort to standardize PET criteria is Positron Emission Tomography Response Criteria in Solid Tumors (PERCIST 1.0) by the European Organisation for Research and Treatment of Cancer and NCI. PERCIST specifies that the percentage of change in metabolic activity from baseline to post-treatment scans be recorded to provide a continuous plot of tumor activity (Sandrasegaran, 2015). However, because of variations in patient activity, carbohydrate intake, blood glucose, and timing, unifying ^{18}F-FDG PET response criteria remains a challenge (Fojo & Bates, 2015).

7. Serum biomarkers
   a) Tumor markers are a group of proteins that can be measured in the blood to indirectly evaluate progression of cancer. These markers are most useful in monitoring response to a treatment or progression of disease. The direction, whether future levels increase or decrease, and the rate of change allow the provider to determine efficacy of treatment. Therefore, it is helpful to obtain baseline tumor markers before the tumor is excised and before the initiation of treatment (Reilly, 2013).
   b) Serum biomarkers differ from the assays determining the presence of an overexpressed or mutated molecular target. The recent investment in the development of predictive markers has reduced the focus on protein biomarkers as an indicator of treatment response relative to older literature (Fojo & Bates, 2015).
8. Circulating tumor cells and circulating tumor DNA are under investigation and may show potential to determine therapeutic response.
   a) The number of circulating tumor cells in the blood has been shown to be prognostic, with higher levels conferring a poor prognosis.
   b) The amount of circulating tumor DNA appears to correlate with tumor burden and increases with stage.
   c) Whether these tests prove to be more accurate than serum biomarkers in determining treatment response remains to be determined (Fojo & Bates, 2015).
9. Immune-related response criteria
   a) A number of new therapeutic options are being studied to harness the immune system in controlling malignancy. These approaches include cytokines, T cells (checkpoint inhibitors), manipulation of T cells, oncolytic viruses, therapies directed at other cell types, and vaccines.
   b) The patterns of response to treatment with immunotherapy agents differ from treatments with molecularly targeted agents or cytotoxic agents in several important respects (Shoushtari, Wolchok, & Hellman, 2018).
      (1) The patient may have transient worsening of disease before the disease stabilizes or the tumor regresses; therefore, caution should be taken in stopping treatment early.
      (2) Treatment response can take longer to become apparent compared with cytotoxic therapy.
      (3) Some patients who do not meet criteria for objective response can have prolonged periods of stable disease that are clinically significant.
   c) Immune-related response criteria have been proposed to properly recognize these nontraditional patterns of response seen with checkpoint inhibitors and some other immunotherapies. The use of these criteria is important because the application of RECIST criteria in patients being treated with checkpoint inhibitors may lead to premature discontinuation of treatment in a patient who will eventually respond to treatment or have prolonged disease (Shoushtari et al., 2018; Wolchok et al., 2009).
      (1) Immune-related complete response: Complete resolution of all lesions, with no new lesions. CR must be confirmed by a second consecutive assessment at least four weeks later.
      (2) Immune-related partial response: A decrease in the total tumor burden of 50% or more compared with baseline, which must be confirmed with second assessment at least four weeks later. This allows for inclusion of progression of some lesions or the appearance of new lesions as long as the total tumor burden meets the response criteria.
      (3) Immune-related stable disease: Tumor does not meet the criteria for either a PR or CR or for progressive disease.
      (4) Immune-related progressive disease: Increase in tumor burden of 25% or more relative to the minimum recorded tumor burden. Must be confirmed by second assessment no less than four

weeks after the initial documentation of an increase in tumor.

10. Patient outcomes: Direct evidence of treatment benefit is derived from clinical trial effectiveness endpoints that measure survival or a meaningful aspect of how a patient feels or functions in daily life (U.S. FDA, 2017b). In the 1970s, FDA approved cancer drugs based on objective response rates that were determined by tumor assessments. However, in the 1980s, FDA determined that cancer drug approval should be based on more direct evidence of clinical benefit, such as improvement in survival, improved tumor-related symptoms, quality of life, or physical functioning (U.S. Department of Health and Human Services, 2007).
    a) Survival data are gathered to assess the efficacy of cancer treatment.
        (1) The starting point for survival measurement may be the date of diagnosis, first visit to the physician or clinic, hospital admission, treatment initiation, or randomization to a clinical trial (Hess, 2017).
        (2) The vital status of each patient is noted as alive, dead, or unknown. The status is recorded at the endpoint of participation in a study, including the completion of the study or when the individual is lost to follow-up or dies (Hess, 2017).
    b) Tumor assessment (U.S. Department of Health and Human Services, 2007)
        (1) Time to progression and progression-free survival have also served as primary endpoints for drug approval. *Time to progression* is defined as time from randomization to progression, whereas *progression-free survival* is defined as the time from randomization until disease progression or death.
        (2) *Disease-free survival* is defined as the time from randomization until recurrence of tumor or death from any cause. This endpoint is most frequently used in the adjuvant setting after definitive surgery or radiation therapy.
        (3) *Objective response rate* refers to the proportion of patients in a study with reduction in tumor burden of a predetermined amount and for a minimum period of time. Response duration is measured from the time of initial response until documented tumor progression. Per FDA, if available, standardization criteria should be used to ascertain response (e.g., RECIST criteria has been considered appropriate).
        (4) *Time to treatment failure* is the endpoint measuring time from randomization to discontinuation of treatment for any reason, including progression, treatment toxicity, or death.
    c) Symptom assessment: Quality of life
        (1) The ASCO Cancer Research Committee stated, "In arriving at goals for clinical trials, both survival and quality of life were considered as important to outcomes that are clinically meaningful for patients" (Stenger, 2014, "Primary Goal," para. 1).
        (2) The committee also stated that symptoms from cancer progression and tolerability of treatment are critically important factors when considering whether a new treatment is associated with a clinically meaningful outcome (Stenger, 2014).
    d) Performance status
        (1) Performance status is the measure of level of functioning in terms of the amount of normal daily activity that patients can maintain to care for themselves and physical ability such as walking and working. Performance status is affected by cancer, complications of cancer, and comorbid conditions (Søgaard, Thomsen, Bossen, Sørensen, & Nørgaard, 2013).
        (2) Assessing performance status is a way for physicians to track changes in a patient's level of functioning as a result of cancer treatment. Documenting performance status using a standardized index allows clinicians to report a patient's response to clinical trials in a consistent manner (ECOG-ACRIN Cancer Research Group, 2016).
        (3) Commonly used measurements of performance status
            (a) Eastern Cooperative Oncology Group (ECOG) score
                i. First published in 1982, also called the WHO or Zubrod score. Key elements of the ECOG scale first appeared in medical literature in 1960 by C. Gordon Zubrod. This rating scale uses scores from 0 to 5, indicating poorer performance status as the score

increases (ECOG-ACRIN Cancer Research Group, 2016).

ii. Researchers worldwide take the ECOG Performance Status into consideration when planning trials to study a new treatment method. This numbering scale is one way to define the population of patients to be studied in the trial so that it can be uniformly reproduced among physicians who enroll patients (ECOG-ACRIN Cancer Research Group, 2016).

(b) The Karnofsky Performance Status Scale was first introduced in 1949 with an index rating between 100 and 0, with higher score indicating better performance (ECOG-ACRIN Cancer Research Group, 2016).

(c) The Lansky Play-Performance Scale for Pediatric Patients is used to classify patients younger than 16 years. The form is completed by parents based on the child's activity over the past week and is repeated over time to assess for changes in performance status (Lansky, List, Lansky, Ritter-Sterr, & Miller, 1987).

(d) Table 4-2 compares the three performance rating scales.

H. Factors affecting treatment response

1. Comorbidity is defined as "the coexistence of disorders in addition to a primary disease of interest" (Sarfati, Koczwara, & Jackson, 2016, p. 338).

a) 40% of patients with cancer have at least one other chronic condition, and 15% have two or more (Sarfati et al., 2016).

b) Comorbidity has consistently been found to have an adverse impact on cancer survival (Sarfati et al., 2016). It can affect cancer survival through its impact on factors such as cancer detection, treatment, and adherence (Søgaard et al., 2013).

c) Patients with comorbidities are less likely to receive adjuvant therapy, more likely to receive a reduced dose, and less likely to complete a course of treatment (Søgaard et al., 2013).

(1) It has been found that 24%–70% of patients with cancer with comorbidity are not treated according to guidelines (Søgaard et al., 2013).

(2) Substantial inconsistency and lack of consensus exist in treatment decisions based on comorbidity (Sarfati et al., 2016).

(3) Factors that may affect treatment decisions in patients with comorbidity include concern about toxicity, patient age, race, and education level (Søgaard et al., 2013).

d) Cancer or its treatment may affect comorbidity outcomes. Cancer therapies can increase the risk of cardiovascular, metabolic, musculoskeletal, and other conditions and can worsen preexisting comorbidities (Sarfati et al., 2016).

2. Performance status: Measuring performance status is useful because it reflects patients' potential ability to tolerate and respond to further treatment. Two patients with similar stages of disease but significantly different performance indexes may have very different outcomes (Reilly, 2013).

3. Tumor burden: According to NCI (n.d.-d), *tumor burden* refers to the number of cancer cells, the size of the tumor, or the amount of cancer in the body. The larger the tumor (sometimes referred to as the bulkiness of disease), the greater the chance for spread and development of metastatic disease. Tumor burden continues to be the most important disease characteristic when determining treatment for patients with Hodgkin lymphoma (Cuccaro et al., 2014).

4. Resistance: Genetic instability of the tumor cell and emergence of drug resistance are currently considered the most significant determination of response (Tortorice, 2018).

a) Temporary or relative resistance is usually a function of the drug's inability to reach the target cell. Causes of temporary resistance include the following (Tortorice, 2018):

(1) Poor blood supply

(2) Anatomic sanctuary sites, such as the testes and central nervous system

(3) Altered pharmacokinetic parameters

(a) *Pharmacokinetics* is defined as the action of the body in response to a drug (Alfarouk et al., 2015).

(b) Pharmacokinetic resistance is a concept that describes the body-related factors that alter a drug's effectiveness so that it does not reach its target or accomplish

Table 4-2. Performance Status Scales

Scale	Grade/Score	Description
Eastern Cooperative Oncology Group (also known as ECOG, Zubrod, or World Health Organization) performance scale	0	Fully active; no performance restrictions
	1	Strenuous physical activity restricted; fully ambulatory and able to carry out light work
	2	Capable of all self-care but unable to carry out any work activities; up and about > 50% of waking hours
	3	Capable of only limited self-care; confined to bed or chair > 50% of waking hours
	4	Completely disabled; cannot carry out any self-care; totally confined to bed or chair
	5	Dead
Karnofsky Performance Status Scale	100	Normal; no complaints; no evidence of disease
	90	Able to carry on normal activity; minor signs or symptoms of disease
	80	Normal activity with effort; some signs or symptoms of disease
	70	Cares for self; unable to carry on normal activity or do active work
	60	Requires occasional assistance but able to care for most needs
	50	Requires considerable assistance and frequent medical care
	40	Disabled; requires special care and assistance
	30	Severely disabled; hospitalization indicated although death not imminent
	20	Hospitalization necessary; very sick; active supportive treatment necessary
	10	Moribund; fatal processes progressing rapidly
	0	Dead
Lansky Play-Performance Scale for Pediatric Patients	100	Fully active; normal
	90	Minor restrictions with strenuous physical activity
	80	Active, but gets tired more quickly
	70	Both greater restriction of and less time spent in active play
	60	Up and around but minimal active play; keeps busy with quieter activities
	50	Lying around much of the day but gets dressed; no active play; participates in all quiet play and activities
	40	Mostly stays in bed; participates in quiet activities
	30	Stuck in bed; needs help even for quiet play
	20	Often sleeping; play is entirely limited to very passive activities
	10	Does not play or get out of bed
	0	Unresponsive

Note. Based on information from ECOG-ACRIN Cancer Research Group, 2016; Michigan Care Management Resource Center, n.d.

its intended goal. The following factors can affect pharmacokinetic resistance (Alfarouk et al., 2015):

i. Absorption: Orally ingested agents for cancer can be affected by the presence or absence of food in the patient's stomach and the presence of permeability glycoprotein, or P-glycoprotein (P-gp), which is found along the gastrointestinal tract. P-gp has been shown to reduce the oral bioavailability of some anticancer drugs.

ii. Distribution: A higher volume of distribution means more drug penetrates into a tissue while it is more diluted in the plasma. Volume of distribution can be affected by gender, weight, plasma proteins, and circadian rhythm.

iii. Metabolism: Cytochrome P450 enzymes are responsible for drug metabolism. Overexpression might lead to resistance due to rapid inactivation of the drug.

iv. Excretion of drugs can be affected by:
- Overexpression of multidrug resistance protein, which is correlated with an increase in biliary excretion
- Renal excretion: The kidney is the primary organ by which drugs are excreted. Changes in glomerular filtration rate based on gender and ethnic differences can have a direct effect on drug availability.

(c) Drug–drug interactions: Coadministration of drugs might result in antagonism such that one drug may counteract or neutralize another. A common example is tamoxifen, which needs to be converted to its active form by the metabolizing enzyme CYP2D6. This same enzyme is inhibited by certain selective serotonin reuptake inhibitors, thus reducing the efficacy of tamoxifen (Alfarouk et al., 2015).

(d) In some conditions, temporary resistance may be reversed by altering drug delivery, dose, or scheduling of drug administration (Tortorice, 2018).

b) Permanent or phenotypic drug resistance is an inheritable mechanism that may result from a genetic mutation or preexisting trait (Tortorice, 2018).

(1) Primary resistance: Present prior to treatment

(2) Secondary resistance: Develops after exposure to the cytotoxic drug

(3) The Goldie-Coldman hypothesis predicts that drug-resistant tumor cell clones survive because of a favorable spontaneous mutation that occurs in approximately one in a million cells. Because 1 g of tumor contains 1×10^9 cells, cancers with high tumor burden contain cells with a tremendous number of mutations, which can contribute to drug resistance. This is the rationale for using combination chemotherapy at specific dose intervals to maximize dose intensity (Gerson, Caimi, William, & Kreger, 2018).

(4) Tumor heterogeneity: Refers to the differences between tumors of the same type in different patients and the genetic differences of the cancer cells within a tumor. Heterogeneity increases the risk for primary or secondary resistance. As cells divide, new mutations emerge. With successive mutations, new cells become resistant (O'Dwyer & Calvert, 2015).

c) Multidrug resistance is observed when tumor cells develop mechanisms to protect themselves against cytotoxic drugs (Tortorice, 2018).

(1) Drug inactivation: Many cancer drugs must undergo metabolic activation to acquire clinical efficacy. However, cancer cells can develop resistance through decreased drug activation. Examples include the following (Housman et al., 2014):

(a) Cytarabine (ara-C) is activated through phosphorylation events that convert it to ara-C triphosphate. Downregulation or mutation in this pathway can produce a

decrease in the activation of ara-C, resulting in ara-C drug resistance in the treatment of acute myeloid leukemia.

(*b*) In patients with ovarian cancer, resistance to platinum-based therapy can occur through drug inactivation by metallothionein and thiol glutathione, which activate the detoxification system.

(2) Drug target alteration: A drug's efficacy is influenced by its molecular target and alterations of this target. In cancers, these target alterations can ultimately lead to drug resistance (Housman et al., 2014).

(*a*) Point mutations are the most common mechanism of resistance to TKIs. The development of resistance against a specific inhibitor can be the result of a preexisting cancer cell subpopulation carrying the mutation or the emergence of new mutations that may affect drug sensitivity (Gerson et al., 2018).

i. Human epidermal growth factor receptor 2 (HER2) is a receptor tyrosine kinase that is overexpressed in 30% of patients with breast cancer, and drug resistance can result after long-term use of inhibitors targeting this kinase (Housman et al., 2014).

ii. Increased response rates to EGFR inhibitors have been reported in certain lung cancers, with EGFR mutations reported to have acquired resistance within one year. The development of an EGFR-T790M gatekeeper mutation was reported in half of all cases (Housman et al., 2014).

iii. Imatinib is a TKI that specifically targets the *BCR-ABL* protein and induces remission in patients with chronic myeloid leukemia. Imatinib resistance can be caused by a point mutation in the *ABL* gene and amplification of the *BCR-ABL* fusion gene (Housman et al., 2014).

(3) Drug efflux: Involves reducing drug accumulation by removing the drug from inside the cancer cell. Members of the adenosine triphosphate–binding cassette (ABC) transporter family include proteins that enable this efflux.

(*a*) ABC transporters are highly expressed in the epithelium of the liver and intestine, where the proteins protect the body by pumping drugs and other harmful molecules into the bile duct and intestinal lumen. While efflux via ABC transporters is a normal physiologic process, it is also a known mechanism of drug resistance in cancer cells (Housman et al., 2014).

(*b*) Multidrug resistance protein 1 (MDR1), which produces P-gp, was the first transporter to be identified and has been studied extensively (Housman et al., 2014).

i. P-gp is part of the ABC superfamily of transporters. It is localized in the plasma protein, where it functions as a drug efflux pump (Gerson et al., 2018).

ii. Recent simplified terminology also refers to P-gp as ABC-B1 transporter (Gerson et al., 2018).

iii. The presence of *MDR1* gene and overexpression of P-gp have been found to be predictors of poor prognosis and shortened survival in patients with acute leukemia, multiple myeloma, and malignant lymphoma (Tortorice, 2018).

(4) DNA reparability: When cells suffer DNA damage, several different pathways can kick in to help repair it, depending on the type of damage. Cells from different people and different tumors vary greatly in their ability to repair DNA damage, and scientists have been pursuing measurements of this ability to predict how patients will respond to DNA-damaging chemotherapy (Nagel et al., 2017).

(5) Cell death inhibition

(a) Tumor suppressor protein p53 is a regulator protein that allows cells with undamaged DNA to proceed into the cell cycle. Following exposure to the DNA damaging agents of cytotoxic therapy, an intact *TP53* gene prevents the tumor cell from entering the cell cycle, leading to apoptosis (Tortorice, 2018).

(b) Mutations in the *TP53* gene are among the most common genetic changes observed in tumor cells and may occur in a least 50% of all tumors. When *TP53* function is lost, the tumor cell survives the apoptotic stimuli, and the disease progresses. The presence of *TP53* mutation usually indicates poorer prognosis (Tortorice, 2018).

5. Biomarkers

a) Certain biomarkers are used as a predictive factor, as they provide information on the likelihood of tumor response to a specific therapeutic regimen. This differs from a protein biomarker used as a prognostic indicator, which provides information during the course of treatment by indicating growth, invasion, or metastatic potential (Chia, 2016).

b) Detecting protein biomarkers for estrogen and progesterone receptors through immunohistochemistry staining technique was one of the earliest applications to find a place in patient management (Franklin, Aisner, Post, Bunn, & Garcia, 2014).

(1) Estrogen receptor and progesterone receptor overexpression: The presence of hormone receptors in breast cancer predict the potential for a clinical response to hormone therapy. Estrogen receptor status is also a prognostic indicator in that patients with hormone receptor positivity generally have a more favorable prognosis (Chia, 2016).

(2) HER2 overexpression

(a) Amplification or overexpression of HER2 occurs in approximately 15%–30% of breast cancers and 10%–30% of gastric/gastroesophageal cancers. It is also seen in cancers of the ovary, endometrium, bladder, lung, colon, and head and neck (Iqbal & Iqbal, 2014).

(b) The assay for HER2 amplification has become a standard part of evaluation of breast cancer, as it identifies patients who may benefit from HER2-directed therapies such as ado-trastuzumab, lapatinib, neratinib, pertuzumab, and trastuzumab (Chia, 2016; Iqbal & Iqbal, 2014). In breast cancer, the term *triple-negative* is commonly used to refer to patients who do not have amplifications of estrogen receptor, progesterone receptor, and HER2.

(c) Although therapies directed against HER2 have revolutionized the treatment of HER2-overexpressing breast and gastric cancers, in other cancers, these therapies have provided disappointing results (Iqbal & Iqbal, 2014).

(d) HER2 overexpression also has prognostic value, as patients whose cancer expresses HER2 have shorter median survival (Chia, 2016) and, as in the case with gastric cancer, correlate with poor outcomes and more aggressive disease (Iqbal & Iqbal, 2014).

(3) Some types of cancer will have a target that can be used to attack the cell. For example, in chronic myeloid leukemia, most patients have the *BCR-ABL* fusion gene (NCI, 2017). Targeted therapies work to attack cancer cells by targeting them.

(4) Receptor mutations

(a) DNA sequencing is a laboratory process used to learn the exact order (or sequence) of the four building blocks that make up DNA and is used to find mutations that may cause diseases such as cancer (NCI, n.d.-b).

(b) The Cancer Genome Atlas is a collaboration between NCI and the National Human Genome Research Institute that resulted in the development of comprehensive maps of the key genomic changes taking place in 33 different types of cancer (NCI, n.d.-a).

(c) Specific mutations in the tyrosine kinase signaling pathway lead to uncontrolled cell proliferation

and tumor formation. By stimulating the downstream intracellular signaling process, these mutations cause accelerated cell proliferation, extended cell survival, and increased angiogenesis. Molecular testing for these mutations can provide guidance in prioritizing therapies specific to these receptors for patients who are most likely to benefit from a targeted agent, as well as identifying those patients who will not benefit from a targeted agent. A number of small molecule TKIs have been designed to block phosphorylation and suppress tumor growth (Franklin et al., 2014).

i. EGFR is an example of a protein receptor within the tyrosine kinase pathway that is expressed at high levels in some non-small cell lung and colon carcinomas.

ii. Other mutations and commonly associated diseases for which targeted therapies are available (Franklin et al., 2014)

- *KRAS*: the absence of the mutation in colon cancer and activating mutations in colon cancer
- *BRAF* activating mutations in melanoma, colon cancer, and lung cancer
- *NRAS* activating mutations in colon cancer and non-small cell lung cancer
- c-*KIT* activating mutations in gastrointestinal stromal tumor
- CD20 antigen overexpression in lymphoma
- *KIT* activating mutations in melanoma
- *ALK* gene rearrangement in non-small cell lung cancer

c) Programmed cell death-ligand 1 (PD-L1) protein is found on both normal and cancer cells.

(1) Overexpression of PD-L1 by tumor cells inactivates the body's immune activity against the cancer cell by binding with the programmed cell death protein 1 (PD-1) antigen on the T cell. By suppressing the T cell, the cancer cell can evade attack by the body's immune system.

(2) Immunotherapy treatments that target either PD-L1 or PD-1 block this binding, keeping PD-L1 from inactivating the T cell, thus boosting the immune system in its response against the cancer cell (Bayer et al., 2017).

(a) PD-1 inhibitors have been shown to be helpful in treating several types of cancer, including melanoma, non-small cell lung cancer, kidney cancer, bladder cancer, head and neck cancer, and Hodgkin lymphoma.

(b) PD-L1 inhibitors have been effective in treating bladder cancer, non-small cell lung cancer, and Merkel cell carcinoma (ACS, 2017).

d) Adherence: Poor adherence to cancer treatment, especially to oral agents, includes misuse, overuse, and underuse. Lack of adherence negatively affects providers' abilities to determine treatment efficacy and effectiveness, contributes to increased healthcare costs, and can lead to worsening of disease and decreased overall patient survival (Atkinson et al., 2016).

I. Adherence

1. As treatments for cancer advance to targeted agents, more patients are taking their chemotherapy orally, resulting in a shift from medications given intravenously in the clinic setting to those taken by mouth and managed at home by patients.
2. Advantages of oral agents for cancer (OACs) for patients and healthcare providers (Tipton, 2015)
   a) Less disruption of work and family life
   b) Potentially less time in the clinic and less travel for patients
   c) Potentially less need for IV access
3. Challenges with the increased use of OACs
   a) Acquisition concerns
   b) Financial burden associated with high co-payment, as most oral oncolytics, with a few exceptions, fall under the patient's prescription drug benefit instead of medical benefit
   c) Patient and family understanding of how to take the medication in a safe manner

d) Absorption issues and interactions with food and other medications

e) Monitoring for adherence and toxicities

f) Geographic/travel barriers

4. *Adherence* is defined as the degree or extent of conformity to the provider's recommendations about day-to-day treatment with respect to timing, dosing, and frequency (Neuss et al., 2016).

a) *Adherence* is the preferred term, as it suggests patient and physician shared decision making, whereas *compliance* is defined as how well the patient behavior matches the prescribed therapy. The term *compliance* is commonly avoided today because of the negative connotation implying healthcare provider authority (Tipton, 2015).

b) Adherence to therapy is correlated with treatment success. Nonadherence to the prescribed therapy is associated with treatment failure and increased healthcare costs. It is believed that to achieve maximum benefit from most treatments, patients need to initiate and continue their treatment as prescribed.

(1) The same factors that may affect patient outcomes may be the same factors causing a patient to discontinue treatment early—for example, poor performance status, negative psychological outlook, and nonadherent health behaviors (Hershman, 2016).

(2) Factors affecting the patient's ability to remain adherent may occur simultaneously and can generally be categorized into the following dimensions as listed in Table 4-3 (Hershman, 2016; Irwin & Johnson, 2015; Ruddy, Mayer, & Partridge, 2009; Spoelstra, 2015):

(a) Personal and patient

(b) Medication/treatment

(c) Healthcare system

5. Measures used to promote adherence: For the patient to have the best possible outcome, healthcare provider intervention is essential to assisting the patient in overcoming adherence concerns. By assessing the patient's risk for nonadherence and identifying barriers, healthcare providers can incorporate measures to improve adherence into the patient's care plan (Irwin & Johnson, 2015).

a) ASCO and ONS have collaborated to define safety standards for the administration of chemotherapy, including measures necessary for safe administration of oral oncolytics.

b) Pretreatment assessment: Prior to patients beginning a new chemotherapy regimen, a comprehensive assessment is completed, including medical history, physical examination, psychosocial assessment, and the patients' and/or caregivers' comprehension of the disease and treatment plan (Neuss et al., 2016).

c) Education: Thorough and ongoing education is key to assisting patients in safely managing their oral chemotherapy in the home setting. With proper education, patients and caregivers are better able to manage the symptoms related to the side effects of treatment, adhere to the prescribed regimen, avoid contraindicated medications and foods, and inquire when questions arise (Spoelstra, 2015). The nursing role in medication teaching also may enhance communication between patients and providers, maximizing medication adherence (Atkinson et al., 2016).

(1) Prior to beginning therapy with an OAC, patients and their family or caregivers should receive comprehensive education about the medication(s) to be prescribed, including the following (Neuss et al., 2016):

Table 4-3. Factors Influencing Adherence

Dimension	Influencing Factor
Personal and patient	Age Emotional state Mental status Health beliefs Educational level Expectations of the treatment results Medication knowledge Social support system Socioeconomic status Alcohol or drug abuse Physical condition and the presence of comorbid conditions Lifestyle: the patient's ability to incorporate regimen into daily routine
Medication and treatment	Complexity of regimen Pill burden Duration of treatment Immediacy and evidence of benefit Side effects Cost
Healthcare system	Relationship with providers Satisfaction with care Cost/insurance coverage Education provided prior to treatment Convenience of clinics

Note. Based on information from Hershman, 2016; Irwin & Johnson, 2015; Ruddy et al., 2009; Spoelstra, 2015.

(a) Drugs to be administered, as well as the schedule and duration of treatment
(b) Short- and long-term side effects of treatment, including instructions on when to stop the drug or contact healthcare providers
(c) Possible drug–drug and drug–food interactions
(d) The plan for missed doses
(e) Safe storage and handling of the OAC in the home, including how to manage unused medication
(f) Safe handling of body secretions and waste in the home
(g) Plans for follow-up, including laboratory tests and provider visits

(2) The Multinational Association of Supportive Care in Cancer (MASCC) has developed the MASCC Oral Agent Teaching Tool to assist healthcare providers in the assessment and education of patients receiving OACs (Rittenberg, Johnson, Kav, Barber, & Lemonde, 2016). Components of the teaching tool are as follows:
(a) Key assessment questions to assess the patient's knowledge of the treatment plan, current medications, and ability to obtain and take an OAC
(b) General patient teaching instructions applicable to all OACs, including storage, handling, disposal, system for remembering to take the OAC, and actions to take if problems occur
(c) Drug-specific information that includes the dose, schedule, side effects, and potential interactions
(d) Evaluation questions that may be asked to assess patients' and caregivers' understanding of the information provided

d) Tools to promote adherence: The nurse is an invaluable resource to educate patients on the various measures and tools available to assist in remembering to take their medication and improve adherence (Burhenn & Smuddle, 2015; Ruddy et al., 2009).
(1) Calendars and diaries with daily medication checklists
(2) Pill boxes as permitted by each OAC storage recommendation
(3) Electronic reminders
(a) Smartphone applications
(b) Electronic alarms
(c) Text messaging
(d) Glowing pill bottles
(e) Electronic patient portal
(4) Establishment of a daily routine for taking the OAC at the same time each day

e) Follow-up phone calls: Studies have shown that patients who receive follow-up calls reported that the calls reinforced their knowledge and understanding of their oral chemotherapy, as well as increased their comfort level in managing and being adherent to their treatment (Bellomo, 2016).

6. Monitoring and assessment
a) Adherence assessment: Addressing patient adherence is a crucial factor in promoting safety and effective treatment of the disease (Rudnitzki & McMahon, 2015).
(1) Criteria for assessing adherence to an oral chemotherapy treatment plan (Neuss et al., 2016)
(a) Confirmation that the patient filled the prescription as written
(b) Inquiry regarding concerns about treatment costs
(c) Verification that the patient understands how to take the OAC as prescribed
(d) Verification that the patient understands what to do in case of missed doses
(e) Assessment for potential toxicity during each clinical encounter and in phone encounters. Studies have shown that adverse effects remain one of the leading causes for nonadherence to oral oncolytics (Salgado et al., 2017).
(2) Methods of adherence monitoring
(a) Direct observation measures, such as watching the patient swallow the medication, measuring urine and serum drug assays, or monitoring biologic markers in the blood, are used infrequently because these methods are impractical or too costly. In addition, laboratory drug assays are only available for certain drugs (Spoelstra & Rittenberg, 2015).
(b) Indirect measurement of adherence implies that the medication has been taken by the patient.

i. Patient self-reporting through diaries, calendars, questionnaires, or electronic patient portals, or asking patients whether they are still taking the medication and if they have missed any doses since their last office visit, is one of the simplest measures of adherence (Spoelstra & Rittenberg, 2015).

ii. Pill counts are objective and easy to perform but may prove unreliable, as patients may discard unused medication instead of taking it as directed (Kreys, 2016).

iii. Electronic drug monitoring systems record the date and time the cap was removed from the bottle. This method can be expensive and requires downloading data from the microchip to compatible software (Kreys, 2016).

iv. Pharmacy records and refill rates may indicate acquisition and possession but do not provide information on actual consumption of the medication.

v. Assessment of patients' clinical response may allow the provider to capture severe nonadherence, although factors other than adherence can affect patient's individual responses (Kreys, 2016).

(3) Using more than one method to measure adherence has been suggested to increase the overall accuracy of the assessment, based on the idea that multiple methods would complement each other by overcoming the individual weaknesses of one measure with the strength of another (Kreys, 2016).

7. Developing an interprofessional process

a) Identify key stakeholders and assign responsibilities to ensure there is no duplication of resources.

(1) Physician/prescriber

(2) Advanced practice provider

(3) Oncology RN

(4) Financial advocate

(5) Pharmacist

(6) Specialty pharmacist

(7) Oral oncology nurse navigator or patient navigator

(8) Patient and caregiver

b) Practice considerations

(1) Communication of the plan for the OAC and collaboration within the interprofessional team is crucial to ensure adequate patient education, engagement, and follow-up (Rudnitzki & McMahon, 2015).

(a) Prescriber notifies the clinical staff of the treatment plan. Maximize the use of technology for e-prescribing and electronic alerts to notify appropriate staff when an oral oncolytic has been ordered (Association of Community Cancer Centers [ACCC], 2016).

(b) Collaborate with the specialty pharmacy through proactive communication and frequent follow-up (ACCC, 2016).

(c) Collaborate with the financial advocate.

i. Screen patients at high risk for financial toxicity.

ii. Obtain preauthorization for insurance reimbursement.

iii. Enroll patients in patient assistance program.

(d) Entire team completes documentation in electronic health record.

(2) Develop a robust patient education program (ACCC, 2016).

(a) Schedule dedicated patient education office visit that includes the following:

i. Assessment of health literacy and patient understanding before reviewing important information

ii. How to take the OAC

iii. Safety measures

iv. Symptom management

v. When to call the office

vi. Adherence tools

vii. Patient teach-back

viii. Informed consent

(b) Ensure patients receive pharmacist counseling with first fill and refills.

(c) Provide ongoing education with each clinical encounter and follow-up call.

(3) Patient monitoring and follow-up

(a) Schedule laboratory, other monitoring (e.g., electrocardiogram), and provider follow-up visits that coordinate with the date the patient started taking the oral oncolytic.

(b) Place phone calls to promote adherence, assess for toxicity concerns, and provide reeducation and support (Spoelstra & Sansoucie, 2015).

(c) Consider other electronic means of communication through patient portals.

(d) Perform medication reconciliation and adherence and toxicity assessments at each office visit (Neuss et al., 2016).

(4) Maximize the use of technology to streamline workflow processes and improve communication (ACCC, 2016).

(a) Computerized physician order entry

(b) Standardized forms or flow sheets to follow when placing outreach calls

(c) Secure electronic fax servers

(d) Integrated electronic health record system and patient portals

(5) Staff development

(a) Develop policies and procedures.

(b) Designate educator for staff.

(c) Create checklists for staff to remind them of key elements required for education.

(d) Ensure education materials are current and comprehensive.

(6) Develop quality outcomes for measuring performance and evaluate the use, compliance, and effectiveness of the policies, procedures, and checklists.

J. Toxicity grading

1. The Common Terminology Criteria for Adverse Events (CTCAE) is a descriptive terminology used for adverse event reporting that has become widely accepted throughout the oncology community as the standard classification and severity grading scale for adverse events in cancer therapy clinical trials and other oncology settings.

a) NCI Cancer Therapy Evaluation Program released version 5.0 in November 2017.

b) An *adverse event* is defined as "any unfavorable and unintended sign (including an abnormal laboratory finding), symptom, or disease temporally associated with the use of a medical treatment or procedure that may or may not be considered related to the medical treatment or procedure" (NCI Cancer Therapy Evaluation Program, 2017, p. 2).

c) The criteria incorporated into this toxicity grading scale are used for management of chemotherapy administration and dosing, as well as in clinical trials to provide standardization and consistency in the definition of treatment-related toxicity (Savarese, 2018).

d) In the realm of clinical trials, the grading system is designed to integrate into information networks for safety data exchange and influence data management for adverse event data collection, analysis, and patient outcomes associated with cancer research and care.

e) *Grade* refers to the severity of the adverse event. The CTCAE displays grades 1 through 5 with unique clinical descriptions of severity for each adverse event based on the general guidelines listed in Table 4-4.

2. A patient-reported outcomes (PRO) version of the CTCAE takes into account the patient's perspective on adverse events that may be underdetected using the existing CTCAE system. A PRO version of the CTCAE has been developed but is not yet in widespread use (Savarese, 2018).

a) PROs are defined as any report of the status of a patient's health condition that comes directly from the patient without interpretation by the clinician (Pirschel, 2017).

b) ONS (n.d.) has established criteria for PRO assessment tools and lists instruments meeting these criteria on its website (www.ons.org/assessment-tools).

(1) The MD Anderson Symptom Inventory is one of the PRO assessment tools accepted by ONS (Cleeland, 2016). The tool is used to assess the severity and effect on daily living of 13 high-frequency or severity symptoms: pain, fatigue, nausea, disturbed sleep, distress, shortness of breath, difficulty remembering, lack of appetite, drowsiness, dry mouth, sadness, vomiting, and numbness/tingling.

(2) Assess for any agent-specific symptoms (e.g., vincristine and peripheral neuropathy, methotrexate and stomatitis).

Table 4-4. Common Terminology Criteria for Adverse Events Grading System

Grade	Severity	Definition
1	Mild	Asymptomatic or mild symptoms; clinical or diagnostic observations only; intervention not indicated.
2	Moderate	Minimal, local, or noninvasive intervention indicated; limiting age-appropriate instrumental activities of daily living (ADL) (e.g., preparing meals, shopping for groceries or clothes, using the telephone, managing money).
3	Severe	Medically significant but not immediately life threatening; hospitalization or prolongation of hospitalization indicated; disabling; limiting self-care ADL (e.g., bathing, dressing, undressing, feeding self, using the toilet, taking medications, and not bedridden).
4	Life threatening	Life-threatening consequences; urgent intervention indicated.
5	Death	Fatality occurs related to the adverse event.

Note. Adapted from *Common Terminology Criteria for Adverse Events* [v.5.0], by National Cancer Institute Cancer Therapy Evaluation Program, 2017. Retrieved from https://ctep.cancer.gov/protocoldevelopment/electronic_applications/docs/CTCAE_v5_Quick_Reference_5x7.pdf.

References

Abeloff, M.D. (1995). Vinorelbine (Navelbine) in the treatment of breast cancer: A summary. *Seminars in Oncology, 22*(2, Suppl. 5), 1–4.

Alfarouk, K.O., Stock, C.-M., Taylor, S., Walsh, M., Muddathir, A.K., Verduzco, D., … Rauch, C. (2015). Resistance to cancer chemotherapy: Failure in drug response from ADME to P-gp. *Cancer Cell International, 15,* 71. https://doi.org/10.1186/s12935-015-0221-1

American Brain Tumor Association. (n.d.). Tumor grade. Retrieved from http://www.abta.org/brain-tumor-information/tumor-grade

American Cancer Society. (2016a). Chemotherapy. Retrieved from https://www.cancer.org/treatment/treatments-and-side-effects/treatment-types/chemotherapy.html

American Cancer Society. (2016b). How is chemotherapy used to treat cancer? Retrieved from https://www.cancer.org/treatment/treatments-and-side-effects/treatment-types/chemotherapy/how-is-chemotherapy-used-to-treat-cancer.html

American Cancer Society. (2017). Immune checkpoint inhibitors to treat cancer. Retrieved from https://www.cancer.org/treatment/treatments-and-side-effects/treatment-types/immunotherapy/immune-checkpoint-inhibitors.html

American Cancer Society. (2018). *Cancer facts and figures 2018.* Atlanta, GA: Author.

American Joint Committee on Cancer. (2017a). *AJCC 8th edition staging.* Retrieved from https://cancerstaging.org/CSE/general/Documents/AJCC%20Staging%20Rules%208th%20Ed.pdf

American Joint Committee on Cancer. (2017b). What is cancer staging? Retrieved from https://cancerstaging.org/references-tools/Pages/What-is-Cancer-Staging.aspx

American Society of Clinical Oncology. (n.d.). Cancer progress timeline. Retrieved from https://www.asco.org/research-progress/cancer-progress-timeline

American Society of Clinical Oncology. (2017). Advance of the year: Immunotherapy 2.0. Retrieved from https://www.asco.org/research-progress/reports-studies/clinical-cancer-advances/advance-year-immunotherapy-20

Amiri-Kordestani, L., Blumenthal, G.M., Xu, Q.C., Zhang, L., Tang, S.W., Ha, L., … Cortazar, P. (2014). FDA approval: Ado-trastuzumab emtansine for the treatment of patients with HER2-positive metastatic breast cancer. *Clinical Cancer Research, 20,* 4436–4441. https://doi.org/10.1158/1078-0432.CCR-14-0012

Anassi, E., & Ndefo, U.A. (2011). Sipuleucel-T (Provenge) injection: The first immunotherapy agent (vaccine) for hormone-refractory prostate cancer. *Pharmacy and Therapeutics, 36,* 197–202.

Association of Community Cancer Centers. (2016). *Steps to success: Implementing oral oncolytics.* Retrieved from https://www.accc-cancer.org/resources/pdf/Implementing-Oral-Oncolytics-final.pdf

Atkinson, T.M., Rodriguez, V.M., Gordon, M., Avildsen, I.K., Emanu, J.C., Jewell, S.T., … Ginex, P.K. (2016). The association between patient-reported and objective oral anticancer medication adherence measures: A systematic review. *Oncology Nursing Forum, 43,* 576–582. https://doi.org/10.1188/16.ONF.576-582

Bayer, V., Amaya, B., Baniewicz, D., Callahan, C., Marsh, L., & McCoy, A.S. (2017). Cancer immunotherapy: An evidence-based overview and implications for practice. *Clinical Journal of Oncology Nursing, 21*(Suppl. 2), 13–21. https://doi.org/10.1188/17.CJON.S2.13-21

Behrend, S.W. (2018). Radiation treatment planning. In C.H. Yarbro, D. Wujcik, & B.H. Gobel (Eds.), *Cancer nursing: Principles and practice* (8th ed., pp. 285–331). Burlington, MA: Jones & Bartlett Learning.

Bellomo, C. (2016). Oral chemotherapy: Patient education and nursing intervention. *Journal of Oncology Navigation and Survivorship, 7.* Retrieved from http://www.jons-online.com/issue-archive/2016-issue/july-2016-vol-7-no-6/oral-chemotherapy-patient-education-and-nursing-intervention

Bender, C.M., Gentry, A.L., Brufsky, A.M., Castillo, F.E., Cohen, S.M., Dailey, M.M., … Sereika, S.M. (2014). Influence of patient and treatment factors on adherence to adjuvant endocrine therapy in breast cancer. *Oncology Nursing Forum, 41,* 274–285. https://doi.org/10.1188/14.ONF.274-285

Block, K.I., Gyllenhaal, C., Lowe, L., Amedei, A., Amin, A.R.M.R., Amin, A., … Zollo, M. (2015). Designing a broad-spectrum integrative approach for cancer prevention and treatment. *Seminars in Cancer Biology, 35*(Suppl.), S276–S304. https://doi.org/10.1016/j.semcancer.2015.09.007

Bonadonna, G., Zambetti, M., & Valagussa, P. (1995). Sequential or alternating doxorubicin and CMF regimens in breast cancer with more than three positive nodes: Ten-year results. *JAMA, 273,* 542–547. https://doi.org/10.1001/jama.1995.03520310040027

Bristol-Myers Squibb Co. (2011, March 25). *FDA approves Yervoy™ (ipilimumab) for the treatment of patients with newly diagnosed or previously-treated unresectable or metastatic melanoma, the deadli-*

est form of skin cancer [Press release]. Retrieved from https://news.bms.com/press-release/rd-news/fda-approves-yervoy-ipilimumab-treatment-patients-newly-diagnosed-or-previousl

Burchenal, J.H. (1977). The historical development of cancer chemotherapy. *Seminars in Oncology, 4,* 135–146.

Burhenn, P.S., & Smuddle, J. (2015). Using tools and technology to promote education and adherence to oral agents for cancer. *Clinical Journal of Oncology Nursing, 19*(Suppl.), 53–59. https://doi.org/10.1188/15.S1.CJON.53-59

Chang, A. (2017). Tumor-treating fields: Nursing implications for an emerging technology. *Clinical Journal of Oncology Nursing, 21,* 302–304. https://doi.org/10.1188/17.CJON.302-304

Chia, S. (2016). Prognostic and predictive factors in metastatic breast cancer. In S.R. Vora (Ed.), *UpToDate.* Retrieved January 31, 2018, from http://www.uptodate.com/contents/prognostic-and-predictive-factors-in-metastatic-breast-cancer

Cleeland, C.S. (2016). *The M.D. Anderson symptom inventory: User guide* (Version 1). Retrieved from https://www.mdanderson.org/documents/Departments-and-Divisions/Symptom-Research/MDASI_userguide.pdf

Cranley, N.M., Curbow, B., George, T.J., Jr., & Christie, J. (2017). Influential factors on treatment decision making among patients with colorectal cancer: A scoping review. *Supportive Care in Cancer, 25,* 2943–2951. https://doi.org/10.1007/s00520-017-3763-z

Cuccaro, A., Bartolomei, F., Cupelli, E., Galli, E., Giachelia, M., & Hohaus, S. (2014). Prognostic factors in Hodgkin lymphoma. *Mediterranean Journal of Hematology and Infectious Diseases, 6,* e2014053. https://doi.org/10.4084/mjhid.2014.053

Dowling, M., McDonagh, B., & Meade, E. (2017). Arthralgia in breast cancer survivors: An integrative review of endocrine therapy. *Oncology Nursing Forum, 44,* 337–349. https://doi.org/10.1188/17.337-349

Doyle-Lindrud, S. (2015a). Proton beam therapy for pediatric malignancies. *Clinical Journal of Oncology Nursing, 19,* 521–523. https://doi.org/10.1188/15.CJON.521-523

Doyle-Lindrud, S. (2015b). Use of robotics in oncology surgery. *Clinical Journal of Oncology Nursing, 19,* 265–266. https://doi.org/10.1188/15.CJON.265-266

Drooger, J.C., van Pelt-Sprangers, J.M., Leunis, C., Jager, A., & de Jongh, F.E. (2016). Neutrophil-guided dosing of anthracycline–cyclophosphamide-containing chemotherapy in patients with breast cancer: A feasibility study. *Medical Oncology, 32,* 113. https://doi.org/10.1007/s12032-015-0550-x

ECOG-ACRIN Cancer Research Group. (2016). ECOG Performance Status. Retrieved from http://ecog-acrin.org/resources/ecog-performance-status

Eggert, J.A. (2018). Biology of cancer. In C.H. Yarbro, D. Wujcik, & B.H. Gobel (Eds.), *Cancer nursing: Principles and practice* (8th ed., pp. 3–24). Burlington, MA: Jones & Bartlett Learning.

Eilber, F.R., Morton, D.L., Eckardt, J., Grant, T., & Weisenburger, T. (1984). Limb salvage for skeletal and soft tissue sarcomas: Multidisciplinary preoperative therapy. *Cancer, 53,* 2579–2584. https://doi.org/10.1002/1097-0142(19840615)53:12<2579::AID-CNCR2820531202>3.0.CO;2-V

Epperla, N., Ahn, K.W., Ahmed, S., Jagasia, M., DiGilio, A., Devine, S.M., … Hamadani, M. (2017). Rituximab-containing reduced-intensity conditioning improves progression-free survival following allogeneic transplantation in B cell non-Hodgkin lymphoma. *Journal of Hematology and Oncology, 10,* 117. https://doi.org/10.1186/s13045-017-0487-y

Farber, S., Diamond, L.K., Mercer, R.D., Sylvester, R.F., Jr., & Wolff, J.A. (1948). Temporary remissions in acute leukemia in children produced by folic acid antagonist, 4-aminopteroylglutamic acid (aminopterin). *New England Journal of Medicine, 238,* 787–793. https://doi.org/10.1056/NEJM194806032382301

Fisher, B., Fisher, E.R., & Redmond, C. (1986). Ten-year results from the National Surgical Adjuvant Breast and Bowel Project (NSABP) clinical trial evaluating the use of L-phenylalanine mustard (L-PAM) in the management of primary breast cancer. *Journal of Clinical Oncology, 4,* 929–941. https://doi.org/10.1200/JCO.1986.4.6.929

Fojo, A.T., & Bates, S.E. (2015). Assessment of clinical response. In V.T. DeVita Jr., T.S. Lawrence, & S.A. Rosenberg (Eds.), *DeVita, Hellman, and Rosenberg's cancer: Principles and practice of oncology* (10th ed., pp. 308–319). Philadelphia, PA: Wolters Kluwer Health.

Franklin, W.A., Aisner, D.L., Post, M.D., Bunn, P.A., & Garcia, M.V. (2014). Pathology, biomarkers, and molecular diagnostics. In J.E. Niederhuber, J.O. Armitage, J.H. Doroshow, M.B. Kastan, & J.E. Tepper (Eds.), *Abeloff's clinical oncology* (5th ed., pp. 226–248) Philadelphia, PA: Elsevier Saunders.

Gerson, S.L., Caimi, P.F., William, B.M., & Kreger, R.J. (2018). Pharmacology and molecular mechanisms of antineoplastic agents for hematologic malignancies. In R. Hoffman, E.J. Benz Jr., L.E. Silverstein, H.E. Heslop, J.I. Weitz, J. Anastasi, … S.A. Abutalib (Eds.), *Hematology: Basic principles and practice* (7th ed., pp. 849–912). https://doi.org/10.1016/B978-0-323-35762-3.00057-3

Gilman, A. (1963). The initial clinical trial of nitrogen mustard. *American Journal of Surgery, 105,* 574–578. https://doi.org/10.1016/0002-9610(63)90232-0

Gilman, A., & Philips, F.S. (1946). The biological actions of therapeutic applications of the B-chloroethyl amines and sulfides. *Science, 103,* 409–436. https://doi.org/10.1126/science.103.2675.409

Gnarra, J.R., Lerman, M.I., Zbar, B., & Linehan, W.M. (1995). Genetics of renal-cell carcinoma and evidence for a critical role for von Hippel-Lindau in renal tumorigenesis. *Seminars in Oncology, 22,* 3–8.

Gosselin, T.K. (2018). Principles of radiation therapy. In C.H. Yarbro, D. Wujcik, & B.H. Gobel (Eds.), *Cancer nursing: Principles and practice* (8th ed., pp. 267–284). Burlington, MA: Jones & Bartlett Learning.

Griffith, N., McBride, A., Stevenson, J.G., & Green, L. (2014). Formulary selection criteria for biosimilars: Considerations for US health-system pharmacists. *Hospital Pharmacy, 49,* 813–825. https://doi.org/10.1310/hpj4909-813

Guy, J.L., & Ingram, B.A. (1996). Medical oncology—The agents. In R. McCorkle, M. Grant, M. Frank-Stromborg, & S.B. Baird (Eds.), *Cancer nursing: A comprehensive textbook* (2nd ed., pp. 359–394). Philadelphia, PA: Saunders.

Gyurkocza, B., & Sandmaier, B.M. (2014). Conditioning regimens for hematopoietic cell transplantation: One size does not fit all. *Blood, 124,* 344–353. https://doi.org/10.1182/blood-2014-02-514778

Haque, W., Verma, V., Butler, E.B., & Teh, B.S. (2017). Patterns of care and outcomes of multi-agent versus single-agent chemotherapy as part of multimodal management of low grade glioma. *Journal of Neuro-Oncology, 133,* 369–375. https://doi.org/10.1007/s11060-017-2443-7

Hassen, E., Eggert, J., & Loud, J.T. (2018). Genetic risk and hereditary cancer syndromes. In C.H. Yarbro, D. Wujcik, & B.H. Gobel (Eds.), *Cancer nursing: Principles and practice* (8th ed., pp. 135–168). Burlington, MA: Jones & Bartlett Learning.

Havrilesky, L.J., Reiner, M., Morrow, P.K., Watson, H., & Crawford, J. (2015). A review of relative dose intensity and survival in patients with metastatic solid tumors. *Critical Reviews in Oncology/Hematology, 93,* 203–210. https://doi.org/10.1016/j.critrevonc.2014.10.006

Hershman, D.L. (2016). Sticking to it: Improving outcomes by increasing adherence. *Journal of Clinical Oncology, 34,* 2440–2442. https://doi.org/10.1200/JCO.2016.67.7336

Hess, K.R. (2017). Cancer survival analysis. In M.B. Amin (Ed.), *AJCC cancer staging manual* (8th ed., pp. 39–45). Chicago, IL: Springer.

Hoskins, K.F., Stopfer, J.E., Calzone, K.A., Merajver, S.D., Rebbeck, T.R., Garber, J.E., & Weber, B.L. (1995). Assessment and counseling for women with a family history of breast cancer. *JAMA, 273,* 577–585. https://doi.org/10.1001/jama.1995.03520310075033

Housman, G., Byler, S., Heerboth, S., Lapinska, K., Longacre, M., Snyder, N., & Sarkar, S. (2014). Drug resistance in cancer: An overview. *Cancers, 6,* 1769–1792. https://doi.org/10.3390/cancers6031769

Hui, D., & Bruera, E. (2016). Integrating palliative care into the trajectory of cancer care. *Nature Reviews Clinical Oncology, 13,* 159–171. https://doi.org/10.1038/nrclinonc.2015.201

Inan, H., Wang, S., Inci, F., Baday, M., Zangar, R., Kesiraju, S., ... Demirci, U. (2017). Isolation, detection, and quantification of cancer biomarkers in HPV-associated malignancies. *Scientific Reports, 7,* 3322. https://doi.org/10.1038/s41598-017-02672-6

International Agency for Research on Cancer. (2017, October 27). Agents classified by the *IARC Monographs,* volumes 1–120. Retrieved from http://monographs.iarc.fr/ENG/Classification

Iqbal, N., & Iqbal, N. (2014). Human epidermal growth factor receptor 2 (HER2) in cancers: Overexpression and therapeutic implications. *Molecular Biology International, 2014,* 852748. https://doi.org/10.1155/2014/852748

Irwin, M., & Johnson, L.A. (2015). Factors influencing oral adherence: Qualitative metasummary and triangulation with quantitative evidence. *Clinical Journal of Oncology Nursing, 19*(Suppl. 3), 6–30. https://doi.org/10.1188/15.S1.CJON.6-30

Jin, S.-F., Fan, Z.-K., Pan, L., & Jin, L.-M. (2017). Gemcitabine-based combination therapy compared with gemcitabine alone for advanced pancreatic cancer: A meta-analysis of nine randomized controlled trials. *Hepatobiliary and Pancreatic Diseases International, 16,* 236–244. https://doi.org/10.1016/S1499-3872(17)60022-5

Kourlaba, G., Dimopoulos, M.A., Pectasides, D., Skarlose, D.V., Gogas, H., Pentheroudakis, G., ... Maniadakis, N. (2015). Comparison of filgrastim and pegfilgrastim to prevent neutropenia and maintain dose intensity of adjuvant chemotherapy in patients with breast cancer. *Supportive Care in Cancer, 23,* 2045–2051. https://doi.org/10.1007/s00520-014-2555-y

Kreamer, K., & Riordan, D. (2015). Targeted therapies for non-small cell lung cancer: An update on the epidermal growth factor receptor and anaplastic lymphoma kinase inhibitors. *Clinical Journal of Oncology Nursing, 19,* 734–742. https://doi.org/10.1188/15.CJON.734-742

Kreys, E. (2016). Measurements of medication adherence: In search of a gold standard. *Journal of Clinical Pathways, 2,* 43–47. Retrieved from http://www.journalofclinicalpathways.com/article/measurements-medication-adherence-search-gold-standard

Lambertini, M., Ceppi, M., Cognetti, F., Cavazzini, G., De Laurentiis, M., De Placido, S., ... Del Mastro, L. (2017). Dose-dense adjuvant chemotherapy in premenopausal breast cancer patients: A pooled analysis of the MIG1 and GIM2 phase III studies. *European Journal of Cancer, 71,* 34–42. https://doi.org/10.1016/j.ejca.2016.10.030

Lansky, S.B., List, M.A., Lansky, L.L., Ritter-Sterr, C., & Miller, D.R. (1987). The measurement of performance in childhood cancer patients. *Cancer, 60,* 1651–1656. https://doi.org/10.1002/1097-0142(19871001)60:7<1651::AID-CNCR2820600738>3.0.CO;2-J

Lea, D.H. (2018). Gene therapy. In C.H. Yarbro, D. Wujcik, & B.H. Gobel (Eds.), *Cancer nursing: Principles and practice* (8th ed., pp. 681–696). Burlington, MA: Jones & Bartlett Learning.

Lester, J. (2018). Surgical oncology. In C.H. Yarbro, D. Wujcik, & B.H. Gobel (Eds.), *Cancer nursing: Principles and practice* (8th ed., pp. 243–266). Burlington, MA: Jones & Bartlett Learning.

Leukemia and Lymphoma Society. (n.d.-a). CLL staging. Retrieved from https://www.lls.org/leukemia/chronic-lymphocytic-leukemia/diagnosis/cll-staging

Leukemia and Lymphoma Society. (n.d.-b). Hodgkin lymphoma staging. Retrieved from https://www.lls.org/lymphoma/hodgkin-lymphoma/diagnosis/hodgkin-lymphoma-staging

Lilley, E.J., Bader, A.M., & Cooper, Z. (2015). A values-based conceptual framework for surgical appropriateness: An illustrative case report. *Annals of Palliative Medicine, 4,* 54–57. https://doi.org/10.3978/j.issn.2224-5820.2015.05.01

Mahon, S.M. (2018). Screening and detection for asymptomatic individuals. In C.H. Yarbro, D. Wujcik, & B.H. Gobel (Eds.), *Cancer nursing: Principles and practice* (8th ed., pp. 111–133). Burlington, MA: Jones & Bartlett Learning.

Marcial, V.A., Pajak, T.F., Kramer, S., Davis, L.W., Stetz, J., Laramore, G.E., ... Brady, L.W. (1988). Radiation Therapy Oncology Group (RTOG) studies in head and neck cancer. *Seminars in Oncology, 15,* 39–60.

Martin, C. (2017). Oncolytic viruses: Treatment and implications for patients with gliomas. *Clinical Journal of Oncology Nursing, 21*(Suppl. 2), 60–64. https://doi.org/10.1188/17.CJON.S2.60-64

Matikas, A., Foukakis, T., & Bergh, J. (2017). Dose intense, dose dense, and tailored dose adjuvant chemotherapy for early breast cancer: An evolution of concepts. *Acta Oncologica, 56,* 1143–1151. https://doi.org/10.1080/0284186X.2017.1329593

McIntyre, K. (2015). An oncology nurses' guide to new targeted agents for metastatic colorectal cancer. *Clinical Journal of Oncology Nursing, 19,* 571–579. https://doi.org/10.1188/15.CJON.571-579

Michigan Care Management Resource Center. (n.d.). Lansky Play-Performance Scale for Pediatric Patients. Retrieved from http://micmrc.org/system/files/Lansky%20Scale.pdf

Miki, Y., Swensen, J., Shattuck-Eidens, D., Futreal, P.A., Harshman, K., Tavtigian, S., ... Skolnick, M.H. (1994). A strong candidate for the breast and ovarian cancer susceptibility gene *BRCA1. Science, 266,* 66–71. https://doi.org/10.1126/science.7545954

Mitra, A.K., Agrahari, V., Mandal, A., Cholkar, K., Natarajan, C., Shah, S., ... Pal, D. (2015). Novel delivery approaches for cancer therapeutics. *Journal of Controlled Release, 219,* 248–268. https://doi.org/10.1016/j.jconrel.2015.09.067

Mokhtari, R.B., Homayouni, T.S., Baluch, N., Morgatskaya, E., Kumar, S., Das, B., & Yeger, H. (2017). Combination therapy in combating cancer. *Oncotarget, 8,* 38022–38043. https://doi.org/10.18632/oncotarget.16723

Muehlbauer, P.M., Callahan, A., Zlott, D., & Dahl, B.J. (2018). Biotherapy. In C.H. Yarbro, D. Wujcik, & B.H. Gobel (Eds.), *Cancer nursing: Principles and practice* (8th ed., pp. 611–651). Burlington, MA: Jones & Bartlett Learning.

Multiple Myeloma Research Foundation. (n.d.). International staging system. Retrieved from https://www.themmrf.org/multiple-myeloma/prognosis/myeloma-stages/international-staging-system

Nagel, Z.D., Kitange, G.J., Gupta, S.K., Joughin, B.A., Chaim, I.A., Mazzucato, P., ... Samson, L.D. (2017). DNA repair capability in multiple pathways predicts chemotherapy resistance in glioblastoma multiforme. *Cancer Research, 77,* 198–206. https://doi.org/10.1158/0008-5472.CAN-16-1151

National Cancer Institute. (n.d.-a). The Cancer Genome Atlas. Retrieved from https://cancergenome.nih.gov

National Cancer Institute. (n.d.-b). DNA sequencing. In *NCI dictionary of cancer terms.* Retrieved from https://www.cancer.gov/publications/dictionaries/cancer-terms?cdrid=753867

National Cancer Institute. (n.d.-c). SEER training modules. Pediatric staging. Retrieved from https://training.seer.cancer.gov/staging/systems/schemes/pediatric.html

National Cancer Institute. (n.d.-d). Tumor burden. In *NCI dictionary of cancer terms.* Retrieved from https://www.cancer.gov/publications/dictionaries/cancer-terms?cdrid=44627

National Cancer Institute. (2013, May 3). Tumor grade. Retrieved from https://www.cancer.gov/about-cancer/diagnosis-staging/prognosis/tumor-grade-fact-sheet

National Cancer Institute. (2015a, March 9). Cancer staging. Retrieved from https://www.cancer.gov/about-cancer/diagnosis-staging/staging

National Cancer Institute. (2015b). Milestones in cancer research and discovery. Retrieved from https://www.cancer.gov/research/progress/250-years-milestones

National Cancer Institute. (2016, December 21). Identifying novel drug combinations to overcome treatment resistance. Retrieved from https://www.cancer.gov/about-cancer/treatment/research/drug-combo-resistance

National Cancer Institute. (2017, November 6). Targeted cancer therapies. Retrieved from https://www.cancer.gov/about-cancer/treatment/types/targeted-therapies/targeted-therapies-fact-sheet

National Cancer Institute Cancer Therapy Evaluation Program. (2017). *Common terminology criteria for adverse events* [v.5.0]. Retrieved from https://ctep.cancer.gov/protocoldevelopment/electronic_applications/docs/CTCAE_v5_Quick_Reference_5x7.pdf

National Toxicology Program. (2016). *Report on carcinogens* (14th ed.). Retrieved from https://ntp.niehs.nih.gov/pubhealth/roc/index-1.html

Neuss, M.N., Gilmore, T.R., Belderson, K.M., Billett, A.L., Conti-Kalchik, T., Harvey, B.E., ... Polovich, M. (2016). 2016 updated American Society of Clinical Oncology/Oncology Nursing Society chemotherapy administration safety standards, including standards for pediatric oncology. *Journal of Oncology Practice, 12,* 1262–1271. https://doi.org/10.1200/JOP.2016.017905

Noonan, K. (2007). Introduction to B-cell disorders. *Clinical Journal of Oncology Nursing, 11*(Suppl. 1), 3–12. https://doi.org/10.1188/07.CJON.S1.3-12

Novartis Pharmaceuticals Corp. (2017, July 13). Novartis CAR-T cell therapy CTL019 unanimously (10-0) recommended for approval by FDA advisory committee to treat pediatric, young adult r/r B-cell ALL. Retrieved from https://www.novartis.com/news/media-releases/novartis-car-t-cell-therapy-ctl019-unanimously-10-0-recommended-approval-fda

O'Dwyer, P.J., & Calvert, A.H. (2015). Platinum analogs. In V.T. DeVita Jr., T.S. Lawrence, & S.A. Rosenberg (Eds.), *DeVita, Hellman, and Rosenberg's cancer: Principles and practice of oncology* (10th ed., pp. 199–207). Philadelphia, PA: Wolters Kluwer Health.

Oncology Nursing Society. (n.d.). Assessment tools. Retrieved from http://www.ons.org/assessment-tools

Oncology Nursing Society. (2014). *Palliative care for people with cancer* [Position statement]. Retrieved from https://www.ons.org/advocacy-policy/positions/practice/palliative-care

Peppercorn, J.M., Smith, T.J., Helft, P.R., DeBono, D.J., Berry, S.R., Wollines, D.S., ... Schnipper, L.E. (2011). American Society of Clinical Oncology statement: Toward individualized care for patients with advanced cancer. *Journal of Clinical Oncology, 29,* 755–760. https://doi.org/10.1200/JCO.2010.33.1744

Perez, E.A. (1995). Review of the preclinical pharmacology and comparative efficacy of 5-hydroxytryptamine-3 receptor antagonists for chemotherapy-induced emesis. *Journal of Clinical Oncology, 13,* 1036–1043. https://doi.org/10.1200/JCO.1995.13.4.1036

Perry, A.R., & Linch, D.C. (1996). The history of bone-marrow transplantation. *Blood Reviews, 10,* 215–219. https://doi.org/10.1016/S0268-960X(96)90004-1

Pirschel, C. (2017, August). Improving patient care through patient-reported outcomes. *ONS Voice, 32*(8), 16–21.

Pritchard, J.R., Bruno, P.M., Gilbert, L.A., Capron, K.L., Lauffenburger, D.A., & Hemann, M.T. (2013). Defining principles of combination drug mechanisms of action. *Proceedings of the National Academy of Sciences of the United States of America, 110,* E170–E179. https://doi.org/10.1073/pnas.1210419110

Raedler, L.A. (2015, March). Keytruda (pembrolizumab): First PD-1 inhibitor approved for previously treated unresectable or metastatic melanoma. *American Health and Drug Benefits, 8*(Special Feature), 96–100. Retrieved from https://www.ncbi.nlm.nih.gov/pmc/articles/PMC4665064

Reilly, P. (2013). Cancer—Integrated naturopathic support. In J.E Pizzorno & M.T. Murray (Eds.), *Textbook of natural medicine* (4th ed., pp. 440–461). St. Louis, MO: Elsevier Churchill Livingstone.

Rittenberg, C.N., Johnson, J., Kav, S., Barber, L., & Lemonde, M. (2016, September 9). MASCC Oral Agent Teaching Tool (MOATT) (Version 1.2). Retrieved from http://www.mascc.org/MOATT

Rowinsky, E.K., Onetto, N., Canetta, R.M., & Arbuck, S.G. (1992). Taxol: The first of the taxanes, an important new class of antitumor agents. *Seminars in Oncology, 19,* 646–662.

Ruddy, K., Mayer, E., & Partridge, A. (2009). Patient adherence and persistence with oral anticancer treatment. *CA: A Cancer Journal for Clinicians, 59,* 56–66. https://doi.org/10.3322/caac.20004

Rudnitzki, T., & McMahon, D. (2015). Oral agents for cancer: Safety challenges and recommendations. *Clinical Journal of Oncology Nursing, 19*(Suppl. 3), 41–46. https://doi.org/10.1188/15.S1.CJON.41-46

Salgado, T.M., Mackler, E., Severson, J.A., Lindsay, J., Batra, P., Petersen, L., & Farris, K.B. (2017). The relationship between patient activation, confidence to self-manage side effects, and adherence to oral oncolytics: A pilot study with Michigan oncology practices. *Supportive Care in Cancer, 25,* 1797–1807. https://doi.org/10.1007/s00520-017-3584-0

Salins, N., Patra, L., Usha Rani, M.R., Lohitashva, S.O., Rao, R., Ramanjulu, R., & Vallath, N. (2016). Integration of early specialist palliative care in cancer care: Survey of oncologists, oncology nurses, and patients. *Indian Journal of Palliative Care, 22,* 258–265. https://doi.org/10.4103/0973-1075.185030

Sandrasegaran, K. (2015). Monitoring gastrointestinal tumor response to therapy. In R.M. Gore & M.S. Levine (Eds.), *Textbook of gastrointestinal radiology* (4th ed., pp. 2295–2305). Philadelphia, PA: Elsevier Saunders.

Sarfati, D., Koczwara, B., & Jackson, C. (2016). The impact of comorbidity on cancer and its treatment. *CA: A Cancer Journal for Clinicians, 66,* 337–350. https://doi.org/10.3322/caac.21342

Saria, M.G., & Kesari, S. (2016). Efficacy and safety of treating glioblastoma with tumor-treating fields therapy. *Clinical Journal of Oncology Nursing, 20*(Suppl. 5), 9–13. https://doi.org/10.1188/16.CJON.S1.9-13

Savarese, D.M.F. (2018). Common terminology criteria for adverse events. In J.S. Tirnauer (Ed.), *UpToDate.* Retrieved January 31, 2018, from http://www.uptodate.com/contents/common-terminology-criteria-for-adverse-events

Shoushtari, A.N., Wolchok, J., & Hellman, M. (2018). Principles of cancer immunotherapy. In M.E. Ross (Ed.), *UpToDate.* Retrieved January 31, 2018, from http://www.uptodate.com/contents/principles-of-cancer-immunotherapy

Smith, J.J., Richmond, E., & Dunn, B.K. (2018). Dynamics of cancer prevention. In C.H. Yarbro, D. Wujcik, & B.H. Gobel (Eds.),

Cancer nursing: Principles and practice (8th ed., pp. 81–110). Burlington, MA: Jones & Bartlett Learning.

Søgaard, M., Thomsen, R.W., Bossen, K.S., Sørensen, H.T., & Nørgaard, M. (2013). The impact of comorbidity on cancer survival: A review. *Clinical Epidemiology, 5*(Suppl.), 3–29. https://doi.org/10.2147/CLEP.S47150

Speyer, J.L., Green, M.D., Kramer, E., Rey, M., Sanger, J., Ward, C., ... Muggia, F. (1988). Protective effect of the bispiperazinedione ICRF-187 against doxorubicin-induced cardiac toxicity in women with advanced breast cancer. *New England Journal of Medicine, 319,* 745–752. https://doi.org/10.1056/NEJM198809223191203

Spoelstra, S.L. (2015). Why patients prescribed oral agents for cancer need training: A case study. *Clinical Journal of Oncology Nursing, 19*(Suppl. 3), 3–5. https://doi.org/10.1188/15.S1.CJON.3-5

Spoelstra, S.L., & Rittenberg, C.N. (2015). Assessment and measurement of medication adherence: Oral agents for cancer. *Clinical Journal of Oncology Nursing, 19*(Suppl. 3), 47–52. https://doi.org/10.1188/15.S1.CJON.47-52

Spoelstra, S.L., & Sansoucie, H. (2015). Putting evidence into practice: Evidence-based interventions for oral agents for cancer. *Clinical Journal of Oncology Nursing, 19*(Suppl. 3), 60–72. https://doi.org/10.1188/15.S1.CJON.60-72

Stenger, M. (2014, May). ASCO committee defines clinically meaningful goals for clinical trials in pancreas, breast, lung, and colorectal cancers. *ASCO Post.* Retrieved from http://www.ascopost.com/issues/may-15-2014/asco-committee-defines-clinically-meaningful-goals-for-clinical-trials-in-pancreas-breast-lung-and-colorectal-cancers

Tajima, H., Makino, I., Ohbatake, Y., Nakanuma, S., Hayashi, H., Nakagawara, H., ... Ohta, T. (2017). Neoadjuvant chemotherapy for pancreatic cancer: Effects on cancer tissue and novel perspectives (Review). *Oncology Letters, 13,* 3975–3981. https://doi.org/10.3892/ol.2017.6008

Tipton, J.M. (2015). Overview of the challenges related to oral agents for cancer and their impact on adherence. *Clinical Journal of Oncology Nursing, 19*(Suppl. 3), 37–40. https://doi.org/10.1188/15.S1.CJON.37-40

Tortorice, P.V. (2018). Cytotoxic chemotherapy: Principles of therapy. In C.H. Yarbro, D. Wujcik, & B.H. Gobel (Eds.), *Cancer nursing: Principles and practice* (8th ed., pp. 375–416). Burlington, MA: Jones & Bartlett Learning.

U.S. Department of Health and Human Services. (2007). *Guidance for industry: Clinical trial endpoints for the approval of cancer drugs and biologics.* Retrieved from https://www.fda.gov/downloads/drugs/guidancecomplianceregulatoryinformation/guidances/ucm071590.pdf

U.S. Food and Drug Administration. (2017a). Biosimilars. Retrieved from https://www.fda.gov/drugs/developmentapprovalprocess/howdrugsaredevelopedandapproved/approvalapplications/therapeuticbiologicapplications/biosimilars/default.htm

U.S. Food and Drug Administration. (2017b). Clinical outcome assessment: Glossary of terms. Retrieved from https://www.fda.gov/Drugs/DevelopmentApprovalProcess/DrugDevelopmentToolsQualificationProgram/ucm370262.htm

U.S. Food and Drug Administration. (2017c). FDA approves first biosimilar for cancer treatment. Retrieved from https://www.fda.gov/Drugs/InformationOnDrugs/ApprovedDrugs/ucm576096.htm

U.S. Food and Drug Administration. (2017d). FDA grants first treatment for rare form of skin cancer. Retrieved from https://www.fda.gov/newsevents/newsroom/pressannouncements/ucm548278.htm

Vioral, A. (2018). Immunology. In C.H. Yarbro, D. Wujcik, & B.H. Gobel (Eds.), *Cancer nursing: Principles and practice* (8th ed., pp. 25–42). Burlington, MA: Jones & Bartlett Learning.

Vogel, W.H. (2018). Diagnostic evaluation, classification, and staging. In C.H. Yarbro, D. Wujcik, & B.H. Gobel (Eds.), *Cancer nursing: Principles and practice* (8th ed., pp. 169–203). Burlington, MA: Jones & Bartlett Learning.

Wolchok, J.D., Hoos, A., O'Day, S., Weber, J.S., Hamid, O., Lebbé, C., ... Hodi, F.S. (2009). Guidelines for the evaluation of immune therapy activity in solid tumors: Immune-related response criteria. *Clinical Cancer Research, 15,* 7412–7420. https://doi.org/10.1158/1078-0432.CCR-09-1624

World Health Organization. (n.d.). WHO definition of palliative care. Retrieved from http://www.who.int/cancer/palliative/definition/en

Wujcik, D. (2018). Targeted therapy. In C.H. Yarbro, D. Wujcik, & B.H. Gobel (Eds.), *Cancer nursing: Principles and practice* (8th ed., pp. 653–680). Burlington, MA: Jones & Bartlett Learning.

Zack, E. (2018). Principles and techniques of bone marrow transplantation. In C.H. Yarbro, D. Wujcik, & B.H. Gobel (Eds.), *Cancer nursing: Principles and practice* (8th ed., pp. 555–590). Burlington, MA: Jones & Bartlett Learning.

Zhang, X.-W., Ma, Y.-X., Sun, Y., Cao, Y.-B., Li, Q., & Xu, C.-A. (2017). Gemcitabine in combination with a second cytotoxic agent in the first-line treatment of locally advanced or metastatic pancreatic cancer: A systematic review and meta-analysis. *Targeted Oncology, 12,* 309–321. https://doi.org/10.1007/s11523-017-0486-5

Zubrod, C.G. (1984). Origins and development of chemotherapy research at the National Cancer Institute. *Cancer Treatment Reports, 68,* 9–19.

CHAPTER 5

Clinical Trials and Drug Development

A. Clinical research
   1. Clinical research involves studies conducted on human beings with the goal of developing knowledge about human health and illness. These studies may involve an individual person or a group of people or may use data or materials from humans (i.e., biospecimens).
   2. Types of clinical research (U.S. Food and Drug Administration [FDA], 2017b)
      a) Patient-oriented research, which involves individuals, their data, or their biospecimens to study
         (1) Mechanisms of human disease
         (2) Treatments or interventions for disease
         (3) Development of technology related to disease
      b) Epidemiologic and behavioral research, which looks at the distribution of disease, the factors that affect health, and how people make health-related decisions
      c) Health services research, which seeks to identify the most effective ways to organize, finance, manage, and deliver high-quality care, reduce medical errors, and improve patient safety
      d) Outcomes research, which identifies healthcare practices and interventions to support more informed patient care decisions
   3. Clinical trials: A clinical trial is one type of patient-oriented research in which the patient (i.e., research participant) is prospectively assigned to an intervention to evaluate the effects of the intervention on health-related biomedical or behavioral outcomes (National Institutes of Health, 2017). Table 5-1 summarizes five types of clinical trials (Ness & Royce, 2017; U.S. FDA, 2017b).
      a) Cancer clinical trials are essential for the identification of new, more effective therapies to improve disease prevention, detection, treatment, and rehabilitation. Clinical trials have

Table 5-1. Types of Clinical Trials

Type of Trial	Description
Prevention	Evaluate the effectiveness of ways to reduce the risk of developing a disease or preventing a disease from returning by one of the following: • "Doing" something (e.g., lifestyle changes, including diet, exercise, or smoking cessation) • "Taking" something (e.g., medications, vitamins, vaccines)
Diagnostic	Develop better tests or procedures to more accurately identify and diagnose a disease or condition (e.g., imaging tests, laboratory tests, tumor markers).
Screening	Assess new or better ways of detecting disease or health conditions earlier in healthy people. Examples include obtaining the following: • Tissue samples • Laboratory tests, including genetic testing • Imaging tests • Physical examinations • Health histories, including family histories and pedigrees
Quality of life	Evaluate measures to improve comfort and quality of life for people with chronic illnesses through better therapies or psychosocial interventions. • Focus can be on the patient, families, or other caregivers. • These are also known as supportive care trials.
Treatment	Test new treatments or devices, new combinations of drugs, or new approaches to surgery or radiation therapy. Treatment trials, especially trials for drugs that are not yet approved for general use (i.e., investigational drugs), are categorized by phases.

Note. Based on information from National Institutes of Health, 2017; Ness & Royce, 2017.

had a significant role in improvement of outcomes for people with cancer. For example, results from breast cancer clinical trials have led to improvements in screening, surgery, chemotherapy, radiation therapy, and hormone therapy with lengthened survival for people with breast cancer.

b) Ideas for clinical trials are generated from both the clinical and basic sciences.
   (1) Many ideas come from basic science research, which increases our understanding about the biology of cancer. Ideas that come from basic science research are first investigated in the laboratory. Treatments with the most promising results are studied in clinical trials.
   (2) Some ideas come from the results of previous clinical research, where new questions are raised as previous ones are answered.
   (3) Ideas for clinical trials also may come from patients and their healthcare providers as they try to determine how to manage their disease and side effects.

c) Patients choose to participate in clinical trials for different reasons. These reasons will depend on each patient's beliefs, culture, disease status, treatment options, and knowledge and perception about clinical trials.
   (1) Understanding individuals' reasons for participating in a clinical trial will help oncology nurses know how to best support them.
   (2) Common reasons for participation (Czaplicki, 2016)
      (a) Access to treatments that patients may not otherwise be able to afford
      (b) Hope that they will be given a better treatment than the current standard
      (c) The desire to contribute to research so that others may benefit in the future
      (d) Following the family's wishes
      (e) Lack of available treatment options

4. The protocol: Clinical research and clinical trials are based on protocols. Protocols ensure that the activities outlined in the research study are carried out in a consistent way that could be repeated. The protocol is written by a team and includes physicians, scientists, statisticians, nurses, and others (e.g., pharmacists). Every protocol should include the same parts, but the order may differ. The basic elements of a protocol are listed in Figure 5-1 (Mitchell & Smith, 2016; Ness & Royce, 2017).
   a) The information included in a clinical trial protocol is used to write orders for study activities, such as tests or procedures and medications to be administered. It also should include instructions of when to contact a member of the research team. The protocol can also provide helpful information about the following:
      (1) Potential or anticipated side effects or adverse events of the intervention and how to treat them
      (2) Administration instructions
         (a) Rate of infusion for study medication
         (b) Pre- and postmedication or hydration needs
         (c) How to treat side effects, including when to hold or reduce dosage of study medication
      (3) Safety assessments, including blood work and physical examinations

Figure 5-1. Basic Sections of a Protocol

- Title page—title of study, version date, local protocol number, name of investigator(s)
- Table of contents
- Abstract—summary of the study background, objectives, eligibility, and design
- Introduction—outlines the objectives and scientific support for the study
- Eligibility assessment and enrollment—describes the patients that can be on the study
  - Inclusion criteria—criteria that a patient must meet to be eligible for the clinical trial
  - Exclusion criteria—reasons that a patient may not be eligible for the clinical trial
- Study implementation—provides information about the study treatment and plan
  - Study design or structure
  - Information about how the intervention will be given
  - Other information or specimens that will be collected
  - What other treatments a patient can or cannot receive while on the study
  - Reason the patient might be taken off the study
  - What needs to be done after the patient goes off the study
- Supportive care—how a patient's symptoms can be managed while the patient is on the study
- Data collection, evaluation, and reporting
  - What types of information about a patient need to be collected
  - How this information needs to be documented and evaluated
- Human subjects protection procedures, including consent and assent
- Drug information, including known or suspected side effects

Note. Based on information from Mitchell & Smith, 2016; Ness & Royce, 2017.

(4) When biospecimens are to be collected
(5) Randomization procedures

5. Protecting research patients: *Good clinical practice* in conducting research refers to a standard that ensures ethical and scientific quality in research with human subjects (i.e., living individuals who volunteer to participate in clinical research). Adherence to the principles of good clinical practice, including adequate human subject protection, is universally recognized as a critical requirement to the conduct of research involving human subjects (Woltz & Moore, 2016). Human subjects are living individuals, their data, and biospecimens. For the purposes of this chapter, human subjects will be referred to as *patients*.
   a) Regulations and guidance documents that affect the conduct of clinical trials are designed to protect patients participating in clinical research and ensure the accuracy of the data being collected. Several groups with regulatory authority are involved in the conduct of clinical trials in the United States.
      (1) The Office for Human Research Protections maintains regulatory oversight and provides advice on ethical and regulatory issues in biomedical and behavioral research that is funded or supported by the U.S. Department of Health and Human Services.
      (2) The U.S. FDA has oversight for product development (e.g., drugs, biologics, devices) regardless of the funding source.
   b) Ethical review of the protocol: All clinical trials must have an ethical review and be approved by an institutional review board (IRB) prior to implementation (Filchner, 2016). If any changes happen in the protocol (i.e., protocol amendment), the IRB would also review the changes prior to implementation.
      (1) The primary responsibility of the IRB is to protect the rights and safety of patients.
      (2) The IRB must decide whether the anticipated benefit, either of new knowledge or of improved health for patients on the clinical trial, justifies the risks that patients may experience.
      (3) The IRB cannot approve research in which the risks are too high in relation to the anticipated benefits.
   c) Informed consent: Informed consent is an ongoing process of communication and understanding between a patient and investigator. As a part of this process, the patient decides whether to voluntarily agree to enter a clinical trial. The informed consent process includes the sharing of information about the nature of the research and evaluation of the patient's comprehension of that information and his or her voluntary decision to participate (Klimaszewski, 2016; National Commission for the Protection of Human Subjects of Biomedical and Behavioral Research, 1979).
      (1) One tool used in the informed consent process is the informed consent document. Common information included on all informed consent documents based on federal regulations are found in Figure 5-2 (Elements of Informed Consent, 2017; General Requirements for Informed Consent, 2009).
      (2) The patient indicates initial agreement by signing an informed consent document. However, this does not mean that the patient must continue in the clinical trial if he or she decides to withdraw for any reason.

6. Roles and responsibilities: The clinical research enterprise is vast and involves many individuals and groups (Ness & Royce, 2017; Schmotzer & Ness, 2016).

Figure 5-2. Common Elements of the Informed Consent Document

- Statement that the clinical trial involves research, including the following:
  - Explanation of the purpose of the research
  - Expected length of participation
  - Description of procedures to be followed
  - Identification of any procedures that are experimental
- Any predictable risks to patients, as well as a statement that the intervention or procedure may cause unforeseeable risks
- Any benefits to patients or others
- Any alternatives to study participation
- How patients' confidentiality will be maintained
- Contact people for questions related to research and the research participants' rights
- Statement that participation is voluntary and that there will be no penalty if patients do not want to participate
- Reason why investigators may stop treating patients on the clinical trial
- Costs for which patients may be responsible
- Whether patients will receive any compensation for participation in the clinical trial
- Statement that patients will be notified of new findings that may affect their decision to continue participation

Note. Based on information from Elements of Informed Consent, 2017; General Requirements for Informed Consent, 2009.

a) Every clinical trial team will have a principal investigator (i.e., individual who is responsible for the overall conduct of the clinical trial) and research participants. The team may also include the following:
   (1) Subinvestigator (or subinvestigators): Individual selected by the principal investigator who provides support for the conduct of a clinical trial
   (2) Study coordinator: Individual responsible for the organization of the day-to-day activities of a clinical trial at a specific site, including gathering data
   (3) Clinical data manager: Individual responsible for organizing and collecting the data required by the protocol

b) Nurses at all levels of education and practice play key roles in clinical research.
   (1) Nurse researcher: The nurse researcher provides leadership in the development, performance, and analysis of clinical research.
   (2) Clinical trial nurse: Clinical trials nursing is a specialty nursing role that focuses on the coordination of clinical trials and the management of patients on those trials. Other titles for this role include clinical research nurse, clinical trials coordinator, and clinical research associate. Specific responsibilities and competencies for the oncology clinical trial nurses have been developed and are available online (see Oncology Nursing Society, 2016).
   (3) Direct care nurses: The primary responsibility of these nurses is the clinical care of patients. Their responsibilities with clinical trials can widely vary but may include patient and caregiver education, finding information about clinical trials for patients, advocating for ethical care, administering the treatments, collecting biospecimens, and monitoring for side effects (Parreco, Ness, Galassi, & O'Mara, 2012; see Tablc 5-2).

B. Drug development process
   1. The drug development process is a highly regulated process involving many steps to prove that a drug or biologic is safe and effective before it is marketed.
   2. The two essential roles in drug development in the United States are the sponsor and the FDA.
      a) Sponsor: The sponsor is responsible for the development of the product (i.e., drug or biologic) and producing the evidence (i.e., safety and efficacy) to FDA. This includes both preclinical activities and clinical activities (Gillogly, Perry, & Westendorp, 2016; U.S. FDA, 2018a; see Table 5-3). Most sponsors are pharmaceutical/biotechnology companies. Other sponsors may include academic medical centers or the National Cancer Institute Cancer Therapy Evaluation Program.
      b) U.S. FDA: FDA reviews the evidence against the standards of excellence (i.e., good clinical practice, good manufacturing practice, and good laboratory practice) to ensure that the product is safe and effective.
   3. Investigational new drug (IND) application: Before beginning the clinical trial, the sponsor must submit an IND application (IND Application, 2017). This process protects clinical trial patients from unreasonable and significant risk.
      a) Information included in the IND application
         (1) Animal study and toxicity data
         (2) Manufacturing information
         (3) Protocols for the clinical trials to be conducted
         (4) Information about the investigator
      b) FDA has 30 days to review the initial IND application before clinical trials may begin. If it finds any potential safety concerns (e.g., patients are exposed to unreasonable or significant risk; not enough information is provided about the trial's risk; the principal investigator is not qualified), the sponsor will need to resolve the concerns to FDA's satisfaction.
      c) The sponsor is responsible for informing FDA about new protocols, amendments to existing protocols, and any serious side effects seen during the trials. This information continues until the sponsor files a marketing application or decides to withdraw the IND.
      d) FDA assigns an IND number, which is often noted in the protocol (e.g., title page, pharmaceutical section).
   4. Clinical testing: FDA will notify the sponsor that the IND is safe to proceed, which means that clinical trials may begin. Clinical trials have three main phases, plus a fourth phase that takes place after a drug enters the market (IND Application, 2017; Ness & Cusack, 2016; see Table 5-4). The sponsor is responsible for ensuring that the clinical trials are monitored for patient safety and quality data.

Table 5-2. Direct Care Nurse Responsibilities When Caring for a Clinical Trial Patient

Research Activity	Responsibilities
Identifying which patients are on a clinical trial	Know how the organization identifies a patient on a clinical trial.
Maintaining the informed consent (IC) process	Locate the signed IC document. Ideally it should be in the patient's medical record, but the location depends on the organization's policy. Read the IC document to learn more about the clinical trial. Support the patient's decision to participate in the clinical trial. Encourage the patient to have others (e.g., family, referring physician) included in discussions about participation in a clinical trial. Encourage patient to read the IC document and other materials about the clinical trial and to ask questions. Assess the patient's comprehension of the study and his or her responsibilities by using open-ended questions. If asked to serve as a witness, know the organization's definition of witness (e.g., witness to the patient's signature or to the actual IC discussion). If unable to answer the patient's questions, contact the principal investigator or other designated member of the research team.
Administering the study drug or intervention	Obtain a copy of the study protocol. Information about the study intervention is in either the study design or pharmaceutical section of the protocol. The medical orders should be consistent with the protocol. Determine if other medications or interventions are needed (e.g., specific hydration before or after chemotherapy administration). Understand the appropriate handling of the drug, including how soon an IV drug needs to be infused after it is mixed. For study medications that the patient will self-administer, reinforce the proper usage, storage, and disposal of the drug and what to do for a missed dose.
Monitoring safety and response to intervention	The types of laboratory and/or imaging studies that will be used to monitor response to the study intervention should be listed in the protocol's study calendar. Assist in the identification of adverse events (AEs). An AE is similar to a side effect or toxicity except with these terms, a relationship to the intervention is implied. In research, the cause of the AE will be determined by the principal investigator and may or may not be related to the study intervention. Avoid asking questions about specific AEs that may be anticipated; these are found in the protocol and the IC document. Instead, ask the patient open-ended questions to help in the identification of AEs. Know when an AE should be reported to the research team and how to contact them.
Performing documentation and data collection	Document all prescription and over-the-counter medications, including complementary and alternative medications. Document the dose, how long the patient has been taking the medication, and the indication for its use. Document study-specific interventions. For IV study drugs, include the start and stop time. Document the AE details: • When the AE started • Description of the AE, which will be used by the research team to indicate its severity • Treatment for the AE • When the AE ended, if known For studies that require biospecimen collection, document the type of sample collected (e.g., blood, saliva), the time the sample was collected, how the sample is to be stored (e.g., room temperature, on ice), and whom to contact to pick up the specimen (e.g., research nurse, research assistant).

Note. Based on information from Parreco et al., 2012.

5. The FDA review process starts with the sponsor submitting a new drug application (NDA) to market the drug (U.S. FDA, 2018a; see Table 5-4).
   a) The NDA should provide the evidence of the drug's safety and effectiveness, the appropriateness of the proposed labeling, and the consistent manufacturing of the drug.
   b) FDA's Center for Drug Evaluation and Research will then review the application against its standards of excellence.
   c) FDA's approval grants a license for interstate commerce.
      (1) A drug is not licensed without a use.
      (2) Each drug is approved for a specific use, which is termed an *indication.*
      (3) A drug may have more than one indication.
   d) The license and description of the safe and effective use of the product is stated in the approved package insert (product label).

Table 5-3. Drug Development Process

Drug Development Stage	Description
Discovery and preclinical testing	Begins in the laboratory to find a chemical compound Completion of laboratory and animal testing to answer essential questions • Drug absorption, distribution, metabolism, and excretion • Potential benefits and mechanisms of action • Determination of the best dosage for a clinical trial • Side effects or adverse events (i.e., toxicity) Manufacturing of the drug • Preliminary stability of the drug • Finding the optimal drug formulation (e.g., oral or IV, additive needed)
Clinical testing	Begins with the submission of the investigational new drug application (NDA) Designing and conducting clinical trials to answer specific research questions Selection of investigators and research sites Monitoring the clinical trials for patient protection and quality data Sharing safety information with investigators Ensuring accountability for all investigational drug supplies
U.S. Food and Drug Administration (FDA) review for approval	Begins with sponsor submission of the NDA to FDA Full review by each NDA reviewer of his or her section of the application (e.g., medical officer and statistician review the clinical data) • Routine inspections of clinical study sites to verify accuracy of the clinical data submitted by the sponsor in the NDA and that no data have been withheld • Facilities where the drug will be manufactured Review of the drug's labeling (also known as the package insert) to ensure appropriate information is communicated to healthcare professionals and patients and assist sponsor in refining the prescribing information Granting of FDA approval Regulatory mechanisms to speed up the review and approval process for drugs that treat serious diseases • Priority review: FDA's goal is to act on the NDA within 6 months. • Breakthrough therapy: Process designed to expedite the development and review of drugs that may demonstrate substantial improvement over available therapy • Accelerated approval: Allows surrogate endpoints (e.g., a laboratory measurement, radiographic image, physical sign) to be used for drug approval to fill an unmet need • Fast track: Facilitates the development and expedited review of drugs

Note. Based on information from Gillogly et al., 2016; U.S. Food and Drug Administration, 2018a, 2018b.

e) When a drug is not used per the prescribing information or indication, this is referred to as *off-label* use.

6. Postapproval: Information about a drug's safety continues to evolve even after FDA approval. Sponsors also may continue the development of the drug for other indications (U.S. FDA, 2018a).
   a) FDA reviews reports of problems with all drugs and can decide if cautions need to be added to prescribing information.
   b) After the initial approval to market a drug, a sponsor may want to add other indications, change the formulation (e.g., IV to oral) or the dosage strengths, or other labeling changes. This requires a submission of a supplement application to the FDA for approval.
7. Generic drugs: Once a new drug is approved, the sponsor (i.e., the company manufacturing the drug) has exclusive rights to market the drug for a period. Once the patent and exclusive marketing rights have expired, other drug manufacturers may develop the drug (U.S. FDA, 2018a).
   a) Generic drugs must have the same dosage, safety, strength, quality, mechanism of action, and prescribing information as the brand name drug.
   b) Bioequivalence studies: Generic drug manufacturers conduct bioequivalence studies and file an abbreviated NDA. Bioequivalence studies include pharmacokinetic, pharmacodynamic, clinical, and in vitro studies.
8. Biologic development: Unlike drugs that are made of pure chemical substances, biologic products (e.g., monoclonal antibodies, vaccines, gene therapy) are made from living organisms and are larger molecules or a mixture of molecules (Buske, Ogura, Kwon, & Yoon, 2017).

Table 5-4. Phases of Clinical Trials

Phase	Description
1	Goal: Determine a dose or dosing schedule that is safe in humans—the maximum tolerated dose (MTD). Studies are small, usually 15–60 patients. Eligible patients may have a variety of cancers but have no available standard therapy options. All patients receive the study drug. Drug doses are increased slowly, and patients are monitored for side effects until the MTD is found. Phase 1 clinical trials help to determine the drug's pharmacokinetics, measuring how the drug is absorbed, distributed, metabolized, and excreted, revealing the following: • Drug dose • Administration schedule • Dose adjustments for certain medical conditions • Possible drug interactions
2	Goal: Evaluate the activity or effectiveness of the drug or regimen and determine if there should be further development of an intervention. Studies are larger in size (e.g., 100–300) and include patients for whom the current standard of care is not effective. In most phase 2 clinical trials, all patients receive the same intervention, including the same dose of the drug being studied (if it is a drug clinical trial). However, different trial designs exist (e.g., adaptive, Bayesian), in which patients may be randomized to one of several treatment groups.
3	Goal: Compare a new drug or treatment to a current standard treatment. Studies include large numbers of patients (e.g., hundreds to thousands) and are conducted at many locations. The standard design for a phase 3 clinical trial is a randomized controlled trial, allowing comparison of a new intervention to the current standard of care. Patients on the clinical trial will be assigned to one of two or more groups: • The treatment group, receiving the new intervention • A control group, receiving either the standard of care or a placebo, if there is no treatment option To ensure study results are due to the intervention, researchers may use the following: • Randomization: Patients are assigned to the study groups with an equal chance of receiving each of the treatment options. • Masking or blinding: Patients and research team members do not know which intervention each patient is receiving.
4	Goal: Further evaluate risks, benefits, and uses in real-life scenarios. Phase 4 trials are follow-up investigations for a drug recently marketed to and available for use by the general public. Studies include very large numbers of patients (e.g., thousands).

Note. Based on information from Investigational New Drug Application, 2017; Ness & Cusack, 2016; U.S. Food and Drug Administration, 2017b.

a) Biologics go through a similar discovery process, laboratory and clinical testing, IND application, and FDA review as drugs. However, the application for approval is referred to as the biologics license application and is reviewed by FDA's Center for Biologics Evaluation and Research.

b) Biosimilars: Biosimilars may be thought of as generic biologic products although they are different than nonbiologic drugs.

(1) Due to the variability of the molecules, it is not possible to develop biosimilars that have the same chemical structure as drugs.

(2) The FDA-approved biologic product is known as the *biologic reference product*. For FDA to approve a biosimilar biologic product, the product must be functionally similar to the reference product.

(3) Biosimilars can be approved for fewer indications and conditions than the approved biologic reference product. Therefore, nurses and other healthcare providers should read the product labeling for uses and routes of administration (Buske et al., 2017; U.S. FDA, 2017a).

References

Buske, C., Ogura, M., Kwon, H.-C., & Yoon, S.W. (2017). An introduction to biosimilar cancer therapeutics: Definitions, rationale for development and regulatory requirements. *Future Oncology, 13*(Suppl. 15), 5–16. https://doi.org/10.2217/fon-2017-0153

Czaplicki, K. (2016). Psychosocial distress. In A.D. Klimaszewski, M.A. Bacon, J.A. Eggert, E. Ness, J.G. Westendorp, & K. Willenberg (Eds.), *Manual for clinical trials nursing* (3rd ed., pp. 303–312). Pittsburgh, PA: Oncology Nursing Society.

Elements of Informed Consent, 21 C.F.R. § 50.25 (2017). Retrieved from http://www.accessdata.fda.gov/scripts/cdrh/cfdocs/cfcfr/CFRSearch.cfm?fr=50.25

Filchner, K. (2016). Protocol review and approval process. In A.D. Klimaszewski, M.A. Bacon, J.A. Eggert, E. Ness, J.G. Westendorp, & K. Willenberg (Eds.), *Manual for clinical trials nursing* (3rd ed., pp. 141–154). Pittsburgh, PA: Oncology Nursing Society.

General Requirements for Informed Consent, 45 C.F.R. § 46.116 (2009). Retrieved from http://www.hhs.gov/ohrp/humansubjects/guidance/45cfr46.html#46.116

Gillogly, D., Perry, P., & Westendorp, J.G. (2016). Drug development. In A.D. Klimaszewski, M.A. Bacon, J.A. Eggert, E. Ness, J.G. Westendorp, & K. Willenberg (Eds.), *Manual for clinical trials nursing* (3rd ed., pp. 13–16). Pittsburgh, PA: Oncology Nursing Society.

Investigational New Drug Application, 21 C.F.R. pt. 312 (2017). Retrieved from http://www.accessdata.fda.gov/scripts/cdrh/cfdocs/cfcfr/CFRSearch.cfm?CFRPart=312&showFR=1

Klimaszewski, A.D. (2016). Informed consent. In A.D. Klimaszewski, M.A. Bacon, J.A. Eggert, E. Ness, J.G. Westendorp, & K. Willenberg (Eds.), *Manual for clinical trials nursing* (3rd ed., pp. 113–125). Pittsburgh, PA: Oncology Nursing Society.

Mitchell, W., & Smith, Z. (2016). Elements of a protocol. In A.D. Klimaszewski, M.A. Bacon, J.A. Eggert, E. Ness, J.G. Westendorp, & K. Willenberg (Eds.), *Manual for clinical trials nursing* (3rd ed., pp. 109–111). Pittsburgh, PA: Oncology Nursing Society.

National Commission for the Protection of Human Subjects of Biomedical and Behavioral Research. (1979, April 18). *The Belmont Report: Ethical principles and guidelines for the protection of human subjects of research.* Retrieved from https://www.hhs.gov/ohrp/regulations-and-policy/belmont-report/index.html

National Institutes of Health. (2017, December). Glossary of common site terms. Retrieved from http://clinicaltrials.gov/ct2/about-studies/glossary#wrapper

Ness, E., & Cusack, G. (2016). Types of clinical research: Experimental. In A.D. Klimaszewski, M.A. Bacon, J.A. Eggert, E. Ness, J.G. Westendorp, & K. Willenberg (Eds.), *Manual for clinical trials nursing* (3rd ed., pp. 23–34). Pittsburgh, PA: Oncology Nursing Society.

Ness, E.A., & Royce, C. (2017). Clinical trials and the clinical trials nurse. *Nursing Clinics of North America, 52,* 133–148. https://doi.org/10.1016/j.cnur.2016.10.005

Oncology Nursing Society. (2016). *2016 oncology clinical trials nurse competencies.* Retrieved from https://www.ons.org/sites/default/files/OCTN_Competencies_FINAL.PDF

Parreco, L.K., Ness, E., Galassi, A., & O'Mara, A.M. (2012). Care of clinical trial participants: What nurses need to know. *American Nurse Today,* 7(6). Retrieved from https://www.americannursetoday.com/care-of-clinical-trial-participants-what-nurses-need-to-know

Schmotzer, G.L., & Ness, E. (2016). The research team. In A.D. Klimaszewski, M.A. Bacon, J.A. Eggert, E. Ness, J.G. Westendorp, & K. Willenberg (Eds.), *Manual for clinical trials nursing* (3rd ed., pp. 77–88). Pittsburgh, PA: Oncology Nursing Society.

U.S. Food and Drug Administration. (2017a, October 23). Biosimilar and interchangeable products. Retrieved from https://www.fda.gov/Drugs/DevelopmentApprovalProcess/HowDrugsareDevelopedandApproved/ApprovalApplications/TherapeuticBiologicApplications/Biosimilars/ucm580419.htm

U.S. Food and Drug Administration. (2017b, May 25). What are the different types of clinical research? Retrieved from https://www.fda.gov/forpatients/clinicaltrials/types/ucm20041762.htm

U.S. Food and Drug Administration. (2018a, January 4). The drug development process. Retrieved from https://www.fda.gov/ForPatients/Approvals/Drugs/default.htm

U.S. Food and Drug Administration. (2018b, January 4). Fast track, breakthrough therapy, accelerated approval, priority review. Retrieved from https://www.fda.gov/ForPatients/Approvals/Fast/ucm20041766.htm

Woltz, P.C., & Moore, A.C. (2016). Good clinical practice. In A.D. Klimaszewski, M.A. Bacon, J.A. Eggert, E. Ness, J.G. Westendorp, & K. Willenberg (Eds.), *Manual for clinical trials nursing* (3rd ed., pp. 67–76). Pittsburgh, PA: Oncology Nursing Society.

SECTION III

Cancer Therapeutics

CHAPTER 6

Chemotherapy

A. Chemotherapy in the treatment of cancer

1. Chemotherapy is the use of chemical agents to treat cancer. The use of chemotherapy dates back to the 1940s when nitrogen mustard was introduced as the first alkylating chemotherapy agent to have activity against cancer. To understand how chemotherapy works, it is important to review the principles of chemotherapy, including the kinetics of cellular growth. For a general overview of cancer treatment strategies, tumor response definitions, drug resistance, and dosing strategies, see Chapter 4.
2. Cellular kinetics: Three types of cells exist simultaneously.
   a) Nondividing and terminally differentiated
   b) Continually proliferating
   c) Resting cells that can be recruited into the cell cycle at any time (e.g., stem cells)
3. Tumor kinetics (Takimoto & Calvo, 2007)
   a) The rate of growth of a tumor is dependent on the following:
      (1) Growth fraction—the proportion of actively dividing cells
      (2) Doubling time—the length of the cell cycle
      (3) Rate of cell loss/death
   b) Tumor doubling time varies with tumor size.
      (1) Larger tumors tend to grow slower because of limited blood and oxygen supply.
      (2) Smaller tumors tend to be more responsive to cytotoxic therapy.
   c) The cell life cycle is a five-stage reproductive process occurring in both normal and malignant cells (see Figure 6-1).
      (1) The most important regulatory components of the cell cycle are cyclins and cyclin-dependent kinase (CDK) enzymes. Cyclins, a family of proteins, activate CDK enzymes and form a complex that promotes cell cycle progression. CDK inhibitors prevent cells from progressing through the cell cycle (Hydbring, Malumbres, & Sicinski, 2016; Malumbres, 2014; Olsen, 2017).
      (2) Chemotherapy agents target different phases of the cell cycle and halt growth and division of cells, leading to cell death. Chemotherapy is administered using a variety of schedules and doses designed to achieve therapeutic goals and based on the principles of cellular kinetics.
4. Phases of the cell cycle
   a) Gap 0 (G_0)
      (1) Resting or dormant phase
      (2) Cells are temporarily out of the cycle and not actively proliferating; however, all other cellular activities occur.
      (3) Cells continue in G_0 until a stimulus causes them to reenter the cell cycle.
      (4) Because they are not actively proliferating, cells in this phase have some protection from exposure to cell cycle–specific chemotherapy agents.

Figure 6-1. The Cell Cycle

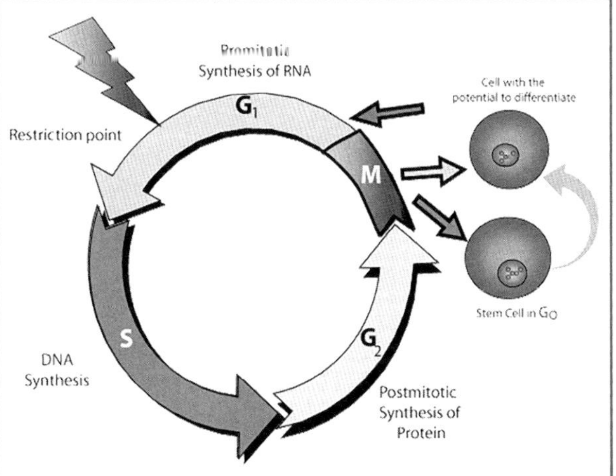

Note. Image courtesy of University of Texas MD Anderson Cancer Center. Used with permission.

b) Gap 1 (G_1)
   (1) Postmitotic phase
   (2) Cells begin the first phase of reproduction and growth by synthesizing the proteins and RNA necessary for cell division.
c) Synthesis (S): DNA is replicated.
d) Gap 2 (G_2)
   (1) Premitotic (or postsynthetic) phase
   (2) The second phase of protein and RNA synthesis occurs.
   (3) Preparation for mitotic spindle formation occurs.
   (4) The cell is now prepared for division.
e) Mitosis (M)
   (1) Cell division occurs.
   (2) Shortest phase of the cell life cycle
   (3) Mitosis results in formation of two daughter cells with exact copies of the parent cell's DNA. Cells either reenter the cell cycle to reproduce or perform the specific functions of the tissue for which they are programmed.

5. Cyclin–CDK complexes (Hydbring et al., 2016; Malumbres, 2014)
   a) Cyclins are cell cycle kinase regulators (e.g., cyclin D).
   b) CDKs are cell cycle kinase inhibitors (e.g., CDK4).
   c) Cyclins and CDKs unite and create complexes that propel the cell through each phase of the cell cycle (e.g., cyclin D–CDK4, cyclin D–CDK6, cyclin E–CDK2 drive G_1).
   d) CDK mutations have been linked to tumor formation (e.g., CDK6 is overexpressed in many hematologic malignancies, glioblastoma, and lung cancer).
   e) Anti-CDK/cyclin inhibitors are being developed and tested in clinical trials as a method to inhibit tumor growth.

B. Classification of chemotherapy agents
1. Drugs are classified according to their pharmacologic action or effect on cell reproduction (see Table 6-1).
2. Cell cycle–specific drugs exert effect within a specific phase of the cell cycle (Tortorice, 2018).
   a) These drugs have the greatest tumor cell kill when given in divided but frequent doses or as a continuous infusion with a short cycle time. This allows the maximum number of cells to be exposed to the drug at the specific time in their life cycle when they are vulnerable to the drug.
   b) Classifications include antimetabolites, plant alkaloids (camptothecins, epipodophyllotoxins, taxanes, and vinca alkaloids), and miscellaneous agents.
3. Cell cycle–nonspecific drugs exert effect in all phases of the cell cycle, including the G_0 (resting) phase (Tortorice, 2018).
   a) Cell cycle–nonspecific drugs may be effective in treating tumors with more slowly dividing cells.
   b) If the cancer is sensitive to the agent used, the drug is incorporated into the cell. The cell kill may not be instantaneous but may occur when the cell attempts to divide.
      (1) Destruction of tumor cells is directly proportional to the amount of drug administered.
      (2) These drugs are given intermittently, allowing the individual to recover from dose-limiting toxicities before the drug is given again.
      (3) The most frequent dose-limiting toxicity is bone marrow suppression.
      (4) In general, the greater the dose of the drug, the greater the cell kill.
   c) Classifications include alkylating agents, antitumor antibiotics, hormone therapies, and nitrosoureas.

C. Chemotherapy classifications (Sparreboom & Baker, 2015)
1. Alkylating agents
   a) First anticancer agents developed
   b) Cell cycle nonspecific
   c) Cause breakage in DNA helix strand, thereby interfering with DNA replication and resulting in cell death
   d) Dose-limiting toxicities include bone marrow suppression, gastrointestinal toxicities, and organ-specific toxicities (e.g., renal and hepatic, dependent on drug and dose; see Figure 6-2).
   e) Other effects include carcinogenic and mutagenic effects and impaired fertility.
   f) Examples: bendamustine, busulfan, cyclophosphamide, cisplatin
2. Antimetabolites
   a) Block DNA and RNA growth by interfering with enzymes (e.g., antifolates, a type of antimetabolite, interfere with the use of folic acid, which is necessary for normal cellular metabolism)
   b) Often divided into the following categories: folate analogs, purine analogs, adenosine analogs, pyrimidine analogs, and substituted ureas (Takimoto & Calvo, 2007)

Table 6-1. Chemotherapy Agents

Classification	Mechanism of Action	Drug	Route	Indications	Side Effects	Nursing Considerations
Alkylating agents	Break DNA helix strand, thereby interfering with DNA replication	Altretamine (Hexalen®)	PO	Ovarian cancer	Dose-limiting toxicities: Neurotoxicity, peripheral neuropathy, myelosuppression Nausea, vomiting, skin rash, hypersensitivity reaction, diarrhea	Do not open capsules. Monitor for progressive neurologic toxicity. Instruct patients to take after meals and at bedtime. Monoamine oxidase inhibitor antidepressants should be avoided because severe orthostatic hypotension may occur. (Eisai Inc., 2009)
		Bendamustine (Treanda®, Bendeka®)	IV	CLL Indolent NHL	Dose-limiting toxicity: Myelosuppression Pyrexia, nausea, vomiting, skin reactions, TLS, hepatotoxicity, irritation to vein	Infuse Treanda over 30–60 minutes. Bendeka may be infused in 10 minutes. Dilute Treanda in 500 ml NS to minimize vein irritation when giving peripherally. Bendamustine may inflame and irritate peripheral veins and can cause skin and tissue damage (irritant and vesicant properties). Monitor closely for infusion reactions (especially in second or subsequent cycles). Dose reduction or discontinuation may be necessary for hematologic toxicities. Take precautions for TLS in high-risk patients. Concomitant use of allopurinol may increase risk of severe skin toxicity. Undiluted Treanda is not compatible with polycarbonate or acrylonitrile-butadiene-styrene. (Cephalon, Inc., 2016; Teva Pharmaceuticals USA, Inc., 2017a)
		Busulfan (IV: Busulfex®; oral: Myleran®)	IV, PO	CML Hematopoietic stem cell transplant preparation	Dose-limiting toxicities: Myelosuppression, pulmonary fibrosis Profound tachycardia, hypertension, chest pain, hyperpigmentation, alopecia, sperm or ovarian suppression, confusion, seizures, mucositis, nausea, vomiting, insomnia, hyperglycemia, blurred vision, second malignancy; increased risk of hepatic sinusoidal obstruction syndrome (previously known as veno-occlusive disease) at AUC > 1,500 mcm × min	Monitor blood counts closely. Withhold oral doses for leukocyte count < 15,000/mm^3. Administer seizure prophylaxis. IV form should be administered through a central line and has been associated with inflammation and pain during infusion. Busulfan is not compatible with polycarbonate. (Aspen Global Inc., 2012a; Otsuka America Pharmaceutical Inc., 2017)

(Continued on next page)

Table 6-1. Chemotherapy Agents *(Continued)*

Classification	Mechanism of Action	Drug	Route	Indications	Side Effects	Nursing Considerations
Alkylating agents *(cont.)*		Carboplatin	IV	Ovarian cancer	Dose-limiting toxicity: Thrombocytopenia Neutropenia (myelosuppression is more pronounced with renal impairment), nausea, vomiting, hypersensitivity reaction, mild alopecia, skin rash	Drug is an irritant. Carboplatin exhibits less renal toxicity than cisplatin. Monitor blood counts closely and reduce the dose per protocol. Drug is most toxic to platelet precursors. Monitor for signs of bleeding. Check creatinine level prior to each dose (for AUC dosing). Have emergency medications available for hypersensitivity reaction, which may occur during any dose of therapy or be delayed. Most patients can be successfully desensitized via a multistep titration. (Teva Parenteral Medicines, Inc., 2016; Winkeljohn & Polovich, 2006)
		Chlorambucil (Leukeran®)	PO	CLL HL NHL	Dose-limiting toxicities: Myelosuppression, skin reactions Ovarian or sperm suppression, nausea, vomiting, secondary malignancy, hyperuricemia, pulmonary fibrosis, seizure (increased risk in children with nephrotic syndrome)	Take on an empty stomach. Use with caution in patients with seizure history and within 1 month of radiation or cytotoxic therapy. (Aspen Global Inc., 2016)
		Cisplatin	IV	Ovarian cancer Testicular cancer Bladder cancer	Dose-limiting toxicities: Severe nephrotoxicity, myelosuppression Severe acute and delayed nausea, vomiting, ototoxicity (tinnitus and high-frequency hearing loss are most common), hyperuricemia, hypersensitivity reaction, hypomagnesemia and other electrolyte abnormalities, peripheral neuropathy	Mannitol (to maximize urine flow) and rigorous hydration (prehydration and post-hydration with NS) may reduce nephrotoxicity. Monitor serum creatinine prior to each dose. Renal function must return to normal before subsequent doses are administered; renal toxicity becomes more prolonged and severe with repeated courses. Potential exists for delayed nausea and vomiting up to 6 days after administration. Consider obtaining a baseline audiogram. Monitor electrolytes and replace as needed. (Teva Parenteral Medicines, Inc., 2015a)

(Continued on next page)

Table 6-1. Chemotherapy Agents *(Continued)*

Classification	Mechanism of Action	Drug	Route	Indications	Side Effects	Nursing Considerations
Alkylating agents *(cont.)*		Cyclophosphamide	IV, PO	Breast cancer Ovarian cancer Multiple myeloma Leukemias Lymphomas Neuroblastoma Retinoblastoma Mycosis fungoides	Dose-limiting toxicities: Hemorrhagic cystitis, myelosuppression Vomiting, nausea, alopecia, may cause a temporary maxillary burning if administered too quickly, secondary malignancy, testicular or ovarian failure High-dose: Acute cardiomyopathy SIADH	Aggressive hydration and frequent bladder emptying can help reduce frequency and severity of bladder toxicity and hemorrhagic cystitis. Mesna may be considered in conjunction with hydration for prevention of hemorrhagic cystitis. Previous or concurrent radiation may increase toxicities. Withhold doses for ANC ≤ 1,500/mm^3 and platelets < 50,000/mm^3. (Baxter Healthcare Corp., 2017; West-Ward Pharmaceuticals Corp., 2016)
		Dacarbazine	IV	Metastatic malignant melanoma HL	Dose-limiting toxicities: Severe neutropenia and thrombocytopenia (with nadir at 2–3 weeks or later) Severe nausea and vomiting for up to 12 hours, anorexia, alopecia, rash, flu-like syndrome (fever, malaise, myalgias), hypotension, hypersensitivity reaction (uncommon), photosensitivity	Dacarbazine is an irritant. Protect solution from light. Flu-like syndrome may occur up to 7 days after drug administration; treat symptoms. (Teva Parenteral Medicines, Inc., 2015b)
		Ifosfamide (Ifex®)	IV	Testicular cancer	Dose-limiting toxicities: Hemorrhagic cystitis, myelosuppression Nausea, alopecia, vomiting, neurotoxicity (somnolence, confusion, hallucinations, depressive psychoses, and encephalopathy), urotoxicity, cardiotoxicity, pulmonary toxicity Methylene blue has been used to treat ifosfamide-induced encephalopathy; reports have shown that the encephalopathy may spontaneously resolve.	Administer over at least 30 minutes. Patient should receive extensive hydration of at least 2 L IV or oral fluid per day. Hemorrhagic cystitis can be severe and can be reduced by the prophylactic use of mesna. (Baxter Healthcare Corp., 2014; Patel, 2006)

(Continued on next page)

Table 6-1. Chemotherapy Agents *(Continued)*

Classification	Mechanism of Action	Drug	Route	Indications	Side Effects	Nursing Considerations
Alkylating agents *(cont.)*		Mechlorethamine (nitrogen mustard, Mustargen®, Valchlor®)	IV, topical, intracavitary	HL NHL CLL CML Polycythemia vera Mycosis fungoides Bronchogenic carcinoma	Severe nausea, vomiting, alopecia, myelosuppression, hyperuricemia, pain or phlebitis at IV site, chills, fever, testicular or ovarian failure Topical: Dermatitis, pruritus, skin infection, ulceration, hyperpigmentation	Drug is a vesicant and irritant. Administer through the side arm of a free-flowing IV. Flush with 125–150 ml NS following infusion to minimize phlebitis. If extravasation occurs, antidote is sodium thiosulfate. Use mechlorethamine as soon after preparation as possible (15–30 minutes); it is extremely unstable. (Actelion Pharmaceuticals US, Inc., 2016; Recordati Rare Diseases Inc., 2013b)
		Melphalan (Alkeran®, Evomela®)	IV, PO	Multiple myeloma Ovarian cancer	Dose-limiting toxicity: Myelosuppression Nausea, vomiting, mucositis, hypersensitivity reactions	Instruct patients to take on an empty stomach. Application of ice chips to oral cavity is recommended during high-dose melphalan administration to prevent oral mucositis (Lilleby et al., 2006). Melphalan has been described as an irritant and a vesicant. Administer over 15–20 minutes into a fast-running IV solution into an injection port on the IV tubing; do not administer by direct injection into a peripheral vein. Alkeran must be administered within 1 hour of reconstitution. Evomela is stable for 4 hours at room temperature. Dose reduce in renal insufficiency (blood urea nitrogen ≥ 30 mg/dl). (ApoPharma USA, Inc., 2016; GlaxoSmithKline, 2012; Lilleby et al., 2006; Spectrum Pharmaceuticals, Inc., 2017)
		Oxaliplatin (Eloxatin®)	IV	Colorectal cancer	Dose-limiting toxicities: Peripheral neuropathy, myelosuppression (not usually severe with single-agent oxaliplatin) Acute, reversible, primary peripheral sensory neuropathy that presents within 1–48 hours, resolves within 14 days, and manifests as paresthesia, dysesthesia, or hypesthesia in hands, feet, oral cavity, and throat; can be aggravated by cold temperatures	Oxaliplatin is not compatible with sodium chloride or other chloride-containing solutions. Flush with D5W following infusion. Persistent (> 14 days) peripheral sensory neuropathy characterized by paresthesias, dysesthesias, and hypesthesias may occur that can interfere with daily activities (writing, buttoning, difficulty walking). Oxaliplatin has been described as an irritant and a vesicant. Monitor for acute, reversible effects and persistent neurotoxicity. Avoid ice to oral cavity during oxaliplatin infusion.

(Continued on next page)

Table 6-1. Chemotherapy Agents *(Continued)*

Classification	Mechanism of Action	Drug	Route	Indications	Side Effects	Nursing Considerations
Alkylating agents *(cont.)*		Oxaliplatin (Eloxatin®) *(cont.)*			Anaphylactic reaction, nausea, vomiting, diarrhea, pulmonary fibrosis, fatigue, fever, increased transaminases and alkaline phosphatase	For 3–4 days after therapy, patients should avoid consuming cold drinks and foods and breathing cold air (cover mouth with scarf). Dose reduce in patients with severe renal impairment (CrCl < 30 ml/min). (Sanofi-Aventis U.S. LLC, 2011)
		Temozolomide (Temodar®)	IV, PO	Refractory anaplastic astrocytoma Newly diagnosed glioblastoma multiforme	Dose-limiting toxicity: Myelosuppression Nausea, vomiting, headache, fatigue, hepatic toxicity, constipation, rash, alopecia	IV: Administer over 90 minutes. PO: Do not open capsules. Instruct patients to take on an empty stomach to decrease risk of nausea and vomiting. Do not administer temozolomide if patients have had an allergic reaction to dacarbazine. Temozolomide is only compatible with 0.9% sodium chloride. Administer *Pneumocystis jiroveci* pneumonia prophylaxis with trimethoprim-sulfamethoxazole in patients receiving temozolomide with radiation therapy for 42-day regimen. Consider bedtime administration for oral dosing to decrease nausea and vomiting. (Merck and Co., Inc., 2017)
		Thiotepa	IV, IT, intravesical, intracavitary, PO	Bladder cancer Breast cancer Ovarian cancer HL NHL	Dose-limiting toxicity: Myelosuppression Fatigue, weakness, fever, hypersensitivity reaction, ovarian or sperm suppression, nausea, vomiting, pain at infusion site, rash, alopecia, skin burn, mucositis, hemorrhagic cystitis	Use with caution in patients with severe renal or hepatic dysfunction. Withhold dose for WBCs < $3,000/mm^3$ or platelets < $150,000/mm^3$. Thiotepa used in the transplant setting can cause severe skin irritation. Frequent showering immediately following and during the first 48 hours after administration helps remove the chemical from the skin. Additionally, avoid tapes and skin adherents during treatment and for 48 hours following administration. Filter through a 0.22 micron filter prior to administration. (West-Ward Pharmaceuticals Corp., 2015b)

(Continued on next page)

Table 6-1. Chemotherapy Agents *(Continued)*

Classification	Mechanism of Action	Drug	Route	Indications	Side Effects	Nursing Considerations
Alkylating agents *(cont.)*		Trabectedin (Yondelis®)	IV	Liposarcoma Leiomyosarcoma	Dose-limiting toxicities: Myelosuppression (neutropenic sepsis), hepatotoxicity, cardiomyopathy Rhabdomyolysis, capillary leak syndrome, nausea, fatigue, vomiting, constipation, decreased appetite, diarrhea, peripheral edema, dyspnea, headache	Drug is administered as a 24-hour continuous infusion and must be given through a central line with a 0.2 micron filter. Trabectedin is a vesicant; extravasation can result in severe tissue injury. Premedicate with 20 mg IV dexamethasone 30 minutes prior to infusion. Dose reduce in patients with hepatic impairment. Trabectedin is metabolized through the CYP3A pathway; use caution when administering concurrently with CYP3A inducers or inhibitors. (Janssen Products, LP, 2015)
Antimetabolites	Azacitidine is believed to cause hypomethylation of DNA and direct cytotoxicity on abnormal hematopoietic cells in the bone marrow. Abnormal cells, including cancer cells, no longer respond to normal growth control mechanisms.	Azacitidine (Vidaza®)	IV, SC	Specific subtypes of MDS	Dose-limiting toxicities: Myelosuppression, elevated SCr, renal failure, hepatic toxicity TLS, nausea, vomiting, diarrhea, fatigue, fever, erythema at injection site, constipation IV only: Petechiae, rigors, weakness, hypokalemia	SC: Resuspend suspension immediately prior to administration by rolling syringe between palms (solution should be uniformly cloudy). Stable at room temperature for 1 hour and under refrigeration for 8 hours (when reconstituted using room-temperature water). Divide doses > 4 ml into two syringes and inject into two separate sites. Administer new injections at least 1 in. from old site. To minimize skin irritation, ensure that the needle is empty of drug and do not expel air into needle before giving the injection. Do not use ice on injection site, as it may decrease drug absorption. IV: Mix in 50–100 ml NS or lactated Ringer's solution only. Infuse over 10–40 minutes. Administration should be completed within 1 hour of reconstitution. Monitor CBC and liver and renal function during therapy. Drug is contraindicated in patients with hypersensitivity to azacitidine or mannitol and those with advanced malignant hepatic tumors. (Celgene Corp., 2016c)

(Continued on next page)

Table 6-1. Chemotherapy Agents *(Continued)*

Classification	Mechanism of Action	Drug	Route	Indications	Side Effects	Nursing Considerations
Antimetabolites *(cont.)*	Most other antimetabolites interfere with one or more enzymes or their reactions that are necessary for DNA synthesis. They affect DNA synthesis by acting as a substitute to the metabolites that would be used in the normal metabolism (e.g., antifolates interfere with the use of folic acid).	Capecitabine (Xeloda®)	PO	Colon cancer Metastatic colorectal cancer Metastatic breast cancer	Dose-limiting toxicities: Diarrhea, palmar-plantar erythrodysesthesia (hand-foot syndrome) Mucositis, nausea, vomiting, myelosuppression, increased bilirubin, fatigue	Patient education regarding importance of reporting toxicity and dose reduction is critical. Drug is contraindicated in patients with known hypersensitivity to 5-FU. Monitor PT/INR closely, as capecitabine increases effect of warfarin. Administer with food and water. Dose reduce if CrCl < 50 ml/min. Uridine triacetate (Vistogard®) is FDA approved for the emergency treatment of 5-FU or capecitabine overdose regardless of the presence of symptoms or in patients who exhibit early-onset (within 96 hours of administration) severe or life-threatening cardiac or CNS toxicity and/or early-onset (within 96 hours of administration) unusually severe adverse reactions (GI toxicities and/or neutropenia). Uridine triacetate is a prodrug of uridine, which competes with 5-fluorouridine triphosphate, a toxic metabolite of 5-FU, for incorporation into RNA during RNA sequencing. (Genentech, Inc., 2016; Wellstat Therapeutics Corp., 2017)
		Cladribine	IV	Hairy cell leukemia	Dose-limiting toxicities: Myelosuppression, neurotoxicity Fever, nausea, vomiting, hypersensitivity reaction, TLS, nephrotoxicity (high-dose therapy)	Use with caution in patients with liver and renal dysfunction. (Fresenius Kabi USA, LLC, 2016b)
		Clofarabine (Clolar®)	IV	Relapsed or refractory ALL in patients aged 1–21	Dose-limiting toxicities: Bone marrow suppression (including anemia, leukopenia, thrombocytopenia, neutropenia, and febrile neutropenia), infection, hepatobiliary toxicity, renal toxicity Nausea, vomiting, diarrhea, rare cases of systemic inflammatory response syndrome/capillary leak syndrome and cardiotoxicity	Continuous IV fluid administration and alkalization of urine during the 5 days of chemotherapy administration is encouraged to reduce risk of TLS and other adverse effects. Discontinue if hypotension develops during the 5 days of administration. Use prophylactic steroids to help prevent systemic inflammatory response syndrome and capillary leak syndrome. Give allopurinol if hyperuricemia is expected. Monitor respiratory status and blood pressure during infusion.

(Continued on next page)

Table 6-1. Chemotherapy Agents *(Continued)*

Classification	Mechanism of Action	Drug	Route	Indications	Side Effects	Nursing Considerations
Antimetabolites *(cont.)*		Clofarabine (Clolar®) *(cont.)*			including tachycardia, pericardial effusion, and left ventricular systolic dysfunction; TLS, headache, pruritus, rash, palmar-plantar erythrodysesthesia	Monitor renal and hepatic function during the days of administration. Dose reduce in patients with renal impairment (< 60 ml/min). Monitor hematologic status closely following treatment. (Genzyme Corp., 2013)
		Cytarabine	IT, IV, SC	ALL AML CML CNS leukemia	Dose-limiting toxicity: Myelosuppression Nausea, vomiting, anorexia, fever, mucositis, diarrhea, hepatic dysfunction, rash, pruritus, localized pain and thrombophlebitis at IV site High-dose (1–3 g/m^2): Cerebellar toxicity, keratitis (treat with dexamethasone ophthalmic drops), dermatologic toxicities	Determine if ordered dose is standard dose or high dose; administer according to institutional guidelines. Toxicities vary depending on rate of high-dose cytarabine administration. Continuous-infusion cytarabine is associated with pulmonary toxicity (fluid overload), and bolus administration is associated with cerebellar toxicities. Specific nursing interventions are warranted for each. See Chapters 17 and 24 for information on pulmonary toxicities and neurotoxicity. For IT administration: Use preservative-free saline. (Mylan Institutional, LLC, 2014a)
		Cytarabine liposomal (DepoCyt®)	IT only	Lymphomatous meningitis	Neurotoxicity, mucositis, chemical arachnoiditis (nausea, vomiting, headache, fever), seizure, nausea, vomiting, constipation, weakness	Do not use in pediatric patients. Administer IT only. Patients should lie flat for 1 hour after lumbar puncture. Monitor closely for immediate toxic reactions. Administer dexamethasone 4 mg BID (PO or IV) for 5 days (start day of cytarabine administration) to decrease symptoms of chemical arachnoiditis. (Sigma-Tau Pharmaceuticals, Inc., 2017)
	Decitabine is believed to cause hypomethylation of DNA and direct cytotoxicity on abnormal hematopoietic cells in the bone marrow. Abnormal cells, including cancer cells, no longer respond to normal growth control mechanisms.	Decitabine (Dacogen®)	IV	MDS	Myelosuppression, fever, fatigue, nausea, cough, diarrhea, hyperglycemia, petechiae, peripheral edema	Prepare using cold infusion fluids and store refrigerated; it is stable for 4 hours. Must be used within 15 minutes if prepared in room-temperature fluids. (Eisai Inc., 2014)

(Continued on next page)

Table 6-1. Chemotherapy Agents *(Continued)*

Classification	Mechanism of Action	Drug	Route	Indications	Side Effects	Nursing Considerations
Antimetabolites *(cont.)*		Floxuridine	Intra-arterial	GI adenocarcinoma with metastasis to liver	Myelosuppression, nausea, vomiting, diarrhea, stomatitis, mucositis, localized erythema, alopecia, photosensitivity, darkening of the veins, abdominal pain, gastritis, enteritis, hepatotoxicity	Do not use in pediatric patients. Floxuridine has been described as an irritant. (Fresenius Kabi USA, LLC, 2016c)
		Fludarabine	IV, PO	CLL	Dose-limiting toxicity: Myelosuppression TLS, nausea, vomiting, diarrhea, rash, neurotoxicity, interstitial pneumonitis, weakness, hemolytic anemia, cough, infection	Administer as a 30-minute infusion. Monitor PFTs. Allopurinol and IV hydration are recommended for newly diagnosed patients with CLL or patients with high tumor burden to prevent TLS. Do not use in combination with pentostatin, because it may cause severe pulmonary toxicity. Use with caution in patients with renal impairment. Tablets may be taken with or without food and must not be chewed. Do not break or crush tablets. (Teva Parenteral Medicines, Inc., 2017b)
	Drug is a combination of a thymidine-based nucleoside analog and a thymidine phosphorylase inhibitor. It incorporates into DNA, interferes with DNA synthesis, and inhibits cell proliferation.	Trifluridine and tipiracil (Lonsurf®)	PO	Previously treated metastatic colorectal cancer	Anemia, neutropenia, fatigue, nausea, vomiting, diarrhea, abdominal pain, pyrexia, embryo-fetal toxicity	Administer 35 mg/m^2 PO twice daily on days 1–5 and days 8–12 of each 28-day cycle. Take within 1 hour after meals 12 hours apart. Round dose to nearest 5 mg increment. Do not administer if ANC $< 50,000/mm^3$ or platelets $< 50,000/mm^3$. (Taiho Oncology, Inc., 2017)

(Continued on next page)

Table 6-1. Chemotherapy Agents *(Continued)*

Classification	Mechanism of Action	Drug	Route	Indications	Side Effects	Nursing Considerations
Antimetabolites *(cont.)*	Nucleoside metabolic inhibitor that interferes with the synthesis of DNA and to a lesser extent inhibits the formation of RNA	5-FU (Adrucil®)	IV, topical	Colorectal cancer Breast cancer Pancreatic cancer Gastric cancer Pancreatic cancer	Dose-limiting toxicities: Mucositis, myelosuppression Nausea, anorexia, vomiting, diarrhea, alopecia, ocular toxicities (e.g., increased lacrimation, photosensitivity), darkening of the veins, dry skin, cardiotoxicity (rare), neurotoxicity, palmar-plantar erythrodysesthesia	Ensure that patients take year-round photosensitivity precautions; encourage sunscreen use if patients must be exposed. Leucovorin often is given concurrently to enhance 5-FU activity. Apply ice chips to the oral cavity 10–15 minutes pre- and post-IV bolus dose of 5-FU to reduce oral mucositis in patients with GI malignancies. Ice chips are not recommended in patients receiving capecitabine or oxaliplatin because of potential discomfort with exposure to coldness. Uridine triacetate (Vistogard) is FDA-approved for the emergency treatment of 5-FU or capecitabine overdose regardless of the presence of symptoms or in patients who exhibit early-onset (within 96 hours of administration) severe or life-threatening cardiac or CNS toxicity and/or early-onset (within 96 hours of administration) unusually severe adverse reactions (GI toxicities and/or neutropenia). Uridine triacetate is a prodrug of uridine, which competes with 5-fluorouridine triphosphate, a toxic metabolite of 5-FU, for incorporation into RNA during RNA sequencing. (Teva Parenteral Medicines, Inc., 2017a; Wellstat Therapeutics Corp., 2017)
		Gemcitabine (Gemzar®)	IV	Pancreatic cancer Breast cancer Ovarian cancer NSCLC	Dose-limiting toxicity: Myelosuppression (especially thrombocytopenia) Nausea, vomiting; flu-like symptoms including fever, headache, arthralgias, and myalgias; rash, peripheral edema, dyspnea, pulmonary toxicity with increased infusion time, hepatotoxicity	Gemcitabine is an irritant. Infuse over 30 minutes; infusion longer than 60 minutes or more than weekly can increase hematologic toxicity. Use with caution in patients with renal impairment. Increased (severe and life-threatening) toxicity may occur when gemcitabine is administered within 7 days of radiation therapy. (Eli Lilly and Co., 2017)
		6-Mercaptopurine (6-MP; Purinethol®)	PO	ALL	Myelosuppression, hepatotoxicity, mucositis, nausea, vomiting, anorexia, hyperuricemia, hyperuricosuria, alopecia, rash, hyperpigmentation	Reduce oral dose by 75% when used concurrently with allopurinol. Instruct patient to take on an empty stomach. (Kantarjian et al., 2000; Mylan Pharmaceuticals Inc., 2013)

(Continued on next page)

Table 6-1. Chemotherapy Agents *(Continued)*

Classification	Mechanism of Action	Drug	Route	Indications	Side Effects	Nursing Considerations
Antimetabolites *(cont.)*		Methotrexate	IM, IT, IV, PO, SC	NHL Leukemia CNS metastasis Lung cancer Breast cancer Head and neck cancer Gestational trophoblastic tumor Osteosarcoma Rheumatoid arthritis Psoriasis Gestational choriocarcinoma Chorioadenoma destruens Hydatidiform mole	Dose-limiting toxicities: Hepatotoxicity, renal toxicity Mucositis, nausea, vomiting, myelosuppression, oral or GI ulceration, pneumonitis, photosensitivity, neurotoxicity associated with high-dose therapy	High-dose methotrexate doses are adjusted for patients with renal dysfunction. High doses must be followed by timely administration of leucovorin and alkaline hydration. Follow dosing schedule carefully. Monitor serum methotrexate levels until ≤ 0.1 mcmol/L. Monitor urine pH and maintain ≥ 7 before and until serum methotrexate levels ≤ 0.05 mcmol/L. Depending on methotrexate clearance, some patients may require additional leucovorin rescue and serum methotrexate monitoring. Instruct patients on strict mouth care. Ensure that patients avoid taking multivitamins with folic acid. Multiple drug interactions (e.g., NSAIDs, alcohol, aspirin, warfarin, aminoglycosides) are possible. Glucarpidase (Voraxaze®) is FDA-approved for patients with delayed methotrexate clearance due to renal impairment. This drug reduces systemic methotrexate levels by rapidly converting methotrexate to glutamate and 4-deoxy-4-amino-N^{10}-methylpteroic acid. (BTG International Inc., 2013; Fresenius Kabi USA, LLC, 2014)
		Nelarabine (Arranon®)	IV	T-cell ALL T-cell lymphoblastic lymphoma	Dose-limiting toxicity: Neurotoxicity Myelosuppression, headache, nausea, vomiting, diarrhea, constipation, cough, fatigue, peripheral neuropathy, dyspnea, neurologic toxicities (somnolence, seizures, ataxia)	Drug is administered as an undiluted IV infusion over 2 hours for adults and 1 hour for pediatrics. Administer with appropriate supportive care medications to prevent hyperuricemia and TLS. Discontinue for ≥ grade 2 neurologic events (severe somnolence, seizure, and peripheral neuropathy). Use caution in patients with renal or hepatic dysfunction. (GlaxoSmithKline, 2014a)

(Continued on next page)

Table 6-1. Chemotherapy Agents *(Continued)*

Classification	Mechanism of Action	Drug	Route	Indications	Side Effects	Nursing Considerations
Antimetabolites *(cont.)*		Pemetrexed (Alimta®)	IV	Mesothelioma Nonsquamous NSCLC	Myelosuppression, fatigue, nausea, vomiting, anorexia, chest pain, and dyspnea. Vitamin supplementation reduces these side effects. Renal and liver toxicity	Infuse over 10 minutes. To reduce treatment-related hematologic and GI toxicities, administer folic acid 400–1,000 mcg PO daily starting 1 week prior to the first cycle and daily for 3 weeks after final cycle. Give vitamin B_{12} injection 1,000 mcg IM 1 week before first cycle and repeat every 9 weeks until treatment is completed. Dexamethasone 4 mg BID for 3 days starting the day before treatment decreases incidence of rash. Monitor CBC on days 8 and 15. Hold treatment if ANC < 1,500/mm^3, platelets < 100,000/mm^3, or CrCl < 45 ml/min. Monitor renal and hepatic function. Concurrent use of NSAIDs may increase the risk of renal damage. (Eli Lilly and Co., 2013)
		Pentostatin (Nipent™)	IV	Hairy cell leukemia	Dose-limiting toxicity: Myelosuppression Acute pulmonary edema, hypotension, fever, chills, nausea, vomiting, rash, renal toxicity, confusion, hepatic enzyme elevation, heightened infection risk, cough, cardiac	Administer with 500–1,000 ml 5% dextrose in ½ NS solution prior to the infusion and an additional 500 ml after infusion. Do not administer with fludarabine, carmustine, etoposide, or high-dose cyclophosphamide. (Hospira, Inc., 2018)
		Pralatrexate (Folotyn®)	IV	Peripheral T-cell lymphoma	Dose-limiting toxicity: Myelosuppression Mucositis, dermatologic reactions, TLS, hepatotoxicity, edema, fatigue, nausea	Drug is administered as an IV push over 3–5 minutes. Consider dose reduction in patients with impaired renal function (estimated glomerular filtration rate < 30 ml/min/1.73 m^2). Prophylactic folic acid and vitamin B_{12} supplements must be given. Supplement patients with vitamin B_{12} 1 mg IM every 8–10 weeks and folic acid 1–1.25 mg PO daily. Monitor liver and renal function. (Allos Therapeutics, 2016)
		Thioguanine (6-TG; Tabloid®)	PO	ANLL	Dose-limiting toxicity: Myelosuppression Hyperuricemia, nausea, hepatotoxicity, diarrhea	Monitor hepatic function. (Aspen Global Inc., 2012b)

(Continued on next page)

Table 6-1. Chemotherapy Agents *(Continued)*

Classification	Mechanism of Action	Drug	Route	Indications	Side Effects	Nursing Considerations
Antitumor antibiotics	Bind with DNA, thereby inhibiting DNA and RNA synthesis	Bleomycin	IM, intrapleural, IV, SC	Malignant pleural effusion Testicular cancer HL NHL Squamous cell cancers of the head and neck, cervix, vulva, and penis	Dose-limiting toxicities: Hypersensitivity or anaphylactic reaction (rare), pulmonary toxicity Hyperpigmentation, alopecia, photosensitivity, renal toxicity, hepatotoxicity, fever, chills, erythema, rash, mucositis	This drug is ordered in units. Bleomycin is not compatible with D5W. Patients with lymphoma have a higher incidence of anaphylaxis after receiving bleomycin than do other patients who receive the drug (usually occurring after the first or second dose). Therefore (per institutional protocol), two test doses of 1–2 units IV, IM, or SC may be administered before the first regular dose of bleomycin in patients with lymphoma. Patients who have received prior bleomycin are at risk for pulmonary toxicity when exposed to oxygen during surgery. Ensure that patients and family members understand the lifelong necessity of disclosing previous use of bleomycin when future needs for anesthesia occur to prevent a fatal episode of pulmonary failure. Because of the dose-related incidence of pulmonary fibrosis, the cumulative lifetime dose should not exceed 400 units. PFTs are recommended at initiation of bleomycin and every 1–2 months thereafter. Consider stopping drug if a 30%–35% decrease from pretreatment values occurs. Acetaminophen and an antihistamine may decrease fever and chills in first 24 hours after administration. Consider dose reductions in patients with CrCl < 50 ml/min. (Fresenius Kabi USA, LLC, 2016a)
		Dactinomycin (Actinomycin-D; Cosmegen®)	IV	Wilms tumor Childhood rhabdomyosarcoma Testicular cancer Ewing sarcoma Gestational trophoblastic disease	Dose-limiting toxicity: Myelosuppression Nausea, vomiting, alopecia, mucositis, diarrhea, ovarian or sperm suppression, radiation recall (hyperpigmentation of previously irradiated areas), sinusoidal obstruction syndrome, renal toxicity, hepatotoxicity	Dactinomycin is a vesicant; extravasation can result in severe tissue injury. Administer through the side port of a free-flowing IV. Dactinomycin is highly toxic and corrosive to soft tissues; inhalation and contact with the eyes must be avoided. This drug may be ordered in micrograms, so check the dose carefully. Dactinomycin is contraindicated in patients with concurrent or recent chicken pox or herpes zoster. Avoid within 2 months of radiation therapy for right-sided Wilms tumor. (Recordati Rare Diseases Inc., 2013a)

(Continued on next page)

Table 6-1. Chemotherapy Agents *(Continued)*

Classification	Mechanism of Action	Drug	Route	Indications	Side Effects	Nursing Considerations
Antitumor antibiotics *(cont.)*		Mitomycin C (Mutamycin®)	Intravesical, IV	Pancreatic cancer Stomach cancer Bladder cancer	Dose-limiting toxicity: Myelosuppression Nausea, vomiting, anorexia, fever, renal toxicity, pulmonary toxicity, fatigue	Drug is purple/blue in color. Mitomycin is a vesicant; extravasation can result in severe tissue injury. Administer through the side port of a free-flowing IV. Nadir occurs within 8 weeks after treatment begins (average of 4 weeks). Acute shortness of breath and bronchospasm can occur very suddenly when this drug is given with a vinca alkaloid. Withhold doses for platelets $< 100,000/mm^3$ or WBCs $< 4,000/mm^3$. Do not use in patients with SCr > 1.7 mg/dl. Hemolytic uremic syndrome has been seen with a single dose ≥ 60 mg. Mitomycin is contraindicated in patients with coagulation disorders. (Accord BioPharma Inc., 2016)
		Mitoxantrone	IV	Prostate cancer ANLL Multiple sclerosis	Dose-limiting toxicities: Myelosuppression, cardiotoxicity (risk increased if patient was treated with other cardiotoxic drugs) Nausea, vomiting, mucositis, alopecia, fever, weakness, hyperuricemia, amenorrhea, blue-green–colored urine, bluish skin or sclera	Drug is blue in color. Mitoxantrone is fatal if given intrathecally. Mitoxantrone is an irritant with vesicant potential. Withhold dose for ANC $< 1,500/mm^3$. Risk of cardiotoxicity with mitoxantrone is less than that with doxorubicin, but prior anthracycline use, chest irradiation, or cardiac disease increases risk. Prior to beginning therapy, evaluate patients for cardiac signs and symptoms, including obtaining multigated acquisition scan, baseline left ventricular ejection fraction, and ECG. Mitoxantrone should not be used in patients with hepatic impairment. (Fresenius Kabi USA, LLC, 2013)

(Continued on next page)

Table 6-1. Chemotherapy Agents *(Continued)*

Classification	Mechanism of Action	Drug	Route	Indications	Side Effects	Nursing Considerations
Antitumor antibiotics: Anthracyclines	Bind with DNA, thereby inhibiting DNA and RNA synthesis	Daunorubicin	IV	ALL in children AML	Dose-limiting toxicities: Myelosuppression, cardiotoxicity Nausea, vomiting, alopecia, hyperuricemia, radiation recall, red-colored urine	Drug is red in color. Daunorubicin is a vesicant; extravasation can result in severe tissue injury. Administer through the side arm of a free-flowing IV. Dose reduce in patients with hepatic or renal impairment. Test patients' cardiac ejection fraction before starting therapy. Total lifetime dose in adults is 550 mg/m^2 in those without cardiovascular risk factors and 400 mg/m^2 in adults receiving chest irradiation. (Halison Pharmaceuticals USA, 2014)
		Daunorubicin and cytarabine liposome (Vyxeos™)	IV	AML	Dose-limiting toxicities: Myelosuppression, cardiotoxicity, hypersensitivity reaction Hemorrhage events, copper overload	Administer over 90 minutes through a central line. Total lifetime daunorubicin dose in adults is 550 mg/m^2 in those without cardiovascular risk factors and 400 mg/m^2 in adults receiving chest irradiation. Vyxeos contains copper gluconate; copper toxicity is possible in patients with Wilson disease. Daunorubicin is a vesicant; extravasation can result in severe tissue injury. (Jazz Pharmaceuticals, Inc., 2017)
		Doxorubicin (Adriamycin®)	IV	Breast cancer ALL AML HL NHL Wilms tumor Neuroblastoma Sarcoma Ovarian cancer Bladder cancer Thyroid cancer Stomach cancer Bronchogenic carcinoma	Dose-limiting toxicities: Myelosuppression, cardiotoxicity, hepatotoxicity Nausea, vomiting, alopecia, mucositis, radiation recall, hyperuricemia, photosensitivity, red-colored urine	Drug is red in color. Doxorubicin is a vesicant; extravasation can result in severe tissue injury. Administer through the side arm of a free-flowing IV or via continuous infusion through a central catheter only. Consider administration of dexrazoxane if extravasation occurs. Dose reduce in patients with elevated serum total bilirubin. Test patients' cardiac ejection fraction before starting therapy. Do not exceed a lifetime cumulative dose of 550 mg/m^2 (450 mg/m^2 if the patient has had prior chest irradiation or concomitant cyclophosphamide treatment). Consider initiating dexrazoxane for cardiac protection in patients who have received a cumulative dose of 300 mg/m^2 and are continuing doxorubicin treatment. (West-Ward Pharmaceuticals Corp., 2015a)

(Continued on next page)

Table 6-1. Chemotherapy Agents *(Continued)*

Classification	Mechanism of Action	Drug	Route	Indications	Side Effects	Nursing Considerations
Antitumor antibiotics: Anthracyclines *(cont.)*		Doxorubicin liposomal (Doxil®)	IV	Ovarian cancer AIDS-related Kaposi sarcoma Multiple myeloma	Dose-limiting toxicities: Myelosuppression, cardiotoxicity, infusion-related reactions Nausea, vomiting, alopecia, mucositis, arrhythmia, amenorrhea, radiation recall, palmar-plantar erythrodysesthesia, hypersensitivity reaction, red-colored urine	Drug is red in color. Doxorubicin liposomal is an irritant with vesicant properties; take caution to avoid extravasation. The same warnings as with conventional doxorubicin apply regarding cardiovascular complications. Do not substitute for doxorubicin. Do not use an in-line filter. (Janssen Products, LP, 2017)
		Epirubicin (Ellence®)	IV	Breast cancer	Dose-limiting toxicities: Myelosuppression, cardiotoxicity Nausea, vomiting, mucositis, diarrhea, alopecia, amenorrhea, infection, hyperuricemia, radiation recall, flushing, red-colored urine	Drug is red in color. Epirubicin is a vesicant; extravasation can result in severe tissue injury. Infuse into the side port of a free-flowing IV. Do not use if baseline ANC is $< 1{,}500/mm^3$. Consider dose reduction in patients with hepatic and severe renal impairment (SCr > 5 mg/dl). Cumulative dosing should not exceed $900\ mg/m^2$. Test patients' cardiac ejection fraction before starting epirubicin therapy. (Pfizer Inc., 2014)
		Idarubicin (Idamycin®)	IV	AML	Dose-limiting toxicities: Myelosuppression, cardiomyopathy Hyperuricemia, nausea, vomiting, alopecia, vein itching, radiation recall, rash, mucositis, diarrhea, severe enterocolitis with perforation, red-colored urine	Drug is red-orange in color. Idarubicin is a vesicant; extravasation can result in severe tissue injury. Inject slowly over 10–15 minutes into free-flowing side-arm infusion. Cardiotoxicity of idarubicin is less than that of daunorubicin. Cumulative doses $> 150\ mg/m^2$ are associated with decreased ejection fraction. Local reactions (hives at injection site) may occur. Consider dose reduction in patients with renal or hepatic impairment. (Pfizer Inc., 2015)
		Valrubicin (Valstar®)	Intravesical	Intravesical therapy of bacillus Calmette-Guérin–refractory in situ bladder cancer	Dysuria, bladder spasm and irritation, urinary incontinence, leukopenia, hyperglycemia; drug may turn the urine red.	Administer via intravesical route only. Do not use in pediatric patients. Valrubicin is a vesicant; extravasation can result in severe tissue injury if perforation of bladder occurs. Use non-PVC, non-DEHP containing tubing. (Endo Pharmaceuticals Solutions Inc., 2017)

(Continued on next page)

Table 6-1. Chemotherapy Agents *(Continued)*

Classification	Mechanism of Action	Drug	Route	Indications	Side Effects	Nursing Considerations
Miscellaneous	Induces cytodifferentiation and decreased proliferation of APL cells in culture and in vivo	All-trans-retinoic acid (ATRA, tretinoin, Vesanoid®)	PO, topical as a cream	Induction of remission in patients with APL characterized by the presence of t(15;17) translocation and/or the presence of PML/RARα gene who are refractory to, or who have relapsed from, anthracycline chemotherapy, or for whom anthracycline-based chemotherapy is contraindicated	Headache, fever, dry skin, bone pain, nausea, vomiting, rash, pruritus, mouth sores, skin and oral membrane dryness, flu-like symptoms, abdominal pain, diarrhea, constipation, leukocytosis, differentiation syndrome (see Chapter 17), bleeding	PO: Patients should take with food. Confirm negative pregnancy test in females within 1 week of starting treatment. Instruct patients to use two forms of contraception during therapy and for 1 month following discontinuation of therapy. (Roche Laboratories Inc., 2008)
	Causes DNA fragmentation and morphologic changes characteristic of apoptosis in NB4 cells and degrades the chimeric PML/RARα protein	Arsenic trioxide (Trisenox®)	IV	APL	Fatigue, prolonged QT interval, APL differentiation syndrome, leukocytosis, headache, nausea, vomiting, diarrhea, abdominal pain, fever, dermatitis, cough, dyspnea, peripheral neuropathy	Use with caution with other agents that prolong QT/QTc interval. Obtain baseline ECG prior to therapy. Ensure QTc interval < 500 ms prior to infusion. QTc intervals should be measured periodically during therapy (e.g., weekly). Use with caution in patients with renal impairment. Monitor electrolytes during therapy. Maintain serum potassium > 4 mEq/L and magnesium > 1.8 mg/dl. Renal or hepatic impairment may increase toxicity risk. Administer over 1–2 hours (may be extended up to 4 hours if acute vasomotor reactions are observed). (Teva Pharmaceuticals USA, Inc., 2016)
	Depletes plasma asparagine, leading to leukemic cell death	Asparaginase *Erwinia chrysanthemi* (Erwinaze®)	IM, IV	ALL	Hypersensitivity reaction (including anaphylaxis), pancreatitis, glucose intolerance, thrombosis, abdominal pain, diarrhea	Keep medications to treat anaphylaxis at bedside. Limit the volume of reconstituted asparaginase at a single injection site to 2 ml; if reconstituted dose to be administered is > 2 ml, use multiple injection sites. When given IV, infuse in 100 ml over 1–2 hours. (Jazz Pharmaceuticals, Inc., 2016)

(Continued on next page)

Table 6-1. Chemotherapy Agents *(Continued)*

Classification	Mechanism of Action	Drug	Route	Indications	Side Effects	Nursing Considerations
Miscellaneous *(cont.)*	Depletes plasma asparagine, leading to leukemic cell death	Pegaspargase (Oncaspar®)	IM, IV	ALL	Pancreatitis, thrombosis, glucose intolerance, coagulopathy, hepatotoxicity, allergic reactions (including anaphylaxis)	When given IM, maximum volume per injection site is 2 ml. When given IV, give over 1–2 hours. (Baxalta US Inc., 2016)
	Acts in S phase as antimetabolite	Hydroxyurea (Hydrea®, Mylocel®)	PO	CML Squamous cell cancer of the head and neck	Dose-limiting toxicity: Myelosuppression Vasculitic toxicities, macrocytosis, nausea, vomiting, diarrhea, renal failure, mucositis, fever, hyperuricemia, rash, alopecia, second malignancies	Do not open capsules. Monitor blood counts weekly. Patients should avoid live vaccines. (Bristol-Myers Squibb Co., 2017b)
	Inhibits adrenal steroid production	Mitotane (Lysodren®)	PO	Adrenocortical cancer	CNS toxicity, adrenal insufficiency/crisis, ovarian macrocysts in premenopausal women, anorexia, nausea, vomiting, mucositis, lethargy, dizziness or vertigo, rash	Monitor PT/INR closely in patients on warfarin therapy. Adrenal steroid replacement is indicated. Consider dose reduction in patients with renal or hepatic impairment. (Bristol-Myers Squibb Co., 2017c)
	May inhibit protein, RNA, and DNA synthesis	Procarbazine (Matulane®)	PO	Stage III and IV HL	Dose-limiting toxicity: Myelosuppression Nausea, vomiting, hepatic dysfunction	Patients should avoid foods high in tyramine, such as aged cheeses, air-dried or cured meats, fava or broad bean pods, tap/draft beer, wine (> 120 ml), vermouth, marmite concentrate, sauerkraut, and soy sauce and other soybean condiments because procarbazine inhibits monoamine oxidase. Patients should avoid alcohol for possible disulfiram-like reaction. (Sigma-Tau Pharmaceuticals, Inc., 2016)
	Inhibits growth phase of microtubules, arresting cell cycle at G_2/M phase	Eribulin (Halaven®)	IV	Metastatic breast cancer Unresectable or metastatic liposarcoma	Dose-limiting toxicities: Neutropenia, peripheral neuropathy Fatigue, alopecia, nausea, constipation, anemia, QTc prolongation	Monitor electrolytes, ECG, and renal and liver function tests. Initiate at lower doses with hepatic or renal insufficiency. Eribulin is not compatible with D5W. (Eisai Inc., 2016)
	Inhibits the enzymatic activity of HDAC	Romidepsin (Istodax®)	IV	Cutaneous and peripheral T-cell lymphoma	Dose-limiting toxicities: Myelosuppression, life-threatening infections QTc prolongation, fatigue, fever, pruritus, nausea, vomiting, anorexia, constipation, diarrhea, TLS	Obtain baseline and periodic ECG. Monitor electrolytes and correct imbalances. (Celgene Corp., 2016b)

(Continued on next page)

Table 6-1. Chemotherapy Agents *(Continued)*

Classification	Mechanism of Action	Drug	Route	Indications	Side Effects	Nursing Considerations
Miscellaneous *(cont.)*	Inhibits the enzymatic activity of HDAC	Vorinostat (Zolinza®)	PO	Cutaneous T-cell lymphoma	Dose-limiting toxicities: Thrombocytopenia, anemia Pulmonary embolism, deep vein thrombosis, nausea, vomiting, diarrhea, hyperglycemia, electrolyte abnormalities, fatigue, anorexia, dysgeusia	Reduce initial dose if bilirubin > 1 × ULN or AST > ULN. Do not use if bilirubin > 3 × ULN. Patients should drink at least 2 L of fluid per day. Monitor CBC, electrolytes, glucose, and SCr every 2 weeks during first 2 months and monthly thereafter. Do not open or crush capsules. Drug may interact with warfarin (increasing PT/INR) and other HDAC inhibitors (e.g., valproic acid; causing severe thrombocytopenia and GI bleeding). (Merck and Co., Inc., 2015)
	Semisynthetic analog of epothilone B; binds to beta-tubulin on microtubules, leading to cell death by blocking cells in mitotic phase of cell division cycle	Ixabepilone (Ixempra®)	IV	Metastatic or locally advanced breast cancer	Dose-limiting toxicities: Peripheral sensory neuropathy, myelosuppression, hypersensitivity reaction Fatigue, myalgia, alopecia, nausea, vomiting, mucositis, diarrhea, musculoskeletal pain	Drug is contraindicated in combination with capecitabine if bilirubin > 1 × ULN or AST or ALT > 2.5 × ULN. Patient may still receive monotherapy ixabepilone. CYP3A4 inhibitors may increase ixabepilone concentration, and CYP3A4 inducers may decrease ixabepilone concentration. Avoid St. John's wort. Premedicate with diphenhydramine (50 mg PO) and ranitidine (150–300 mg PO) 1 hour prior to dose to decrease risk of hypersensitivity reaction. Use non-PVC, non-DEHP bags and tubing; solution is only stable for 6 hours. Administer through a 0.2–1.2 micron in-line filter. Infuse over 3 hours. (R-Pharm US, LLC, 2016)
	Inhibits protein synthesis and is independent of direct Bcr-Abl binding	Omacetaxine (Synribo®)	SC	CML in chronic or accelerated phase with resistance and/or intolerance to 2 or more tyrosine kinase inhibitors	Dose-limiting toxicity: Myelosuppression Thrombocytopenia with bleeding risk, hyperglycemia, nausea, vomiting, diarrhea, alopecia, fatigue	Some patients may self-administer at home. Monitor patient for bleeding. Rotate injection sites. (Teva Pharmaceuticals USA, Inc., 2017b)

(Continued on next page)

Table 6-1. Chemotherapy Agents *(Continued)*

Classification	Mechanism of Action	Drug	Route	Indications	Side Effects	Nursing Considerations
Nitrosoureas	Break DNA helix, interfering with DNA replication; cross the blood–brain barrier	Carmustine (BiCNU®)	Implantation (Gliadel® wafer), IV	HL NHL CNS tumors Multiple myeloma	Dose-limiting toxicities: Myelosuppression, pulmonary toxicity Nausea, vomiting, renal toxicity Gliadel-specific toxicities: Seizures, intracranial hypertension, meningitis, impaired neurosurgical wound healing	Nadir occurs 4–6 weeks after therapy starts. Because of delayed toxicity, successive treatments usually are given no more frequently than once every 6–8 weeks. Rapid infusion may cause burning along the vein and flushing of the skin (infuse over at least 2 hours). Long-term therapy can result in irreversible pulmonary fibrosis, which may present as an insidious cough and dyspnea or sudden respiratory failure. Use non-PVC, non-DEHP bags and tubing. Cumulative dose of 1,400 mg/m^2 should not be exceeded because of pulmonary toxicity. (Arbor Pharmaceuticals, LLC, 2015; Heritage Pharmaceuticals Inc., 2017)
		Lomustine (Gleostine®)	PO	CNS and brain tumors HL	Dose-limiting toxicity: Myelosuppression (delayed, dose related, and cumulative) Pulmonary toxicity, secondary malignancies, hepatotoxicity, nephrotoxicity, nausea, vomiting, alopecia, fatigue, visual disturbances	Because of delayed myelosuppression, do not repeat the dose more than once every 6 weeks. Only 1 dose should be dispensed per treatment cycle. Patients should take on an empty stomach. Monitor PFTs, LFTs, and renal function. (NextSource Biotechnology, LLC, 2016)
		Streptozocin (Zanosar®)	IV	Metastatic islet-cell pancreatic carcinoma	Dose-limiting toxicity: Renal toxicity Myelosuppression, nausea, vomiting, hypoglycemia, proteinuria, hepatotoxicity, confusion, lethargy, depression	Streptozocin is an irritant. Nephrotoxicity may be dose limiting. This drug may alter glucose metabolism in some patients. (Teva Parenteral Medicines, Inc., 2007)
Plant alkaloids: Camptothecins	Act in S phase; inhibit topoisomerase I; cause double-strand DNA changes	Irinotecan	IV	Metastatic colorectal cancer	Dose-limiting toxicity: Diarrhea Myelosuppression, hypersensitivity reaction, alopecia, fever, nausea, vomiting	Irinotecan is an irritant; exfoliative dermatitis may occur. This drug can cause early and late diarrhea, which can be dose limiting. Early diarrhea can occur within 24 hours of administration and generally is cholinergic. Consider prophylactic or therapeutic (0.25–1 mg) IV or SC. Patients should receive antiemetic premedications: 10 mg dexamethasone and a 5-HT_3 blocker at least 30 minutes prior to administration. (Hospira, Inc., 2017)

(Continued on next page)

Table 6-1. Chemotherapy Agents *(Continued)*

Classification	Mechanism of Action	Drug	Route	Indications	Side Effects	Nursing Considerations
Plant alkaloids: Camptothecins *(cont.)*	Inhibit topoisomerase I	Irinotecan liposomal (Onivyde®)	IV	In combination with 5-fluorouracil and leucovorin for the treatment of metastatic adenocarcinoma of the pancreas after disease progression following gemcitabine therapy	Interstitial lung disease, diarrhea, fatigue, nausea, vomiting, stomatitis, pyrexia	Administer IV over 90 minutes 70 mg/m² every 2 weeks. Recommended dose for patient homozygous for UGT1A1*28 is 50 mg/m² every 2 weeks. Premedicate with a corticosteroid and an antiemetic 30 minutes prior to administration. (Ipsen Biopharmaceuticals, Inc., 2017)
		Topotecan (Hycamtin®)	IV, PO	Metastatic ovarian cancer Cervical cancer SCLC	Dose-limiting toxicity: Myelosuppression Diarrhea, alopecia, nausea, vomiting, fatigue, interstitial lung disease	Do not administer to patients with baseline ANC < 1,500/mm³ or platelets > 100,000/mm³. Consider dose reduction in patients with renal impairment. (GlaxoSmithKline, 2014b, 2015)
Plant alkaloids: Epipodophyllotoxins	Induce irreversible blockade of cells in premitotic phases of cell cycle (late G_2 and S phases); interfere with topoisomerase II enzyme reaction	Etoposide (VP-16, Toposar®, VePesid®); etoposide phosphate (Etopophos®)	IV, PO	Testicular cancer SCLC	Dose-limiting toxicity: Myelosuppression Hypersensitivity reaction, nausea, vomiting, alopecia, anorexia, hypotension	Do not administer via rapid IV infusion or IV push. Infuse over 30–60 minutes to avoid hypotension. Prior to use, dilute the drug to a final concentration of 0.2–0.4 mg/ml to avoid precipitation. Use non-PVC, non-DEHP bags and tubing. Monitor for crystallization during infusion. If a patient has an allergic reaction to etoposide, premedicate with diphenhydramine. Consider dose reduction in patients with renal impairment. (Bristol-Myers Squibb Co., 2017a; Mylan Pharmaceuticals Inc., 2016; Teva Parenteral Medicines, Inc., 2012)
		Teniposide	IV	Induction therapy in childhood ALL	Dose-limiting toxicity: Myelosuppression Hypersensitivity reaction, anaphylaxis, nausea, vomiting, mucositis, diarrhea, alopecia	Drug may cause an allergic reaction. Do not administer via rapid infusion. Infuse over 30–60 minutes to avoid hypotension. Use non-PVC, non-DEHP bags and tubing. Contraindicated in patients with history of reactions to teniposide or other drugs formulated in polyoxyl 35 castor oil (a solvent). Consider dose reduction in patients with renal or hepatic impairment. (WG Critical Care, LLC, 2015)

(Continued on next page)

Table 6-1. Chemotherapy Agents *(Continued)*

Classification	Mechanism of Action	Drug	Route	Indications	Side Effects	Nursing Considerations
Plant alkaloids: Taxanes	Stabilize microtubules, inhibiting cell division; effective in G_2 and M phases	Cabazitaxel (Jevtana®)	IV	Hormone-refractory metastatic prostate cancer	Hypersensitivity reaction, myelosuppression, fatigue, diarrhea, nausea, vomiting, peripheral neuropathy	Withhold dose for ANC < 1,500/mm³. Premedicate as follows to prevent hypersensitivity reaction, including anaphylaxis, at least 30 minutes before treatment: IV diphenhydramine 25 mg, dexamethasone 8 mg, and ranitidine 50 mg. Administer over 1-hour infusion through a 0.2 micron in-line filter. Use non-PVC bags and tubing. Do not use in patients with severe hepatic impairment (total bilirubin > 3 × ULN). (Sanofi-Aventis U.S. LLC, 2016)
		Docetaxel (Taxotere®)	IV	Breast cancer NSCLC Hormone-refractory prostate cancer Gastric adenocarcinoma Squamous cell carcinoma of the head and neck	Myelosuppression, febrile neutropenia, hypersensitivity reaction, fluid retention, alopecia, skin and nail changes, nausea, vomiting, neurotoxicity	Premedicate as follows to reduce the severity of hypersensitivity reaction and fluid retention: Dexamethasone 8 mg PO BID for 3 days, beginning 1 day prior to docetaxel treatment and continuing for the day of treatment and 1 day after. Docetaxel extravasation may cause local pain, edema, erythema, and hyperpigmentation at infusion site. Do not administer if bilirubin > ULN or AST and/or ALT > 1.5 × ULN with alkaline phosphatase > 2.5 × ULN. Withhold dose for ANC < 1,500/mm³. Do not use PVC tubing or bags to administer docetaxel. Administer over 1-hour infusion. (Sanofi-Aventis U.S. LLC, 2015)
		Paclitaxel	IV	Breast cancer Ovarian cancer NSCLC AIDS-related Kaposi sarcoma	Dose-limiting toxicities: Hypersensitivity reaction (dyspnea, hypotension, angioedema, urticaria), myelosuppression, peripheral neuropathy Alopecia, facial flushing, myalgia, mucositis, diarrhea, nausea	Paclitaxel is an irritant and potential vesicant. Extravasation may lead to local pain, edema, and erythema at infusion site. Paclitaxel is contraindicated in patients with history of reactions to paclitaxel or other drugs formulated in polyoxyl 35 castor oil (a solvent). Patients should be premedicated to minimize reaction risk: Dexamethasone, diphenhydramine, and ranitidine prior to infusion. Premedication dosages and frequency may vary per specific regimens. Reactions occur more frequently with first or second doses; consider reducing premedications with subsequent doses.

(Continued on next page)

Table 6-1. Chemotherapy Agents *(Continued)*

Classification	Mechanism of Action	Drug	Route	Indications	Side Effects	Nursing Considerations
Plant alkaloids: Taxanes *(cont.)*		Paclitaxel *(cont.)*				Do not use in patients with solid tumor who have baseline ANC < 1,500/mm³ or in patients with AIDS-related Kaposi sarcoma who have baseline ANC < 1,000/mm³. Withhold subsequent doses until counts recover to these levels. Filter paclitaxel with a 0.2 micron in-line filter. Use non-PVC, non-DEHP bags and tubing to administer paclitaxel. Consider dose reduction in patients with renal or hepatic impairment. To prevent severe myelosuppression, give paclitaxel before platinum-containing drugs. (Mylan Institutional, LLC, 2014b)
		Paclitaxel protein-bound particles; albumin-bound (Nab-paclitaxel; Abraxane®)	IV	Metastatic breast cancer NSCLC Metastatic adenocarcinoma of the pancreas	Dose-limiting toxicities: Myelosuppression, sensory neuropathy Sepsis, pneumonitis, hypersensitivity reaction, alopecia, anemia, myalgia/arthralgia, nausea, vomiting, diarrhea Toxicities may be enhanced with hepatic insufficiency.	Premedication is generally not required. Withhold dose for grade 3–4 peripheral neuropathy; resume only with grade 1 or complete resolution. Withhold dose for ANC < 1,500/mm³. (Celgene Corp., 2016a)
Plant alkaloids: Vinca alkaloids	Act in late G_2 phase, blocking DNA production, and in M phase, preventing cell division	Vinblastine	IV	HL NHL Mycosis fungoides Testicular cancer Kaposi sarcoma Histiocytosis Breast cancer	Dose-limiting toxicities: Myelosuppression, constipation, neurotoxicity, peripheral neuropathy, jaw pain Alopecia Toxicities may be enhanced with hepatic insufficiency.	Drug is fatal if given via routes other than IV. Vinblastine is a vesicant; extravasation can result in severe tissue injury. Administer via a minibag through the side port of a free-flowing IV. Generally, neurotoxicity occurs less frequently with vinblastine than with vincristine; however, it is rare and usually reversible. (Fresenius Kabi USA, LLC, 2016d)

(Continued on next page)

Table 6-1. Chemotherapy Agents *(Continued)*

Classification	Mechanism of Action	Drug	Route	Indications	Side Effects	Nursing Considerations
Plant alkaloids: Vinca alkaloids *(cont.)*		Vincristine	IV	ALL HL NHL Neuroblastoma Wilms tumor Rhabdomyosarcoma	Dose-limiting toxicity: Neurotoxicity Alopecia, peripheral neuropathy, constipation, paralytic ileus, renal toxicity, hepatotoxicity, hypersensitivity reaction	Drug is fatal if given via routes other than IV. Vincristine is a vesicant; extravasation can result in severe tissue injury. Administer via a minibag through the side port of a free-flowing IV. Neurotoxicity is cumulative; conduct a neurologic evaluation before each dose. Withhold dose if severe paresthesia, motor weakness, or other abnormality develops. Reduce dose in the presence of significant liver disease. Stool softeners and/or a stimulant laxative may help to prevent severe constipation. (Hospira, Inc., 2013)
	Liposome-encapsulated vincristine alters microtubular structure and function.	Vincristine liposomal (Marqibo®)	IV	PH– ALL in second or greater relapse whose disease has progressed after 2 or more anti-leukemic regimens	Fatigue, nausea, pyrexia, myelosuppression, neurologic toxicity, TLS, liver toxicity, constipation, embryo-fetal toxicity	Vincristine liposomal is a vesicant; extravasation can result in severe tissue injury. Drug is fatal if given via routes other than IV. Administer 2.25 mg/m² IV over 1 hour every 7 days. (Talon Therapeutics, Inc., 2016)
		Vinorelbine (Navelbine®)	IV	NSCLC	Dose-limiting toxicities: Myelosuppression, hepatic toxicity, severe constipation and bowel obstruction, neurologic toxicity (peripheral neuropathy), pulmonary toxicity and respiratory failure. Nausea, vomiting, alopecia	Vinorelbine is fatal if given via routes other than vesicant intravenously. Vinorelbine is an irritant with vesicant potential. Extravasation can result in severe tissue injury. Administer via a minibag through the side port of a free-flowing IV. Flush with 75–125 ml solution after completion of vinorelbine administration to prevent phlebitis. (Pierre Fabre Pharmaceuticals, Inc., 2014)

Note. For drugs listed as vesicants or irritants, refer to Chapter 13.

AIDS—acquired immunodeficiency syndrome; ALL—acute lymphoblastic leukemia; ALT—alanine aminotransferase; AML—acute myeloid leukemia; ANC—absolute neutrophil count; ANLL—acute nonlymphocytic leukemia; APL—acute promyelocytic leukemia; AST—aspartate aminotransferase; AUC—area under the plasma concentration versus time curve; BID—twice daily; CBC—complete blood count; CLL—chronic lymphocytic leukemia; CML—chronic myeloid leukemia; CNS—central nervous system; CrCl—creatinine clearance; DEHP—di(2-ethylhexyl) phthalate; D5W—5% dextrose in water; DNA—deoxyribonucleic acid; ECG—electrocardiogram; FDA—U.S. Food and Drug Administration; 5-FU—5-fluorouracil; GI—gastrointestinal; G_2—gap 2; HDAC—histone deacetylase; HL—Hodgkin lymphoma; IM—intramuscular; INR—international normalized ratio; IT—intrathecal; IV—intravenous; LFTs—liver function tests; M—mitosis; MDS—myelodysplastic syndrome; ms—millisecond; NHL—non-Hodgkin lymphoma; NS—normal saline; NSAID—nonsteroidal anti-inflammatory drug; NSCLC—non-small cell lung cancer; PFTs—pulmonary function tests; PML—promyelocytic leukemia; PO—by mouth; PT—prothrombin time; PVC—polyvinyl chloride; QTc—QT interval corrected; RAR—retinoic acid receptor; RNA—ribonucleic acid; S—synthesis; SC—subcutaneous; SCLC—small cell lung cancer; SCr—serum creatinine; SIADH—syndrome of inappropriate antidiuretic hormone secretion; TLS—tumor lysis syndrome; ULN—upper limit of normal; WBC—white blood cell

Figure 6-2. Potential Side Effects and Toxicities of Chemotherapy by System

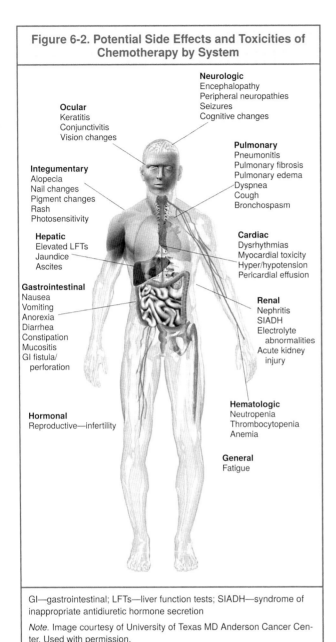

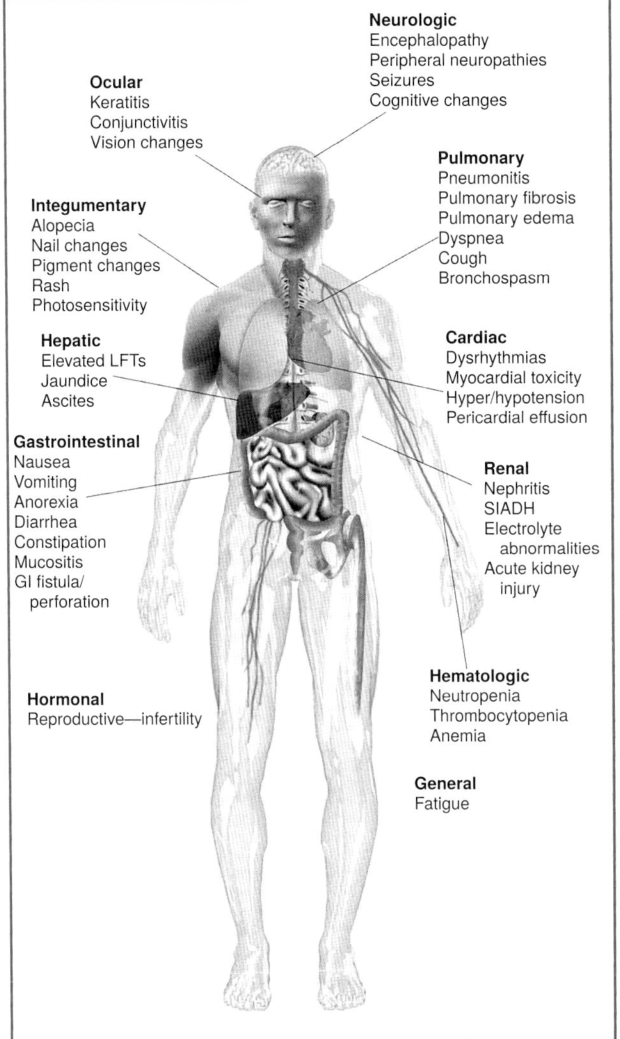

GI—gastrointestinal; LFTs—liver function tests; SIADH—syndrome of inappropriate antidiuretic hormone secretion

Note. Image courtesy of University of Texas MD Anderson Cancer Center. Used with permission.

c) Tumors with a high growth rate, or a high percentage of cells in the S phase, are the most susceptible to antimetabolites (Olsen, 2017). Normal cells with high division rates, such as gastrointestinal mucosal and bone marrow cells, are sensitive to antimetabolites. This results in mucositis, diarrhea, and myelosuppression.

d) Examples: capecitabine, cytarabine, 5-fluorouracil, gemcitabine, methotrexate

3. Antitumor antibiotics (Olsen, 2017)

a) Interfere with DNA synthesis by binding with DNA at various points, preventing RNA synthesis

b) Myelosuppression, gastrointestinal toxicities, and alopecia are common.

c) A number of these agents are cardiotoxic or pulmonary toxic.

d) Examples: doxorubicin, bleomycin, epirubicin, mitoxantrone

4. Miscellaneous agents

a) Drugs in this category have a unique mechanism of action and side effect profile. They cannot be grouped with other chemotherapy agents.

b) Examples: asparaginase, arsenic, vorinostat

(1) Asparaginase is an enzyme derived from bacteria (*Escherichia coli* or *Erwinia chrysanthemi*) that depletes circulating levels of asparagine, resulting in cell death.

(2) Arsenic is a differentiating agent that causes fragmented changes in the DNA, leading to apoptosis. It inhibits the self-renewal of leukemia cells due to free radical formation (Olsen, 2017).

5. Nitrosoureas

a) A distinct group of drugs that have the capacity to cross the blood–brain barrier (high lipid solubility); sometimes categorized with alkylating agents

b) Cause breakage in DNA helix strand, thereby interfering with DNA replication and resulting in cell death

c) Dose-limiting toxicities include bone marrow suppression, gastrointestinal toxicities, and organ-specific toxicities (e.g., renal and hepatic, dependent on drug and dose).

d) Other effects include carcinogenic and mutagenic effects and impaired fertility.

e) Examples: carmustine, lomustine, streptozocin

6. Plant alkaloids

a) Camptothecins

(1) Semisynthetic analogs of the alkaloid camptothecin from the Chinese ornamental tree *Camptotheca acuminata*

(2) Target topoisomerase I, an enzyme necessary for DNA synthesis, which causes DNA damage and cell death

(3) Diarrhea and myelosuppression are the most common dose-limiting toxicities of irinotecan, and myelosuppression is the most common dose-limiting toxicity of topotecan.

(4) Examples: irinotecan, topotecan

b) Epipodophyllotoxins

(1) Antimicrotubule agent derived from the *Podophyllum peltatum*, or mandrake, plant

(2) Induce irreversible blockage of cells in premitotic phases of cell cycle (late G_2 and S phases); interfere with topoisomerase II enzyme reaction
(3) Dose-limiting toxicity includes myelosuppression with a nadir of 10–14 days. Mild to moderate nausea, vomiting, mucositis, and alopecia also can occur with this class and are dose dependent.
(4) Other effects include carcinogenic and mutagenic effects.

c) Taxanes
(1) Semisynthetic derivatives of precursors from yew plants
(2) Stabilize microtubules, inhibiting cell division; effective in G_2 and M phases
(3) Common side effects include infusion reactions, peripheral neuropathy, myelosuppression, arthralgias, and myalgias. Docetaxel is associated with edema and nail changes.

d) Vinca alkaloids
(1) Derived from the *Vinca rosea*, or periwinkle, plant
(2) Depolymerize microtubules and destroy mitotic spindles
(3) Myelosuppression (except vincristine) and neurologic and hepatic toxicities are common.
(4) Drugs in this category are vesicants.
(5) Drugs in this category are fatal if given into the central nervous system.

D. Combination chemotherapy principles
1. Benefits
a) Maximum cell kill within dose limits
b) Broader coverage to overcome resistant cell lines
2. Drug selection for combination chemotherapy
a) Are active as single agents
b) Have differing mechanisms of action making them synergistic
c) Have differing dose-limiting toxicities to allow therapeutic doses to be tolerated
d) Have differing patterns of resistance
e) Should be used at optimal schedule and dose
f) Should be given at consistent intervals

References

Accord BioPharma Inc. (2016). *Mutamycin® (mitomycin)* [Package insert]. Durham, NC: Author.

Actelion Pharmaceuticals US, Inc. (2016). *Valchlor® (mechlorethamine)* [Package insert]. South San Francisco, CA: Author.

Allos Therapeutics. (2016). *Folotyn® (pralatrexate)* [Package insert]. Westminster, CO: Author.

ApoPharma USA, Inc. (2016). *Alkeran® (melphalan)* [Package insert]. Rockville, MD: Author.

Arbor Pharmaceuticals, LLC. (2015). *Gliadel® (carmustine)* [Package insert]. Atlanta, GA: Author.

Aspen Global Inc. (2012a). *Myleran® (busulfan)* [Package insert]. Grand Bay, Mauritius: Author.

Aspen Global Inc. (2012b). *Tabloid® (thioguanine)* [Package insert]. Grand Bay, Mauritius: Author.

Aspen Global Inc. (2016). *Leukeran® (chlorambucil)* [Package insert]. Grand Bay, Mauritius: Author.

Baxalta US Inc. (2016). *Oncaspar® (pegaspargase)* [Package insert]. Westlake Village, CA: Author.

Baxter Healthcare Corp. (2014). *Ifex® (ifosfamide)* [Package insert]. Deerfield, IL: Author.

Baxter Healthcare Corp. (2017). *Cyclophosphamide* [Package insert]. Deerfield, IL: Author.

Bristol-Myers Squibb Co. (2017a). *Etopophos® (etoposide phosphate)* [Package insert]. Princeton, NJ: Author.

Bristol-Myers Squibb Co. (2017b). *Hydrea® (hydroxyurea)* [Package insert]. Princeton, NJ: Author.

Bristol-Myers Squibb Co. (2017c). *Lysodren® (mitotane)* [Package insert]. Princeton, NJ: Author.

BTG International Inc. (2013). *Voraxaze® (glucarpidase)* [Package insert]. Brentwood, TN: Author.

Celgene Corp. (2016a). *Abraxane® (paclitaxel protein-bound particles for injectable suspension)* [Package insert]. Summit, NJ: Author.

Celgene Corp. (2016b). *Istodax® kit (romidepsin)* [Package insert]. Summit, NJ: Author.

Celgene Corp. (2016c). *Vidaza® (azacitidine)* [Package insert]. Summit, NJ: Author.

Cephalon, Inc. (2016). *Treanda® (bendamustine HCl)* [Package insert]. Frazer, PA: Author.

Eisai Inc. (2009). *Hexalen® (altretamine)* [Package insert]. Woodcliff Lake, NJ: Author.

Eisai Inc. (2014). *Dacogen® (decitabine for injection)* [Package insert]. Woodcliff Lake, NJ: Author.

Eisai Inc. (2016). *Halaven® (eribulin mesylate)* [Package insert]. Woodcliff Lake, NJ: Author.

Eli Lilly and Co. (2013). *Alimta® (pemetrexed for injection)* [Package insert]. Indianapolis, IN: Author.

Eli Lilly and Co. (2017). *Gemzar® (gemcitabine for injection)* [Package insert]. Indianapolis, IN: Author.

Endo Pharmaceuticals Solutions Inc. (2017). *Valstar® (valrubicin)* [Package insert]. Malvern, PA: Author.

Fresenius Kabi USA, LLC. (2013). *Mitoxantrone* [Package insert]. Lake Zurich, IL: Author.

Fresenius Kabi USA, LLC. (2014). *Methotrexate* [Package insert]. Lake Zurich, IL: Author.

Fresenius Kabi USA, LLC. (2016a). *Bleomycin* [Package insert]. Lake Zurich, IL: Author.

Fresenius Kabi USA, LLC. (2016b). *Cladribine injection* [Package insert]. Lake Zurich, IL: Author.

Fresenius Kabi USA, LLC. (2016c). *Floxuridine* [Package insert]. Lake Zurich, IL: Author.

Fresenius Kabi USA, LLC. (2016d). *Vinblastine sulfate* [Package insert]. Lake Zurich, IL: Author.

Genentech, Inc. (2016). *Xeloda® (capecitabine)* [Package insert]. South San Francisco, CA: Author.

Genzyme Corp. (2013). *Clolar® (clofarabine injection)* [Package insert]. Cambridge, MA: Author.

GlaxoSmithKline. (2012). *Alkeran® (melphalan)* [Package insert]. Research Triangle Park, NC: Author.

GlaxoSmithKline. (2014a). *Arranon® (nelarabine)* [Package insert]. Research Triangle Park, NC: Author.

GlaxoSmithKline. (2014b). *Hycamtin® (topotecan hydrochloride capsule)* [Package insert]. Research Triangle Park, NC: Author.

GlaxoSmithKline. (2015). *Hycamtin® (topotecan hydrochloride injection)* [Package insert]. Research Triangle Park, NC: Author.

Halison Pharmaceuticals USA. (2014). *Daunorubicin hydrochloride* [Package insert]. Princeton, NJ: Author.

Heritage Pharmaceuticals Inc. (2017). *BiCNU® (carmustine)* [Package insert]. Eatontown, NJ: Author.

Hospira, Inc. (2013). *Vincristine sulfate* [Package insert]. Lake Forest, IL: Author.

Hospira, Inc. (2017). *Irinotecan hydrochloride* [Package insert]. Lake Forest, IL: Author.

Hospira, Inc. (2018). *Nipent™ (pentostatin)* [Package insert]. Lake Forest, IL: Author.

Hydbring, P., Malumbres, M., & Sicinski, P. (2016). Non-canonical functions of cell-cycle cyclins and cyclin-dependent kinases. *Nature Reviews Molecular Cell Biology, 17,* 280–292. https://doi.org/10.1038/nrm.2016.27

Ipsen Biopharmaceuticals Inc. (2017). *Onivyde® (irinotecan liposome injection)* [Package insert]. Basking Ridge, NJ: Author.

Janssen Products, LP. (2015). *Yondelis® (trabectedin)* [Package insert]. Horsham, PA: Author.

Janssen Products, LP. (2017). *Doxil® (doxorubicin hydrochloride liposome injection)* [Package insert]. Horsham, PA: Author.

Jazz Pharmaceuticals, Inc. (2016). *Erwinaze® (asparaginase Erwinia chrysanthemi)* [Package insert]. Palo Alto, CA: Author.

Jazz Pharmaceuticals, Inc. (2017). *Vyxeos™ (daunorubicin and cytarabine) liposome* [Package insert]. Palo Alto, CA: Author.

Kantarjian, H.M., O'Brien, S., Smith, T.L., Cortes, J., Giles, F.J., Beran, M., ... Freireich, E.J. (2000). Results of treatment with hyper-CVAD, a dose-intensive regimen, in adult acute lymphocytic leukemia. *Journal of Clinical Oncology, 18,* 547–561. https://doi.org/10.1200/JCO.2000.18.3.547

Lilleby, K., Garcia, P., Gooley, T., McDonnell, P., Taber, R., Holmberg, L., ... Bensinger, W. (2006). A prospective, randomized study of cryotherapy during administration of high-dose melphalan to decrease the severity and duration of oral mucositis in patients with multiple myeloma undergoing autologous peripheral blood stem cell transplantation. *Bone Marrow Transplantation, 37,* 1031–1035. https://doi.org/10.1038/sj.bmt.1705384

Malumbres, M. (2014). Cyclin-dependent kinases. *Genome Biology, 15,* 122. https://doi.org/10.1186/gb4184

Merck and Co., Inc. (2015). *Zolinza® (vorinostat)* [Package insert]. Whitehouse Station, NJ: Author.

Merck and Co., Inc. (2017). *Temodar® (temozolomide)* [Package insert]. Whitehouse Station, NJ: Author.

Mylan Institutional, LLC. (2014a). *Cytarabine* [Package insert]. Rockford, IL: Author.

Mylan Institutional, LLC. (2014b). *Paclitaxel* [Package insert]. Rockford, IL: Author.

Mylan Pharmaceuticals Inc. (2013). *Purinethol® (mercaptopurine)* [Package insert]. Morgantown, WV: Author.

Mylan Pharmaceuticals Inc. (2016). *Etoposide* [Package insert]. Morgantown, WV: Author.

NextSource Biotechnology, LLC. (2016). *Gleostine® (lomustine)* [Package insert]. Miami, FL: Author.

Olsen, M. (2017). Chemotherapy. In J. Eggert (Ed.), *Cancer basics* (2nd ed., pp. 197–219). Pittsburgh, PA: Oncology Nursing Society.

Otsuka America Pharmaceutical Inc. (2017). *Busulfex® (busulfan)* [Package insert]. Rockville, MD: Author.

Patel, P.N. (2006). Methylene blue for management of ifosfamide-induced encephalopathy. *Annals of Pharmacotherapy, 40,* 299–303. https://doi.org/10.1345/aph.1G114

Pfizer Inc. (2014). *Ellence® (epirubicin hydrochloride)* [Package insert]. New York, NY: Author.

Pfizer Inc. (2015). *Idamycin® (idarubicin hydrochloride)* [Package insert]. New York, NY: Author.

Pierre Fabre Pharmaceuticals, Inc. (2014). *Navelbine® (vinorelbine tartrate)* [Package insert]. Parsippany, NJ: Author.

Recordati Rare Diseases Inc. (2013a). *Cosmegen® (dactinomycin)* [Package insert]. Lebanon, NJ: Author.

Recordati Rare Diseases Inc. (2013b). *Mustargen® (mechlorethamine)* [Package insert]. Lebanon, NJ: Author.

Roche Laboratories Inc. (2008). *Vesanoid® (tretinoin)* [Package insert]. Nutley, NJ: Author.

R-Pharm US, LLC. (2016). *Ixempra® (ixabepilone)* [Package insert]. Princeton, NJ: Author.

Sanofi-Aventis U.S. LLC. (2011). *Eloxatin® (oxaliplatin)* [Package insert]. Bridgewater, NJ: Author.

Sanofi-Aventis U.S. LLC. (2015). *Taxotere® (docetaxel for injection)* [Package insert]. Bridgewater, NJ: Author.

Sanofi-Aventis U.S. LLC. (2016). *Jevtana® (cabazitaxel)* [Package insert]. Bridgewater, NJ: Author.

Sigma-Tau Pharmaceuticals, Inc. (2016). *Matulane® (procarbazine hydrochloride)* [Package insert]. Gaithersburg, MD: Author.

Sigma-Tau Pharmaceuticals, Inc. (2017). *DepoCyt® (cytarabine liposome injection)* [Package insert]. Gaithersburg, MD: Author.

Sparreboom, A., & Baker, S.D. (2015). Pharmacokinetics and pharmacodynamics of anticancer drugs. In V.T. DeVita Jr., T.S. Lawrence, & S.A. Rosenberg (Eds.), *DeVita, Hellman, and Rosenberg's cancer: Principles and practice of oncology* (10th ed., pp. 174–182). Philadelphia, PA: Wolters Kluwer Health.

Spectrum Pharmaceuticals, Inc. (2017). *Evomela® (melphalan)* [Package insert]. Irvine, CA: Author.

Taiho Oncology, Inc. (2017). *Lonsurf® (trifluridine and tiripacil)* [Package insert]. Princeton, NJ: Author.

Takimoto, C., & Calvo, E. (2007). Principles of oncologic pharmacotherapy. Retrieved from http://www.cancernetwork.com/articles/principles-oncologic-pharmacotherapy

Talon Therapeutics, Inc. (2016). *Marqibo® (vincristine sulfate liposome injection)* [Package insert]. Irvine, CA: Author.

Teva Parenteral Medicines, Inc. (2007). *Zanosar® (streptozocin)* [Package insert]. Irvine, CA: Author.

Teva Parenteral Medicines, Inc. (2012). *Toposar® (etoposide injection)* [Package insert]. Irvine, CA: Author.

Teva Parenteral Medicines, Inc. (2015a). *Cisplatin* [Package insert]. North Wales, PA: Author.

Teva Parenteral Medicines, Inc. (2015b). *Dacarbazine* [Package insert]. North Wales, PA: Author.

Teva Parenteral Medicines, Inc. (2016). *Carboplatin* [Package insert]. North Wales, PA: Author.

Teva Parenteral Medicines, Inc. (2017a). *Adrucil® (fluorouracil injection, USP)* [Package insert]. Irvine, CA: Author.

Teva Parenteral Medicines, Inc. (2017b). *Fludarabine phosphate* [Package insert]. North Wales, PA: Author.

Teva Pharmaceuticals USA, Inc. (2016). *Trisenox®* (*arsenic trioxide*) [Package insert]. North Wales, PA: Author.

Teva Pharmaceuticals USA, Inc. (2017a). *Bendeka® (bendamustine hydrochloride)* [Package insert]. North Wales, PA: Author.

Teva Pharmaceuticals USA, Inc. (2017b). *Synribo® (omacetaxine mepesuccinate)* [Package insert]. North Wales, PA: Author.

Tortorice, P.V. (2018). Cytotoxic chemotherapy: Principles of therapy. In C.H. Yarbro, D. Wujcik, & B.H. Gobel (Eds.), *Cancer nursing: Principles and practice* (8th ed., pp. 375–416). Burlington, MA: Jones & Bartlett Learning.

Wellstat Therapeutics Corp. (2017). *Vistogard® (uridine triacetate)* [Package insert]. Rockville, MD: Author.

West-Ward Pharmaceuticals Corp. (2015a). *Adriamycin® (doxorubicin hydrochloride injection, USP)* [Package insert]. Eatontown, NJ: Author.

West-Ward Pharmaceuticals Corp. (2015b). *Thiotepa for injection, USP* [Package insert]. Eatontown, NJ: Author.

West-Ward Pharmaceuticals Corp. (2016). *Cyclophosphamide* [Package insert]. Eatontown, NJ: Author.

WG Critical Care, LLC. (2015). *Teniposide injection* [Package insert]. Paramus, NJ: Author.

Winkeljohn, D., & Polovich, M. (2006). Carboplatin hypersensitivity reactions. *Clinical Journal of Oncology Nursing, 10,* 595–598. https://doi.org/10.1188/06.CJON.595-598

CHAPTER 7

Hormone Therapy

A. Hormone therapy in the treatment of cancer
   1. Hormonal manipulations are used in the treatment of a number of cancers that are hormone sensitive. Prostate and breast cancers are the prime examples. To a lesser degree, endocrine treatment is also used for adrenal, ovarian, thyroid, and androgen-sensitive salivary cancers.
   2. Most current endocrine treatments involve decreasing levels of a specific hormone in the body by interfering with its release, blocking other hormones that trigger its production and release, blocking hormone receptors, or destroying the hormone entirely.
   3. Although effective in prolonging survival, hormone treatments have side effects that can affect an individual's quality of life and are associated with physiologic changes that may increase the risk for other health conditions.
   4. This section will provide a brief overview of cancers treated with endocrine therapy, describe categories of hormones used in cancer treatment, identify associated side effects and health risks (see Figure 7-1), and discuss implications for nursing care. See Table 7-1 for additional drug-specific information.

B. Cancers treated with hormone therapy
   1. Hormone therapies are most often used to treat prostate and breast cancers. These are the most commonly diagnosed cancers in men and women, respectively (American Cancer Society [ACS], 2018). Although both types of cancer exist in a hormonal milieu, differences exist in mechanisms and response to hormone therapy.
   2. Hormone therapy in specific cancers
      a) Prostate cancer
         (1) Androgens (i.e., testosterone and dihydrotestosterone) are hormones that are essential for normal prostate function, as well as prostate cancer growth. They bind with and activate the androgen receptor, which, in turn, activates expression of genes that promote prostate cell growth.
         (2) Androgens are synthesized in the prostate tissue from dehydroepiandrosterone (DHEA) and by the adrenal glands, in addition to the testicles (Labrie, 2015).

Figure 7-1. Potential Side Effects and Toxicities of Hormone Therapy by System

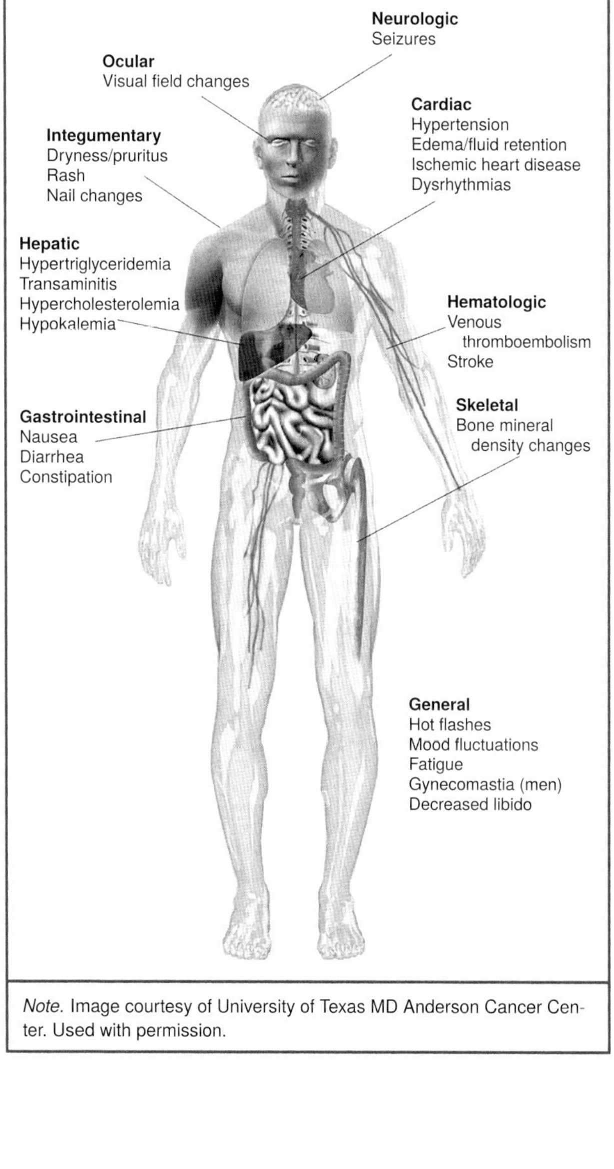

Note. Image courtesy of University of Texas MD Anderson Cancer Center. Used with permission.

Table 7-1. Hormone Therapy Agents

Classification	Drug	Route/Dosing	Indications	Side Effects	Nursing Considerations
Adrenolytics	Mitotane (Lysodren®)	0.5–2 g PO daily, titrated up every 1–2 weeks to serum concentrations between 14–20 mg/L	Adrenal cancer	Anorexia, nausea, diarrhea, transaminitis, hypercholesterolemia, hypothyroidism, glucocorticoid excess	Administer in 3–4 divided daily doses. Cerebellar ataxia and other neurologic symptoms may develop with concentrations > 20 mg/L.
Antiandrogens	Apalutamide (Erleada™)	240 mg PO daily	Prostate cancer	GI effects (nausea, diarrhea), fatigue, decreased appetite, seizures, falls/fracture, hypertension	Patients should receive an LHRH agonist or antagonist concurrently or should have had bilateral orchiectomy prior to initiation of therapy. Men should be counseled not to donate sperm during treatment and for 3 months following the last dose of apalutamide. CYP drug interactions are possible.
	Bicalutamide (Casodex®)	50 mg PO daily	Prostate cancer	Hepatotoxicity, GI effects (nausea, diarrhea, constipation), fatigue	Drug can be added to LHRH agonist/antagonist therapy after progression or used temporarily to prevent symptoms of tumor flare. Bicalutamide offers better tolerance and once-daily dosing compared to nilutamide and flutamide. CYP drug interactions are possible.
	Enzalutamide (Xtandi®)	160 mg PO daily	Prostate cancer	GI effects (nausea, diarrhea), fatigue, seizures	Enzalutamide is a pure androgen receptor signaling inhibitor that is used alone or with prednisone only in the castration-refractory prostate cancer setting. CYP drug interactions are possible.
	Flutamide (Eulexin®)	250 mg PO every 8 hours	Prostate cancer	Hepatotoxicity, GI effects (nausea, diarrhea, constipation), fatigue	Drug can be added to LHRH agonist/antagonist therapy after progression or used temporarily to prevent symptoms of tumor flare. CYP drug interactions are possible.

(Continued on next page)

Table 7-1. Hormone Therapy Agents *(Continued)*

Classification	Drug	Route/Dosing	Indications	Side Effects	Nursing Considerations
Antiandrogens *(cont.)*	Nilutamide (Nilandron®)	300 mg PO daily for 30 days, then 150 mg daily thereafter	Prostate cancer	Hepatotoxicity, GI effects (nausea, diarrhea, constipation), fatigue, visual field changes, disulfiram-like reaction	Drug can be added to LHRH agonist/antagonist therapy after progression or used temporarily to prevent symptoms of tumor flare. CYP drug interactions are possible.
Aromatase inhibitors	Anastrozole (Arimidex®)	1 mg PO daily	Breast cancer	Arthralgias/myalgias, decreased BMD, fatigue, hot flashes, CVD (HTN, edema, ischemic heart disease), hypercholesterolemia, VTE	If adverse effects are intolerable, another aromatase inhibitor may be given. Drug is used in postmenopausal patients or premenopausal patients with ovarian ablation. Breast cancer must be HR positive.
	Exemestane (Aromasin®)	25 mg PO daily	Breast cancer	Arthralgias/myalgias, decreased BMD, fatigue, hot flashes, CVD (HTN, edema, ischemic heart disease), hypercholesterolemia, VTE	If adverse effects are intolerable, another aromatase inhibitor may be given. Drug is used in postmenopausal patients or premenopausal patients with ovarian ablation. Breast cancer must be HR positive.
	Letrozole (Femara®)	2.5 mg PO daily	Breast cancer	Arthralgias/myalgias, decreased BMD, fatigue, hot flashes, CVD (HTN, edema, ischemic heart disease), hypercholesterolemia, VTE	If adverse effects are intolerable, another aromatase inhibitor may be given. Drug is used in postmenopausal patients or premenopausal patients with ovarian ablation. Breast cancer must be HR positive.
CYP17 inhibitors	Abiraterone (Zytiga®)	1,000 mg PO daily	Prostate cancer	HTN, fluid retention, hypokalemia, transaminitis, hypertriglyceridemia, fatigue	Administer with prednisone 5 mg twice daily to mitigate symptoms of mineralocorticoid excess. Administer on an empty stomach. CYP and P-gp drug interactions are possible.
	Ketoconazole (Nizoral®)	400 mg PO 3 times daily	Prostate cancer	Black box warnings: Severe hepatotoxicity, QTc prolongation Diarrhea, gynecomastia, fatigue, dizziness	Administer with soda or other acidic beverage for better absorption. Administer with oral hydrocortisone 20 mg every morning and 10 mg every evening to simulate physiologic adrenocorticoid release. CYP and P-gp drug interactions are possible.

(Continued on next page)

Table 7-1. Hormone Therapy Agents *(Continued)*

Classification	Drug	Route/Dosing	Indications	Side Effects	Nursing Considerations
Estrogen receptor antagonists/ selective estrogen receptor downregulators	Fulvestrant (Faslodex®)	Loading: 500 mg IM days 1, 15, and 29 Maintenance: 500 mg IM every 4 weeks	Breast cancer	Injection site pain, hot flashes, musculoskeletal weakness	Each dose is administered as two 250 mg (5 ml) injections over 1–2 minutes. Breast cancer must be HR positive.
LHRH agonists	Goserelin (Zoladex®)	3.6 mg SC every 4 weeks 10.8 mg SC every 12 weeks (prostate only)	Breast cancer Prostate cancer	Injection site pain, mood changes, hot flashes, decreased libido, musculoskeletal weakness, decreased BMD, CVD (QTc prolongation, heart failure), gynecomastia (men)	Temporary tumor flare (bladder outlet obstruction, bone pain, neurologic symptoms) may occur within first few weeks after initial dose secondary to initial increases in estradiol or testosterone levels. Breast cancer must be HR positive.
	Leuprolide (Lupron Depot®, Eligard®)	Breast: 3.75 mg IM every 4 weeks Prostate • 7.5 mg SC or IM every 4 weeks • 22.5 mg SC or IM every 12 weeks • 30 mg SC or IM every 16 weeks • 45 mg SC or IM every 24 weeks	Breast cancer Prostate cancer	Injection site pain, mood changes, hot flashes, decreased libido, musculoskeletal weakness, decreased BMD, CVD (QTc prolongation, heart failure), gynecomastia (men)	SC leuprolide (Eligard) is approved by the U.S. Food and Drug Administration for prostate cancer only. Temporary tumor flare (bladder outlet obstruction, bone pain, neurologic symptoms) may occur within first few weeks after initial dose secondary to initial increases in estradiol or testosterone level. Breast cancer must be HR positive.
	Triptorelin (Trelstar®)	3.75 mg IM every 4 weeks 7.5 mg IM every 12 weeks 11.25 mg IM every 24 weeks	Prostate cancer	Injection site pain, mood changes, hot flashes, decreased libido, musculoskeletal weakness, decreased BMD, CVD (QTc prolongation, heart failure), gynecomastia (men)	Temporary tumor flare (bladder outlet obstruction, bone pain, neurologic symptoms) may occur within first few weeks after initial dose secondary to initial increases in estradiol or testosterone levels.
LHRH antagonists	Degarelix (Firmagon®)	Loading: 240 mg SC once Maintenance: 80 mg SC every 4 weeks	Prostate cancer	Injection site pain, mood changes, hot flashes, decreased libido, musculoskeletal weakness, decreased BMD, CVD (QTc prolongation, heart failure), gynecomastia (men)	Administer immediately after reconstitution. Loading dose is administered as two 120 mg (2 ml) injections. Maintenance dose is administered as single 3 ml injection.

(Continued on next page)

Table 7-1. Hormone Therapy Agents *(Continued)*

Classification	Drug	Route/Dosing	Indications	Side Effects	Nursing Considerations
Selective estrogen receptor modulators	Tamoxifen (Nolvadex®)	Breast: 20 mg PO daily Endometrial: 40 mg PO daily (one 20 mg dose twice daily)	Breast cancer Endometrial cancer	Black box warnings: Stroke, pulmonary embolism, uterine malignancies Hyperlipidemia, BMD changes (increased in postmenopausal patients, decreased in premenopausal patients), hot flashes, mood changes	Certain SSRIs may reduce tamoxifen efficacy. Citalopram, escitalopram, and venlafaxine are preferred in lieu of other SSRIs. If adverse effects are intolerable, another selective estrogen receptor modulator may be given. Drug can be used in pre- or postmenopausal patients. Maximum duration of treatment is 5 years.

BMD—bone mineral density; CVD—cardiovascular disease; CYP—cytochrome P450; GI—gastrointestinal; HR—hormone receptor; HTN—hypertension; IM—intramuscular; LHRH—luteinizing hormone–releasing hormone; P-gp—P-glycoprotein; QTc—QT interval corrected; SC—subcutaneous; SSRIs—selective serotonin reuptake inhibitors; VTE—venous thromboembolism

Note. Based on information from AbbVie Inc., 2014; Actavis Pharma, Inc., 2014; Astellas Pharma US, Inc., 2016; AstraZeneca Pharmaceuticals LP, 2010, 2015, 2016, 2017; Bristol-Myers Squibb Co., 2017; Concordia Pharmaceuticals, Inc., 2017; Fassnacht et al., 2011; Fay et al., 2014; Ferring Pharmaceuticals, Inc., 2017; Janssen Pharmaceutical Companies, 2013, 2017, 2018; National Comprehensive Cancer Network, 2017, 2018a, 2018b; Novartis Pharmaceuticals Corp., 2014; Pfizer Inc., 2016; Tolmar Pharmaceuticals, Inc., 2016; van Slooten et al., 1984; Veytsman et al., 2009.

(3) Androgen suppression early in prostate cancer development effectively slows the growth of prostate cancer cells. This can be accomplished by bringing circulating testosterone to castrate levels through orchiectomy or a variety of medications. In the mid-1900s, Charles Huggins discovered that orchiectomy dramatically decreased the progression of metastatic prostate cancer. However, the development of medications that alter hormonal levels has led to a decline in orchiectomy for the treatment of prostate cancer (ACS, 2014; Rove & Crawford, 2014).

(4) Over time, men become resistant to hormone therapy as prostate cancers lose their androgen sensitivity. This results in resurgence in the growth and proliferation of prostate cancer cells and what is referred to as *castration-resistant* or *hormone-refractory* prostate cancer (Penning, 2014).

b) Breast cancer

(1) Hormone receptor (HR)-positive breast cancer is the most common type of breast cancer. It grows in response to action by estrogen and/or progesterone.

(2) Estrogen receptor (ER)-positive breast cancer accounts for approximately 70% of all breast cancers (Lumachi, Brunello, Maruzzo, Basso, & Basso, 2013).

(3) In general, the goal of hormone therapy is to decrease concentrations of estrogens and progestins or prevent the interaction with their receptors; however, treatment is highly dependent on whether a woman is pre- or postmenopausal and the HR status (American Society of Clinical Oncology, 2016).

c) Ovarian, endometrial, and uterine cancers

(1) Epithelial ovarian cancer is the most commonly diagnosed ovarian cancer and is usually seen in postmenopausal women. Although hormone replacement therapy is not used to directly treat ovarian cancer, numerous studies suggest that it can be safely used to treat severe menopausal symptoms postoperatively and may improve overall survival and quality of life (Eeles et al., 2015; Li, Ding, & Qiu, 2015).

(2) Research exploring androgen receptors, ERs, and progesterone receptors (PRs) as possible targets for ovarian cancer is ongoing (Burke et al., 2014; Eeles et al., 2015; Fenlon, 2015).

(3) Endometrial carcinoma is the most common uterine cancer, followed by uterine sarcoma.

(4) Progestins are commonly used as conservative hormone therapy in women who wish to preserve fertility and those who are poor surgical candidates. Additionally, some evidence suggests that combination therapy with tamoxifen and medroxyprogesterone may improve survival (Burke et al., 2014).

d) Adrenal cancer

(1) Adrenocortical carcinoma is rare, occurring mainly in adults. More than half of adrenocortical carcinoma symptoms are caused by oversecretion of adrenal hormones by the tumor.

(2) Although primary treatment is resection, adrenolytic antihormone therapy is used for unresectable or widely metastatic tumors (National Cancer Institute, 2018).

e) Thyroid cancer

(1) Usual treatment of thyroid cancer is through thyroid ablation followed by replacement of thyroid hormones (Fenlon, 2015).

(2) Although complete thyroid-stimulating hormone suppression has been used in the past to limit recurrence, emerging evidence suggests that this may be unnecessary, especially for those who have had excellent or indeterminate response to initial treatment (Freudenthal & Williams, 2017; Haugen et al., 2016).

f) Pituitary tumors: Removal of the pituitary gland results in the need to regulate and replace pituitary hormone for the rest of the individual's life (Fenlon, 2015).

C. Hormone treatment categories

1. Luteinizing hormone–releasing hormone (LHRH) antagonists and agonists

a) These are primarily used to treat breast and prostate cancer. Mounting evidence indicates that giving these agents concurrently with radiation therapy in patients with prostate cancer improves overall survival in select nonmetastatic stages of disease (Juloori, Shah, Stephans, Vassil, & Tendulkar, 2016; Lei et al., 2015; Roach, 2014; Sun, Wang, Yang, & Ma, 2014).

b) LHRH antagonists immediately block the release of LHRH from the hypothalamus, which prevents the release of luteinizing hormone (LH) and follicle-stimulating hormone (FSH) from the anterior pituitary gland. LHRH agonists produce an initial increase in LH and FSH, which translates to increased testosterone concentrations (flare). Concentrations gradually reach castrate levels within two to four weeks, as LHRH release slows significantly in response to downregulation of LHRH receptors in the anterior pituitary (Crawford & Hou, 2009; Rove & Crawford, 2014).

c) Symptoms of tumor flare, specifically urinary retention and pain, result from the increased growth of prostate cancer cells at active disease sites. This is prevented by adding a nonsteroidal antiandrogen. Other side effects of LHRH agonists include decreased bone mineral density, increased insulin resistance, dyslipidemia, increased visceral fat deposition, erectile dysfunction, decreased libido, neurocognitive changes, and depression (Rove & Crawford, 2014; Thompson & Easton, 2001). Although a pooled analysis of studies showed that men receiving LHRH antagonist therapy, compared with LHRH agonists, had fewer urinary tract infections (5% vs. 8%) and better progression-free survival at one year (66% vs. 54.7%), no differences in cardiovascular or metabolic effects were demonstrated (Klotz et al., 2014). LHRH agonists and antagonists share a very similar side effect profile.

d) LHRH agonists work similarly when used to treat breast cancer. These agents also downregulate ovarian production of estrogen by preventing the release of LH. An estrogen flare similar to a testosterone flare occurs at the beginning of treatment (Fenlon, 2015). LHRH agonists are used in the adjuvant setting for women with ER- or PR-positive premenopausal breast cancer with or without tamoxifen to reduce recurrence and preserve ovarian function (National Comprehensive Cancer Network® [NCCN®], 2018a).

e) NCCN guidelines for breast cancer only recommend select LHRH agonists (leuprolide, goserelin) for the treatment of breast cancer. The guidelines for prostate cancer state that LHRH antagonists (degarelix) and agonists (leuprolide, goserelin, triptorelin) may be used interchangeably when androgen deprivation therapy is indicated (NCCN, 2018a, 2018b).

f) Nursing implications

(1) Recent literature has shown that men are particularly susceptible to some of the cardiovascular and metabolic adverse effects from LHRH agonist and

antagonist therapy (Levine et al., 2010). Nurses should educate men and their families on the increased risk for diabetes, heart attack, hypertension, weight gain, visceral fat deposition, loss of lean muscle mass, and bone fracture. Additionally, men can suffer from declines in psychosocial health, namely neurocognitive dysfunction and depression, which can sometimes be exacerbated by erectile dysfunction, hot flashes, and gynecomastia.

(2) Counseling and social work services should be made available for the evaluation of psychosocial health. Referral for medical services should be made for dyslipidemia or other cardiac issues, impaired glucose (abnormal blood glucose, increased A1c), and evaluation of bone mineral density, pain management, and nutrition as necessary. It is important to include the patient's family and/or caregivers in the overall management plan.

(3) Women will experience menopausal symptoms and should be monitored for these. Although estrogen supplementation is not recommended, nurses can assist women with other interventions to relieve symptoms. Metabolic syndrome and bone mineral density should also be regularly monitored.

2. Antiandrogens

a) Antiandrogens are indicated in prostate cancer and are used to mitigate tumor flare with LHRH agonist or antagonist therapy.

b) Antiandrogens are also added to LHRH agonist or antagonist therapy after disease progression in a concept called *combined androgen blockade* (CAB). Although CAB has been shown to achieve more complete suppression of circulating testosterone and improve survival, it is associated with more adverse events and poorer quality of life (Rove & Crawford, 2014).

c) Antiandrogens block the effects of testosterone and dihydrotestosterone at their target receptors in tissues. As a result, they do not reduce serum concentrations of androgens and are not often used as single agents to treat prostate cancer (Actavis Pharma, Inc., 2014; AstraZeneca Pharmaceuticals LP, 2015; Concordia Pharmaceuticals, Inc., 2017; NCCN, 2018b).

d) Adverse effects of antiandrogens include diarrhea and transaminitis. Nilutamide is also associated with visual field changes and disulfiram-like reactions. Because of the latter, patients should be educated to avoid alcohol consumption while on therapy (Actavis Pharma, Inc., 2014; AstraZeneca Pharmaceuticals LP, 2015; Concordia Pharmaceuticals, Inc., 2017).

e) Enzalutamide, a next-generation antiandrogen, inhibits several steps in the androgen receptor signaling process and much more potently binds to the androgen receptor. It is given alone or in combination with prednisone exclusively in the castration-resistant prostate cancer setting (Astellas Pharma US, Inc., 2016; Semenas, Dizeyi, & Persson, 2013).

f) Apalutamide, another next-generation antiandrogen, shares a mechanism similar to that of enzalutamide. It is approved by the U.S. Food and Drug Administration specifically for nonmetastatic castration-resistant prostate cancer in combination with LHRH agonist/antagonist therapy or in patients who have undergone prior orchiectomy (Janssen Pharmaceutical Companies, 2017).

g) Although bicalutamide, flutamide, and nilutamide can be used interchangeably in CAB or to minimize symptoms from tumor flare, bicalutamide offers better tolerance than nilutamide and the advantage of once-daily dosing (AstraZeneca Pharmaceuticals LP, 2015).

3. CYP17 inhibitors

a) Ketoconazole and abiraterone are indicated in prostate cancer after progression on LHRH agonist or antagonist therapy (Janssen Pharmaceutical Companies, 2013, 2017). Abiraterone is more widely used in the castration-refractory prostate cancer setting (NCCN, 2018b).

b) These agents decrease extragonadal production of androgens by inhibiting the CYP17 enzyme. This action blocks the formation of DHEA from pregnenolone, thereby inhibiting the synthesis of androgens. Most extragonadal production of testosterone occurs in the adrenal glands through steroid hormone biosynthesis pathways for which cholesterol is the precursor molecule (Janssen Pharmaceutical Companies, 2013, 2017; Labrie, 2015; Sewer & Li, 2008).

c) Ketoconazole and abiraterone are associated with transaminitis and mineralocorticoid excess. Symptoms of mineralocorticoid excess include hyperkalemia and fluid retention. These agents should not be used in patients with New York Heart Association class III or IV heart failure. To mitigate symptoms of mineralocorticoid excess and hypothalamus-pituitary-adrenal axis suppression, these agents should be given with low-dose oral corticosteroids (Janssen Pharmaceutical Companies, 2013, 2017; NCCN, 2018b).

4. ER antagonists/selective estrogen receptor downregulators
   a) Fulvestrant is indicated for the treatment of metastatic ER-positive breast cancer alone or in combination with palbociclib (AstraZeneca Pharmaceuticals LP, 2017; Elguero, Patel, & Liu, 2014).
   b) Fulvestrant binds to ER and degrades it. Both actions render circulating estrogen unable to exert its effects on breast cancer cells (AstraZeneca Pharmaceuticals LP, 2017; Dean, 2007; Litsas, 2011).
   c) Fulvestrant is fairly well tolerated and is occasionally associated with injection site pain and hot flashes (AstraZeneca Pharmaceuticals LP, 2017).
5. Aromatase inhibitors (AIs)
   a) These agents are also used in the treatment of ER-positive breast cancer in pre- and postmenopausal women (Nourmoussavi et al., 2017).
   b) In premenopausal women, concomitant ovarian ablation with LHRH agonist therapy is recommended in the adjuvant, recurrent, or metastatic settings (Gradishar et al., 2015; NCCN, 2018a; Nourmoussavi et al., 2017).
   c) AIs are also used to treat ER-positive breast cancer in men. Therapy in men should be guided by treatment recommendations for AIs in postmenopausal women (Maugeri-Saccà et al., 2014; NCCN, 2018a; Zagouri et al., 2015).
   d) AIs are classified as steroidal (type 1) or nonsteroidal (type 2) and inhibit the conversion of aromatase, which is the enzyme that converts androgens to estrogen. Steroidal AIs bind aromatase irreversibly. They inhibit the enzyme by binding covalently to the site of aromatase. Nonsteroidal AIs (e.g., anastrozole, letrozole) bind reversibly (Ahmad et al., 2015; Dean, 2007). The blockade of aromatase is dependent on the continuous presence of the inhibitor, and aromatase will begin to release in its absence (Ahmad et al., 2015).
   e) Adverse effects of these agents include menopausal symptoms, decreased bone mineral density, and musculoskeletal disorders (Dean, 2007). AIs can also be used for treatment of selected stages of endometrial cancer (Gao, Wang, Tian, Zhu, & Xue, 2014).
6. Selective estrogen receptor modulators (SERMs)
   a) These drugs are used to treat ER-positive breast cancer and endometrial cancer. SERMs have both estrogenic and antiestrogen properties (Fenlon, 2015) and are tissue specific (Komm & Mirkin, 2014).
   b) SERMs downregulate and block ERs to varying degrees in different tissues (Komm & Mirkin, 2014). In addition to breast cancer, SERMs can be used to treat osteoporosis and menopausal symptoms (Komm & Mirkin, 2014).
   c) SERMs have been associated with increased risk of deep vein thrombosis or pulmonary embolism (Adomaityte, Farooq, & Qayyum, 2008). They have also been associated with development of uterine malignancies, hyperlipidemia, and menopausal symptoms (AstraZeneca Pharmaceuticals LP, 2016; Dean, 2007; Komm & Mirkin, 2014; Nourmoussavi et al., 2017).
   d) SERMs can be used in men and pre- or postmenopausal women in the adjuvant, recurrent, or metastatic breast cancer settings. The duration of therapy with SERMs in the adjuvant setting is highly dependent on menopausal status and whether a patient has been treated with an AI. Generally, treatment lasts 5–10 years, and within that time frame, patients can be transitioned to or from AI therapy based on menopausal status and tolerance (Early Breast Cancer Trialists Collaborative Group, 2015; Komm & Mirkin, 2014; Mirkin & Pickar, 2015; NCCN, 2018a). Third- and fourth-generation SERMs are being explored to prevent breast cancer in high-risk women (Komm & Mirkin, 2014; Li et al., 2015).
   e) Nursing implications
      (1) Blocking or eliminating estrogen will cause premature menopause in premenopausal women and heightened or renewed symptoms in postmenopausal women.
      (2) SERMs may put women at higher risk for endometrial cancer and deep vein thrombosis. Adherence is challenging for patients on AIs and SERMs because of the discomfort of symptoms, such as

hot flashes, cognitive changes, fatigue, myalgias and arthralgias, and physical changes (Huober et al., 2014; Lombard et al., 2016).

(3) Nurses can provide education and support to women undergoing this treatment. Additionally, some women benefit from participation in support groups with other women.

7. Adrenolytics

a) Drug therapy with mitotane is indicated in unresectable or metastatic adrenocortical cancer or as adjuvant treatment following complete resection.

b) Although its mechanism has not entirely been elucidated, mitotane acts within the adrenal cortex as a cytotoxic agent. As a result, it affects malignant and nonmalignant adrenocortical tissues.

c) Mitotane is associated with nausea, vomiting, diarrhea, ataxia, amnesia, confusion, and suppression of hormones synthesized and released from the adrenal cortex (i.e., corticosteroids) (Bristol-Myers Squibb Co., 2017).

d) Nursing implications

(1) Both therapeutic and toxic effects are correlated with plasma concentration, requiring close monitoring and supportive management of adverse effects with the use of hydrocortisone, antiemetics, and antidiarrheals.

(2) Thyroid and androgen supplementation may also be necessary. Serum hormone concentrations should be assessed at least every three months in patients receiving mitotane. Patients should be educated about adherence to mitotane therapeutic drug monitoring and other follow-up to limit the risk of drug discontinuation due to toxicity (Kerkhofs, Ettaieb, Hermsen, & Haak, 2015).

References

AbbVie Inc. (2014). *Lupron Depot® (leuprolide acetate)* [Package insert]. North Chicago, IL: Author.

Actavis Pharma, Inc. (2014). *Flutamide* [Package insert]. Parsippany, NJ: Author.

Adomaityte, J., Farooq, M., & Qayyum, R. (2008). Effect of raloxifene therapy on venous thromboembolism in postmenopausal women. A meta-analysis. *Thrombosis and Haemostasis, 99,* 338–342. https://doi.org/10.1160/TH07-07-0468

Ahmad, A., Ginnebaugh, K.R., Yin, S., Bollig-Fischer, A., Reddy, K.B., & Sarkar, F.H. (2015). Functional role of miR-10b in tamoxifen resistance of ER-positive breast cancer cells through down-regulation of HDAC4. *BMC Cancer, 15,* 540. https://doi.org/10.1186/s12885-015-1561-x

American Cancer Society. (2014). Evolution of cancer treatments: Hormone therapy. Retrieved from https://www.cancer.org/cancer/cancer-basics/history-of-cancer/cancer-treatment-hormone-therapy.html

American Cancer Society. (2018). *Cancer facts and figures 2018.* Atlanta, GA: Author.

American Society of Clinical Oncology. (2016, February 16). Hormonal therapy for early-stage hormone receptor-positive breast cancer. Retrieved from http://www.cancer.net/research-and-advocacy/asco-care-and-treatment-recommendations-patients/hormonal-therapy-early-stage-hormone-receptor-positive-breast-cancer

Astellas Pharma US, Inc. (2016). *Xtandi® (enzalutamide)* [Package insert]. Northbrook, IL: Author.

AstraZeneca Pharmaceuticals LP. (2010). *Arimidex® (anastrozole)* [Package insert]. Wilmington, DE: Author.

AstraZeneca Pharmaceuticals LP. (2015). *Casodex® (bicalutamide)* [Package insert]. Wilmington, DE. Author.

AstraZeneca Pharmaceuticals LP. (2016). *Nolvadex® (tamoxifen citrate)* [Package insert]. Wilmington, DE: Author.

AstraZeneca Pharmaceuticals LP. (2017). *Faslodex® (fulvestrant)* [Package insert]. Wilmington, DE: Author.

Bristol-Myers Squibb Co. (2017). *Lysodren® (mitotane)* [Package insert]. Princeton, NJ: Author.

Burke, W.M., Orr, J., Leitao, M., Salom, E., Gehrig, P., Olawaiye, A.B., … Abu Shahin, F. (2014). Endometrial cancer: A review and current management strategies: Part II. *Gynecologic Oncology, 134,* 393–402. https://doi.org/10.1016/j.ygyno.2014.06.003

Concordia Pharmaceuticals, Inc. (2017). *Nilandron® (nilutamide)* [Package insert]. Saint Michael, Barbados: Author.

Crawford, E.D., & Hou, A.H. (2009). The role of LHRH antagonists in the treatment of prostate cancer. *Oncology, 23,* 626–630.

Dean, A. (2007). Hormone treatment for breast cancer. *Cancer Nursing Practice, 6,* 35–39. https://doi.org/10.7748/cnp2007.02.6.1.35.c4191

Early Breast Cancer Trialists Collaborative Group. (2015). Aromatase inhibitors versus tamoxifen in early breast cancer: Patient-level meta-analysis of the randomised trials. *Lancet, 386,* 1341–1352. https://doi.org/10.1016/S0140-6736(15)61074-1

Eeles, R.A., Morden, J.P., Gore, M., Mansi, J., Glees, J., Wenczi, M., … Bliss, J.M. (2015). Adjuvant hormone therapy may improve survival in epithelial ovarian cancer: Results of the AHT randomized trial. *Journal of Clinical Oncology, 33,* 4138–4144. https://doi.org/10.1200/JCO.2015.60.9719

Elguero, S., Patel, B., & Liu, J.H. (2014). Misperception of estrogen activity in patients treated with an estrogen receptor antagonist. *American Journal of Obstetrics and Gynecology, 211,* e1–e2. https://doi.org/10.1016/j.ajog.2014.05.038

Fassnacht, M., Libé, R., Kroiss, M., & Allolio, B. (2011). Adrenocortical carcinoma: A clinician's update. *Nature Reviews Endocrinology, 7,* 323–355. https://doi.org/10.1038/nrendo.2010.235

Fay, A.P., Elfiky, A., Teló, G.H., McKay, R.R., Kaymakcalan, M., Nguyen, P.L., … Choueiri, T.K. (2014). Adrenocortical carcinoma: The management of metastatic disease. *Critical Reviews in Oncology/Hematology, 92,* 123–132. https://doi.org/10.1016/j.critrevonc.2014.05.009

Fenlon, D. (2015). Endocrine therapies. In J. Corner & C. Bailey (Eds.), *Cancer nursing: Care in context* (2nd ed., pp. 360–370). Hoboken, NJ: Wiley-Blackwell.

Ferring Pharmaceuticals, Inc. (2017). *Firmagon® (degarelix)* [Package insert]. Parsippany, NJ: Author.

Freudenthal, B., & Williams, G.R. (2017). Thyroid stimulating hormone suppression in the long-term follow-up of differentiated thyroid cancer. *Clinical Oncology, 5,* 325–328. https://doi.org/10.1016/j.clon.2016.12.011

Gao, C.W., Wang, Y., Tian, W., Zhu, Y., & Xue, F. (2014). The therapeutic significance of aromatase inhibitors in endometrial carcinoma. *Gynecologic Oncology, 134,* 190–195. https://doi.org/10.1016/j.ygyno.2014.04.060

Gradishar, W.J., Anderson, B.O., Balassanian, R., Blair, S.L., Burstein, H.J., Cyr, A., … Kumar, R. (2015). NCCN Guidelines® Insights: Breast cancer, version 1.2016. *Journal of the National Comprehensive Cancer Network, 13,* 1475–1485. Retrieved from http://www.jnccn.org/content/13/12/1475.long

Haugen, B.R., Alexander, E.K., Bible, K.C., Doherty, G.M., Mandel, S.J., Nikiforov, Y.E., … Wartofsky, L. (2016). 2015 American Thyroid Association management guidelines for adult patients with thyroid nodules and differentiated thyroid cancer: The American Thyroid Association Guidelines Task Force on Thyroid Nodules and Differentiated Thyroid Cancer. *Thyroid, 26,* 1–133. https://doi.org/10.1089/thy.2015.0020

Huober, J., Cole, B.F., Rabaglio, M., Giobbie-Hurder, A., Wu, J., Ejlertsen, B., … Thürlimann, B. (2014). Symptoms of endocrine treatment and outcome in the BIG 1-98 study. *Breast Cancer Research and Treatment, 143,* 159–169. https://doi.org/10.1007/s10549-013-2792-7

Janssen Pharmaceutical Companies. (2013). *Nizoral® (ketoconazole)* [Package insert]. Titusville, NJ: Author.

Janssen Pharmaceutical Companies. (2017). *Zytiga® (abiraterone acetate)* [Package insert]. Horsham, PA: Author.

Janssen Pharmaceutical Companies. (2018). *Erleada™ (apalutamide)* [Package insert]. Horsham, PA: Author.

Juloori, A., Shah, C., Stephans, K., Vassil, A., & Tendulkar, R. (2016). Evolving paradigm of radiotherapy for high-risk prostate cancer: Current consensus and continuing controversies. *Prostate Cancer, 2016,* 1–12. https://doi.org/10.1155/2016/2420786

Kerkhofs, T.M.A., Ettaieb, M.H.T., Hermsen, I.G.C., & Haak, H.R. (2015). Developing treatment for adrenocortical carcinoma. *Endocrine-Related Cancer, 22,* R325–R338. https://doi.org/10.1530/ERC-15-0318

Klotz, L., Miller, K., Crawford, E.D., Shore, N., Tombal, B., Karup, C., … Persson, B.-E. (2014). Disease control outcomes from analysis of pooled individual patient data from five comparative randomised clinical trials of degarelix versus luteinizing hormone-releasing hormone agonists. *European Urology, 66,* 1101–1108. https://doi.org/10.1016/j.eururo.2013.12.063

Komm, B.S., & Mirkin, S. (2014). An overview of current and emerging SERMs. *Journal of Steroid Biochemistry and Molecular Biology, 143,* 207–222. https://doi.org/10.1016/j.jsbmb.2014.03.003

Labrie, F. (2015). Combined blockade of testicular and locally made androgens in prostate cancer: A highly significant medical progress based upon intracrinology. *Journal of Steroid Biochemistry and Molecular Biology, 145,* 144–156. https://doi.org/10.1016/j.jsbmb.2014.05.012

Lei, J., Rudolph, A., Moysich, K.B., Rafiq, S., Behrens, S., Goode, E.L., … Chang-Claude, J. (2015). Assessment of variation in immunosuppressive pathway genes reveals *TGFBR2* to be associated with prognosis of estrogen receptor-negative breast cancer after chemotherapy. *Breast Cancer Research, 17,* 18. https://doi.org/10.1186/s13058-015-0522-2

Levine, G.N., D'Amico, A.V., Berger, P., Clark, P.E., Eckel, R.H., Keating, N.H., … Zakai, N. (2010). Androgen-deprivation therapy in prostate cancer and cardiovascular risk: A science advisory from the American Heart Association, American Cancer Society, and American Urological Association: Endorsed by the American Society for Radiation Oncology. *CA: A Cancer Journal for Clinicians, 60,* 194–201. https://doi.org/10.3322/caac.20061

Li, D., Ding, C.-Y., & Qiu, L.-H. (2015). Postoperative hormone replacement therapy for epithelial ovarian cancer patients: A systematic review and meta-analysis. *Gynecologic Oncology, 139,* 355–362. https://doi.org/10.1016/j.ygyno.2015.07.109

Litsas, G. (2011). Nursing perspectives on fulvestrant for the treatment of postmenopausal women with metastatic breast cancer. *Clinical Journal of Oncology Nursing, 15,* 674–681. https://doi.org/10.1188/11.CJON.674-681

Lombard, J.M., Zdenkowski, N., Wells, K., Beckmore, C., Reaby, L., Forbes, J.F., & Chirgwin, J. (2016). Aromatase inhibitor induced musculoskeletal syndrome: A significant problem with limited treatment options. *Supportive Care in Cancer, 24,* 2139–2146. https://doi.org/10.1007/s00520-015-3001-5

Lumachi, F., Brunello, A., Maruzzo, M., Basso, U., & Basso, S.M.M. (2013). Treatment of estrogen receptor-positive breast cancer. *Current Medical Chemistry, 20,* 596–604. https://doi.org/10.2174/092986713804999303

Maugeri-Saccà, M., Barba, M., Vici, P., Pizzuti, L., Sergi, D., De Maria, R., & Di Lauro, L. (2014). Aromatase inhibitors for metastatic male breast cancer: Molecular, endocrine, and clinical considerations. *Breast Cancer Research and Treatment, 147,* 227–235. https://doi.org/10.1007/s10549-014-3087-3

Mirkin, S., & Pickar, J.H. (2015). Selective estrogen receptor modulators (SERMs): A review of clinical data. *Maturitas, 80,* 52–57. https://doi.org/10.1016/j.maturitas.2014.10.010

National Cancer Institute. (2018). Adrenocortical carcinoma treatment (PDQ®) [Health professional version]. Retrieved from https://www.cancer.gov/types/adrenocortical/hp/adrenocortical-treatment-pdq

National Comprehensive Cancer Network. (2017). *NCCN Clinical Practice Guidelines in Oncology (NCCN Guidelines®): Uterine neoplasms* [v.1.2018]. Retrieved from https://www.nccn.org/professionals/physician_gls/pdf/uterine.pdf

National Comprehensive Cancer Network. (2018a). *NCCN Clinical Practice Guidelines in Oncology (NCCN Guidelines®): Breast cancer* [v.4.2017]. Retrieved from https://www.nccn.org/professionals/physician_gls/pdf/breast.pdf

National Comprehensive Cancer Network. (2018b). *NCCN Clinical Practice Guidelines in Oncology (NCCN Guidelines®): Prostate cancer* [v.1.2018]. Retrieved from https://www.nccn.org/professionals/physician_gls/pdf/prostate.pdf

Novartis Pharmaceuticals Corp. (2014). *Femara® (letrozole)* [Package insert]. East Hanover, NJ: Author.

Penning, T.M. (2014). Androgen biosynthesis in castration-resistant prostate cancer. *Endocrine-Related Cancer, 21,* T67–T78. https://doi.org/10.1530/ERC-14-0109

Pfizer Inc. (2016). *Aromasin® (exemestane)* [Package insert]. New York, NY: Author.

Roach, M., 3rd. (2014). Current trends for the use of androgen deprivation therapy in conjunction with radiotherapy for patients with unfavorable intermediate-risk, high-risk, localized, and locally advanced prostate cancer. *Cancer, 120,* 1620–1629. https://doi.org/10.1002/cncr.28594

Rove, K.O., & Crawford, E.D. (2014). Traditional androgen ablation approaches to advanced prostate cancer: New insights. *Canadian Journal of Urology, 21,* 14–21.

Semenas, J., Dizeyi, N., & Persson, J.L. (2013). Enzalutamide as a second generation antiandrogen for treatment of advanced prostate cancer. *Drug Design, Development and Therapy, 7,* 875–881. https://doi.org/10.2147/DDDT.S45703

Sewer, M.B., & Li, D. (2008). Regulation of steroid hormone biosynthesis by the cytoskeleton. *Lipids, 43,* 1109–1115. https://doi.org/10.1007/s11745-008-3221-2

Sun, Y., Wang, C., Yang, H., & Ma, X. (2014). The effect of estrogen on the proliferation of endometrial cancer cells is mediated by ERRγ through AKT and ERK1/2. *European Journal of Cancer Prevention, 23,* 418–424. https://doi.org/10.1097/CEJ.0000000000000052

Thompson, D., & Easton, D. (2001). Variation in cancer risks, by mutation position, in BRCA2 mutation carriers. *American Journal of Human Genetics, 68,* 410–419. https://doi.org/10.1086/318181

Tolmar Pharmaceuticals, Inc. (2016). *Eligard® (leuprolide)* [Package insert]. Fort Collins, CO: Author.

van Slooten, H., Moolenaar, A.J., van Seter, A.P., & Smeenk, D. (1984). The treatment of adrenocortical carcinoma with *o,p'*-DDD: Prognostic simplications of serum level monitoring. *European Journal of Cancer and Clinical Oncology, 20,* 47–53. https://doi.org/10.1016/0277-5379(84)90033-6

Veytsman, I., Nieman, L., & Fojo, T. (2009). Management of endocrine manifestations and the use of mitotane as a chemotherapeutic agent for adrenocortical carcinoma. *Journal of Clinical Oncology, 27,* 4619–4629. https://doi.org/10.1200/JCO.2008.17.2775

Zagouri, F., Sergentanis, T.N., Azim, H.A., Jr., Chrysikos, D., Dimopoulos, M.-A., & Psaltopoulou, T. (2015). Aromatase inhibitors in male breast cancer: A pooled analysis. *Breast Cancer Research and Treatment, 151,* 141–147. https://doi.org/10.1007/s10549-015-3356-9

CHAPTER 8

Targeted Therapy

A. Targeted therapies in the treatment of cancer
   1. Molecularly targeted anticancer agents selectively target molecular pathways, as opposed to traditional cytotoxic chemotherapy agents that target DNA, tubulin, or cell division machinery (Parulekar & Eisenhauer, 2004).
      a) A growing number of unique molecular targets have been identified within cancer cells, resulting in the discovery of novel agents, many of which are oral.
      b) The oral route allows for continuous administration of lower doses of agents, which may be primarily cytostatic in nature, versus traditional cytotoxic agents for which episodic delivery allows for bone marrow recovery (Weingart et al., 2008).
      c) See Table 8-1 for a list of targeted therapies. Agents that target primarily immune pathways (e.g., cytotoxic T-lymphocyte antigen 4) and extracellular molecular markers (e.g., CD20) are discussed in Chapter 10.
   2. Tyrosine kinase inhibitors (TKIs): Tyrosine kinases direct many cellular functions, including cell signaling, growth, and division. These enzymes may be overly active in some cancer cells, and inhibition of them may stop cancer cell growth (National Cancer Institute, n.d.). See Figure 8-1 for a diagram of the basic principles of tyrosine kinases and Figure 8-2 for a depiction of epidermal growth factor receptor (EGFR) and vascular endothelial growth factor receptor pathways. When a TKI is introduced within these pathways, the enhanced activity is inhibited, leading to decreased cell proliferation (Simmons, 2012).
   3. Agents by primary molecular target
      a) Anaplastic lymphoma kinase (ALK) inhibitors: The fusion between echinoderm microtubule-associated protein-like 4 (EML4) and ALK is an oncogene present in 3%–5% of patients with non-small cell lung cancer, most commonly younger patients, never- or light-smokers with adenocarcinoma, and those without *EGFR* and *KRAS* mutations. EML4 is essential for microtubule formation. ALK belongs to the family of insulin receptor kinases. The fusion point for EML4 and ALK is variable; however, all lead to ALK phosphorylation and activation of RAS/RAF/MEK, PI3K-mTOR, and JAK/STAT pathways. Inhibition of ALK can vary based on the fusion variant (Karachaliou et al., 2017). Examples: alectinib, brigatinib, ceritinib, crizotinib.
      b) *BCR-ABL* tyrosine kinase inhibitors: The *BCR-ABL* protein has the ability to develop into a mutant form that is resistant to some formulations of *BCR-ABL* TKIs. Patients taking these medications for chronic myeloid leukemia require long-term therapy. Data demonstrate the need for adherence monitoring, as patients who are adherent have better early response and/or long-term outcomes (Cuellar, Vozniak, Rhodes, Forcello, & Olszta, 2018). Examples: imatinib, bosutinib, dasatinib, nilotinib, ponatinib.
      c) BRAF V600E mutation inhibitors and MEK inhibitors: The mitogen-activated protein (MAP) kinase signaling pathway mediates cell proliferation and differentiation. When BRAF is mutated, this leads to constitutive activation of signaling via this pathway. The BRAF V600E mutation is present in 40%–60% of melanomas. Inhibition of BRAF and MEK in patients with this mutation in metastatic melanoma has improved progression-free survival and overall survival (Devji, Levine, Neupane, Beyene, & Xie, 2017). Examples: dabrafenib, vemurafenib (BRAF inhibitors); cobimetinib, trametinib (MEK inhibitors).
      d) B-cell receptor pathway inhibitors: A normal B cell is activated when an antigen binds to member receptors, leading to activation of two main pathways, Bruton tyrosine kinase (BTK) and phosphoinositide 3-kinase (PI3K). These ultimately lead to stimulation of the

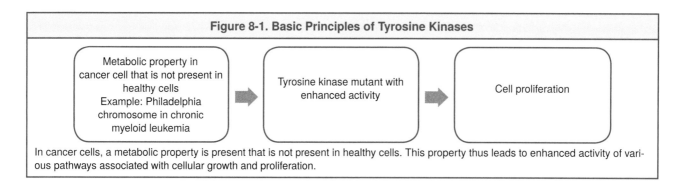

Figure 8-1. Basic Principles of Tyrosine Kinases

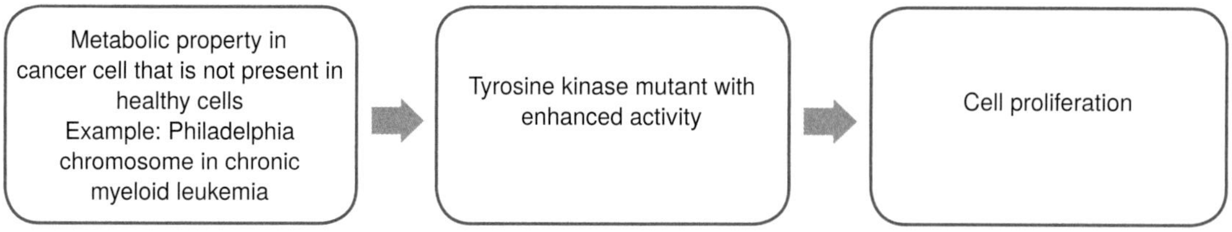

In cancer cells, a metabolic property is present that is not present in healthy cells. This property thus leads to enhanced activity of various pathways associated with cellular growth and proliferation.

growth and survival of B cells and mediate B-cell migration and trafficking (Aw & Brown, 2017). Inhibition of these pathways in B-cell malignancies leads to decreased cell proliferation. Examples: acalabrutinib, ibrutinib (BTK inhibitors); idelalisib (PI3Kδ inhibitor).

e) CDK inhibitors: D-type cyclins (D1, D2, and D3) are overexpressed in some cancers, leading to activation of CDK. Inhibition of cyclin D3 and CDK6 complexes leads to accumulation of reactive oxygen species and subsequent apoptosis (Wang et al., 2017). Examples: abemaciclib, palbociclib, ribociclib.

f) EGFR inhibitors: Activation of EGFR leads to tyrosine phosphorylation and activation of multiple downstream pathways, including MAP kinase, PI3K/AKT, and JAK/STAT. Alterations of EGFR signaling in carcinomas lead to tumorigenesis, proliferation, survival, and angiogenesis. TKIs inhibit this pathway by binding to the adenosine triphosphate–binding pocket of the intracellular kinase domain. Mutations to this binding site are believed to lead to tumor resistance to these agents (Neal & Sequist, 2011). Examples: afatinib, erlotinib, gefitinib, lapatinib, osimertinib, vandetanib.

g) Epigenetic mechanisms

(1) These include DNA methylation, histone modifications, and noncoding RNA deregulation (Eckschlager, Plch, Stiborova, & Hrabeta, 2017).

(2) Histone deacetylase (HDAC) inhibitors: Different HDAC enzymes are expressed in different malignancy types, leading specific HDAC inhibitors to work in specific tumor types. Histones are modified by acetylation to play a role in gene expression via epigenetic regulation. This mechanism controls transcription of approximately 2%–10% of genes (Eckschlager et al., 2017). Examples: belinostat, panobinostat, romidepsin, vorinostat.

h) FMS-like tyrosine kinase 3 (FLT3) inhibitors: FLT3 is a tyrosine kinase receptor that plays a critical role in normal hematopoiesis. This is the most frequently mutated gene in acute myeloid leukemia; the presence of an FLT3–internal tandem duplication (known as FLT3-ITD) mutation adversely affects prognosis for patients (Hospital et al., 2017). Examples: midostaurin, sorafenib.

i) Hedgehog pathway inhibitors: The Hedgehog pathway is critical for embryonic and stem cell development. This pathway includes multiple potential targets for inhibition, including SMO, PTCH1, and others. Ultimately, activation of this pathway leads to cell fate determinants of tissue patterning, cell proliferation, and cell survival regulators—all of which are regulated by components acting in positive or negative feedback loops. This pathway plays a role in a multitude of cancer types (Wu, Zhang, Sun, McMahon, & Wang, 2017). Examples: sonidegib, vismodegib.

j) Janus kinase-2 (JAK2) inhibitors: The JAK2 V617F mutation is present in 95% of patients with polycythemia vera, 65% of patients with myelofibrosis, and 55% of patients with essential thrombocythemia. This mutation leads to the activation of JAK2 signaling. JAK2 signaling is also required for normal hematopoietic stem cell function. Therefore, ideal targets will be for only JAK2 V617F mutations. Non–mutation-specific inhibitors exhibit cytopenias as the primary toxicity and the most common reason for treatment discontinuation (Hobbs, Rozelle, & Mullally, 2017). Examples: ruxolitinib, tofacitinib.

k) Mammalian target of rapamycin (mTOR) kinase inhibitors: The PI3K/AKT/mTOR pathway regulates cellular growth and survival; deregulation of this pathway is associated with a high risk of poor-prognosis can-

Figure 8-2. Epidermal Growth Factor Receptor and Vascular Endothelial Growth Factor Receptor Pathways

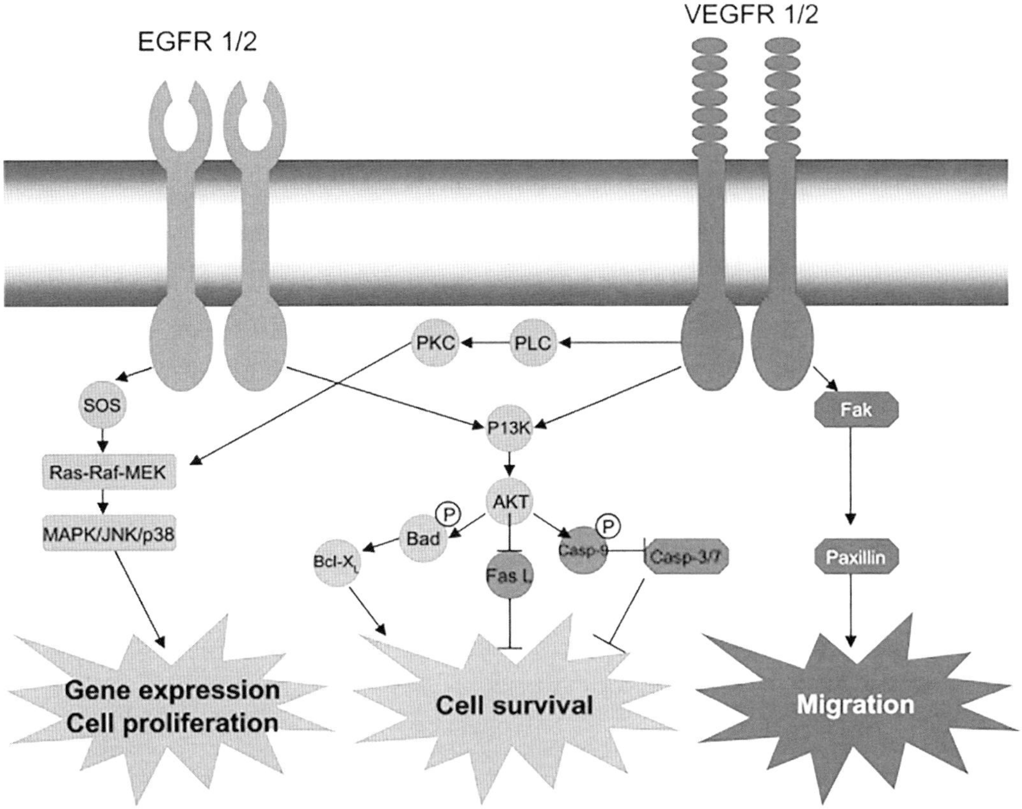

Examples of targeted pathways. In these pathways, the extracellular receptor is activated, leading to a cascade of events resulting in enhanced gene expression, cell proliferation, cell survival, and migration.

EGFR—epidermal growth factor receptor; VEGFR—vascular endothelial growth factor receptor

Note. From "Growth Factor Receptors and Apoptosis Regulators: Signaling Pathways, Prognosis, Chemosensitivity and Treatment Outcomes of Breast Cancer," by S. Sarkar and M. Mandal, 2009, *Breast Cancer: Basic and Clinical Research, 3,* p. 52. Copyright 2009 by The Authors, licensee Libertas Academia Ltd.; distributed under CC BY 2.0 (http://www.creativecommons.org/licenses/by/2.0), which permits unrestricted use, distribution, and reproduction, provided the original work is properly cited.

cers. The activation of mTOR is a convergence point leading to phosphorylation events that ultimately result in cell growth and proliferation, angiogenesis, and prevention of apoptosis (Chen, Doyle, Takebe, Timmer, & Ivy, 2011). Examples: everolimus, temsirolimus.

l) Mediators of apoptosis Bcl-2: The Bcl-2 family of proteins consists of both antiapoptotic and proapoptotic proteins. This network regulates the mitochondrial apoptotic response, allowing for reaction to stimuli and preventing unwanted cell death in normal cell functioning. Overexpression of antiapoptotic Bcl-2 family proteins occurs via a variety of mechanisms in many different tumor types. Conversely, decreased expression of proapoptotic Bcl-2 family proteins also facilitates tumor formation and growth (Hata, Engelman, & Faber, 2015). Example: venetoclax.

m) Poly(ADP-ribose) polymerase (PARP) inhibitors: PARP allows for base excision repair of DNA in the case of single-strand DNA breaks. In the absence of PARP, these single-strand breaks progress to double-strand breaks, which may be poorly repaired, especially in tumors with mutations in *BRCA1* or *BRCA2* (del Rivero & Kohn, 2017). Examples: olaparib, rucaparib.

n) Proteasome inhibitors: The ubiquitin-proteasome pathway regulates fundamental processes, including apoptosis, cell growth and proliferation, DNA repair, unfolded protein response, and immune response. The proteasome is composed of two structures, the 20S proteasome and the 19S regulatory subunit. They form a complex referred to as a 26S proteasome (Espinoza-Delgado, Chiaramonte, Swerdlow, & Wright, 2011).

Second-generation agents in this class (carfilzomib, ixazomib) attempt to overcome resistance mechanisms and increase tolerability, particularly with respect to peripheral neuropathy (Schlafer, Shah, Panjic, & Lonial, 2017). Examples: bortezomib, carfilzomib (parenteral); ixazomib (oral).

o) Thrombopoietin (TPO) receptor agonists: TPO is the key cytokine that stimulates platelet production. First-generation peptide-based TPO agonists were associated with development of antibodies. Second-generation TPO mimetics have been developed to avoid this antibody production. These agents bind to the TPO receptor to stimulate pathways for platelet production, including JAK2/STAT (Rodeghiero & Carli, 2017). Examples: romiplostim (parenteral); eltrombopag (oral).

p) Vascular endothelial growth factor (VEGF) inhibitors: The VEGF pathway is an essential component of angiogenesis, the recruitment of new blood vessels to a tumor as it grows. Tumor hypoxia induces VEGF expression. While normal tissues lack angiogenesis, significant toxicities have been noted with VEGF pathway inhibitors, potentially as a result of off-target effects in the normal vasculature (Wisinkski & Gradishar, 2011). Examples: axitinib, lenvatinib, pazopanib, sorafenib, sunitinib, ziv-aflibercept.

q) Multiple kinase targets: These agents target multiple kinase pathways, leading to alterations in cell proliferation. The exact primary target is unknown. Examples: cabozantinib, regorafenib.

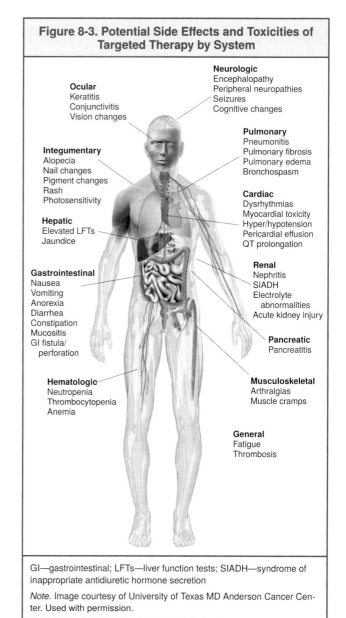

Figure 8-3. Potential Side Effects and Toxicities of Targeted Therapy by System

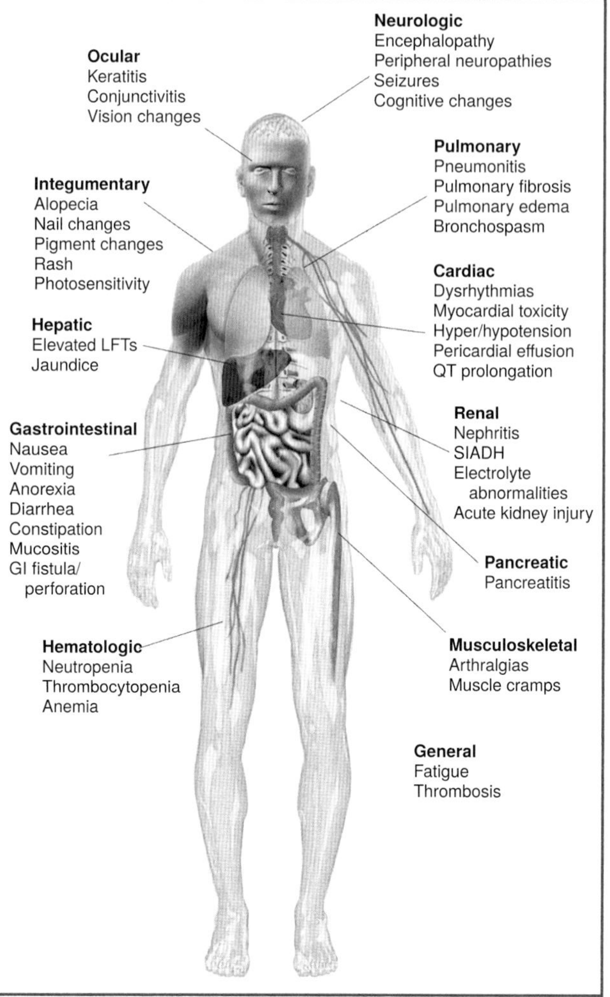

GI—gastrointestinal; LFTs—liver function tests; SIADH—syndrome of inappropriate antidiuretic hormone secretion

Note. Image courtesy of University of Texas MD Anderson Cancer Center. Used with permission.

B. Adverse effects of targeted therapies

1. In contrast to cytotoxic agents, targeted therapies interfere with specific pathways in cancer cells, with little or no effect on normal tissues. Consequently, they have a nontraditional side effect profile compared to cytotoxic agents (Priestman, 2012).
2. Table 8-1 and Figure 8-3 include notable side effects for the different targeted agents. These include acneform rash, cardiotoxicity, hepatotoxicity, hypertension, metabolic abnormalities (hyperglycemia, hyperlipidemia), and others as noted.

C. Drug–drug interactions

1. Cytochrome P450 (CYP) enzymes are expressed primarily in the liver and are responsible for the metabolism of drugs. Although more than 50 of these enzymes exist, 6 of them metabolize 90% of drugs (CYP1A2, CYP2C9, CYP2C19, CYP2D6, CYP3A4, and CYP3A5).
2. Drugs can inhibit or induce these enzymes, leading to drug–drug interactions. The clinical outcome of these interactions can be adverse reactions or therapeutic failures from over- or underexposure to the intended medication. For example, ritonavir is a strong inhibitor of CYP3A4. When a drug that is metabolized by CYP3A4 is administered with ritonavir, patients experience decreased metabolism and overexposure to that drug (Lynch & Price, 2017).
3. Many TKIs undergo metabolism via CYP pathways, leading to a high propensity for drug–drug interactions. Table 8-1 includes specifics to avoid interactions.

Table 8-1. Targeted Therapies

Drug	Mechanism of Action	Route	Indications	Side Effects	Nursing Considerations
Abemaciclib (Verzenio™)	Inhibits cyclin-dependent kinases 4 and 6 (CDK4 and CDK6), which promote cell cycle progression and cell proliferation, leading to apoptosis	PO	In combination with fulvestrant for HR-positive, HER2-negative advanced or metastatic breast cancer in patients with disease progression following endocrine therapy Monotherapy for HR-positive, HER2-negative advanced or metastatic breast cancer in patients with disease progression following endocrine therapy and prior chemotherapy in the metastatic setting	Diarrhea, hepatotoxicity, venous thromboembolism, neutropenia, nausea, abdominal pain, infections, fatigue, anemia, leukopenia, decreased appetite, vomiting, headache, thrombocytopenia	Patients should take twice daily with or without food at approximately the same time each day. If patients vomit or miss a dose, they should take the next dose at its scheduled time. Patients should swallow tablets whole and not chew, crush, or split them or take tablets that are broken, cracked, or otherwise not intact. Dosing varies if given as monotherapy or in combination with fulvestrant. Concomitant use with CYP3A4/5 inhibitors, including grapefruit juice, or inducers may alter exposure to abemaciclib and should be avoided. Dose modifications are required in severe hepatic impairment. Dose modifications are required based on the severity of the adverse reaction. At the first sign of a loose stool, patients should start antidiarrheal therapy (e.g., loperamide), increase oral fluids, and notify their healthcare provider for further instructions. Women of reproductive potential should use contraception during treatment and for 3 weeks following completion of therapy. (Eli Lilly and Company, 2017)
Acalabrutinib (Calquence®)	Inhibits Bruton tyrosine kinase, which is a signaling molecule of the B-cell antigen receptor, leading to inhibition of malignant B-cell proliferation	PO	Mantle cell lymphoma after at least 1 prior therapy	Hemorrhage, infections, anemia, neutropenia, thrombocytopenia, second primary malignancies, atrial fibrillation and flutter, headache, diarrhea, fatigue, myalgia, bruising	Patients should take every 12 hours, swallowing whole with water, with or without food. Capsules should not be chewed, broken, or opened. If patients miss a dose by more than 3 hours, they should skip it and take the next dose at its regular time. They should not make up missed doses. Concomitant use with CYP3A4/5 inhibitors, including grapefruit juice, or inducers may alter exposure to acalabrutinib and should be avoided. Avoid coadministration with PPIs. Stagger dosing with H_2 antagonists and antacids by at least 2 hours. Advise patients to use sun protection. (AstraZeneca Pharmaceuticals LP, 2017a)

(Continued on next page)

Table 8-1. Targeted Therapies *(Continued)*

Drug	Mechanism of Action	Route	Indications	Side Effects	Nursing Considerations
Afatinib (Gilotrif®)	Binds to the tyrosine kinase domain of EGFR, HER2, and HER4, leading to inhibition of autophosphorylation and downregulation of signaling pathways	PO	Metastatic NSCLC in patients whose tumors have EGFR exon 19 deletions or exon 21 (L858R) substitution mutations Metastatic squamous NSCLC progressing after platinum-based chemotherapy	Diarrhea, cutaneous reactions, rash, acneform dermatitis, ILD, hepatotoxicity, ventricular dysfunction, keratitis, stomatitis, paronychia, dry skin, decreased appetite, nausea, vomiting, pruritus	Patients should take at least 1 hour before or 2 hours after a meal once daily. They should not take a missed dose within 12 hours of the next dose. Concomitant use with P-gp inhibitors or inducers may alter exposure to afatinib and should be avoided. If concomitant use cannot be avoided, dose adjustment of afatinib should be made. Dose modifications are required in severe renal impairment. Diarrhea may be severe enough to lead to dehydration and renal failure. Patients should take an antidiarrheal agent (e.g., loperamide) at the onset of diarrhea until loose bowel movements cease for 12 hours. Contact lens use increases the risk of keratitis and ulceration. Advise patients to minimize sun exposure and use broad-spectrum sunscreen. (Boehringer Ingelheim Pharmaceuticals, Inc., 2016)
Alectinib (Alecensa®)	TKI that targets ALK and RET to decrease tumor cell viability in cell lines harboring ALK fusions, amplifications, or activating mutations	PO	ALK-positive, metastatic NSCLC in patients who have progressed on or are intolerant to crizotinib	Hepatotoxicity (elevated AST, ALT, or bilirubin), ILD, bradycardia, myalgia, CPK elevation, fatigue, constipation, edema	Patients should take every 12 hours with food. Do not open or dissolve contents of the capsule. If patients miss or vomit a dose, they should take the next dose at the scheduled time. Monitor heart rate and blood pressure regularly. Advise patients to report any changes in heart or blood pressure medication. Advise patients to minimize sun exposure and use broad-spectrum sunscreen during treatment and for at least 7 days after discontinuation. Women of reproductive potential should use contraception during treatment and for 1 week following completion of therapy. Men should use contraception during treatment and for 3 months following completion of therapy. (Genentech, Inc., 2016a)

(Continued on next page)

Table 8-1. Targeted Therapies *(Continued)*

Drug	Mechanism of Action	Route	Indications	Side Effects	Nursing Considerations
Axitinib (Inlyta®)	Inhibits tyrosine kinases, including VEGFRs, leading to interferences with tumor angiogenesis, growth, and progression	PO	Advanced RCC after failure of 1 prior systemic therapy	Hypertension including hypertensive crisis, arterial and venous thromboembolism, hemorrhage, GI perforation, GI fistula formation, hypothyroidism, proteinuria, elevated LFTs, cardiac failure, RPLS, diarrhea, fatigue, decreased appetite, nausea, dysphonia, hand-foot syndrome, weight loss, vomiting, asthenia, constipation	Patients should take every 12 hours, swallowing whole with a glass of water, with or without food. Concomitant use with CYP3A4/5 inhibitors, including grapefruit juice, or inducers may alter exposure to axitinib and should be avoided. If patients have moderate hepatic impairment, the dose should be adjusted. No data are available for severe hepatic impairment. Dosing should be held beginning at least 24 hours before surgery because of risk of impaired wound healing. Time to restart therapy is based on clinical judgment. Do not use in patients with untreated brain metastasis or recent active GI bleeding because of risk of hemorrhage. (Pfizer Inc., 2014)
Belinostat (Beleodaq®)	Inhibits HDAC, causing accumulation of acetylated histones and other proteins, leading to cell cycle arrest and apoptosis of transformed cells	IV	Relapsed or refractory peripheral T-cell lymphoma	Thrombocytopenia, leukopenia (neutropenia and lymphopenia), anemia, infections (e.g., pneumonia, sepsis), hepatotoxicity, TLS, nausea, fatigue, pyrexia, vomiting	Infuse IV over 30 minutes with a 0.22 mcm in-line filter. If infusion pain or other symptoms potentially attributable to the infusion occur, infusion time may be extended to 45 minutes. The infusion bag with drug solution may be stored at room temperature for up to 36 hours, including infusion time. Avoid concomitant administration with strong inhibitors of UGT1A1. Avoid use in patients with moderate or severe hepatic dysfunction and severe renal dysfunction. Dose adjustments for hematologic toxicity should be based on the nadir counts in the preceding cycle. ANC and platelets should recover prior to starting the subsequent cycle. (Spectrum Pharmaceuticals, Inc., 2017)

(Continued on next page)

Table 8-1. Targeted Therapies *(Continued)*

Drug	Mechanism of Action	Route	Indications	Side Effects	Nursing Considerations
Bortezomib (Velcade®)	Inhibits chymotrypsin-like activity of 26S proteasome, resulting in disruption of cellular homeostatic mechanisms that can lead to cell death	IV, SC	Multiple myeloma Mantle cell lymphoma	Peripheral neuropathy, neuralgia, hypotension, cardiac failure, pulmonary toxicity, nausea, vomiting, diarrhea, constipation, fatigue, thrombocytopenia, neutropenia, RPLS, TLS, hepatotoxicity, rash, pyrexia, anorexia	For IV administration, a 3- to 5-second bolus IV injection is used. For SC injection, the administration site should be rotated in the thigh or abdomen. Select new site at least 1 inch from old site and avoid tender or bruised areas. Drug is fatal if given intrathecally. Reconstitute only with NS. Use reconstituted solution within 8 hours. Concentrations of SC (2.5 mg/ml) and IV (1 mg/ml) doses are different, and final volume depends on calculated dose. Concomitant use with CYP3A4 inhibitors, including grapefruit juice, or inducers may alter exposure to bortezomib. Patients on an oral antidiabetic agent require close monitoring of their blood glucose and may need adjustment of their antidiabetic medication. If patients have moderate or severe hepatic impairment, dosing should be adjusted. Monitor hydration status and treat as necessary. Prior to starting each cycle, platelets, ANC, and hemoglobin should be assessed for potential dose adjustment. (Millennium Pharmaceuticals, Inc., 2017)
Bosutinib (Bosulif®)	Inhibits *BCR-ABL* tyrosine kinase created by the Ph+ genetic abnormality, inhibiting proliferation, and induces apoptosis in *BCR-ABL*+ cell lines	PO	Ph+ CML in chronic phase Chronic, accelerated, or blast phase Ph+ CML that is resistant or intolerant to other therapies	Diarrhea, nausea, vomiting, abdominal pain, thrombocytopenia, anemia, hepatotoxicity, fluid retention presenting as pericardial effusion, pulmonary edema, peripheral edema, rash, respiratory tract infections, pyrexia, fatigue, cough, headache	Patients should take daily with food. Do not crush or cut tablets. If patients miss a dose beyond 12 hours, they should skip the dose and take the usual dose on the following day. Concomitant use with CYP3A4 inhibitors, including grapefruit juice, or inducers may alter exposure to bosutinib. Use of proton pump inhibitors may reduce bosutinib concentration and is not recommended. Use of antacids or H_2 antagonists should be separated from bosutinib administration by more than 2 hours. Monitor liver transaminases and hold dose if elevations > 5 × ULN occur. Discontinue if bilirubin elevations > 2 × ULN or alkaline phosphatase elevations occur. Hold dosing and adjust dose if severe or persistent thrombocytopenia or neutropenia occurs. Hold dosing if other clinically significant moderate or severe nonhematologic toxicities occur, then restart once symptoms abate. (Pfizer Inc., 2017a)

(Continued on next page)

Table 8-1. Targeted Therapies *(Continued)*

Drug	Mechanism of Action	Route	Indications	Side Effects	Nursing Considerations
Brigatinib (Alunbrig®)	Multikinase inhibitor that targets ALK, IGF-1R, FLT3, and ROS1, which inhibits subsequent downstream signaling proteins	PO	ALK-positive metastatic NSCLC in patients who have progressed on or are intolerant to crizotinib	ILD/pneumonitis, hypertension, bradycardia, visual disturbance, CPK elevation, pancreatic enzyme elevation, hyperglycemia	Patients should take once daily with or without food. Tablets should be taken whole and not crushed or chewed. Dose should be increased on day 7 if tolerated. If brigatinib therapy is interrupted for 14 days or longer, resume treatment at lower starting dose. If patients miss or vomit a dose, they should skip the dose and take the usual dose the following day. Concomitant use with CYP3A4 inhibitors, including grapefruit juice, or inducers may alter exposure to brigatinib. Dose modifications are required based on the severity of the adverse reaction. Discontinue in patients unable to tolerate 60 mg daily. Hormonal contraceptives may be ineffective because of decreased exposure when used concurrently with brigatinib. Women of reproductive potential should use contraception during treatment and for 4 months following completion of therapy. Men should use contraception during treatment and for 3 months following completion of therapy. (Takeda Pharmaceuticals Co., 2017)
Cabozantinib (Cometriq® [capsules]; Cabometyx® [tablets])	Inhibits tyrosine kinase activity of multiple receptor kinases involved with oncogenesis, metastasis, tumor angiogenesis, and maintenance of the tumor microenvironment	PO	Capsules: Progressive, metastatic, medullary thyroid cancer Tablets: Advanced RCC in patients who have received prior antiangiogenic therapy	Black box: Perforations and fistulas, hemorrhage Thrombotic events (e.g., myocardial infarction, cerebral infarction), wound complications, hypertension, osteonecrosis of the jaw, hand-foot syndrome, proteinuria, RPLS, diarrhea, stomatitis, weight loss, decreased appetite, nausea, fatigue, oral pain, hair color changes, dysgeusia, abdominal pain, constipation; increased AST, ALT, and alkaline phosphatase; lymphopenia, hypocalcemia, neutropenia, thrombocytopenia, hypophosphatemia, hyperbilirubinemia	DO NOT substitute capsules for tablets or vice versa. Patients should take once daily. Drug should not be taken with food. Patients should not eat at least 2 hours before and 1 hour after taking cabozantinib. Capsules should be swallowed whole and not opened. Missed doses should not be taken within 12 hours of the next dose. Concomitant use with CYP3A4 inhibitors, including grapefruit juice, or inducers and MRP2 inhibitors may alter exposure to cabozantinib. Dose adjustments are required in patients with hepatic impairment. Dose modifications are required based on the severity of the adverse reaction. Discontinue in patients unable to tolerate 60 mg daily (thyroid cancer) or 20 mg daily (RCC). Treatment with cabozantinib should be held at least 28 days prior to scheduled surgery, including dental surgery, and resumed based on clinical assessment of wound healing. Women of reproductive potential should use contraception during treatment and for 4 months following completion of therapy. (Exelixis, Inc., 2016a, 2016b)

(Continued on next page)

Table 8-1. Targeted Therapies *(Continued)*

Drug	Mechanism of Action	Route	Indications	Side Effects	Nursing Considerations
Carfilzomib (Kyprolis®)	Binds to and inhibits the 20S proteasome, resulting in antiproliferative and antiapoptotic activities	IV	In combination with dexamethasone or lenalidomide plus dexamethasone for relapsed or refractory multiple myeloma in patients who have received 1–3 prior lines of therapy Single agent for relapsed or refractory multiple myeloma in patients who have received at least 1 prior line of therapy	Cardiac failure or ischemia, acute renal failure, TLS, pulmonary toxicity (acute respiratory distress syndrome, acute respiratory failure, acute diffuse infiltrative pulmonary disease), pulmonary hypertension, dyspnea, hypertension including hypertensive crisis, venous thromboembolism, infusion reactions, hemorrhage, thrombocytopenia, anemia, hepatotoxicity and hepatic failure, thrombotic microangiopathy, RPLS, fatigue, nausea, pyrexia, dyspnea, diarrhea, headache, cough, peripheral edema, insomnia, muscle spasm, upper respiratory tract infection, hypokalemia	Administer IV over 10 minutes or 30 minutes depending on the dosage regimen. If patient's body surface area exceeds 2.2 m^2, calculate the dose based on a body surface area of 2.2 m^2. Give patients hydration prior to and following administration as needed. Recommended hydration includes oral fluids (30 ml/kg at least 48 hours before cycle 1, day 1) and IV fluids (250–500 ml of appropriate fluid). Premedicate with dexamethasone PO/IV prior to each dose during the first cycle and in subsequent cycles if infusion reactions occur. Premedication should be given at least 30 minutes, but no more than 4 hours, prior to all doses. Do not administer mixed with other IV medications. Infusion line should be flushed with NS or D5W before and after administration of carfilzomib. Store unopened vials in refrigerator. Reconstituted product is stable for 24 hours under refrigeration or 4 hours at room temperature. Adjust dose for mild or moderate hepatic impairment. Antiviral prophylaxis should be considered in patients with a history of herpes zoster infection. Thromboprophylaxis should be administered in patients receiving concurrent therapy with dexamethasone or lenalidomide. Increased fatal and serious toxicities may occur when drug is given in combination with melphalan and prednisone in newly diagnosed transplant-ineligible patients. (Onyx Pharmaceuticals, Inc., 2017)

(Continued on next page)

Table 8-1. Targeted Therapies *(Continued)*

Drug	Mechanism of Action	Route	Indications	Side Effects	Nursing Considerations
Ceritinib (Zykadia®)	Kinase inhibitor that targets ALK, IGF-1R, INSR, and ROS1, inhibiting proliferation of ALK-dependent cancer cells	PO	ALK-positive, metastatic NSCLC	Diarrhea, nausea, vomiting, abdominal pain, hepatotoxicity, ILD/pneumonitis, QT interval prolongation, hyperglycemia, bradycardia, pancreatitis, fatigue, decreased appetite, weight loss	Patients should take once daily with food. If patients miss a dose, they should make up that dose unless the next dose is due within 12 hours. If vomiting occurs, patients should not take an additional dose. Concomitant use with CYP3A4 inhibitors, including grapefruit juice, or inducers may alter exposure to ceritinib. Avoid use of ceritinib with CYP3A4 or CYP2C9 substrates (e.g., fentanyl, warfarin). If patients have moderate or severe hepatic impairment, dose should be adjusted. Dose modifications are required based on the severity of the adverse reaction. Discontinue in patients unable to tolerate 300 mg daily. Monitor heart rate and blood pressure regularly. Advise patients to report any changes in heart or blood pressure medication. Women of reproductive potential should use contraception during treatment and for 6 months following completion of therapy. Men should use contraception during treatment and for 3 months following completion of therapy. (Novartis Pharmaceuticals Corp., 2017j)
Cobimetinib (Cotellic®)	Reversible inhibitor of kinases in the RAS/RAF/MEK/ERK pathway, leading to inhibition of tumor cell growth	PO	Unresectable or metastatic melanoma with BRAF V600E or V600K mutation in combination with vemurafenib	New primary malignancies (cutaneous and noncutaneous), hemorrhage, cardiomyopathy, severe skin rash, retinopathy/retinal vein occlusion, hepatotoxicity, rhabdomyolysis, photosensitivity, diarrhea, nausea, pyrexia, vomiting, CPK elevation, hypophosphatemia, lymphopenia, hyponatremia	Patients should take once daily, with or without food, for the first 21 days of a 28-day cycle. If patients miss or vomit a dose, they should skip the dose and take the usual dose on the following day. Concomitant use with CYP3A4 inhibitors, including grapefruit juice, or inducers may alter exposure to cobimetinib. Dose modifications are required based on the severity of the adverse reaction. Discontinue in patients unable to tolerate 20 mg daily. Evaluate LVEF before treatment, after 1 month of treatment, then every 3 months during treatment. Advise patients to minimize sun exposure and use broad-spectrum sunscreen and lip balm (SPF $\geq$ 30). Women of reproductive potential should use contraception during treatment and for 2 weeks following completion of therapy. (Genentech, Inc., 2016b)

(Continued on next page)

Table 8-1. Targeted Therapies *(Continued)*

Drug	Mechanism of Action	Route	Indications	Side Effects	Nursing Considerations
Copanlisib (Aliqopa™)	Inhibits PI3K with inhibitory activity predominantly against PI3Kα and PI3Kδ isoforms expressed in malignant B cells, leading to induction of tumor cell death by apoptosis and inhibition of proliferation of malignant B-cell lines	IV	Relapsed follicular lymphoma in patients who have received at least 2 prior systemic therapies	Infections, hyperglycemia, hypertension, noninfectious pneumonitis, neutropenia, severe cutaneous reactions, diarrhea, decreased general strength and energy, leukopenia, nausea, lower respiratory tract infections, thrombocytopenia	Administer IV over 60 minutes. The single-dose vial should be reconstituted with 4.4 ml of 0.9% NaCl solution using a 5 ml syringe. Further dilute the appropriate dosage amount of the reconstituted solution in 100 ml 0.9% NaCl solution. Store reconstituted solution in the vial or diluted solution in the infusion bag in the refrigerator for up to 24 hours. Allow product to return to room temperature before use. Avoid exposure of diluted solution to direct sunlight. Concomitant use with CYP3A4 inhibitors, including grapefruit juice, or inducers may alter exposure to copanlisib. Dose modifications are required based on the severity of the adverse reaction. Consider PJP prophylaxis for populations at risk. Blood glucose levels typically peak 5–8 hours following infusion and subsequently decline to baseline in most patients. Blood pressure typically remains elevated for 6–8 hours following the infusion. Women and men of reproductive potential should use contraception during treatment and for 1 month following completion of therapy. (Bayer HealthCare Pharmaceuticals Inc., 2017a)
Crizotinib (Xalkori®)	Inhibits multiple tyrosine kinases, including ALK, HGFR, ROS1, and RON, which reduces tumor cell proliferation and survival	PO	Locally advanced or metastatic ALK-positive NSCLC Metastatic NSCLC in patients whose tumors are ROS1 positive	Hepatotoxicity, ILD/pneumonitis, QT prolongation, bradycardia, vision loss, nausea, diarrhea, vomiting, edema, constipation, neutropenia, fatigue, anorexia, upper respiratory tract infection, dizziness, neuropathy	Patients should take twice daily with or without food. Capsules should be swallowed whole and not crushed, chewed, or opened. If patients miss a dose, they should make up that dose unless the next dose is due within 6 hours. If vomiting occurs after taking a dose, patients should take the next dose at the regular time. Concomitant use with CYP3A4 inhibitors, including grapefruit juice, or inducers may alter exposure to crizotinib. Avoid use of crizotinib with CYP3A4 substrates (e.g., fentanyl, midazolam). Dose adjustment is required with severe renal impairment. Dose modifications are required based on the severity of the adverse reaction. Discontinue in patients unable to tolerate 250 mg daily. Monitor and correct for hypomagnesemia and hypokalemia to reduce risk of QT prolongation. Do not use in patients with hypokalemia, hypomagnesemia, or long QT syndrome.

(Continued on next page)

Table 8-1. Targeted Therapies *(Continued)*

Drug	Mechanism of Action	Route	Indications	Side Effects	Nursing Considerations
Crizotinib (Xalkori®) *(cont.)*					Monitor heart rate and blood pressure regularly. Advise patients to report any changes in heart or blood pressure medication. Women of reproductive potential should use contraception during treatment and for 45 days following completion of therapy. Men should use contraception during treatment and for 90 days following completion of therapy. (Pfizer Inc., 2017d)
Dabrafenib (Tafinlar®)	Inhibits some mutated forms of BRAF kinases to inhibit tumor cell growth *Note. Dabrafenib and trametinib target two different kinases in the RAS/RAF/MEK/ERK pathway, leading to greater inhibition of tumor growth.*	PO	Single agent for patients with unresectable or metastatic melanoma with BRAF V600E mutation Combination with trametinib for patients with unresectable or metastatic melanoma with BRAF V600E mutation or V600K mutation Combination with trametinib for patients with NSCLC with BRAF V600E mutation Combination with trametinib for anaplastic thyroid cancer with BRAF V600E mutations	New primary malignancies (cutaneous and noncutaneous), tumor promotion in BRAF wild-type melanoma, hemorrhage, cardiomyopathy, uveitis, febrile reactions (pyrexia), serious to mild skin rash, hyperglycemia, hemolytic anemia, hyperkeratosis, headache, arthralgia, papilloma, alopecia, hand-foot syndrome, cough, fatigue, nausea, vomiting, diarrhea, dry skin, anorexia, edema, chills, dyspnea	Patients should take twice daily approximately 12 hours apart and at least 1 hour before or 2 hours after a meal. Patients should not take a missed dose within 6 hours of the next dose. Do not open, crush, or break the capsules. Concomitant use with CYP3A4 or CYP2C8 inhibitors, including grapefruit juice, or inducers may alter exposure to dabrafenib. Avoid use of dabrafenib with CYP3A4, CYP2C8, CYP2C9, CYP2C19, or CYP2B6 substrates (e.g., warfarin) because of loss of efficacy of these agents. Dose modifications are required based on the severity of the adverse reaction. Discontinue in patients unable to tolerate at least 50 mg twice daily. Assess LVEF before initiation, one month after initiation, and then at intervals of 2–3 months while on treatment. For patients who develop a severe febrile reaction or fever associated with complications, administer antipyretics as secondary prophylaxis when resuming dabrafenib. Administer corticosteroids for at least 5 days for second or subsequent development of pyrexia if temperature does not return to baseline within 3 days of onset. Hormonal contraceptives may be ineffective because of decreased exposure when used concurrently with dabrafenib. Advise women of reproductive potential to use nonhormonal contraception during treatment and for at least 2 weeks following completion of therapy. (Novartis Pharmaceuticals Corp., 2017f)

(Continued on next page)

Table 8-1. Targeted Therapies *(Continued)*

Drug	Mechanism of Action	Route	Indications	Side Effects	Nursing Considerations
Dasatinib (Sprycel®)	Inhibits multiple tyrosine kinases, including *BCR-ABL*, SRC family, c-KIT, EPHA2, and PDGFR-beta	PO	Ph+ CML in chronic phase Chronic, accelerated, or myeloid or lymphoid blast phase Ph+ CML with resistance or intolerance to prior therapy including imatinib Ph+ ALL with resistance or intolerance to prior therapy	Myelosuppression/bleeding events, fluid retention including pleural effusions, cardiac dysfunction, pulmonary arterial hypertension, QT prolongation, dermatologic toxicities, TLS, diarrhea, headache, fatigue, dyspnea, nausea, musculoskeletal pain	Patients should take once daily with or without food either in the morning or in the evening. Do not crush or cut tablets. Use with caution in patients taking anticoagulants. Concomitant use with CYP3A4 inhibitors, including grapefruit juice, or inducers may alter exposure to dasatinib and should be avoided. If concomitant use cannot be avoided, dose adjustment of dasatinib should be made. Use of proton pump inhibitors or H_2 antagonists may reduce dasatinib concentration and is not recommended. Use of antacids should be separated from administration of dasatinib by ≥ 2 hours. Elevation of transaminases or bilirubin, hypocalcemia, and hypophosphatemia may occur. Hypocalcemia may require oral calcium supplements. (Bristol-Myers Squibb Co., 2017)
Eltrombopag (Promacta®)	TPO receptor agonist that interacts with the transmembrane domain of the human TPO receptor and initiates signaling cascades that induce proliferation and differentiation from bone marrow progenitor cells	PO	Thrombocytopenia with chronic immune (idiopathic) thrombocytopenia in patients who have had an insufficient response to corticosteroids, immunoglobulins, or splenectomy Thrombocytopenia with chronic hepatitis C to allow initiation and maintenance of interferon-based therapy Severe aplastic anemia with an insufficient response to immunosuppressive therapy	Black box: In patients with chronic hepatitis C, eltrombopag in combination with interferon and ribavirin may increase the risk of hepatic decompensation. Hepatotoxicity, thrombotic/thromboembolic complications, nausea, diarrhea, upper respiratory tract infection, vomiting, increased ALT, myalgia, urinary tract infection, nasopharyngitis, anemia, pyrexia, fatigue, headache, decreased appetite, influenza-like illness, asthenia, insomnia, cough, pruritus, chills, myalgia, alopecia, peripheral edema, cataracts	Patients should take once daily on an empty stomach 1 hour before or 2 hours after a meal. Do not crush tablets and mix with food or liquids. Prior to using the oral suspension, patients or caregivers must receive proper education on dosing, preparation, and administration. Administer the oral suspension immediately after preparation. Discard any suspension not administered within 30 minutes of preparation. Prepare with water only. DO NOT use hot water. When switching between the tablet and oral suspension, assess platelet counts for 2 weeks, then change to monthly monitoring. Dose modification may be necessary for patients with mild, moderate, or severe hepatic impairment and some patients of East Asian ancestry. Adjust dose to maintain a platelet count ≥ 50,000/mm^3. DO NOT exceed 75 mg/day. Patients should take 2 hours before or 4 hours after any medications or products containing polyvalent cations (e.g., antacids, calcium-rich foods, mineral supplements). Use caution when coadministering with substrates of OATP1B1 or BCRP. (Novartis Pharmaceuticals Corp., 2017d)

(Continued on next page)

Table 8-1. Targeted Therapies *(Continued)*

Drug	Mechanism of Action	Route	Indications	Side Effects	Nursing Considerations
Enasidenib (Idhifa®)	Inhibits the IDH2 enzyme, leading to decreased 2-hydroxyglutarate levels and induction of myeloid differentiation	PO	Relapsed or refractory AML with an IDH2 mutation	Black box: Differentiation syndrome (symptoms: fever, dyspnea, acute respiratory distress, pulmonary infiltrates, pleural or pericardial effusions, rapid weight gain or peripheral edema, lymphadenopathy, bone pain, and hepatic, renal, and multiorgan dysfunction) Embryo-fetal toxicity, nausea, vomiting, diarrhea, elevated bilirubin, decreased appetite, TLS, noninfectious leukocytosis	Patients should take once daily with or without food at approximately the same time each day. If a dose is vomited, missed, or not taken at the usual time, administer the dose as soon as possible on the same day, and return to the normal schedule the following day. Patients should not take 2 doses to make up for the missed dose. Do not split or crush tablets; instruct patients to swallow whole with a cup of water. Keep the bottle tightly closed. Store in the original bottle (with a desiccant canister) to protect from moisture. If no disease progression or unacceptable toxicity, treat for a minimum of 6 months to allow time for clinical response. If differentiation syndrome is suspected, initiate oral or IV corticosteroids (e.g., dexamethasone 10 mg every 12 hours). Taper only after resolution of symptoms. If patients require intubation or ventilator support or renal dysfunction is present for more than 48 hours after initiation of corticosteroids, interrupt enasidenib until symptoms are no longer severe. Use caution when coadministering substrates of various CYP enzymes. Hormonal contraceptives may be ineffective because of decreased exposure when used concurrently with enasidenib. Women and men of reproductive potential should use contraception during treatment and for 1 month following completion of therapy. (Celgene Corp., 2017)
Erlotinib (Tarceva®)	Inhibits autophosphorylation of tyrosine kinase associated with EGFR, inhibiting further downstream signaling	PO	Metastatic NSCLC whose tumors express EGFR exon 19 deletions or exon 21 (L858R) substitution mutations for first-line, maintenance, or second or greater treatment following at least 1 prior chemotherapy regimen First-line treatment for locally advanced, unresectable, or metastatic pancreatic cancer in combination with gemcitabine	ILD (dyspnea, cough, fever), renal failure, hepatotoxicity, GI perforations, bullous and exfoliative skin disorders, ocular disorders, hemorrhage in combination with warfarin, rash, diarrhea, anorexia, fatigue, nausea, vomiting In patients with pancreatic cancer: cerebrovascular accident, microangiopathic hemolytic anemia	Patients should take once daily on an empty stomach at least 1 hour before or 2 hours after food. Concomitant use with CYP3A4 and CYP1A2 inhibitors, including grapefruit juice, or inducers may alter exposure to erlotinib. Cigarette smoking may decrease erlotinib concentrations; avoid concomitant use. Drugs that increase gastric pH decrease erlotinib concentrations. For PPIs, avoid concomitant use. For H_2 antagonists, take erlotinib 10 hours after H_2 antagonist. For antacids, separate dosing by several hours. Monitor LFTs and consider dose reductions. Regularly monitor INR in patients receiving warfarin. Monitor for GI bleeding and elevated INR. Diarrhea can be managed using loperamide. Women of reproductive potential should use contraception during treatment and for at least 1 month following completion of therapy. (Genentech, Inc., 2016d)

(Continued on next page)

Table 8-1. Targeted Therapies *(Continued)*

Drug	Mechanism of Action	Route	Indications	Side Effects	Nursing Considerations
Everolimus (Afinitor®, Afinitor Disperz® tablets for oral suspension)	Binds to FKBP12 intracellular protein and inhibits mTOR, which is a serine-threonine kinase downstream of the PI3K/AKT pathway, resulting in reduced cell proliferation and angiogenesis	PO	Postmenopausal women with advanced HR-positive, HER2-negative breast cancer in combination with exemestane after patients have failed treatment with letrozole or anastrozole Progressive NET of pancreatic origin and progressive, well-differentiated, nonfunctional NETs of lung or GI origin that are unresectable, locally advanced, or metastatic Advanced RCC after failed treatment with sunitinib or sorafenib Renal angiomyolipoma and tuberous sclerosis complex not requiring surgery Tuberous sclerosis complex in patients who have subependymal giant cell astrocytoma that requires therapeutic intervention but cannot be resected *Note: Afinitor Disperz is indicated for tuberous sclerosis complex with subependymal giant cell astrocytoma only. Everolimus branded as Zortress® is indicated to prevent rejection in solid organ transplant recipients.*	Noninfectious pneumonitis, infections, angioedema, oral ulceration/stomatitis, renal failure, impaired wound healing, proteinuria, hyperglycemia, hyperlipidemia, anemia, neutropenia, thrombocytopenia, rash, fatigue, diarrhea, edema, abdominal pain, nausea, fever, asthenia, cough, headache, decreased appetite, respiratory tract infection	Patients should take drug at the same time each day and consistently either with or without food. Tablets should be swallowed whole with a full glass of water. Do not break or crush tablets. Patients with tuberous sclerosis complex who have subependymal giant cell astrocytoma only: Dosing should be adjusted to maintain trough concentrations of 5–15 ng/ml. Trough levels should be monitored routinely using the same assay and laboratory throughout treatment. Measure trough concentrations 2 weeks after starting treatment and with changes in dose, interacting drugs, hepatic function, body size, or dosage form (oral tablets or tablets for oral suspension). Dose modifications are required based on the severity of the adverse reaction. Concomitant use with CYP3A4 inhibitors, including grapefruit juice, or inducers may alter exposure to everolimus. Concomitant use with P-gp inhibitors, such as verapamil or diltiazem, may alter exposure to everolimus. Disperz tablets can be used to prepare an oral suspension. • Prepare oral suspension in 25 ml of water only, immediately prior to use, and discard if not administered within 60 minutes. Prepared doses should not exceed 10 mg. If higher doses are required, prepare a second dose. Once tablets are added to water, allow 3 minutes for suspension to form, stir gently, and have patients drink. After administration, add 25 ml additional water to the same glass and stir with the same spoon to suspend any remaining particles, and administer to patient. • Oral suspension may be administered using a 10 ml oral syringe in doses not to exceed 10 mg per syringe. Draw 5 ml of water and 4 ml of air into the syringe. Place the filled syringe tip up into a container for 3 minutes until the tablets are in suspension. Invert the syringe 5 times prior to administration. After dosing via an oral syringe, rinse the syringe with 5 ml of water to capture remaining drug particles, and administer to patient. Patients should avoid live vaccines and close contact with those who have received live vaccines. Adjust dose for hepatic impairment. Women of reproductive potential should use contraception during treatment and for at least 8 weeks following completion of therapy. (Novartis Pharmaceuticals Corp., 2016a)

(Continued on next page)

Table 8-1. Targeted Therapies *(Continued)*

Drug	Mechanism of Action	Route	Indications	Side Effects	Nursing Considerations
Gefitinib (Iressa®)	Inhibits autophosphorylation of tyrosine kinase associated with EGFR, inhibiting further downstream signaling	PO	First-line metastatic NSCLC in patients whose tumors express EGFR exon 19 deletions or exon 21 (L858R) substitution mutations	ILD, hepatotoxicity, GI perforation, diarrhea, ocular disorders including keratitis, bullous and exfoliative skin disorders, hemorrhage in patients taking warfarin, skin reactions	Patients should take once daily with or without food. They should not take a missed dose within 12 hours of the next dose. For patients who have difficulty swallowing solids, immerse gefitinib in 4–8 oz of water and stir for approximately 15 minutes. Have patients drink immediately or administer through nasogastric tube. Rinse the container with 4–8 oz of water and have patients drink immediately or administer through the nasogastric tube. Concomitant use with CYP3A4 inhibitors, including grapefruit juice, or inducers may alter exposure to gefitinib. Regularly monitor INR in patients receiving warfarin. Monitor for GI bleeding and elevated INR. Drugs that increase gastric pH decrease gefitinib concentrations. For PPIs, take gefitinib 12 hours after the last dose or 12 hours before the next dose of the PPI. For H_2 antagonists, take gefitinib 6 hours after or 6 hours before H_2 antagonist or an antacid. Women of reproductive potential should use contraception during treatment and for at least 2 weeks following completion of therapy. (AstraZeneca Pharmaceuticals LP, 2015)
Ibrutinib (Imbruvica®)	Inhibits Bruton tyrosine kinase, which is a signaling molecule of the B-cell antigen receptor, leading to inhibition of malignant B-cell proliferation	PO	Patients with mantle cell lymphoma who have received at least 1 prior therapy CLL/SLL with 17p deletion Waldenström macroglobulinemia Patients with marginal zone lymphoma who require systemic therapy and have received at least 1 prior anti-CD20-based therapy Graft-versus-host disease	Hemorrhage, infections (e.g., progressive multifocal leukoencephalopathy, PML), thrombocytopenia, neutropenia, anemia, atrial fibrillation, hypertension, second primary malignancies, TLS, diarrhea, musculoskeletal pain, rash, nausea, bruising, fatigue, pyrexia	Patients should take once daily with a glass of water. Capsules should not be opened, broken, or chewed. If patients miss a dose, they should take it as soon as possible on the same day with a return to the normal schedule on the next day. Concomitant use with CYP3A4 inhibitors, including grapefruit juice, or inducers may alter exposure to ibrutinib. Coadministration of P-gp or BCRP substrates (e.g., digoxin, methotrexate) will increase their blood concentrations. Avoid use in patients with moderate or severe baseline hepatic impairment. Dose modifications are required based on the severity of the adverse reaction. Discontinue in patients unable to tolerate after 3 dose changes. Secondary to hemorrhage risk, consider withholding ibrutinib for at least 3–7 days pre- and postsurgery. Women and men of reproductive potential should use contraception during treatment and for at least 1 month following completion of therapy. (Pharmacyclics LLC & Janssen Biotech, Inc., 2017)

(Continued on next page)

Table 8-1. Targeted Therapies *(Continued)*

Drug	Mechanism of Action	Route	Indications	Side Effects	Nursing Considerations
Idelalisib (Zydelig®)	Inhibits PI3Kδ, which is expressed in normal and malignant B cells, leading to apoptosis and inhibited cell proliferations via chemotaxis, adhesion, and reduced cell viability	PO	Relapsed CLL in combination with rituximab in patients for whom rituximab alone would be considered appropriate therapy because of other comorbidities Relapsed follicular B-cell NHL in patients who have received at least 2 prior systemic therapies Relapsed SLL in patients who have received at least 2 prior systemic therapies	Black box: Hepatotoxicity, diarrhea, colitis, pneumonitis, infections, intestinal perforation Cutaneous reactions, anaphylaxis, neutropenia, diarrhea, fatigue, nausea, cough, pyrexia, abdominal pain, pneumonia, rash, neutropenia, increased AST/ALT	Patients should take twice daily with or without food and swallow tablets whole. Concomitant use with CYP3A4 inhibitors, including grapefruit juice, or inducers may alter exposure to idelalisib. Avoid use of idelalisib with CYP3A4 substrates (e.g., fentanyl). Dose modifications are required based on the severity of the adverse reaction. Discontinue in patients unable to tolerate at least 100 mg twice daily. Consider PJP prophylaxis. Diarrhea caused by idelalisib responds poorly to antimotility agents. Corticosteroids may be needed to resolve diarrhea or pneumonitis. (Gilead Sciences, Inc., 2016)
Imatinib mesylate (Gleevec®)	Inhibits *BCR-ABL* tyrosine kinase created by the Ph+ genetic abnormality, inhibiting proliferation and inducing apoptosis in *BCR-ABL*+ cell lines; also inhibits PDGF, SCF, and c-KIT	PO	Newly diagnosed Ph+ CML in chronic phase Ph+ CML in blast crisis, accelerated phase, or chronic phase after failure of interferon-alfa therapy Relapsed or refractory Ph+ ALL MDS/myeloproliferative diseases associated with *PDGFR* gene rearrangements ASM without D816V c-KIT mutation or unknown c-KIT mutation status Hypereosinophilic syndrome and/or chronic eosinophilic leukemia in patients who have the FIP1L1-PDGFRα fusion kinase or unknown fusion kinase status Unresectable, recurrent, or metastatic dermatofibrosarcoma protuberans KIT (CD117)-positive unresectable or metastatic malignant GIST Adjuvant treatment of resected KIT (CD117)-positive GIST	Edema, fluid retention, effusions, neutropenia, thrombocytopenia, anemia, cardiomyopathy/cardiogenic shock, hepatotoxicity, hemorrhage, GI perforations, dermatologic toxicities, hypothyroidism, growth retardation (children and preadolescents), TLS, nausea, vomiting, muscle cramps, musculoskeletal pain, diarrhea, rash, fatigue, abdominal pain	Patients should take with a meal and a full glass of water. Dosing may be once or twice daily. For patients unable to swallow tablets, tablets may be dissolved in a glass of water or apple juice immediately before administration. Use 50 ml for a 100 mg tablet and 200 ml for a 400 mg tablet. Concomitant use with CYP3A4 or CYP2D6 inhibitors, including grapefruit juice, or inducers may alter exposure to imatinib. Avoid use of imatinib with CYP3A4 or CYP2D6 substrates. Patients requiring anticoagulation should receive low-molecular-weight or standard heparin and not warfarin because of high propensity of drug–drug interactions. Dose modifications are required in patients with severe hepatic impairment and moderate or severe renal impairment. Weigh patients frequently and monitor for signs and symptoms of fluid retention. In patients with high eosinophil levels, consider prophylactic use of systemic steroid for 1–2 weeks concurrently with initiation of imatinib. (Novartis Pharmaceuticals Corp., 2017a)

(Continued on next page)

Table 8-1. Targeted Therapies *(Continued)*

Drug	Mechanism of Action	Route	Indications	Side Effects	Nursing Considerations
Ixazomib (Ninlaro®)	Reversible proteasome inhibitor leading to apoptosis of myeloma cells	PO	In combination with lenalidomide and dexamethasone for the treatment of patients with multiple myeloma who have received at least 1 prior therapy	Thrombocytopenia, diarrhea, constipation, nausea, vomiting, peripheral neuropathy, peripheral edema, rash, hepatotoxicity, back pain	Patients should take on days 1, 8, and 15 of a 28-day cycle at approximately the same time and with water at least 1 hour before or 2 hours after food. Capsules should not be crushed, chewed, or opened. Drug should be stored in the original packaging and not removed until just prior to taking. If a dose is delayed or missed, the dose should only be taken if the next scheduled dose is ≥ 72 hours away. If vomiting occurs, do not repeat the dose. Concomitant use with CYP3A4 inducers may alter exposure to ixazomib. Dose modifications are required in patients with moderate or severe hepatic impairment and severe renal impairment. Assess hematologic parameters prior to initiating a new cycle. Consider antiviral prophylaxis to decrease risk of herpes zoster reactivation. Hormonal contraceptives may be ineffective when used concurrently. Advise women of reproductive potential to use nonhormonal contraception during treatment and for at least 90 days after the final dose. (Millennium Pharmaceuticals, Inc., 2015)
Lapatinib (Tykerb®)	4-Anilinoquinazoline kinase inhibitor of the intracellular tyrosine kinase domains of both EGFR and HER2	PO	In combination with capecitabine for treatment of patients with advanced or metastatic breast cancer whose tumors overexpress HER2 and who have received prior therapy including an anthracycline, a taxane, and trastuzumab In combination with letrozole in postmenopausal women with HR-positive metastatic breast cancer that overexpresses HER2 for whom hormone therapy is indicated	Black box: Hepatotoxicity Decreased LVEF, diarrhea, ILD/pneumonitis, QT prolongation, cutaneous reactions, hand-foot syndrome, nausea, rash, vomiting, fatigue	Patients should take once daily at least 1 hour before or 1 hour after a meal. Do not divide the daily dose. However, capecitabine should be taken with a meal or within 30 minutes after a meal. If a dose is missed, the patient should not double the dose the following day. Concomitant use with CYP3A4, CYP2C8, or P-gp inhibitors, including grapefruit juice, or inducers may alter exposure to lapatinib. Avoid use of lapatinib with CYP3A4, CYP2C8, or P-gp substrates. Dose modifications are required in patients with severe hepatic impairment. Confirm normal LVEF before beginning drug. Lapatinib should be discontinued in patients if LVEF drops below lower limits of normal. Diarrhea may be managed with antidiarrheal agents (e.g., loperamide); replace fluids and electrolytes if severe. Monitor and correct for hypomagnesemia and hypokalemia to reduce risk of QT prolongation. (Novartis Pharmaceuticals Corp., 2017h)

(Continued on next page)

Table 8-1. Targeted Therapies *(Continued)*

Drug	Mechanism of Action	Route	Indications	Side Effects	Nursing Considerations
Lenvatinib (Lenvima®)	TKI of primarily VEGF receptors, which includes angiogenesis, tumor growth, and cancer progression	PO	As a single agent for locally recurrent or metastatic, progressive, radioactive iodine–refractory differentiated thyroid cancer Advanced RCC in combination with everolimus following 1 prior antiangiogenic therapy	Hypertension, cardiac failure, arterial thromboembolic events, hepatotoxicity, proteinuria, diarrhea, renal failure and impairment, GI perforation and fistula formation, QT interval prolongation, hypocalcemia, RPLS, hemorrhagic events, thyroid dysfunction, fatigue, headache, vomiting, nausea, decreased appetite, hand-foot syndrome, abdominal pain, dysphonia, arthralgia/myalgia, stomatitis, peripheral edema, cough, dyspnea, weight loss	Patients should take once daily at the same time with or without food. The capsule should be swallowed whole or dissolved in small glass of liquid. Patient instructions for dissolving the drug: Measure 1 tablespoon of water or apple juice and put the capsules into the liquid without breaking or crushing them. Leave the capsules in the liquid for at least 10 minutes. Stir for at least 3 minutes. Drink the mixture. After drinking, add a new tablespoon of liquid to the glass, swirl a few times and drink the contents. If a dose is missed and cannot be taken within 12 hours, patients should skip that dose. Dose modifications are required in patients with severe hepatic impairment or severe renal impairment. Diarrhea may be managed with antidiarrheal agents (e.g., loperamide) and hydration as needed. Control blood pressure prior to initiating therapy. Women of reproductive potential should use contraception during treatment and for at least 2 weeks following completion of therapy. (Eisai Inc., 2017)
Midostaurin (Rydapt®)	Inhibits multiple receptor tyrosine kinases, primarily FLT3 receptor signaling, inducing apoptosis in FLT3-expressing cells	PO	Newly diagnosed AML that is FLT3 mutation–positive in combination with standard cytarabine and daunorubicin induction and cytarabine consolidation ASM, systemic mastocytosis with associated hematologic neoplasm, or mast cell leukemia	Pulmonary toxicity (ILD/pneumonitis), febrile neutropenia, nausea, mucositis, vomiting, headache, petechiae, musculoskeletal pain, epistaxis, device-related infection, hyperglycemia, upper respiratory tract infection, diarrhea, edema, abdominal pain, fatigue, constipation, pyrexia, dyspnea	Patients should take twice daily approximately every 12 hours with food. Do not open or crush the capsules. For AML, take on days 8–21 of each cycle of induction or consolidation. If patients miss or vomit a dose, they should not make up the dose. Concomitant use with CYP3A4 inhibitors, including grapefruit juice, or inducers may alter exposure to midostaurin. Administer a prophylactic antiemetic prior to each dose. For systemic mastocytosis, dosing should be adjusted based on toxicity parameters. Women and men of reproductive potential should use contraception during treatment and for at least 4 months following completion of therapy. (Novartis Pharmaceuticals Corp., 2017e)

(Continued on next page)

Table 8-1. Targeted Therapies *(Continued)*

Drug	Mechanism of Action	Route	Indications	Side Effects	Nursing Considerations
Neratinib (Nerlynx®)	Inhibits EGFR, HER2, and HER4 in EGFR- and HER2-expressing carcinoma cell lines, leading to inhibition of tumor growth	PO	Extended adjuvant treatment of early-stage HER2-overexpressed/amplified breast cancer to follow adjuvant trastuzumab-based therapy	Diarrhea, hepatotoxicity, nausea, abdominal pain, fatigue, vomiting, rash, stomatitis, decreased appetite, muscle spasms, dyspepsia, AST/ALT elevations, nail disorder, dry skin, abdominal distension, weight loss, urinary tract infection	Patients should take once daily at approximately the same time with food and swallow tablets whole. Tablets should not be chewed, crushed, or split. If a dose is missed, do not replace the missed dose. Resume with the next scheduled daily dose. Concomitant use with CYP3A4 inhibitors, including grapefruit juice, or inducers may alter exposure to neratinib. Concomitant use with P-gp substrates may alter exposure to the P-gp substrate. Avoid concomitant use with PPIs and H_2 antagonists. Separate by 3 hours from antacid dosing. Dose adjustment is required in patients with severe hepatic impairment. Dose modifications are required based on the severity of the adverse reaction. Initiate loperamide with the first dose of neratinib and continue during first 2 cycles (56 days) of treatment. Titrate to 1–2 bowel movements per day. Refer to package insert for specific loperamide prophylaxis dosing recommendations. With severe diarrhea, initiate fluids and electrolytes as needed. Women of reproductive potential should use contraception during treatment and for 1 month following completion of therapy. Men should use contraception during treatment and for 3 months following completion of therapy. (Puma Biotechnology, Inc., 2017)
Nilotinib (Tasigna®)	Binds to and stabilizes the inactive conformation of *BCR-ABL*, the kinase produced by Ph	PO	Newly diagnosed Ph+ CML in chronic phase Chronic and accelerated phase Ph+ CML in patients who are resistant or intolerant to prior therapy including imatinib	Black box: QT prolongation, sudden death Myelosuppression, cardiac and arterial vascular occlusive events, pancreatitis and elevated serum lipase, hepatotoxicity, electrolyte abnormalities (hypophosphatemia, hypokalemia, hyperkalemia, hypocalcemia, hyponatremia), TLS, hemorrhage, fluid retention, nausea, rash, headache, fatigue, pruritus, vomiting, diarrhea, cough, constipation, arthralgia, nasopharyngitis, pyrexia, night sweats	Patients should take twice daily at 12-hour intervals. No food should be consumed for at least 2 hours before the dose and 1 hour after. Patients should take capsules whole with water. For patients unable to swallow capsules, the contents may be mixed in 1 teaspoon of applesauce and taken within 15 minutes. Concomitant use with CYP3A4 inhibitors, including grapefruit juice, or inducers may alter exposure to nilotinib. Dose reduction may be necessary if inhibitors must be given, and the QTc should be monitored closely. Avoid concomitant use of drugs known to prolong QT interval. Dose modifications are required based on the severity of the adverse reaction. Monitor and correct for hypomagnesemia and hypokalemia to reduce risk of QT prolongation. Do not use in patients with hypokalemia, hypomagnesemia, or long QT syndrome. Obtain ECG at baseline, 7 days after initiation, and periodically to monitor QTc. (Novartis Pharmaceuticals Corp., 2017g)

(Continued on next page)

Table 8-1. Targeted Therapies *(Continued)*

Drug	Mechanism of Action	Route	Indications	Side Effects	Nursing Considerations
Niraparib (Zejula®)	Inhibits PARP enzymes, which play a role in DNA repair, leading to DNA damage, apoptosis, and cell death	PO	Recurrent epithelial ovarian, fallopian tube, or primary peritoneal cancer in patients who had complete or partial response to platinum-based chemotherapy	MDS/AML, bone marrow suppression, cardiovascular events, thrombocytopenia, anemia, neutropenia, leukopenia, palpitations, nausea, constipation, vomiting, abdominal pain/distension, mucositis/stomatitis, diarrhea, dyspepsia, dry mouth, fatigue/asthenia, decreased appetite, urinary tract infection, AST/ALT elevation, myalgia, back pain, arthralgia, headache, dizziness, dysgeusia, insomnia, anxiety, nasopharyngitis, dyspnea, cough, rash, hypertension	Patients should take once daily at approximately the same time with or without food. Capsules should be swallowed whole. Bedtime administration may help with managing nausea. If patients miss or vomit a dose, they should take the next dose at the next regularly scheduled time rather than taking an additional dose. Dose modifications are required based on the severity of the adverse reaction. Discontinue in patients unable to tolerate at least 100 mg daily. Treatment should start no more than 8 weeks following platinum-containing chemotherapy. Women of reproductive potential should use contraception during treatment and for at least 6 months following completion of therapy. (Tesaro, Inc., 2017)
Olaparib (Lynparza®)	Inhibits PARP enzymes that are involved in normal cellular homeostasis such as DNA transcription, cell cycle regulation, and DNA repair	PO	Maintenance treatment of recurrent epithelial ovarian, fallopian tube, or primary peritoneal cancer in patients in complete or partial response to platinum-based chemotherapy Deleterious or suspected deleterious germline *BRCA*-mutated advanced ovarian cancer in patients who have been treated with ≥ 3 prior lines of chemotherapy Breast cancer with deleterious or suspected deleterious germline *BRCA*-mutated, HER2-negative metastatic disease who have been treated with chemotherapy; in HR-positive disease, patients should have received endocrine therapy or be considered inappropriate for endocrine therapy	MDS/AML, pneumonitis, anemia, nausea, fatigue, vomiting, diarrhea, dysgeusia, dyspepsia, headache, decreased appetite, nasopharyngitis/pharyngitis/upper respiratory tract infection, cough, arthralgia/musculoskeletal pain, myalgia, back pain, dermatitis/rash, abdominal pain/discomfort, elevated serum creatinine, mean corpuscular volume elevation, leukopenia, neutropenia, thrombocytopenia	Patients should take twice daily with or without food and swallow capsule whole. Capsules should not be chewed, dissolved, or opened. If patients miss a dose, they should take the next dose at the next regularly scheduled time. Concomitant use with CYP3A4 inhibitors, including grapefruit juice, or inducers may alter exposure to olaparib. Dose adjustment is required in patients with moderate renal impairment. Women of reproductive potential should use contraception during treatment and for at least 6 months following completion of therapy. (AstraZeneca Pharmaceuticals LP, 2018)

(Continued on next page)

Table 8-1. Targeted Therapies *(Continued)*

Drug	Mechanism of Action	Route	Indications	Side Effects	Nursing Considerations
Osimertinib (Tagrisso®)	Inhibits EGFR by binding irreversibly to certain mutant forms (T790M, L858R, and exon 19 deletion)	PO	Metastatic EGFR T790M mutation-positive NSCLC in patients who have progressed on or after EGFR TKI therapy	ILD/pneumonitis, QTc prolongation, cardiomyopathy, keratitis, diarrhea, rash, dry skin, nail toxicity, fatigue	Patients should take once daily with or without food. If a dose is missed, patients should take the next dose at the next regularly scheduled time. In patients with difficulty swallowing tablets, disperse tablet in 60 ml of noncarbonated water only. Stir until tablet is dispersed into small pieces (the tablet will not completely dissolve) and swallow immediately. Do not crush, heat, or ultrasonicate during preparation. Rinse the container with 120–240 ml water and immediately drink. If administered via nasogastric tube, disperse in 15 ml of water and use an additional 15 ml to transfer any residue to a syringe. Administer this 30 ml immediately with appropriate water flushes (approximately 30 ml). Concomitant use with CYP3A4 inducers may alter exposure to osimertinib. Assess LVEF at baseline. Women of reproductive potential should use contraception during treatment and for 6 weeks following completion of therapy. Men should use contraception during treatment and for 4 months following completion of therapy. (AstraZeneca Pharmaceuticals LP, 2017b)
Palbociclib (Ibrance®)	Inhibits CDK4 and CDK6, leading to reduced cellular proliferation by blocking progression of the cell cycle from G_1 into S phase	PO	HR-positive, HER2-negative, advanced or metastatic breast cancer in combination with an aromatase inhibitor as initial endocrine-based therapy in postmenopausal women or fulvestrant in women with disease progression following endocrine therapy	Neutropenia, infections, leukopenia, fatigue, nausea, stomatitis, anemia, diarrhea, thrombocytopenia, rash, vomiting, decreased appetite, asthenia, pyrexia	Patients should take once daily with food at approximately the same time for 21 days followed by 7 days off treatment. Concomitant use with CYP3A4 inhibitors, including grapefruit juice, or inducers may alter exposure to palbociclib. CYP3A4 substrates may need dose reductions when used in combination with palbociclib. Women of reproductive potential should use contraception during treatment and for 3 weeks following completion of therapy. Men should use contraception during treatment and for 3 months following completion of therapy. (Pfizer Inc., 2017b)

(Continued on next page)

Table 8-1. Targeted Therapies *(Continued)*

Drug	Mechanism of Action	Route	Indications	Side Effects	Nursing Considerations
Panobinostat (Farydak®)	Inhibits HDAC, resulting in increased acetylation of histone proteins, inducing cell cycle arrest and/or apoptosis of cells	PO	In combination with bortezomib and dexamethasone for multiple myeloma in patients who have received at least 2 prior regimens, including bortezomib and an immunomodulatory agent	Black box: Severe diarrhea, cardiotoxicities Hemorrhage, hepatotoxicity, diarrhea, fatigue, nausea, peripheral edema, decreased appetite, pyrexia, vomiting, hypophosphatemia, hypokalemia, hyponatremia, increased creatinine, thrombocytopenia, lymphopenia, leukopenia, neutropenia, anemia	Patients should take every other day for 3 doses per week during weeks 1 and 2 of each 21-day cycle. Drug should be taken at approximately the same time each day with or without food and capsules swallowed whole with a cup of water. Capsules should not be opened, crushed, or chewed. If patients miss a dose beyond 12 hours, they should skip the dose and take the usual dose on the following day. If patients vomit a dose, they should skip the dose and take the usual dose on the following day. Patients should receive 8 cycles with potential for an additional 8 cycles for a total duration of 16 cycles. Concomitant use with CYP3A4 inhibitors, including grapefruit juice, or inducers may alter exposure to panobinostat. CYP2D6 substrates may need dose reductions when used in combination with panobinostat. Avoid concomitant use with antiarrhythmic drugs and QT-prolonging drugs. Dose adjustment is required in patients with hepatic impairment. Dose modifications are required based on the severity of the adverse reaction. Discontinue in patients unable to tolerate at least 10 mg given 3 times per week. At the first sign of diarrhea, patients should be treated with antidiarrheal medications (e.g., loperamide). Consider prophylactic antiemetics. Women of reproductive potential should use contraception during treatment and for 3 months following completion of therapy. Men should use contraception during treatment and for 6 months following completion of therapy. (Novartis Pharmaceuticals Corp., 2016b)

(Continued on next page)

Table 8-1. Targeted Therapies *(Continued)*

Drug	Mechanism of Action	Route	Indications	Side Effects	Nursing Considerations
Pazopanib (Votrient®)	Inhibits VEGFRs with tyrosine kinase activity, which interferes with tumor angiogenesis, growth, and progression	PO	Advanced RCC Advanced soft tissue sarcoma in patients who have received prior chemotherapy	Black box: Hepatotoxicity QTc prolongation, LVEF dysfunction, hemorrhage, arterial and venous thromboembolism, thrombotic microangiopathy including thrombotic thrombocytopenic purpura and hemolytic uremic syndrome, ILD/pneumonitis, GI perforation, GI fistula formation, RPLS, hypertension, hypothyroidism, proteinuria, infection, diarrhea, hair color changes, nausea, anorexia, vomiting, fatigue, decreased appetite, tumor pain, dysgeusia, headache, musculoskeletal pain, myalgia, GI pain, dyspnea	Patients should take once daily at least 1 hour before or 2 hours after a meal. Do not crush tablets. If a dose is missed beyond 12 hours, the patient should skip the dose and take the usual dose on the following day. Concomitant use of CYP3A4 inhibitors, including grapefruit juice, and inducers may alter exposure to pazopanib. Concomitant use of substrates of CYP3A4, CYP2D6, or CYP2C8 is not recommended. Concomitant use of PPIs or H_2 antagonists is not recommended; consider short-acting antacids instead. Concomitant use with simvastatin may increase risk of ALT elevations. Measure LFTs before start of pazopanib use and monitor at least monthly during the first 4 months of treatment, then periodically thereafter. Use with caution in patients with a history of QT prolongation or concomitantly using other drugs that prolong QT interval. Stop use of pazopanib at least 7 days prior to planned surgery, and restart based on clinical judgment. Dose adjustment is required in patients with moderate or severe hepatic impairment. Women and men of reproductive potential should use contraception during treatment and for 2 weeks following completion of therapy. (Novartis Pharmaceuticals Corp., 2017i)
Ponatinib (Iclusig®)	TKI of *BCR-ABL* and T315I-mutated *BCR-ABL*	PO	Chronic, accelerated, or blast phase CML or Ph+ ALL in patients for whom no other TKI is indicated T315I-positive CML (chronic, accelerated, or blast phase) or T315I-positive Ph+ ALL	Black box: Arterial occlusion, venous thromboembolism, heart failure, hepatotoxicity Hypertension, pancreatitis, neuropathy, ocular toxicity, hemorrhage, fluid retention, cardiac arrhythmias, myelosuppression, TLS, RPLS, impaired wound healing, GI perforation, abdominal pain, rash, constipation, headache, dry skin, fatigue, pyrexia, arthralgia, nausea, diarrhea, increased lipase, vomiting, myalgia, pain in extremities	Patients should take once daily with or without food and swallow tablets whole. Dose adjustment is required in patients with hepatic impairment. Concomitant use of CYP3A4 inhibitors, including grapefruit juice, and inducers may alter exposure to ponatinib. Dose modifications are required based on the severity of the adverse reaction. Discontinue in patients unable to tolerate at least 15 mg daily. Ponatinib is available only through a restricted distribution program including 1 approved pharmacy. Women of reproductive potential should use contraception during treatment and for 3 weeks following completion of therapy. (Ariad Pharmaceuticals, Inc., 2016)

(Continued on next page)

Table 8-1. Targeted Therapies *(Continued)*

Drug	Mechanism of Action	Route	Indications	Side Effects	Nursing Considerations
Regorafenib (Stivarga®)	Inhibits multiple membrane-bound and intracellular kinases involved in oncogenesis, tumor angiogenesis, metastasis, and tumor immunity	PO	Metastatic colorectal cancer previously treated with other therapies including a fluoropyrimidine, oxaliplatin, irinotecan, anti-VEGF therapy, and anti-EGFR therapy (if RAS wild type) Locally advanced, unresectable, or metastatic GIST following previous treatment with imatinib and sunitinib Hepatocellular carcinoma previously treated with sorafenib	Black box: Hepatotoxicity Infections, hemorrhage, GI perforation or fistula, dermatologic toxicities, hypertension, cardiac ischemia and infarction, RPLS, wound healing complications, pain, hand-foot skin reactions, anorexia, dysphonia, hyperbilirubinemia, fever, mucositis, weight loss, nausea	Patients should take once daily at the same time each day for the first 21 days of a 28-day cycle. Tablets should be swallowed whole with a low-fat meal containing less than 600 calories and less than 30% fat. If a dose is missed, patients should skip the dose and take the usual dose on the following day. Concomitant use with CYP3A4 inhibitors, including grapefruit juice, or inducers may alter exposure to regorafenib. Concomitant use may increase exposure to BCRP substrates. Dose modifications are required based on the severity of the adverse reaction. Discontinue 2 weeks prior to surgery. The decision to restart should be based on clinical judgment of wound healing. Women and men of reproductive potential should use contraception during treatment and for 2 months following completion of therapy. (Bayer HealthCare Pharmaceuticals Inc., 2017b)
Ribociclib (Kisqali®)	Inhibits CDK4 and CDK6, leading to arrest in the G_1 phase of the cell cycle and reduced cell proliferation	PO	Combination with an aromatase inhibitor as initial endocrine-based therapy for the treatment of postmenopausal women with HR-positive, HER2-negative advanced or metastatic breast cancer	QTc prolongation, hepatobiliary toxicity, neutropenia, nausea, fatigue, diarrhea, leukopenia, alopecia, vomiting, constipation, headache, back pain	Patients should take once daily at the same time each day, preferably the morning, with or without food for 21 days followed by 7 days off treatment. Patients should swallow tablets whole and not take tablets that are broken, cracked, or otherwise not intact. If patients miss or vomit a dose, they should skip the dose and take the usual dose on the following day. Concomitant use of CYP3A4 inhibitors, including grapefruit juice, and inducers may alter exposure to ribociclib. CYP3A4 substrates may need dose reductions when used in combination with ribociclib. Avoid concomitant use of drugs known to prolong the QT interval. Correct any electrolyte abnormalities prior to starting therapy to avoid QT prolongation. Dose adjustment is required in patients with moderate or severe hepatic impairment. Dose modifications are required based on the severity of the adverse reaction. Discontinue in patients unable to tolerate at least 200 mg daily. Women of reproductive potential should use contraception during treatment and for 3 weeks following completion of therapy. (Novartis Pharmaceuticals Corp., 2017b)

(Continued on next page)

Table 8-1. Targeted Therapies *(Continued)*

Drug	Mechanism of Action	Route	Indications	Side Effects	Nursing Considerations
Romidepsin (Istodax®)	Inhibits HDAC, leading to the accumulation of acetylated histones, inducing cell cycle arrest and apoptosis of some cancer cell lines	IV	Cutaneous T-cell lymphoma in patients who have received 1 prior systemic therapy Peripheral T-cell lymphoma in patients who have received at least 1 prior therapy	Thrombocytopenia, leukopenia (neutropenia and lymphopenia), anemia, infections, ECG changes (QT prolongation), TLS, nausea, fatigue, vomiting, anorexia	Administer over 4 hours. Closely monitor patients on concurrent warfarin therapy. The single-dose vial should be reconstituted with 2.2 ml of the supplied diluent. The reconstituted solution is 5 mg/ml. The patient-specific dose should be diluted in 500 ml NS and is stable for 24 hours at room temperature. Concomitant use of CYP3A4 inhibitors, including grapefruit juice, and inducers may alter exposure to romidepsin. Monitor INR more frequently in patients receiving concurrent warfarin therapy. Dose modifications may be necessary in patients with moderate or severe hepatic impairment. Correct hypokalemia and hypomagnesemia before administration. (Celgene Corp., 2016)
Romiplostim (Nplate®)	Binds to and activates the TPO receptor to increase platelet production, a mechanism akin to endogenous TPO	SC	Thrombocytopenia in patients with chronic immune thrombocytopenia who have had an insufficient response to corticosteroids, immunoglobulins, or splenectomy	Progression to AML in patients with MDS, thrombotic/thromboembolic complications, formation of neutralizing antibodies, arthralgia, dizziness, insomnia, myalgia, pain in extremities, abdominal pain, shoulder pain, dyspepsia, paresthesia, headache	Calculate the dose and reconstitute with the correct volume of sterile water for injection. Gently swirl and invert the vial to reconstitute. Do not shake during reconstitution; protect reconstituted solution from light. Administer reconstituted solution within 24 hours. The administered volume may be very small. Use a syringe with graduations to 0.01 ml. Discard any unused portions of the vial. Adjust dose weekly based on platelet counts. Do not exceed the maximum weekly dose of 10 mcg/kg. Do not dose if platelets exceed 400,000/mm^3. Treatment should only be used in patients whose degree of thrombocytopenia and clinical condition increase the risk for bleeding. Do not use to normalize platelet counts. (Amgen Inc., 2017)
Rucaparib (Rubraca®)	Inhibits PARP, which plays a role in DNA repair, resulting in DNA damage, apoptosis, and cell death	PO	Monotherapy for deleterious *BRCA* mutation (germline or somatic)–associated ovarian cancer in patients who have been treated with at least 2 chemotherapies	MDS/AML, nausea, fatigue, vomiting, anemia, abdominal pain, dysgeusia, constipation, decreased appetite, diarrhea, dyspnea, increased creatinine, increased AST/ALT, lymphopenia, hyperlipidemia, thrombocytopenia, neutropenia	Patients should take twice daily approximately 12 hours apart with or without food. If patients miss or vomit a dose, they should skip the dose and take the next scheduled dose. Advise patients to use appropriate sun protection because of increased susceptibility to sunburn. Women of reproductive potential should use contraception during treatment and for 6 months following completion of therapy. (Clovis Oncology, Inc., 2017)

(Continued on next page)

Table 8-1. Targeted Therapies *(Continued)*

Drug	Mechanism of Action	Route	Indications	Side Effects	Nursing Considerations
Ruxolitinib (Jakafi®)	Inhibits JAK1 and JAK2, which mediate cytokines and growth factors responsible for hematopoiesis and immune function	PO	Intermediate- or high-risk myelofibrosis, including primary myelofibrosis, post–polycythemia vera myelofibrosis, and post–essential thrombocytopenia myelofibrosis Polycythemia vera in patients with an inadequate response or intolerance to hydroxyurea	Thrombocytopenia, anemia, neutropenia, infections (tuberculosis, herpes zoster, hepatitis B), nonmelanoma skin cancer, hyperlipidemia, bruising, dizziness, headache	Patients should take twice daily with or without food. If patients miss a dose, they should skip the dose and take the next scheduled dose. If patients are unable to swallow the tablets, ruxolitinib may be mixed to a suspension by adding the tablet to 40 ml of water and stirring for 10 minutes before administration via nasogastric tube, followed by a flush with 75 ml of water. Administer the suspension within 6 hours of preparation. Concomitant use of CYP3A4 inhibitors, including grapefruit juice, and inducers may alter exposure to ruxolitinib. Dose modifications may be necessary in patients with moderate or severe hepatic or renal impairment. The starting dose is based on a patient's current platelet count; monitor CBC every 2–4 weeks until the dose is stabilized, then as needed. Based on indication, duration of therapy, and CBC results, doses may be increased or decreased according to response. When discontinuing therapy for reasons other than thrombocytopenia, a gradual taper by 5 mg twice daily each week should occur. Sudden interruption of therapy can lead to symptom exacerbation. Assess lipid parameters approximately 8–12 weeks following initiation. (Incyte Corp., 2016)
Sonidegib (Odomzo®)	Inhibits Hedgehog pathway by binding to and inhibiting Smoothened, a transmembrane protein involved in Hedgehog signal transduction	PO	Locally advanced basal cell carcinoma that has recurred following surgery or radiation therapy or in patients who are not candidates for surgery or radiation therapy	Black box: Embryo-fetal toxicity Musculoskeletal adverse reactions/pain, muscle spasms, alopecia, dysgeusia, fatigue, nausea, diarrhea, weight loss, decreased appetite, myalgia, abdominal pain, headache, pain, vomiting, pruritus	Patients should take once daily on an empty stomach at least 1 hour before or 2 hours after a meal. If patients miss a dose, they should resume dosing with the next scheduled dose. Concomitant use of CYP3A4 inhibitors, including grapefruit juice, and inducers may alter exposure to sonidegib. Advise patients to not donate blood for at least 20 months after the last dose. Verify pregnancy status prior to starting therapy. Women of reproductive potential should use contraception during treatment and for 20 months following completion of therapy. Men should use contraception during treatment and for 8 months following completion of therapy. (Sun Pharmaceutical Industries, Inc., 2017)

(Continued on next page)

Table 8-1. Targeted Therapies *(Continued)*

Drug	Mechanism of Action	Route	Indications	Side Effects	Nursing Considerations
Sorafenib (Nexavar®)	Inhibits multiple kinases thought to be involved in tumor cell signaling, angiogenesis, and apoptosis	PO	Unresectable hepatocellular carcinoma Advanced RCC Locally recurrent or metastatic, progressive, differentiated thyroid carcinoma refractory to radioactive iodine treatment	Cardiac ischemia and/or infarction, bleeding, hypertension, dermatologic toxicities, GI perforation, prolongation of QT interval, hepatitis, impairment of thyroid-stimulating hormone suppression, diarrhea, fatigue, infection, alopecia, hand-foot skin reaction, rash, weight loss, decreased appetite, nausea, GI and abdominal pain, hemorrhage	Patients should take twice daily without food at least 1 hour before or 2 hours after a meal. Use with carboplatin and paclitaxel is contraindicated in patients with squamous cell lung cancer because of increased risk of mortality. Sorafenib may increase activity of warfarin if taken concomitantly. Concomitant use of CYP3A4 inducers may alter exposure to sorafenib. Temporary interruption is recommended in patients undergoing major surgical procedures. Women and men of reproductive potential should use contraception during treatment and for 2 weeks following completion of therapy. (Bayer HealthCare Pharmaceuticals Inc., 2013)
Sunitinib (Sutent®)	Inhibits multiple receptor tyrosine kinases, including PDGFR, VEGFR, KIT, FLT3, CSF-1R and RET, leading to decreases in tumor cell proliferation and reduction of tumor angiogenesis	PO	GIST after disease progression while on imatinib or intolerance to imatinib Advanced RCC Adjuvant treatment of RCC with high risk of recurrence following nephrectomy Progressive, well-differentiated, unresectable, locally advanced, or metastatic pancreatic NETs	Hepatotoxicity including liver failure, cardiovascular events including myocardial ischemia/infarction and left ventricular dysfunction, QT prolongation and torsades de pointes, hypertension, hemorrhagic events, TLS, thrombotic microangiopathy, proteinuria, dermatologic toxicities, thyroid dysfunction, hypoglycemia, osteonecrosis of the jaw, impaired wound healing, adrenal hemorrhage, fatigue, asthenia, fever, diarrhea, nausea, mucositis/stomatitis, vomiting, dyspepsia, abdominal pain, constipation, hypertension, peripheral edema, rash, hand-foot syndrome, skin discoloration, dry skin, hair color changes, altered taste, headache, back pain, arthralgia, extreme pain, cough, dyspnea, anorexia, bleeding	Patients should take daily with or without food. The utilization of an off-treatment period varies based on indication. Concomitant use with CYP3A4 inhibitors, including grapefruit juice, or inducers may alter exposure to sunitinib. Obtain baseline LVEF prior to initiation of sunitinib, especially in patients with cardiac risk factors. Monitor and correct for hypomagnesemia and hypokalemia to reduce risk of QT prolongation. Consider preventive dentistry prior to treatment. Avoid invasive dental procedures, especially in patients receiving concurrent bisphosphonates. Temporary interruption of therapy is recommended during major surgical procedures. (Pfizer Inc., 2015)

(Continued on next page)

Table 8-1. Targeted Therapies *(Continued)*

Drug	Mechanism of Action	Route	Indications	Side Effects	Nursing Considerations
Temsirolimus (Torisel®)	Binds to the intracellular protein FKBP12, resulting in inhibition of mTOR, causing an interruption of cell division	IV	Advanced RCC	Hypersensitivity reaction, hyperglycemia, hyperlipidemia, infections (PJP), ILD, bowel perforation, renal failure, abnormal wound healing, rash, asthenia, mucositis, nausea, edema, anorexia, anemia, hypertriglyceridemia, elevated alkaline phosphatase, elevated serum creatinine, lymphopenia, hypophosphatemia, thrombocytopenia, elevated AST, leukopenia	Administer over 30–60 minutes. Premedicate with prophylactic IV diphenhydramine 25–50 mg (or similar antihistamine) approximately 30 minutes before the start of each dose. To treat hypersensitivity reaction, stop infusion and treat with an antihistamine (such as diphenhydramine) if not previously administered and/or an H_2 antagonist (IV famotidine or ranitidine) approximately 30 minutes before restarting. Temsirolimus may then be started at a lower infusion rate (up to 60 minutes) following a 30–60-minute observation period. Store drug in refrigerator and protect from light. Vial content must first be diluted with enclosed diluent before diluting the resultant solution with 250 ml NS. Prepare temsirolimus in PVC-free, non-DEHP glass bottles or infusion bags (polypropylene, polyolefin) and use polyethylene-lined tubing. Protect prepared product from light and administer through an in-line filter of < 5 microns within 6 hours after dilution in NS. Concomitant use of CYP3A4 inhibitors, including grapefruit juice, and inducers may alter exposure to temsirolimus. Dose-limiting toxicities were observed in combination with sunitinib. Angioedema has been reported in combination with angiotensin-converting enzyme inhibitors or calcium channel blockers. Dose modifications are required in patients with mild hepatic impairment, and drug is contraindicated in patients with bilirubin > 1.5 × ULN. Hyperglycemia and hyperlipidemia are likely and may require treatment. Monitor glucose and lipid profiles. Patients with central nervous system tumors or receiving additional anticoagulation may be at increased risk for bleeding. Because of the risk for abnormal wound healing, use with caution in the perioperative period. Patients should avoid receiving live vaccines and having close contact with those who have received live vaccines. Bowel perforations may occur; promptly evaluate for fever, abdominal pain, bloody stools, and acute abdominal pain. Older adult patients may be more likely to experience certain adverse reactions, including diarrhea, edema, and pneumonia. Monitor renal function at baseline and throughout treatment. Women and men of reproductive potential should use contraception during treatment and for 3 months following completion of therapy. (Pfizer Inc., 2017c)

(Continued on next page)

Table 8-1. Targeted Therapies *(Continued)*

Drug	Mechanism of Action	Route	Indications	Side Effects	Nursing Considerations
Tofacitinib (Xeljanz®)	Inhibits JAKs, preventing phosphorylation and activation of signal transducers and activators of transcription that modulate intracellular activity, including gene expression	PO	Moderately to severely active rheumatoid arthritis in patients with inadequate response or intolerance to methotrexate as monotherapy or in combination with methotrexate or other nonbiologic disease-modifying antirheumatic drugs	Black box: Serious infections (tuberculosis, bacterial, invasive fungal, viral, other opportunistic infections), lymphoma, and other malignancies GI perforations, lymphocytosis, neutropenia, anemia, increased AST/ALT, lipid elevations, increased serum creatinine, upper respiratory tract infection, headache, diarrhea, nasopharyngitis	Patients should take once daily (extended-release formulation) or twice daily with or without food and should not crush, split, or chew extended-release tablets. Avoid live vaccines. Concomitant use of CYP3A4 or CYP2C19 inhibitors, including grapefruit juice, and inducers may alter exposure to tofacitinib. Dose adjustment is required in patients with moderate or severe hepatic or renal impairment. Test patients for tuberculosis prior to initiating therapy. (Pfizer Inc., 2016)
Trametinib (Mekinist®)	Reversible inhibitor of MEK1 and MEK2, which are upstream regulators of the extracellular signal-related kinase pathway that promotes cellular proliferation	PO	Single agent for unresectable or metastatic melanoma with BRAF V600E or V600K mutation Combination with dabrafenib for unresectable or metastatic melanoma with BRAF V600E mutation Combination with dabrafenib for metastatic NSCLC with BRAF V600E mutation	New primary malignancies (cutaneous and noncutaneous), hemorrhage, colitis and GI perforation, venous thromboembolism, cardiomyopathy, ocular toxicities, ILD/pneumonitis, serious febrile reactions, serious skin toxicity, hyperglycemia, rash, diarrhea, lymphedema, pyrexia, nausea, chills, vomiting, hypertension, peripheral edema, fatigue, dry skin, anorexia, edema, cough, dyspnea	Patients should take once daily at least 1 hour before or 2 hours after a meal. Dose modifications are required based on the severity of the adverse reaction. Discontinue in patients unable to tolerate at least 1 mg daily. Following the first febrile reaction, administer antipyretics as secondary prophylaxis. Administer corticosteroids for at least 5 days for second or subsequent development of pyrexia if temperature does not return to baseline within 3 days of onset. Women of reproductive potential should use contraception during treatment and for 4 months following completion of therapy. (Novartis Pharmaceuticals Corp., 2017c)

(Continued on next page)

Table 8-1. Targeted Therapies *(Continued)*

Drug	Mechanism of Action	Route	Indications	Side Effects	Nursing Considerations
Vandetanib (Caprelsa®)	Inhibits VEGFR and EGFR tyrosine kinase activity that interferes with oncogenesis, metastasis, tumor angiogenesis, and maintenance of the tumor microenvironment	PO	Symptomatic or progressive, unresectable, locally advanced or metastatic medullary thyroid cancer	Black box: QT prolongation, torsades de pointes, sudden death Skin reactions, skin photosensitivity, ILD, ischemic cardiovascular events, hemorrhage, heart failure, diarrhea, hypothyroidism, hypertension, RPLS, diarrhea/colitis, rash, acne, nausea, headache, upper respiratory tract infection, anorexia, abdominal pain	Patients should take once daily with or without food. Do not crush tablets. If patients are unable to swallow tablets, tablets can be dispersed in 2 oz of water, stirred for approximately 10 minutes, and then swallowed immediately. Any residue in the glass should be mixed with 4 oz of additional water and swallowed. The tablets will not dissolve completely. If a dose is missed, the dose can be taken up to 12 hours prior to the next dose. Concomitant use with CYP3A4 inducers, including grapefruit juice, may decrease exposure to vandetanib and should be avoided. Dose modifications are required for moderate or severe renal impairment. Do not use in patients with moderate or severe hepatic impairment. Vandetanib increases concentrations of metformin and digoxin; use caution and closely monitor for toxicities. Vandetanib is available only through a restricted distribution program requiring certification of prescribers and pharmacies. Use is contraindicated in patients with congenital QT prolongation. Monitor and correct for hypocalcemia, hypomagnesemia, and hypokalemia to reduce risk of QT prolongation. Avoid concomitant use of drugs that prolong QT interval or perform more frequent ECG monitoring if use is unavoidable. Instruct patients to wear sunscreen and protective clothing when exposed to sun. Women of reproductive potential should use contraception during treatment and for 4 months following completion of therapy. (Sanofi Genzyme, 2016)

(Continued on next page)

Table 8-1. Targeted Therapies *(Continued)*

Drug	Mechanism of Action	Route	Indications	Side Effects	Nursing Considerations
Vemurafenib (Zelboraf®)	Inhibits the mutated form of BRAF serine/threonine kinase, which is constitutively activated in the mutated forms, causing cell proliferation in the absence of growth factors normally required for proliferation	PO	Unresectable or metastatic melanoma with BRAF V600E mutation Erdheim-Chester disease with BRAF V600 mutation	New primary cutaneous malignancies, new noncutaneous squamous cell carcinoma, other malignancies, hypersensitivity reactions, skin reactions, QT prolongation, hepatotoxicity, photosensitivity, serious ophthalmologic reactions, arthralgia, alopecia, pruritus, fatigue, nausea, skin papilloma, radiation recall	Patients should take approximately every 12 hours with or without food. Tablets should not be crushed or chewed. If patients miss a dose, they can take it up to 4 hours prior to the next dose. If a dose is vomited, patients should take the next scheduled dose, not an additional dose. Concomitant use with CYP3A4 inhibitors, including grapefruit juice, and inducers may alter exposure to vemurafenib. Avoid use of vemurafenib with CYP1A2 or P-gp substrates. Do not use in wild-type BRAF melanoma because of the risk for increased cell proliferation. Patients should receive a dermatologic evaluation prior to starting vemurafenib and then every 2 months thereafter until 6 months post-therapy because of the risk of new primary cutaneous malignancies. Dose modifications are required based on the severity of the adverse reaction. Discontinue in patients unable to tolerate at least 480 mg twice daily. Monitor and correct for hypocalcemia, hypomagnesemia, and hypokalemia to reduce risk of QT prolongation. ECG should be obtained at baseline, 15 days after the start of treatment, monthly during the first 3 months of treatment, and then at least every 3 months thereafter. Avoid use in patients with a QTc > 500 ms, and hold therapy if QTc exceeds this time during treatment. Instruct patients to avoid sun exposure and wear protective clothing and use broad-spectrum sunscreen and lip balm (SPF ≥ 30) when outdoors. Increases in transaminase and bilirubin occurred in a majority of patients receiving concurrent ipilimumab. Women of reproductive potential should use contraception during treatment and for 2 weeks following completion of therapy. (Genentech, Inc., 2017)
Venetoclax (Venclexta®)	Inhibits Bcl-2, an antiapoptotic product	PO	CLL with 17p deletion in patients who have received at least 1 prior therapy	TLS, neutropenia, diarrhea, nausea, anemia, upper respiratory tract infection, thrombocytopenia, fatigue	Patients should take once daily with a meal and water at approximately the same time each day. Tablets should not be chewed, crushed, or broken. The dose should be increased according to a weekly ramp-up schedule over 5 weeks. If patients miss a dose by more than 8 hours or vomit, they should take the next regularly scheduled dose at the usual time. Concomitant use with CYP3A4 or P-gp inhibitors, including grapefruit juice, or inducers may alter exposure to venetoclax. P-gp substrates should be taken at least 6 hours before venetoclax.

(Continued on next page)

Table 8-1. Targeted Therapies *(Continued)*

Drug	Mechanism of Action	Route	Indications	Side Effects	Nursing Considerations
Venetoclax (Venclexta®) *(cont.)*					Concurrent use of CYP3A4 inhibitors during the ramp-up phase is contraindicated. Administer TLS prophylaxis. Patients with high tumor burden are recommended to be admitted for administration of the first dose of weeks 1 and 2. Do not administer live attenuated vaccines prior to, during, or after treatment. Women of reproductive potential should use contraception during treatment and for 30 days following completion of therapy. (AbbVie Inc., 2016)
Vismodegib (Erivedge®)	Inhibits the Hedgehog pathway via binding to and inhibiting Smoothened, a transmembrane protein involved in Hedgehog signal transduction	PO	Metastatic basal cell carcinoma or locally advanced basal cell carcinoma that has advanced following surgery or in patients who are not candidates for surgery or radiation therapy	Black box: Embryo-fetal toxicity Premature fusion of epiphyses, muscle spasm, alopecia, dysgeusia, weight loss, fatigue, nausea, diarrhea, anorexia, constipation, arthralgia, vomiting, ageusia	Patients should take once daily with or without food and swallow capsules whole. Capsules should not be crushed or chewed. If patients miss a dose, they should take the next regularly scheduled dose at the usual time. Because of teratogenicity, determine pregnancy status of women of childbearing age within 7 days prior to starting therapy. Inform male patients of fetal risk and instruct on use of contraception during treatment. Patients may not donate blood during treatment and for at least 24 months after completing treatment. Men should not donate semen during treatment and for 3 months after therapy. Women of reproductive potential should use contraception during treatment and for 24 months after the final dose. Men should use contraception during treatment for 3 months following completion of therapy. (Genentech, Inc., 2016c)
Vorinostat (Zolinza®)	Inhibits HDAC, leading to accumulation of acetyl groups on histone lysine residues, resulting in cell cycle arrest and/or apoptosis	PO	Cutaneous manifestations of cutaneous T-cell lymphoma in patients who have progressive, persistent, or recurrent disease following 2 systemic therapies	Pulmonary embolism/deep vein thrombosis, thrombocytopenia, anemia, nausea, vomiting, diarrhea, hyperglycemia, clinical chemistry abnormality (creatinine, magnesium, calcium), GI bleeding, fatigue, anorexia, dysgeusia	Patients should take once daily with food. Do not open or crush the capsules. Use with other HDAC inhibitors (e.g., valproic acid) increases the risk for GI bleeding. Use in combination with warfarin may lead to elevated INR. Monitor INR frequently. Dose modifications are required for mild, moderate, or severe hepatic impairment. Patients may require antiemetics, antidiarrheals, fluid, and electrolytes. (Merck and Co., Inc., 2015)

(Continued on next page)

Table 8-1. Targeted Therapies *(Continued)*

Drug	Mechanism of Action	Route	Indications	Side Effects	Nursing Considerations
Ziv-aflibercept (Zaltrap®)	Acts as a soluble receptor and binds to VEGF-A, VEGF-B, and placental growth factor (known as PIGF), leading to inhibition of neovascularization and decreased vascular permeability	IV	In combination with 5-fluorouracil, leucovorin, and irinotecan in patients with metastatic colorectal cancer that is resistant or progressing following treatment with oxaliplatin-based therapy	Black box: Hemorrhage, GI perforation, impaired wound healing Fistula formation, hypertension, arterial thromboembolic events (e.g., transient ischemic attack, cerebrovascular accident, angina), proteinuria, nephrotic syndrome, thrombotic microangiopathy, neutropenia, infection, diarrhea, dehydration, RPLS, increases in AST/ALT, weight loss, anorexia, epistaxis, abdominal pain, dysphonia, elevated serum creatinine, headache	Administer infusions over 1 hour through a 0.2 micron polyethersulfone filter prior to any of the other drugs used in the chemotherapy regimen. Store in refrigerator and keep vials in original container until time of use to protect from light. Do not use with filters made from polyvinylidene fluoride or nylon. Do not use product if solution is anything other than clear/colorless to pale yellow in color. Discard unused product following initial one-time access into vial. Dilute in NS or D5W to a concentration of 0.6 to 8 mg/ml. Do not administer combined with other IV medications in the same infusion bag or IV line. Diluted solution may be stored under refrigeration for up to 24 hours and at room temperature for up to 8 hours. Hold dosing at least 4 weeks prior to elective surgery and do not resume for at least 4 weeks following major surgery and until the wound is fully healed. Hold dosing if recurrent or severe hypertension occurs and restart at a lower dose once blood pressure is controlled. Monitor urine protein and hold dosing if proteinuria > 2 g/24 hours; restart once proteinuria < 2 g/24 hours. Dose reduction is recommended for recurrent proteinuria > 2 g/24 hours. Women and men of reproductive potential should use contraception during treatment and for 3 months following completion of therapy. (Sanofi-Aventis U.S. LLC, 2016)

Note. For hazardous oral medications, additional precautions should be taken to prevent exposure when handling or manipulating. Refer to Chapter 12, Safe Handling of Hazardous Drugs.

ALK—anaplastic lymphoma kinase; ALL—acute lymphoblastic leukemia; ALT—alanine transaminase; AML—acute myeloid leukemia; ANC—absolute neutrophil count; ASM—aggressive systemic mastocytosis; AST—aspartate transaminase; BCRP—breast cancer resistance protein; *BRCA*—breast cancer gene; CBC—complete blood count; CLL—chronic lymphocytic leukemia; CML—chronic myeloid leukemia; CPK—creatine phosphokinase; DEHP—di(2-ethylhexyl) phthalate; D5W—5% dextrose in water; ECG—electrocardiogram; EGFR—epidermal growth factor receptor; FLT3—FMS-like tyrosine kinase 3; GI—gastrointestinal; GIST—gastrointestinal stromal tumor; HDAC—histone deacetylase; HER—human epidermal growth factor receptor; HGFR—hepatocyte growth factor receptor; HR—hormone receptor; H_2—histamine; IDH2—isocitrate dehydrogenase 2; IGF-1R—insulin-like growth factor 1 receptor; ILD—interstitial lung disease; INR—international normalized ratio; INSR—insulin receptor; IV—intravenous; JAK—janus kinase; LFTs—liver function tests; LVEF—left ventricular ejection fraction; MDS—myelodysplastic syndrome; mTOR—mammalian target of rapamycin; NaCl—sodium chloride; NET—neuroendocrine tumor; NHL—non-Hodgkin lymphoma; NS—normal saline; NSCLC—non-small cell lung cancer; PARP—poly(ADP-ribose) polymerase; PDGF—platelet-derived growth factor; PDGFR—platelet-derived growth factor receptor; P-gp—P-glycoprotein; Ph—Philadelphia chromosome; PI3K—phosphoinositide 3-kinase; PJP—*Pneumocystis jiroveci* pneumonia; PO—by mouth; PPI—proton pump inhibitor; PVC—polyvinyl chloride; RCC—renal cell carcinoma; RPLS—reversible posterior leukoencephalopathy syndrome; SC—subcutaneous; SCF—stem cell factor; SLL—small lymphocytic lymphoma; SPF—sun protection factor; TKI—tyrosine kinase inhibitor; TLS—tumor lysis syndrome; TPO—thrombopoietin; ULN—upper limit of normal; VEGF—vascular endothelial growth factor; VEGFR—vascular endothelial growth factor receptor

References

AbbVie Inc. (2016). *Venclexta® (venetoclax)* [Package insert]. North Chicago, IL: Author.

Amgen Inc. (2017). *Nplate® (romiplostim)* [Package insert]. Thousand Oaks, CA: Author.

Ariad Pharmaceuticals, Inc. (2016). *Iclusig® (ponatinib)* [Package insert]. Cambridge, MA: Author.

AstraZeneca Pharmaceuticals LP. (2015). *Iressa® (gefitinib)* [Package insert]. Wilmington, DE: Author.

AstraZeneca Pharmaceuticals LP. (2017a). *Calquence® (acalabrutinib)* [Package insert]. Wilmington, DE: Author.

AstraZeneca Pharmaceuticals LP. (2017b). *Tagrisso® (osimertinib)* [Package insert]. Wilmington, DE: Author.

AstraZeneca Pharmaceuticals LP. (2018). *Lynparza® (olaparib)* [Package insert]. Wilmington, DE: Author.

Aw, A., & Brown, J.R. (2017). Current status of Bruton's tyrosine kinase inhibitor development and use in B-cell malignancies. *Drugs and Aging, 34,* 509–527. https://doi.org/10.1007/s40266-017-0468-4

Bayer HealthCare Pharmaceuticals Inc. (2013). *Nexavar® (sorafenib)* [Package insert]. Whippany, NJ: Author.

Bayer HealthCare Pharmaceuticals Inc. (2017a). *Aliqopa™ (copanlisib)* [Package insert]. Whippany, NJ: Author.

Bayer HealthCare Pharmaceuticals Inc. (2017b). *Stivarga® (regorafenib)* [Package insert]. Whippany, NJ: Author.

Boehringer Ingelheim Pharmaceuticals, Inc. (2016). *Gilotrif® (afatinib)* [Package insert]. Ridgefield, CT: Author.

Bristol-Myers Squibb Co. (2017). *Sprycel® (dasatinib)* [Package insert]. Princeton, NJ: Author.

Celgene Corp. (2016). *Istodax® (romidepsin)* [Package insert]. Summit, NJ: Author.

Celgene Corp. (2017). *Idhifa® (enasidenib)* [Package insert]. Summit, NJ: Author.

Chen, H.X., Doyle, A.L., Takebe, N., Timmer, W.C., & Ivy, P.S. (2011). Signaling inhibitors: IGFR, PI3K pathway, embryonic signaling inhibitors, and mitotic kinase inhibitors. In B.A. Chabner & D.L. Longo (Eds.), *Cancer chemotherapy and biotherapy: Principles and practice* (5th ed., pp. 547–576). Philadelphia, PA: Lippincott Williams & Wilkins.

Clovis Oncology, Inc. (2017). *Rubraca® (rucaparib)* [Package insert]. Boulder, CO: Author.

Cuellar, S., Vozniak, M., Rhodes, J., Forcello, N., & Olszta, D. (2018). BCR-ABL1 tyrosine kinase inhibitors for the treatment of chronic myeloid leukemia. *Journal of Oncology Pharmacy Practice, 24,* 433–452. https://doi.org/10.1177/1078155217710553

del Rivero, J., & Kohn, E.C. (2017). PARP inhibitors: The cornerstone of DNA repair-targeted therapies. *Oncology, 31,* 265–273.

Devji, T., Levine, O., Neupane, B., Beyene, J., & Xie, F. (2017). Systemic therapy for previously untreated advanced BRAF-mutated melanoma: A systematic review and network meta-analysis of randomized clinical trials. *JAMA Oncology, 7,* 366–373. https://doi.org/10.1001/jamaoncol.2016.4877

Eckschlager, T., Plch, J., Stiborova, M., & Hrabeta, J. (2017). Histone deacetylase inhibitors as anticancer drugs. *International Journal of Molecular Sciences, 18,* 1414. https://doi.org/10.3390/ijms18071414

Eisai Inc. (2017). *Lenvima® (lenvatinib)* [Package insert]. Woodcliff Lake, NJ: Author.

Eli Lilly and Company. (2017). *Verzenio™ (abemaciclib)* [Package insert]. Indianapolis, IN: Author.

Espinoza-Delgado, I., Chiaramonte, M.G., Swerdlow, R.D., & Wright, J.J. (2011). Proteasome inhibitors. In B.A. Chabner & D.L. Longo (Eds.), *Cancer chemotherapy and biotherapy: Principles and practice* (5th ed., pp. 421–441). Philadelphia, PA: Lippincott Williams & Wilkins.

Exelixis, Inc. (2016a). *Cabometyx® (cabozantinib)* [Package insert]. South San Francisco, CA: Author.

Exelixis, Inc. (2016b). *Cometriq® (cabozantinib)* [Package insert]. South San Francisco, CA: Author.

Genentech, Inc. (2016a). *Alecensa® (alectinib)* [Package insert]. South San Francisco, CA: Author.

Genentech, Inc. (2016b). *Cotellic® (cobimetinib)* [Package insert]. South San Francisco, CA: Author.

Genentech, Inc. (2016c). *Erivedge® (vismodegib)* [Package insert]. South San Francisco, CA: Author.

Genentech, Inc. (2016d). *Tarceva® (erlotinib)* [Package insert]. South San Francisco, CA: Author.

Genentech, Inc. (2017). *Zelboraf® (vemurafenib)* [Package insert]. South San Francisco, CA: Author.

Gilead Sciences, Inc. (2016). *Zydelig® (idelalisib)* [Package insert]. Foster City, CA: Author.

Hata, A.N., Engelman, J.A., & Faber, A.C. (2015). The BCL2 family: Key mediators of the apoptotic response to targeted anticancer therapeutics. *Cancer Discovery, 5,* 475–487. https://doi.org/10.1158/2159-8290.CD-15-0011

Hobbs, G.S., Rozelle, R.S., & Mullally, A. (2017). The development and use of Janus kinase 2 inhibitors for the treatment of myeloproliferative neoplasms. *Hematology/Oncology Clinics of North America, 31,* 613–626. https://doi.org/10.1016/j.hoc.2017.04.002

Hospital, M.-A., Green, A.S., Maciel, T.T., Moura, I.C., Leung, A.Y., Bouscary, D., & Tamburini, J. (2017). FLT3 inhibitors: Clinical potential in acute myeloid leukemia. *OncoTargets and Therapy, 10,* 607–615. https://doi.org/10.2147/OTT.S103790

Incyte Corp. (2016). *Jakafi® (ruxolitinib)* [Package insert]. Wilmington, DE: Author.

Karachaliou, N., Santarpia, M., Gonzalez Cao, M., Teixido, C., Sosa, A.E., Berenguer, J., ... Rosell, R. (2017). Anaplastic lymphoma kinase inhibitors in phase I and phase II clinical trials for non-small cell lung cancer. *Expert Opinion on Investigational Drugs, 26,* 713–722. https://doi.org/10.1080/13543784.2017.1324572

Lynch, T., & Price, A. (2017). The effect of cytochrome P450 metabolism on drug response, interactions and adverse effects. *American Family Physician, 76,* 391–396.

Merck and Co., Inc. (2015). *Zolinza® (vorinostat)* [Package insert]. Whitehouse Station, NJ: Author.

Millennium Pharmaceuticals, Inc. (2015). *Ninlaro® (ixazomib)* [Package insert]. Cambridge, MA: Author.

Millennium Pharmaceuticals, Inc. (2017). *Velcade® (bortezomib)* [Package insert]. Cambridge, MA: Author.

National Cancer Institute. (n.d.). Tyrosine kinase inhibitor. In *NCI dictionary of cancer terms.* Retrieved from https://www.cancer.gov/publications/dictionaries/cancer-terms?cdrid=44833

Neal, J.W., & Sequist, L.V. (2011). Epidermal growth factor receptor inhibitors. In B.A. Chabner & D.L. Longo (Eds.), *Cancer chemotherapy and biotherapy: Principles and practice* (5th ed., pp. 511–516). Philadelphia, PA: Lippincott Williams & Wilkins.

Novartis Pharmaceuticals Corp. (2016a). *Afinitor® (everolimus tablets for oral administration) and Afinitor® Disperz® (everolimus tablets for oral suspension)* [Package insert]. East Hanover, NJ: Author.

Novartis Pharmaceuticals Corp. (2016b). *Farydak® (panobinostat)* [Package insert]. East Hanover, NJ: Author.

Novartis Pharmaceuticals Corp. (2017a). *Gleevec® (imatinib mesylate)* [Package insert]. East Hanover, NJ: Author.

Novartis Pharmaceuticals Corp. (2017b). *Kisqali® (ribociclib)* [Package insert]. East Hanover, NJ: Author.

Novartis Pharmaceuticals Corp. (2017c). *Mekinist® (trametinib)* [Package insert]. East Hanover, NJ: Author.

Novartis Pharmaceuticals Corp. (2017d). *Promacta® (eltrombopag)* [Package insert]. East Hanover, NJ: Author.

Novartis Pharmaceuticals Corp. (2017e). *Rydapt® (midostaurin)* [Package insert]. East Hanover, NJ: Author.

Novartis Pharmaceuticals Corp. (2017f). *Tafinlar® (dabrafenib)* [Package insert]. East Hanover, NJ: Author.

Novartis Pharmaceuticals Corp. (2017g). *Tasigna® (nilotinib)* [Package insert]. East Hanover, NJ: Author.

Novartis Pharmaceuticals Corp. (2017h). *Tykerb® (lapatinib)* [Package insert]. East Hanover, NJ: Author.

Novartis Pharmaceuticals Corp. (2017i). *Votrient® (pazopanib)* [Package insert]. East Hanover, NJ: Author.

Novartis Pharmaceuticals Corp. (2017j). *Zykadia® (ceritinib)* [Package insert]. East Hanover, NJ: Author.

Onyx Pharmaceuticals, Inc. (2017). *Kyprolis® (carfilzomib)* [Package insert]. South San Francisco, CA: Author.

Parulekar, W.R., & Eisenhauer, E.A. (2004). Phase I trial design for solid tumor studies of targets, non-cytotoxic agents: Theory and practice. *Journal of the National Cancer Institute, 96,* 990–997. https://doi.org/10.1093/jnci/djh182

Pfizer Inc. (2014). *Inlyta® (axitinib)* [Package insert]. New York, NY: Author.

Pfizer Inc. (2015). *Sutent® (sunitinib malate)* [Package insert]. New York, NY: Author.

Pfizer Inc. (2016). *Xeljanz® (tofacitinib)* [Package insert]. New York, NY: Author.

Pfizer Inc. (2017a). *Bosulif® (bosutinib)* [Package insert]. New York, NY: Author.

Pfizer Inc. (2017b). *Ibrance® (palbociclib)* [Package insert]. New York, NY: Author.

Pfizer Inc. (2017c). *Torisel® (temsirolimus)* [Package insert]. New York, NY: Author.

Pfizer Inc. (2017d). *Xalkori® (crizotinib)* [Package insert]. New York, NY: Author.

Pharmacyclics LLC & Janssen Biotech, Inc. (2017). *Imbruvica® (ibrutinib)* [Package insert]. Sunnyvale, CA, and Horsham, PA: Authors.

Priestman, T. (2012). *Cancer chemotherapy in clinical practice.* https://doi.org/10.1007/978-0-85729-727-3

Puma Biotechnology, Inc. (2017). *Nerlynx® (neratinib)* [Package insert]. Los Angeles, CA: Author.

Rodeghiero, F., & Carli, G. (2017). Beyond immune thrombocytopenia: The evolving role of thrombopoietin receptor agonists. *Annals of Hematology, 96,* 1421–1434. https://doi.org/10.1007/s00277-017-2953-6

Sanofi-Aventis U.S. LLC. (2016). *Zaltrap® (ziv-aflibercept)* [Package insert]. Cambridge, MA: Author.

Sanofi Genzyme. (2016). *Caprelsa® (vandetanib)* [Package insert]. Cambridge, MA: Author.

Schlafer, D., Shah, K.S., Panjic, E.H., & Lonial, S. (2017). Safety of proteasome inhibitors for treatment of multiple myeloma. *Expert Opinion on Drug Safety, 16,* 167–183. https://doi.org/10.1080/14740338.2017.1259310

Simmons, M.A. (2012). *Pharmacology: An illustrated review.* New York, NY: Thieme Medical Publishers.

Spectrum Pharmaceuticals, Inc. (2017). *Beleodaq® (belinostat)* [Package insert]. Irvine, CA: Author.

Sun Pharmaceutical Industries, Inc. (2017). *Odomzo® (sonidegib)* [Package insert]. Cranbury, NJ: Author.

Takeda Pharmaceuticals Co. (2017). *Alunbrig® (brigatinib)* [Package insert]. Cambridge, MA: Author.

Tesaro, Inc. (2017). *Zejula® (niraparib)* [Package insert]. Waltham, MA: Author.

Wang, H., Nicolay, B.N., Chick, J.M., Gao, X., Geng, Y., Ren, H., … Sicinski, P. (2017). The metabolic function of cycle D3-CDK6 kinase in cancer cell survival. *Nature, 546,* 426–430. https://doi.org/10.1038/nature22797

Weingart, S.N., Brown, E., Pach, P.B., Eng, K., Johnson, S.A., Kuzel, T.M., … Walters, R.S. (2008). NCCN Task Force report: Oral chemotherapy. *Journal of the National Comprehensive Cancer Network, 6*(Suppl. 3), S1–S14.

Wisinkski, K.B., & Gradishar, W.J. (2011). Inhibitors of tumor angiogenesis. In B.A. Chabner & D.L. Longo (Eds.), *Cancer chemotherapy and biotherapy: Principles and practice* (5th ed., pp. 495–510). Philadelphia, PA: Lippincott Williams & Wilkins.

Wu, F., Zhang, Y., Sun, B., McMahon, A.P., & Wang, Y. (2017). Hedgehog signaling: From basic biology to cancer therapy. *Cell Chemical Biology, 24,* 252–280. https://doi.org/10.1016/j.chembiol.2017.02.010

CHAPTER 9

Principles of the Immune System

A. Overview of immunology
   1. Current advances in immunotherapy utilize existing immune pathways and cellular mechanisms as a therapeutic approach to the treatment and prevention of cancer. Basic knowledge of the immune system and immune response to tumor cells is essential to understand the clinical application of immunotherapy, the use of the body's own immune system mechanisms to treat cancer.
   2. The immune system (see Figure 9-1) is a highly specialized and adaptive system of barriers, organs, cells, and molecules that guards an individual by providing the following (Abbas, Lichtman, & Pillai, 2016):
      a) Protection: Defense against foreign pathogens (i.e., bacteria, viruses, fungi, and parasites)
      b) Homeostasis: Elimination of damaged or dead cells and initiation of tissue repair
      c) Surveillance: Identification of foreign or nonself substances; inhibition of tumor growth

B. Types of immune response
   1. An immune response is the reaction of the immune system against a foreign substance, or antigen (e.g., bacteria). The immune system consists of two types of immunity: innate and adaptive (Actor, 2014; see Table 9-1).
   2. Innate, also known as natural or native immunity (see Figure 9-2)
      a) Innate immunity is the first line of defense and is essential for inducing a nonspecific response to a pathogen or foreign substance (Actor, 2014). It does not generate immunologic memory.
      b) Components of innate immunity (Actor, 2014)
         (1) Physical barriers (skin and mucous membranes)
         (2) Mechanical barriers (coughing, sneezing, and blinking)
         (3) Chemical barriers (tears, acidic pH, and sweat)
         (4) Inflammatory barriers (vascular fluid leakage)
         (5) Complement activation (plasma proteins mark pathogens for destruction)
         (6) Acute-phase protein production (recruit phagocytes to site of infection or tissue injury)
         (7) Production of large granular lymphocytes (kill and digest pathogens)

Figure 9-1. Primary and Secondary Lymphoid Organs

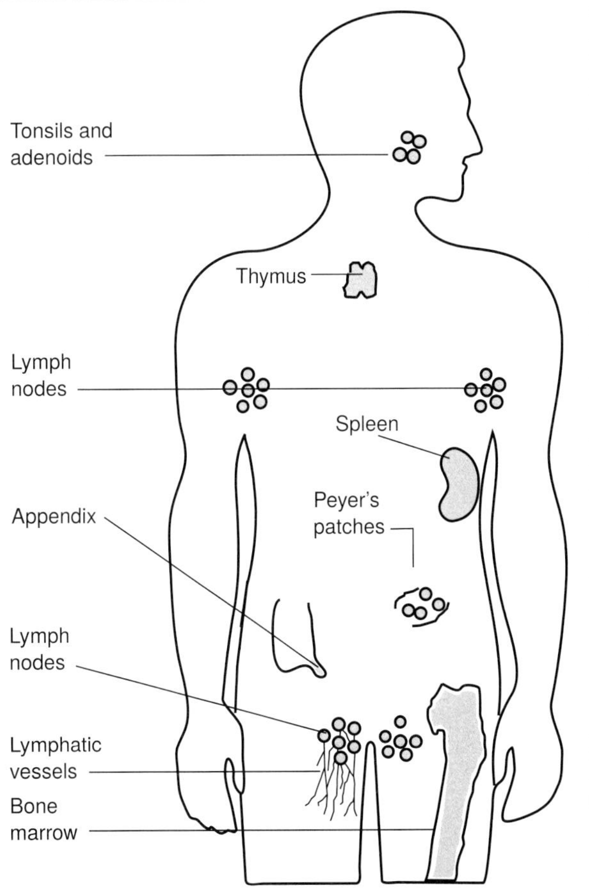

Table 9-1. Innate and Adaptive Immune Responses

Immune Response	Mechanism of Action	Cells Primarily Involved
Innate	Primary line of defense Nonspecific No memory	Neutrophils Monocytes, macrophages Large granular lymphocytes (natural killer cells)
Adaptive	Secondary line of defense Specific memory	Lymphocytes T cells (in cell-mediated immunity) B cells (in humoral immunity)

Note. Based on information from Paul, 2013.

3. Adaptive or acquired immunity
   a) Adaptive immunity is the secondary line of defense and involves immunologic memory, specificity, and collaboration of B and T cells (Medina, 2016).
   b) Three types of adaptive immunity (see Figure 9-2)
      (1) Humoral immunity: B lymphocytes, memory B cells, and plasma cells mediate humoral immunity. The result is the production of immunoglobulins (Igs), or antibodies (Actor, 2014).
      (2) Cell-mediated immunity: This type of immunity is mediated by T cells and their cytokine products. It does not involve an antibody but rather cytotoxic T cells and helper T cells (TH1 or TH2) (Actor, 2014; Annunziato, Romagnani, & Romagnani, 2015).
      (3) Regulatory T cells (Tregs), also known as suppressor T cells (Hall, 2015): Tregs limit the activity of other immune effector cells.
         (a) Major role is to prevent the onset of immunity to normal tissue of the body and limit the inflammatory response that can occur with infections.
         (b) Absence of Tregs may trigger inflammatory disorders primarily involving the bowel, skin, and liver.

Figure 9-2. The Innate and Adaptive Immune Response

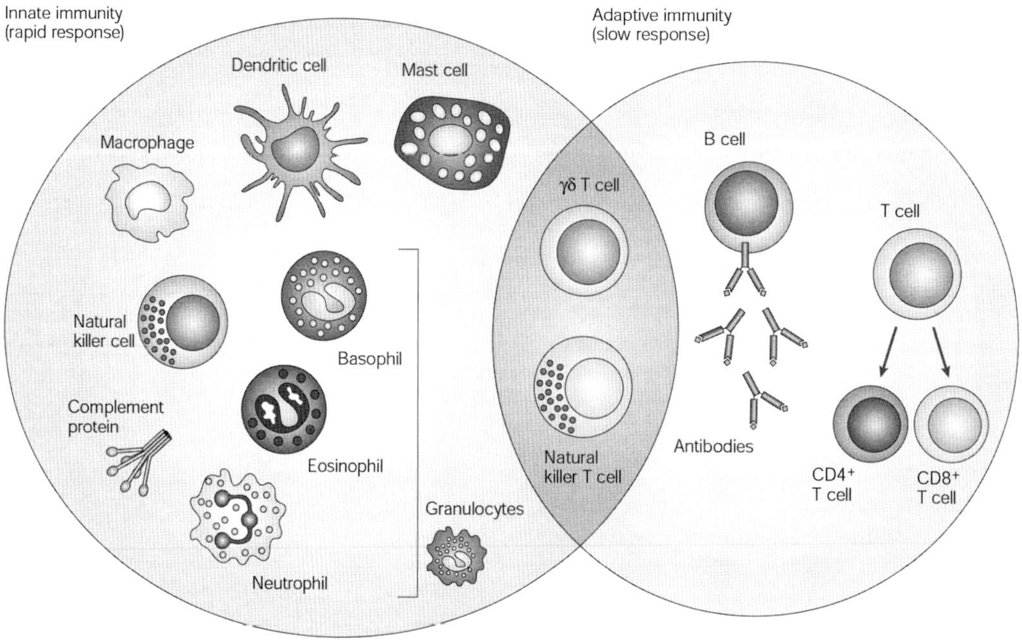

The innate immune response functions as the first line of defense against infection. It consists of soluble factors, such as complement proteins, and diverse cellular components including granulocytes (basophils, eosinophils and neutrophils), mast cells, macrophages, dendritic cells and natural killer cells. The adaptive immune response is slower to develop, but manifests as increased antigenic specificity and memory. It consists of antibodies, B cells, and CD4+ and CD8+ T lymphocytes. Natural killer T cells and γδ T cells are cytotoxic lymphocytes that straddle the interface of innate and adaptive immunity.

Note. From "Cytokines in Cancer Pathogenesis and Cancer Therapy," by G. Dranoff, 2004, *Nature Reviews Cancer, 4,* p. 13. Copyright 2004 by Springer Nature. Reprinted with permission.

C. Organs of the immune system (Actor, 2014; Ruddle, 2014)
   1. The immune system consists of primary and secondary lymphoid organs.
   2. Primary lymphoid organs are bone marrow and thymus. They are sites of lymphocyte development and differentiation.
   3. Secondary lymphoid organs include lymph nodes, spleen, Peyer's patches, adenoids, tonsils, and mucosa-associated lymphoid tissue. They are sites of antigen-driven proliferation and lymphocyte maturation.

D. Cells of the immune system (see Figure 9-3)
   1. The immune response involves the intricate interaction of a number of cells and proteins. Cells are widely categorized by their progenitor bone marrow cell lines (Actor, 2014; see Figure 14-1).
   2. Myeloid cells arise from the myeloid stem cell line, which also gives rise to red blood cells and platelets (Weiskopf et al., 2016).
      a) Myeloid immune cells are called *granulocytes* and include neutrophils, eosinophils, and basophils.
      b) Neutrophils are the first responders, phagocytosing infection and initiating inflammation.
   3. Lymphoid cells arise from the lymphoid stem cell line and include effector cell functions (Actor, 2014).
      a) T cells
         (1) Helper T cells: These cells coordinate the immune response and cell-mediated immunity; they are required to maintain cytotoxic T-cell responses and express CD4.
            (a) TH1 cells are necessary for activating macrophages and are involved in the production of certain antibody isotypes.
            (b) TH2 cells are effective activators of B cells, particularly in primary responses.
         (2) Cytotoxic T cells: These cells kill foreign cells, virally infected cells, or cells with new surface antigens. Cytotoxic T cells express CD8.
         (3) Tregs/suppressor T cells: These cells interfere with the development of an immune reaction when recognizing an antigen. Their primary role is to modulate the severity of inflammation produced by infection and prevent autoimmunity; they may be involved in malignancy.
         (4) Memory T cells: These cells recognize specific antigens and induce recall responses.
      b) B lymphocytes give rise to plasma cells and memory cells (Actor, 2014).
         (1) Plasma cells manufacture antibodies (or Igs) specific to an initiating antigen.
            (a) Their function is to enhance effector cell functions. The majority of peripheral blood antibodies are IgG, which enhances phagocytosis of antigen by macrophages, monocytes, polymorphonuclear cells, and some lymphocytes.
            (b) IgM is the first antibody produced in response to an antigen.

Figure 9-3. Cells of the Immune System

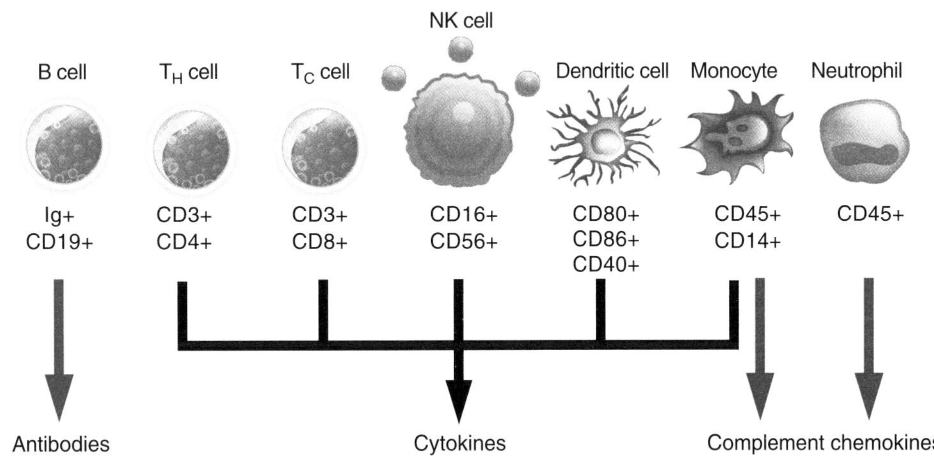

CD—cluster of differentiation; Ig—immunoglobulin; NK—natural killer; T_C—cytotoxic T cell; T_H—helper T cell

(c) IgA is present in body secretions and helps to prevent infections at sites where the environment interacts with the body, such as the nose and lungs.

(d) IgD is present in small amounts in normal serum. The exact biologic function is unclear; however, IgD may have some antibody function for penicillin, diphtheria, and insulin.

(e) IgE exists in trace amounts in normal serum and is associated with immediate hypersensitivity reactions. IgE antibodies are generated when combined with certain antigens, thus activating the release of histamine from mast cells.

(2) Memory cells recognize a specific antigen and can survive for a long period of time after clearance of the primary infestation. They can quickly produce antigen-specific antibodies upon reexposure (Kurosaki, Kometani, & Ise, 2015).

c) Natural killer (NK) cells: These cells are cytotoxic to tumor cells and virally infected autologous cells by producing substances that can bind to and destroy foreign invaders without having to identify a specific antigen. NK cells identify foreign substances by their lack of identifying surface molecules (Marcus et al., 2014).

d) NKT cells: These cells have markers of both NK and T cells (Marcus et al., 2014).

E. Immune system proteins and receptors

1. Several components of the immune system direct immune cells to desired target sites of immune activity and also mediate response with the goal of limiting autoimmunity.

2. Checkpoint molecules: Checkpoint molecules contribute to inhibition of T-cell immune responses (Beatty & Gladney, 2015; Ott, Hodi, & Robert, 2013; Pardoll, 2012; Zitvogel & Kroemer, 2012).

a) Cytotoxic T-lymphocyte antigen 4 (CTLA-4): CTLA-4 ligands bind to antigen-presenting cells, downregulating T-cell activity. CTLA-4 expression decreases the activation of T cells, as well as sends inhibitory signals to the T cell. CTLA-4 is expressed by activated CD8+ cells, but the primary role of CTLA-4 is diminishing helper T-cell activity and enhancing Tregs' immunosuppressive activity.

b) Programmed cell death protein 1 (PD-1): PD-1 is an inhibitory receptor on T cells that interacts with its ligand, programmed cell death-ligand 1 (PD-L1). PD-1/PD-L1 interaction inhibits T-cell proliferation and cytotoxic function, induces T-cell regulatory function, and induces T-cell apoptosis. PD-L1 overexpression has been observed in several tumor types and is correlated with poor prognosis.

3. Epidermal growth factor receptors (EGFRs; Keith & Abueg, 2015; Lemmon, Schlessinger, & Ferguson, 2014; Normanno et al., 2006)

a) Function and structure

(1) EGFRs are membrane-bound surface proteins (tyrosine kinase receptors) consisting of three components: an extracellular portion that binds circulating growth factors such as epidermal growth factors, a transmembrane portion, and an intracellular portion that interacts with cell signal transduction pathways.

(2) EGFRs communicate extracellular growth signals via the internal cell signal transduction pathways to the cell nucleus, ultimately causing gene activation.

(3) EGFR activation (termed *dimerization*) occurs through interaction with circulating growth factors or by interaction with a neighboring EGFR.

(4) EGFRs are a member of the ErbB family of membrane-bound tyrosine kinase receptors. The members are EGFR (ErbB1), HER2 (ErbB2), HER3 (ErbB3), and HER4 (ErbB4).

b) EGFRs are often mutated or overexpressed in malignant tumors. EGFR mutations result in EGFR pathway activation in the absence of the appropriate extracellular growth signal, resulting in unregulated tumor growth.

c) EGFRs are common targets of immunotherapy and targeted therapies.

(1) Monoclonal antibodies target the surface-bound portion of EGFRs, inducing immune-mediated cellular toxicity and halting cell signal transduction.

(2) Small molecule tyrosine kinase inhibitors disrupt the interaction between molecules of the cell signal transduction pathways.

4. Cytokines: Cytokines are glycoprotein products of immune cells such as lymphocytes and mac-

rophages. Cytokines are produced in response to T-cell activation and mediate effector defense functions. Cytokines (e.g., interleukins [ILs], interferon) themselves usually are not cytotoxic (Iwasaki & Medzhitov, 2015).

5. Chemokines: Known as chemotactic cytokines, these protein molecules regulate leukocyte migration and are key organizers of cell distribution in both immune and inflammatory responses (Griffith, Sokol, & Luster, 2014).

F. Phases of immune response (Abbas et al., 2016; Actor, 2014)

1. Antigen recognition: Circulating antibodies recognize a foreign antigen, which activates the immune system.
2. Lymphocyte activation: B or T cells are activated to proliferate and differentiate into effector lymphocytes.
3. Effector phase: Foreign antigen is inactivated or destroyed.
4. Contraction: During this phase, T-cell expansion is inhibited or activated cells are eliminated by apoptosis, facilitating the immune system's return to a resting state and limiting tissue damage and chronic inflammation.
5. Memory: Lymphocytes that survive the immune response become memory cells that can recognize a former antigen and initiate a rapid response.

G. Immune interaction with targets

1. The immune system interacts with the body by recognizing and evaluating various characteristic structures on circulating cells.
2. Targeted therapies and immunotherapies use the structures to identify their targets.
   a) Cluster of differentiation (CD) markers are commonly expressed on cell surfaces, especially on immune cells. These CD markers (e.g., CD4, CD20) are associated with certain immune functions.
   b) Membrane-bound receptors (e.g., EGFR) mediate the interaction of the cell with circulating growth factors.
   c) Antigens are molecular structures that are recognized by and can stimulate the immune system.
   d) Antigen-presenting cells (e.g., macrophages, B cells, dendritic cells) efficiently present antigen to T cells; only dendritic cells are capable of initiating a primary immune response.
      (1) Antigen presentation must occur in the presence of inflammatory factors to generate immune response. Antigen presentation in the absence of a noninflammatory environment can result in immune tolerance.
      (2) Tumors manipulate antigen presentation as a mechanism of tumor escape.

H. Tumor escape mechanisms

1. *Immune surveillance* refers to the process "whereby the immune system identifies cancerous and/or precancerous cells and eliminates them before they can cause harm" (Swann & Smyth, 2007, p. 1137). When immune surveillance fails, tumor formation occurs (Beatty & Gladney, 2015; Swann & Smyth, 2007).
2. Theories of tumor escape mechanisms (Beatty & Gladney, 2015; Coulie, Van den Eynde, van der Bruggen, & Boon, 2014; Demaria, 2013; Motz & Coukos, 2013; Teng, Kershaw, & Smyth, 2013)
   a) Altered immunogenicity: Tumor antigens are either cell surface molecules that function as targets for antibody responses or are intracellular molecules that are presented within the context of major histocompatibility complex (MHC) molecules capable of T-cell recognition. Alterations to antigen recognition or presentation dampen immune response.
      (1) Tumor recognized as self: Tumors express surface antigens that are also expressed on self-cells.
      (2) Neoantigens are products of acquired gene mutations resulting in altered antigen expression on the tumor cell surface, allowing the antigen to go unrecognized by the humoral immune system.
      (3) MHC molecule loss or alteration blunts cell-mediated immune response.
      (4) The peptide epitope (antigen) that binds to the MHC molecule and is recognized by T cells is lost or mutated.
      (5) Antibodies produced as part of the immune response cause antigens to enter the tumor cell or leave it completely. This further limits immune cells' ability to recognize the tumor cell as nonself.
   b) Acquired deficiencies to immune sensitivity
      (1) These include age- and disease-associated alterations, such as decreased or increased apoptosis and signaling defects of T cells.
      (2) Immunologic aging or immunosenescence causes a decline in the follow-

ing: numbers of naïve T cells; generation of cytotoxic T cells, hematopoietic stem cells, phagocytes, and NK cells; production of IL-2; signal transduction of lymphocytes; and humoral immunity. It also results in decreased antigen response and proliferation, increased number of memory T cells, and a potentially decreased number of functional Tregs.

c) Tumors develop adaptive mechanisms to evade immune detection.

(1) Tumors create a microenvironment rich in suppressive interactions that downregulate immune response. Immune interactions occurring in the tumor microenvironment can result in immune suppression rather than immune activation (Beatty & Gladney, 2015; Demaria, 2013; Motz & Coukos, 2013; Teng et al., 2013).

(a) The tumor itself produces substances that alter or inhibit the body's immune response. Examples include transforming growth factor-beta, IL-10, and adenosine, which limit T-cell toxicity functions.

(b) Tumors can overexpress receptors or immune checkpoints (e.g., CTLA-4, PD-1, lymphocyte activation gene 3 [known as LAG3]), which inhibit T-cell activity.

(c) Tumors recruit Tregs. Tregs' interaction with tumor antigen results in sustained immune tolerance and T-cell suppression.

(d) Tumors fail to give off inflammatory warning signals to stimulate an immune response. T-cell interaction in the absence of inflammatory signals results in sustained immune tolerance.

(2) *Immunoediting* is the development of an immune-resistant tumor mass resulting from prior exposure to immune attack. Three phases lead to its development (Chen & Mellman, 2013; Mittal, Gubin, Schreiber, & Smyth, 2014; Swann & Smyth, 2007; Teng et al., 2013).

(a) In the elimination phase, cellular and humoral immune cells eliminate highly immunogenic tumor cells. Cells with low immunogenicity survive.

(b) Tumor cells with low immunogenicity are ignored by a tolerant immune system during the equilibrium phase.

(c) The tumor mass is allowed to grow and spread unchecked in the escape phase.

I. Angiogenesis (Bielenberg & Zetter, 2015; Rajabi & Mousa, 2017; Zhao & Adjei, 2015)

1. Angiogenesis is the development of new blood vessels. It is a complex, multistep process required for a host of normal functions, including wound healing, tissue repair, reproduction, growth, and development.
2. Under normal circumstances, angiogenesis is tightly controlled by a balance of stimulators and inhibitors.
3. In malignant angiogenesis, that balance is disrupted, leading to irregular molecular and cellular events that contribute to tumor neovascularization.
4. In the context of tumors, *angiogenesis* refers to the growth of new vessels within a tumor. The new vessels develop from the existing vascular network and provide a blood supply for the tumor.
5. Tumors are initially antiangiogenic; the angiogenic switch converts the tumor to a proangiogenic state that leads to the development of new blood vessels.

a) Hypoxia activates intracellular molecules, including the hypoxia-inducible factor-1 (HIF-1) complex. HIF-1 activation causes upregulation of proangiogenic factors, including vascular endothelial growth factor (VEGF), platelet-derived growth factor, and nitric oxide synthase. HIF-1 is essential in inducing the angiogenic switch.

b) VEGF and basic fibroblast growth factor are circulating growth factors known to induce angiogenesis. Their presence has been reported to correlate with extent of disease, clinical status, and survival.

c) Endothelial cells line the vasculature of normal tissues. In a resting state, they provide a homeostatic barrier that prevents the uncontrolled extravasation of intravascular components and inhibits coagulation.

d) When a tumor begins to grow in normal tissue, tumor cells release factors that elicit responses from the surrounding endothelium. The result is vascular growth from normal tissue in the tumor.

e) Neovascularization contributes to tumor invasion and metastasis.

(1) Tumor vasculature is permeable and disorganized with a weak basement membrane. These conditions facilitate the migration of endothelial cells.

(2) VEGF can cause accumulation of endothelial cells and stimulate further tumor angiogenesis.

(3) Blood flow in tumors is sluggish, thus inducing hypoxia and acidosis. Tumor hypoxia further induces tumor angiogenesis.

(4) Hypoxia and acidosis may contribute to chemotherapy and radiation therapy resistance because of lack of oxygen.

6. Other molecular pathways involved in tumor angiogenesis

a) Matrix metalloproteinases are involved in degrading the extracellular matrix components. In angiogenesis, matrix metalloproteinases invade the extracellular matrix via new vessel formation and lead to proliferation and migration of tumor cells (Cathcart, Pulkoski-Gross, & Cao, 2015).

b) Tumor angiogenesis also affects the Notch receptor pathway. Notch surface cell receptors are involved in cell fate, differentiation, and proliferation. Vascular endothelial cells express certain Notch receptors. One type is needed for the vascular development of embryos but also is upregulated in tumor vasculature. This process may be VEGF mediated (Dimova, Popivanov, & Djonov, 2014).

c) The tyrosine kinase pathway is another receptor involved in angiogenesis. This pathway is associated with VEGF receptors (VEGFR1, VEGFR2, and VEGFR3) and Tie receptors (Tie1 and Tie2) (Jeltsch, Leppänen, Saharinen, & Alitalo, 2013). Both types of receptors play a key role in the generation of blood and lymphatic vessels during embryonic development and tumor angiogenesis.

J. Therapeutic uses for immunotherapeutic agents

1. Cure, when used as a primary or adjuvant therapy
2. Improve overall response or increase disease-free survival when used in conjunction with conventional therapies
3. Control or stabilize disease
4. Maintain or enhance quality of life
5. Function in a supportive care capacity by decreasing the severity of toxicities associated with other therapeutic modalities (e.g., hematopoietic growth factors can mitigate chemotherapy-associated cytopenias)

References

Abbas, A.K., Lichtman, A.H., & Pillai, S. (2016). *Basic immunology: Functions and disorders of the immune system* (5th ed.). St. Louis, MO: Elsevier Saunders.

Actor, J.K. (2014). *Introductory immunology: Basic concepts for interdisciplinary applications.* Cambridge, MA: Elsevier Academic Press.

Annunziato, F., Romagnani, C., & Romagnani, S. (2015). The 3 major types of innate and adaptive cell-mediated effector immunity. *Journal of Allergy and Clinical Immunology, 135,* 626–635. https://doi.org/10.1016/j.jaci.2014.11.001

Beatty, G.L., & Gladney, W.L. (2015). Immune escape mechanisms as a guide for cancer immunotherapy. *Clinical Cancer Research, 21,* 687–692. https://doi.org/10.1158/1078-0432.CCR-14-1860

Bielenberg, D.R., & Zetter, B.R. (2015). The contribution of angiogenesis to the process of metastasis. *Cancer Journal, 21,* 267–273. https://doi.org/10.1097/PPO.0000000000000138

Cathcart, J., Pulkoski-Gross, A., & Cao, J. (2015). Targeting matrix metalloproteinases in cancer: Bringing new life to old ideas. *Genes and Diseases, 2,* 26–34. https://doi.org/10.1016/j.gendis.2014.12.002

Chen, D.S., & Mellman, I. (2013). Oncology meets immunology: The cancer-immunity cycle. *Immunity, 39,* 1–10. https://doi.org/10.1016/j.immuni.2013.07.012

Coulie, P.G., Van den Eynde, B.J., van der Bruggen, P., & Boon, T. (2014). Tumor antigens recognized by T lymphocytes: At the core of cancer immunotherapy. *Nature Reviews Cancer, 14,* 136–146. https://doi.org/10.1038/nrc3670

Demaria, S. (2013). Immune escape: Immunosuppressive networks. In G.C. Prendergast & E.M. Jaffee (Eds.), *Cancer immunotherapy: Immune suppression and tumor growth* (2nd ed., pp. 149–164). https://doi.org/10.1016/B978-0-12-394296-8.00011-7

Dimova, I., Popivanov, G., & Djonov, V. (2014). Angiogenesis in cancer—General pathways and their therapeutic implications. *Journal of B.U.ON., 19,* 15–21.

Griffith, J.W., Sokol, C.L., & Luster, A.D. (2014). Chemokines and chemokine receptors: Positioning cells for host defense and immunity. *Annual Review of Immunology, 32,* 659–702. https://doi.org/10.1146/annurev-immunol-032713-120145

Hall, B.M. (2015). T cells: Soldiers and spies—The surveillance and control of effector T cells by regulatory T cells. *Clinical Journal of the American Society of Nephrology, 10,* 2050–2064. https://doi.org/10.2215/CJN.06620714

Iwasaki, A., & Medzhitov, R. (2015). Control of adaptive immunity by the innate immune system. *Nature Immunology, 16,* 343–353. https://doi.org/10.1038/ni.3123

Jeltsch, M., Leppänen, V.-M., Saharinen, P., & Alitalo, K. (2013). Receptor tyrosine kinase-mediated angiogenesis. *Cold Spring Harbor Perspectives in Biology, 5*(9). https://doi.org/10.1101/cshperspect.a009183

Keith, B., & Abueg, K.D. (2015). Nursing implications of targeted therapies and biotherapy. In J.K. Itano (Ed.), *Core curriculum for oncology nursing* (5th ed., pp. 251–267). St. Louis, MO: Elsevier.

Kurosaki, T., Kometani, K., & Ise, W. (2015). Memory B cells. *Nature Reviews Immunology, 15,* 149–159. https://doi.org/10.1038/nri3802

Lemmon, M.A., Schlessinger, J., & Ferguson, K.M. (2014). The EGFR family: Not so prototypical receptor tyrosine kinases. *Cold Spring Harbor Perspectives in Biology, 6,* a020768. https://doi.org/10.1101/cshperspect.a020768

Marcus, A., Gowen, B.G., Thompson, T.W., Iannello, A., Ardolino, M., Deng, W., ... Raulet, D.H. (2014). Recognition of tumors by the innate immune system and natural killer cells. In F.W. Alt (Ed.), *Advances in immunology: Vol. 122* (pp. 91–128). https://doi.org/10.1016/B978-0-12-800267-4.00003-1

Medina, K.L. (2016). Overview of the immune system. In S.J. Pittock & A. Vincent (Eds.), *Handbook of Clinical Neurology: Vol. 133. Autoimmune neurology* (pp. 61–76). https://doi.org/10.1016/B978-0-444-63432-0.00004-9

Mittal, D., Gubin, M.M., Schreiber, R.D., & Smyth, M.J. (2014). New insights into cancer immunoediting and its three component phases—elimination, equilibrium and escape. *Current Opinion in Immunology, 27,* 16–25. https://doi.org/10.1016/j.coi.2014.01.004

Motz, G.T., & Coukos, G. (2013). Deciphering and reversing tumor immune suppression. *Immunity, 39,* 61–73. https://doi.org/10.1016/j.immuni.2013.07.005

Normanno, N., De Luca, A., Bianco, C., Strizzi, L., Mancino, M., Maiello, M.R., ... Salomon, D.S. (2006). Epidermal growth factor receptor (EGFR) signaling in cancer. *Gene, 366,* 2–16. https://doi.org/10.1016/j.gene.2005.10.018

Ott, P.A., Hodi, F.S., & Robert, C. (2013). CTLA-4 and PD-1/PD-L1 blockade: New immunotherapeutic modalities with durable clinical benefit in melanoma patients. *Clinical Cancer Research, 19,* 5300–5309. https://doi.org/10.1158/1078-0432.CCR-13-0143

Pardoll, D.M. (2012). The blockade of immune checkpoints in cancer immunotherapy. *Nature Reviews Cancer, 12,* 252–264. https://doi.org/10.1038/nrc3239

Paul, W.E. (2013). The immune system. In W.E. Paul (Ed.), *Fundamental immunology* (7th ed., pp. 1–22). Philadelphia, PA: Wolters Kluwer Health/Lippincott Williams & Wilkins.

Rajabi, M., & Mousa, S. (2017). The role of angiogenesis in cancer treatment. *Biomedicines, 5,* 34. https://doi.org/10.3390/biomedicines5020034

Ruddle, N.H. (2014). Lymphatic vessels and tertiary lymphoid organs. *Journal of Clinical Investigation, 124,* 953–959. https://doi.org/10.1172/JCI71611

Swann, J.B., & Smyth, M.J. (2007). Immune surveillance of tumors. *Journal of Clinical Investigation, 117,* 1137–1146. https://doi.org/10.1172/JCI31405

Teng, M.W.L., Kershaw, M.H., & Smyth, M.J. (2013). Cancer immunoediting: From surveillance to escape. In G.C. Prendergast & E.M. Jaffee (Eds.), *Cancer immunotherapy: Immune suppression and tumor growth* (2nd ed., pp. 85–99). https://doi.org/10.1016/B978-0-12-394296-8.00007-5

Weiskopf, K., Schnorr, P.J., Pang, W.W., Chao, M.P., Chhabra, A., Seita, J., ... Weissman, I.L. (2016). Myeloid cell origins, differentiation, and clinical implications. *Microbiology Spectrum, 4*(5). https://doi.org/10.1128/microbiolspec.MCHD-0031-2016

Zhao, Y., & Adjei, A.A. (2015). Targeting angiogenesis in cancer therapy: Moving beyond vascular endothelial growth factor. *Oncologist, 20,* 660–673. https://doi.org/10.1634/theoncologist.2014-0465

Zitvogel, L., & Kroemer, G. (2012). Targeting PD-1/PD-L1 interactions for cancer immunotherapy. *OncoImmunology, 1,* 1223–1225. https://doi.org/10.4161/onci.21335

CHAPTER 10

Immunotherapy

A. Immunotherapy in the treatment of cancer
   1. Immunotherapy uses the patient's own immune system to manage or eradicate diverse cancer types (Farkona, Diamandis, & Blaustig, 2016). Therapeutic approaches engage underlying pathophysiologic mechanisms of the immune system to target cellular pathways associated with tumor development and growth, as well as to attack the malignancy itself (see Chapter 9).
   2. Six categories of immunotherapeutic approaches are presented in this chapter: checkpoint inhibitors, chimeric antigen receptor (CAR) T-cell immunotherapy, cytokines, immunomodulators, monoclonal antibodies (mAbs; including radioimmunotherapy [RIT]), and oncolytic viral therapies.

B. Categories of immunotherapeutic approaches
   1. Checkpoint inhibitors
      a) Pathophysiology: The immune system utilizes inhibitory and stimulatory pathways and immune checkpoints to regulate the process of identification and elimination of abnormal cells. Cancer cells use a different mechanism to disrupt these pathways and avoid recognition (Bayer et al., 2017). Immune checkpoint inhibitors block the proteins that help moderate the immune system and prevent T lymphocytes from recognizing and killing cancer cells. With this action blocked, T cells are released and can elicit an immune response against cancer cells. Several checkpoint inhibitors have been approved for the treatment of cancer, including anti–cytotoxic T-lymphocyte antigen (CTLA-4), anti–programmed cell death protein 1 (PD-1), and anti–programmed cell death-ligand 1 (PD-L1) (Pardoll, 2012).
      b) Mechanism of action
         (1) CTLA-4: First-in-class checkpoint inhibitor. CTLA is a receptor found on T cells that is engaged by its ligand B7 to prevent overactivation. Blockade of CTLA allows for continued T-cell activation, thus enhancing antitumor responses (Bayer et al., 2017). Example: ipilimumab.
         (2) PD-1: PD-1 is an inhibitory pathway present on activated T cells. PD-1 binds to the PD-L1 ligand, disrupting immune surveillance and antitumor responses. Checkpoint inhibitors targeting PD-1 can disrupt this process, thereby allowing for continued T-cell activation and tumor surveillance and elimination (Sosman, 2017). Examples: nivolumab, pembrolizumab.
         (3) PD-L1: PD-L1 can be found on tumor cells. It has an affinity for binding to PD-1 and B7 receptors, which inhibits T-cell activation and ongoing antitumor responses by immune surveillance. Blocking of PD-L1 can help restore immune activity (Chen, Irving, & Hodi, 2012). Examples: atezolizumab, avelumab, durvalumab.
      c) Indications: Indications for checkpoint inhibitors are rapidly expanding and include both solid tumor and hematologic malignancies. Indications by agent, as of the date of publication, are presented in Table 10-1.
      d) Administration: Checkpoint inhibitors are administered via IV infusion.
      e) Toxicities: Based on the mechanism of action, toxicities associated with checkpoint inhibitors are termed *immune-related adverse events* (irAEs). These events are often driven by an inflammatory response to immune-mediated activity resulting in inflammation within one or more organ system (Gordon et al., 2017; Postow & Wolchok, 2018; Villadolid & Amin, 2015).
         (1) Early recognition of irAEs is critical to safe and effective management, which may include the use of immunosuppressive agents. Patients and caregivers should be educated on irAEs, including signs and symptoms and management.

Table 10-1. Immunotherapy Agents

Classification	Mechanism of Action	Drug	Route	Indications	Side Effects	Nursing Considerations
Checkpoint inhibitors: CTLA-4	Binds to and blocks the interaction of CTLA-4 with its ligands	Ipilimumab (Yervoy®)	IV	Unresectable or metastatic melanoma Adjuvant melanoma	Fatigue, headache, skin toxicity (dermatitis), weight loss, GI toxicities (colitis, diarrhea), elevated LFTs, endocrinopathies, hepatitis, pneumonitis	For unresectable or metastatic melanoma: Administer 3 mg/kg IV, with an in-line filter, over 90 minutes every 3 weeks for a total of 4 doses. For adjuvant melanoma: Administer 10 mg/kg IV over 90 minutes every 3 weeks for a total of 4 doses followed by 10 mg/kg every 12 weeks for up to 3 years or until disease recurrence or unacceptable toxicity. Monitor for irAEs and follow management algorithms for dose modifications. Advise patients to report dermatologic reactions, liver toxicities, and GI toxicities. (Bristol-Myers Squibb Co., 2017b)
Checkpoint inhibitors: PD-1	Inhibits PD-1 immune checkpoint protein	Nivolumab (Opdivo®)	IV	Unresectable or metastatic melanoma Metastatic NSCLC Renal cell carcinoma Classical Hodgkin lymphoma Squamous cell carcinoma of the head and neck Urothelial carcinoma	Fatigue, malaise, peripheral neuropathy, GI toxicities, elevated LFTs, increased creatinine, electrolyte imbalances, weakness, anemia, neutropenia, thrombocytopenia, myalgia, upper respiratory tract infection, cough, febrile reaction	Administer 240 mg as an IV infusion, with an in-line filter, over 30 minutes every 2 weeks until disease progression or unacceptable toxicity for all indications or 480 mg as an IV infusion, with an in-line filter, over 30 minutes every 4 weeks until disease progression or unacceptable toxicity approved for all toxicities except microsatellite instability–high or mismatch repair–deficient metastatic colorectal cancer. Monitor for irAEs (including liver and kidney toxicities, colitis, and electrolyte imbalances) and follow management algorithms for dose modifications. (Bristol-Myers Squibb Co., 2017a)
	Binds to and blocks PD-1 with its ligands (PD-L1 and PD-L2)	Pembrolizumab (Keytruda®)	IV	Melanoma NSCLC Head and neck cancer Classical Hodgkin lymphoma Urothelial carcinoma Microsatellite instability–high cancer	Fatigue, skin rash, hyperglycemia, metabolic imbalances (hypomagnesemia, hypocalcemia, hypophosphatemia, hypokalemia), GI toxicities (vomiting), urinary tract infection, anemia, lymphocytopenia, thrombocytopenia, elevated LFTs, myalgia, increased serum creatinine, fever	Adults: 200 mg flat dose as an IV infusion over 30 minutes every 3 weeks Pediatrics: 2 mg/kg as an IV infusion over 30 minutes every 3 weeks Administer 2 mg/kg as an IV infusion over 30 minutes every 3 weeks. Monitor for irAEs and follow management algorithms for dose modifications. (Merck and Co. Inc., 2016)

(Continued on next page)

Table 10-1. Immunotherapy Agents *(Continued)*

Classification	Mechanism of Action	Drug	Route	Indications	Side Effects	Nursing Considerations
Checkpoint inhibitors: PD-L1	Inhibits PD-L1 interactions with PD-1 and B7-1 receptors	Atezolizumab (Tecentriq®)	IV	Locally advanced or metastatic urothelial carcinoma Metastatic NSCLC	Fatigue, hypoalbuminemia, hyponatremia, decreased appetite, nausea, constipation, urinary tract infection, increased serum alkaline phosphatase, increased serum AST, increased serum ALT, antibody development, infection, musculoskeletal pain, fever, pneumonitis	Administer 1,200 mg as an IV infusion mixed in 0.9% sodium chloride only, with or without an in-line filter over 60 minutes every 3 weeks until disease progression or unacceptable toxicity. Monitor for infusion-related reactions. If first infusion is tolerated, all subsequent infusions may be delivered over 30 minutes. Do not administer as an IV push or bolus. Monitor for irAEs and follow management algorithms for dose modifications. Advise patients to report symptoms of liver toxicities, infection, and neurologic and endocrine effects. (Genentech, Inc., 2017c)
	Binds to PD-L1 on T cells and blocks the interaction of PD-L1 with PD-1 and B7-1 receptors	Avelumab (Bavencio®)	IV	Merkel cell carcinoma Metastatic urothelial carcinoma (or locally advanced with progression during or after platinum-containing therapy or within 12 months of neoadjuvant or adjuvant treatment with platinum-containing chemotherapy)	Peripheral edema, fatigue, skin rash, diarrhea, nausea, decreased appetite, lymphocytopenia, anemia, increased serum AST, increased serum ALT, musculoskeletal pain, infusion-related reaction, pneumonitis, colitis, hepatitis, adrenal insufficiency, hypo- and hyperthyroidism, diabetes mellitus, nephritis	Premedicate with an antihistamine and acetaminophen prior to each of first 4 infusions. Administer 10 mg/kg IV infusion over 60 minutes once every 2 weeks until disease progression or unacceptable toxicity. Use an in-line filter for administration. Monitor for irAEs and follow management algorithms for dose modifications. Advise patients to report liver, pulmonary, and dermatologic toxicities. (EMD Serono, Inc., 2017)
	Inhibits PD-L1 interactions with the PD-1 and CD80 receptors	Durvalumab (Imfinzi®)	IV	Locally advanced or metastatic urothelial carcinoma Stage III unresectable NSCLC	Common: Fatigue, constipation, infection, decreased appetite, nausea, peripheral edema, urinary tract infection, musculoskeletal pain Serious: Immune-mediated pneumonitis, hepatitis, colitis, endocrinopathies (including adrenal insufficiency, hypophysitis, or type 1 diabetes mellitus), nephritis, infection, infusion-related reactions	Administer 10 mg/kg as an IV infusion over 60 minutes with an in-line filter every 2 weeks. Monitor for infusion-related reactions. Monitor for irAEs and follow management algorithms for dose modifications. Advise patients to report symptoms of infection, liver toxicity, and endocrine abnormalities. Drug may be withheld for moderate irAEs and permanently discontinued for severe or life-threatening irAEs. (AstraZeneca Pharmaceuticals LP, 2017)

(Continued on next page)

Table 10-1. Immunotherapy Agents *(Continued)*

Classification	Mechanism of Action	Drug	Route	Indications	Side Effects	Nursing Considerations
CAR T-cell immunotherapy	Binds to CD19-expressing cancer cells and normal B cells, activating downstream signaling cascades that lead to T-cell activation and secretion of inflammatory cytokines and chemokines that contribute to the death of CD19-expressing cells	Axicabtagene ciloleucel (Yescarta®)	IV	Relapsed or refractory large B-cell lymphoma (including diffuse large B-cell lymphoma not otherwise specified or arising from follicular lymphoma, primary mediastinal large B-cell lymphoma, or high-grade B-cell lymphoma) after 2 or more lines of systemic therapy	CRS, fever, hypotension, encephalopathy, tachycardia, fatigue, headache, decreased appetite, chills, diarrhea, febrile neutropenia, infections, nausea, hypoxia, tremor, cough, vomiting, dizziness, constipation, cardiac arrhythmias	Target dose is 2×10^6 CAR-positive viable T cells per kg body weight, with a maximum of 2×10^8 CAR-positive viable T cells (but is ultimately based on the number of CAR-positive viable T cells). Lymphodepleting regimen of cyclophosphamide 500 mg/m² and fludarabine 30 mg/m² should be administered on the fifth, fourth, and third day before axicabtagene ciloleucel; do not use a leukocyte-depleting filter. Premedicate with acetaminophen 650 mg PO and an H_1-antihistamine 12.5 mg IV or PO approximately 1 hour before infusion. Axicabtagene ciloleucel must be thawed at approximately 37°C prior to infusion and is viable at room temperature for 3 hours. After infusion is complete, the tubing should be flushed with NS to ensure all product is administered. Monitor for hypersensitivity reaction during infusion, as well as for signs of infection and prolonged cytopenias following infusion. Tocilizumab (an IL-6 receptor antagonist) IV over 60 minutes may be administered to manage severe or life-threatening CRS associated with CAR T-cell treatment. Patients should be monitored for at least 7 days in the hospital for toxicities and should remain within close proximity to the treating institution for at least 4 weeks following infusion. Hypogammaglobulinemia may occur and should be managed with replacement therapy. Drug is for autologous use only. Avoid prophylactic use of systemic corticosteroids, which may interfere with the activity of axicabtagene ciloleucel. (Kite Pharma, Inc., 2017)

(Continued on next page)

Table 10-1. Immunotherapy Agents *(Continued)*

Classification	Mechanism of Action	Drug	Route	Indications	Side Effects	Nursing Considerations
CAR T-cell immunotherapy *(cont.)*	Reprograms autologous T cells with a transgene encoding a CAR to identify and eliminate CD19-expressing malignant and normal cells	Tisagenlecleucel (Kymriah®)	IV	B-cell precursor acute lymphoblastic leukemia in individuals aged 25 years or younger Adults with relapsed or refractory large B-cell lymphoma after 2 or more lines of systemic therapy	CRS (fever, myalgias, fatigue, nausea, headaches, hypotension, capillary leak), intracranial hemorrhage, cardiac arrest, cardiac failure, hypogammaglobulinemia, infection, pyrexia, decreased appetite, encephalopathy, bleeding, tachycardia, vomiting, diarrhea, hypoxia, acute kidney injury, delirium	Administer as an IV infusion at 10–20 ml/min (adjusted by age and volume). The volume in the infusion bag ranges 10–50 ml. Do not use a leukocyte-depleting filter. Prime prior to and rinse following infusion with NS. Monitor patients for hypersensitivity during infusion and for signs and symptoms of CRS and neurotoxicity, both of which may be life threatening. Tocilizumab (an IL-6 receptor antagonist) IV over 60 minutes may be administered to manage severe or life-threatening CRS associated with CAR T-cell treatment. Because of prolonged cytopenias following infusion, patients are at an elevated risk for infection several weeks after treatment. Hypogammaglobinemia may occur and should be managed with replacement therapy. Patients should be advised not to drive or operate heavy machinery for up to 8 weeks following treatment. (Novartis Pharmaceuticals Corp., 2017a)
Cytokines: Growth factors	Stimulates erythropoiesis through interaction with progenitor stem cells to release RBCs	Darbepoetin (Aranesp®)	IV, SC	Treatment of anemia in patients with nonmyeloid malignancies due to effects of chemotherapy	Common: Fatigue, edema, nausea, vomiting, diarrhea, fever, dyspnea Serious: If Hgb > 11 g/dl, increased mortality, risk of MI, stroke, and thromboembolism; pneumonia, dehydration, fever, vomiting, dyspnea, death	Do not initiate therapy if Hgb ≥ 10 g/dl. Once-weekly dosage: Initial dosage is 2.25 mcg/kg SC weekly or 150 mcg/week. For titration, adjust dosage to maintain the lowest Hgb level needed to avoid RBC transfusions. Discontinue after completion of chemotherapy or if no response after 8 weeks of therapy (manufacturer dosage). Every-2-week dosage: 300 mcg SC every 2 weeks Every-3-week dosage: Initial dosage is 500 mcg SC every 3 weeks. For titration, adjust dosage to maintain the lowest Hgb level needed to avoid RBC transfusions. Discontinue after completion of chemotherapy or if no response after 8 weeks of therapy (manufacturer dosage).

(Continued on next page)

Table 10-1. Immunotherapy Agents *(Continued)*

Classification	Mechanism of Action	Drug	Route	Indications	Side Effects	Nursing Considerations
Cytokines: Growth factors *(cont.)*		Darbepoetin (Aranesp®) *(cont.)*				Hgb should be tested weekly until it has stabilized and then monthly thereafter. Administer supplemental iron during therapy to replenish or maintain iron stores (transferrin saturation should be ≥ 20% and ferritin ≥ 100 mcg/L). (Amgen Inc., 2017a)
	Stimulates erythropoiesis by the same mechanisms as endogenous erythropoietin	Epoetin alfa (Procrit®)	IV, SC	Treatment of chemotherapy-induced anemia	Common: Joint, muscle, and bone pain; fever, cough, dizziness, hyperglycemia, chills, rash, nausea, vomiting, trouble sleeping, itching, headache, respiratory infection, weight loss, depression, muscle spasms, redness and pain at injection site, leukopenia, hypokalemia Serious: If Hgb > 11, increased mortality, risk of MI, stroke, and thromboembolism; risk of tumor progression or recurrence; hypertension, seizures, lack or loss of Hgb response; pure red cell aplasia; serious allergic reactions, severe cutaneous reactions	Recommended dosing is 150 units/kg SC 3 times per week until completion of a chemotherapy course, or 40,000 units SC weekly until completion of a chemotherapy course. Pediatric patients (5–18 years): Dosage is 600 units/kg IV weekly until completion of a chemotherapy course. Do not shake or dilute. Protect from light. Discard unused portions of preservative-free drug; multidose vials may be stored at 36°F–46°F for up to 21 days. Initiate only if Hgb < 10 g/dl. Drug should not be used in patients receiving hormonal agents, biologic products, or radiation therapy, unless also receiving chemotherapy. Drug is also contraindicated in patients in whom anemia can be managed with transfusion. (Amgen Inc., 2017b)

(Continued on next page)

Table 10-1. Immunotherapy Agents *(Continued)*

Classification	Mechanism of Action	Drug	Route	Indications	Side Effects	Nursing Considerations
Cytokines: Growth factors *(cont.)*	Acts on hematopoietic cells by binding to specific cell surface receptors, thereby stimulating proliferation, differentiation, commitment, and end-cell functional activation, specifically stimulating neutrophil production; is a short-acting drug, so an immediate response will be seen in CBC	Filgrastim (G-CSF; Neupogen®)	SC	Prophylaxis of chemotherapy-induced febrile neutropenia in patients after a bone marrow transplant Prophylaxis of chemotherapy-induced febrile neutropenia in patients treated for nonmyeloid malignancies Chronic neutropenic disorders Myelosuppression due to radiation	Common: Rash, diarrhea, anemia, bone pain, headache, cough, dyspnea, epistaxis, fatigue, fever, pain Serious: Capillary leak syndrome, vasculitis of the skin, myelodysplastic syndrome, sickle cell anemia with crisis, anaphylaxis, hypersensitivity reaction, glomerulonephritis, ARDS, splenic rupture, Stevens-Johnson syndrome	Drug will be given daily until desired ANC is achieved. For prophylaxis of febrile neutropenia in patients with nonmyeloid malignancies undergoing myeloablative chemotherapy followed by marrow transplantation: Administer 10 mcg/kg/day as an IV infusion lasting no longer than 24 hours, starting at least 24 hours after chemotherapy and bone marrow infusion. For prophylaxis of febrile neutropenia in patients with nonmyeloid malignancies following myelosuppressive chemotherapy: Administer 5 mcg/kg SC or IV daily, starting at least 24 hours after chemotherapy. For prophylaxis of febrile neutropenia in patients with AML receiving chemotherapy: Administer 5 mcg/kg SC or IV daily, starting at least 24 hours after chemotherapy. For radiation injury of bone marrow or acute exposure to myelosuppressive radiation doses: Administer 10 mcg/kg SC as a single daily dose, starting as soon as possible after suspected or confirmed exposure to radiation dose > 2 Gy; do not delay administration if a CBC is unavailable; continue until ANC > 1,000/mm^3 for 3 consecutive CBCs obtained approximately every third day or ANC > 10,000/mm^3 after radiation-induced nadir. Educate patients on possible side effects. Monitor CBC, kidney function, and for side effects listed. Bone pain does not occur frequently, but if it occurs, pretreat with loratadine to help with bone pain. Nonsteroidal anti-inflammatory drugs or analgesics can also be used unless contraindicated. (Amgen Inc., 2016b; Romeo et al., 2014)

(Continued on next page)

Table 10-1. Immunotherapy Agents *(Continued)*

Classification	Mechanism of Action	Drug	Route	Indications	Side Effects	Nursing Considerations
Cytokines: Growth factors *(cont.)*	Binds to the human keratinocyte growth factor receptor to promote proliferation, differentiation, and migration of epithelial cells	Palifermin (rHuKG-CSF; Kepivance®)	IV	To decrease incidence and duration of severe oral mucositis in patients undergoing myelotoxic therapy with HSCT support	Common: Skin toxicities (rash, edema, erythema, pruritus), fever, GI events, respiratory complications, pain, arthralgias, dysesthesias, hypertension Serious: Potential for stimulation of tumor growth	Dosage is 60 mcg/kg/day IV bolus for 3 consecutive days before myelotoxic therapy (the third dose should be given 24–48 hours prior to starting myelotoxic therapy) and 3 consecutive days after myelotoxic therapy (first of these doses should be administered after, but on the same day of, hematopoietic stem cell infusion and at least 7 days after most recent dose of palifermin); a total of 6 doses is given. Reconstitute only with sterile water; administer 3 consecutive days before and after myelotoxic therapy. Do NOT shake vigorously or agitate the vial. Protect from light. Do NOT filter. Discard after 1 hour at room temperature. (Swedish Orphan Biovitrum, 2011)
	Acts on hematopoietic cells by stimulating proliferation, differentiation, commitment, and end-cell functional activation, specifically stimulating neutrophil production; pegylated characteristic of Neulasta decreases the half-life and therefore 1 dose per chemotherapy cycle is adequate to enhance neutrophil recovery	Pegfilgrastim (pegylated G-CSF; Neulasta®)	SC	Prophylaxis of chemotherapy-induced neutropenia Treatment of febrile neutropenia and radiation injury of bone marrow	Common: Bone pain, pain in limb Serious: Capillary leak syndrome, leukocytosis, splenic rupture, sickle cell anemia with crisis, anaphylaxis, glomerulonephritis, ARDS	For patients with cancer receiving myelosuppressive chemotherapy: Dosage is 6 mg SC once per chemotherapy cycle; do not administer between 14 days prior to and 24 hours after the administration of chemotherapy. May take about 7 days to see effect on CBC. For patients acutely exposed to myelosuppressive doses of radiation: Dosage is 6 mg SC for 2 doses, administered 1 week apart. Administer first dose as soon as possible after suspected or confirmed exposure to myelosuppressive doses of radiation, and a second dose 1 week after. Educate patients on possible side effects. Monitor CBC, kidney function, and for side effects listed. Pretreat with loratadine to help with bone pain (Romeo et al., 2014). Neulasta Onpro® is an OBI device that is placed on the body the last day of chemotherapy. It is not recommended to use for acute radiation injury. It auto-injects the medication 24 hours after placement. It is

(Continued on next page)

Table 10-1. Immunotherapy Agents *(Continued)*

Classification	Mechanism of Action	Drug	Route	Indications	Side Effects	Nursing Considerations
Cytokines: Growth factors *(cont.)*		Pegfilgrastim (pegylated G-CSF; Neulasta®) *(cont.)*				imperative to call the oncologist if the autoinjector does not deliver the dose. The OBI should be disposed of in a sharps container once the dose has been administered. It takes about 45 minutes to administer a full dose via the OBI. Educate patients to avoid bumping the OBI, putting lotions and creams around the OBI, using hot tubs, bathtubs, or saunas, and exposing the OBI to direct sunlight. (Amgen Inc., 2016a)
	Triggers proliferation and differentiation of hematopoietic progenitor cells, primarily neutrophils, monocytes/macrophages, and myeloid-derived dendritic cells; may also stimulate polymorphonuclear neutrophils to block the growth of tumor cells and increase the cytotoxic activity of monocytes against certain types of neoplastic cells	Sargramostim (GM-CSF; Leukine®)	IV, SC	AML Myeloid reconstitution after allogeneic or autologous bone marrow transplantation Mobilization and myeloid reconstitution in autologous HSCT	Common: Chest pain, peripheral edema, pruritus, rash, hypercholesterolemia, hypomagnesemia, metabolic disease, weight loss, abdominal pain, diarrhea, dysphagia, GI hemorrhage, hematemesis, nausea, vomiting, increased bilirubin level, arthralgia, bone pain, asthenia, intraocular hemorrhage, anxiety, elevated serum blood urea nitrogen, pharyngitis, fever, malaise, rigor Serious: Capillary leak syndrome, cardiac dysrhythmia, pericardial effusion, cerebral hemorrhage, renal failure	AML: Neutrophil recovery, following induction chemotherapy: Dosage is 250 mcg/m²/day IV over 4 hours beginning on or about day 11 or 4 days following the completion of induction chemotherapy if day 10 bone marrow is hypoplastic (< 5% blasts). Continue sargramostim until the ANC is > 1,500/mm³ for 3 consecutive days or for a maximum of 42 days. If a second cycle of induction chemotherapy is required, administer sargramostim approximately 4 days following completion of chemotherapy if bone marrow is hypoplastic with < 5% blasts. Discontinue if leukemic regrowth occurs. Allogeneic bone marrow transplantation, myeloid reconstitution: Dosage is 250 mcg/m²/day IV over 2 hours; begin 2–4 hours after bone marrow infusion and continue until ANC is > 1,500/mm³ for 3 consecutive days. Do not administer sooner than 24 hours after the last dose of chemotherapy/radiation therapy or until post–marrow infusion ANC is < 500/mm³. Discontinue if blast cells appear or disease progression occurs. Autologous bone marrow transplantation, myeloid reconstitution: Dosage is 250 mcg/m²/day IV over 2 hours, begin 2–4 hours after bone marrow infusion and not less than 24 hours after the last dose of

(Continued on next page)

Table 10-1. Immunotherapy Agents *(Continued)*

Classification	Mechanism of Action	Drug	Route	Indications	Side Effects	Nursing Considerations
Cytokines: Growth factors *(cont.)*		Sargramostim (GM-CSF; Leukine®) *(cont.)*				chemotherapy or radiation therapy. Do not administer until post–marrow infusion ANC is < 500/mm³. Continue until ANC is > 1,500/mm³ for 3 consecutive days. Discontinue if blast cells appear or disease progression occurs. Autologous peripheral blood HSCT, following myeloablative chemotherapy: Dosage is 250 mcg/m²/day IV over 24 hours or SC once daily; begin immediately following peripheral blood progenitor cell infusion and continue until ANC is > 1,500/mm³ for 3 consecutive days. Bone marrow transplant dose, delay, or failure of myeloid engraftment: Dosage is 250 mcg/m²/day IV over 2 hours for 14 days; repeat after 7 days off therapy if engraftment has not occurred. After an additional 7 days, a third course of 500 mcg/m²/day IV for 14 days may be administered if engraftment still has not occurred. Discontinue if blast cells appear or disease progression occurs. Monitor CBC, renal and liver function, and for side effects listed. Assess for and educate patients on signs and symptoms of infection. Monitor electrolytes in patients with nausea, vomiting, or diarrhea. Notify MD of any sign or symptom of graft failure. (Sanofi-Aventis U.S. LLC, 2013)

(Continued on next page)

Table 10-1. Immunotherapy Agents *(Continued)*

Classification	Mechanism of Action	Drug	Route	Indications	Side Effects	Nursing Considerations
Cytokines: Growth factors *(cont.)*	Binds to G-CSF receptors and stimulates proliferation of neutrophils	Tbo-filgrastim (Granix®)	SC	Patients with nonmyeloid malignancies undergoing myelosuppressive treatment associated with prolonged neutropenia	Common: Bone pain, myalgia, headache, vomiting, acute febrile neutrophilic dermatosis, cutaneous vasculitis, thrombocytopenia Serious: Splenic rupture, ARDS, capillary leak syndrome, potential for tumor growth stimulatory effects	Administer no earlier than 24 hours following and not within 24 hours prior to the administration of myelosuppressive chemotherapy. Prefilled syringe is for single use only; recommended injection sites include abdomen, front of middle thigh, upper outer areas of buttocks, and upper back area of upper arms. Bone pain is common and may be treated with analgesics unless otherwise contraindicated; pretreatment with loratadine can be used to help with bone pain. Advise patients to report pain in the left upper quadrant of the abdomen or left shoulder, as these may be signs of splenic enlargement or rupture. (Romeo et al., 2014; Teva Pharmaceuticals, 2014)
Cytokines: Interferons (IFNs)	Stimulates secretion of proteins in response to foreign invasion in the body, which activates a cascade, suppressing cell proliferation, enhancing phagocytic activity of macrophages, augmenting specific cytotoxicity of lymphocytes for target cells, and inhibiting viral replication in virus-infected cells	IFN alfa-2b (Intron® A)	IM, IV, SC, and intralesional; depends on disease being treated	Chronic myeloid leukemia Hairy cell leukemia Follicular lymphoma Cutaneous T-cell lymphoma Melanoma Renal cell carcinoma Carcinoid tumors	Common: Alopecia, decreased weight, abdominal pain, diarrhea, decreased appetite, anorexia, nausea, vomiting, neutropenia, increased liver enzymes, arthralgia, myalgia, asthenia, headache, depression, fatigue, fever, flu-like symptoms, shivering Serious: Cardiac dysrhythmia, cardiomyopathy, hypotension, MI, supraventricular arrhythmia, tachycardia, Raynaud disease, vasculitis, GI hemorrhage, pancreatitis, anemia, aplastic anemia, thrombocytopenia, hepatic encephalopathy, liver failure, functional vision loss, optic disc edema, optic neuritis, retinal hemorrhage, retinopathy, thrombosis of retinal vein or artery, suicidal thoughts, suicide, obliterative bronchiolitis, pneumonia, pneumonitis, pneumothorax, PE, pulmonary hypertension, pulmonary infiltrate, sarcoidosis	Induction dosage is 20 million IU/m² IV 5 consecutive days/week for 4 weeks; maintenance dosage is 10 million IU/m² SC 3 times/week for 48 weeks. Monitor CBC, liver panel, thyroid function studies (TSH/T4), and for side effects listed. Discuss depression and always ask patients if they are having suicidal or homicidal thoughts. (Merck and Co., Inc., 2015a)

(Continued on next page)

Table 10-1. Immunotherapy Agents *(Continued)*

Classification	Mechanism of Action	Drug	Route	Indications	Side Effects	Nursing Considerations
Cytokines: Interferons (IFNs) *(cont.)*	Exact mechanism unknown, but the functions of IFN are suppression of cell proliferation, antiviral activity, and immune-modulating effects, such as augmentation of macrophage phagocytic activity	IFN alfa-2b (pegylated; Sylatron™)	SC	Adjuvant treatment of melanoma	Common: Alopecia, injection site reaction, decreased appetite, anorexia, nausea, vomiting, increased liver enzymes, arthralgia, myalgia, headache, fatigue, rigor Serious: Bundle branch block, cardiomyopathy, hypotension, MI, supraventricular arrhythmia, ventricular tachycardia, colitis, pancreatitis, anemia, thrombocytopenia, encephalopathy, blindness or vision impairment, optic neuritis, retinal hemorrhage, thrombosis of retinal vein, aggressive behavior, bipolar disorder, depression, hallucinations, homicidal thoughts, suicidal thoughts, suicide	Dosage is 6 mcg/kg/week SC for 8 doses, then 3 mcg/kg/week SC for up to 5 years; premedicate with acetaminophen 500–1,000 mg PO 30 minutes prior to first dose and as needed for subsequent doses. Monitor CBC, liver panel, thyroid function studies (TSH/T4), and for side effects listed. Discuss depression and always ask patients if they are having suicidal or homicidal thoughts. (Merck and Co., Inc., 2015b)
	Binds to a different cell surface receptor and is classified as a type 2 IFN; enhances oxidative metabolism of macrophages, antibody-dependent cellular cytotoxicity, activation of NK cells, and expression of Fc receptors and major histocompatibility antigens	IFN gamma (Actimmune®)	SC	To reduce frequency and severity of serious infections associated with chronic granulomatous disease To delay time to disease progression in patients with severe malignant osteopetrosis	Common: Flu-like symptoms, fever, chills, myalgia, fatigue, neutropenia, thrombocytopenia, liver enzyme elevation, rash, diarrhea, vomiting, nausea, arthralgia Serious: Exacerbations of underlying cardiac disease, hepatic insufficiency, pancreatitis with death, asthenia, chest pain, upper respiratory tract infection, muscle spasm, pain, confusion, depression, hallucination, mental status decrease, atopic dermatitis, urticaria	Administer SC at a dose of 50 mcg/m^2 for patients whose body surface area is > 0.5 m^2 and 1.5 mcg/kg for patients whose body surface area is ≤ 0.5 m^2 three times weekly. Monitor CBC, chemistries, and urinalysis prior to and every 3 months following treatment. Monitor LFTs and renal function studies. Assess for signs and symptoms of infection. Report new symptoms immediately. Symptoms will be most intense in the beginning and can wane in intensity as treatment continues. (HZNP USA Inc., 2015)

(Continued on next page)

Table 10-1. Immunotherapy Agents *(Continued)*

Classification	Mechanism of Action	Drug	Route	Indications	Side Effects	Nursing Considerations
Cytokines: ILs	Exact mechanism unknown, but causes induction of lymphokine-activated killer cells, NK cells, and IFN gamma production; inhibits tumor growth by stimulating growth and activity of T cells and B lymphocytes	Aldesleukin (IL-2; Proleukin®)	IV	Metastatic melanoma Metastatic renal cell carcinoma	Common: Hypotension, peripheral edema, tachycardia, vasodilation, pruritus, rash, diarrhea, loss of appetite, nausea, vomiting, anemia, thrombocytopenia, hyperbilirubinemia, asthenia, confusion, somnolence, oliguria, elevated serum creatinine, dyspnea, fever, infections, malaise, shivering Serious: Capillary leak syndrome, hypotension, MI, supraventricular tachycardia, ventricular tachycardia, acute renal failure, anuria, ARDS, apnea, intubation, respiratory failure, fever, sepsis	Dosing is weight based: 600,000 IU/kg (0.037 mg/kg) IV every 8 hours for 14 doses; repeat after a rest period of 9 days. Drug must be administered in a center that has cardiac monitoring capability and intensive care if needed. Monitor for acute signs of infection and for side effects listed. Monitor weight; urine output and bowel movements; and blood pressure, heart rate, temperature, respiratory rate, and oxygen saturation while receiving therapy. Administer supportive medications for side effects. Patients need central line access while on high-dose therapy because they will need IV medications to support blood pressure. These pressor support medications have vesicant properties. (Prometheus Laboratories Inc., 2012)
	Thrombopoietic growth factor that directly stimulates proliferation of hematopoietic stem cells and megakaryocyte progenitor cells and induces megakaryocyte maturation, resulting in increased platelet production	Oprelvekin (IL-11; Neumega®)	SC	To prevent severe thrombocytopenia and reduce the need for platelet transfusions following myelosuppressive chemotherapy in adult patients with nonmyeloid malignancies who are at high risk for severe thrombocytopenia	Common: Rash, candidiasis, nausea, oral candidiasis, vomiting, dizziness, fatigue, headache, blurred vision, conjunctival hyperemia, dyspnea Serious: Atrial arrhythmia, body fluid retention, cardiomegaly, edema, increased plasma volume, palpitations, syncope, tachyarrhythmia, ventricular arrhythmia, hypokalemia, febrile neutropenia, anaphylaxis, cerebral artery occlusion, optic disc edema, pleural effusion	Dosage is 50 mcg/kg SC once daily for 14–21 days or until postnadir platelet count is > 50,000/mm^3. Monitor CBC; goal is platelet count > 50,000/mm^3. Monitor renal function. Educate patients to report fluid retention. Monitor for side effects listed. (Wyeth Pharmaceuticals Inc., 2009)

(Continued on next page)

Table 10-1. Immunotherapy Agents *(Continued)*

Classification	Mechanism of Action	Drug	Route	Indications	Side Effects	Nursing Considerations
Miscellaneous: Autologous cellular immunotherapy	Precise mechanism of action unknown; autologous peripheral blood mononuclear cells, including antigen-presenting cells (dendritic cells), are incubated with recombinant fusion protein antigen, which contains both PAP and GM-CSF; designed to induce an immune response against prostate cancer	Sipuleucel-T (Provenge®)	IV	Treatment of asymptomatic or minimally symptomatic metastatic castrate-resistant (hormone-refractory) prostate cancer	Common: Chills, fatigue, fever, back pain, nausea, joint aches, headache Serious: Hemorrhagic and ischemic stroke, deep vein thrombosis, PE	Dose is a minimum of 50 million autologous CD54+ cells activated with PAP-GM-CSF, suspended in 250 ml of lactated Ringer's solution. Course of therapy is 3 complete doses. Each infusion is preceded by a leukapheresis procedure approximately 3 days prior. Administer over 60 minutes; do not use a filter. Drug must be administered within 3 hours once brought to room temperature. Premedicate 30 minutes prior to infusion with acetaminophen and an antihistamine to reduce or mitigate transfusion reactions. Monitor patients for acute infusion reactions within 1 day of infusion, which include fever, chills, dyspnea, hypoxia, bronchospasm, nausea, vomiting, fatigue, hypertension, and tachycardia. Use universal precautions when handling because of potential risk of transmitting infectious diseases. (Dendreon Corp., 2014)
Miscellaneous: Hematopoietic stem cell mobilizers	Inhibits CXCR4 chemokine receptor and blocks binding of SDF-1α, resulting in leukocytosis and increased circulating hematopoietic progenitor cells	Plerixafor (Mozobil®)	SC	Mobilization of hematopoietic stem cells for autologous collection in patients with non-Hodgkin lymphoma and multiple myeloma	Common: Diarrhea, nausea, fatigue, injection site reaction, headache, arthralgia, dizziness, vomiting Serious: Thrombocytopenia, splenic enlargement or rupture, anaphylactic shock or hypersensitivity	G-CSF 10 mcg/kg is administered once daily for 4 days prior to first evening dose of plerixafor and on each day prior to apheresis. Drug may cause mobilization of leukemic cells; monitor platelet counts for signs of thrombocytopenia, which can occur with use. Assess for signs of splenic enlargement and rupture, including left upper quadrant or scapular pain. Drug was teratogenic in animal studies and should be avoided in women who are or may become pregnant. (Genzyme Corp., 2017)

(Continued on next page)

Table 10-1. Immunotherapy Agents *(Continued)*

Classification	Mechanism of Action	Drug	Route	Indications	Side Effects	Nursing Considerations
Miscellaneous: Immunomodulators	Analog of thalidomide that inhibits its proliferation and induces apoptosis of malignant hematopoietic cells; immunomodulatory effects include activation and increase in number of T and NK cells.	Lenalidomide (Revlimid®)	PO	Multiple myeloma, in combination with dexamethasone Multiple myeloma, as maintenance following autologous HSCT Transfusion-dependent anemia due to myelodysplastic syndromes associated with a deletion 5q abnormality with or without additional cytogenetic abnormalities Relapsed or progressed mantle cell lymphoma after 2 prior therapies, 1 of which included bortezomib	Common: Diarrhea, anemia, constipation, peripheral edema, neutropenia, fatigue, back pain, nausea, asthenia, insomnia, hypokalemia, rash, cataracts, lymphopenia, dyspnea, deep vein thrombosis, hyperglycemia, leukopenia Serious: Embryo-fetal toxicity, hematologic toxicity, venous and arterial thromboembolism, increased mortality in patients with chronic lymphocytic leukemia, second primary malignancies, hepatotoxicity, severe cutaneous reactions (e.g., Stevens-Johnson syndrome), tumor lysis syndrome, tumor flare reactions, impaired stem cell mobilization, thyroid disorders, early mortality in patients with mantle cell lymphoma	Dosing is the following: • Multiple myeloma (combination therapy): 25 mg once daily on days 1–21 of repeated 28-day cycles, in combination with dexamethasone • Multiple myeloma (maintenance therapy following autologous HSCT): 10 mg once daily continuously on days 1–28 of repeated 28-day cycles • Myelodysplastic syndrome: 10 mg once daily • Mantle cell lymphoma: 25 mg once daily on days 1–21 of repeated 28-day cycles Drug is available in 2.5, 5, 10, 15, 20, and 25 mg capsules. Drug should be taken orally at the same time each day with or without food; advise patients that capsules should be swallowed whole with water and should not be opened, broken, or chewed. Drug is teratogenic and should not be used in women who are or may become pregnant. Women should avoid pregnancy for at least 4 weeks before beginning therapy; during therapy, including dose interruptions; and for at least 4 weeks after therapy. Obtain 2 negative pregnancy tests prior to initiating therapy. Men receiving therapy should use a latex or synthetic condom when having intercourse with women of childbearing potential during treatment and for 4 weeks after taking lenalidomide. Lenalidomide is only available under a risk evaluation and mitigation strategy program. Monitor digoxin plasma levels because of increased C_{max} and area under the plasma concentration versus time curve with concomitant lenalidomide therapy. Patients taking concomitant therapies, such as erythropoietin-stimulating agents or estrogen-containing therapies, may have an increased risk of thrombosis. Patients must not donate blood during treatment and for 1 month following treatment. (Celgene Corp., 2017a)

(Continued on next page)

Table 10-1. Immunotherapy Agents *(Continued)*

Classification	Mechanism of Action	Drug	Route	Indications	Side Effects	Nursing Considerations
Miscellaneous: Immunomodulators *(cont.)*	Analog of thalidomice that inhibits proliferation and induces apoptosis of malignant hematopoietic cells	Pomalidomide (Pomalyst®)	PO	Multiple myeloma in patients who have received at least 2 prior therapies, including lenalidomide and bortezomib, and have demonstrated disease progression on or within 60 days of completion of the last therapy	Common: Fatigue, asthenia, neutropenia, anemia, constipation, nausea, diarrhea, dyspnea, upper respiratory tract infection, back pain, pyrexia Serious: Embryo-fetal toxicities, venous thromboembolism, hematologic toxicity, hypersensitivity reactions, dizziness, confusion, neuropathy, risk of second primary malignancies	Dosing is 4 mg/day taken on days 1–21 of repeated 28-day cycles until disease progression, in combination with dexamethasone. Drug is available in 1, 2, 3, and 4 mg capsules. Advise patients that capsules should be swallowed whole with water, with or without food, and should not be opened, broken, or chewed. Avoid use in patients with serum creatinine > 3 mg/dl. Patients should avoid pregnancy for at least 4 weeks before beginning therapy; during therapy, including dose interruptions; and for at least 4 weeks after therapy. Obtain 2 negative pregnancy tests prior to initiating therapy. Men receiving therapy should use a latex or synthetic condom when having intercourse with women of childbearing potential during treatment and for 28 days after taking pomalidomide. Patients must not donate blood during treatment and for 1 month following treatment. Drug is only available under a risk evaluation and mitigation strategy program. (Celgene Corp., 2016)
	Not fully understood; possesses immunomodulatory, anti-inflammatory, and anti-angiogenic properties	Thalidomide (Thalomid®)	PO	Newly diagnosed multiple myeloma, in combination with dexamethasone	Common: Fatigue, hypocalcemia, edema, constipation, peripheral neuropathy, dyspnea, muscle weakness, leukopenia, neutropenia, rash/desquamation, confusion, anorexia, nausea, anxiety/agitation, asthenia, tremor, fever, weight loss, thrombosis/embolism, motor neuropathy, weight gain, dizziness, dry skin Serious: Ischemic heart disease in patients treated in combination with dexamethasone; dizziness and orthostatic hypotension, neutropenia, thrombocytopenia, bradycardia, Stevens-Johnson	Dosing is 200 mg once daily in combination with dexamethasone 40 mg/day on days 1–4, 9–12, and 17–20 every 28 days. Drug is available in 50, 100, 150, and 200 mg capsules. Administer once daily with water, preferably at bedtime and at least 1 hour after a meal. Drug is teratogenic; avoid use in pregnant women and women of childbearing potential. Patients should avoid pregnancy for at least 4 weeks before beginning therapy; during therapy, including dose interruptions; and for at least 4 weeks after therapy. Obtain 2 negative pregnancy tests prior to initiating therapy. Men receiving therapy should use a latex or synthetic condom when having intercourse with women of childbearing potential during

(Continued on next page)

Table 10-1. Immunotherapy Agents *(Continued)*

Classification	Mechanism of Action	Drug	Route	Indications	Side Effects	Nursing Considerations
Miscellaneous: Immunomodulators *(cont.)*		Thalidomide (Thalomid®) *(cont.)*			syndrome, toxic epidermal necrolysis, seizures, tumor lysis syndrome, hypersensitivity reaction, increased HIV viral load	treatment and for 28 days after taking thalidomide. Examine patients every 3 months for signs of peripheral neuropathy. Patients must not donate blood during treatment and for 1 month following treatment. (Celgene Corp., 2017b)
Monoclonal antibodies: Chimeric	Targets the CD30 antigen and delivers a drug called monomethyl auristatin E, or MMAE	Brentuximab vedotin (anti-CD30 antibody; Adcetris®)	IV	Lymphoma	Peripheral neuropathy, fatigue, rash, GI toxicities, neutropenia, anemia, upper respiratory tract infection, cough, fever, infusion-related reactions	Recommended dosage is 1.8 mg/kg up to 180 mg IV over 30 minutes every 3 weeks. Dose reduce in patients with mild hepatic impairment. Monitor liver enzymes and bilirubin. Monitor CBC, with intervention if grade 3 or higher neutropenia occurs. Advise patients to report symptoms of pulmonary toxicity, hepatotoxicity, and dermatologic toxicity. Store reconstituted vials or diluted solution at 2°C–8°C and use within 24 hours. Do not administer as an IV push or bolus. (Truven Health Analytics, 2017)
	Blocks the binding of ligands to EGFR	Cetuximab (anti-EGFR antibody; Erbitux®)	IV	Colorectal cancer Head and neck cancers	Fatigue, pain, peripheral neuropathy, headache, insomnia, weight loss, skin toxicities (e.g., acneform rash, nail changes), hypomagnesemia, dehydration, GI toxicities, elevated LFTs, weakness, dyspnea, cough, fever, pharyngitis, infusion-related reactions	Administer 400 mg/m² initial dose as a 120-minute IV infusion. Maintenance dosage is 250 mg/m² weekly over 60 minutes (maximum infusion rate is 10 mg/min). Initiate cetuximab 1 week prior to start of radiation. Complete cetuximab 1 hour prior to platinum-based therapy with 5-fluorouracil and FOLFIRI (leucovorin, 5-fluorouracil, and irinotecan). Administer with a 0.22 micrometer in-line filter. Premedicate with an H_1 antagonist. Monitor serum electrolytes (e.g., magnesium, potassium, calcium). Monitor for dermatologic toxicities and advise patients to wear sunscreen. Monitor for preexisting cardiac disease or worsening or new cardiac symptoms. Preparations are stable for 12 hours at 2°C–8°C or for 8 hours at 20°C–25°C. Do not administer as an IV push or bolus. (Truven Health Analytics, 2017)

(Continued on next page)

Table 10-1. Immunotherapy Agents *(Continued)*

Classification	Mechanism of Action	Drug	Route	Indications	Side Effects	Nursing Considerations
Monoclonal antibodies: Chimeric *(cont.)*	Binds to GD2 on neuroblastoma cells, resulting in cell lysis	Dinutuximab (anti-GD2 antibody; Unituxin®)	IV	Neuroblastoma	Hypotension, capillary leak syndrome, pain, urticaria, hyponatremia, hypokalemia, hypoalbuminemia, hypocalcemia, hypophosphatemia, increased ALT, vomiting, diarrhea, increased serum AST, thrombocytopenia, lymphocytopenia, anemia, neutropenia, severe infusion-related reactions, fever, hypoxia	Administer 17.5 mg/m²/day IV over 10–20 hours for 4 consecutive days for up to 5 cycles. Premedicate with an analgesic, antiemetic, antihistamine, antipyretic, and IV hydration with NS. Monitor peripheral blood counts and serum electrolytes. Advise patients to report symptoms of electrolyte dysfunctions, eye disorders, thrombocytopenia, neutropenia, and worsening neuropathy. Store for up to 4 hours at 2°C–8°C prior to administration. Do not administer as an IV push or bolus. (Truven Health Analytics, 2017)
	Binds to the antigen CD20	Rituximab (anti-CD20 antibody; Rituxan®)	IV	Chronic lymphocytic leukemia Non-Hodgkin lymphoma	Fatigue, chills, neuropathy, nausea, lymphocytopenia, anemia, infection, weakness, infusion-related reactions, tumor lysis syndrome	Administer 375 mg/m² IV for non-Hodgkin lymphoma. Administer 375 mg/m² in first cycle and 500 mg/m² in cycles 2–6 for chronic lymphocytic leukemia. With first administration, use stepped-up dosing: 50 mg on day 1, 150 mg on day 2, and the remainder of the 375 mg/m² on day 3. Pretreat with acetaminophen and an antihistamine prior to each infusion. Monitor renal function and CBC. Advise patients to avoid vaccines. Administration of non-live vaccines should take place at least 4 weeks prior to 2-week treatment. Instruct patients to report any skin toxicities. If patients have a history of hepatitis B, advise them to report any signs or symptoms of an active infection. Store diluted solution at 2°C–8°C for up to 24 hours. Do not administer as an IV push or bolus. (Truven Health Analytics, 2017)

(Continued on next page)

Table 10-1. Immunotherapy Agents *(Continued)*

Classification	Mechanism of Action	Drug	Route	Indications	Side Effects	Nursing Considerations
Monoclonal antibodies: Chimeric *(cont.)*	Binds to the antigen CD20 and is combined with hyaluronidase human	Rituximab and hyaluronidase (Rituxan Hycela™)	SC	Chronic lymphocytic leukemia Non-Hodgkin lymphoma	Neutropenia, anemia, hypersensitivity reaction, nausea, constipation, diarrhea, fatigue, tumor lysis syndrome, bowel obstruction or perforation, embryo-fetal toxicities	All patients receive at least one full dose of rituximab IV before receiving SC dose of Rituxan Hycela. Chronic lymphocytic leukemia: 1,600 mg rituximab and 26,800 units hyaluronidase human. Administer SC over 7 minutes. Non-Hodgkin lymphoma: 1,400 mg rituximab and 23,400 units hyaluronidase human. Administer SC over 5 minutes. Premedicate with acetaminophen and antihistamine before each dose. Consider premedication with corticosteroid. (Genentech, Inc., 2017b)
Monoclonal antibodies: Human	Binds to CD38	Daratumumab (anti-CD38 antibody; Darzalex®)	IV	Multiple myeloma	Fatigue, nausea, lymphocytopenia, neutropenia, anemia, back pain, cough, fever, infusion-related reactions	Administer 16 mg/kg IV. Use a 0.22 or 0.2 mcm in-line filter. Titrate per package insert based on volume and dose. Administer weekly for 8 doses (weeks 1–8), then every 2 weeks (weeks 9–24), and then every 4 weeks (starting week 25) until disease progression. Pretreat with dexamethasone 20 mg plus an oral antipyretic and oral or IV antihistamine. Interference with serologic testing: Daratumumab binds to CD38 on RBCs and results in a positive indirect Coombs test. A type and screen must be done for all patients prior to starting therapy. Positive Coombs test may occur up to 6 months after last administration. Notify transfusion center that the patient has received daratumumab. Educate patients to report symptoms of infection and easy bruising or bleeding. Do not administer as an IV push or bolus. (Truven Health Analytics, 2017)
	Binds to RANKL and blocks its interaction with RANK	Denosumab (anti-RANK antibody; Prolia®, Xgeva®)	SC	Prolia: Increases bone mass and treats osteoporosis Xgeva: Bone metastasis	Osteonecrosis of the jaw, hypocalcemia, hypophosphatemia, dyspnea, infusion-related reactions	Prolia: Administer SC 60 mg every 6 months. Xgeva: Administer SC 120 mg every 4 weeks. Monitor calcium levels. Assess for and advise patients to report symptoms of osteonecrosis of the jaw or hypocalcemia. (Truven Health Analytics, 2017)

(Continued on next page)

Table 10-1. Immunotherapy Agents *(Continued)*

Classification	Mechanism of Action	Drug	Route	Indications	Side Effects	Nursing Considerations
Monoclonal antibodies: Human *(cont.)*	Binds to and prevents the ligand binding of EGFR	Necitumumab (anti-EGFR antibody; Portrazza®)	IV	Lung cancer	Skin toxicity, rash, hypomagnesemia, hypocalcemia, hypophosphatemia, hypokalemia, vomiting, infusion-related reactions	Administer 800 mg as an IV infusion over 60 minutes on days 1 and 8 of each 21-day cycle. Monitor serum electrolytes. Advise patients to report symptoms of thromboembolic events and to wear sunscreen and report dermatologic toxicities. Educate patients to report symptoms of hypomagnesemia. (Truven Health Analytics, 2017)
	Binds to CD20 antigen on B cells	Ofatumumab (anti-CD20 antibody; Arzerra®)	IV	Leukemia	Neutropenia, infection, pneumonia, infusion-related reactions	Administer as an IV infusion. Dosing is dependent on stage and treatment history; see package insert. Titrate per package insert. Premedicate with acetaminophen, an IV or oral antihistamine, and an IV corticosteroid. Monitor CBC and neurologic function. Advise patients to report symptoms of myelosuppression. If patients have a history of hepatitis B, instruct them to report any signs or symptoms of an active infection. Start infusion within 12 hours of preparation, and discard after 24 hours. Once drug is diluted, store at 2°C–8°C. Do not administer as an IV push or bolus. (Truven Health Analytics, 2017)
	Binds to PDGFR-α, blocking it	Olaratumab (anti-PDGFR-α antibody; Lartruvo™)	IV	Sarcoma	Fatigue, neuropathy, alopecia, nausea, mucositis, vomiting, diarrhea, decreased appetite, abdominal pain, musculoskeletal pain, lymphocytopenia, neutropenia, hyperglycemia, hypokalemia, hypophosphatemia, thrombocytopenia, prolonged activated partial thromboplastin time, infusion-related reactions	Administer at 15 mg/kg over 60 minutes as an IV infusion on days 1 and 8 of each 21-day cycle. Premedicate with an antihistamine IV prior to drug on day 1 of cycle 1. Administer for first 8 cycles with doxorubicin for patients with sarcoma. Instruct patients to report symptoms of infusion-related reactions. Allow refrigerated solution to come to room temperature prior to infusion. Diluted solution may be stored up to 24 hours at 2°C–8°C and up to an additional 4 hours at room temperature. Do not administer as an IV push or bolus. (Truven Health Analytics, 2017)

(Continued on next page)

Table 10-1. Immunotherapy Agents *(Continued)*

Classification	Mechanism of Action	Drug	Route	Indications	Side Effects	Nursing Considerations
Monoclonal antibodies: Human *(cont.)*	Blocks the binding of ligands to EGFR	Panitumumab (anti-EGFR; Vectibix®)	IV	Colorectal cancer	Fatigue, skin toxicity (acneform dermatitis, pruritus, erythema, rash, exfoliation, paronychia, dry skin, fissures; occurred in 90% of patients and were grade 3 or higher in 15% of patients), ocular toxicity, nausea, diarrhea, vomiting, dyspnea, pulmonary fibrosis/interstitial lung disease, infusion-related reactions	Administer 6 mg/kg every 14 days as an IV infusion. If dose < 1,000 mg, infuse over 60 minutes; if dose > 1,000 mg, infuse over 90 minutes. Administer using a low-protein-binding 0.2 mm or 0.22 mm in-line filter. Monitor electrolytes. Monitor for ocular toxicities (keratitis or ulcerative keratitis) and dermatologic toxicities. Advise patient to limit sun exposure. Use the diluted solution within 6 hours of dilution if stored at room temperature or within 24 hours if stored at 2°C–8°C. Do not administer as an IV push or bolus. (Truven Health Analytics, 2017)
	Binds to VEGFR2 and prevents ligands from binding	Ramucirumab (anti-VEGFR2 antibody; Cyramza®)	IV	Colorectal cancer Lung cancer Gastric cancer	Hypertension (> 15%), proteinuria, infusion-related reactions	Administer 8–10 mg/kg IV infusion over 60 minutes; schedule is specific to cancer type. Administer with sodium chloride only. Administer with a protein-sparing 0.22 micron filter. Premedicate with IV H_1 antagonist. If patients had a prior grade 1 or 2 infusion reaction, also premedicate with dexamethasone and acetaminophen. Monitor blood pressure and discontinue if patients experience severe and uncontrolled hypertension. Monitor urine protein levels and thyroid function. Withhold drug prior to surgery and until wound is healed. Monitor for signs and symptoms of bleeding. Drug may cause fetal harm when administered to pregnant women. Women should use contraception during treatment and for 3 months after the last dose. Use diluted solution within 24 hours if stored at 2°C–8°C or within 4 hours if stored at room temperature. Do not administer as an IV push or bolus. (Eli Lilly and Co., 2017; Truven Health Analytics, 2017)

(Continued on next page)

Table 10-1. Immunotherapy Agents *(Continued)*

Classification	Mechanism of Action	Drug	Route	Indications	Side Effects	Nursing Considerations
Monoclonal antibodies: Humanized	Targets HER2 and delivers a drug called DM-1	Ado-trastuzumab emtansine (anti-HER2 antibody conjugated with emtansine; Kadcyla™)	IV	Breast cancer	Fatigue, headache, peripheral neuropathy, hypokalemia, GI toxicities, thrombocytopenia, anemia, neutropenia, hemorrhage, elevated LFTs, myalgias, epistaxis, infusion-related reactions	Administer 3.6 mg/kg as an IV infusion every 21 days. Give first infusion over 90 minutes followed by at least 90 minutes observation following initial dose due to risk of infusion reactions. If initial dose is tolerated, subsequent infusions can be given over 30 minutes followed by 30 minutes of observation. Use an in-line filter during administration. Monitor platelet counts. Monitor for signs and symptoms of neurotoxicity, and assess for acute hepatotoxicity, cardiac dysfunction, pneumonitis, thrombocytopenia, and extravasation and infusion site reactions. Administer immediately after preparation or within 24 hours if refrigerated. Do not administer as an IV push or bolus. (Truven Health Analytics, 2017)
	Targets the CD52 antigen on leukemia cells	Alemtuzumab (anti-CD52 antibody; Campath®)	IV	Leukemia	Headache, fatigue, rash, thyroid disease, nausea, lymphocytopenia, antibody development, infection, infusion-related reactions, nasopharyngitis, fever	Initiate at a dose of 3 mg IV over 2 hours daily. When 3 mg IV is tolerated, the dose can be escalated to 10 mg and then up to the maintenance dose of 30 mg IV daily. The maintenance dose is administered 3 times per week for 12 weeks. Premedicate with an antihistamine and acetaminophen, with or without anti-infectives. Determine history of varicella or varicella zoster virus vaccination prior to administration. Monitor CBC and platelets. Advise patient to report symptoms of infection or signs of thyroid disorder. Do not administer as an IV push or bolus. (Truven Health Analytics, 2017)

(Continued on next page)

Table 10-1. Immunotherapy Agents *(Continued)*

Classification	Mechanism of Action	Drug	Route	Indications	Side Effects	Nursing Considerations
Monoclonal antibodies: Humanized *(cont.)*	Binds to VEGF and prevents it from binding with its receptors	Bevacizumab (anti-VEGF antibody; Avastin®)	IV	Breast cancer Cervical cancer Colorectal cancer Fallopian tube cancer Glioblastoma Lung cancer Ovarian cancer Primary peritoneal cancer Renal cell cancer	Hypertension, fatigue, pain, headache, abdominal pain, constipation, diarrhea, nausea, vomiting, loss of appetite, hyperglycemia, proteinuria, hemorrhage, leukopenia, upper respiratory tract infection, epistaxis, dyspnea, infusion-related reactions	Administer 5–10 mg/kg as an IV infusion every 2–3 weeks depending on cancer type. Monitor blood pressure and urine protein. Advise patient to use reliable contraception and to report signs of thrombotic events and GI perforation. Diluted solution may be stored at 2°C–8°C for up to 8 hours. Do not administer as an IV push or bolus. Do not administer within 28 days before or after surgery. (Truven Health Analytics, 2017)
	Binds to complement protein C5 to inhibit the formation of the terminal complement complex C5b-9 to mediate intravascular hemolysis	Eculizumab (anti-CD5 antibody; Soliris®)	IV	Hemolysis associated with paroxysmal nocturnal hemoglobinuria Atypical hemolytic uremic syndrome	Headache, nasopharyngitis, back pain, nausea, increased risk of meningococcal infections, infusion-related reactions	For paroxysmal nocturnal hemoglobinuria: Administer 600 mg over 35 minutes IV every 7 days for first 4 weeks, then 900 mg for the fifth dose 7 days later, then 900 mg every 14 days thereafter. For atypical hemolytic uremic syndrome: Administer 900 mg over 35 minutes IV every 7 days for first 4 weeks, then 1,200 mg for the fifth dose 7 days later, then 1,200 mg every 14 days thereafter. Monitor CBC and serum lactate dehydrogenase levels. Administer by IV infusion over 35 minutes. If the infusion is slowed for infusion-related reactions, the total infusion time should not exceed 2 hours. Do not use in patients with unresolved serious *Neisseria meningitides* infection or those who are currently not vaccinated against it. Vaccinate patients at least 2 weeks in advance of first dose of eculizumab. Revaccinate according to medical guidelines for vaccine use. (Truven Health Analytics, 2017)

(Continued on next page)

Table 10-1. Immunotherapy Agents *(Continued)*

Classification	Mechanism of Action	Drug	Route	Indications	Side Effects	Nursing Considerations
Monoclonal antibodies: Humanized *(cont.)*	Binds to SLAMF7 on myeloma cells and activates NK cell cytotoxicity	Elotuzumab (anti-SLAMF7 antibody; Empliciti™)	IV	Multiple myeloma	Bradycardia, tachycardia, altered blood pressure, fatigue, peripheral neuropathy, hyperglycemia, hypocalcemia, hypoalbuminemia, decreased serum bicarbonate, hyperkalemia, diarrhea, constipation, decreased appetite, lymphocytopenia, leukopenia, thrombocytopenia, increased serum alkaline phosphatase, infection, cough, nasopharyngitis, upper respiratory tract infection, pneumonia, fever, infusion-related reactions	Administer 10 mg/kg IV every week, with an in-line filter, for first 2 cycles, then every 2 weeks thereafter. Premedicate with an oral or IV antihistamine, an oral H_2 antagonist, and acetaminophen 600–1,000 mg PO, and dexamethasone. Monitor liver function. Instruct patients to report symptoms of infection and signs of electrolyte imbalances. Complete infusion within 24 hours of reconstitution. Do not administer as an IV push or bolus. (Truven Health Analytics, 2017)
	Binds to CD33 antigen on leukemia cells	Gemtuzumab ozogamicin (anti-CD33 antibody; Mylotarg™)	IV	Leukemia	Abdominal pain, anorexia, chills, constipation, diarrhea, dyspnea, esophagitis, fever, headache, hyperbilirubinemia, hypokalemia, infection, nausea, mucositis, vomiting, weakness, infusion-related reactions	Administer 2–6 mg/kg IV over 2 hours, with an in-line filter, depending on leukemia type. Premedicate with acetaminophen 650 mg PO and an antihistamine. Monitor platelet counts. Advise patient to report signs of infection, GI toxicities, and hypokalemia. Infuse immediately. Do not administer as an IV push or bolus. (Truven Health Analytics, 2017)
	Binds to CD22 and is conjugated with a cytotoxic agent	Inotuzumab ozogamicin (Besponsa®)	IV	Relapsed or refractory B-cell precursor acute lymphoblastic leukemia in adults	Myelosuppression, infusion-related reactions, QT interval prolongation, embryo-fetal toxicity, fatigue, liver toxicity	Administer IV over 1 hour: • Day 1: 0.8 mg/m² • Day 8: 0.5 mg/m² • Day 15: 0.5 mg/m² Premedicate with corticosteroid, antipyretic, and antihistamine prior to administration. Monitor for at least 1 hour after infusion for infusion reactions. (Wyeth Pharmaceuticals Inc., 2018)

(Continued on next page)

Table 10-1. Immunotherapy Agents *(Continued)*

Classification	Mechanism of Action	Drug	Route	Indications	Side Effects	Nursing Considerations
Monoclonal antibodies: Humanized *(cont.)*	Binds to CD20, eventually leading to cell death	Obinutuzumab (anti-CD20 antibody; Gazyva®)	IV	Leukemia Lymphoma	Hypophosphatemia, hypocalcemia, hyperkalemia, hyponatremia, hypoalbuminemia, lymphocytopenia, leukopenia, anemia, elevated LFTs, infection, decreased creatinine clearance, increased serum creatinine, cough, infusion-related reactions	Administer for 6 cycles: 100 mg IV on day 1, cycle 1; 900 mg on day 2, cycle 1; 1,000 mg on days 8 and 15 of cycle 1; and 1,000 mg on day 1 of cycles 2–6. See package insert for titration guidelines. Premedicate with acetaminophen 650–1,000 mg, dexamethasone 20 mg IV or methylprednisolone 80 mg IV, and an antihistamine for cycle 1. For all subsequent infusions, premedicate with acetaminophen 650–1,000 mg. Monitor CBC and electrolytes. Patients should avoid live vaccines. Instruct patients to report liver and kidney toxicity symptoms. May store at 2°C–8°C for up to 24 hours. Do not administer as an IV push or bolus. (Truven Health Analytics, 2017)
	Targets HER2 protein on breast cancer cells	Pertuzumab (anti-HER2 antibody; Perjeta®)	IV	Breast cancer	Weakness, myalgias, neutropenia, anemia, diarrhea, nausea, vomiting, alopecia, rash, fatigue, headache, left ventricular cardiac dysfunction, infusion-related reactions	Administer initial dose of 840 mg IV over 60 minutes, then 420 mg every 3 weeks over 30–60 minutes. Monitor LVEF and for cardiac failure/dysfunction symptoms. Administer immediately or store at 2°C–8°C for 24 hours. Do not administer as an IV push or bolus. (Truven Health Analytics, 2017)
	Targets HER2 protein on breast cancer cells	Trastuzumab (anti-HER2 antibody; Herceptin®)	IV	Breast cancer Gastric cancer	Decreased LVEF, pain, chills, headache, diarrhea, nausea, vomiting, abdominal pain, weakness, cough, dyspnea, fever, infusion-related reactions	Administer initial dose of 2–8 mg/kg IV. Dose depends on cancer type. Monitor LVEF and for cardiac failure/dysfunction symptoms. Drug may be stored at 2°C–8°C for no more than 24 hours prior to use. Do not administer as an IV push or bolus. (Truven Health Analytics, 2017)

(Continued on next page)

Table 10-1. Immunotherapy Agents *(Continued)*

Classification	Mechanism of Action	Drug	Route	Indications	Side Effects	Nursing Considerations
Monoclonal antibodies: Murine	Binds to CD19 on precursor B cells and to CD3 on the surface of T cells	Blinatumomab (anti-CD19/CD3 antibody; Blincyto®)	IV	Leukemia	Edema, hypertension, neurotoxicity, headache, rash, hypokalemia, nausea, vomiting, abdominal pain, anemia, thrombocytopenia, neutropenia, leukopenia, febrile neutropenia, elevated serum ALT, infection, fever, infusion-related reactions	Treatment course consists of up to 2 cycles for induction, followed by 3 additional cycles of consolidation, and up to 4 cycles of continued therapy. Administer 5–28 mcg/m^2 IV based on weight and cycle. Dosage is weight and cycle based. Premedicate with dexamethasone 20 mg an hour prior to first dose of each cycle, prior to a step dose (such as cycle 1, day 8), and when restarting an infusion after an interruption of ≥ 4 hours. Instruct patients to refrain from driving while blinatumomab is infusing. Hospitalization is recommended for first 9 days of first cycle and first 2 days of the second cycle. Patients should be aware of the neurotoxicity effects and avoid activities that require mental alertness or coordination for first dose. Instruct patients to report these neurologic toxicities, as well as symptoms of infection and pancreatitis. Advise patients not to change pump settings and to alert healthcare worker immediately if pump malfunctions. Reconstituted solution may be stored at room temperature for 4 hours or at 2°C–8°C for 24 hours. Do not administer as an IV push or bolus. (Truven Health Analytics, 2017)

(Continued on next page)

Table 10-1. Immunotherapy Agents *(Continued)*

Classification	Mechanism of Action	Drug	Route	Indications	Side Effects	Nursing Considerations
Monoclonal antibodies: Radioimmuno-therapy	IgG1 kappa murine mAb conjugated with yttrium-90 (^{90}Y), targeting CD20 on cells	^{90}Y-ibritumomab tiuxetan (Zevalin®)	IV	Relapsed or refractory follicular B-cell or low-grade non-Hodgkin lymphoma Follicular lymphoma in patients who achieved a complete or partial response to first-line chemotherapy	Hematologic toxicity is the major side effect; onset may be delayed and duration prolonged (cytopenias have persisted 12 weeks postadministration). Fatigue, nasopharyngitis, nausea, abdominal pain, asthenia, cough, diarrhea, and pyrexia are also common. Severe infusion reactions have occurred with rituximab, as a component of the therapeutic regimen; premedications should be given before rituximab. See prescribing information for side effects attributable to rituximab. Secondary leukemias and myelodysplastic syndrome have been reported in 1%–7% of patients (Casadei et al., 2016; Stefoni et al., 2016). Severe cutaneous and mucocutaneous reactions: Erythema multiforme, Stevens-Johnson syndrome, toxic epidermal necrolysis, and exfoliative and bullous dermatitis have been reported.	^{90}Y-ibritumomab tiuxetan is administered on a specific regimen that includes "pretargeting" of the tissues with the mAb rituximab first, followed by the radiolabeled isotope. Patients receive rituximab 250 mg/m^2 on day 1. On day 7, 8, or 9, a second dose of rituximab 250 mg/m^2 is administered, followed by the ^{90}Y-ibritumomab tiuxetan. If platelet count ≥ 150,000/mm^3: Within 4 hours after rituximab infusion, administer 0.4 mCi/kg (14.8 MBq/kg) ^{90}Y-ibritumomab tiuxetan IV. If platelet count ≥ 100,000/mm^3 but ≤ 149,000/mm^3 in patients with relapsed or refractory disease: Within 4 hours after rituximab infusion, administer 0.3 mCi/kg (11.1 MBq/kg) ^{90}Y-ibritumomab tiuxetan IV. Monitor CBC weekly for up to 3 months after administration. Instruct patients to use effective contraception methods during treatment and for 12 months postadministration because of potential gonadal toxicity. Pregnancy should be avoided, and women should discontinue breastfeeding. The ability to generate an immune response to vaccines after administration has not been established, nor has the safety of administration of live vaccines. It is recommended that patients not receive live vaccines. (Spectrum Pharmaceuticals, Inc., 2013)

(Continued on next page)

Table 10-1. Immunotherapy Agents *(Continued)*

Classification	Mechanism of Action	Drug	Route	Indications	Side Effects	Nursing Considerations
Oncolytic viral therapy	Replicates within tumors to produce the immune-stimulatory protein GM-CSF, causing tumor lysis and promoting an antitumor response	Talimogene laherparepvec (Imlygic®)	SC (intralesional injection)	Metastatic melanoma	Immune-mediated: Fever, malaise, chills, nausea, vomiting, headache, elevated liver enzymes, injection site pain, autoimmune vitiligo	Protect the drug from light. Administer via injection into cutaneous, subcutaneous, or nodal lesions at a starting dose of up to a maximum of 4 ml at a concentration of 10^6 (1 million) PFU/ml. Subsequent doses should be administered up to 4 ml of talimogene laherparepvec at a concentration of 10^8 (100 million) PFU/ml. Wear personal protective equipment when administering and clean all surfaces that may have come in contact with agent with a virucidal agent. Immunocompromised individuals should NOT administer the drug, change dressings, or have contact with body fluids. Monitor injection site for necrosis or ulceration, cellulitis, and infection; keep injection site covered for at least a week after each treatment. Women of childbearing potential should use effective contraception during treatment. Caregivers should wear protective gloves when assisting patients in applying or changing occlusive dressings. Dispose of dressings and cleaning materials used for the site in a sealed plastic bag and dispose in household waste. (Amgen Inc., 2015; Hoffner et al., 2016)

ALT—alanine aminotransferase; AML—acute myeloid leukemia; ANC—absolute neutrophil count; ARDS—acute respiratory distress syndrome; AST—aspartate aminotransferase; CAR—chimeric antigen receptor; CBC—complete blood count; CD—cluster of differentiation; CRS—cytokine release syndrome; CTLA-4—cytotoxic T-lymphocyte antigen 4; EGFR—epidermal growth factor receptor; G-CSF—granulocyte–colony-stimulating factor; GD2—ganglioside; GI—gastrointestinal; GM-CSF—granulocyte macrophage–colony-stimulating factor; HER2—human epidermal growth factor receptor 2; Hgb—hemoglobin; HSCT—hematopoietic stem cell transplantation; IFN—interferon; IL—interleukin; IM—intramuscular; irAEs—immune-related adverse events; IV—intravenous; LFTs—liver function tests; LVEF—left ventricular ejection fraction; MI—myocardial infarction; NK—natural killer; NS—normal saline; NSCLC—non-small cell lung cancer; OBI—on-body injector; PAP—prostatic acid phosphatase; PDGFR—platelet-derived growth factor receptor; PD-L1—programmed cell death-ligand 1; PD-L2—programmed cell death-ligand 2; PD-1—programmed cell death protein 1; PE—pulmonary embolism; PFUs—plaque-forming units; PO—by mouth; RANK—receptor activator of nuclear factor kappa-B; RANKL—receptor activator of nuclear factor kappa-B ligand; RBC—red blood cell; rHu—recombinant human; SC—subcutaneous; SLAMF7—signaling lymphocytic activation molecule family member 7; T4—thyroxine; TSH—thyroid-stimulating hormone; VEGF—vascular endothelial growth factor; VEGFR—vascular endothelial growth factor receptor

(2) Most commonly observed irAEs (see Figure 10-1)
   (a) Gastrointestinal: Diarrhea, colitis
   (b) Pulmonary: Pneumonitis
   (c) Dermatologic: Rash, pruritus
   (d) Endocrine: Hypophysitis, hyper- or hypothyroidism
   (e) Renal: Nephritis

(3) Management: Management of irAEs entails assessment, pharmacologic management, and potential holding or withdrawal of the causative agent. Several organizations, such as the American Society of Clinical Oncology, the National Comprehensive Cancer Network, the Society for Immunotherapy of Cancer, and the European Society for Medical Oncology (Brahmer et al., 2018; Haanen et al., 2017), have published clinical guidelines for checkpoint inhibitor–related irAEs. General recommendations include the following (Brahmer et al., 2018):
   (a) Grade 1 toxicities can generally be managed while continuing checkpoint inhibitor therapy (with the exception of certain neurologic and hematologic toxicities).
   (b) Grade 2 toxicities generally require holding checkpoint inhibitors until grade 1 or lower toxicity levels are achieved. Corticosteroids may be introduced for toxicity management.
   (c) Grade 3 toxicities require the checkpoint inhibitors be held, and high-dose corticosteroid therapy over six weeks is recommended. Checkpoint inhibitors should be restarted cautiously, if at all.
   (d) Grade 4 toxicities typically require permanent discontinuation of checkpoint inhibitors.

f) Education (Bayer et al., 2017)
   (1) Patients should be educated prior to the start and throughout the duration of therapy about the potential toxicities associated with immunotherapy.
   (2) Patients should be educated about how to manage irAEs associated with therapy and when to present to the hospital or emergency department for further assessment.
   (3) Patients should be aware of food and beverages that can exacerbate gastrointestinal inflammation and may need to implement dietary changes in the event of immune-mediated colitis (Brahmer et al., 2018).

2. CAR T-cell immunotherapy
   a) Pathophysiology: CARs (also referred to as *immune effector cells*) are synthetic, genetically engineered receptors consisting of signal domains and an extracellular recognition domain derived from either murine or humanized antibodies (Maus, Grupp, Porter, & June, 2014; Tasian & Gardner, 2015).
      (1) CAR T-cell therapy uses tumor-specific antigen recognition to target specific malignancies.
      (2) Cells can be autologous (collected from the patient during leukapheresis) or

Figure 10-1. Potential Side Effects and Toxicities of Immunotherapy by System

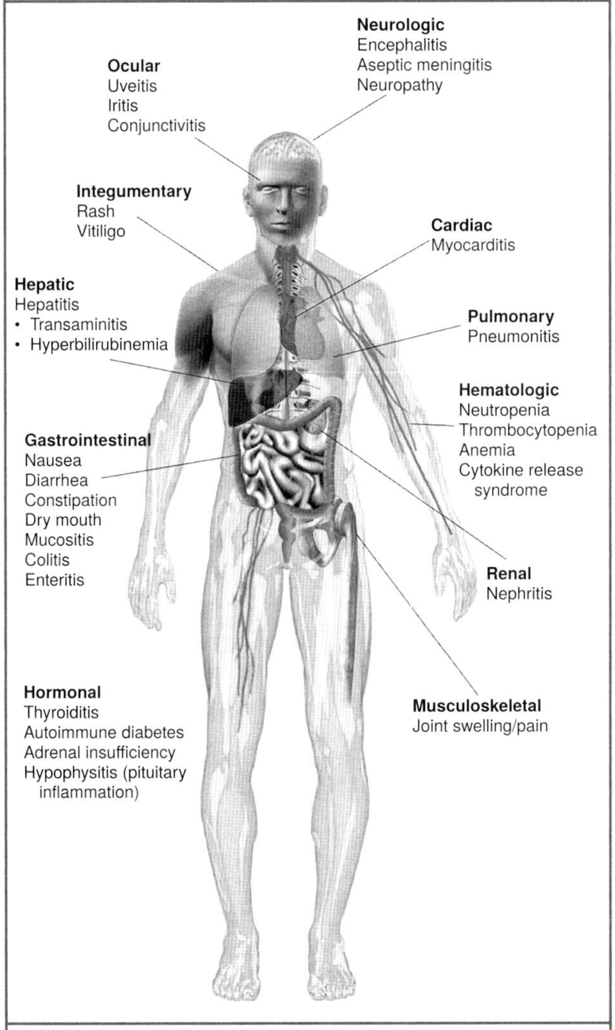

Note. Image courtesy of University of Texas MD Anderson Cancer Center. Used with permission.

allogeneic (collected from a healthy donor during leukapheresis).

(3) T cells are extracted and expanded, or multiplied by millions, in a laboratory setting (Callahan, Baniewicz, & Ely, 2017).

(4) The cells are then reinfused, targeting malignant cells through activation of T-cell memory, which also has the capacity for surveillance (Singh, Frey, Grupp, & Maude, 2016).

(5) A benefit of this type of therapy is persistence of the cells—the ability of the modified T cells to continue to target any cells with the specific antigen indefinitely (Grupp, 2014).

b) Mechanism of action

(1) Two agents are U.S. Food and Drug Administration (FDA) approved: axicabtagene ciloleucel and tisagenlecleucel.

(2) In their current FDA-approved format, CAR T cells function by targeting the CD19 antigen, which is highly present in individuals with acute lymphoblastic leukemia (National Cancer Institute, 2017).

(3) CD19 is highly expressed throughout B-cell development from the early pro-B-cell stage through mature B cells (Maude, Teachey, Porter, & Grupp, 2015).

(4) CAR T cells link an anti-CD19 single-chain variable fragment derived from an antibody to cells expressing the CD19 antigen (Maude, Shpall, & Grupp, 2014).

c) Indications: CAR T-cell immunotherapy has been FDA approved for the treatment of relapsed or refractory B-cell acute lymphoblastic leukemia in pediatric and young adult patients (Novartis Pharmaceuticals Corp., 2017b). In October 2017, FDA also approved a second cell-based gene therapy for certain types of refractory or relapsed large B-cell lymphoma, including diffuse large B-cell lymphoma, primary mediastinal large B-cell lymphoma, high-grade B-cell lymphoma, and B-cell lymphoma arising from follicular lymphoma, in adult patients after two other lines of treatment for the disease (Kite Pharma, Inc., 2017; U.S. FDA, 2017).

d) Collaborative management

(1) Administration: IV infusion (Bayer et al., 2017). At the time of infusion, nursing responsibilities include administration of premedications if ordered, as well as careful monitoring of vital signs and signs and symptoms of infusion reactions.

(2) Monitoring: After infusion, frequent nursing assessments are vital to ensure patient safety.

(a) Monitoring includes frequent vital signs; assessment for pain, infection, and neurologic status changes; and laboratory assessments for inflammatory biomarkers, organ toxicities, and coagulopathies.

(b) Early recognition of changes could help prevent or aid in earlier intervention for more serious side effects, such as severe cytokine release syndrome (CRS) and cerebral edema.

(c) Frequent follow-up with the patient's physician for the first several weeks after infusion is important for monitoring of blood counts and overall health.

(d) Other tests that may be performed with less frequency include bone marrow aspirates and biopsies and radiologic imaging.

(e) Patients who received CAR T-cell infusion through a clinical trial may be asked to participate in long-term follow-up to monitor for persistence of the CAR T cells, adverse events, and disease relapse or other autoimmune or hematologic disorders, such as B-cell aplasia (McConville et al., 2017).

e) Toxicities

(1) CD19 is present on both healthy and malignant cells, both of which are targeted by CAR T-cell therapy (Grupp, 2014). This results in the expected side effect of B-cell aplasia. This may be managed with IV immunoglobulin replacement therapy to help provide antibodies to prevent infection. Treatment for this toxicity may be needed for several years following CAR T-cell therapy (National Cancer Institute, 2017).

(2) Serious and potentially fatal neurotoxicities are associated with CAR T-cell therapy. Hallmark signs include confusion, aphasia, and seizures; therefore, neurologic assessment is imperative.

(3) CRS is the most common toxicity of CAR T-cell therapy and includes symptoms of fever, myalgias, fatigue, nausea, headaches, hypotension, and capillary leak (Maude, Barrett, Teachey, & Grupp, 2014). Actemra® (tocilizumab), an interleukin (IL)-6 receptor blockade, is approved for the treatment and management of severe CRS (Genentech, Inc., 2017a).

(*a*) The hallmark of CRS is elevated inflammatory cytokines caused by immune activation, with patients demonstrating dramatic IL-6 levels following CAR T-cell infusion. Tocilizumab has exhibited almost immediate reversal of CRS (Bonifant, Jackson, Brentjens, & Curran, 2016).

(*b*) Dosing of tocilizumab: Weight based

i. Weight less than 30 kg
- Usual dosage: 12 mg/kg IV infusion over 60 minutes, alone or in combination with corticosteroids
- Repeat dosage: If no improvement in signs and symptoms, may give up to three additional doses at least eight hours apart

ii. Weight greater than 30 kg
- Usual dosage: 8 mg/kg IV infusion over 60 minutes, alone or in combination with corticosteroids
- Repeat dosage: If no improvement in signs and symptoms, may give up to three additional doses at least eight hours apart
- Maximum dosage: 800 mg/IV infusion

(*c*) Administration of tocilizumab

i. May be used alone or in combination with corticosteroids

ii. Allow tocilizumab infusion to reach room temperature prior to infusion. Administer over 60 minutes using an infusion set. Do not administer as an IV push or bolus.

(*d*) Assessment (Truven Health Analytics, 2017)

i. Assess lipid parameters at approximately four to eight weeks following initiation of therapy and every 24 weeks.

ii. Evaluate for tuberculosis risk factors, and test for latent tuberculosis prior to initiation.

iii. Evaluate new-onset abdominal symptoms for development of gastrointestinal perforation.

f) Education

(1) Prior to infusion of CAR T cells, nurses should focus on patient education, including caregiver requirements, financial implications, infection prevention, and emergency management.

(2) Ensure that patients and caregivers are aware of potential toxicities, particularly CRS and neurotoxicities. Educate patients and caregivers on the signs and symptoms of these presentations and how they will be managed if they occur.

(3) Educate patients on the need for adherence to long-term follow-up and toxicity management once discharged from direct patient care.

3. Cytokines

a) Pathophysiology: Cytokines are small protein molecules released by different cells throughout the body, aiding with communication between the cells of the immune system (Lee & Margolin, 2011).

(1) They can be further classified based on the proximity of the signaling cell to the target cell (Owen, Punt, & Stranford, 2013).

(*a*) Endocrine action requires the cytokine to transmit its signal via the blood circulation to its distant target.

(*b*) Paracrine action is when the cytokine signal has to diffuse through tissue fluids across an immunologic synapse.

(*c*) Autocrine action is when a cell receives a signal from a cytokine within its own membrane receptors.

(2) Cytokines generally are activated by a stimulus and induce responses by binding to specific receptors (Owen et al., 2013).

(a) Cells expressing receptors for specific cytokines can be activated or inhibited, either of which alters the immune effector function.
(b) Some cytokines are pleiotropic: they can induce different outcomes based on the nature of the target cell.

b) Mechanism of action (Lee & Margolin, 2011; Owen et al., 2013)
(1) Cytokines affect the growth and differentiation of white blood cells, red blood cells, platelets, and other cells that regulate immune and inflammatory responses within the body.
(2) Cytokines may enhance cytotoxic activity and secrete additional cytokines, resulting in amplification of immune response.
(a) This enhanced immune response stimulates proliferation or activation and recruitment of additional immune effector cells.
(b) This is also known as the *cascade effect*, in which one cytokine reaches its receptor on the target cell and then that cell produces one or more additional cytokines.
(3) Cytokines can exact proinflammatory, anti-inflammatory, and regulatory functions in the immune system, such as hematopoiesis and wound healing.
(4) Cytokines can send signals that inhibit or promote cell death.
(5) Cytokines include a variety of chemokines—a small group of cytokines that help mobilize immune cells toward specific sites in the body. These include interleukins, interferons, tumor necrosis factors, and growth factors.
(6) Cytokines regulate antibody production, the functions of B and T cells, and interactions with antigen-presenting cells and natural killer cells.

c) Indications: Cytokines have diverse indications (see Table 10-1) based on agent categories grouped as follows (National Cancer Institute, 2013):
(1) Hematopoietic growth factors
(a) Stimulate growth, differentiation, and maturation of target cells
(b) The stimulating growth factors that are commonly used in patients with cancer are isolated to stimulate red blood cells, platelets, and white blood cells. Table 10-1 lists the currently used FDA-approved drugs. Examples: epoetin alfa, filgrastim.
(2) Interferons (Parker, Rautela, & Hertzog, 2016)
(a) Currently utilized as antineoplastic and antiviral therapies. This chapter focuses on only the currently FDA-approved antitumor therapies.
(b) Interferon is part of the cell's defense mechanism against viruses and other foreign substances. It was discovered in the 1950s when scientists saw that it "interfered" with viral replication and growth.
(c) Interferon inhibits B-lymphocyte (B-cell) activation, enhances T-lymphocyte (T-cell) activity, and increases the cellular destruction capability of natural killer cells.
(d) Three forms of interferon exist: alpha, beta, and gamma. Interferon alpha and interferon beta can be produced by any cell exposed to the virus, whereas interferon gamma is only secreted by natural killer cells and T lymphocytes (Owen et al., 2013). Examples: interferon alfa-2b, peginterferon alfa-2b (alpha); interferon beta; interferon gamma.
(3) Interleukins
(a) Interleukins are naturally occurring proteins secreted by cells as a response to a stimulus, such as an infection. Once interleukins are bound to a receptor, a cascade effect is created of signals that regulate growth, differentiation, and motility of cells (Ardolino, Hsu, & Raulet, 2015).
(b) They were discovered in the 1970s and named *interleukins* because, with the minimal knowledge available at that time, it appeared they were made by leukocytes and acted on other leukocytes. Further discoveries revealed they are created by many different cells and provide a variety of functions (Owen et al., 2013).

(c) There are now 37 known interleukins, and each of them functions differently with receptors on a variety of cells (Akdis et al., 2011). Examples: aldesleukin (IL-2), oprelvekin (IL-11).

(4) Unfortunately, naturally occurring growth factors also exist that, when overproduced in the body, can contribute to the progression of cancer. One example is vascular endothelial growth factor, which stimulates endothelial cells to increase production, penetrate tumors, and aid in angiogenesis, which allows the tumor access to nutrients to grow and progress (Vacchelli et al., 2014).

d) Collaborative management

(1) Administration: Cytokines have diverse administration routes, which are listed by agent in Table 10-1.

(2) Monitoring

(a) Interferons: Monitor laboratory values, specifically white blood cells, hemoglobin, platelets, and kidney and liver function. Assess for injection site redness versus infection or cellulitis.

(b) Interleukins: Monitor laboratory values, including complete blood count and kidney and liver function (Prometheus Laboratories Inc., 2012).

e) Toxicities: Cytokine toxicities vary by agent and are listed in Table 10-1.

f) Education

(1) Patients might be reluctant to discuss side effects because they are concerned of dose reductions or delays. Ask specific questions related to the drug therapy they are taking so that management of toxicities can be started quickly and appropriately.

(2) Educate patients and caregivers to report new symptoms to their provider immediately.

(a) Interferons (Merck and Co., Inc., 2015a, 2015b): Nausea, vomiting, loss of appetite, weight loss, hair loss, dry skin/rash, and fatigue are anticipated side effects. Notify providers of any depression and suicidal thoughts or plan. Avoid alcohol use.

(b) Interleukins (Prometheus Laboratories Inc., 2012): Possible side effects include diarrhea, worsening rash with or without itching, cough, shortness of breath, swelling of the extremities, chest pain, tachycardia, yellowing of the skin and eyes, bloated feeling, abdominal distension, loss of appetite, and headache.

i. Use unscented, dye-free creams to help with rash.

ii. Document weight daily while on therapy, and notify team of a 10% loss or gain.

(3) Be aware that immunotherapy, especially agents that stimulate cytokines, can potentially cause ongoing overstimulation of the immune system, so these side effects might require lifelong management.

(4) Counsel patients on avoidance of pregnancy during all therapies. Include information on reliable contraception methods such as intrauterine devices, oral contraceptive pills, condoms, and spermicide.

4. Immunomodulators

a) Pathophysiology: Immunomodulators are a class of agents with immunomodulatory, antiangiogenic, or antineoplastic properties primarily targeting pathways related to multiple myeloma (e.g., thalidomide).

b) Mechanism of action: Cereblon, a human protein encoded by the *CRBN* gene, has recently been identified as the primary target for this class of agents, as it is involved in the downregulation of interferon regulatory factor 4, tumor necrosis factor-alpha, and T-cell immunomodulatory activity (Zhu, Kortuem, & Stewart, 2012). Examples: lenalidomide, pomalidomide, thalidomide.

c) Indications: Indications for immunomodulators include primarily hematologic malignancies (see Table 10-1).

d) Collaborative management

(1) Administration: Routes include oral administration. Drug-specific administration is outlined in Table 10-1 (Celgene Corp., 2016, 2017a, 2017b). This class of agents is highly teratogenic; therefore, safe handling by providers, patients, and caregivers is important.

(2) Monitoring: Prior to the start of therapy, pregnancy screening (two tests) in women of childbearing potential is imperative.

e) Toxicities: See Table 10-1.
f) Education: Appropriate contraception should be used up to four weeks before and after treatment.

5. Monoclonal antibodies
   a) Pathophysiology: Monoclonal antibodies are laboratory-made substances that mimic antibodies produced naturally by the human body as a part of the immune system response (El Miedany, 2015).
      (1) Bind with proteins and antigens
      (2) Four types (see Figure 10-2)
         (a) Murine: Made from mice (suffix: -omab). Examples: blinatumomab, yttrium-90 (^{90}Y)-ibritumomab tiuxetan.
         (b) Chimeric: Part mouse and part human (suffix: -ximab). Examples: brentuximab, cetuximab, dinutuximab, rituximab.
         (c) Humanized: Small portions of mouse antibodies are attached to human antibodies (suffix: -zumab). Examples: ado-trastuzumab emtansine, alemtuzumab, bevacizumab, eculizumab, elotuzumab, gemtuzumab ozogamicin, obinutuzumab, pertuzumab, trastuzumab.
         (d) Human: Completely human antibodies (suffix: -umab). Examples: daratumumab, denosumab, necitumumab, ofatumumab, olaratumab, panitumumab, ramucirumab.
   b) Mechanism of action
      (1) Monoclonal antibodies function in one of three manners (Johnson, 2015).
         (a) One method involves the mAb's ability to bind to cancer cells that contain tumor antigens. The antigens then prompt apoptosis (unconjugated antibodies).
         (b) Another involves the particular mAb's ability to bind to a receptor, blocking any antigens that would fuel cancer growth (unconjugated antibodies).
         (c) Lastly, special antibodies can be conjugated to an element that is toxic to cancer cells (chemotherapy, radiation, or another toxin). These antibodies can then be used to destroy tumor cells (conjugated antibodies).
      (2) Unconjugated antibodies (American Cancer Society, 2016)
         (a) Most common mAbs
         (b) Work alone (versus conjugated antibodies, which join with a drug or particle)
         (c) Can work by stimulating a person's immune response by binding to cancer cells and mimicking a marker so that the body's own immune system will destroy it. An example is alemtuzumab, which can be used as treatment for chronic lymphocytic leukemia. This mAb binds to CD52 antigens, thus drawing the immune cells to destroy them.
         (d) Other mAbs can work by blocking the antigens on cancer cells that can help cancer spread. An example is trastuzumab, which can be used as treatment for breast cancer. This mAb binds to the HER2 protein, impairing its functionality.
      (3) Conjugated antibodies

Figure 10-2. Types of Monoclonal Antibodies

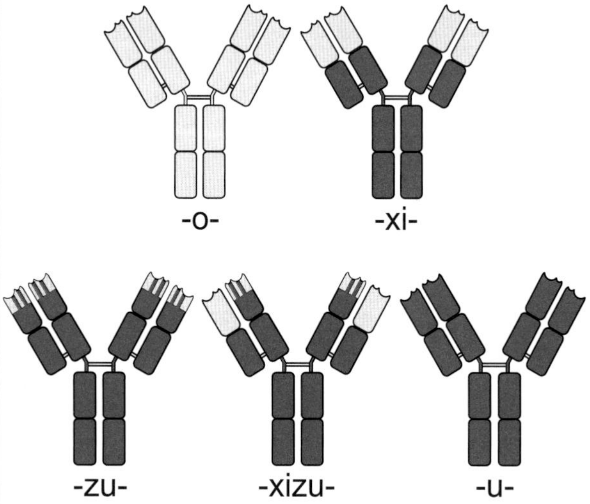

Comparison of monoclonal antibodies (dark—human, light—nonhuman):
- Top row: mouse, chimeric
- Bottom row: humanized, chimeric/humanized, human

The substems according to the nomenclature of monoclonal antibodies are shown below each antibody.

Note. From "Chimeric and Humanized Antibodies," by Anypodetos, 2010. Retrieved from https://en.wikipedia.org/wiki/File:Chimeric_and_humanized_antibodies.svg#file. This work has been released into the public domain by its author, Anypodetos at English Wikipedia. Anypodetos grants anyone the right to use this work for any purpose, without any conditions, unless such conditions are required by law.

(a) Work by being combined with a chemotherapy agent or radioactive particle
   i. Monoclonal antibodies deliver the conjugated agent straight to cancer cells in the body. An example is ado-trastuzumab emtansine, which can be used as treatment for breast cancer. It is attached to DM1, a chemotherapy agent, and targets the HER2 protein.
   ii. Monoclonal antibodies attach directly to cancer cell surface antigens so that the conjugated agent can be directly delivered.

(b) Targeted radionuclide therapy and RIT
   i. Pathophysiology: Targeted radionuclide therapy is a treatment modality in which a therapeutic radionuclide (radioactive isotope) is conjugated with a carrier molecule (e.g., mAbs or peptides) and, after administration, delivers a therapeutic dose of ionizing radiation for curative intent, disease control, or palliation (Chatal & Hoefnagel, 1999; Dash, Chakraborty, Pillai, & Knapp, 2015).
   ii. RIT is a form of targeted radionuclide therapy that uses mAbs conjugated to therapeutic radionuclides.
      - Once deposited in tissue, these radionuclides decay and emit radiation to specific cells or an organ. Radiation induces damage directly, by causing single- and double-strand DNA breaks, crosslinks, and DNA base damage, and indirectly, by the creation of free radicals. Free radicals can form harmful compounds and initiate chemical reactions within a cell, leading to mutations, altered function, or cell death.
      - RIT delivers a highly concentrated absorbed radiation dose to the targeted cells, sparing surrounding normal tissue (Yeong, Cheng, & Ng, 2014). This is particularly helpful when conventional radiation cannot be used because of unacceptable toxicities to healthy tissue, as with widely disseminated disease or tumors located close to sensitive organs (Pouget, Lozza, Deshayes, Boudousq, & Navarro-Teulon, 2015).
      - Tumor response is highly dependent on the amount of tissue being irradiated, the radiosensitivity of the tissue, the cell proliferation rate, genetics, and the microenvironment of the cell (Larson, Carrasquillo, Cheung, & Press, 2015; Pouget et al., 2015).
   iii. Mechanism of action
      - The only RIT agent that currently is FDA approved and commercially available is ^{90}Y-ibritumomab tiuxetan.
      - RIT mAbs target specific antigens on the tumor cell, and once they are bound, radiation is delivered to the tumor. The uptake of radioactivity by tissues differs and is dependent on the number and heterogeneous expression of antigens on the targeted cell, as well as immunoreactivity of the conjugated mAb. Extensive angiogenesis and poor vasculature of the tumor may prevent delivery of the radionuclide (Gill, Falzone, Du, & Vallis, 2017; Pouget et al., 2015).
      - RIT mAbs may also directly induce apoptosis

and synergize with cytotoxic effects caused by radionuclides; this allows for both immunologic and radiobiologic cytotoxicity and higher antitumor efficacy (Kraeber-Bodéré et al., 2015).

- Clinical trials are evaluating the feasibility and potential improved efficacy of combining RIT with chemotherapy, immunotherapy, external beam radiation therapy, and other therapeutic strategies, including regional delivery and hematopoietic stem cell support (Jurcic et al., 2016).

c) Indications: Indications for mAbs include both solid tumor and hematologic malignancies.

(1) RIT is sometimes used with hematologic malignancies such as leukemia and lymphoma, which are very radiosensitive tumors. Solid tumors are more radioresistant and require 5–10-fold radiation doses (Larson et al., 2015; Pouget et al., 2015).

(2) Monoclonal antibodies can also be used for other nonmalignant conditions not discussed in this text. See Table 10-1 for specific indications.

d) Collaborative management

(1) Administration: Includes both IV and SC administration (see Table 10-1).

(a) Although several agents have been tested for safety as treatment during pregnancy (e.g., bevacizumab, rituximab, trastuzumab), most were found to have the potential for harm during fetal development. Therefore, treatment with mAbs should be avoided during pregnancy (Sarno, Mancari, Azim, Colombo, & Peccatori, 2013).

(b) RIT is administered on a specific regimen, which may include "pretargeting" of the tissues with an unconjugated mAb (e.g., rituximab) first, followed by the radiolabeled isotope. Pretargeting is a strategy to decrease toxicity to normal tissue while enhancing radiation dose to tumor. This is achieved by separating the tumor antigen targeting phase from the radioisotope delivery phase (Patra, Zarschler, Pietzsch, Stephan, & Gasser, 2016).

i. ^{90}Y-ibritumomab tiuxetan can safely be administered in the outpatient setting with few discharge instructions and minimal risk of radiation exposure to others.

ii. Because the primary route of elimination of ^{90}Y-ibritumomab tiuxetan is through the kidneys, urine and other body fluids should be flushed down the toilet and any spills cleaned up. Linens contaminated with body fluids should be washed separately. Handwashing should be emphasized.

(2) Monitoring

(a) Assessment with complete blood count, urinalysis, thyroid function testing, and pregnancy testing, along with cardiovascular and pulmonary assessments, is recommended prior to the start of therapy (Gharwan & Groninger, 2016).

(b) Monitor for acute infusion reactions.

(c) Monitor for acute and long-term system-related toxicities, which may include cardiac, renal, and dermatologic toxicities, as well as myelosuppression and thromboembolic events (Gharwan & Groninger, 2016).

e) Toxicities

(1) Common side effects include allergic-type reactions (e.g., hives, pruritus) and flu-like symptoms (e.g., fatigue, headache, muscle ache, chills, fever, nausea, vomiting, diarrhea) (Gharwan & Groninger, 2016).

(2) More severe toxicities include prolonged cytopenias and cardiotoxicity (Gharwan & Groninger, 2016).

(3) With the use of murine (mouse) mAbs, the immune system can recognize the mouse antibody as foreign and develop antibodies against the mAb, called *human anti-mouse antibod-*

ies (HAMAs). A HAMA response can cause rapid clearance of the therapeutic mAb from the circulation, reducing uptake by tumor (DeNardo, Knox, & Gamo, 2010).

(*a*) Considerable variability exists in the development of a HAMA response among patients. In some patients, HAMAs can be detected as soon as one week after infusion and may persist for months or years, precluding additional mAb infusions (DeNardo et al., 2010).

(*b*) Patients with hematologic malignancies are less likely to form HAMAs because of the inherent immunosuppressive nature of hematologic malignancies (Larson et al., 2015).

(*c*) Symptoms can range from a mild rash to a more severe reaction including anaphylaxis and may occur within two to three weeks after the first mAb administration and within hours or days after a repeated administration (DeNardo et al., 2010).

(4) Drug-specific toxicities are listed in Table 10-1.

f) Education: Patients should use precautions to prevent pregnancy during and following treatment according to drug-specific recommendations.

g) RIT-specific considerations

(1) Administration

(*a*) RIT involves a multidisciplinary coordinated approach by hematology oncologist, nurses, a radiation oncologist, physicists and dosimetrists, pharmacists, and nuclear medicine personnel (Iwamoto, Haas, & Gosselin, 2012).

(*b*) Minimize radiation exposure to patients and clinicians consistent with institutional radiation safety practices and patient management procedures (Spectrum Pharmaceuticals, Inc., 2013). Radiation safety precautions will depend on the specific isotope used.

(*c*) For clinicians, safety precautions include standard universal precautions with an addition of acrylic shielding during administration.

(2) Monitoring: Monitor for any signs of infusion or allergic reaction, such as urticaria, respiratory or cardiac abnormalities, and any symptoms of extravasation during the infusion.

(3) Education

(*a*) Patients should be educated on specific side effects, safety, and self-care measures relative to the agent used (Spectrum Pharmaceuticals, Inc., 2013).

(*b*) The ability to generate an immune response to vaccines after ^{90}Y-ibritumomab tiuxetan has not been established, nor has the safety of administration of live vaccines. It is recommended that patients not receive live vaccines (Spectrum Pharmaceuticals, Inc., 2013).

6. Oncolytic viral therapies

a) Pathophysiology: Oncolytic viral immunotherapy is a viral targeted therapy that directly kills cancer cells by causing tumor death, producing tumor-toxic cytokines or antitumor host immune responses (see Table 10-1). Two types of oncolytic viral immunotherapies are nonpathogenic (harmless to humans) and pathogenic (requiring genetic modification for use) (Prestwich et al., 2008).

b) Mechanism of action

(1) The only FDA-approved agent is talimogene laherparepvec (Imlygic®).

(2) Four mechanisms of action thought to exist with oncolytic viral immunotherapies (Wollmann, Ozduman, & van den Pol, 2012)

(*a*) Viral cell receptor response: Viral cell receptor responses target viral-specific cell surface receptors that are overexpressed in cancer cells.

(*b*) Cytokine release: Cytokine release is seen with double-stranded RNA viruses that cause antiviral cellular activation of cytokines that promote apoptosis, such as influenza.

(*c*) Nuclear replication: Nuclear replication of cancer cells can be disrupted by certain double-stranded DNA viruses that have been genetically modified to target tumor DNA synthesis.

(*d*) Extracellular immune response: Extracellular immune responses or antitumor host immune responses are activated with the introduction of specific viruses working synergistically to kill cancer cells.

c) Indications: Oncolytic viral immunotherapies, including adenoviruses, herpes simplex virus, measles virus, Newcastle disease virus, reovirus, vaccinia virus, and vesicular stomatitis virus, are being investigated in clinical trials across a wide array of cancer types (Eager & Nemunaitis, 2011; Msaouel, Opyrchal, Domingo Musibay, & Galanis, 2013). However, the only FDA-approved indication at the time of this publication is metastatic melanoma.

d) Collaborative management
  (1) Administration: Intralesional injection for metastatic melanoma (see Table 10-1 for more information)
    (a) Safe handling (Hoffner, Iodice, & Gasal, 2016)
      i. Change needle after each injection to avoid infection.
      ii. Apply sterile gauze to the site for at least 30 seconds after injection.
      iii. Discard gloves immediately after injection, and perform hand hygiene. After donning a new set of gloves, apply an absorbent pad and dry occlusive dressing to the site.
    (b) Immunocompromised individuals (e.g., caregivers) should not handle, administer, or care for the injection site of the drug.
  (2) Monitoring: Monitor for injection site pain and irritation.

e) Toxicities: Fever, malaise, chills, nausea, vomiting, headache, elevated liver enzymes, injection site pain, autoimmune vitiligo

f) Education
  (1) Counsel patients and caregivers on using standard precautions when changing dressings, including safe disposal (placing soiled dressings in a sealed bag).
  (2) To prevent possible viral infections, counsel patients on avoiding young children and immunocompromised individuals during treatment.

C. General patient and family education
1. Convey to patients and families that immunotherapy is *not* chemotherapy and that it works differently within the body (Brahmer et al., 2018).
2. Inform patients and families that immune response may continue even after discontinuation of the drug (Brahmer et al., 2018).
3. Instruct patients to inform their provider of any new medications or dietary supplements introduced during therapy (Bayer et al., 2017).
4. Educate patients about side effects and potential toxicities unique to immunotherapies (Bayer et al., 2017).
5. Educate patients on when to present to the hospital or emergency department for toxicity management (Bayer et al., 2017).
6. Encourage patients to carry a card identifying the type of immunotherapy they are receiving (see Figure 10-3). This can be useful if presenting for care in an emergency department, clinic, or other primary provider outside the cancer care setting (Brahmer et al., 2018).

References

Akdis, M., Burgler, S., Crameri, R., Eiwegger, T., Fujita, H., Gomez, E., … Akdis, C.A. (2011). Interleukins, from 1 to 37, and interferon-γ: Receptors, functions, and roles in diseases. *Journal of Allergy and Clinical Immunology, 127,* 701–721.e70. https://doi.org/10.1016/j.jaci.2010.11.050

American Cancer Society. (2016). Monoclonal antibodies to treat cancer. Retrieved from https://www.cancer.org/treatment/treatments-and-side-effects/treatment-types/immunotherapy/monoclonal-antibodies.html

Amgen Inc. (2015). *Imlygic® (talimogene laherparepvec)* [Package insert]. Thousand Oaks, CA: Author.

Amgen Inc. (2016a). *Neulasta® (pegfilgrastim injection)* [Package insert]. Thousand Oaks, CA: Author.

Amgen Inc. (2016b). *Neupogen® (filgrastim injection)* [Package insert]. Thousand Oaks, CA: Author.

Amgen Inc. (2017a). *Aranesp® (darbepoetin alfa)* [Package insert]. Thousand Oaks, CA: Author.

Amgen Inc. (2017b). *Procrit® (epoetin alfa)* [Package insert]. Thousand Oaks, CA: Author.

Ardolino, M., Hsu, J., & Raulet, D.H. (2015). Cytokine treatment in cancer immunotherapy. *Oncotarget, 6,* 19346–19347. https://doi.org/10.18632/oncotarget.5095

AstraZeneca Pharmaceuticals LP. (2017). *Imfinzi® (durvalumab)* [Package insert]. Wilmington, DE: Author.

Bayer, V., Amaya, B., Baniewicz, D., Callahan, C., Marsh, L., & McCoy, A.S. (2017). Cancer immunotherapy: An evidence-based overview and implications for practice. *Clinical Journal of Oncology Nursing, 21*(Suppl. 2), 13–21. https://doi.org/10.1188/17.CJON.S2.13-21

Bonifant, C.L., Jackson, H.J., Brentjens, R.J., & Curran, K.J. (2016). Toxicity and management in CAR T-cell therapy. *Molecular Therapy Oncolytics, 3,* 16011. https://doi.org/10.1038/mto.2016.11

Brahmer, J.R., Lacchetti, C., Schnieder, B.J., Atkins, M.B., Brassil, K.J., Caterino, J.M., … Thompson, J.A. (2018). Management of immune-related adverse events in patients treated with immune checkpoint inhibitor therapy: American Society of Clinical Oncology clinical practice guideline. *Journal of Clinical Oncology, 36,* 1714–1768. https://doi.org/10.1200/JCO.2017.77.6385

Figure 10-3. Wallet Card for Patients Receiving Immunotherapy

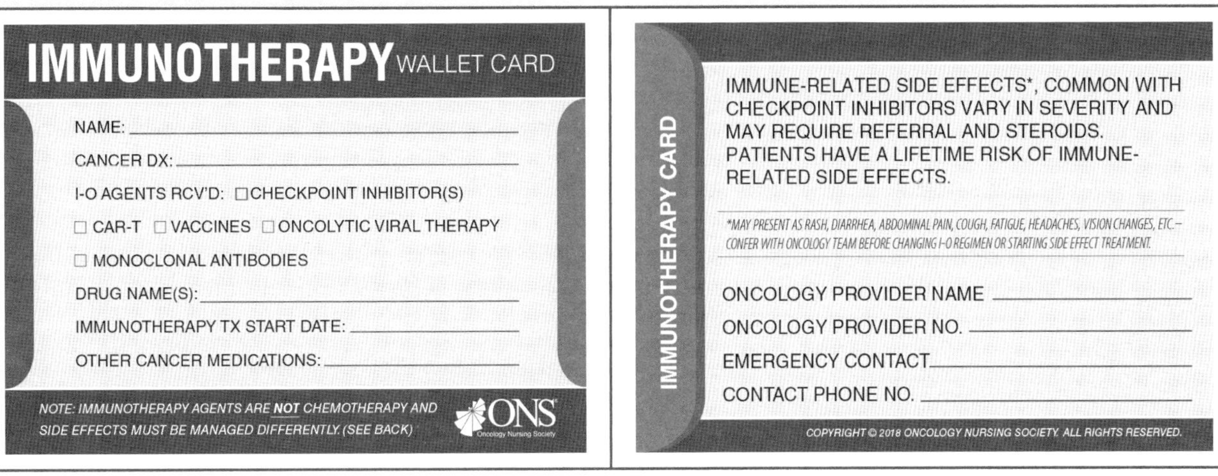

Note. Copyright 2018 by Oncology Nursing Society. Used with permission. For more information and to order cards, visit www.ons.org/practice-resources/cancer-therapies/immunotherapy-resources.

Bristol-Myers Squibb Co. (2017a). *Opdivo® (nivolumab)* [Package insert]. Retrieved from https://packageinserts.bms.com/pi/pi_opdivo.pdf

Bristol-Myers Squibb Co. (2017b). *Yervoy® (ipilimumab)* [Package insert]. Retrieved from https://packageinserts.bms.com/pi/pi_yervoy.pdf

Callahan, C., Baniewicz, D., & Ely, B. (2017). CAR T-cell therapy: Pediatric patients with relapsed and refractory acute lymphoblastic leukemia. *Clinical Journal of Oncology Nursing, 21*(Suppl. 2), 22–28. https://doi.org/10.1188/17.CJON.S2.22-28

Casadei, B., Pellegrini, C., Pulsoni, A., Annechini, G., De Renzo, A., Stefoni, V., ... Zinzani, P.L. (2016). 90-Yttrium-ibritumomab tiuxetan consolidation of fludarabine, mitoxantrone, rituximab in intermediate/high-risk follicular lymphoma: Updated long-term results after a median follow-up of 7 years. *Cancer Medicine, 5,* 1093–1097. https://doi.org/10.1002/cam4.684

Celgene Corp. (2016). *Pomalyst® (pomalidomide)* [Package insert]. Summit, NJ: Author.

Celgene Corp. (2017a). *Revlimid® (lenalidomide)* [Package insert]. Summit, NJ: Author.

Celgene Corp. (2017b). *Thalomid® (thalidomide)* [Package insert]. Summit, NJ: Author.

Chatal, J.-F., & Hoefnagel, C.A. (1999). Radionuclide therapy. *Lancet, 354,* 931–935. https://doi.org/10.1016/S0140-6736(99)06002-X

Chen, D.S., Irving, B.A., & Hodi, F.S. (2012). Molecular pathways: Next-generation immunotherapy—Inhibiting programmed death-ligand 1 and programmed death-1. *Clinical Cancer Research, 18,* 6580–6587. https://doi.org/10.1158/1078-0432.CCR-12-1362

Dash, A., Chakraborty, S., Pillai, M.R.A., & Knapp, F.F., Jr. (2015). Peptide receptor radionuclide therapy: An overview. *Cancer Biotherapy and Radiopharmaceuticals, 30,* 47–71. https://doi.org/10.1089/cbr.2014.1741

DeNardo, S.J., Knox, S.J., & Gamo, I.A. (2010). Tumor-targeted radioisotope therapy. In R.T. Hoppe, T.L. Phillips, & M. Roach III (Eds.), *Leibel and Phillips textbook of radiation oncology* (3rd ed., pp. 1544–1563). Philadelphia, PA: Elsevier Saunders.

Dendreon Corp. (2014). *Provenge® (sipuleucel-T)* [Package insert]. Seattle, WA: Author.

Eager, R.M., & Nemunaitis, J. (2011). Clinical development directions in oncolytic viral therapy. *Cancer Gene Therapy, 18,* 305–317. https://doi.org/10.1038/cgt.2011.7

Eli Lilly and Co. (2017). *Cyramza® (ramucirumab solution)* [Package insert]. Indianapolis, IN: Author.

El Miedany, Y. (2015). MABS: Targeted therapy tailored to the patients need. *British Journal of Nursing, 24*(Suppl. 16a), S4–S13. https://doi.org/10.12968/bjon.2015.24.Sup16a.S4

EMD Serono, Inc. (2017). *Bavencio® (avelumab)* [Package insert]. Rockland, MA: Author.

Farkona, S., Diamandis, E.P., & Blaustig, I.M. (2016). Cancer immunotherapy: The beginning of the end of cancer? *BMC Medicine, 14,* 73. https://doi.org/10.1186/s12916-016-0623-5

Genentech, Inc. (2017a). *Actemra® (tocilizumab)* [Package insert]. South San Francisco, CA: Author.

Genentech, Inc. (2017b). *Rituxan Hycela™ (rituximab and hyaluronidase human)* [Package insert]. South San Francisco, CA: Author.

Genentech, Inc. (2017c). *Tecentriq® (atezolizumab)* [Package insert]. South San Francisco, CA: Author.

Genzyme Corp. (2017). *Mozobil® (plerixafor)* [Package insert]. Cambridge, MA: Author.

Gharwan, H., & Groninger, H. (2016). Kinase inhibitors and monoclonal antibodies in oncology: Clinical implications. *Nature Reviews Clinical Oncology, 13,* 209–227. https://doi.org/10.1038/nrclinonc.2015.213

Gill, M.R., Falzone, N., Du, Y., & Vallis, K.A. (2017). Targeted radionuclide therapy in combined-modality regimens. *Lancet Oncology, 18,* e414–e423. https://doi.org/10.1016/S1470-2045(17)30379-0

Gordon, R., Kasler, M.K., Stasi, K., Shames, Y., Errante, M., Ciccolini, K., ... Fischer-Cartlidge, E. (2017). Checkpoint inhibitors: Common immune-related adverse events and their management. *Clinical Journal of Oncology Nursing, 21*(Suppl. 2), 45–52. https://doi.org/10.1188/17.CJON.S2.45-52

Grupp, S.A. (2014). Advances in T-cell therapy for ALL. *Best Practice and Research Clinical Haematology, 27,* 222–228. https://doi.org/10.1016/j.beha.2014.10.014

Haanen, J.B.A.G., Carbonnel, F., Robert, C., Kerr, K.M., Peters, S., Larkin, J., & Jordan, K. (2017). Management of toxicities from immunotherapy: ESMO Clinical Practice Guidelines for diagnosis, treatment and follow-up. *Annals of Oncology, 28*(Suppl. 4), iv119–iv142. https://doi.org/10.1093/annonc/mdx225

Hoffner, B., Iodice, G.M., & Gasal, E. (2016). Administration and handling of talimogene laherparepvec: An intralesional oncolytic immunotherapy for melanoma. *Oncology Nursing Forum, 43,* 219–226. https://doi.org/10.1188/16.ONF.219-226

HZNP USA Inc. (2015). *Actimmune® (interferon gamma-1b)* [Package insert]. Roswell, GA: Author.

Iwamoto, R.R., Haas, M.L., & Gosselin, T.K. (Eds.). (2012). *Manual for radiation oncology nursing practice and education* (4th ed.). Pittsburgh, PA: Oncology Nursing Society.

Johnson, M. (2015). Monoclonal antibodies. In K. Fust (Ed.), *The Gale encyclopedia of cancer: A guide to cancer and its treatments* (4th ed., pp. 1160–1161). Retrieved from http://link.galegroup.com/apps/doc/CX3620800387/GVRL?u=txshracd2617&sid=GVRL&xid=6d1c171c

Jurcic, J.G., Wong, J.Y.C., Knox, S.J., Wahl, D.R., Rosenblat, T.L., & Meredith, R.F. (2016). Targeted radionuclide therapy. In L.L. Gunderson & J.E. Tepper (Eds.), *Clinical radiation oncology* (4th ed., 399–418.e14). https://doi.org/10.1016/B978-0-323-24098-7.00022-8

Kite Pharma, Inc. (2017). *Yescarta® (axicabtagene ciloleucel)* [Package insert]. Santa Monica, CA: Author.

Kraeber-Bodéré, F., Rousseau, C., Bodet-Milin, C., Mathieu, C., Guérard, F., Frampas, E., … Barbet, J. (2015). Tumor immunotargeting using innovative radionuclides. *International Journal of Molecular Sciences, 16,* 3932–3954. https://doi.org/10.3390/ijms16023932

Larson, S.M., Carrasquillo, J.A., Cheung, N.-K., & Press, O.W. (2015). Radioimmunotherapy of human tumours. *Nature Reviews Cancer, 15,* 347–360. https://doi.org/10.1038/nrc3925

Lee, S., & Margolin, K. (2011). Cytokines in cancer immunotherapy. *Cancers, 3,* 3856–3893. https://doi.org/10.3390/cancers3043856

Maude, S.L., Barrett, D., Teachey, D.T., & Grupp, S.A. (2014). Managing cytokine release syndrome associated with novel T cell-engaging therapies. *Cancer Journal, 20,* 119–122. https://doi.org/10.1097/PPO.0000000000000035

Maude, S.L., Shpall, E.J., & Grupp, S.A. (2014). Chimeric antigen receptor T-cell therapy for ALL. *Hematology: American Society of Hematology Education Program Book, 2014,* 559–564. https://doi.org/10.1182/asheducation-2014.1.559

Maude, S.L., Teachey, D.T., Porter, D.L., & Grupp, S.A. (2015). CD19-targeted chimeric antigen receptor T-cell therapy for acute lymphoblastic leukemia. *Blood, 125,* 4017–4023. https://doi.org/10.1182/blood-2014-12-580068

Maus, M.V., Grupp, S.A., Porter, D.L., & June, C.H. (2014). Antibody-modified T cells: CARs take the front seat for hematologic malignancies. *Blood, 123,* 2625–2635. https://doi.org/10.1182/blood-2013-11-492231

McConville, H., Harvey, M., Callahan, C., Motley, L., Difilippo, H., & White, C. (2017). CAR T-cell therapy effects: Review of procedures and patient education [Online exclusive]. *Clinical Journal of Oncology Nursing, 21,* E79–E86. https://doi.org/10.1188/17.CJON.E79-E86

Merck and Co., Inc. (2015a). *Intron® A (interferon alfa-2b, recombinant)* [Package insert]. Whitehouse Station, NJ: Author.

Merck and Co., Inc. (2015b). *Sylatron™ (peginterferon alfa-2b)* [Package insert]. Whitehouse Station, NJ: Author.

Merck and Co., Inc. (2016). *Keytruda® (pembrolizumab)* [Package insert]. Whitehouse Station, NJ: Author.

Msaouel, P., Opyrchal, M., Domingo Musibay, E., & Galanis, E. (2013). Oncolytic measles virus strains as novel anti-cancer agents. *Expert Opinion on Biological Therapy, 13,* 483–502. https://doi.org/10.1517/14712598.2013.749851

National Cancer Institute. (2013). Biological therapies for cancer. Retrieved from https://www.cancer.gov/about-cancer/treatment/types/immunotherapy/bio-therapies-fact-sheet

National Cancer Institute. (2017). CAR T cells: Engineering patients' immune cells to treat their cancers. Retrieved from https://www.cancer.gov/about-cancer/treatment/research/car-t-cells

Novartis Pharmaceuticals Corp. (2017a). *Kymriah® (tisagenlecleucel)* [Package insert]. East Hanover, NJ: Author.

Novartis Pharmaceuticals Corp. (2017b). Novartis CAR-T cell therapy CTL019 unanimously (10-0) recommended for approval by FDA advisory committee to treat pediatric, young adult r/r B-cell ALL. Retrieved from https://www.novartis.com/news/media-releases/novartis-car-t-cell-therapy-ctl019-unanimously-10-0-recommended-approval-fda

Owen, J.A., Punt, J., & Stranford, S.A., with Jones, P.P. (2013). *Kuby immunology* (7th ed.). New York, NY: W.H. Freeman & Co.

Pardoll, D.M. (2012). The blockade of immune checkpoints in cancer immunotherapy. *Nature Reviews Cancer, 12,* 252–264. https://doi.org/10.1038/nrc3239

Parker, B.S., Rautela, J., & Hertzog, P.J. (2016). Antitumour actions of interferons: Implications for cancer therapy. *Nature Reviews Cancer, 16,* 131–144. https://doi.org/10.1038/nrc.2016.14

Patra, M., Zarschler, K., Pietzsch, H.-J., Stephan, H., & Gasser, G. (2016). New insights into the pretargeting approach to image and treat tumours. *Chemical Society Reviews, 45,* 6415–6431. https://doi.org/10.1039/C5CS00784D

Postow, M., & Wolchok, J. (2018). Toxicities associated with checkpoint inhibitor immunotherapy. In M.E. Ross (Ed.), *UpToDate.* Retrieved March 2, 2018, from http://www.uptodate.com/contents/toxicities-associated-with-checkpoint-inhibitor-immunotherapy

Pouget, J.-P., Lozza, C., Deshayes, E., Boudousq, V., & Navarro-Teulon, I. (2015). Introduction to radiobiology of targeted radionuclide therapy. *Frontiers in Medicine, 2,* 12. https://doi.org/10.3389/fmed.2015.00012

Prestwich, R.J., Harrington, K.J., Pandha, H.S., Vile, R.G., Melcher, A.A., & Errington, F. (2008). Oncolytic viruses: A novel form of immunotherapy. *Expert Review of Anticancer Therapy, 8,* 1581–1588. https://doi.org/10.1586/14737140.8.10.1581

Prometheus Laboratories Inc. (2012). *Proleukin® (aldesleukin)* [Package insert]. San Diego, CA: Author.

Romeo, C., Li, Q., & Copeland, L. (2014). Severe pegfilgrastim-induced bone pain completely alleviated with loratadine: A case report. *Journal of Oncology Pharmacy Practice, 21,* 301–304. https://doi.org/10.1177/1078155214527858

Sanofi-Aventis U.S. LLC. (2013). *Leukine® (sargramostim)* [Package insert]. Bridgewater, NJ: Author.

Sarno, M.A., Mancari, R., Azim, H.A., Colombo, N., & Peccatori, F.A. (2013). Are monoclonal antibodies a safe treatment for cancer during pregnancy? *Immunotherapy, 5,* 733–741. https://doi.org/10.2217/imt.13.64

Singh, N., Frey, N.V., Grupp, S.A., & Maude, S.L. (2016). CAR T cell therapy in acute lymphoblastic leukemia and potential for chronic lymphocytic leukemia. *Current Treatment Options in Oncology, 17,* 28. https://doi.org/10.1007/s11864-016-0406-4

Sosman, J.A. (2017). Immunotherapy of advanced melanoma with immune checkpoint inhibition. In M.E. Ross (Ed.), *UpToDate.* Retrieved March 2, 2018, from https://www.uptodate.com/contents/immunotherapy-of-advanced-melanoma-with-immune-checkpoint-inhibition

Spectrum Pharmaceuticals, Inc. (2013). *Zevalin® (ibritumomab tiuxetan)* [Package insert]. Irvine, CA: Author.

Stefoni, V., Casadei, B., Bottelli, C., Gaidano, G., Ciochetto, C., Cabras, M.G., … Zinzani, P.L. (2016). Short-course R-CHOP followed by ^{90}Y-ibritumomab tiuxetan in previously untreated high-risk elderly diffuse large B-cell lymphoma patients: 7-year long-term results. *Blood Cancer Journal, 6,* e425. https://doi.org/10.1038/bcj.2016.29

Swedish Orphan Biovitrum. (2011). *Kepivance® (palifermin)* [Package insert]. Stockholm, Sweden: Author.

Tasian, S., & Gardner, R. (2015). CD19-redirected chimeric antigen receptor-modified T cells: A promising immunotherapy for children and adults with B-cell acute lymphoblastic leukemia (ALL). *Therapeutic Advances in Hematology, 6,* 228–241. https://doi.org/10.1177/2040620715588916

Teva Pharmaceuticals. (2014). *Granix® (tbo-filgrastim)* [Package insert]. North Wales, PA: Author.

Truven Health Analytics. (2017). Micromedex® Solutions [Web application]. Retrieved from http://www.micromedexsolutions.com/micromedex2/librarian

U.S. Food and Drug Administration. (2017, October 18). *FDA approves CAR-T cell therapy to treat adults with certain types of large B-cell lymphoma* [Press release]. Retrieved from https://www.fda.gov/NewsEvents/Newsroom/PressAnnouncements/ucm581216.htm

Vacchelli, E., Aranda, F., Obrist, F., Eggermont, A., Galon, J., Cremer, I., ... Galluzzi, L. (2014). Trial watch: Immunostimulatory cytokines in cancer therapy. *OncoImmunology, 3,* E29030. https://doi.org/10.4161/onci.29030

Villadolid, J., & Amin, A. (2015). Immune checkpoint inhibitors in clinical practice: Update on management of immune-related toxicities. *Translational Lung Cancer Research, 4,* 560–575. https://doi.org/10.3978/j.issn.2218-6751.2015.06.06

Wollmann, G., Ozduman, K., & van den Pol, A.N. (2012). Oncolytic virus therapy for glioblastoma multiforme: Concepts and candidates. *Cancer Journal, 18,* 69–81. https://doi.org/10.1097/PPO.0b013e31824671c9

Wyeth Pharmaceuticals Inc. (2009). *Neumega® (oprelvekin)* [Package insert]. Philadelphia, PA: Author.

Wyeth Pharmaceuticals Inc. (2018). *Besponsa® (inotuzumab ozogamicin)* [Package insert]. Philadelphia, PA: Author.

Yeong, C.-H., Cheng, M.-H., & Ng, K.-H. (2014). Therapeutic radionuclides in nuclear medicine: Current and future prospects. *Journal of Zhejiang University Science B, 15,* 845–863. https://doi.org/10.1631/jzus.B1400131

Zhu, Y.X., Kortuem, K.M., & Stewart, A.K. (2012). Molecular mechanism of action of immune-modulatory drugs thalidomide, lenalidomide and pomalidomide in multiple myeloma. *Leukemia and Lymphoma, 54,* 683–687. https://doi.org/10.3109/10428194.2012.728597

SECTION IV

Treatment Administration and Safety

CHAPTER 11

Administration Considerations

A. Components of safe and effective administration of cancer therapies
   1. A comprehensive pretreatment assessment
   2. System safeguards to prevent errors and manage emergencies
   3. Dose calculations and verification processes
   4. Evidence-based practices for all routes of chemotherapy, targeted therapy, and immunotherapy administration
   5. Refer to Chapter 1 for nursing scope and standards, professional education, policy and procedure requirements, and an overview of antineoplastic medication safety. Chapter 12 reviews safe handling precautions to be followed during administration of hazardous drugs (HDs). Chapter 13 discusses infiltration, extravasation, and infusion-related complications.

B. Pretreatment
   1. A thorough assessment of the patient, patient history, and cancer treatment plan (including orders and treatment notes) with proactive interventions can prevent adverse reactions and errors.
      a) The assessment should be performed for all routes of chemotherapy, targeted therapy, and immunotherapy, including those given via the oral route.
      b) Assess information specific to the agent (see Tables 6-1, 8-1, and 10-1 in earlier chapters) and route of administration.
      c) Assess for risk factors for potential adverse reactions, review laboratory values, identify potential interactions with concurrent treatments and medications, and determine if it is appropriate to treat the patient.
      d) Review all information and identify questions and concerns that require discussion or collaboration with the patient's provider.
   2. Before the administration of a new treatment regimen, review the patient's medical record for the following elements (Neuss et al., 2016):
      a) The patient's cancer diagnosis, stage, and current cancer status
      b) The cancer treatment plan, including goals of therapy, medications, and duration of treatment
         (1) Goals of therapy include chemoprevention, cure, control, or palliation. Electronic documentation systems often have a location for the prescriber to document goals on the cancer treatment plan. Some informed consent documents include goals of treatment.
         (2) For curative therapy, the duration is often a set number of cycles. However, for metastatic disease, treatment may continue until disease progression or toxicity or the decision is made to decline or terminate treatment.
      c) The planned frequency of office visits and patient monitoring appropriate for treatment plan
         (1) The National Comprehensive Cancer Network® (NCCN®, www.nccn.org) has disease-specific guidelines and chemotherapy order templates that include suggested patient monitoring for cancer type and stage (e.g., type and timing of imaging) and treatment regimen (toxicity monitoring).
         (2) See Appendix C for an example of a chemotherapy order template.
      d) Risk factors for adverse reactions (NCCN, 2018a, 2018b, 2018c, 2018g), such as the following examples:
         (1) Patients with rapidly growing cancers, such as small cell lung cancer, aggressive forms of lymphoma, and acute leukemia, have an increased risk for tumor lysis syndrome at the initiation of treatment.
         (2) Patient populations with an increased risk for acute infusion reactions
            (a) Patients with B-cell lymphomas and leukemia with high circulating blast counts (greater than

25,000/mm³) or who have bulky disease are at increased risk for cytokine release infusion reactions with the initiation of treatment with anti-CD20 antibodies, such as rituximab (Genentech, Inc., 2016).

(b) Patients with *BRCA1* or *BRCA2* mutations associated with breast or ovarian cancer have been shown to have a higher incidence of hypersensitivity reactions to carboplatin, and reactions may occur at a lower cumulative dose (Galvão, Phillips, Giavina-Bianchi, & Castells, 2017; Moon et al., 2013).

(3) Hematologic malignancies or bone marrow involvement increases the risk for myelosuppression from chemotherapy (NCCN, 2017b).

e) The patient's cancer treatment history, which could contribute to toxicities for the planned therapy. Examples include the following:

(1) Radiation recall, characterized by an acute inflammatory reaction confined to previously irradiated sites, can be triggered by the administration of systemic agents (e.g., doxorubicin) after radiation (Burris & Hurtig, 2010). It can occur months or even years after radiation.

(2) Prior treatment with an anthracycline antitumor antibiotic can increase the patient's risk for congestive heart failure if other potentially cardiotoxic therapies are planned (Smith et al., 2010). Review cumulative dose of all drugs in this category. See Table 6-1 in Chapter 6 for cumulative dose information for each anthracycline drug and Chapter 16 for information on cardiotoxicity.

f) The patient's medical history, including comorbidities

(1) Assess for noncancer diagnoses and treatments that could potentially adversely affect the patient's cancer therapy or outcome.

(2) Comorbidity index scoring systems have been developed to capture the complexity of comorbidities and assign a score (Sarfati et al., 2014; Wass, Hitz, Schaffrath, Müller-Tidow, & Müller, 2016).

(3) Examples of comorbidities that can affect cancer therapies

(a) Alcohol and substance abuse is associated with numerous medical problems, including liver disease, pancreatitis, and peripheral neuropathy. Alcohol abuse has been found to adversely affect prognosis in patients with head and neck cancers receiving chemotherapy (Mayne, Cartmel, Kirsh, & Goodwin, 2009).

(b) Congestive heart failure may preclude treatment with anthracycline antitumor antibiotics and HER2/neu receptor antibodies (Smith et al., 2010).

(c) Diabetes: Poor glycemic control in patients with cancer has been associated with development of adverse events such as neutropenia, infections, and mortality (Hershey & Hession, 2017; Peairs et al., 2011).

i. Blood glucose can be more difficult to control in patients receiving steroids as part of their chemotherapy treatment plan, as steroids can increase blood glucose (Hershey & Hession, 2017).

ii. Patients with complications from diabetes have been found to have more than twice the risk for chemotherapy-related neuropathy compared to patients without diabetes (Hershman et al., 2016).

(d) Liver disease: Underlying disease can alter hepatic drug metabolism and cause higher or prolonged drug levels with resultant increased toxicity and worsening hepatic function (Kasi et al., 2015).

i. Patients receiving immunosuppressant agents, including select chemotherapy, targeted therapy, and immunotherapy agents, are at increased risk for hepatitis B reactivation (Paul et al., 2016). See Tables 6-1, 8-1, and 10-1 and Chapter 18 for more information.

ii. All patients should be asked if they have a personal history of hepatitis B (Hwang et al.,

2015; Lok & McMahon, 2009; Reddy, Beavers, Hammond, Lim, & Falck-Ytter, 2015; Weinbaum et al., 2008).

(e) Renal failure: Many chemotherapy, targeted therapy, and immunotherapy agents are excreted primarily by the kidneys. Impaired renal function can lead to alterations in pharmacokinetics, elevated blood levels of drugs, and increased toxicity (Khoury & Steele, 2017). Hemodialysis can remove some chemotherapy and immunotherapy agents from the bloodstream (Kuo & Craft, 2015). Collaborate with a nephrologist, oncologist, and pharmacist to determine if dose adjustments are needed and to determine appropriate timing to avoid drug removal from dialysis.

g) Medication history

(1) Review the patient's current medications.

(2) Verify that the patient has been prescribed supportive medications. Verify that the patient understands the purpose, dosing, administration instructions, and schedule of all medications.

(a) Provide the patient with written and verbal information, and a schedule (as appropriate).

(b) Examples of supportive medications

i. Antibiotics, antifungals, and antiviral agents: NCCN has published guidelines for infection prophylaxis for various regimens, based on the risk for infection (NCCN, 2017b).

ii. Antidiarrheal agents: Patients receiving capecitabine, 5-fluorouracil, irinotecan, and other agents with an increased risk for diarrhea should be prescribed antidiarrheal agents, such as loperamide (Shaw & Taylor, 2012).

iii. Antiemetics: Several studies have indicated that adherence to postchemotherapy antiemetics, especially dexamethasone, is low, with resulting increased incidence of nausea and vomiting (Chan, Low, & Yap, 2012). Patient education has shown to improve adherence and decrease the incidence of nausea and vomiting (Chan et al., 2012; Hendricks, 2015).

(3) Drug interactions: Identify any medication interactions, including over-the-counter medications. Be aware of common antineoplastic drug–drug interactions and food–drug interactions and have access to resources for safe nursing practice. Numerous online resources, such as Lexicomp®, are available to check for interactions. Examples of potential interactions are detailed below (Segal et al., 2014; van Leeuwen et al., 2013).

(a) CYP3A4 inhibitors and inducers: Some anticancer agents are metabolized through the cytochrome P450 enzymes in the liver, especially CYP3A4. Many non-anticancer medications and herbs can inhibit or induce this enzyme and affect drug levels.

i. CYP3A4 inducers decrease the level of the cancer drug, making it less effective.

ii. CYP3A4 inhibitors increase the concentration of the drug and contribute to increased toxicities.

iii. Strong CYP3A4 inducers and inhibitors should be avoided in patients if the anticancer agent is metabolized by that pathway. When avoidance is not possible, some medications have specific dosing recommendations that should be followed.

iv. A significant interaction can occur when chemotherapy or immunotherapy agents that are CYP3A4 inhibitors are used with opioids that are also CYP3A4 inhibitors, such as fentanyl (Janssen Pharmaceuticals, Inc., 2017). Fatal overdoses of fentanyl have been reported. This also can occur when chemotherapy or immunotherapy agents that are CYP3A4 inducers are discontinued.

(*b*) QT-prolonging medications: Prolonged QT intervals can place patients at risk for life-threatening ventricular arrhythmias, such as torsades de pointes. The risk is increased in patients receiving more than one QT-prolonging agent. The Arizona Center for Education and Research on Therapeutics, a federally funded program, maintains a list of medications that can prolong QT intervals at https://crediblemeds.org.

i. Examples of antineoplastic agents that can prolong QT intervals include arsenic trioxide, eribulin, capecitabine, dasatinib, lapatinib, and sunitinib (Kloth et al., 2015).

ii. Significant nonantineoplastic medication classifications that can prolong QT intervals are antipsychotics, 5-HT_3 antiemetics, antibiotics, antifungals, and antiarrhythmics. Methadone, an analgesic frequently used for patients with cancer, can also prolong QT intervals.

(*c*) Potentially nephrotoxic medications, such as nonsteroidal anti-inflammatory drugs (NSAIDs), can potentiate renal toxicity in patients receiving nephrotoxic chemotherapy, such as cisplatin (Sato et al., 2016). Caution should be used when administering NSAIDs to patients with mild to moderate renal insufficiency who are receiving pemetrexed (Eli Lilly and Co., 2017).

h) Immunizations: Before starting therapy, assess the patient's immunization status.

(1) Patients with hematologic and solid tumor malignancies should receive the inactivated influenza virus annually (Centers for Disease Control and Prevention, 2018; Rubin et al., 2014).

(2) Inactivated vaccines can be administered safely to people with altered immunocompetence (Centers for Disease Control and Prevention, 2018; Rubin et al., 2014).

(3) Except for the inactivated influenza vaccine, vaccination during chemotherapy or radiation therapy should be avoided if possible because antibody response might be suboptimal (Centers for Disease Control and Prevention, 2018; Rubin et al., 2014).

(4) Live vaccines should be avoided (Centers for Disease Control and Prevention, 2018; Rubin et al., 2014). If the patient recently received a live virus, contact the provider.

(5) Review vaccination recommendations, as they change frequently. Current recommendations are available from the Centers for Disease Control and Prevention and the Infectious Diseases Society of America (see Centers for Disease Control and Prevention, 2018; Rubin et al., 2014).

i) Complementary and alternative therapies: Review the use of complementary and alternative therapies and assess for any interactions with planned therapy.

(1) *Alternative care* refers to nontraditional treatment intervention used in place of conventional medicine. Although there is anecdotal evidence addressing the benefits, it has not been subjected to the type of rigorous testing for safety and efficacy for the intended use (U.S. National Library of Medicine, 2018).

(2) *Complementary health approaches* refers to a group of diverse medical and healthcare systems, practices, and products used together with conventional medicine or usual care and are not used as alternative or in place of conventional medicine (U.S. National Library of Medicine, 2018).

(3) Complementary health approaches include natural products (herbs [botanicals], vitamins, and minerals), essential oils (including aromatherapy), and mind–body practices (e.g., acupuncture, acupressure, chiropractic and osteopathic manipulation, healing touch, hypnotherapy, massage, meditation, movement therapies).

(4) Assess for interactions and potential adverse reactions of herbs, vitamins, minerals, and other supple-

ments. Memorial Sloan Kettering Cancer Center has a mobile and web application that can be used as a guide to herbs called "About Herbs" (www.mskcc.org/cancer-care/diagnosis-treatment/symptom-management/integrative-medicine/herbs). Another resource is Natural Medicines, which can be found at http://info.therapeuticresearch.com/natural-medicines-learn-more.

j) Age-related factors

(1) Note the patient's age. Assess potential issues associated with various age groups.

(2) Cancer occurs more commonly in older adults; 87% of all cancers in the United States are diagnosed in people 50 years of age and older (American Cancer Society, 2018).

(a) Challenges regarding adequate and safe dosing for older patients include inadequate representation in oncology trials; higher risk of treatment-related toxicity due to alterations in drug metabolism, distribution, and excretion; comorbidities; frequent use of concurrent medications; and other physiologic effects of the natural aging process, such as decreased marrow reserves (Lichtman et al., 2016; Scher & Hurria, 2012; Walko & McLeod, 2014). NCCN (2017a) has guidelines for treating older adults with cancer.

(b) Chronologic age may not correlate with physiologic impairment and decline in functional reserve, both of which vary substantially among individuals. Therefore, treatment in older adults should focus on the extent of comorbidity and functional status rather than chronologic age (Pallis et al., 2010).

(c) Cognitive impairment or decline may affect comprehension and adherence to therapies and can occur at any age. Studies investigating adherence to oral cancer therapies in older adults have been conflicting. Some studies have indicated decreased adherence, whereas others have found no significant difference in adherence rates (Demissie, Silliman, & Lash, 2001; Patridge et al., 2010; Partridge, Wang, Winer, & Avorn, 2003; Silliman et al., 2002; see Chapter 24).

(d) Polypharmacy, which is more common in older adult patients, increases the risk for drug interactions (Balducci, Goetz-Parten, & Steinman, 2013).

(3) Pediatric oncology: Safe administration of chemotherapy in pediatric patients requires a specialized knowledge set. The Association of Pediatric Hematology/Oncology Nurses provides resources for pediatric oncology nurses. For more information, see www.aphon.org.

k) Physical examination

(1) A complete physical examination should be documented in the patient's medical record.

(2) Review prior to the initiation of a new therapy.

(3) Note any abnormalities and use as a comparison for future assessments.

l) Pregnancy status: As appropriate, assess the patient's pregnancy status.

(1) Pregnancy testing is recommended prior to treatment; however, few formal guidelines exist regarding pregnancy screening protocols, and there is a lack of consensus regarding the frequency of testing (Neuss et al., 2016).

(a) Inclusion criteria for testing prior to chemotherapy are most often cited in the literature as "women of childbearing age."

(b) Exclusion criteria for testing should take into consideration the patient's age, prior tubal ligation or hysterectomy, and laboratory tests confirming menopause.

(c) Use of prechemotherapy checklists and orders for point-of-care pregnancy tests has been found to improve screening rates (Rogers, Kolarich, & Markham, 2017).

(2) If the patient is pregnant: Consensus guidelines for cancer chemotherapy during pregnancy have been developed (Koren et al., 2013; Lishner et al., 2016).

(a) The patient should be managed by an interprofessional team, including the oncologist, the maternal

fetal medicine team, and psychological, social, and spiritual support team members, as indicated or requested (Koren et al., 2013; Lishner et al., 2016).

(b) Risk to the fetus is dependent on the gestational age and the planned agents to be administered (Koren et al., 2013; Lishner et al., 2016; National Toxicology Program, 2013).

(c) Chemotherapy during the first trimester may increase the risk of spontaneous abortions, fetal death, and major congenital malformation (Koren et al., 2013; Lishner et al., 2016; National Toxicology Program, 2013).

(d) Effects depend on the drug, dose, time of administration, and cumulative exposure (Koren et al., 2013; Lishner et al., 2016; National Toxicology Program, 2013).

(e) Administration of chemotherapy during the second and third trimesters has not been associated with major congenital malformations but may increase the risk for intrauterine growth retardation, low birth weight, and stillbirth (Koren et al., 2013; Lishner et al., 2016; National Toxicology Program, 2013).

m) Allergies and history of infusion reactions (see Chapter 13)

(1) Patients with multiple allergies have an increased risk for anaphylaxis (Simons, 2008).

(2) Review any past infusion reactions (e.g., hypersensitivity, cytokine release syndrome) for the grade of the reaction, symptoms, onset, course of progression, interventions, patient response, and time to resolution of symptoms. A thorough history of previous reactions is one of the most important risk assessment tools when administering chemotherapy or immunotherapy (Vogel, 2010).

(a) Documentation tools and grading systems should be integrated into electronic health records to better identify patients who have had reactions (Andrews, 2017). See Chapter 13 for grading criteria for infusion reactions.

(b) For many agents, the grade of the previous reaction is used to order future premedications, infusion rates, and infusion volumes. Previous reactions also may require a change in location of treatment (inpatient versus outpatient) and increased nurse-to-patient ratio, depending on the severity of the reaction.

(3) Verify that emergency equipment and supplies, including oxygen, are available and functional and that staff are aware of their location. Chemotherapy chairs should be capable of changing to the supine position if needed.

n) Initial psychosocial assessment

(1) Use a standardized tool, such as a distress screening tool, to assess psychosocial concerns (Neuss et al., 2016; Pirl et al., n.d.).

(2) The American College of Surgeons Commission on Cancer (Ferris & Takanishi, 2014) implemented mandatory distress screening as criteria for accreditation.

(3) *Distress* has been defined as "a multifactorial unpleasant experience of a psychological (i.e., cognitive, behavioral, emotional), social, spiritual, and/or physical nature that may interfere with the ability to cope effectively with cancer, its physical symptoms, and its treatment" (NCCN, 2018e, p. DIS-2).

(4) It "extends along a continuum, ranging from common normal feelings of vulnerability, sadness, and fears to problems that can become disabling, such as depression, anxiety, panic, social isolation, and existential and spiritual crisis" (NCCN, 2018e, p. DIS-2).

(5) The NCCN Distress Thermometer is a tool used to screen for distress (NCCN, 2018e; see Appendix F).

(a) The patient is asked to rate distress on a 0–10 scale, with 0 representing no distress and 10 representing extreme distress. If the score exceeds the distress threshold, a clinician trained in distress screening should evaluate the cause of distress and ensure that a referral to a clinician qualified to address distress is completed (NCCN, 2018e).

(b) Ideally, screening should occur at every medical visit. At minimum, distress screening should occur at the initial visit, at appropriate intervals, and as clinically indicated (e.g., changes in disease status, such as recurrence and progression).

(c) For additional information regarding distress management, see NCCN (2018e).

(6) Regardless of the tool used for distress screening, assess the following:

(a) Family structure and dynamics, living conditions, and caregivers

(b) Transportation, financial, or insurance issues. Patients receiving sedating premedications or opioids will need transportation to and from treatment.

(c) Religious beliefs or spiritual concerns that may affect dietary and other requirements and restrictions

o) Patient and caregiver comprehension of the disease and planned treatment (see Chapter 3)

(1) Use teach-back strategies to assess comprehension (Agency for Healthcare Research and Quality, 2015; Portz & Johnston, 2014).

(2) *Teach-back* refers to a method to assess understanding by asking patients to state in their own words the information they have been taught.

(3) Using teach-back strategies for assessing comprehension in patients receiving oral chemotherapy has been found to improve patient adherence to treatment (Bellomo, 2016).

p) Informed consent: Verify that the informed consent document has been completed and is accurate and current (see Chapter 2).

3. At each clinical encounter related to treatment (e.g., office visit prior to treatment, hospitalization for inpatient treatment, infusion visit), assess the following (Neuss et al., 2016):

a) Performance status: Performance status is a measure of the patient's functional capacity, including the ability to perform activities of daily living (Neuss et al., 2016).

(1) Performance status is used as a predictor of patient tolerance and response to treatment (Jang et al., 2014).

(2) Different tools used to assess performance status include the Eastern Cooperative Oncology Group scale and the Karnofsky Performance Status Scale (see Chapter 4).

(3) The literature reports conflicting data regarding the reliability of performance status measurements, with variable levels of interrater reliability (Chow et al., 2016).

(4) The American Society of Clinical Oncology (ASCO) recommends against the use of chemotherapy in patients with solid tumors who have an Eastern Cooperative Oncology Group performance score of 3 or above, demonstrated no benefit from prior evidence-based interventions, are not eligible for a clinical trial, and have no strong evidence supporting the clinical value of further anticancer treatment (Schnipper et al., 2013).

b) Vital signs: Monitor vital signs before each treatment.

(1) Assess for abnormal vital signs (e.g., increased temperature, which could indicate an infection) and adverse reactions to previous doses (e.g., bevacizumab can cause hypertension).

(2) Use as a baseline for agents with a potential for infusion reactions.

c) Height and weight: Monitor the patient's height and weight at least weekly when the patient is present in the healthcare setting (Neuss et al., 2016). The following are recommended by the Institute for Safe Medication Practices [ISMP], 2018):

(1) Accurate, measured height and weight are imperative for correct dosing of weight-based drugs.

(2) One of the most commonly reported medication errors related to dose is inaccurate height and weight.

(3) Avoid the use of stated or estimated height or weight or a weight from a previous encounter.

(4) Measure and document the patient's weight in metric units.

(5) Place a conversion chart near all scales so that patients and caregivers can be told the weight in pounds, when requested.

(6) If purchasing scales, buy scales that measure in kilograms or can be locked out to measure in metric units only.

(7) Computer screens and IV infusion pumps should prompt patient weight in metric units only.

d) Physical examination: Perform an assessment prior to each treatment.

(1) Assessment should include but not be limited to orientation, level of consciousness, signs of infection, nutritional status, indicators of pain, toxicities from previous doses, and any change that may preclude the patient from treatment (e.g., new onset of tachycardia, arrhythmia, shortness of breath, syncope).

(2) Perform a focused assessment based on the potential adverse reactions of the agents to be administered.

(3) For patients with vascular access devices, assess patency, including a blood return, and for signs of complications.

(4) Notify the provider for any signs of infection.

(a) The treatment plan and assessment findings are considered in the decision to hold or continue therapy.

(b) For example, the provider may elect to proceed with treatment in a patient with an uncomplicated urinary tract infection who is receiving a nonmyelosuppressive agent.

e) Symptom assessment: Assess patient symptoms using an evidence-based patient reporting tool.

(1) Patient-reported outcomes are recommended as the preferred method to screen for symptoms because of underdetection of symptoms by healthcare providers (Pirschel, 2017). *Patient-reported outcomes* are defined as any report of a patient's health condition that comes directly from the patient without interpretation by the clinician (Pirschel, 2017).

(2) The Oncology Nursing Society (ONS) has established criteria for patient-reported outcome assessment tools and lists instruments that meet these criteria on its website (www.ons.org/assessment-tools).

f) Toxicity grading: Grade any toxicities found during the physical examination and symptom assessment (Neuss et al., 2016).

(1) Grading is used to standardize communication among healthcare providers. Toxicity grades can be included as parameters to withhold, delay, or dose reduce treatment. They are also included as part of clinical trials.

(2) The National Cancer Institute Cancer Therapy Evaluation Program's Common Terminology Criteria for Adverse Events tool is available online at https://ctep.cancer.gov/protocolDevelopment/electronic_applications/ctc.htm.

g) Laboratory values: Review laboratory values prior to each treatment.

(1) Laboratory tests ordered are specific for the agent, regimen, and the individual patient. They may be ordered to calculate doses (e.g., serum creatinine for carboplatin), assess for toxicities from prior treatments (e.g., myelosuppression), and ensure that the agent will be adequately metabolized and excreted (e.g., doxorubicin and total bilirubin).

(2) Determine if the values meet predetermined parameters, which can be included on the treatment orders (ISMP, 2010) or listed in a policy or procedure. Parameters to hold the agent or reduce the dose are depend on the goals of therapy, the regimen, and the patient.

(3) Examples of laboratory tests that may be ordered

(a) Complete blood count and differential: Evaluate the absolute neutrophil count and platelet count to determine if the dose should be delayed or reduced.

i. Parameters for holding therapy should be defined by the practice or prescriber. This can be done based on the individual patient via a specific provider order or a regimen guideline that is approved for a specific diagnosis. For example, in patients with solid tumors, a parameter to hold treatment or clarify with the prescriber might be an absolute neutrophil count of less than 1,500/mm^3 and platelet count less than 100,000/mm^3.

ii. The red blood cell count, hemoglobin, and hematocrit should be evaluated to determine if the patient is anemic; however, anemia is often not an indication to hold chemotherapy.

(b) Serum creatinine and creatinine clearance

i. Serum creatinine and creatinine clearance are used to calculate doses of carboplatin.

ii. Many agents such as carboplatin, cisplatin, cyclophosphamide, and pemetrexed are excreted in the urine (Perazella, 2012). These agents require dose reduction for impaired renal function because renal impairment can cause delayed excretion and increased toxicities.

iii. Renal function is also monitored to assess for nephrotoxicity from agents such as cisplatin, high-dose methotrexate, and mitomycin C (Perazella, 2012).

iv. Immune checkpoint inhibitors can cause renal damage, including tubulointerstitial nephritis and immune complex glomerulonephritis (Izzedine et al., 2017).

(c) Total bilirubin and liver function tests

i. Many agents are metabolized and cleared from the body by the liver; therefore, dose reductions may be needed for patients with impaired hepatic function (Kistler, 2013).

ii. Some chemotherapy and immunotherapy agents can also cause hepatotoxicity (Grigorian & O'Brien, 2014).

(d) Electrolytes, including calcium, magnesium, and potassium: Nephrotoxic agents such as cisplatin can cause electrolyte wasting (Anand & Nikhil, 2015). The most common individual abnormality reported with cisplatin is hypomagnesemia, with incidences reported as high as 91.8% of patients (Anand & Nikhil, 2015).

(e) Hepatitis B core antibody and surface antigen testing: Hepatitis B reactivation can occur in immunocompromised patients, including those receiving chemotherapy, targeted therapy, and immunotherapy agents (Paul et al., 2016). Numerous guidelines exist regarding who should be tested and the type of testing that should be done (Hwang et al., 2015; Lok & McMahon, 2009; Reddy et al., 2015; Rubin et al., 2014; Weinbaum et al., 2008).

i. The Centers for Disease Control and Prevention recommends prechemotherapy hepatitis B screening for all patients receiving cytotoxic or immunosuppressive therapy (Weinbaum et al., 2008).

ii. ASCO recommends screening only for individuals at high risk for hepatitis B infection (e.g., patient or parents born in a high-prevalence region, injection drug user, household or sexual contact with a person who is hepatitis B surface antigen–positive), those who have planned treatment with a hematopoietic stem cell transplantation, or those going to receive treatment with an anti-CD20 antibody (Hwang et al., 2015).

iii. All guidelines recommend testing in patients receiving anti-CD20 antibodies, such as rituximab (Hwang et al., 2015; Lok & McMahon, 2009; Reddy et al., 2015; Weinbaum et al., 2008).

(f) Thyroid function tests: Immune checkpoint inhibitors, such as nivolumab, ipilimumab, and pembrolizumab, can cause endocrinopathies, such as hypothyroidism (Rossi et al., 2016). Monitor thyroid function tests throughout treatment with immunotherapy drugs that may be associated with endocrine disorders.

h) Diagnostic tests: Review results of diagnostic tests pertinent to the specific agent.

(1) Cardiac testing

(a) Echocardiogram

i. Patients receiving anthracycline antitumor antibiotics (e.g., doxorubicin) should have a baseline echocardiogram to evaluate left ventricular ejection fraction (Plana et al., 2014). Recommendations to repeat echocardiograms are dependent on the agent and cumulative dose.

ii. Product labeling for trastuzumab recommends the following in the adjuvant setting: echocardiogram at baseline, every three months during treatment, and every six months for two years following the completion of treatment (Genentech, Inc., 2017a). If trastuzumab is held because of a decrease in left ventricular ejection fraction, patients should have repeat monitoring four weeks after discontinuation (Genentech, Inc., 2017a).

(b) Electrocardiogram: A baseline electrocardiogram should be done before initiating agents with a potential to prolong QT intervals to monitor for potential life-threatening arrhythmias (Hartkopf Smith, 2012). The frequency of follow-up electrocardiograms varies with the agent. The corrected QT, known as QTc, takes into account the patient's heart rate.

(2) Pulmonary testing

(a) Pulmonary function tests may be ordered prior to initiating bleomycin and at intervals throughout treatment; however, effectiveness in detecting changes from bleomycin is controversial (Roncolato et al., 2016). Spirometry and diffusing capacity for carbon monoxide are typically ordered.

(b) Some recommendations advocate chest x-rays or computed tomography scans at intervals throughout bleomycin treatment (Khan, Nagarajaiah, & Irion, 2016).

i) Psychosocial concerns: Assess psychosocial concerns at each visit.

(1) NCCN recommends completion of distress screening at every medical visit, including chemotherapy and immunotherapy treatments (NCCN, 2018e; see Appendix F). At a minimum, NCCN recommends distress screening at the initial visit and at appropriate intervals, including with any change in disease status, progression, or treatment-related complications.

(2) ASCO/ONS Chemotherapy Administration Safety Standards recommend psychosocial assessment with each cycle and more frequently as indicated (Neuss et al., 2016).

j) Allergies and previous treatment-related reactions: Review and update at each visit (see B.2.*m*).

k) Review and update medication list at each visit (see B.2.*g*).

C. Chemotherapy, targeted therapy, and immunotherapy dosing

1. The dose calculation should include the calculation methodology, variables used to calculate the dose, frequency at which the variables are reevaluated, and changes in the values that prompt confirmation of dosing (Neuss et al., 2016).

2. Different methods of dosing may be used to calculate doses, depending on the agent and regimen ordered.

a) Fixed dosing (flat dosing): Dosing not based on the patient's height and/or weight. Many oral agents are prescribed as fixed doses. Be aware of agents that may be ordered as fixed doses or based on body surface area (BSA)—for example, bleomycin flat dose of 30 units or BSA dose of 10 units/m^2. Confirm with a reference if the agents in the regimen include fixed doses or doses based on BSA or weight alone.

b) Weight-based dosing: Dosing is expressed as dose of drug per unit of body weight (e.g., mg/kg).

c) BSA dosing: Most chemotherapy agents are dosed using the patient's BSA (m^2).

(1) The BSA is a function of height and weight and can be calculated using a variety of formulas, including the Du Bois and Du Bois formula and the Mosteller formula (see Figure 11-1).

(2) The calculated BSA is then multiplied by the dose in mg/m^2, mcg/m^2, or g/

Figure 11-1. Calculating Chemotherapy Dose Using Body Surface Area

Formulas to calculate estimated body surface area (BSA)
- Du Bois and Du Bois: BSA (m^2) = Weight $(kg)^{0.425}$ × Height $(cm)^{0.725}$ × 0.007184
- Mosteller (metric): BSA (m^2) = $\sqrt{((\text{Height (cm)} \times \text{Weight (kg)})/3{,}600)}$

To calculate the total dose of chemotherapy or immunotherapy
Calculated BSA (m^2) × dose in mcg/m^2, mg/m^2, or g/m^2 = total dose of chemotherapy

Example
The patient is 157.48 cm tall and weighs 60 kg. She is scheduled to receive paclitaxel 80 mg/m^2 IV.
- Using the Mosteller formula, calculate the BSA.
  - Multiply height and weight using metric units.
    157.48 cm × 60 kg = 9,448.8
  - Divide the total by 3,600.
    9,448.8 / 3,600 = 2.6246
  - Using a calculator, determine the square root.
    Square root = 1.62 m^2
- Calculate the total dose by multiplying the body surface by the dose ordered in mg/m^2.
  1.62 m^2 × 80 mg/m^2 = 129.6 mg

Note. Based on information from Du Bois & Du Bois, 1916; Mosteller, 1987.

m^2 to determine the total dose of the agent to be administered.

(3) The underlying assumption for dosing based on BSA is that BSA is a more reliable indicator than using weight alone for predicting pharmacokinetics. However, BSA dosing does not take into account factors such as gender and age.

(4) In most situations, there is no significant difference between doses calculated using different BSA formulas (Faisal, Tang, Tiley, & Kukard, 2016). However, different formulas may produce different results for patients who have extremes of height and weight (Faisal et al., 2016; Fancher, Sacco, Gwin, Gormley, & Mitchell, 2016).

(5) The Mosteller equation has the advantage of being easily performed using any calculator with a square root function.

d) Carboplatin and area under the plasma concentration versus time curve (AUC) dosing: Carboplatin is dosed using AUC-based dosing, which refers to the amount of drug exposure over time or the total drug concentration in plasma over a period of time.

(1) AUC dosing takes into account age, gender, weight, and renal function.

(2) Carboplatin drug clearance is strongly correlated with renal function.

(3) Carboplatin doses are determined by first calculating the creatinine clearance and then calculating the total dose of carboplatin by using the Calvert formula (see Figure 11-2). The AUC is prescribed in the treatment plan and usually ranges from 2 (low dose) to 6 (higher dose).

(a) To calculate the patient's creatinine clearance: An estimated creatinine clearance is most often used, rather than an actual glomerular filtration rate (24-hour urine for creatinine clearance).

(b) A variety of formulas are used to calculate creatinine clearance, with the Cockcroft-Gault being the most common in the United States. Different formulas can yield different results (Nagao et al., 2005).

(c) To calculate creatinine clearance using the Cockcroft-Gault formula, obtain the patient's age, gender, weight in kilograms, and a recent serum creatinine (see Figure 11-3). The formula may not be accurate in patients with rapidly changing serum creatinine levels (Gaguski & Karcheski, 2011).

Figure 11-2. Calculating Carboplatin Dose Using the Calvert Formula

Dose of carboplatin (mg) = (target AUC) × (GFR + 25)
Total dose calculated is in mg, not mg/m^2.

AUC—area under the plasma concentration versus time curve; GFR—glomerular filtration rate

Note. Based on information from Calvert et al., 1989.

Figure 11-3. Calculating Glomerular Filtration Rate Using the Cockcroft-Gault Formula

Males

$$\text{estCrCl (ml/min)} = \frac{(140 - \text{age}) \times (\text{weight in kg})}{72 \times \text{serum creatinine (mg/dl)}}$$

Females

$$\text{estCrCl (ml/min)} = \frac{(140 - \text{age}) \times (\text{weight in kg}) \times (0.85)}{72 \times \text{serum creatinine (mg/dl)}}$$

estCrCl—estimated creatinine clearance

Note. Based on information from Cockcroft & Gault, 1976.

(*d*) The National Cancer Institute Cancer Therapy Evaluation Program (2010) recommends capping estimated serum creatinine clearance at 125 ml/min to prevent overdosing and dose capping carboplatin based on AUC (see Figure 11-4).

(*e*) If variance exists between the prescribed dose and the recalculated dose, clarify with the prescriber whether the actual, adjusted, or ideal weight was used when calculating creatinine clearance and whether an adjusted serum creatinine was used.

(*f*) The Gynecologic Oncology Group (2011) has established additional criteria to standardize carboplatin calculations; these criteria are included in the calculator (available to Gynecologic Oncology Group members) on its website.

e) Pharmacogenomics and chemotherapy dosing

(1) Pharmacogenomics combines the science of how drugs work (pharmacology) and the science of the human genome (genomics) to determine drug selection and drug doses (Weiss, 2008).

(2) Irinotecan is an example of pharmacogenomic-based dosing. Some individuals with a genetic variant in UGT1A1 might not be able to eliminate irinotecan from their bodies as rapidly as others, leading to severe diarrhea and severe neutropenia (Pfizer Inc., 2016). Patients with this variant may need to receive lower doses of the drug.

3. Dosing and obesity

a) Controversy has existed regarding dosing for obese patients. Concerns voiced were fears of toxicity versus compromising disease-free survival in the curative setting. ASCO (Griggs et al., 2012) has developed formalized guidelines to address this issue.

b) Actual weight (full weight–based doses) is recommended when calculating doses for obese and morbidly obese patients with cancer, especially when the goal of treatment is cure (Griggs et al., 2012). An adult with a body mass index (BMI) of 30 kg/m^2 or greater is considered obese; an adult with a BMI greater than 40 kg/m^2 (or greater than 35 kg/m^2 with comorbid conditions) is considered morbidly obese (Griggs et al., 2012).

c) Furlanetto et al. (2016) found a higher rate of severe toxicities in obese patients receiving dose-dense chemotherapy according to unadjusted BSA. The investigators found no difference in disease-free survival between the obese and nonobese groups in this randomized controlled trial. The authors concluded that a dose adjustment should be performed in obese patients to prevent serious complications.

4. Dosing and underweight patients

a) No formal guidelines exist addressing dosing of underweight patients, those with low BMI, or those with sarcopenia (low skeletal mass).

b) In a study examining prescribing practices, Anglada-Martínez et al. (2014) found that

Figure 11-4. Calculating Carboplatin Dose Capping Using Estimated Creatinine Clearance

Dose of carboplatin (mg) = (target AUC) × (estCrCl + 25)

estCrCl capped at 125 ml/min

Maximum doses for sample target AUCs

- Target AUC 6: Maximum carboplatin dose = 6 × (125 + 25) = 900 mg
- Target AUC 5: Maximum carboplatin dose = 5 × (125 + 25) = 750 mg
- Target AUC 4: Maximum carboplatin dose = 4 × (125 + 25) = 600 mg

AUC—area under the plasma concentration versus time curve; estCrCl—estimated creatinine clearance

Note. Based on information from Calvert et al., 1989; Smart, 2011.

almost 100% of respondents used actual body weight when calculating doses for cachectic patients.

5. Dose rounding
   a) Be aware of dose rounding policies and practices when calculating and verifying doses.
   b) Institutional dose rounding policies often allow dose rounding at 5% or 10% of the prescribed therapy. Policies may also differentiate between chemotherapy and immunotherapy doses, the intent of therapy (e.g., cure vs. palliation), and whether doses can be rounded up, down, or both. Some institutions may not dose round for pediatric patients. Clinical trials may specify the accepted percentage for dose rounding.
   c) Hematology/Oncology Pharmacy Association (2017) recommendations
      (1) Monoclonal antibodies, other immunotherapies, and traditional cytotoxic chemotherapy: Dose round to the nearest vial size within 10% of the prescribed dose.
      (2) Monoclonal antibodies with conjugated (attached) cytotoxic agents: Apply dose rounding to the cytotoxic component of the agent. It can be rounded to the nearest vial size within 10% of the prescribed dose.
      (3) Oral chemotherapy: Use one dose strength and round the final dose, when possible, to simplify dosing for patients.
      (4) Dose rounding can be used for both curative and palliative therapy as long as the rounding does not influence clinical safety or effectiveness.

D. Verification
1. The healthcare setting should have established processes for verification and clearly defined steps to take when discrepancies arise (Neuss et al., 2016). *Verification* refers to determining the accuracy of the prescribed therapy, prepared medication, patient identification, and pump settings, if applicable.
2. Verification should occur prior to administration for all routes of chemotherapy, targeted therapy, and immunotherapy, including the oral route.
   a) Independent dual verification (i.e., independent double-checks) is a process in which a second person conducts an independent verification of the accuracy of the prescribed therapy, without telling his or her findings to the other verifier until both have completed the process (ISMP Canada, 2005). Checklists may help promote a consistent process (White et al., 2010; see Appendix D for an example).
   b) Verify the accuracy of the following information on the treatment plan.
      (1) Verify a minimum of two patient identifiers per institutional policy, such as name, date of birth, and medical record number. Do not use room or chair numbers as patient identifiers (Neuss et al., 2016).
      (2) Compare the treatment plan (orders) with a reference for doses, routes, and schedule. For example, a treatment plan (orders) for dose-dense doxorubicin and cyclophosphamide that includes orders for doxorubicin 60 mg/m^2 IV and cyclophosphamide 600 mg/m^2 IV every two weeks for a total of four cycles is compared with a reference, which confirms the doses, routes, and schedule. Never verify accuracy by comparing to previous patient doses, as they may have been changed because of patient toxicities or other factors.
      (3) Confirm the accuracy of the treatment plan cycle and day number.
         (a) Compare the date on patient orders, the date of planned therapy, and previously administered doses (e.g., the patient is scheduled for cycle 12 of weekly paclitaxel, but the nurse notes from the medical record that patient has received 10 doses).
         (b) Confirm that the appropriate interval has occurred between treatments (e.g., seven days).
      (4) Compare the height and weight on the treatment plan with current, measured height and weight. Use only metric units of measurement (ISMP, 2018).
      (5) For BSA-dosed medications: Recalculate the BSA based on the current, measured height and weight (see Figure 11-1). Compare the recalculated BSA with the BSA on the treatment plan. Recalculate the total dose and compare with the prescribed dose.
      (6) For carboplatin: Recalculate the patient's creatinine clearance. Using the Calvert formula, recalculate the total dose (see Figure 11-2). Compare the recalculated dose with the prescribed dose.

(7) For weight-based medications: Recalculate the total dose.

(8) For fixed-dose medications: Compare the prescribed dose with a reference.

(9) Verify the route of administration, sequence of administration, and the duration of infusion, if applicable. The sequence in which chemotherapy and immunotherapy are given may affect the pharmacokinetics and pharmacodynamics of the agents (Modlin & Mancini, 2011). However, it is not always known if a specific sequence of treatment results in better outcomes. Modlin and Mancini (2011) developed tables to guide staff who administer therapy where evidence for sequencing exists.

(10) Verify the compatibility of any IV solutions and medications used during administration.

(11) Confirm that supportive care treatments are ordered and are appropriate to the regimen (e.g., premedications, hydration, growth factors, rescue agents, medications to manage infusion reactions).

(12) Clarify any discrepancies with the prescriber before initiating treatment. Common reasons for discrepancies include inaccurate height and weight and use of different formulas for calculating BSA or creatinine clearance.

3. Check the prepared medication.
   a) Compare the medication and label with the treatment plan (orders) and verify the following:
      (1) Patient name, date of birth, and any other identifier as established in institutional policy
      (2) Medication name and total dose
      (3) Diluent type and total volume (as appropriate)
      (4) Expiration date and time
   b) Appearance and physical integrity of the medication and medication container (e.g., clarity, leaking)
   c) Any special labelling (e.g., hazardous medication, for intravenous use only, protect from light)
4. Verification of the patient, medication, and pump programming at the bedside (or chairside): Immediately prior to administration, the following should be verified by two practitioners approved by the healthcare setting:
   a) Patient's stated name and date of birth and any other established patient identifiers with the patient's wristband (sticker or other method of patient identification), the medication label, and the treatment plan (orders)
   b) Compare the medication name, dose, route, and schedule on the label with the treatment plan (orders).
5. Include the patient as part of the verification process.
   a) Patient involvement: Involve patients and families in the medication verification process by providing them with the medication names, schedule, potential adverse reactions, and indications for when to notify their healthcare provider.
   b) Encourage patients to alert their nurse to clarify any possible discrepancies (e.g., "I thought today was my last chemotherapy, not next week," "Is it OK for me to get my 5-fluorouracil if I've been having diarrhea six to eight times a day?") (Agency for Healthcare Research and Quality, 2018; Hartkopf Smith, 2009a; Schwappach, Hochreutener, & Wernli, 2010).
   c) Research indicates that involving patients in their care can lead to measurable improvements in safety (Maurer, Dardess, Carman, Frazier, & Smeeding, 2012).
   d) Scan patients' wristbands and medications, if this technology is available. Studies have indicated that scanning decreases the risk of medication errors (Bonkowski et al., 2013; Seibert, Maddox, Flynn, & Williams, 2014).
   e) Verify any infusion pump programming with the treatment plan (orders) and reference (Neuss et al., 2016).
6. Continuous infusions in the inpatient settings: If an infusion was initiated by another nurse, the nurse assuming the care of the patient should verify the drug, dose, date, patient, and pump settings for infusion during shift handoff to prevent possible propagation of a previous error.
7. When chemotherapy is administered in the home by a healthcare provider, verify the drug, dose, date, patient, and pump settings for infusion. A second identifier, such as a driver's license, should be used to confirm the patient's identity (Neuss et al., 2016).

E. Routes of chemotherapy, immunotherapy, and targeted therapy administration
   1. Oral route
      a) Oral cancer treatments have experienced a rapid increase over the past 10 years, with

new cytotoxic agents, small molecule inhibitors, and other targeted therapies. The oral route presents unique challenges for oncology nurses and patients as treatment shifts from clinician-administered therapy in a healthcare setting to self-administration.

b) Pretreatment assessment (in addition to the general pretreatment assessment) (Neuss et al., 2016; ONS, 2016)
   (1) Financial/insurance coverage for the medication and available pharmaceutical company assistance programs
   (2) Method and/or location the patient will obtain the medication (e.g., specialty pharmacy, drop shipment)
   (3) The patient's ability to swallow and retain pills (e.g., dysphagia, strictures, presence of gastrostomy or jejunostomy tube, mucositis, esophageal strictures, vomiting)
   (4) The patient's ability to read labels, instructions, and calendars
   (5) The patient's ability to open medication bottles or packages
   (6) The patient's ability to comprehend instructions regarding dosing, schedules, and indications for when to hold the medication and notify the healthcare provider.
   (7) Possible food–drug interactions, drug–drug interactions, and supplement–drug interactions

c) System safeguards to prevent errors and manage emergencies (also see Chapters 1, 12, and 13)
   (1) Independent practitioners who are determined to be qualified by the healthcare setting should sign oral chemotherapy, targeted therapy, and immunotherapy orders for the treatment of cancer (Neuss et al., 2016).
   (2) Information to include in prescriptions or orders for oral chemotherapy, targeted therapies, and immunotherapy (Neuss et al., 2016; ONS, 2016)
      (a) Patient name, date of birth, and any institution-specific identifiers
      (b) Full generic name of medication
      (c) Drug dose and calculation methodology (e.g., mg/m^2)
      (d) Schedule of administration
      (e) Drug quantity to be dispensed and number of refills, with zero as the acceptable default value. A time limitation to refills helps ensure appropriate evaluation at predetermined intervals.
      (f) Any special instructions
   (3) Institutional policies should address the process for continuation of oral chemotherapy, targeted therapy, and immunotherapy when patients are admitted to the hospital.
      (a) In many settings, patients may be admitted by a hospitalist or other non-oncologist. The potential for error exists if the therapy is continued as part of a home medication list, although it may be contraindicated for the patient's current condition (Booth, Booth, & Crawford, 2011; Schleisman & Mahon, 2015).
      (b) Prior to giving an oral chemotherapy, targeted therapy, or immunotherapy agent in the inpatient setting as a continuation of home therapy, verify that the agent was ordered by a licensed independent practitioner who is determined to be qualified by the healthcare setting and that the therapy has been determined to be appropriate to continue and at the same dose.

d) Dosing: When possible, one dose strength of pill should be used and rounded to the final dose (Hematology/Oncology Pharmacy Association, 2017).

e) Verification: See section D.

f) Administration
   (1) Do not crush hazardous oral antineoplastics outside of a containment primary engineering control. If the patient is unable to take oral medication, discuss an alternative route with the oncologist or use strategies for safe administration (Polovich & Olsen, 2018; see Chapter 12).
   (2) For intact oral tablets, capsules, or pills designated as hazardous, wear one pair of gloves tested for use with HDs. A mask with a face shield and double gloves should be worn if there is a potential for sprays, aerosols, or splattering of the agent, such as with liquid oral HDs (Polovich & Olsen, 2018).

g) Other considerations
   (1) The institution or practice should determine a process to assess and track

patient adherence to oral cancer therapy (Neuss et al., 2016; ONS, 2016).

(2) Strategies to encourage adherence include calendars or daily medication checklists, pill diaries, electronic reminders, and text messages (Burhenn & Smuddle, 2015; ONS, 2016; Rodriguez, Utate, Joseph, & St. Victor, 2017; Spoelstra & Sansoucie, 2015; see Chapter 4).

(3) Set up routine appointments to monitor patients' response to therapy, including follow-up laboratory testing.

(4) Information to include in patient education (ONS, 2016)

(a) Drug name, dose, and schedule, including calendar as appropriate

(b) How the drug will be obtained

(c) Potential side effects, management, and indications for when to notify the healthcare provider

(d) Safe storage and handling

(e) Disposal of unused medication (e.g., drug drop-off sites that accept hazardous medications)

(f) Food, drug, and supplement interactions

(g) Plan for missed doses

(h) Schedule of appointments for monitoring

(i) Process for refills

2. Subcutaneous (SC) and intramuscular (IM) routes

a) Few chemotherapy, targeted, and immunotherapy agents are ordered via the SC or IM route. Select hormonal agents used as antineoplastics are administered via these routes. See Tables 6-1, 7-1, 8-1, and 10-1 for a listing of drugs given via these routes.

b) Pretreatment assessment in addition to the general pretreatment assessment

(1) Assess for adequate subcutaneous or muscle sites.

(2) Review any coagulation values and other risks for bleeding and bruising.

c) System safeguards to prevent errors and manage emergencies: Never administer vesicants by the SC or IM route.

d) Dosing: Depending on the total volume of the syringe, the medication may have to be divided into several syringes.

(1) The maximum volume for IM injections varies according to muscle mass and the muscle used, with the deltoid muscle ranging 0.5–2 ml, the dorsogluteal 4 ml, and the vastus lateralis 5 ml (Hopkins & Arias, 2013).

(2) The maximum volume for SC injections varies according to the amount of subcutaneous muscle and the location of injection, with a volume range of 2–3 ml (Ferruccio et al., 2016). An exception is rituximab and hyaluronidase human (Genentech, Inc., 2017b), for which the total volume of SC injection is 11.7 ml or 13.4 ml, depending on the dose. The addition of hyaluronidase, an enzyme that increases that distribution and absorption of locally injected substances, permits the large volume of the SC injection. Care must be taken to ensure this formulation is not given IV.

e) Verification: See section D.

f) Administration

(1) For SC and IM medications designated as hazardous (Polovich & Olsen, 2018)

(a) Wear two pair of gloves and a gown that have been tested for use with HDs. Wear a mask with face protection if splashing is possible (see Chapter 12).

(b) Use closed-system drug-transfer devices (CSTDs) attached between the syringe and needle when possible (Polovich & Olsen, 2018).

(c) If air bubbles are noted in the syringe, do not express unless in a containment primary engineering control (Polovich & Olsen, 2018; see Chapter 12).

(2) Use the smallest gauge needle possible.

(3) Review product literature for any specific instructions regarding the site of SC or IM injection. For example, instructions for bortezomib specify injection into the thigh or abdomen (Millennium Pharmaceuticals, Inc., 2017).

(4) Avoid scarred areas.

(5) Rotate sites.

(6) Clean the site with antiseptic and allow to dry completely prior to injection.

(7) For IM injections (Sisson, 2015)

(a) Usual sites for delivering an IM injection include the deltoid, vastus lateralis, ventrogluteal, and dorsogluteal muscles.

(b) The deltoid, vastus lateralis, and ventrogluteal sites are recommended because these sites are far-

ther from major blood vessels and nerves. Aspiration is not required for these sites.

(c) Aspiration is still advised when injecting into the dorsogluteal muscle because of its proximity to the gluteal artery.

(8) Inject medication at the prescribed rate.

(9) Dispose of any unused supplies in appropriate waste container.

(10) Other considerations: Following administration, assess for pain, swelling, induration, hemorrhage, erythema, pruritus, and rash.

3. IV route

a) IV administration is one of the most common routes of administration. Medications can be administered by the following methods, depending on the agent and regimen: IV push, short-term infusion, or continuous IV infusion.

b) Pretreatment assessment/actions in addition to the general pretreatment assessment

(1) Evaluate the patient's venous access. Determine if it is appropriate or adequate for the prescribed therapy.

(a) Consider the agents to be administered; their vesicant, irritant or nonvesicant properties; the prescribed method of administration; and the overall duration of therapy.

(b) Refer to ONS's *Access Device Standards of Practice for Oncology Nursing* (Camp-Sorrell & Matey, 2017).

(2) Identify risk factors for extravasation if the treatment regimen includes a vesicant (see Chapter 13).

(3) Review and confirm the sequence of medication administration.

c) System safeguards to prevent errors and manage emergencies (also see Chapters 12 and 13)

(1) The institution or practice should define a process to manage overfill, especially for continuous infusions (ISMP, 2013b).

(a) Commercially available bags of standard IV solutions (e.g., normal saline) often contain overfill (e.g., a 1,000 ml bag of normal saline could potentially contain 1,100 ml, but the bag may still be labeled as 1,000 ml). Some institutions add the medication to the bag without concern for overfill, others may withdraw a volume equal to the medication, some may withdraw the drug volume and overfill volume prior to admixture, and some may start with an empty bag to mix an exact total volume (ISMP, 2013b).

(b) Nurses must be aware of the method used at their healthcare setting, as it can affect the duration of the infusion and the concentration of the medication.

(2) Vinca alkaloids: Strategies that should be implemented to prevent errors from inadvertent administration of vinca alkaloids into cerebrospinal fluid (NCCN, n.d.)

(a) Administer vinca alkaloids in a minibag (IV piggyback [IVPB]). Never administer using an IV pump when administering through a peripheral IV catheter. Do not administer in a syringe in facilities where intrathecal medications are administered.

(b) Label all vinca alkaloid bags "FOR INTRAVENOUS USE ONLY—FATAL IF GIVEN BY OTHER ROUTES."

(c) Never dispense vinca alkaloids to an area where intrathecal medications are administered.

(d) Never give vinca alkaloids in the same treatment room as intrathecal medications.

(3) Ambulatory infusion pumps

(a) To prevent errors, prescribers should order 5-fluorouracil and other continuous infusion antineoplastics in single, daily doses with directions to infuse continuously over a specific number of days (e.g., 750 mg/m^2 IV over 24 hours days 1, 2, 3, 4, 5) (ISMP, 2015a).

(b) Numerous errors have been reported regarding home infusions of 5-fluorouracil, often related to prescribing errors and pump programming errors (ISMP, 2015a, 2015b). A common error reported is confusing the *dose per day* with the *total dose to be infused over multiple days* (ISMP, 2015a, 2015b). This can result in fatal errors.

(c) Use infusion pumps with dose error reduction software, when possible (ISMP, 2015b, 2018).

(d) The information the pharmacist or nurse needs to program the pump is displayed clearly on the medication label (ISMP, 2015a, 2015b).

(e) Information to include in patient and caregiver education (ISMP, 2015a)

i. Total dose they are to receive, the length of time the infusion should last, and instruction to routinely check that the pump is not infusing too fast

ii. Troubleshooting alarms and infusion pump malfunction

iii. Steps to follow if tubing becomes disconnected, a spill occurs, or a port needle becomes dislodged

iv. 24-hour contact information for questions and problems

(f) The institution or practice must establish a process to address patients who present to emergency departments and inpatient areas with ambulatory pumps with an antineoplastic infusing. Often, healthcare providers in these areas are not familiar with all the ambulatory pumps in use, and patients who use these devices may be ill informed, leading to serious errors (ISMP, 2015a, 2015b).

d) Dosing: See section C.

e) Verification

(1) Verify any infusion pump programming with another provider (Neuss et al., 2016).

(2) Continuous infusions in inpatient settings: If an infusion was initiated by another nurse, the nurse assuming the care of the patient should verify the infusion during shift handoff to prevent possible propagation of a previous error.

(3) When chemotherapy is administered in the home by a healthcare provider, a second identifier, such as a driver's license, should be used to confirm the patient's identity (Neuss et al., 2016).

f) Administration

(1) Equipment

(a) IV tubing selection

i. Standardize the use of IV tubings.

ii. Use IV tubings with Luer-lock connections.

iii. For hazardous medications, use CSTDs (Polovich & Olsen, 2018; see Chapter 12). Some manufacturers incorporate these devices as part of the IV tubing.

iv. Minimal research exists to support the most effective IV tubing setup for parenteral antineoplastic medication administration (Wiley, 2017). Select IV tubings and setups that do the following:

- Provide minimal waste remaining in the IV tubing after the medication is completed, thus providing the maximum dose of medication to the patient and a minimal amount of hazardous waste that requires disposal
- Permit the least amount of manipulation of the system, thus decreasing the risk of infection for the patient and decreasing the risk of hazardous waste exposure for the healthcare provider
- Allow for emergency response if administering a drug that can cause hypersensitivity reaction or anaphylaxis. The main IV line should contain a compatible carrier solution that can be turned on immediately after stopping the drug the patient is reacting to.

v. Some medications require DEHP-free tubing (see Tables 6-1, 8-1, and 10-1). DEHP is a plasticizer added to polyvinyl chloride plastic to make it flexible. Select agents cause leaching of DEHP, which may be harmful to patients.

vi. Some medications require an in-line filter (see Tables 6-1, 8-1, and 10-1 and drug package inserts).

vii. For medications designated as hazardous, wear two pair of gloves and a gown that have been tested for use with HDs. Wear a mask with face protection if splashing is possible (Polovich & Olsen, 2018; see Chapter 12).

(b) Use IV pumps with dose error reduction software, when possible, for the administration of infusions of chemotherapy, targeted therapies, and immunotherapy, excluding peripheral administration of vesicants (ISMP, 2018).

i. Do not rely on pump alarms to detect IV infiltration or extravasation.

ii. IV pumps with dose error reduction software are preferred because they include medication dosing guidelines, concentrations, dose limits, and advisories (Infusion Nurses Society, 2016; ISMP, 2018; Orto, Hendrix, Griffith, & Shaikewitz, 2015).

iii. Pumps with dose error reduction software should never replace the use of independent double-checks (ISMP, 2009).

iv. *Infusion interoperability* is the ability of an infusion pump to receive and transmit information in near real-time with the electronic health record. Medication orders and parameters automatically program the infusion pump. The pump can then send back infusion status and history to the electronic health record.

v. Infusion interoperability should never replace the use of independent double-checks (ISMP, 2009).

(2) Peripheral venous access

(a) Do not use peripheral IV sites for the administration of vesicants given as continuous infusions. When administering vesicants via a peripheral IV site, limit the infusion time to 30–60 minutes and remain with the patient during the entire infusion.

(b) Venipuncture

i. Avoid the use of established IV sites that are more than 24 hours old.

ii. No clear evidence exists to support the use of a new venipuncture site versus one less than 24 hours old for the administration of vesicants. Regardless, thoroughly assess the site for patency, including blood return, and complications before and during drug administration.

iii. Choose veins that are large, smooth, and pliable.

iv. Sites to avoid

- Ventral surface of the hand
- Joints and areas near joints
- Antecubital fossa
- Lower extremities
- Areas distal to a recent venipuncture, including laboratory draws
- Areas of impaired circulation or lymph node drainage
- Areas with decreased sensation (e.g., peripheral neuropathy)

v. No definitive guidelines exist regarding venipuncture, including vesicant administration, for patients who have had a sentinel lymph node biopsy.

vi. Ultrasound-guided peripheral catheter insertion in deep veins in the upper arms may be associated with an increased incidence of undetected infiltration and extravasation. Staff skilled in ultrasound-guided IV insertion must ensure that sufficient catheter length is threaded into the vein to prevent catheter dislodgment during patient movement. Nurses should assess the vein frequently for signs and symptoms of infiltration (Infusion Nurses Society, 2016).

vii. Avoid the use of metal needles, as they may increase the risk of infiltration or extravasation (Mackey, 2017a).

viii. Perform venipuncture according to institutional policy and procedure. If unsuccessful, restart IV using a different site on the opposite arm, if possible, or proximal to the previous puncture site.

ix. Apply transparent dressing to the insertion site and secure the catheter. Ensure visualization of peripheral IV entrance site.

x. Ensure securement of the peripheral IV to help prevent dislodgment. In a study examining 673 vesicant extravasations and irritant infiltrations, one of the most common etiologies was patient movement and subsequent dislodgment (Jackson-Rose et al., 2017).

xi. Educate the patient to report unusual tugging on tubing or IV, discomfort, swelling, or pain during administration of therapy.

xii. Confirm and document a blood return and absence of signs and symptoms of infiltration prior to and every 2–5 ml during IV push administration of vesicant chemotherapy. Do not administer vesicants in the absence of a blood return or if other signs or symptoms of extravasation are present.

xiii. Observe for swelling, pain, burning, tightness, cool skin, skin color change, and changes in flow rate. If infiltration occurs, immediately stop infusion. For vesicant extravasation, see Chapter 13. If additional drug remains to be administered, place a new IV at a different site on the opposite arm, if possible, or proximal to previous venipuncture sites and the infiltration.

(3) Midline catheters

(a) Midlines are defined as peripheral IV catheters that are greater than three inches in length and terminate in the axillary vein in the upper arm (Cope, 2017; Infusion Nurses Society, 2016). Midlines can be placed with or without ultrasound guidance.

(b) Do not use for continuous infusions of vesicants (Cope, 2017).

(c) Ultrasound-guided peripheral catheter insertion in deep veins in the upper arms may be associated with an increased incidence of undetected infiltration and extravasation. Staff skilled in ultrasound-guided IV insertion must ensure that sufficient catheter length is threaded into the vein to prevent catheter dislodgment during patient movement. Nurses should assess the vein frequently for signs and symptoms of infiltration (Infusion Nurses Society, 2016).

(d) The use of midline catheters for administering IV push or intermittent infusions of vesicants is controversial. Caution is recommended with midlines because of the risk of undetected extravasation, as the vein may be deeper than a traditional short peripheral IV (Cope, 2017).

(e) Confirm and document a blood return and absence of signs and symptoms of infiltration prior to and every 2–5 ml during IV push administration of vesicant chemotherapy. Do not administer vesicants in the absence of a blood return.

(4) Central venous access devices: These include percutaneous subclavian or jugular catheters, tunneled catheters, peripherally inserted central catheters, and implanted ports.

(a) Indications include patients receiving continuous infusion of vesicants, vesicant infusions of longer than 60 minutes, complex treatment regimens in which frequent access is necessary, and poor or limited patient venous access.

(b) Central venous access devices should be used for patients receiving home infusions of chemotherapy via ambulatory infusion pumps.

(c) Ideally, central venous catheter tip location should be at the distal third of the superior vena cava or cavoatrial junction (Infusion Nurses Society, 2016; Mackey, 2017b).

(d) Assess for signs and symptoms of malposition or occlusion prior to administration of cancer therapy. Do not proceed if any of the following are present, and contact provider:

i. Absent or sluggish blood return
ii. Change in color of blood from lumen(s)
iii. Difficulty flushing or IV does not flow freely
iv. Atrial or ventricular arrhythmias
v. Pain, edema, or strange sensations in neck, shoulder, chest, or back
vi. Gurgling or rushing sound on the side of the central venous access device, which could indicate tip malposition in jugular vein
vii. Neurologic changes or paresthesias

(e) Follow institutional guidelines for troubleshooting and declotting procedures and/or dye study, as indicated.

(f) For implanted ports, access the port with noncoring needle. Select the appropriate needle length based on the depth of the port. Stabilize the needle with tape and transparent dressing or securement device to help prevent dislodgment and possible infiltration during medication administration. Inspect the insertion site for evidence of needle dislodgment, leakage of IV fluid, or edema during infusions.

(g) For all central venous access devices, use a transparent dressing to ensure visualization of the site during administration. Gauze may be used to stabilize the needle wings as long as the insertion site is not covered (Infusion Nurses Society, 2016).

(5) IV push method

(a) Refer to institutional guidelines and drug references for the recommended rate of administration. In addition, take into account the status of the patient's veins or type of venous access.

(b) Although there are limited published evidence reviews or research supporting the superiority of the free flow (side-arm technique) versus the direct push method, the side-arm technique allows for constant dilution of vesicant during administration, which may decrease the severity of an extravasation injury.

(c) Side-arm technique for administration of IV push

i. Hang a primary IV line with a solution compatible with the IV push medications.
ii. Allow the primary IV solution to run freely, without using an infusion pump.
iii. Flush vascular access device with a saline prefilled syringe at the closest side port to the patient to ensure patency and lack of signs and symptoms of infiltration.
iv. Use a transparent dressing over the site to visualize signs and symptoms of vesicant extravasation or infiltration.
v. Assess for blood return and signs of infiltration (e.g., pain, burning, leaking, or swelling at catheter insertion site).
vi. Two methods for verification of blood return
    - Aspirate with a syringe at the lowest Y-site and clamp off fluid from the bag.

- Use gravity to check by lowering the IV bag below the patient's IV site.

vii. Attach the syringe of the antineoplastic to the injection port closest to the patient on the primary IV tubing using a CSTD (Polovich & Olsen, 2018).

viii. Slowly administer the medication. Allow the primary IV solution to run continuously, to dilute the medication.

ix. Assess for blood return every 2–5 ml.

x. Continuously assess the site for signs and symptoms of infiltration or extravasation.

xi. If multiple medications are administered, flush with the primary IV solution between each drug and at the completion of the infusion.

xii. Stop administration immediately for signs or symptoms of infiltration or extravasation. (e.g., pain, burning, redness, edema, any patient-reported discomfort). It is important to distinguish between extravasation and flare reaction or radiation recall (see Chapter 13 for management of vesicant extravasation or irritant infiltration).

(d) Direct IV push method

i. A primary IV line with dilution is not used.

ii. Establish venous access as outlined previously.

iii. Flush the vascular access device with a saline prefilled syringe to ensure patency and lack of signs and symptoms of infiltration (e.g., no pain, no leaking, no swelling at IV site).

iv. Use a transparent dressing over the site.

v. Ensure that blood return is present prior to direct IV push.

vi. Slowly administer the antineoplastic through a syringe using a CSTD (Polovich & Olsen, 2018).

vii. Assess for blood return every 2–5 ml during administration.

viii. Stop administration immediately for signs and symptoms of infiltration.

ix. Disconnect the medication syringe, and reconnect another flush syringe using a CSTD.

x. Flush the line.

(6) Short-term/minibag (e.g., IVPB)

(a) Hang a primary IV tubing, and prime with a solution compatible with the medications to be administered.

(b) Flush the vascular access device with a saline prefilled syringe at the closest side port to the patient to ensure patency and lack of signs and symptoms of infiltration.

(c) Assess for blood return and other signs of patency (e.g., no pain, no leaking, no swelling at IV site).

(d) Attach the minibag of medication to the injection port on the primary IV tubing using a CSTD (Polovich & Olsen, 2018).

(e) Refer to medication orders, institutional guidelines, or drug references for the recommended rate of administration. The rate of administration of the agent may vary according to the prescribed regimen.

(f) For <u>nonvesicant</u> short-term/minibag (IVPB) infusions

i. Insert the medication tubing into the Y-site above or below the IV pump, depending on the agent or institutional procedure, using a CSTD (Polovich & Olsen, 2018).

ii. Infuse as ordered and/or per institutional guidelines or drug reference.

iii. Assess for signs and symptoms of infiltration.

iv. If multiple agents are administered, flush with the primary IV solution between each agent and at the completion of the infusion.

(*g*) For <u>vesicant</u> short-term/minibag infusions

i. Peripheral IV administration
- Do not use an infusion pump for administration of vesicants through a peripheral IV.
- Administer by gravity through a free-flowing primary IV line using a CSTD (Polovich & Olsen, 2018).
- Remain with the patient during the entire infusion.
- Use a transparent dressing to visualize the IV site.
- Limit administration to ≤ 30 minutes.
- Verify blood return before, every five minutes during, and after the infusion is complete.
- See Chapter 13 for more information on taxanes.

ii. Administer all vinca alkaloids as a short-term/minibag infusion (IV minibag) (ISMP, 2016; NCCN, n.d.; Neuss et al., 2016).

iii. Numerous studies have indicated the risk of extravasation is less than 0.05% when vinca alkaloids are administered using the following method (Gilbar & Carrington, 2006; Hartkopf-Smith & Hughes-McNally, 2012; Nurgat et al., 2015).
- Vinca alkaloids should be prepared as a minibag infusion (e.g., 25–50 ml).
- Do not use an IV pump when administering vesicants through a peripheral IV.
- Administer by gravity through a free-flowing primary IV line using a CSTD (Polovich & Olsen, 2018).
- Remain with the patient during the entire infusion.
- Use a transparent dressing to visualize the IV site.
- Infuse over 5–15 minutes.
- Assess for blood return during any vesicant administration via a short-term infusion before, every five minutes during, and after the infusion is complete.
- Closely monitor for signs and symptoms of extravasation, such as swelling, loss of blood return, and patient's report of pain or burning sensation. Confirming extravasation of vesicants during chemotherapy administration can be difficult because manifestations can vary from no immediate signs to pain, swelling, and loss of blood return.
- Stop administration immediately for signs and symptoms of infiltration and extravasation. See Chapter 13 for management of vesicant extravasation.

(7) Continuous infusions

(*a*) Assess for blood return and other signs of patency prior to, during, and after drug administration according to institutional policy (e.g., no pain, no leaking, no swelling at IV site).

(*b*) Hang a primary IV tubing with a solution compatible with the medications to be administered (excluding home infusions using ambulatory infusion pumps).

(*c*) Use an IV pump (ISMP, 2018; Polovich & Olsen, 2018). Administer via a programmable infusion pump using dose error–reduction software in both inpatient and outpatient areas (ISMP, 2018).

(*d*) Connect chemotherapy, targeted therapy, or immunotherapy tubing into primary IV, as per institutional policy. Use a CSTD for administration of HDs (Polovich & Olsen, 2018).

(*e*) Infuse as ordered and/or per institutional guidelines or drug reference.

(*f*) Assess for signs and symptoms of infiltration.

(g) For continuous infusions of vesicants

i. Always infuse through a central venous access device.

ii. Assess for blood return and other signs and symptoms of extravasation prior to initiating the infusion, at periods specified by institutional policy, and at the completion.

iii. Check for blood return and other signs and symptoms of extravasation if there are any indications that the pump is not flowing (e.g., pump alarm for occlusion, infusion rate appears to be too slow) and at the completion of therapy.

iv. Use a transparent dressing over the site to visualize signs and symptoms of extravasation.

v. Stop administration immediately for signs and symptoms of infiltration and extravasation. See Chapter 13 for management of vesicant extravasation.

4. Intraperitoneal

a) Intraperitoneal chemotherapy is the administration of chemotherapy directly into the peritoneal cavity via an external catheter or port.

(1) It is most frequently used for ovarian cancer, as the most common route of spread for this cancer is within the peritoneal cavity (NCCN, 2018f).

(2) Compared with IV chemotherapy, intraperitoneal administration permits a several-fold increase in drug concentration within the abdominal cavity (Dedrick, Myers, Bungay, & DeVita, 1978).

(3) For ovarian cancer, IV chemotherapy is administered in conjunction with intraperitoneal chemotherapy to treat systemic disease (NCCN, 2018f).

(4) The most commonly administered intraperitoneal agents for ovarian cancer are cisplatin and paclitaxel (NCCN, 2018f).

b) Pretreatment assessment in addition to the general assessment prior to chemotherapy

(1) Verify the type of device (implanted intraperitoneal port vs. external intraperitoneal catheter) and location in intraperitoneal space by reviewing operative notes or imaging.

(2) Assess for signs and symptoms of access device complications (Rogers, 2017).

(a) Exit site infection: Fever, chills, drainage, erythema, tenderness at site

(b) For tunneled catheters, tunnel infection: inflammation appearing along the tunnel line

(c) Leakage, bleeding, drainage at exit site

(d) Presence or absence of ascites. If patient has ascites, discuss with prescriber if ascites should be drained prior to chemotherapy in order to promote comfort and tolerance (Rogers, 2017).

(3) Baseline respiratory status: Note any shortness of breath.

(4) Signs and symptoms of peritonitis: Fever, chills, abdominal pain

(5) Abdominal pain, cramping, diarrhea

(6) Peripheral neuropathy from previous doses of platinum or taxane chemotherapy. Report any peripheral neuropathy. Intraperitoneal chemotherapy may be held for worsening peripheral neuropathy.

(7) Renal function: Check serum creatinine and creatinine clearance prior to cisplatin.

c) System safeguards to prevent errors and manage emergencies

(1) Clearly label lines as *intraperitoneal* and *intravenous* to prevent accidental administration of medications via the wrong route (ISMP, 2013a).

(2) When administering medications and fluids, trace all catheters and lines from the access site into the patient's body (ISMP, 2013a).

(3) Route IV tubing and intraperitoneal tubing to different sides of the bed or chair.

(4) Infuse intraperitoneal fluids through tubing without injection ports (Rogers, 2017).

(5) Intraperitoneal administration of paclitaxel and cisplatin has potential to cause hypersensitivity reactions, including anaphylaxis. Ensure that emergency medications are available (NCCN, 2018f).

d) Dosing: Intraperitoneal dosing is based on the disease, regimen, patient-specific factors, and presence of toxicities. Care must be taken to verify dosing of intraperitoneal and IV chemotherapy when administered in the same regimen.

e) Verification: Immediately prior to administration, verify that the agent to be administered is intraperitoneal and that the tubing and line it is connected to is the intraperitoneal access device.

f) Administration

(1) Ask the patient to void prior to starting the procedure and report difficulty with voiding or a lack of urine output.

(2) Obtain intravascular access for administration of IV fluids (e.g., prior to administration of intraperitoneal cisplatin).

(3) Access the patient's intraperitoneal port.

(a) Apply topical anesthetic, if requested.

(b) Use strict sterile technique and maximum barrier precautions when accessing an intraperitoneal port (Rogers, 2017).

(c) Instruct the patient to lie flat for port access, if possible.

(d) Use a noncoring needle. If the location of the port is the lower ribs, where there may be more subcutaneous tissue, a longer needle may be needed. Patient anatomy will often dictate provider placement.

(e) A blood return should not occur if aspiration is attempted, as the tip of the catheter is in the peritoneal space. If the patient has ascites, peritoneal fluid may be withdrawn (often straw colored, sometimes blood tinged). Often, intraperitoneal ports will not yield a specimen (Rogers, 2017).

(f) Flush with 10–20 ml normal saline (Rogers, 2017). Assess for signs and symptoms of infiltration, including pain, burning, and leaking of fluid.

(g) Apply a sterile, transparent dressing.

(4) Place the patient in a semi-Fowler position. A flat position during infusion may increase pressure on the diaphragm, causing respiratory compromise and gastrointestinal upset.

(5) Administer IV premedications and IV hydration as ordered.

(6) No definitive recommendations can be made regarding the warming of intraperitoneal fluid prior to administration (Rogers, 2017). Patients may tolerate room-temperature fluids better than cold ones.

(7) Wear two pair of gloves and a gown that have been tested for use with HDs. Wear a mask with face protection if splashing is possible (Polovich & Olsen, 2018; see Chapter 12).

(8) Chemotherapy is often mixed in one liter of fluid and followed by an additional liter of normal saline. If the patient experiences discomfort and fullness, the second liter of intraperitoneal fluid (normal saline) is often discontinued (Anastasia, 2012).

(9) Infuse intraperitoneal fluids by gravity using a CSTD as rapidly as the patient will tolerate (Anastasia, 2012; Polovich & Olsen, 2018; Potter & Held-Warmkessel, 2008).

(a) The fluid should flow freely and is often infused over 60–180 minutes. If the infusion will not run within this time period, notify the prescriber, as the catheter may be malpositioned, have a fibrin sheath, or the tip may be located in a pocket formed from bowel adhesions located in the intraperitoneal cavity (Anastasia, 2012; Potter & Held-Warmkessel, 2008; Rogers, 2017).

(b) Infusion of intraperitoneal chemotherapy by an infusion pump can cause needle dislodgment and infiltration (Potter & Held-Warmkessel, 2008).

(c) Slow the intraperitoneal infusion for complaints of discomfort, dyspnea, or leaking around the intraperitoneal device site (Anastasia, 2012; Potter & Held-Warmkessel, 2008; Rogers, 2017).

(10) After the infusion is complete, instruct the patient to turn from side to side every 15–30 minutes for 1–2 hours to facilitate drug distribution (Anastasia, 2012; Potter & Held-Warmkessel, 2008).

(11) Disconnect the tubing. Flush with a minimum of 20 ml normal saline and discontinue the port needle. No definitive recommendations can be made regarding the use of heparin (Rogers, 2017).

(12) The infused fluid is not drained and will absorb over several days to a week (Potter & Held-Warmkessel, 2008).

(13) Assess for the following throughout the intraperitoneal infusion and after completion (Anastasia, 2012; Potter & Held-Warmkessel, 2008; Rogers, 2017):

(a) Signs and symptoms of a hypersensitivity reaction

(b) Signs and symptoms of fluid overload

(c) Dyspnea

(d) Abdominal pain or discomfort

(e) Failure of the intraperitoneal fluids to infuse freely by gravity (Anastasia, 2012; Rogers, 2017)

i. Line placement and patency may need to be confirmed by a dye study with fluoroscopy.

ii. Alteplase for catheter clearance has been used to clear fibrin.

(f) Leaking around the port needle site or external catheter exit site (Anastasia, 2012; Rogers, 2017)

i. Verify needle placement.

ii. Excessive pressure from ascites can cause leaking around the catheter or needle.

(g) In the event of extravasation (evidenced by abdominal pain and delayed erythema, often as the result of port malfunction or port flipping) or intraperitoneal port malfunction, discontinue intraperitoneal therapy and notify authorized prescriber immediately.

(h) For patients on cisplatin, monitor magnesium levels, and replace as ordered.

(i) For patients with significant nausea or vomiting who are unable to self-hydrate, consider scheduling return visits for IV hydration.

g) Other considerations: Heated intraperitoneal chemotherapy (HIPEC)

(1) HIPEC is intraoperative delivery of heated chemotherapy into the intraperitoneal space. It is administered following cytoreductive surgery with the goal of eradicating microscopic disease. Hyperthermia is used to increase uptake of the chemotherapy into the cancer cells (González-Moreno, González-Bayon, & Ortega-Pérez, 2012; Neuwirth, Alexander, & Karakousis, 2016).

(2) HIPEC has been used for a variety of intraperitoneal cancers, including appendiceal cancer, peritoneal mesothelioma, and colon cancer (González-Moreno et al., 2012; Neuwirth et al., 2016).

(3) Agents used during HIPEC include carboplatin, cisplatin, 5-fluorouracil, irinotecan, mitomycin C, and oxaliplatin (González-Moreno et al., 2012; Neuwirth et al., 2016).

(4) The HIPEC procedure is performed after the cytoreductive surgery is completed. The surgeon places intraperitoneal catheters and temperature probes into the intraperitoneal space. The chemotherapy is heated by a perfusion machine and continuously circulates the chemotherapy throughout the intraperitoneal cavity, often for two hours.

(5) All personnel who administer HDs via the intraperitoneal route must wear double gloves and a gown during IV administration of HDs, as well as a mask with face protection if there is a potential for spilling, splashing, or aerosols (Polovich & Olsen, 2018). See Chapter 12.

(6) The patient is often "rocked" back and forth during the procedure. After the completion of the procedure, the chemotherapy is drained, and the catheters removed.

(7) The patient is then transferred to the intensive care unit and usually hospitalized until recovery.

(8) Complications from the procedure include nausea, vomiting, pain, bleeding, ileus, anastomotic leaks, bowel perforations, and infection (Cianos, LaFe-

ver, & Mills, 2013; González-Moreno et al., 2012).

(9) Although nurses do not administer the actual chemotherapy intraoperatively, they play an important role in the prevention and management of complications related to this procedure (Dell, Held-Warmkessel, Jakubek, & O'Mara, 2014).

5. Intrathecal, lumbar puncture

a) Intrathecal chemotherapy is the administration of chemotherapy directly into the intrathecal space by a lumbar puncture. The goal of intrathecal chemotherapy is the prophylaxis or treatment of malignant cells within sites that cannot be reached by systemic chemotherapy because of the blood–brain barrier (NCCN, 2018c).

(1) Indications for prophylactic intrathecal chemotherapy include acute lymphoblastic leukemia (NCCN, 2018a) and Burkitt lymphoma (NCCN, 2018c).

(2) Intrathecal chemotherapy is also used for leptomeningeal metastasis (meningeal carcinomatosis) that can occur from the spread of leukemia, lymphoma, and solid tumors such as breast, lung, and gastrointestinal cancers (NCCN, 2018a, 2018c).

(a) The leptomeninges are two tissue linings, the arachnoid and pia mater, that cover the brain and spinal cord. The layers encase the arachnoid space, which contains the cerebrospinal fluid.

(b) Cancer cells can enter the cerebrospinal fluid by numerous routes, including the blood, the meninges, and extension from spinal metastases.

(3) Few chemotherapy agents can safely be given into the intrathecal space. The most commonly used agents are cytarabine arabinoside and methotrexate (Gabay, Thakkar, Stachnik, Woelich, & Villano, 2012).

b) Pretreatment assessment

(1) Assess the patient's risk for bleeding. An increased risk for bleeding places the patient at risk for an epidural hematoma and possible paralysis from the lumbar puncture (Balaban, Veneziano, Cartabuke, & Tobias, 2016; Nair, 2016).

(a) Review the patient's laboratory values for bleeding risk (platelets, coagulation studies) and follow institutional guidelines.

(b) Review the patient's medication list. Determine if the patient has been on any anticoagulants or NSAIDs.

i. Obtain information regarding the dose, route, and date and time of last administration.

ii. The American Society of Regional Anesthesia and Pain Medicine, the European Society of Regional Anaesthesia and Pain Therapy, the American Academy of Pain Medicine, the International Neuromodulation Society, the North American Neuromodulation Society, and the World Institute of Pain (Narouze et al., 2015) have established guidelines for procedures involving the spine, such as lumbar puncture, for patients on antiplatelet and anticoagulant medications. The guidelines include specific details related to when anticoagulants should be held and restarted in relation to a lumbar puncture.

(2) Review if the patient has any abnormalities of the lumbar vertebrae or would have difficulty maintaining the position required for the procedure.

(3) Clarify with the prescriber whether cerebrospinal fluid specimens should be drawn and sent (e.g., cytology, cell count, glucose, protein, tumor markers).

(4) Conduct a neurologic assessment to establish baseline orientation, level of consciousness, presence or absence of headaches, history of seizures, and numbness, tingling, or pain in lower extremities.

c) System safeguards to prevent errors and manage emergencies: This section applies to both the intrathecal and intraventricular routes.

(1) Work with the interprofessional team to establish policies and procedures related to anticoagulants, coagulation studies, and lumbar puncture.

(2) Work with an interprofessional team to prevent fatal chemotherapy errors related to the inadvertent administration of vinca alkaloids via a route other than IV (Hartkopf Smith, 2009b).
  (a) Since the approval of vincristine in the 1960s, more than 125 deaths have been reported in the United States and abroad from the accidental administration of vinca alkaloids into the intrathecal space (NCCN, n.d.).
  (b) Many patients receive IV vincristine as part of their chemotherapy regimen, which also includes chemotherapy given into the intrathecal or intraventricular space. In most reports of accidental intrathecal administration, the syringe of vincristine was accidentally administered into the cerebrospinal fluid, instead of the intended medication.
  (c) Administration of vinca alkaloids, such as vincristine, given via this route can cause severe neurologic toxicity, including coma and death (Reddy, Brown, & Nanda, 2011).
  (d) More than 27 years ago, the United States Pharmacopeial Convention developed requirements for manufacturers and pharmacies to label doses of vincristine with warnings. However, instances of accidental injection of vincristine continued to occur.
  (e) Strategies to prevent errors (NCCN, n.d.)
    i. Vincristine and other vinca alkaloids must only be given intravenously in a minibag (e.g., IVPB).
    ii. Never dispense vinca alkaloids to an area where intrathecal or intraventricular medications are administered.
    iii. Never give vinca alkaloids in the same treatment room as intrathecal or intraventricular medications.
    iv. Healthcare providers who prescribe, prepare, and administer intrathecal or intraventricular chemotherapy must receive specialized educational programs that include safe handling of HDs.
    v. Institutions should establish a list of drugs that can be given intrathecally or intraventricularly.
    vi. Orders for intrathecal chemotherapy should be separate from IV chemotherapy orders.
    vii. Order and deliver intrathecal or intraventricular chemotherapy as close as possible to the time of administration.
    viii. Package and transport intrathecal and intraventricular chemotherapy separately from IV and other drugs.
    ix. Intrathecal and intraventricular chemotherapy should not be stored in patient care areas.
    x. Time-out procedures should be conducted immediately preceding intrathecal and intraventricular chemotherapy administration.

d) Dosing: Depending on the regimen, the agent may be administered once, twice, or three times a week. The duration and frequency of treatment are often dependent on whether the goal is prophylaxis or treatment.

e) Verification
  (1) Verify that the patient's coagulation studies meet institutional parameters for a lumbar puncture.
  (2) Verify that the patient is not receiving anticoagulants or that they have been stopped for the necessary amount of time before the lumbar puncture, per institutional standards.
  (3) Immediately preceding the procedure
    (a) Perform a time-out procedure.
    (b) Verify with the practitioner performing the procedure (e.g., oncologist, radiologist, advanced practice provider) the following information:
      i. The medication to be administered is safe to administer by the intrathecal route.
      ii. The medication is not a vinca alkaloid or bortezomib.

iii. The medication is mixed with preservative-free normal saline or Elliotts B® solution.

f) Administration

(1) Intrathecal chemotherapy via a lumbar puncture may be administered at the bedside, in the ambulatory care center, or in interventional radiology or fluoroscopy depending on the health-care setting.

(2) It may be administered by an oncology physician, a radiologist, an advanced practice provider, or a physician assistant.

(3) Refer to state and institutional policies regarding the role of advanced practice nurses in administering intrathecal chemotherapy by a lumbar puncture.

(4) All personnel who administer HDs via a lumbar puncture must wear two pair of gloves (outer gloves are sterile) and a gown that have been tested for use with HDs. Wear a mask with face protection (see Chapter 12). A plastic-backed absorbent pad should be placed under the site where the needle enters the spine and the syringe connection (Polovich & Olsen, 2018).

(5) Use strict sterile technique and sterile barrier precautions (e.g., mask, sterile field, sterile gloves).

(a) The use of a mask decreases the transfer of *Streptococcus salivarius*, bacteria that can cause meningitis, to the treatment field (Shewmaker et al., 2010).

(b) Cleanse the skin prior to needle puncture with an antiseptic (Aiello-Laws & Rutledge, 2008; Elledge, 2017). The use of chlorhexidine gluconate is controversial. Current package labeling states it is contraindicated because of the risk of meningitis (Sviggum et al., 2012). If chlorhexidine is used as a disinfectant for intrathecal chemotherapy administration, it must dry completely prior to needle puncture. Proponents of its use state it has a more rapid onset of action, extended duration of effect, rare drug resistance, and little evidence to support its role in the development of meningitis (Sviggum et al., 2012).

(c) If the syringe containing the medication is not sterile, once a person touches it, that hand is not sterile (Aiello-Laws & Rutledge, 2008; Elledge, 2017). If the syringe containing the medication is sterile, the label on the medication must also be sterile (Aiello-Laws & Rutledge, 2008). For nonsterile syringes, the provider should access the cerebrospinal fluid with sterile gloves and then administer intrathecal medication without touching the sterile access site (Polovich & Olsen, 2018).

(6) The needle and infusion syringe and tubing should be discarded in an appropriate hazardous waste container (Polovich & Olsen, 2018).

g) Other considerations: Post–dural puncture headache is a common complication of lumbar punctures. A systematic review assessed the efficacy of prolonged bedrest versus immediate ambulation and found a lack of evidence to support routine bedrest after dural puncture. The role of fluid supplementation after dural puncture requires further study (Arevalo-Rodriguez, Ciapponi, Roqué i Figuls, Muñoz, & Bonfill Cosp, 2016).

6. Intraventricular (e.g., Ommaya reservoir)

a) Intraventricular chemotherapy is the administration of chemotherapy into the lateral ventricle of the brain—a network of communicating cavities filled with cerebrospinal fluid. Intraventricular administration is an alternative to administering intrathecal chemotherapy by lumbar puncture.

(1) Administration of vinca alkaloids, such as vincristine, given via this route can cause severe neurologic toxicity, including coma and death (Reddy et al., 2011).

(2) Ventricular reservoirs (Ommaya reservoirs) consist of a silicone dome and a catheter. A neurosurgeon surgically places the dome under the scalp (subcutaneous), and the catheter is threaded into the lateral ventricle of the brain (Volkov, Filis, & Vrionis, 2017).

(a) The reservoir volume of the dome ranges from 1.5–2.5 ml (Elledge, 2017). The catheter length varies, as it is trimmed to fit within the frontal horn of the lateral ventricle of the brain (Elledge, 2017).

(*b*) Ventricular reservoirs can be used for the administration of medications, including chemotherapy, and for sampling of cerebrospinal fluid.

(*c*) Ventricular reservoirs with an attached shunt with on-off flushing reservoirs: Some ventricular reservoirs have an attached shunt with an on-off flushing reservoir. Finger pressure on a specific component of the device can open and close the shunting system, thus controlling the flow of cerebrospinal fluid (Palejwala et al., 2014; Volkov et al., 2017). These types of reservoirs are used to drain cerebrospinal fluid, usually into the peritoneal space. When chemotherapy is administered, the shunting system is closed. After a set time (e.g., four hours), the shunt is reopened (Volkov et al., 2017).

b) Pretreatment assessment/actions

(1) Prior to accessing and using a ventricular reservoir, verify it is within the scope of practice by the state board of nursing and institutional policy.

(2) Prior to using a new ventricular reservoir

(*a*) Confirm that postoperative imaging was completed to confirm reservoir placement, flow patency, and cerebrospinal fluid flow (Elledge, 2017).

(*b*) Flow studies identify areas of obstruction that could prevent chemotherapy from being distributed equally, with resultant increased toxicity and decreased efficacy.

(*c*) Discuss with the provider when the ventricular access can be used. Practices vary from the day of placement to multiple days after placement (Elledge, 2017).

(*d*) Verify the type of ventricular access. Administration and management of patients with ventricular reservoirs with an attached shunt with on-off flushing reservoirs are not addressed in these recommendations.

(3) Assess vital signs.

(4) Assess neurologic history and status to serve as a baseline, including but not limited to orientation, level of consciousness, headaches, and seizures.

(5) Assess for signs of infection over the ventricular reservoir.

(6) Clip—not shave—the hair over the ventricular reservoir.

(7) Clarify with the prescriber whether specimens should be drawn and sent (e.g., cytology, cell count, glucose, protein, tumor markers).

c) System safeguards to prevent errors and manage emergencies: Follow system safeguards listed for the intrathecal route.

d) Dosing: Depending on the regimen, the agent may be administered once, twice, or three times a week (NCCN, 2018a, 2018c). The duration of treatment is dependent on whether the goal is prophylaxis or treatment.

e) Verification immediately preceding the procedure

(1) Perform a time-out procedure.

(2) Verify with another chemotherapy-qualified nurse, pharmacist, or physician the following information:

(*a*) The medication to be administered is safe to administer by the intraventricular route.

(*b*) The medication is not a vinca alkaloid or bortezomib.

(*c*) The medication is mixed with preservative-free normal saline or Elliotts B solution.

f) Administration

(1) No consistent recommendations can be made regarding the patient's position during the procedure. Aiello-Laws and Rutledge (2008) recommended a supine position. Place a plastic-backed absorbent pad under the site where the needle enters the reservoir if feasible.

(2) All personnel who administer HDs via this route must wear two pair of gloves and a gown that have been tested for use with HDs. Wear a mask with face protection (Polovich & Olsen, 2018; see Chapter 12).

(3) Use strict sterile technique and sterile barrier precautions (e.g., mask, sterile field, sterile gloves).

(*a*) The use of a mask decreases the transfer of *Streptococcus salivarius*, bacteria that can cause meningitis, to the treatment field (Shewmaker et al., 2010).

(b) If the syringe containing the medication is not sterile, once a person touches it, that hand is not sterile (Aiello-Laws & Rutledge, 2007; Elledge, 2017). If the syringe containing the medication is sterile, the label on the medication must also be sterile (Aiello-Laws & Rutledge, 2008). For nonsterile syringes, the provider should access the cerebrospinal fluid with sterile gloves and then administer intrathecal medication without touching the sterile access site (Polovich & Olsen, 2018).

(4) Cleanse the reservoir with an antiseptic (Aiello-Laws & Rutledge, 2008; Elledge, 2017). The use of chlorhexidine gluconate is controversial. Current package labeling states it is contraindicated because of the risk of meningitis (Sviggum et al., 2012). If chlorhexidine is used as a disinfectant for intraventricular chemotherapy administration, it must dry completely prior to accessing reservoir. Proponents of its use state it is has a more rapid onset of action, extended duration of effect, rare drug resistance, and little evidence to support its role in the development of meningitis (Sviggum et al., 2012).

(5) Use a 25-gauge or smaller butterfly (Aiello-Laws & Rutledge, 2008; Elledge, 2017) attached to an empty syringe (equal to the volume of the chemotherapy syringe). Some practices recommend the use of a stopcock. Never use a vacutainer (Aiello-Laws & Rutledge, 2008).

(6) Palpate the reservoir. Pump the reservoir three to four times to fill the reservoir with cerebrospinal fluid.

(7) Insert the butterfly at a 45°–90° angle into the ventricular reservoir. Once it is inside the dome of the reservoir, decreased resistance should be felt.

(8) Aspirate. If blood is present, stop and withdraw needle. If blood is not present, slowly withdraw cerebrospinal fluid equal to the volume of chemotherapy to be administered (Aiello-Laws & Rutledge, 2008; Elledge, 2017).

(9) Examine the cerebrospinal fluid. If it is cloudy or bloody, do not proceed. Discontinue the procedure and notify the healthcare provider. Anticipate orders to send a specimen for tests.

(10) If the cerebrospinal fluid is clear, slowly administer the chemotherapy.

(11) Flush with reserved cerebrospinal fluid or preservative-free normal saline (Aiello-Laws & Rutledge, 2008; Elledge, 2017).

(12) Remove the needle.

(13) Apply pressure with a sterile gauze.

(14) Pump the reservoir three to five times. This distributes the medication into the cerebrospinal fluid.

(15) Apply a sterile dressing.

(16) Postprocedure care

(a) No consistent recommendations can be made regarding the patient's position following the procedure.

(b) Take vital signs.

(c) Assess for complications, including headache, nausea, vomiting, seizures, and change in neurologic status.

g) Other considerations: Patient education

(1) Instruct the patient to notify the healthcare provider if headache, nausea, vomiting, neck stiffness, or other neurologic symptoms develop.

(2) Instruct the patient to avoid trauma to the ventricular reservoir site.

7. Intravesical (bladder)

a) Intravesical chemotherapy is the regional administration of chemotherapy directly into the bladder. The medication is administered through a catheter and can be done intraoperatively, immediately postoperatively, and weekly in the outpatient area.

(1) Indications include superficial, non–muscle-invasive bladder cancer (NCCN, 2018d).

(2) Commonly used agents include bacillus Calmette-Guérin (BCG), epirubicin, mitomycin C, and valrubicin (NCCN, 2018d).

b) Pretreatment assessment

(1) Vital signs

(2) Urinalysis prior to each treatment, assessing for urinary tract infection (American Urological Association & Society of Urologic Nurses and Associates, 2015)

(a) If bacteriuria is present on high-power field or greater than five white blood cells are present on high-power field and/or gross

hematuria is noted and the patient is symptomatic, hold treatment.
  - *(b)* Notify the prescriber.
  - *(c)* Send urine for culture, as ordered.
  - *(d)* Discuss findings with the prescribing clinician. Microscopic hematuria only or isolated white blood cells in an otherwise asymptomatic patient should not preclude treatment.
- (3) Gross hematuria
- (4) History of difficult or painful catheterization
- (5) Signs and symptoms of urinary frequency, inability to hold urine
- (6) For BCG: BCG is a live, attenuated form of tuberculosis. Assess for the following contraindications to treatment (American Urological Association & Society of Urologic Nurses and Associates, 2015):
  - *(a)* Within 14 days following bladder or prostatic surgery, including biopsy
  - *(b)* Within 14 days following traumatic catheterization
  - *(c)* Traumatic catheterization or gross hematuria day of treatment
  - *(d)* Active tuberculosis
  - *(e)* Immunosuppressed patients with congenital or acquired immune deficiency, whether due to concurrent disease (e.g., AIDS, leukemia, lymphoma), cancer therapy (e.g., cytotoxic drugs, radiation), or immunosuppressive therapy (e.g., corticosteroids)
  - *(f)* Symptomatic urinary tract infection
  - *(g)* Fever

c) System safeguards to prevent errors and manage emergencies: See Chapter 12 for safe handling precautions with HDs.

d) Dosing: The dosing, duration, and frequency are dependent on individual patient factors and the regimens prescribed.

e) Verification: See section D.

f) Administration (American Urological Association & Society of Urologic Nurses and Associates, 2015; Washburn, 2007)
- (1) For postoperative patients, obtain an order to discontinue any continuous bladder irrigations for a minimum of one hour before treatment.
- (2) All personnel who administer HDs via the bladder must wear two pair of gloves and a gown that have been tested for use with HDs. Wear a face shield and mask (Polovich & Olsen, 2018; see Chapter 12).
- (3) Place the patient in a supine position and place a plastic-backed pad under the patient's hips.
- (4) If the patient has had difficult or painful catheterizations in the past, apply a topical anesthetic as ordered.
- (5) Using sterile technique, place a urethral catheter and drain urine.
- (6) Place a catheter plug at the end of the catheter until ready to administer the chemotherapy or immunotherapy.
- (7) Syringes or bags of medication should have an attached CSTD for administration and disposal of body fluids. Some manufacturers of CSTDs also make adapters for catheters. The adapters consist of a cap, tubing, and slip connection that fits into the urethral catheter. The CSTD at the end of the syringe or tubing can be attached to the cap on the adapter (Polovich & Olsen, 2018).
- (8) Inject or infuse the chemotherapy or immunotherapy at the prescribed rate. Slow the injection or infusion if the patient reports discomfort or bladder spasms.
- (9) If the patient is able to retain the medication for two hours, remove the catheter. If not, leave the catheter in place and plug the end.
- (10) Instruct the patient to hold the medication and to not void for two hours (American Urological Association & Society of Urologic Nurses and Associates, 2015; Washburn, 2007).
- (11) Instruct the patient to rotate every 15–30 minutes from side to back to other side. This distributes the medication throughout the bladder (American Urological Association & Society of Urologic Nurses and Associates, 2015; Washburn, 2007).
- (12) After two hours, the patient may void. Instruct male patients to sit while voiding, rather than standing, for six hours following the administration of the agent to prevent splashing of the medication (American Urological Association & Society of Urologic Nurses and Associates, 2015; Washburn, 2007).

(13) Assess for pain, burning, spasms, and difficulty in retaining the urine for two hours. A rare side effect is extravasation during the administration of a vesicant agent, which can result in severe pelvic pain (Nieuwenhuijzen, Bex, & Horenblas, 2003).

(14) If a catheter and drainage bag are in place, contain the entire intact urinary drainage system in a sealable bag, and discard it in the designated HD waste container (Polovich & Olsen, 2018).

g) Other considerations: Patient education (American Urological Association & Society of Urologic Nurses and Associates, 2015; Washburn, 2007)

(1) Restrict intake of fluid, caffeine, and diuretics beginning four hours before the procedure.

(2) Following the procedure

(a) Sit when voiding for six hours following the procedure to prevent splashing.

(b) Increase fluid to dilute the urine.

(c) Wash any splashing on skin with soap and water.

(d) Wear a condom during intercourse until therapy is completed.

(e) For BCG, place two cups of bleach in the toilet after each void for six hours following the procedure. Let bleach sit in the toilet for 15 minutes. Cover the toilet, and flush twice.

(f) Common side effects include low-grade fever, urinary frequency and urgency, burning with urination, and fatigue.

(g) Remove clothes if contaminated with urine, and wash separately.

8. Intra-arterial

a) Intra-arterial chemotherapy delivers high concentrations of medication directly to the tumor with decreased systemic exposure (Royal, 2013). For all methods of delivery, the intra-arterial catheter is threaded directly into the artery that feeds the tumor.

(1) Indications for intra-arterial chemotherapy are varied; it has been used for cancers of the brain (carotid arterial chemotherapy), liver (intra-arterial ports, programmable intra-arterial pumps, and transarterial hepatic chemoembolization), and limbs, such as with sarcomas (Abdalla et al., 2013; Arai et al., 2015; Deschamps et al., 2010; Guillaume et al., 2010; Liu, Cui, Guo, Li, & Zeng, 2014; Matthews, Snell, & Coats, 2006).

(2) Agents administered intra-arterially are dependent on the indication but can include cisplatin, 5-fluorouracil, floxuridine, irinotecan, and mitomycin C (Abdalla et al., 2013; Arai et al., 2015; Deschamps et al., 2010; Guillaume et al., 2010; Liu et al., 2014).

(3) Intra-arterial chemotherapy can be delivered by temporary percutaneous catheters, intra-arterial ports, programmable intra-arterial pumps, or, in surgery or interventional radiology, transarterial hepatic chemoembolization.

b) Pretreatment assessment/actions

(1) Prior to the placement of any type of arterial catheter, an angiogram or similar dye study is done to confirm location and arterial blood flow and to assess for complications.

(2) When temporary percutaneous catheters are used, assess peripheral circulation of the affected extremity to serve as a baseline (e.g., color, pulse, temperature).

(3) Review any laboratory values as indicated for the procedure, such as complete blood count and differential, coagulation studies, hepatic function tests, and renal function tests.

c) System safeguards to prevent errors and manage emergencies

(1) Clearly label external lines as *intra-arterial* and *intravenous* to prevent accidental administration of medications via the wrong route (ISMP, 2013a).

(2) When administering medications and fluids, trace all catheters and lines from the access site into the patient's body (ISMP, 2013a).

(3) Route intra-arterial tubing and IV tubing to different sides of the bed or chair.

(4) Infuse any intra-arterial fluids through tubing without injection ports (Hartkopf Smith, 2017).

(5) Immediately prior to administration, reclarify if the medication is ordered to be given intravenously or intra-arterially.

(6) Use Luer-lock connections on tubing, and tape all connections securely (Hartkopf Smith, 2017).

(7) For temporary percutaneous catheters, immobilize the extremity as indicated to prevent accidental catheter dislodgment (Hartkopf Smith, 2017).

d) Dosing: The dosing, duration, and frequency are dependent on individual patient factors and the regimens prescribed.

e) Verification: Verify the location of the catheter tip by reviewing imaging or operative reports.

f) Administration

(1) All personnel who administer HDs via this route must wear two pair of gloves and a gown that have been tested for use with HDs. Wear a mask with face protection (Polovich & Olsen, 2018; see Chapter 12).

(2) Temporary percutaneous catheters

(a) Temporary percutaneous catheters have been used for regional limb perfusions, carotid artery infusions, and hepatic artery infusions (Hartkopf Smith, 2017).

(b) They are often placed in radiology. The catheter may remain in place for minutes, hours, or several days.

(c) The most common insertion sites are the brachial and femoral arteries (Abdalla et al., 2013; Basile, Carrafiello, Ierardi, Tsetis, & Brountzos, 2012).

(d) Depending on the location and duration of infusion, the patient may have activity restrictions and limb immobilization.

(e) Place all infusions on a pump.

(f) Assess vital signs, circulation, and for hematoma during the infusion and for at least two hours after the catheter is discontinued.

(3) Intra-arterial ports: Intra-arterial ports have been used for hepatic arterial infusions, most often connected to an ambulatory infusion pump (Deschamps et al., 2010).

(a) The portal body is placed subcutaneously, and the port catheter is threaded into the designated artery.

(b) Ambulatory infusion pumps have been used for the delivery of medication.

(c) Currently, no ports manufactured in the United States are specifically designed for intra-arterial administration of chemotherapy.

(4) Programmable, implanted intra-arterial pumps: Hepatic artery infusion pumps are used to administer chemotherapy for colon cancer that has metastasized to the liver (Parks & Routt, 2015).

(a) The chemotherapy commonly infused through an intra-arterial pump is 5-fluorodeoxyuridine.

(b) At the time of this publication, an implanted pump is approved for this indication—the Codman® 3000 implantable constant-flow infusion pump (Codman & Shurtleff, Inc., 2003). The pump is connected to an arterial catheter threaded into the hepatic artery.

i. Always verify the type and model of pump before administering chemotherapy.

ii. For the Codman 3000 pump

- The pump is inserted in surgery or interventional radiology. It is placed in a subcutaneous pocket, and the catheter is threaded into the hepatic artery.
- The pump rate is constant and cannot be programmed. To change the dose of medication, the concentration is changed.
- Always verify the rate of administration by reviewing the product information. The rate varies with the pump model and individual patient characteristics.
- Always verify the reservoir volume before administering medication. The volume varies with the model.
- Both boluses and continuous infusions can be used. A different needle is used for each.
- Pumps generally must be refilled every two weeks. A common schedule is two weeks of chemotherapy then two weeks of heparinized saline.

- A special, straight non-coring needle is used to access the septum in the pump. Refer to specific pump instructions for more information on the procedure.

9. Intrapleural route
   a) Treatment for patients with malignant pleural tumors (e.g., pleural mesothelioma) and other malignant effusions resulting from a variety of cancer types (e.g., lung, breast, pancreatic) includes chemotherapy, thoracentesis, pleurodesis with a sclerosing agent, insertion of an indwelling pleural drainage catheter, surgical procedures, and radiation (Feller-Kopman et al., 2018). Multiple agents, including chemotherapy and antibiotics, have been used as sclerosing agents in patients with a malignant pleural effusion; however, medical-grade talc is considered the safest and most effective agent (Clive, Jones, Bhatnagar, Preston, & Maskell, 2016). For patients in whom chemical pleurodesis has failed or those with a nonexpandable lung, an indwelling pleural catheter is recommended (Feller-Kopman et al., 2018).
      (1) Ability to instill agent directly into the pleural area where primary or metastatic tumor resides
      (2) Palliation of symptoms (e.g., dyspnea on exertion) for patients with malignant pleural effusions
   b) Pretreatment assessment in addition to the general assessment prior to chemotherapy
      (1) Requires insertion of a thoracotomy tube
      (2) The effusion fluid is completely drained from the pleural cavity before instillation of the agent, and daily drainage is less than 150 ml (Cope, 2018).
   c) System safeguards to prevent errors and manage emergencies: Intrapleural chemotherapy administration must be performed by an authorized prescriber.
   d) Dosing: The sclerosing agent is dissolved in 100–150 ml of normal saline.
   e) Verification: See section D.
   f) Administration
      (1) Use personal protective equipment if agent being instilled is hazardous.
      (2) Maintain aseptic technique.
      (3) Allow the agent to remain for the prescribed dwell time if applicable. If fluid is drained and the agent was hazardous, handle fluid using appropriate personal protective equipment and waste disposal (Polovich & Olsen, 2018).
      (4) Observe for signs and symptoms of respiratory distress, pneumothorax, infection, and pain.

References

Abdalla, E.K., Bauer, T.W., Chun, Y.S., D'Angelica, M., Kooby, D.A., & Jarnagin, W.R. (2013). Locoregional surgical and interventional therapies for advanced colorectal liver metastases: Expert consensus statements. *HPB, 15,* 119–130. https://doi.org/10.1111/j.1477-2574.2012.00597.x

Agency for Healthcare Research and Quality. (2015, February). Use the teach-back method: Tool #5. Retrieved from https://www.ahrq.gov/professionals/quality-patient-safety/quality-resources/tools/literacy-toolkit/healthlittoolkit2-tool5.html

Agency for Healthcare Research and Quality. (2018). Engaging patients and families in their health care. Retrieved from https://www.ahrq.gov/professionals/quality-patient-safety/patient-family-engagement/index.html

Aiello-Laws, L., & Rutledge, D.N. (2008). Management of adult patients receiving intraventricular chemotherapy for the treatment of leptomeningeal metastasis. *Clinical Journal of Oncology Nursing, 12,* 429–435. https://doi.org/10.1188/08.CJON.429-435

American Cancer Society. (2018). *Cancer facts and figures 2018.* Atlanta, GA: Author.

American Urological Association & Society of Urologic Nurses and Associates. (2015). *Intravesical administration of therapeutic medication* [Policy statement]. Retrieved from http://www.auanet.org/guidelines/intravesical-administration-of-therapeutic-medication

Anand, A.S., & Nikhil, S. (2015). Incidence and spectrum of electrolyte disturbances in cisplatin based chemotherapy. *International Journal of Research in Medical Sciences, 3,* 3824–3829. https://doi.org/10.18203/2320-6012.ijrms20151450

Anastasia, P. (2012). Intraperitoneal chemotherapy for ovarian cancer. *Oncology Nursing Forum, 39,* 346–349. https://doi.org/10.1188/12.ONF.346-349

Andrews, A. (2017). Project aims to prevent future infusion-related reactions. *Oncology Nurse-APN/PA, 10*(2). Retrieved from http://www.theoncologynurse.com/top-issues/2017-issues/may-2017-vol-10-no-2/17111-project-aims-to-prevent-future-infusion-related-reactions

Anglada-Martínez, H., Riu-Viladoms, G., do Pazo-Oubiña, F., Molas-Ferrer, G., Mangues-Bafalluy, I., Codina-Jané, C., & Creus-Baró, N. (2014). Dosing of chemotherapy in obese and cachectic patients: Results of a national survey. *International Journal of Clinical Pharmacy, 36,* 589–595. https://doi.org/10.1007/s11096-014-9942-9

Arai, Y., Aoyama, T., Inaba, Y., Okabe, H., Ihaya, T., Kichikawa, K., … Saji, S. (2015). Phase II study on hepatic arterial infusion chemotherapy using percutaneous catheter placement techniques for liver metastases from colorectal cancer (JFMC28 study). *Asia-Pacific Journal of Clinical Oncology, 11,* 41–48. https://doi.org/10.1111/ajco.12324

Arevalo-Rodriguez, I., Ciapponi, A., Roqué i Figuls, M., Muñoz, L., & Bonfill Cosp, X. (2016). Posture and fluids for preventing post-dural puncture headache. *Cochrane Database of Systematic Reviews, 2016*(3). https://doi.org/10.1002/14651858.CD009199.pub3

Balaban, O., Veneziano, G., Cartabuke, R.S., & Tobias, J.D. (2016). Central nervous system hemorrhage following lumbar puncture for intrathecal chemotherapy in a pediatric oncology patient. *Journal of Medical Cases, 7,* 461–466. https://doi.org/10.14740/jmc2656w

Balducci, L., Goetz-Parten, D., & Steinman, M.A. (2013). Polypharmacy and the management of the older cancer patient. *Annals of Oncology, 24*(Suppl. 7), vii36–vii40. https://doi.org/10.1093/annonc/mdt266

Basile, A., Carrafiello, G., Ierardi, A.M., Tsetis, D., & Brountzos, E. (2012). Quality-improvement guidelines for hepatic transarterial chemoembolization. *Cardiovascular and Interventional Radiology, 35,* 765–774. https://doi.org/10.1007/s00270-012-0423-z

Bellomo, C. (2016). Oral chemotherapy: Patient education and nursing intervention. *Journal of Oncology Navigation and Survivorship, 7.* Retrieved from http://www.jons-online.com/issue-archive/2016-issue/july-2016-vol-7-no-6/oral-chemotherapy-patient-education-and-nursing-intervention

Bonkowski, J., Carnes, C., Melucci, J., Mirtallo, J., Prier, B., Reichert, E., … Weber, R. (2013). Effect of barcode-assisted medication administration on emergency department medication errors. *Academic Emergency Medicine, 20,* 801–806. https://doi.org/10.1111/acem.12189

Booth, J.A., Booth, C., & Crawford, S.M. (2011). Inappropriate continuation of medication when patients are admitted acutely: The example of capecitabine [Letter to the editor]. *Clinical Medicine, 11,* 511. https://doi.org/10.7861/clinmedicine.11-5-511

Burhenn, P.S., & Smuddle, J. (2015). Using tools and technology to promote education and adherence to oral agents for cancer. *Clinical Journal of Oncology Nursing, 19*(Suppl. 3), 53–59. https://doi.org/10.1188/15.S1.CJON.53-59

Burris, H.A., III, & Hurtig, J. (2010). Radiation recall with anticancer agents. *Oncologist, 15,* 1227–1237. https://doi.org/10.1634/theoncologist.2009-0090

Calvert, A.H., Newell, D.R., Gumbrell, L.A., O'Reilly, S., Burnell, M., Boxall, F.E., … Wiltshaw, E. (1989). Carboplatin dosage: Prospective evaluation of a simple formula based on renal function. *Journal of Clinical Oncology, 7,* 1748–1756.

Camp-Sorrell, D., & Matey, L. (Eds.). (2017). *Access device standards of practice for oncology nursing.* Pittsburgh, PA: Oncology Nursing Society.

Centers for Disease Control and Prevention. (2018). Vaccine recommendations and guidelines of the ACIP. Altered immunocompetence. Retrieved from https://www.cdc.gov/vaccines/hcp/acip-recs/general-recs/immunocompetence.html

Chan, A., Low, X.H., & Yap, K.Y.-L. (2012). Assessment of the relationship between adherence with antiemetic drug therapy and control of nausea and vomiting in breast cancer patients receiving anthracycline-based chemotherapy. *Journal of Managed Care and Specialty Pharmacy, 18,* 385–394. https://doi.org/10.18553/jmcp.2012.18.5.385

Chow, R., Chiu, N., Bruera, E., Krishnan, M., Chiu, L., Lam, H., … Chow, E. (2016). Inter-rater reliability in performance status assessment among health care professionals: A systematic review. *Annals of Palliative Medicine, 5,* 83–92. https://doi.org/10.21037/apm.2016.03.02

Cianos, R., LaFever, S., & Mills, N. (2013). Heated intraperitoneal chemotherapy in appendiceal cancer treatment. *Clinical Journal of Oncology Nursing, 17,* 84–87. https://doi.org/10.1188/13.CJON.84-87

Clive, A.O., Jones, H.E., Bhatnagar, R., Preston, N.J., & Maskell, N. (2016). Interventions for the management of malignant pleural effusions: A network meta-analysis. *Cochrane Database of Systematic Reviews, 2016*(5). https://doi.org/10.1002/14651858.CD010529.pub2

Cockcroft, D.W., & Gault, M.H. (1976). Prediction of creatinine clearance from serum creatinine. *Nephron, 16,* 31–41. https://doi.org/10.1159/000180580

Codman & Shurtleff, Inc. (2003). *Codman® 3000 implantable constant-flow infusion pump.* Retrieved from http://www.codmanpumps.com/PDFs/Chemo03.pdf

Cope, D.G. (2017). Midline catheters. In D. Camp-Sorrell & L. Matey (Eds.), *Access device standards of practice for oncology nursing* (pp. 37–43). Pittsburgh, PA: Oncology Nursing Society.

Cope, D.G. (2018). Malignant effusions. In C.H. Yarbro, D. Wujcik, & B.H. Gobel (Eds.), *Cancer nursing: Principles and practice* (8th ed., pp. 995–1010). Burlington, MA: Jones & Bartlett Learning.

Dedrick, R.L., Myers, C.E., Bungay, P.M., & DeVita, V.T., Jr. (1978). Pharmacokinetic rationale for peritoneal drug administration in the treatment of ovarian cancer. *Cancer Treatment Reports, 62,* 1–11.

Dell, D.D., Held-Warmkessel, J., Jakubek, P., & O'Mara, T. (2014). Care of the open abdomen after cytoreductive surgery and hyperthermic intraperitoneal chemotherapy for peritoneal surface malignancies. *Oncology Nursing Forum, 41,* 438–441. https://doi.org/10.1188/14.ONF.438-441

Demissie, S., Silliman, R.A., & Lash, T.L. (2001). Adjuvant tamoxifen: Predictors of use, side effects, and discontinuation in older women. *Journal of Clinical Oncology, 19,* 322–328. https://doi.org/10.1200/JCO.2001.19.2.322

Deschamps, F., Rao, P., Teriitehau, C., Hakime, A., Malka, D., Boige, V., … De Baere, T. (2010). Percutaneous femoral implantation of an arterial port catheter for intraarterial chemotherapy: Feasibility and predictive factors of long-term functionality. *Journal of Vascular and Interventional Radiology, 21,* 1681–1688. https://doi.org/10.1016/j.jvir.2010.08.003

Du Bois, D., & Du Bois, E.F. (1916). A formula to estimate the approximate surface area if height and weight be known. *Archives of Internal Medicine, 17,* 863–871. https://doi.org/10.1001/archinte.1916.00080130010002

Eli Lilly and Co. (2017). *Alimta® (pemetrexed for injection)* [Package insert]. Indianapolis, IN: Author.

Elledge, C.M. (2017). Intraventricular access devices. In D. Camp-Sorrell & L. Matey (Eds.), *Access device standards of practice for oncology nursing* (pp. 113–117). Pittsburgh, PA: Oncology Nursing Society.

Faisal, W., Tang, H.-M., Tiley, S., & Kukard, C. (2016). Not all body surface area formulas are the same, but does it matter? *Journal of Global Oncology, 2,* 436–437. https://doi.org/10.1200/JGO.2016.005876

Fancher, K.M., Sacco, A.J., Gwin, R.C., Gormley, L.K., & Mitchell, C.B. (2016). Comparison of two different formulas for body surface area in adults at extremes of height and weight. *Journal of Oncology Pharmacy Practice, 22,* 690–695. https://doi.org/10.1177/1078155215599669

Feller-Kopman, D.J., Reddy, C.B., DeCamp, M.M., Diekemper, R.L., Gould, M.K., Henry, T., … Balekian, A.A. (2018). Management of malignant pleural effusions. An official ATS/STS/STR clinical practice guideline. *American Journal of Respiratory and Critical Care Medicine, 198,* 839–849. https://doi.org/10.1164/rccm.201807-1415ST

Ferris, L.W., & Takanishi, D. (2014, September 2). Accreditation Committee clarifications for standards 3.1 patient navigation process and 3.2 psychosocial distress screening. *CoC Source.* Retrieved from https://www.facs.org/publications/newsletters/coc-source/special-source/standard3132

Ferruccio, L.F., Murray, C., Yee, K.W., Incekol, D., Lee, R., Paisley, E., & Ng, P. (2016). Tolerability of Vidaza (azacitidine) subcutaneous administration using a maximum volume of 3 ml per injection. *Journal of Oncology Pharmacy Practice, 22,* 605–610. https://doi.org/10.1177/1078155215598854

Furlanetto, J., Eiermann, W., Marmé, F., Reimer, T., Reinisch, M., Schmatloch, S., … Möbus, V. (2016). Higher rate of severe toxicities in obese patients receiving dose-dense (dd) chemotherapy according to unadjusted body surface area: Results of the prospectively randomized GAIN study. *Annals of Oncology, 27,* 2053–2059. https://doi.org/10.1093/annonc/mdw315

Gabay, M.P., Thakkar, J.P., Stachnik, J.M., Woelich, S.K., & Villano, J.L. (2012). Intra-CSF administration of chemotherapy medications. *Cancer Chemotherapy and Pharmacology, 70,* 1–15. https://doi.org/10.1007/s00280-012-1893-z

Gaguski, M.E., & Karcheski, T. (2011). Dosing done right: A review of common chemotherapy calculations. *Clinical Journal of Oncology Nursing, 15,* 471–473. https://doi.org/10.1188/11.CJON.471-473

Galvão, V.R., Phillips, E., Giavina-Bianchi, P., & Castells, M.C. (2017). Carboplatin-allergic patients undergoing desensitization: Prevalence and impact of BRCA 1/2 mutation. *Journal of Allergy and Clinical Immunology: In Practice, 5,* 816–818. https://doi.org/10.1016/j.jaip.2016.08.012

Genentech, Inc. (2016). *Rituxan® (rituximab)* [Package insert]. South San Francisco, CA: Author.

Genentech, Inc. (2017a). *Herceptin® (trastuzumab)* [Package insert]. South San Francisco, CA: Author.

Genentech, Inc. (2017b). *Rituxan Hycela™ (rituximab and hyaluronidase human)* [Package insert]. South San Francisco, CA: Author.

Gilbar, P.J., & Carrington, C.V. (2006). The incidence of extravasation of vinca alkaloids supplied in syringes or mini-bags. *Journal of Oncology Pharmacy Practice, 12,* 113–118. https://doi.org/10.1177/1078155206070448

González-Moreno, S., González-Bayon, L., & Ortega-Pérez, G. (2012). Hyperthermic intraperitoneal chemotherapy: Methodology and safety considerations. *Surgical Oncology Clinics, 21,* 543–557. https://doi.org/10.1016/j.soc.2012.07.001

Griggs, J.J., Mangu, P.B., Anderson, H., Balaban, E.P., Dignam, J.J., Hryniuk, W.M., … Lyman, G.H. (2012). Appropriate chemotherapy dosing for obese adult patients with cancer: American Society of Clinical Oncology clinical practice guideline. *Journal of Clinical Oncology, 30,* 1553–1561. https://doi.org/10.1200/JCO.2011.39.9436

Grigorian, A., & O'Brien, C.B. (2014). Hepatotoxicity secondary to chemotherapy. *Journal of Clinical and Translational Hepatology, 2,* 95–102. https://doi.org/10.14218/JCTH.2014.00011

Guillaume, D.J., Doolittle, N.D., Gahramanov, S., Hedrick, N.A., Delashaw, J.B., & Neuwelt, E.A. (2010). Intra-arterial chemotherapy with osmotic blood-brain barrier disruption for aggressive oligodendroglial tumors: Results of a phase I study. *Neurosurgery, 66,* 48–58. https://doi.org/10.1227/01.NEU.0000363152.37594.F7

Gynecologic Oncology Group. (2011, Spring). Updated FAQ's for dosing of carboplatin. *Gynecologic Oncology Group Newsletter,* pp. 2, 4. Retrieved from http://www.gog.org/Spring2011newsletter.pdf

Hartkopf Smith, L. (2009a). National Patient Safety Goal #13: Patients' active involvement in their own care: Preventing chemotherapy extravasation. *Clinical Journal of Oncology Nursing, 13,* 233–234. https://doi.org/10.1188/09.CJON.233-234

Hartkopf Smith, L. (2009b). Preventing intrathecal chemotherapy errors: One institution's experience. *Clinical Journal of Oncology Nursing, 13,* 344–346. https://doi.org/10.1188/09.CJON.344-346

Hartkopf Smith, L. (2012). Torsade de pointes, prolonged QT intervals, and patients with cancer. *Clinical Journal of Oncology Nursing, 16,* 125–128. https://doi.org/10.1188/12.CJON.125-128

Hartkopf Smith, L. (2017). Arterial access devices. In D. Camp-Sorrell & L. Matey (Eds.), *Access device standards of practice for oncology nursing* (pp. 105–112). Pittsburgh, PA: Oncology Nursing Society.

Hartkopf-Smith, L., & Hughes-McNally, C. (2012). Is the administration of vinca alkaloids by minibag infusion a safe risk mitigation strategy to prevent intrathecal chemotherapy errors? [Abstract 1289572]. *Oncology Nursing Forum, 39,* E158. https://doi.org/10.1188/12.ONF.E157-E225

Hematology/Oncology Pharmacy Association. (2017). *Dose rounding of biologic and cytotoxic anticancer agents* [Position statement]. Retrieved from https://www.nccn.org/professionals/OrderTemplates/PDF/HOPA.pdf

Hendricks, C.B. (2015). Improving adherence with oral antiemetic agents in patients with breast cancer receiving chemotherapy. *Journal of Oncology Practice, 11,* 216–218. https://doi.org/10.1200/JOP.2015.004234

Hershey, D.S., & Hession, S. (2017). Chemotherapy and glycemic control in patients with type 2 diabetes and cancer: A comparative case analysis. *Asia-Pacific Journal of Oncology Nursing, 4,* 224–232. https://doi.org/10.4103/apjon.apjon_22_17

Hershman, D.L., Till, C., Wright, J.D., Awad, D., Ramsey, S.D., Barlow, W.E., … Unger, J. (2016). Comorbidities and risk of chemotherapy-induced peripheral neuropathy among participants 65 years or older in Southwest Oncology Group clinical trials. *Journal of Clinical Oncology, 34,* 3014–3022. https://doi.org/10.1200/JCO.2015.66.2346

Hopkins, U., & Arias, C.Y. (2013, February 22). Large-volume IM injections: A review of best practices. *Oncology Nurse Advisor.* Retrieved from http://www.oncologynurseadvisor.com/chemotherapy/large-volume-im-injections-a-review-of-best-practices/article/281208

Hwang, J.P., Somerfield, M.R., Alston-Johnson, D.E., Cryer, D.R., Feld, J.J., Kramer, B.S., … Artz, A.S. (2015). Hepatitis B virus screening for patients with cancer before therapy: American Society of Clinical Oncology provisional clinical opinion update. *Journal of Clinical Oncology, 33,* 2212–2220. https://doi.org/10.1200/JCO.2015.61.3745

Infusion Nurses Society. (2016). *Infusion therapy standards of practice.* Norwood, MA: Author.

Institute for Safe Medication Practices. (2009). *Proceedings from the ISMP summit on the use of smart infusion pumps: Guidelines for safe implementation and use.* Retrieved from https://www.ismp.org/tools/guidelines/smartpumps/printerversion.pdf

Institute for Safe Medication Practices. (2010). *ISMP's guidelines for standard order sets.* Retrieved from http://www.ismp.org/tools/guidelines/standardordersets.pdf

Institute for Safe Medication Practices. (2013a, June 13). Administering a saline flush "site unseen" can lead to a wrong route error. *ISMP Medication Safety Alert! Acute Care.* Retrieved from https://www.ismp.org/resources/administering-saline-flush-site-unseen-can-lead-wrong-route-error

Institute for Safe Medication Practices. (2013b, November 14). Understanding and managing IV container overfill. *ISMP Medication Safety Alert! Acute Care.* Retrieved from https://www.ismp.org/newsletters/acutecare/showarticle.aspx?id=63

Institute for Safe Medication Practices. (2015a, June 18). Accidental overdoses involving fluorouracil infusions. *ISMP Medication Safety Alert! Acute Care.* Retrieved from http://www.ismp.org/newsletters/acutecare/showarticle.aspx?id=111

Institute for Safe Medication Practices. (2015b, November 19). Managing hospitalized patients with ambulatory pumps: Findings from an ISMP survey—part 1. *ISMP Medication Safety Alert! Acute Care.* Retrieved from http://www.ismp.org/newsletters/acutecare/showarticle.aspx?id=125

Institute for Safe Medication Practices. (2016). *ISMP guidelines for safe preparation of compounded sterile preparations.* Retrieved from https://www.ismp.org/Tools/guidelines/IVSummit/IVCGuidelines.pdf

Institute for Safe Medication Practices. (2018). *2018–2019 targeted medication safety best practices for hospitals.* Retrieved from http://www.ismp.org/tools/bestpractices/TMSBP-for-Hospitals.pdf

Institute for Safe Medication Practices Canada. (2005). Lowering the risk of medication errors: Independent double checks. *ISMP Canada Safety Bulletin, 5,* 1–2. Retrieved from http://www.ismp-canada.org/download/safetyBulletins/ISMPCSB2005-01.pdf

Izzedine, H., Mateus, C., Boutros, C., Robert, C., Rouvier, P., Amoura, Z., & Mathian, A. (2017). Renal effects of immune checkpoint inhibitors. *Nephrology Dialysis Transplantation, 32,* 936–942. https://doi.org/10.1093/ndt/gfw382

Jackson-Rose, J., Del Monte, J., Groman, A., Dial, L.S., Atwell, L., Graham, J., ... Rice, R.D. (2017). Chemotherapy extravasation: Establishing a national benchmark for incidence among cancer centers. *Clinical Journal of Oncology Nursing, 21,* 438–445. https://doi.org/10.1188/17.CJON.438-445

Jang, R.W., Caraiscos, V.B., Swami, N., Banerjee, S., Mak, E., Kaya, E., ... Zimmermann, C. (2014). Simple prognostic model for patients with advanced cancer based on performance status. *Journal of Oncology Practice, 10,* e335–e341. https://doi.org/10.1200/JOP.2014.001457

Janssen Pharmaceuticals, Inc. (2017). *Duragesic® (fentanyl transdermal system) for transdermal administration* [Package insert]. Titusville, NJ: Author.

Kasi, P.M., Thanarajasingam, G., Finnes, H.D., Villasboas Bisneto, J.C., Hubbard, J.M., & Grothey, A. (2015). Chemotherapy in the setting of severe liver dysfunction in patients with metastatic colorectal cancer. *Case Reports in Oncological Medicine, 2015.* https://doi.org/10.1155/2015/420159

Khan, A.N., Nagarajaiah, C.P., & Irion, K.L. (2016, July 7). Imaging in drug-induced lung disease. Retrieved from http://emedicine.medscape.com/article/357574-overview

Khoury, C.C., & Steele, D.J.R. (2017, January 15). The challenges of treating cancer patients on hemodialysis, or with chronic kidney disease. *Oncology, 31,* 40–44. Retrieved from http://www.cancernetwork.com/oncology-journal/challenges-treating-cancer-patients-hemodialysis-or-chronic-kidney-disease

Kistler, C.A. (2013, October 21). Elevated liver function tests and chemotherapy. *Cancer Therapy Advisor.* Retrieved from http://www.cancertherapyadvisor.com/general-oncology/elevated-liver-function-tests-and-chemotherapy/article/317204/

Kloth, J.S.L., Pagani, A., Verboom, M.C., Malovini, A., Napolitano, C., Kruit, W.H.J., ... Mathijssen, R.H.J. (2015). Incidence and relevance of QTc-interval prolongation caused by tyrosine kinase inhibitors. *British Journal of Cancer, 112,* 1011–1016. https://doi.org/10.1038/bjc.2015.82

Koren, G., Carey, N., Gagnon, R., Maxwell, C., Nulman, I., & Senikas, V. (2013). Cancer chemotherapy and pregnancy. *Journal of Obstetrics and Gynaecology Canada, 35,* 263–278. https://doi.org/10.1016/S1701-2163(15)30999-3

Kuo, J.C., & Craft, P.S. (2015). Administration of chemotherapy in patients on dialysis. *Anti-Cancer Drugs, 26,* 779–784. https://doi.org/10.1097/CAD.0000000000000243

Lichtman, S.M., Cirrincione, C.T., Hurria, A., Jatoi, A., Theodoulou, M., Wolff, A.C., ... Muss, H.B. (2016). Effect of pretreatment renal function on treatment and clinical outcomes in the adjuvant treatment of older women with breast cancer: Alliance A171201, an ancillary study of CALGB/CTSU 49907. *Journal of Clinical Oncology, 34,* 699–705. https://doi.org/10.1200/JCO.2015.62.6341

Lishner, M., Avivi, I., Apperley, J.F., Dierickx, D., Evens, A.M., Fumagalli, M., ... Amant, F. (2016). Hematologic malignancies in pregnancy: Management guidelines from an international consensus meeting. *Journal of Clinical Oncology, 34,* 501–508. https://doi.org/10.1200/JCO.2015.62.4445

Liu, C., Cui, Q., Guo, J., Li, D., & Zeng, Y. (2014). Intra-arterial intervention chemotherapy for sarcoma and cancerous ulcer via an implanted pump. *Pathology and Oncology Research, 20,* 229–234. https://doi.org/10.1007/s12253-013-9673-6

Lok, A.S.F., & McMahon, B.J. (2009). Chronic hepatitis B: Update 2009. *Hepatology, 50,* 661–662. https://doi.org/10.1002/hep.23190

Mackey, H.T. (2017a). Short-term peripheral intravenous catheters. In D. Camp-Sorrell & L. Matey (Eds.), *Access device standards of practice for oncology nursing* (pp. 25–35). Pittsburgh, PA: Oncology Nursing Society.

Mackey, H.T. (2017b). Tunneled central venous catheters. In D. Camp-Sorrell & L. Matey (Eds.), *Access device standards of practice for oncology nursing* (pp. 59–64). Pittsburgh, PA: Oncology Nursing Society.

Matthews, E., Snell, K., & Coats, H. (2006). Intra-arterial chemotherapy for limb preservation in patients with osteosarcoma: Nursing implications. *Clinical Journal of Oncology Nursing, 10,* 581–589. https://doi.org/10.1188/06.CJON.581-589

Maurer, M., Dardess, P., Carman, K.L., Frazier, K., & Smeeding, L. (2012). *Guide to patient and family engagement: Environmental scan report* (AHRQ Publication No.12-0042-EF). Retrieved from https://psnet.ahrq.gov/resources/resource/24664/guide-to-patient-and-family-engagement-environmental-scan-report

Mayne, S.T., Cartmel, B., Kirsh, V., & Goodwin, W.J., Jr. (2009). Alcohol and tobacco use prediagnosis and postdiagnosis, and survival in a cohort of patients with early stage cancers of the oral cavity, pharynx, and larynx. *Cancer Epidemiology, Biomarkers and Prevention, 18,* 3368–3374. https://doi.org/10.1158/1055-9965.EPI-09-0944

Millennium Pharmaceuticals, Inc. (2017). *Velcade® (bortezomib)* [Package insert]. Cambridge, MA: Author.

Modlin, R., & Mancini, J. (2011). Chemotherapy administration sequence: A review of the literature and creation of a sequencing chart. *Journal of Hematology Oncology Pharmacy, 1,* 17–25. Retrieved from http://jhoponline.com/jhop-issue-archive/2011-issues/march-vol-1-no-1/13240-top-13240

Moon, D.H., Lee, J.-M., Noonan, A.M., Annunziata, C.M., Minasian, L., Houston, N., ... Kohn, E.C. (2013). Deleterious BRCA1/2 mutation is an independent risk factor for carboplatin hypersensitivity reactions. *British Journal of Cancer, 109,* 1072–1078. https://doi.org/10.1038/bjc.2013.389

Mosteller, R.D. (1987). Simplified calculation of body-surface area. *New England Journal of Medicine, 317,* 1098. https://doi.org/10.1056/NEJM198710223171717

Nagao, S., Fujiwara, K., Imafuku, N., Kagawa, R., Kozuka, Y., Oda, T., ... Kohno, I. (2005). Difference of carboplatin clearance estimated by the Cockroft-Gault, Jelliffe, Modified-Jelliffe, Wright or Chatelut formula. *Gynecologic Oncology, 99,* 327–333. https://doi.org/10.1016/j.ygyno.2005.06.003

Nair, A. (2016). Implications of intrathecal chemotherapy for anaesthesiologists: A brief review. *Scientifica, 2016.* https://doi.org/10.1155/2016/3759845

Narouze, S., Benzon, H.T., Provenzano, D.A., Buvanendran, A., De Andres, J., Deer, T.R., ... Huntoon, M.A. (2015). Interventional spine and pain procedures in patients on antiplatelet and anticoagulant medications (second edition): Guidelines from the American Society of Regional Anesthesia and Pain Medicine, the European Society of Regional Anaesthesia and Pain Therapy, the American Academy of Pain Medicine, the International Neuromodulation Society, the North American Neuromodulation Society, and the World Institute of Pain. *Regional Anesthesia and Pain Medicine.* Advance online publication. https://doi.org/10.1097/AAP.0000000000000223

National Cancer Institute Cancer Therapy Evaluation Program. (2010, October 22). Follow-up for information letter regarding AUC-based dosing of carboplatin. Retrieved from https://ctep.cancer.gov/content/docs/carboplatin_information_letter.pdf

National Comprehensive Cancer Network. (n.d.). Just Bag It! NCCN Campaign for Safe Vincristine Handling. Retrieved from https://www.nccn.org/justbagit

National Comprehensive Cancer Network. (2017a). *NCCN Clinical Practice Guidelines in Oncology (NCCN Guidelines®): Older adult oncology* [v.2.2017]. Retrieved from https://www.nccn.org/professionals/physician_gls/default.aspx#senior

National Comprehensive Cancer Network. (2017b). *NCCN Clinical Practice Guidelines in Oncology (NCCN Guidelines®): Prevention and treatment of cancer-related infections* [v.1.2018]. Retrieved from https://www.nccn.org/professionals/physician_gls/pdf/infections.pdf

National Comprehensive Cancer Network. (2018a). *NCCN Clinical Practice Guidelines in Oncology (NCCN Guidelines®): Acute lymphoblastic leukemia* [v.1.2018]. Retrieved from https://www.nccn.org/professionals/physician_gls/pdf/all.pdf

National Comprehensive Cancer Network. (2018b). *NCCN Clinical Practice Guidelines in Oncology (NCCN Guidelines®): Acute myeloid leukemia* [v.1.2018]. Retrieved from https://www.nccn.org/professionals/physician_gls/pdf/aml.pdf

National Comprehensive Cancer Network. (2018c). *NCCN Clinical Practice Guidelines in Oncology (NCCN Guidelines®): B-cell lymphomas: Diffuse large B-cell lymphoma and follicular lymphoma* [NCCN Evidence Blocks™, v.7.2017]. Retrieved from https://www.nccn.org/professionals/physician_gls/pdf/b-cell_blocks.pdf

National Comprehensive Cancer Network. (2018d). *NCCN Clinical Practice Guidelines in Oncology (NCCN Guidelines®): Bladder cancer* [v.2.2018]. Retrieved from https://www.nccn.org/professionals/physician_gls/pdf/bladder.pdf

National Comprehensive Cancer Network. (2018e). *NCCN Clinical Practice Guidelines in Oncology (NCCN Guidelines®): Distress management* [v.2.2018]. Retrieved from https://www.nccn.org/professionals/physician_gls/pdf/distress.pdf

National Comprehensive Cancer Network. (2018f). *NCCN Clinical Practice Guidelines in Oncology (NCCN Guidelines®): Ovarian cancer including fallopian tube cancer and primary peritoneal cancer* [v.2.2018]. Retrieved from https://www.nccn.org/professionals/physician_gls/pdf/ovarian.pdf

National Comprehensive Cancer Network. (2018g). *NCCN Clinical Practice Guidelines in Oncology (NCCN Guidelines®): Small cell lung cancer* [v.2.2018]. Retrieved from https://www.nccn.org/professionals/physician_gls/pdf/sclc.pdf

National Toxicology Program. (2013). *NTP monograph: Developmental effects and pregnancy outcomes associated with cancer chemotherapy use during pregnancy.* Retrieved from https://ntp.niehs.nih.gov/ntp/ohat/cancer_chemo_preg/chemopregnancy_monofinal_508.pdf

Neuss, M.N., Gilmore, T.R., Belderson, K.M., Billett, A.L., Conti-Kalchik, T., Harvey, B.E., … Polovich, M. (2016). 2016 updated American Society of Clinical Oncology/Oncology Nursing Society chemotherapy administration safety standards, including standards for pediatric oncology. *Journal of Oncology Practice, 12,* 1262–1271. https://doi.org/10.1200/JOP.2016.017905

Neuwirth, M.G., Alexander, H.R., & Karakousis, G.C. (2016). Then and now: Cytoreductive surgery with hyperthermic intraperitoneal chemotherapy (HIPEC), a historical perspective. *Journal of Gastrointestinal Oncology, 7,* 18–28. https://doi.org/10.3978%2Fj.issn.2078-6891.2015.106

Nieuwenhuijzen, J.A., Bex, A., & Horenblas, S. (2003). Unusual complication after immediate postoperative intravesical mitomycin C instillation. *European Urology, 43,* 711–712. https://doi.org/10.1016/S0302-2838(03)00151-9

Nurgat, Z.A., Smythe, M., Al-Jedai, A., Ewing, S., Rasheed, W., Belgaumi, A., … Aljurf, M. (2015). Introduction of vincristine mini-bags and an assessment of the subsequent risk of extravasation. *Journal of Oncology Pharmacy Practice, 21,* 339–347. https://doi.org/10.1177/1078155214531803

Oncology Nursing Society. (2016). *Oral adherence toolkit.* Retrieved from https://www.ons.org/sites/default/files/ONS_Toolkit_ONLINE.pdf

Orto, V., Hendrix, C.C., Griffith, B., & Shaikewitz, S.T. (2015). Implementation of a smart pump champions program to decrease potential patient harm. *Journal of Nursing Care Quality, 30,* 138–143. https://doi.org/10.1097/NCQ.0000000000000090

Palejwala, S.K., Stidd, D.A., Skoch, J.M., Gupta, P., Lemole, G.M., Jr., & Weinand, M.E. (2014). Use of a stop-flow programmable shunt valve to maximize CNS chemotherapy delivery in a pediatric patient with acute lymphoblastic leukemia. *Surgical Neurology, 5*(Suppl. 4), S273–S277. https://doi.org/10.4103/2152-7806.139381

Pallis, A.G., Fortpied, C., Wedding, U., Van Nes, M.C., Penninckx, B., Ring, A., … Wildiers, H. (2010). EORTC Elderly Task Force position paper: Approach to the older cancer patient. *European Journal of Cancer, 46,* 1502–1513. https://doi.org/10.1016/j.ejca.2010.02.022

Parks, L., & Routt, M. (2015). Hepatic artery infusion pump in the treatment of liver metastases. *Clinical Journal of Oncology Nursing, 19,* 316–320. https://doi.org/10.1188/15.CJON.316-320

Partridge, A.H., Archer, L., Kornblith, A.B., Gralow, J., Grenier, D., Perez, E., … Muss, H. (2010). Adherence and persistence with oral adjuvant chemotherapy in older women with early-stage breast cancer in CALGB 49907: Adherence companion study 60104. *Journal of Clinical Oncology, 28,* 2418–2422. https://doi.org/10.1200/JCO.2009.26.4671

Partridge, A.H., Wang, P.S., Winer, E.P., & Avorn, J. (2003). Nonadherence to adjuvant tamoxifen therapy in women with primary breast cancer. *Journal of Clinical Oncology, 21,* 602–606. https://doi.org/10.1200/JCO.2003.07.071

Paul, S., Saxena, A., Terrin, N., Viveiros, K., Balk, E.M., & Wong, J.B. (2016). Hepatitis B virus reactivation and prophylaxis during solid tumor chemotherapy: A systematic review and meta-analysis. *Annals of Internal Medicine, 164,* 30–40. https://doi.org/10.7326/M15-1121

Peairs, K.S., Barone, B.B., Snyder, C.F., Yeh, H.-C., Stein, K.B., Derr, R.L., … Wolff, A.C. (2011). Diabetes mellitus and breast cancer outcomes: A systematic review and meta-analysis. *Journal of Clinical Oncology, 29,* 40–46. https://doi.org/10.1200/JCO.2009.27.3011

Perazella, M.A. (2012). Onco-nephrology: Renal toxicities of chemotherapeutic agents. *Clinical Journal of the American Society of Nephrology, 7,* 1713–1721. https://doi.org/10.2215/CJN.02780312

Pfizer Inc. (2016). *Camptosar® (irinotecan hydrochloride injection)* [Package insert]. New York, NY: Author.

Pirl, W.F., Braun, I.M., Deshields, T.L., Fann, J.R., Fulchers, C.D., Greer, J.A., … Bardwell, W.A. (n.d.). *Implementing screening for distress: The joint position statement from the American Psychosocial Oncology Society, Association of Oncology Social Work and Oncology Nursing Society.* Retrieved from https://www.ons.org/sites/default/files/Implementing%20Screening%20for%20Distress.pdf

Pirschel, C. (2017). Improving cancer care through patient-reported outcomes. *ONS Voice, 32*(8), 16–21. Retrieved from https://voice.ons.org/news-and-views/improving-oncology-care-with-pros

Plana, J.C., Galderisi, M., Barac, A., Ewer, M.S., Ky, B., Scherrer-Crosbie, M., … Lancellotti, P. (2014). Expert consensus for multimodality imaging evaluation of adult patients during and after cancer therapy: A report from the American Society of Echocardiography and the European Association of Cardiovascular Imaging. *European Heart Journal—Cardiovascular Imaging, 15,* 1063–1093. https://doi.org/10.1093/ehjci/jeu192

Polovich, M., & Olsen, M.M. (Eds.). (2018). *Safe handling of hazardous drugs* (3rd ed.). Pittsburgh, PA: Oncology Nursing Society.

Portz, D., & Johnston, M.P. (2014). Implementation of an evidence-based education practice change for patients with cancer. *Clinical Journal of Oncology Nursing, 18*(Suppl. 5), 36–40. https://doi.org/10.1188/14.CJON.S2.36-40

Potter, K.L., & Held-Warmkessel, J. (2008). Intraperitoneal chemotherapy for women with ovarian cancer: Nursing care and consideration. *Clinical Journal of Oncology Nursing, 12,* 265–271. https://doi.org/10.1188/08.CJON.265-271

Reddy, G.K., Brown, B., & Nanda, A. (2011). Fatal consequences of a simple mistake: How can a patient be saved from inadvertent intrathecal vincristine? *Clinical Neurology and Neurosurgery, 113,* 68–71. https://doi.org/10.1016/j.clineuro.2010.08.008

Reddy, K.R., Beavers, K.L., Hammond, S.P., Lim, J.K., & Falck-Ytter, Y.T. (2015). American Gastroenterological Association Institute guideline on the prevention and treatment of hepatitis B virus reactivation during immunosuppressive drug therapy. *Gastroenterology, 148,* 215–219. https://doi.org/10.1053/j.gastro.2014.10.039

Rodriguez, G., Utate, M.A., Joseph, G., & St. Victor, T. (2017). Oral chemotherapy adherence: A novel nursing intervention using an electronic health record workflow. *Clinical Journal of Oncology Nursing, 21,* 165–167. https://doi.org/10.1188/17.CJON.165-167

Rogers, B.K., Kolarich, A., & Markham, M.J. (2017). Implementing pregnancy screening prior to chemotherapy: A quality improvement initiative [Abstract]. *Journal of Clinical Oncology, 35*(Suppl. 15). https://doi.org/10.1200/JCO.2017.35.15_suppl.e18274

Rogers, M. (2017). Intraperitoneal catheters. In D. Camp-Sorrell & L. Matey (Eds.), *Access device standards of practice for oncology nursing* (pp. 131–138). Pittsburgh, PA: Oncology Nursing Society.

Roncolato, F.T., Chatfield, M., Houghton, B., Toner, G., Stockler, M., Thomson, D., … Grimison, P. (2016). The effect of pulmonary function testing on bleomycin dosing in germ cell tumours. *Internal Medicine, 46,* 893–898. https://doi.org/10.1111/imj.13158

Rossi, E., Sgambato, A., De Chiara, G., Casaluce, F., Losanno, T., Sacco, P.C., … Gridelli, C. (2016). Endocrinopathies induced by immune-checkpoint inhibitors in advanced non-small cell lung cancer. *Expert Review of Clinical Pharmacology, 9,* 419–428. https://doi.org/10.1586/17512433.2016.1133289

Royal, R.E. (2013). Principles of isolated limb perfusion. In S.T. Kee, D.C. Madoff, & R. Murthy (Eds.), *Clinical interventional oncology* (pp. 26–38). St. Louis, MO: Elsevier Saunders.

Rubin, L.G., Levin, M.J., Ljungman, P., Davies, E.G., Avery, R., Tomblyn, M., … Kang, I. (2014). 2013 IDSA clinical practice guideline for vaccination of the immunocompromised host. *Clinical Infectious Diseases, 58,* e44–e100. https://doi.org/10.1093/cid/cit684

Sarfati, D., Gurney, J., Stanley, J., Salmond, C., Crampton, P., Dennett, E., … Pearce, N. (2014). Cancer-specific administrative data–based comorbidity indices provided valid alternative to Charlson and National Cancer Institute indices. *Journal of Clinical Epidemiology, 67,* 586–595. https://doi.org/10.1016/j.jclinepi.2013.11.012

Sato, K., Watanabe, S., Ohtsubo, A., Shoji, S., Ishikawa, D., Tanaka, T., … Narita, I. (2016). Nephrotoxicity of cisplatin combination chemotherapy in thoracic malignancy patients with CKD risk factors. *BMC Cancer, 16,* 222. https://doi.org/10.1186/s12885-016-2271-8

Scher, K.S., & Hurria, A. (2012). Under-representation of older adults in cancer registration trials: Known problem, little progress. *Journal of Clinical Oncology, 30,* 2036–2038. https://doi.org/10.1200/JCO.2012.41.6727

Schleisman, A., & Mahon, S.M. (2015). Preventing chemotherapy errors with comprehensive medication assessment. *Clinical Journal of Oncology Nursing, 19,* 532–534. https://doi.org/10.1188/15.CJON.532-534

Schnipper, L.E., Lyman, G.H., Blayney, D.W., Hoverman, J.R., Raghavan, D., Wollins, D.S., & Schilsky, R.L. (2013). American Society of Clinical Oncology 2013 top five list in oncology. *Journal of Clinical Oncology, 31,* 4362–4370. https://doi.org/10.1200/JCO.2013.53.3943

Schwappach, D.L.B., Hochreutener, M.-A., & Wernli, M. (2010). Oncology nurses' perceptions about involving patients in the prevention of chemotherapy administration errors [Online exclusive]. *Oncology Nursing Forum, 37,* E84–E91. https://doi.org/10.1188/10.ONF.E84-E91

Segal, E.M., Flood, M.R., Mancini, R.S., Whiteman, R.T., Friedt, G.A., Kramer, A.R., & Hofstetter, M.A. (2014). Oral chemotherapy food and drug interactions: A comprehensive review of the literature. *Journal of Oncology Practice, 10,* e255–e268. https://doi.org/10.1200/JOP.2013.001183

Seibert, H.H., Maddox, R.R., Flynn, E.A., & Williams, C.K. (2014). Effect of barcode technology with electronic medication administration record on medication accuracy rates. *American Journal of Health-System Pharmacy, 71,* 209–218. https://doi.org/10.2146/ajhp130332

Shaw, C., & Taylor, L. (2012). Treatment-related diarrhea in patients with cancer. *Clinical Journal of Oncology Nursing, 16,* 413–417. https://doi.org/10.1188/12.CJON.413-417

Shewmaker, P.L., Gertz, R.E., Jr., Kim, C.Y., de Fijter, S., DiOrio, M., Moore, M.R., & Beall, B.W. (2010). *Streptococcus salivarius* meningitis case strain traced to oral flora of anesthesiologist. *Journal of Clinical Microbiology, 48,* 2589–2591. https://doi.org/10.1128/JCM.00426-10

Silliman, R.A., Guadagnoli, E., Rakowski, W., Landrum, M.B., Lash, T.L., Wolf, R., … Mor, V. (2002). Adjuvant tamoxifen prescription in women 65 years and older with primary breast cancer. *Journal of Clinical Oncology, 20,* 2680–2688. https://doi.org/10.1200/JCO.2002.08.137

Simons, F.E.R. (2008). Anaphylaxis. *Journal of Allergy and Clinical Immunology, 121*(Suppl. 2), S402–S407. https://doi.org/10.1016/j.jaci.2007.08.061

Sisson, H. (2015). Aspirating during the intramuscular injection procedure: A systematic literature review. *Journal of Clinical Nursing, 24,* 2368–2375. https://doi.org/10.1111/jocn.12824

Smart, M. (2011). Oncology update. *Oncology Nursing Forum, 38,* 93–94. https://doi.org/10.1188/11.ONF.93-94

Smith, L.A., Cornelius, V.R., Plummer, C.J., Levitt, G., Verrill, M., Canney, P., & Jones, A. (2010). Cardiotoxicity of anthracycline agents for the treatment of cancer: Systematic review and meta-analysis of randomised controlled trials. *BMC Cancer, 10,* 337. https://doi.org/10.1186/1471-2407-10-337

Spoelstra, S.L., & Sansoucie, H. (2015). Putting evidence into practice: Evidence-based interventions for oral agents for cancer. *Clinical Journal of Oncology Nursing, 19,* 60–72. https://doi.org/10.1188/15.S1.CJON.60-72

Sviggum, H.P., Jacob, A.K., Arendt, K.W., Mauermann, M.L., Horlocker, T.T., & Hebl, J.R. (2012). Neurologic complications after chlorhexidine antisepsis for spinal anesthesia. *Regional Anesthesia and Pain Medicine, 37,* 139–144. https://doi.org/10.1097/AAP.0b013e318244179a

U.S. National Library of Medicine. (2018). Complementary and alternative medicine. In *Collection development manual of the National Library of Medicine*. Retrieved from https://www.nlm.nih.gov/tsd/acquisitions/cdm/subjects24.html

van Leeuwen, R.W., Brundel, D.H.S., Neef, C., van Gelder, T., Mathijssen, R.H.J., Burger, D.M., & Jansman, F.G.A. (2013). Prevalence of potential drug-drug interactions in cancer patients treated with oral anticancer drugs. *British Journal of Cancer, 108,* 1071–1078. https://doi.org/10.1038/bjc.2013.48

Vogel, W.H. (2010). Infusion reactions: Diagnosis, assessment, and management [Online exclusive]. *Clinical Journal of Oncology Nursing, 14,* E10–E21. https://doi.org/10.1188/10.CJON.E10-E21

Volkov, A.A., Filis, A.K., & Vrionis, F.D. (2017). Surgical treatment for leptomeningeal disease. *Cancer Control, 24,* 47–53. https://doi.org/10.1177/107327481702400107

Walko, C.M., & McLeod, H.L. (2014). Personalizing medicine in geriatric oncology. *Journal of Clinical Oncology, 32,* 2581–2586. https://doi.org/10.1200/JCO.2014.55.9047

Washburn, D.J. (2007). Intravesicular antineoplastic therapy following transurethral resection of bladder tumors: Nursing implications from the operating room to discharge. *Clinical Journal of Oncology Nursing, 11,* 553–559. https://doi.org/10.1188/07.CJON.553-559

Wass, M., Hitz, F., Schaffrath, J., Müller-Tidow, C., & Müller, L.P. (2016). Value of different comorbidity indices for predicting outcome in patients with acute myeloid leukemia. *PLOS ONE, 11,* e0164587. https://doi.org/10.1371/journal.pone.0164587

Weinbaum, C.M., Williams, I., Mast, E.E., Wang, S.A., Finelli, L., Wasley, A., ... Ward, J.W. (2008). Recommendations for identification and public health management of persons with chronic hepatitis B virus infection. *MMWR Recommendations and Reports, 57*(RR-8), 1–20. Retrieved from https://www.cdc.gov/mmwr/preview/mmwrhtml/rr5708a1.htm

Weiss, P.A. (2008). Can chemotherapy dosing be individualized? *Clinical Journal of Oncology Nursing, 12,* 975–977. https://doi.org/10.1188/08.CJON.975-977

White, R.E., Trbovich, P.L., Easty, A.C., Savage, P., Trip, K., & Hyland, S. (2010). Checking it twice: An evaluation of checklists for detecting medication errors at the bedside using a chemotherapy model. *Quality and Safety in Health Care, 19,* 562–567. https://doi.org/10.1136/qshc.2009.032862

Wiley, K. (2017, May 23). What special considerations are needed when setting up IV chemotherapy? *ONS Voice.* Retrieved from https://voice.ons.org/news-and-views/administering-iv-chemotherapy-treatments

CHAPTER 12

Safe Handling of Hazardous Drugs

A. Safe handling and disposal of hazardous drugs (HDs)
   1. Many drugs used in the treatment of cancer are hazardous to healthcare workers (HCWs). The term *hazardous* describes drugs that require special handling because occupational exposure may cause adverse health effects. These effects occur because of the inherent toxicities of the drugs (American Society of Health-System Pharmacists [ASHP], 2006; National Institute for Occupational Safety and Health [NIOSH], 2004).
   2. According to the Occupational Safety and Health Administration (OSHA, 2016), a safe level of occupational exposure to HDs is unknown. HCWs who handle HDs are likely exposed to multiple agents on any given day, and no reliable method for monitoring work-related exposure exists.
   3. Therefore, it is imperative that those who work with HDs adhere to practices designed to minimize occupational exposure.

B. Definition of HDs
   1. In 1990, ASHP (then known as the American Society of Hospital Pharmacists) provided the first definition of HDs, which consisted of the first five characteristics; NIOSH (2004, 2010, 2012, 2016b) refined the definition by adding the sixth.
   2. Drugs are considered hazardous if they demonstrate one or more of the following characteristics in humans or animals:
      a) Carcinogenicity
      b) Teratogenicity or developmental toxicity in a fetus
      c) Reproductive toxicity
      d) Organ toxicity at low doses
      e) Genotoxicity
      f) New drugs similar in structure or toxicity to drugs classified as hazardous using the preceding criteria

C. Potential adverse health effects associated with occupational exposure to antineoplastic agents
   1. An increased occurrence of cancer in exposed nurses and other HCWs. Published evidence regarding cancer among occupationally exposed nurses and other HCWs (Blair et al., 2001; Hansen & Olsen, 1994; Levin, Holly, & Seward, 1993; Martin, 2005; Petralia, Dosemeci, Adams, & Zahm, 1999) is limited because of the failure to connect exposure to health outcomes. The International Agency for Research on Cancer (2018) publishes independent assessments of the carcinogenic risks of chemicals and has identified 11 antineoplastic drugs and several combination chemotherapy regimens as known human carcinogens. Other antineoplastic agents are classified as probable or possible carcinogens (see Table 12-1).
   2. Structural defects in a fetus following occupational HD exposure during pregnancy (Hemminki, Kyyrönen, & Lindbohm, 1985; Peelen, Roeleveld, Heederik, Kromhout, & de Kort, 1999). No studies of congenital malformations have been done that report data collected after 2000 (Connor, Lawson, Polovich, & McDiarmid, 2014).
   3. Adverse reproductive outcomes, including miscarriage (Lawson et al., 2012), infertility (Fransman et al., 2007; Martin, 2005), preterm births, and learning disabilities in offspring of nurses exposed to HDs during pregnancy (Martin, 2005)
   4. Chromosomal damage (Buschini et al., 2013; Villarini et al., 2011), chromosomal aberrations (El-Ebiary, Abuelfadl, & Sarhan, 2013; McDiarmid, Oliver, Roth, Rogers, & Escalante, 2010; McDiarmid, Rogers, & Oliver, 2014; Moretti et al., 2015; Santovito, Cervella, & Delpero, 2014), and increased frequency of micronuclei (Bouraoui et al., 2011; El-Ebiary et al., 2013; Ladeira et al., 2014; Moretti et al., 2015; Villarini et al., 2016) in HCWs following exposure to HDs
   5. Acute symptoms such as hair loss, abdominal pain, fatigue, nausea, nasal irritation or sores, contact dermatitis, allergic reactions, skin injury, and eye injury (Baykal, Seren, & Sokmen, 2009;

Table 12-1. Antineoplastic Agents Classified as Carcinogens

Exposure Risk	Antineoplastic Drugs
Group 1: Carcinogenic to humans	Arsenic trioxide Azathioprine Busulfan Chlorambucil Cyclophosphamide Etoposide Etoposide in combination with cisplatin Melphalan MOPP (mechlorethamine hydrochloride, vincristine, procarbazine, and prednisone) Other combined chemotherapy including alkylating agents Semustine Tamoxifen Thiotepa Treosulfan
Group 2A: Probably carcinogenic to humans	Azacitidine Carmustine Cisplatin Doxorubicin Lomustine Nitrogen mustard Procarbazine Teniposide
Group 2B: Possibly carcinogenic to humans	Amsacrine Bleomycin Dacarbazine Daunorubicin Mitomycin Mitoxantrone Streptozocin

Note. Based on information from International Agency for Research on Cancer, 2018.

Constantinidis et al., 2011; Meyer & Skov, 2010) and changes in blood work (Caciari et al., 2012) among exposed HCWs

D. Potential adverse health effects associated with occupational exposure to immunotherapeutic agents

1. Limited data are available regarding the effects of occupational exposure to these agents. It is unclear whether the criteria in the definition of HDs are adequate for protein-based or bioengineered drugs (Halsen & Krämer, 2011; NIOSH, 2016b). Novel viral-based therapies require contact isolation and the use of personal protective equipment (PPE) for infection prevention because patients may shed the viruses (Martin, 2017).
2. Most biologic agents do not affect DNA and thus do not cause genetic changes.
3. Antiangiogenic agents (e.g., thalidomide, lenalidomide) pose a risk to fetuses (Celgene Corp., 2017a, 2017b).
4. Several targeted agents meet one or more of the criteria in the NIOSH definition of HDs and should be handled as hazardous (e.g., handled with PPE and not crushed). Refer to the most recent NIOSH publication for a list of these agents (NIOSH, 2016b).
5. Monoclonal antibodies (mAbs): Harm from occupational exposure to mAbs is minimal because of the low likelihood of internalizing the large molecules through the usual exposure routes (Halsen & Krämer, 2011).
   a) NIOSH does not list all drugs in the classification of mAbs as hazardous; instead, each drug is compared to the criteria in the definition of HDs.
   b) Pertuzumab is hazardous because of embryo-fetal death (NIOSH, 2016b).
   c) Conjugated mAbs are hazardous because of the attached radioactive isotopes (e.g., tositumomab) or toxins (e.g., ado-trastuzumab, brentuximab vedotin, gemtuzumab ozogamicin).
   d) Based on mechanism of action, some mAbs, including alemtuzumab, bevacizumab, cetuximab, panitumumab, rituximab, and trastuzumab, may cause developmental toxicity (Halsen & Krämer, 2011); however, NIOSH does not classify these agents as HDs.

E. *NIOSH List of Antineoplastic and Other Hazardous Drugs in Healthcare Settings, 2016*

1. NIOSH provides a list of HDs, as well as periodic updates, at www.cdc.gov/niosh/topics/hazdrug.
2. The list is divided into three groups:
   a) Group 1 is antineoplastic drugs that meet one or more of the criteria for HDs. This group includes chemotherapy agents, targeted agents, and other biologic drugs used in cancer treatment.
   b) Group 2 is nonantineoplastic drugs that meet one or more of the criteria for HDs. This group includes drugs from several categories, including immunosuppressant agents, antivirals, several anticonvulsants, estrogens, progestins, and androgens.
   c) Group 3 is nonantineoplastic drugs with primarily reproductive effects. These are drugs from different classifications that are harmful to men and women who are actively try-

ing to conceive, and women who are pregnant or breastfeeding.

F. Routes of occupational exposure
1. Absorption through skin or mucous membranes following direct drug contact or contact with surfaces or objects that are contaminated with HDs
   a) Many studies reported measurable levels of cytotoxic agents in the urine of HCWs, most likely from dermal absorption (Connor et al., 2010; Friese et al., 2014; Hama, Fukushima, Hirabatake, Hashida, & Kataoka, 2012; Hon, Teschke, Shen, Demers, & Venners, 2015; Miyake, Iwamoto, Tanimura, & Okuda, 2013; Ndaw, Denis, Marsan, d'Almeida, & Robert, 2010; Pieri et al., 2010; Ramphal, Bains, Vaillancourt, Osmond, & Barrowman, 2014; Sabatini, Barbieri, Lodi, & Violante, 2012; Sottani, Porro, Comelli, Imbriani, & Minoia, 2010; Sugiura, Asano, Kinoshita, Tanimura, & Nabeshima, 2011; Yoshida et al., 2011).
   b) Multiple studies have documented contamination of surfaces with HDs in drug preparation areas, drug administration areas, and patient care areas (Berruyer, Tanguay, Caron, Lefebvre, & Bussières, 2015; Bussières, Tanguay, Touzin, Langlois, & Lefebvre, 2012; Chu, Hon, Danyluk, Chua, & Astrakianakis, 2012; Connor et al., 2010; Kopp, Schierl, & Nowak, 2013; Ladeira et al., 2014; Maeda et al., 2010; Miyake et al., 2013; Moretti et al., 2015; Ramphal et al., 2014; Sottani, Porro, Imbriani, & Minoia, 2012; Sugiura et al., 2011; Villarini et al., 2011; Yoshida et al., 2011). These findings indicate that nurses may be exposed if they do not wear PPE when touching surfaces contaminated with HD residue.
   c) Several researchers have reported drug contamination on the outside of drug vials when delivered by the manufacturers (Connor et al., 2005; Fleury-Souverain, Nussbaumer, Mattiuzzo, & Bonnabry, 2014; Hama et al., 2012; Kopp et al., 2013; Schierl, Herwig, Pfaller, Groebmair, & Fischer, 2010). Cyclophosphamide, 5-fluorouracil, ifosfamide, and platinum have been detected on vial exteriors using various sampling techniques. These findings indicate that HCWs may be exposed if they do not wear PPE while handling unopened drug vials.
2. Injection from needlesticks or contaminated sharps (ASHP, 2006; NIOSH, 2004)
3. Inhalation of drug aerosols, dust, or droplets (Fent, Durgam, & Mueller, 2014; Kiffmeyer et al., 2002).
4. Ingestion of contaminated food, beverages, or tobacco products, or other hand-to-mouth behavior (NIOSH, 2004)

G. Hierarchy of hazard controls aimed at reducing worker exposure (NIOSH, 2016a)
1. Elimination of the hazard: The highest level of protection from a hazardous exposure is to eliminate the hazard or substitute a less toxic substance for the hazardous material, but this is not feasible with drug therapy.
2. Engineering controls: The second highest level of protection is the use of engineering controls—machines or equipment—that isolate or contain the hazard to reduce worker exposure. Examples include biosafety cabinets (BSCs) and closed-system drug-transfer devices (CSTDs).
3. Administrative controls: This third level of protection includes safe handling policies, procedures, work practices, and education and training of those responsible for HD handling.
4. PPE: The lowest level of protection, consisting of garments that provide barriers to protect workers from HDs, places the primary responsibility for protection on the worker.

H. Guidelines regarding PPE
1. Apparel
   a) Gloves: Wear two pair of disposable gloves that are powder free (U.S. Food and Drug Administration [FDA], 2018) and have been tested for use with HDs.
      (1) FDA requires permeation testing for gloves to be labeled as appropriate for use with chemotherapy.
      (2) The ASTM International (2013) standard D6978 involves permeation testing with chemotherapy drugs from several chemical classes.
      (3) Gloves that prevent HD permeation for a minimum of 30 minutes should be worn.
      (4) Test results are printed on the glove box or are available from the manufacturer.
      (5) Several types of materials, such as latex, neoprene, nitrile, and polyurethane, are used to make chemotherapy gloves.
      (6) Tested latex gloves provide protection but should be used with caution because of the potential for latex sensitivity.
      (7) Inspect gloves for physical defects before use.

(8) Remove and discard gloves immediately after use; if a tear, puncture, or known drug contact occurs; or after 30 minutes of wear (ASHP, 2006; NIOSH, 2004; U.S. Pharmacopeial Convention [USP], 2017).

(9) Wearing double gloves, with one pair under and one pair over the gown cuff, and carefully removing them reduces the opportunity for exposure (NIOSH, 2008).

(10) Remove outer gloves first, turning them inside out to prevent the contaminated outer surfaces from touching the inner gloves.

(11) Remove the inner gloves last after discarding all contaminated items and PPE. Do not reuse gloves.

b) Gowns: Wear a disposable, lint-free gown made of a low-permeability fabric, such as polyethylene-coated materials (Connor, 2006; USP, 2017).

(1) The gown should have a solid front, long sleeves, tight cuffs, and back closure.

(2) Discard the gown when it is knowingly contaminated, before leaving HD handling areas, and when finished with HD handling.

(3) Gowns are meant for single use.

(4) Used gowns should not be hung up or reapplied after removal. Single-use gowns prevent transfer of drug contamination to the environment and the worker's clothing (NIOSH, 2008).

c) Respirators: Wear a NIOSH-approved filtering facepiece respirator, such as a fit-tested N95, or a powered air-purifying respirator when inhalation exposure is possible (NIOSH, 2016c).

(1) Two examples are when administering an aerosolized HD or cleaning an HD spill.

(2) If gases or vapors are present, wear a chemical cartridge-type respirator (USP, 2017).

(3) Consult the drug-specific safety data sheet (SDS) for the type of respirator appropriate for the situation. Surgical masks do not provide respiratory protection from HD aerosols.

d) Eye and face protection: Wear goggles and face shield or a combination of goggles, mask, and face shield that provides splash protection whenever HD splashing is possible.

(1) Examples of situations where eye and face protection is necessary include when administering HDs in an operating room, working at or above eye level, or when cleaning up a spill (USP, 2017).

(2) When eye and face protection is worn, remove it after the gown, while still wearing the inner gloves.

2. Situations requiring PPE: Wear PPE whenever HDs might be released into the environment. NIOSH recommends that gowns and gloves be worn for all HD handling activities, and that eye, face, and respiratory protection be used when splashing or inhalation exposure is possible. The only exception is for administering an intact tablet or capsule provided in a unit-dose package, in which case a single pair of chemotherapy-tested gloves is sufficient (NIOSH, 2016b). The following situations require PPE (NIOSH, 2004):

a) Handling HD vials, ampules, or packaging materials

b) Introducing or withdrawing needles or dispensing pins from HD vials

c) Transferring drugs from HD vials to other containers using needles or dispensing pins and syringes

d) Opening ampules of HDs

e) Administering HDs by any route

f) Handling HD leakage from tubing, syringe, and connection sites

g) Discontinuing infusions of HDs

h) Disposing of HDs and items contaminated by HDs

i) Handling the body fluids of a patient who has received HDs recently

j) Cleaning HD spills

k) Touching any surface that is potentially contaminated with HD residue

I. Storage and labeling

1. In clinical areas

a) Store chemotherapy drug containers in a designated location that limits exposure of HCWs and provides appropriate storage conditions (e.g., temperature, light).

b) Use a distinct label on all HD containers to indicate the hazardous nature of the contents (OSHA, 2016).

c) Have access to instructions (e.g., SDSs) regarding what to do in the event of accidental HD exposure.

d) Check HD containers before taking them from the storage area to ensure that the packaging is intact and to detect any leakage or breakage.

2. Patient instructions for HD safety in the home (Polovich & Olsen, 2018; see Figure 12-1)

Figure 12-1. Safe Management of Chemotherapy in the Home

You are getting medicine used to treat cancer (chemotherapy, or "chemo"). You must be careful to make sure other people do not accidentally touch the drugs or your body waste for a time after treatment. This form teaches you and your family how to protect others from the chemo and how to handle the waste from the chemo in your home.

Chemo Drugs Are Dangerous
Chemo drugs are strong chemicals. Only patients who need chemo for treatment should take or touch the drugs. Items that touch the medicines (such as syringes and needles) are contaminated with chemo. Regardless of how you take the medicines, chemo remains in your body for many hours and sometimes days after your treatment. Your body will get rid of the drugs in your urine or stool. Traces of chemo also may be present in vomit.

Disposal of Chemo
Dispose of items contaminated with chemo separately from other trash. If required, the company supplying your medicines and equipment will give you a hard plastic container labeled with "Chemotherapy Waste" or a similar warning. Place equipment and gloves that have touched chemo into this container after use. If the waste is too large to fit in the plastic container, place it in a separate plastic bag and seal it tightly with rubber bands. Place sharp objects in the hard plastic container. The company will tell you who will pick up the disposal container.

Body Waste
You may use the toilet (septic tank or sewer) as usual. Flush twice with the lid closed for 48 hours after receiving chemo. Wash your hands well with soap and water afterward, and wash your skin if urine or stool gets on it. Pregnant women, children, and pets should avoid touching chemo or contaminated waste.

Laundry
Wash your clothing or linen normally unless they become soiled with chemo or body fluids, such as urine, stool, or vomit. If that happens, put on disposable gloves and handle the laundry carefully to avoid getting chemo on your skin. If you do not have a washer, place soiled items in a plastic bag until they can be washed.

Skin Care
Chemo spilled on skin may be irritating. If this happens, thoroughly wash the area with soap and water, then dry. If redness lasts for more than one hour or if a rash occurs, call your doctor. To prevent chemo from being absorbed through the skin, wear gloves when working with chemo, chemo-soiled equipment, or waste.

Eye Care
If any chemo splashes into your eyes, flush them with water for 10–15 minutes and notify your doctor.

Questions and Answers
Is it safe for family members to have contact with me during my chemo treatment?
Yes. Eating together, enjoying favorite activities, hugging, and kissing are all safe.

Is it safe for my family to use the same toilet as I do?
Yes. As long as you clean any chemo waste from the toilet seat, sharing is safe.

What should I do if I do not have control of my bladder or bowels?
Use a disposable, plastic-backed pad, diaper, or sheet to soak up urine or stool. Change immediately when soiled, and wash skin with soap and water. If you have an ostomy, your caregiver should wear gloves when emptying or changing the bags. Discard disposable ostomy supplies in the chemo waste container.

What if I use a bedpan, urinal, or commode?
Your caregiver should wear gloves when emptying body wastes. Rinse the container with water after each use, and wash it with soap and water at least once a day.

What if I vomit?
Your caregiver should wear gloves when emptying the basin. Rinse the container with water after each use, and wash it with soap and water at least once a day.

Is it safe to be sexually active during my treatment?
Ask your doctor or your nurse this question. Traces of chemo may be present in vaginal fluid and semen for up to 48 hours after treatment. Special precautions may be necessary.

(Continued on next page)

Figure 12-1. Safe Management of Chemotherapy in the Home *(Continued)*

How should I store chemo at home?
You should store chemo and equipment in a safe place, out of reach of children and pets. Do not store chemo in the bathroom, as high humidity may damage the drugs. Check medicine labels to see if your chemo should be kept in the refrigerator or away from light. Be sure all medicines have complete labels.

Is it safe to dispose of chemo in the trash?
No. Chemo waste is dangerous and requires separate handling. If you are receiving IV chemo at home, you should have received a special waste container for the chemo and equipment. This includes used syringes, needles, tubing, bags, cassettes, and vials. This container should be hard plastic and labeled with "Chemotherapy Waste" or a similar warning. Follow disposal instructions from your healthcare team.

Can I travel with my chemo?
Yes. Usually, traveling is no problem. Some chemo requires special storage (such as refrigeration), so you may need to make special arrangements. Check with your nurse, doctor, or medicine supplier for further instructions. Regardless of your means of travel (airplane, car, or other), always seal your chemo drugs in a plastic bag.

What should I do if I spill some chemotherapy?
You will have a spill kit if you are receiving IV chemo at home. In the event of a chemo spill, open the spill kit and put on two pairs of gloves, the mask, gown, and goggles. Absorb the spill with the disposable sponge. Clean the area with soap and water. Dispose of all the materials—including gloves, mask, gown, and goggles—in the chemo waste container.

a) Keep HDs out of reach of children and pets.
b) Store HDs in containers that provide protection from puncture or breakage.
c) Label HD containers to indicate the hazardous nature of their contents.
d) Provide instructions listing the procedure for handling a damaged HD container.
e) Store HDs in an area free of moisture and temperature extremes. Some HDs may require refrigeration.
f) Provide HD spill kits and instructions for their use.
g) Give verbal and written instructions about handling and storage of HDs, disposing of HD waste, and what to do with unused drug.

J. Safe handling precautions during compounding
1. Maintain sterile technique during the preparation of parenteral drugs. USP (2015) General Chapter 797 describes standards for the preparation of sterile products, including HDs. The environment in which sterile HD preparation takes place must meet all requirements for ventilation, including air exchanges per hour, particle counts, and negative pressure. See USP (2015) for the full standards.
2. Chemotherapy drugs
a) Prepare sterile cytotoxic drugs in a containment primary engineering control (C-PEC) that protects parenteral doses from microbial contamination and the environment from HD contamination (ASHP, 2006; NIOSH, 2004; USP, 2015, 2017). The two main types of C-PECs are BSCs and compounding aseptic containment isolators (CACIs).
(1) A BSC has an open front, inward airflow that creates an air barrier to prevent HD contaminants from escaping, and HEPA-filtered airflow to minimize bacterial contamination of sterile preparations.
(2) A CACI is an enclosed cabinet that does not allow air exchange with the environment except through a HEPA filter, with attached sleeves and gloves through which the operator performs drug manipulations.
(3) Requirements for C-PECs
(a) Must be located in a containment secondary engineering control, which is an area that is physically separate from other preparation areas and is at negative pressure to an adjacent ante area (USP, 2017)
(b) Must eliminate exhaust through a HEPA filter and be vented to the outside (ASHP, 2006; NIOSH, 2004; USP, 2017)
(c) Must be used by individuals trained to employ techniques that reduce contamination
(d) Must be cleaned, decontaminated, and disinfected at the end of drug preparation or immediately if a spill occurs (USP, 2017)
(e) Must be serviced according to the manufacturer's recommendations
(f) Must be recertified after relocation, repair, filter replacement, and/or every six months (National

Sanitation Foundation, 2016; OSHA, 2016)

(g) The exhaust fan of a BSC must operate continuously (ASHP, 2006; National Sanitation Foundation, 2016; USP, 2017) except when the BSC is being repaired or moved. After the fan has been off, the BSC should be decontaminated before use.

b) When unsterile HDs are being prepared, such as oral drugs that require compounding or crushing, a separate C-PEC should be used (NIOSH, 2016b; USP, 2017). For occasional use, the same C-PEC designated for sterile preparations may be used, but it must be decontaminated, cleaned, and disinfected afterward (USP, 2017).

c) Wash hands before donning PPE.

d) Wear chemotherapy-tested PPE.

e) If desired, place a sterile, plastic-backed, absorbent pad on the work surface.

f) Limit the number of items placed in the C-PEC to avoid interfering with airflow (ASHP, 2006).

g) Use safe technique when opening ampules (ASHP, 2006).

(1) Clear fluid from the ampule neck.
(2) Tilt the ampule away from yourself.
(3) Wrap gauze or an alcohol pad around the neck of the ampule.
(4) Break the ampule in the direction away from yourself.
(5) Use a filtered needle to withdraw fluid.

h) When reconstituting drugs from vials, avoid pressure buildup, which can result in the release of drug aerosols. A CSTD is recommended (USP, 2017). According to NIOSH (2004), a CSTD is "a drug transfer device that mechanically prohibits the transfer of environmental contaminants into the system and the escape of hazardous drug or vapor concentrations outside the system" (p. 44). CSTDs are supplementary engineering controls and do not eliminate the need for a C-PEC or PPE (NIOSH, 2004; USP, 2017).

i) Use tubing and syringes with Luer-lock fittings.

j) Avoid filling syringes more than three-fourths full (ASHP, 2006). An overfilled syringe may separate from the plunger end.

k) Spike IV bags and prime tubing with compatible fluid before adding cytotoxic drugs (ASHP, 2006; OSHA, 2016) or use a CSTD to minimize leakage and exposure (Harrison, Peters, & Bing, 2006; Sessink, Connor, Jorgenson, & Tyler, 2011; Sessink, Trahan, & Coyne, 2013; Siderov, Kirsa, & McLauchlan, 2010; Yoshida et al., 2013). Glass IV bottles should not be used for HDs because of the need for venting and the potential for breakage, both of which can result in exposure.

l) Other activities that should not be performed outside of a C-PEC

(1) Expelling air from an HD-filled syringe
(2) Spiking IV bags containing HDs with IV tubing
(3) Priming IV tubing with HDs
(4) Crushing HD tablets

m) Place a label on each HD container that says "Cytotoxic Drug" or a similar distinct warning.

n) Wipe the outside of the HD container (e.g., syringe, IV bag) with a moistened wipe before placing it in a sealable bag for transport. The act of wiping the final preparation will physically remove surface contamination (ASHP, 2006). Discard the wipe as contaminated waste. Avoid transferring HD contaminants to the outside of the transport bag.

o) Dispose of all material that has come into contact with an HD in a waste container designated for cytotoxic waste.

p) Remove and discard outer gloves, all other PPE, then the inner gloves.

q) Wash hands with soap and water before touching anything or leaving the work area.

3. Immunotherapy drugs

a) Use safe handling precautions (e.g., C-PEC, CSTD, PPE) for immunotherapy agents that are considered hazardous (NIOSH, 2016b).

b) A nuclear pharmacist prepares radiolabeled mAbs for infusion. Federal and state laws require that radiation safety warning signs be placed to designate the areas in which radioisotopes are stored or used (Iwamoto, Haas, & Gosselin, 2012).

K. Transporting HDs (OSHA, 2016)

1. Transport syringes containing HDs in a sealed container with the Luer-lock end of the syringe capped. Do not transport syringes with attached needles.
2. Select a transport receptacle that can contain HD spillage if dropped (e.g., a leakproof, zipper-lock bag), and add impervious packing material as necessary to avoid damage during transport.
3. Label the outermost HD receptacle with a distinct label to indicate that its contents are hazardous.

4. Do not transport parenteral antineoplastic drugs or any liquid HDs in a pneumatic tube (USP, 2017).
5. Ensure that whoever transports HDs has access to a spill kit and is trained in HD spill cleanup.

L. Safe handling precautions during administration (ASHP, 2006; OSHA, 2016; Polovich & Olsen, 2018; USP, 2017; see Appendix G)
1. Always wear chemotherapy-tested PPE.
2. Work below eye level.
3. Ensure that a spill kit and chemotherapy waste container are available.
4. Use a CSTD when the dosage form allows.
5. When a CSTD cannot be used, place a disposable, absorbent, plastic-backed pad on the work area to absorb any drug that may spill.
6. Use needles, syringes, and tubing with Luer-lock connectors.
7. Do not use glass bottles for HDs.
8. If priming occurs at the administration site, prime IV tubing with a fluid that does not contain the HD or by using the backflow method.
9. After IV drug administration, remove the IV container with the tubing attached (NIOSH, 2004; Polovich & Olsen, 2018). Do not remove the spike from IV containers to reuse tubing.
10. If using secondary tubing to administer sequential HDs, use a CSTD at the port above the pump so that the tubing can be safely disconnected and discarded with each subsequent dose.
11. Use detergent and water or cleansing wipes to wipe surfaces that come into contact with HDs (Polovich & Olsen, 2018).
12. Discard all HD-contaminated material and PPE in a designated chemotherapy waste container.

M. Special precautions for radioimmunotherapy (RIT)
1. Special precautions are necessary to protect HCWs from exposure while caring for patients receiving RIT. Radiation protection standards and regulations are determined by the U.S. Nuclear Regulatory Commission, FDA (radiopharmaceuticals), and state radiation regulatory agencies.
2. Occupational radiation exposure should be kept as low as reasonably achievable. This requires close collaboration between the healthcare team and the radiation safety officer (RSO). Three factors help provide protection (Iwamoto et al., 2012):
   a) Time: Limit the amount of time spent near the radioactive source. Radiation exposure is directly proportional to the amount of time spent near the source. After a patient receives RIT, the patient is considered the radioactive source.
   b) Distance: Maximize the amount of space between personnel and the radioactive source. Radiation exposure decreases as the distance from the radioactive source increases.
   c) Shielding: Add a protective barrier between the radioactive source and personnel. The type of shielding used depends on the type of radiation.
3. Radiation monitoring devices are used to measure occupational exposure.
   a) Monitoring of personnel: HCW monitoring is required by law whether a patient is treated as an inpatient or outpatient.
      (1) A film badge is the most widely used monitoring device. Each person caring for a patient receiving radiation therapy should be assigned a film badge that is only worn within the work environment, is changed according to institutional guidelines, and is not shared with anyone else (Iwamoto et al., 2012).
      (2) A dosimeter is another kind of radiation monitoring device. It can be a personal device or one that is shared after being reset.
   b) Monitoring of the environment: Environmental monitoring is done with a survey meter that reacts to the presence of ionizing particles. After a course of inpatient RIT is completed and before the room is cleaned, the RSO surveys the room, linens, and trash.

N. Handling a patient's body fluids
1. After HDs
   a) In general, safe handling precautions are recommended when handling a patient's body fluids for at least 48 hours after drug administration; however, some HDs may be present in excreta longer. For example, cyclophosphamide was present in the urine of patients for up to five days (Yuki, Ishida, & Sekine, 2015). If information about longer excretion time is known, use precautions for the entire time that HDs are likely to be present. Patients receiving oral HDs are expected to have HD residue in their excreta the entire time they are on the therapy and for at least 48 hours after the last dose.
   b) Wear double chemotherapy-tested gloves and a disposable gown when handling the blood,

emesis, urine, and feces of a patient after receiving HDs. Wear a face shield if splashing is possible (NIOSH, 2016b).

c) For an incontinent patient, clean the patient's skin well with each diaper change. Apply a protective barrier ointment to the skin of the patient's diaper area to decrease the chance of skin irritation from contact with drug metabolites (Polovich & Olsen, 2018).

d) Flush the toilet with the lid down after disposing of excreta from a patient who has received HDs. When a lid is not present, cover the open toilet with a plastic-backed pad to prevent splashing or release of aerosols during flushing. There is no research to support the effectiveness of double flushing in reducing contamination, but this may be helpful with low-volume-per-flush toilets (Polovich & Olsen, 2018).

2. After RIT (Iwamoto et al., 2012)

a) Institute standard precautions (gloves and gown) when handling the patient's body fluids (e.g., sweat, saliva, urine, feces, blood, semen, vaginal fluid). The duration of precautions varies depending on the radionuclide's half-life.

b) Consult the RSO or nuclear pharmacist for precautions based on the specific radioisotope.

O. Handling a patient's linens

1. After HDs (Polovich & Olsen, 2018)

a) To the extent possible, preclude the need for laundering linens and clothing by using disposable linens or leakproof pads to contain HD-contaminated body fluids.

b) Handle HD-contaminated bed linens and clothing while wearing PPE as follows:

(1) In the hospital setting

(a) Handle contaminated linens with PPE and place into a leakproof bag.

(b) In most institutions, all linens are handled as contaminated by laundry personnel before washing.

(2) In the home setting (Polovich & Olsen, 2018; see Figure 12-1)

(a) Wearing gloves, place contaminated linens into a washable pillowcase, and keep separate from other items.

(b) Machine wash linens and cloth diapers twice with regular detergent, separately from other household items.

(c) Discard disposable diapers in plastic bags to prevent leakage.

(d) Discard used gloves in a chemotherapy waste container or household trash based on local requirements.

2. After RIT (Iwamoto et al., 2012)

a) If body fluids are present, use standard precautions when handling the linens of a patient who has received RIT.

b) Keep linens in the hospital room until surveyed and cleared by the RSO or nuclear pharmacist.

P. Disposal of HDs and materials contaminated with HDs

1. In the hospital setting (NIOSH, 2004)

a) Place soft contaminated materials into a sealable, leakproof bag or a rigid chemotherapy waste container marked with a brightly colored label that indicates the hazardous nature of the contents.

b) Use puncture-proof containers for sharp or breakable items. Dispose of needles and syringes intact; do not break or recap needles or crush syringes.

c) Seal containers when full.

d) Do not dispose of drug-contaminated items in infectious waste (red) containers. Some facilities autoclave these materials (NIOSH, 2004; Smith, 2002), which does not deactivate HDs.

e) Follow institutional policy regarding disposal of partial doses of HDs when administration is interrupted. Some drugs (e.g., chlorambucil, cyclophosphamide) must be discarded as hazardous waste in designated containers if the container is not empty (Residues of Hazardous Waste in Empty Containers, 2011).

f) Only housekeeping personnel who have received instruction in safe handling procedures should handle chemotherapy waste containers. These personnel should wear gowns with cuffs and a back closure and two pairs of disposable chemotherapy-tested gloves.

2. In the home setting (Polovich & Olsen, 2018; see Figure 12-1)

a) Some agencies that provide HDs arrange for proper disposal of contaminated equipment.

b) Follow all the instructions applicable to the hospital setting except those related to handling the filled waste container (if provided).

c) Designate an area away from children and pets where filled containers are placed for pickup.

d) Follow county and state regulations regarding the disposal of chemotherapy waste.

Q. Procedures following acute HD exposure
1. Accidents, improper technique, faulty equipment, or negligence in C-PEC operation can lead to exposure.
2. Initial interventions
a) In the event of skin exposure: Remove any contaminated garments and immediately wash contaminated skin with soap and water. Refer to the SDS for agent-specific interventions.
b) In case of eye exposure: Immediately flush the eye with saline solution or water for at least 15 minutes (ASHP, 2006), then seek emergency treatment. Ideally, each area where HDs are handled should contain an eyewash station. An acceptable alternative is a sterile saline IV container connected to IV tubing.
c) In the event of inhalation exposure, move away from the area of exposure as quickly as possible. Depending on the severity of symptoms, seek emergency treatment from an employee health professional or emergency department. Refer to the SDS for agent-specific interventions.
d) For accidental ingestion, do not induce vomiting unless indicated in the SDS. Depending on the severity of symptoms, seek emergency treatment from an employee health professional or emergency department. Refer to the SDS for agent-specific interventions.
3. Reporting (Polovich & Olsen, 2018)
a) Employee exposure: Report HD exposure to the employee health department or as institutional policy requires.
b) Patient exposure: Report the exposure as institutional policy requires. In addition, inform the patient's healthcare providers.

R. Spill management
1. HD spills: Spills result in contamination of the environment and are a source of exposure for HCWs and others; therefore, HD spills must be contained and cleaned up as soon as possible (USP, 2017). Consider any HD leak greater than a few drops a spill. Spill kits must be available wherever HDs are stored, transported, prepared, or administered (see Figure 12-2). Train everyone who is responsible for spill management in spill cleanup. Because a qualified person must be available for spill cleanup whenever HDs are handled (USP, 2017), many organizations train all HD handlers. Some facilities may choose to designate a hazardous materials response team to clean up large spills (OSHA, 2004). In case of a spill involving an HD, follow these procedures.

Figure 12-2. Contents of an Antineoplastic Spill Kit

- 2 pairs of disposable chemical-protective gloves
- 1 pair of heavy utility gloves
- Low-permeability, disposable protective garments (coveralls or gown and shoe covers)
- Face shield
- Respirator
- Absorbent, plastic-backed sheets or spill pads
- Disposable towels (3–4)
- At least 2 sealable thick plastic hazardous waste disposal bags with an appropriate warning label
- A disposable scoop for collecting glass fragments and sharps
- A puncture-resistant container for glass fragments

Note. Based on information from American Society of Health-System Pharmacists, 2006.

a) Assess the spill to determine the need for additional help with cleanup.
b) Immediately post signs warning others of the hazardous spill to prevent them from exposure.
c) Don two pairs of chemotherapy-tested gloves, a disposable gown, and a face shield. Wear shoe covers if the spill is on the floor.
d) Wear a NIOSH-approved respirator that is appropriate for the spilled agent (OSHA, 2016).
e) Use items in the spill kit to contain the spill, such as absorbent pads, cloths, or spill control pillows.
f) Clean up the spill according to its location and type. Access the SDS for the spilled agent to determine if a deactivator is recommended (Gonzalez & Massoomi, 2010).
(1) To clean up a spill on a hard surface (ASHP, 2006)
(a) Wipe up liquids using absorbent pads or spill control pillows. Wipe up solids using wet absorbent pads.
(b) Pick up glass fragments using a small scoop or utility gloves worn over chemotherapy gloves. Do not use hands to pick up sharps. Place all sharps in a puncture-proof container.
(c) Place puncture-proof container and contaminated materials into a leakproof waste bag. Seal the bag. Place the sealed bag inside another bag, appropriately labeled as chemotherapy waste. For the moment, leave the outer bag open.
(d) Wash the spill area thoroughly, from least contaminated to most contaminated areas, using deter-

gent and, if recommended in the SDS, sodium hypochlorite solution (bleach) or a peroxide-based solution, based on the surface material and the spilled agent. These solutions reduce HD contamination on surfaces, but no one product removes all residue. If using bleach, allow contact with the surface for at least 30 seconds and follow with a neutralizer (e.g., 1% sodium thiosulfate). Rinse twice with clean water.

(*e*) Use fresh detergent solution to wash any reusable items used to clean up the spill and items located in the spill area. Use clean water to rinse the washed items. Repeat the washing and rinsing.

(*f*) Remove PPE and discard disposable items in the unsealed chemotherapy waste disposal bag.

(*g*) Seal the outer disposal bag and place it in a puncture-proof chemotherapy waste container.

(*h*) Follow institutional or manufacturer guidelines regarding cleaning or maintenance of equipment (e.g., an IV pump).

(*i*) Dispose of all material used in the cleanup process as contaminated waste according to institutional policy and federal, state, and local laws (ASHP, 2006).

(2) To clean up a spill on a carpeted surface (note that carpet is not recommended in HD administration areas) (ASHP, 2006)

(*a*) Don PPE, including a NIOSH-approved respirator.

(*b*) Use absorbent powder, not absorbent towels, to absorb the spill.

(*c*) Use a small vacuum with a HEPA filter (Gonzalez & Massoomi, 2010), reserved for HD cleanup only, to remove the powder. Dispose of the collection bag as chemotherapy waste. Clean the outside of the vacuum before storing.

(*d*) Clean the carpet as usual.

(*e*) Follow guidelines for a spill on a hard surface to clean and dispose of other contaminated items.

(3) To clean up a spill in a BSC or CACI (ASHP, 2006)

(*a*) Clean the spill according to the guidelines for a spill on a hard surface. Complete cleanup by rinsing the surface with sterile saline for irrigation.

(*b*) Include the drain spillage trough in the cleaning and decontamination efforts.

(*c*) If the spill contaminated the HEPA filter: Seal the open front of the BSC in plastic. Label any type of C-PEC as contaminated equipment. Schedule a C-PEC service technician to change the HEPA filter. Ensure that the C-PEC is not used before the filter is replaced.

(4) To clean up a spill in the home setting: See Figure 12-3.

Figure 12-3. Spill Kit Procedure for Home Use

If any chemotherapy ("chemo") spills, you need to clean it up as soon as possible. Spilled drugs can be harmful to people who do not need them for treatment.

1. Do not touch the spilled drug with bare hands.
2. Open the spill kit and put two gloves on each hand.
3. Put on the gown so that it closes in back.
4. Put on the face shield and respirator mask.
5. Use the spill pads or towels to control spill by putting them around the puddle to form a "V."
6. Soak up as much of the spilled drug as possible.
7. Put the pads or towels right into a plastic waste bag from the spill kit. Do not put them down anywhere.
8. Use the scoop to pick up any broken glass and place it in the box from the spill kit. Put the box in the plastic bag.
9. While still wearing the gloves, gown, face shield, and mask, wash the area with dishwashing or laundry detergent and water and disposable cloths or paper towels. Put the used cloths in the plastic waste bag.
10. Rinse the area with clean water using clean cloths. Place all used cloths in the plastic waste bag.
11. Remove the face shield, mask, gown, and then the gloves. Place them in the plastic bag and close it.
12. Place the first plastic bag into a second plastic bag and close it.
13. Wash your hands with soap and water.
14. If the spill occurs on sheets or clothing, handle them with gloves and wash them separately from other laundry. Wash clothing or bed linen soiled with body wastes in the same manner.
15. Call the home health nurse, clinic, or doctor's office promptly to report the spill. They will let you know about plans to replace the spilled chemo to complete treatment. They will also arrange to pick up the waste material or tell you where to bring it for proper disposal.

Note. Based on information from National Institute for Occupational Safety and Health, 2004.

From "Home Chemotherapy Safety Procedures," by C. Blecke, 1989, *Oncology Nursing Forum, 16,* p. 721. Copyright 1989 by Oncology Nursing Society. Adapted with permission.

g) Report and document HD spills according to institutional policy: For any spill greater than a few drops, complete a report about the spill and forward it to those specified by institutional policy (ASHP, 2006). Document the following:
   (1) Name of the drug
   (2) Approximate volume of spill
   (3) How the spill occurred
   (4) Spill management procedures followed
   (5) The names of personnel, patients, and others exposed to the spill
   (6) A list of personnel notified of the spill

2. Radioactive spills: In case of a spill of a radiolabeled mAb or contamination with the radioactive body fluid of a patient recently treated with RIT (Iwamoto et al., 2012)
   a) Restrict access to the area and contact the RSO immediately. Never try to clean the area or touch the radioactive source. Adhere to the principles of time, distance, and shielding discussed previously.
   b) Follow other applicable U.S. Nuclear Regulatory Commission guidelines.

S. Requirements for policies regarding the handling of HDs

1. Occupational Safety and Health Standards (2004) require that employers provide a safe or healthful workplace. Employers must implement policies and procedures related to the safe handling of HDs. Policies should address all aspects of handling these hazardous chemicals to protect employees, patients, customers, and the environment from contamination.
2. Such policies must do the following (NIOSH, 2004; USP, 2017):
   a) Outline procedures to ensure the safe storage, transport, administration, and disposal of hazardous agents.
   b) Describe the procedure for identifying new HDs and updating the list of HDs used in the facility.
   c) Require that all employees who handle HDs wear PPE.
   d) Mandate that HDs be prepared in a BSC or CACI (USP, 2017).
   e) Prohibit staff from eating, drinking, smoking, chewing gum, using tobacco, storing food, and applying cosmetics in areas where HDs are prepared or administered.
   f) Mandate initial training for all employees who prepare, transport, or administer HDs or care for patients receiving these drugs prior to assuming these responsibilities, and require retraining at least annually.
   g) Require training to include the risks of exposure and appropriate procedures for minimizing exposure. The policy should describe how training is documented (OSHA, 2012; USP, 2017).
   h) Require that documents such as SDSs are available to HCWs who handle HDs.
   i) Describe the procedures for management of HD spills.
   j) Set forth a plan for medical surveillance of personnel handling HDs.
   k) Ensure that employees of reproductive capability acknowledge in writing that they have been informed of the risks of HD exposure around pregnancy (USP, 2017).
   l) Address HD handling for workers who are actively trying to conceive or who are pregnant or breastfeeding.
      (1) Even when all recommended precautions are used, the potential for accidental exposure cannot be eliminated (Connor et al., 2010; Schierl, Böhlandt, & Nowak, 2009; Siderov et al., 2010; Turci et al., 2011).
      (2) Developing fetuses and newborn infants may be more susceptible to harm from certain HDs. Therefore, an additional level of protection is recommended for those most vulnerable to the reproductive and developmental effects of HDs (Connor et al., 2014).
      (3) Employers must allow employees who are actively trying to conceive or who are pregnant or breastfeeding to refrain from activities that may expose them and their infant to reproductive health hazards such as chemical, physical, or biologic agents (OSHA, 2016).
      (4) Alternative duty that does not include HD preparation or administration must be made available upon request to both men and women in the aforementioned situations or who have other medical reasons for avoiding exposure to HDs.
      (5) The employee has the responsibility of notifying the employer of the specific situation (e.g., preconception, pregnancy, breastfeeding). The American College of Occupational and Environmental Medicine provides guidelines for reproductive hazard management (Meyer, McDiarmid, Diaz, Baker, & Hieb, 2016).

m) Define quality improvement programs that monitor compliance with safe handling policies and procedures.

References

American Society of Health-System Pharmacists. (2006). ASHP guidelines on handling hazardous drugs. *American Journal of Health-System Pharmacy, 63,* 1172–1193. https://doi.org/10.2146/ajhp050529

American Society of Hospital Pharmacists. (1990). ASHP technical assistance bulletin on handling cytotoxic and hazardous drugs. *American Journal of Hospital Pharmacy, 47,* 1033–1049.

ASTM International. (2013). *Standard practice for assessment of resistance of medical gloves to permeation by chemotherapy drugs* (ASTM D6978-05[2013]). https://doi.org/10.1520/D6978-05R13

Baykal, U., Seren, S., & Sokmen, S. (2009). A description of oncology nurses' working conditions in Turkey. *European Journal of Oncology Nursing, 13,* 368–375. https://doi.org/10.1016/j.ejon.2009.04.004

Berruyer, M., Tanguay, C., Caron, N.J., Lefebvre, M., & Bussières, J.F. (2015). Multicenter study of environmental contamination with antineoplastic drugs in 36 Canadian hospitals: A 2013 follow-up study. *Journal of Occupational and Environmental Hygiene, 12,* 87–94. https://doi.org/10.1080/15459624.2014.949725

Blair, A., Zheng, T., Linos, A., Stewart, P.A., Zhang, Y.W., & Cantor, K.P. (2001). Occupation and leukemia: A population-based case–control study in Iowa and Minnesota. *American Journal of Industrial Medicine, 40,* 3–14. https://doi.org/10.1002/ajim.1066

Bouraoui, S., Brahem, A., Tabka, F., Mrizek, N., Saad, A., & Elghezal, H. (2011). Assessment of chromosomal aberrations, micronuclei and proliferation rate index in peripheral lymphocytes from Tunisian nurses handling cytotoxic drugs. *Environmental Toxicology and Pharmacology, 31,* 250–257. https://doi.org/10.1016/j.etap.2010.11.004

Buschini, A., Villarini, M., Feretti, D., Mussi, F., Dominici, L., Zerbini, I., ... Poli, P. (2013). Multicentre study for the evaluation of mutagenic/carcinogenic risk in nurses exposed to antineoplastic drugs: Assessment of DNA damage. *Occupational and Environmental Medicine, 70,* 789–794. https://doi.org/10.1136/oemed-2013-101475

Bussières, J.-F., Tanguay, C., Touzin, K., Langlois, É., & Lefebvre, M. (2012). Environmental contamination with hazardous drugs in Quebec hospitals. *Canadian Journal of Hospital Pharmacy, 65,* 428–435. https://doi.org/10.4212/cjhp.v65i6.1190

Caciari, T., Casale, T., Tomei, F., Samperi, I., Tomei, G., Capozzella, A., ... Rosati, M.V. (2012). Exposure to antineoplastic drugs in health care and blood chemistry parameters. *La Clinica Terapeutica, 163,* e387–e392.

Celgene Corp. (2017a). *Revlimid® (lenalidomide)* [Package insert]. Summit, NJ: Author.

Celgene Corp. (2017b). *Thalomid® (thalidomide)* [Package insert]. Summit, NJ: Author.

Chu, W.C., Hon, C.-Y., Danyluk, Q., Chua, P.P.S., & Astrakianakis, G. (2012). Pilot assessment of the antineoplastic drug contamination levels in British Columbian hospitals pre- and post-cleaning. *Journal of Oncology Pharmacy Practice, 18,* 46–51. https://doi.org/10.1177/1078155211402106

Connor, T.H. (2006). Personal protective equipment for use in handling hazardous drugs. *Pharmacy Purchasing and Products, 3*(9), 2–6. Retrieved from http://www.pppmag.com/documents/V3N9/2-6.pdf

Connor, T.H., DeBord, D.G., Pretty, J.R., Oliver, M.S., Roth, T.S., Lees, P.S., ... McDiarmid, M.A. (2010). Evaluation of antineoplastic drug exposure of health care workers at three university-based US cancer centers. *Journal of Occupational and Environmental Medicine, 52,* 1019–1027. https://doi.org/10.1097/JOM.0b013e3181f72b63

Connor, T.H., Lawson, C.C., Polovich, M., & McDiarmid, M.A. (2014). Reproductive health risks associated with occupational exposures to antineoplastic drugs in health care settings: A review of the evidence. *Journal of Occupational and Environmental Medicine, 56,* 901–910. https://doi.org/10.1097/JOM.0000000000000249

Connor, T.H., Sessink, P.J.M., Harrison, B.R., Pretty, J.R., Peters, B.G., Alfaro, R.M., ... Dechristoforo, R. (2005). Surface contamination of chemotherapy drug vials and evaluation of new vial-cleaning techniques: Results of three studies. *American Journal of Health-System Pharmacy, 62,* 475–484.

Constantinidis, T.C., Vagka, E., Dallidou, P., Basta, P., Drakopoulos, V., Kakolyris, S., & Chatzaki, E. (2011). Occupational health and safety of personnel handling chemotherapeutic agents in Greek hospitals. *European Journal of Cancer Care, 20,* 123–131. https://doi.org/10.1111/j.1365-2354.2009.01150.x

El-Ebiary, A.A., Abuelfadl, A.A., & Sarhan, N.I. (2013). Evaluation of genotoxicity induced by exposure to antineoplastic drugs in lymphocytes of oncology nurses and pharmacists. *Journal of Applied Toxicology, 33,* 196–201. https://doi.org/10.1002/jat.1735

Fent, K.W., Durgam, S., & Mueller, C. (2014). Pharmaceutical dust exposure at pharmacies using automatic dispensing machines: A preliminary study. *Journal of Occupational and Environmental Hygiene, 11,* 695–705. https://doi.org/10.1080/15459624.2014.918983

Fleury-Souverain, S., Nussbaumer, S., Mattiuzzo, M., & Bonnabry, P. (2014). Determination of the external contamination and cross-contamination by cytotoxic drugs on the surfaces of vials available on the Swiss market. *Journal of Oncology Pharmacy Practice, 20,* 100–111. https://doi.org/10.1177/1078155213482683

Fransman, W., Roeleveld, N., Peelen, S., de Kort, W., Kromhout, H., & Heederik, D. (2007). Nurses with dermal exposure to antineoplastic drugs: Reproductive outcomes. *Epidemiology, 18,* 112–119. https://doi.org/10.1097/01.ede.0000246827.44093.c1

Friese, C.R., McArdle, C., Zhao, T., Sun, D., Spasojevic, I., Polovich, M., & McCullagh, M.C. (2014). Antineoplastic drug exposure in an ambulatory setting: A pilot study. *Cancer Nursing, 38,* 111–117. https://doi.org/10.1097/NCC.0000000000000143

Gonzalez, R., & Massoomi, F. (2010). Manufacturers' recommendations for handling spilled hazardous drugs. *American Journal of Health-System Pharmacy, 67,* 1985–1986. https://doi.org/10.2146/ajhp100137

Halsen, G., & Krämer, I. (2011). Assessing the risk to health care staff from long-term exposure to anticancer drugs—The case of monoclonal antibodies. *Journal of Oncology Pharmacy Practice, 17,* 68–80. https://doi.org/10.1177/1078155210376847

Hama, K., Fukushima, K., Hirabatake, M., Hashida, T., & Kataoka, K. (2012). Verification of surface contamination of Japanese cyclophosphamide vials and an example of exposure by handling. *Journal of Oncology Pharmacy Practice, 18,* 201–206. https://doi.org/10.1177/1078155211419543

Hansen, J., & Olsen, J.H. (1994). Cancer morbidity among Danish female pharmacy technicians. *Scandinavian Journal of Work, Environment and Health, 20,* 22–26. https://doi.org/10.5271/sjweh.1433

Harrison, B.R., Peters, B.G., & Bing, M.R. (2006). Comparison of surface contamination with cyclophosphamide and fluorouracil using a closed-system drug transfer device versus standard preparation techniques. *American Journal of Health-System Pharmacy, 63,* 1736–1744. https://doi.org/10.2146/ajhp050258

Hemminki, K., Kyyrönen, P., & Lindbohm, M.L. (1985). Spontaneous abortions and malformations in the offspring of nurses exposed to anaesthetic gases, cytotoxic drugs, and other potential hazards in hospitals, based on registered information of outcome. *Journal of Epidemiology and Community Health, 39,* 141–147. https://doi.org/10.1136/jech.39.2.141

Hon, C.-Y., Teschke, K., Shen, H., Demers, P.A., & Venners, S. (2015). Antineoplastic drug contamination in the urine of Canadian healthcare workers. *International Archives of Occupational and Environmental Health, 88,* 933–941. https://doi.org/10.1007/s00420-015-1026-1

International Agency for Research on Cancer. (2018, January 26). *Agents classified by the* IARC Monographs, *volumes 1–120.* Retrieved from http://monographs.iarc.fr/ENG/Classification/ClassificationsGroupOrder.pdf

Iwamoto, R.R., Haas, M.L., & Gosselin, T.K. (Eds.). (2012). *Manual for radiation oncology nursing practice and education* (4th ed.). Pittsburgh, PA: Oncology Nursing Society.

Kiffmeyer, T.K., Kube, C., Opiolka, S., Schmidt, K.G., Schöppe, G., & Sessink, P.J.M. (2002). Vapour pressures, evaporation behaviour and airborne concentrations of hazardous drugs: Implications for occupational safety. *Pharmaceutical Journal, 268,* 331–337.

Kopp, B., Schierl, R., & Nowak, D. (2013). Evaluation of working practices and surface contamination with antineoplastic drugs in outpatient oncology health care settings. *International Archives of Occupational and Environmental Health, 86,* 47–55. https://doi.org/10.1007/s00420-012-0742-z

Ladeira, C., Viegas, S., Pádua, M., Gomes, M., Carolino, E., Gomes, M.C., & Brito, M. (2014). Assessment of genotoxic effects in nurses handling cytostatic drugs. *Journal of Toxicology and Environmental Health, Part A: Current Issues, 77,* 879–887. https://doi.org/10.1080/15287394.2014.910158

Lawson, C.C., Rocheleau, C.M., Whelan, E.A., Hibert, E.N.L., Grajewski, B., Spiegelman, D., & Rich-Edwards, J.W. (2012). Occupational exposures among nurses and risk of spontaneous abortion. *American Journal of Obstetrics and Gynecology, 206,* 327.e321–327.e328. https://doi.org/10.1016/j.ajog.2011.12.030

Levin, L.I., Holly, E.A., & Seward, J.P. (1993). Bladder cancer in a 39-year-old female pharmacist. *JNCI: Journal of the National Cancer Institute, 85,* 1089–1091. https://doi.org/10.1093/jnci/85.13.1089

Maeda, S., Miyawaki, K., Matsumoto, S., Oishi, M., Miwa, Y., & Kurokawa, N. (2010). Evaluation of environmental contaminations and occupational exposures involved in preparation of chemotherapeutic drugs. *Yakugaku Zasshi, 130,* 903–910. https://doi.org/10.1248/yakushi.130.903

Martin, C. (2017). Oncolytic viruses: Treatment and complications for patients with gliomas. *Clinical Journal of Oncology Nursing, 21*(Suppl. 2), 60–64. https://doi.org/10.1188/17.CJON.S2.60-64

Martin, S. (2005). Chemotherapy handling and effects among nurses and their offspring [Abstract of paper presented at the Oncology Nursing Society 30th Annual Congress, April 28–May 1, 2005, Orlando, FL]. *Oncology Nursing Forum, 32,* 425–426.

McDiarmid, M.A., Oliver, M.S., Roth, T.S., Rogers, B., & Escalante, C. (2010). Chromosome 5 and 7 abnormalities in oncology personnel handling anticancer drugs. *Journal of Occupational and Environmental Medicine, 52,* 1028–1034. https://doi.org/10.1097/JOM.0b013e3181f73ae6

McDiarmid, M.A., Rogers, B., & Oliver, M.S. (2014). Chromosomal effects of non-alkylating drug exposure in oncology personnel. *Environmental and Molecular Mutagenesis, 55,* 369–374. https://doi.org/10.1002/em.21852

Meyer, H.W., & Skov, P.S. (2010). Occupational rhinosinusitis due to etoposide, an antineoplastic agent. *Scandinavian Journal of Work, Environment and Health, 36,* 266–267. https://doi.org/10.5271/sjweh.2903

Meyer, J.D., McDiarmid, M., Diaz, J.H., Baker, B.A., & Hieb, M. (2016). Reproductive and developmental hazard management. *Journal of Occupational and Environmental Medicine, 58,* e94–e102. https://doi.org/10.1097/JOM.0000000000000669

Miyake, T., Iwamoto, T., Tanimura, M., & Okuda, M. (2013). Impact of closed-system drug transfer device on exposure of environment and healthcare provider to cyclophosphamide in Japanese hospital. *SpringerPlus, 2,* 273. https://doi.org/10.1186/2193-1801-2-273

Moretti, M., Grollino, M.G., Pavanello, S., Bonfiglioli, R., Villarini, M., Appolloni, M., ... Monarca, S. (2015). Micronuclei and chromosome aberrations in subjects occupationally exposed to antineoplastic drugs: A multicentric approach. *International Archives of Occupational and Environmental Health, 88,* 683–695. https://doi.org/10.1007/s00420-014-0993-y

National Institute for Occupational Safety and Health. (2004). *Preventing occupational exposure to antineoplastic and other hazardous drugs in health care settings* (DHHS [NIOSH] Publication No. 2004-165). Retrieved from http://www.cdc.gov/niosh/docs/2004-165

National Institute for Occupational Safety and Health. (2008, October). *Personal protective equipment for health care workers who work with hazardous drugs* (DHHS [NIOSH] Publication No. 2009-106). Retrieved from http://www.cdc.gov/niosh/docs/wp-solutions/2009-106/pdfs/2009-106.pdf

National Institute for Occupational Safety and Health. (2010). *NIOSH list of antineoplastic and other hazardous drugs in healthcare settings 2010* (DHHS [NIOSH] Publication No. 2010-167). Retrieved from http://www.cdc.gov/niosh/docs/2010-167/pdfs/2010-167.pdf

National Institute for Occupational Safety and Health. (2012). *NIOSH list of antineoplastic and other hazardous drugs in healthcare settings 2012* (DHHS [NIOSH] Publication No. 2012-150). Retrieved from http://www.cdc.gov/niosh/docs/2012-150/pdfs/2012-150.pdf

National Institute for Occupational Safety and Health. (2016a). Hierarchy of controls. Retrieved from http://www.cdc.gov/niosh/topics/hierarchy

National Institute for Occupational Safety and Health. (2016b). *NIOSH list of antineoplastic and other hazardous drugs in healthcare settings, 2016* (DHHS [NIOSH] Publication No. 2016-161). Retrieved from http://www.cdc.gov/niosh/docs/2016-161/default.html

National Institute for Occupational Safety and Health. (2016c). Respirator trusted-source information. Section 3: Ancillary respirator information. Retrieved from http://www.cdc.gov/niosh/npptl/topics/respirators/disp_part/respsource3healthcare.html#e

National Sanitation Foundation. (2016). *Biosafety cabinetry: Design, construction, performance, and field certification: Annex E.* Retrieved from http://www.nsf.org/newsroom_pdf/NSF_49-2016_Annex_E.pdf

Ndaw, S., Denis, F., Marsan, P., d'Almeida, A., & Robert, A. (2010). Biological monitoring of occupational exposure to 5-fluorouracil: Urinary α-fluoro-β-alanine assay by high performance liquid chromatography tandem mass spectrometry in health care personnel. *Journal of Chromatography B: Analytical Technologies in the Biomedical and Life Sciences, 878,* 2630–2634. https://doi.org/10.1016/j.jchromb.2010.02.011

Occupational Safety and Health Administration. (2012). Side-by-side comparison of OSHA's existing Hazard Communication

Standard (HCS 1994) vs. the revised Hazard Communication Standard (HCS 2012). Retrieved from http://www.osha.gov/dsg/hazcom/side-by-side.html

Occupational Safety and Health Administration. (2016). Controlling occupational exposure to hazardous drugs. Retrieved from www.osha.gov/SLTC/hazardousdrugs/controlling_occex_hazardousdrugs.html

Occupational Safety and Health Standards, 29 C.F.R. pt. 1910 (2004). Retrieved from https://www.gpo.gov/fdsys/pkg/CFR-2004-title29-vol5/pdf/CFR-2004-title29-vol5-subtitleB-chapXVII.pdf

Peelen, S., Roeleveld, N., Heederik, D., Kromhout, H., & de Kort, W. (1999). *Reproductie-toxische effecten bij ziekenhuispersoneel* [Toxic effects on reproduction in hospital personnel]. Amsterdam, Netherlands: Elsevier.

Petralia, S.A., Dosemeci, M., Adams, E.E., & Zahm, S.H. (1999). Cancer mortality among women employed in health care occupations in 24 U.S. states, 1984–1993. *American Journal of Industrial Medicine, 36,* 159–165. https://doi.org/10.1002/(SICI)1097-0274(199907)36:1<159::AID-AJIM23>3.0.CO;2-K

Pieri, M., Castiglia, L., Basilicata, P., Sannolo, N., Acampora, A., & Miraglia, N. (2010). Biological monitoring of nurses exposed to doxorubicin and epirubicin by a validated liquid chromatography/fluorescence detection method. *Annals of Occupational Hygiene, 54,* 368–376. https://doi.org/10.1093/annhyg/meq006

Polovich, M., & Olsen, M.M. (Eds.). (2018). *Safe handling of hazardous drugs* (3rd ed.). Pittsburgh, PA: Oncology Nursing Society.

Ramphal, R., Bains, T., Vaillancourt, R., Osmond, M.H., & Barrowman, N. (2014). Occupational exposure to cyclophosphamide in nurses at a single center. *Journal of Occupational and Environmental Medicine, 56,* 304–312. https://doi.org/10.1097/JOM.0000000000000097

Residues of Hazardous Waste in Empty Containers, 40 C.F.R. § 261.7 (2011). Retrieved from http://www.gpo.gov/fdsys/pkg/CFR-2011-title40-vol26/pdf/CFR-2011-title40-vol26-sec261-7.pdf

Sabatini, L., Barbieri, A., Lodi, V., & Violante, F.S. (2012). Biological monitoring of occupational exposure to antineoplastic drugs in hospital settings. *La Medicina del Lavoro, 103,* 394–401.

Santovito, A., Cervella, P., & Delpero, M. (2014). Chromosomal damage in peripheral blood lymphocytes from nurses occupationally exposed to chemicals. *Human and Experimental Toxicology, 33,* 897–903. https://doi.org/10.1177/0960327113512338

Schierl, R., Böhlandt, A., & Nowak, D. (2009). Guidance values for surface monitoring of antineoplastic drugs in German pharmacies. *Annals of Occupational Hygiene, 53,* 703–711. https://doi.org/10.1093/annhyg/mep050

Schierl, R., Herwig, A., Pfaller, A., Groebmair, S., & Fischer, E. (2010). Surface contamination of antineoplastic drug vials: Comparison of unprotected and protected vials. *American Journal of Health-System Pharmacy, 67,* 428–429. https://doi.org/10.2146/ajhp080621

Sessink, P.J.M., Connor, T.H., Jorgenson, J.A., & Tyler, T.G. (2011). Reduction in surface contamination with antineoplastic drugs in 22 hospital pharmacies in the US following implementation of a closed-system drug transfer device. *Journal of Oncology Pharmacy Practice, 17,* 39–48. https://doi.org/10.1177/1078155210361431

Sessink, P.J.M., Trahan, J., & Coyne, J.W. (2013). Reduction in surface contamination with cyclophosphamide in 30 US hospital pharmacies following implementation of a closed-system drug transfer device. *Hospital Pharmacy, 48,* 204–212. https://doi.org/10.1310/hpj4803-204

Siderov, J., Kirsa, S., & McLauchlan, R. (2010). Reducing workplace cytotoxic surface contamination using a closed-system drug transfer device. *Journal of Oncology Pharmacy Practice, 16,* 19–25. https://doi.org/10.1177/1078155209352543

Smith, C.A. (2002, November/December). Managing pharmaceutical waste—What pharmacists should know. *Journal of the Pharmacy Society of Wisconsin, 5,* 17–22.

Sottani, C., Porro, B., Comelli, M., Imbriani, M., & Minoia, C. (2010). An analysis to study trends in occupational exposure to antineoplastic drugs among health care workers. *Journal of Chromatography B: Analytical Technologies in the Biomedical and Life Sciences, 878,* 2593–2605. https://doi.org/10.1016/j.jchromb.2010.04.030

Sottani, C., Porro, B., Imbriani, M., & Minoia, C. (2012). Occupational exposure to antineoplastic drugs in four Italian health care settings. *Toxicology Letters, 213,* 107–115. https://doi.org/10.1016/j.toxlet2011.03.028

Sugiura, S.-I., Asano, M., Kinoshita, K., Tanimura, M., & Nabeshima, T. (2011). Risks to health professionals from hazardous drugs in Japan: A pilot study of environmental and biological monitoring of occupational exposure to cyclophosphamide. *Journal of Oncology Pharmacy Practice, 17,* 14–19. https://doi.org/10.1177/1078155209358632

Turci, R., Minoia, C., Sottani, C., Coghi, R., Severi, P., Castriotta, C., ... Imbriani, M. (2011). Occupational exposure to antineoplastic drugs in seven Italian hospitals: The effect of quality assurance and adherence to guidelines. *Journal of Oncology Pharmacy Practice, 17,* 320–332. https://doi.org/10.1177/1078155210381931

U.S. Food and Drug Administration. (2018, February 1). Medical device bans. Retrieved from https://www.fda.gov/medicaldevices/safety/medicaldevicebans/default.htm

U.S. Pharmacopeial Convention. (2015). USP General Chapter <797> Pharmaceutical compounding—Sterile preparations. In *The United States Pharmacopeia–National Formulary* (USP 38–NF 33). Rockville, MD: Author.

U.S. Pharmacopeial Convention. (2017). USP General Chapter <800> Hazardous drugs—Handling in healthcare settings. In *The United States Pharmacopeia–National Formulary* (USP 40–NF 35, Second Supplement). Retrieved from http://www.usp.org/sites/default/files/usp/document/our-work/healthcare-quality-safety/general-chapter-800.pdf

Villarini, M., Dominici, L., Piccinini, R., Fatigoni, C., Ambrogi, M., Curti, G., ... Moretti, M. (2011). Assessment of primary, oxidative and excision repaired DNA damage in hospital personnel handling antineoplastic drugs. *Mutagenesis, 26,* 359–369. https://doi.org/10.1093/mutage/geq102

Villarini, M., Gianfredi, V., Levorato, S., Vannini, S., Salvatori, T., & Moretti, M. (2016). Occupational exposure to cytostatic/antineoplastic drugs and cytogenetic damage measured using the lymphocyte cytokinesis-block micronucleus assay: A systematic review of the literature and meta-analysis. *Mutation Research/Reviews in Mutation Research, 770*(Pt. A), 35–45. https://doi.org/10.1016/j.mrrev.2016.05.001

Yoshida, J., Koda, S., Nishida, S., Nakano, H., Tei, G., & Kumagai, S. (2013). Association between occupational exposure and control measures for antineoplastic drugs in a pharmacy of a hospital. *Annals of Occupational Hygiene, 57,* 251–260. https://doi.org/10.1093/annhyg/mes061

Yoshida, J., Koda, S., Nishida, S., Yoshida, T., Miyajima, K., & Kumagai, S. (2011). Association between occupational exposure levels of antineoplastic drugs and work environment in five hospitals in Japan. *Journal of Oncology Pharmacy Practice, 17,* 29–38. https://doi.org/10.1177/1078155210380485

Yuki, M., Ishida, T., & Sekine, S. (2015). Secondary exposure of family members to cyclophosphamide after chemotherapy of outpatients with cancer: A pilot study. *Oncology Nursing Forum, 42,* 665–671. https://doi.org/10.1188/15.ONF.42-06AP

CHAPTER 13

Infusion-Related Complications

A. Complications during or shortly after parenteral administration of cancer treatment (Pérez Fidalgo et al., 2012)
   1. Infiltration: Passage or escape of intravenously administered drugs into the tissue
   2. Vesicant extravasation: Inadvertent leakage of drugs capable of causing tissue damage into the subcutaneous or subdermal tissue or other unintended sites (e.g., pleural space)
   3. Irritation: A localized inflammatory reaction at the infusion or injection site
   4. Flare reaction: A local allergic reaction along a vein caused by irritating drugs
   5. Infusion reactions: Reactions mediated by the immune system (e.g., hypersensitivity, anaphylaxis, cytokine release syndrome [CRS])

B. Extravasation
   1. Pathophysiology: Occurs as a result of one of two major mechanisms
      a) DNA-binding vesicants: The vesicant binds to nucleic acids in the DNA of healthy cells in the tissue, causing cell death. The dead cells release complexes, which are taken up by adjacent healthy cells. This process of cellular uptake of extracellular substances creates a continuing cycle of tissue damage as the DNA-binding vesicant is retained and recirculated in the tissue for a long period of time (Luedke, Kennedy, & Rietschel, 1979). Examples of DNA-binding vesicants include anthracyclines (daunorubicin, doxorubicin, epirubicin, idarubicin), dactinomycin, mitomycin, mitoxantrone, and trabectedin (Kreidieh, Moukadem, & El Saghir, 2016; Theman et al., 2015).
      b) Non-DNA-binding vesicants: The vesicant does not bind to cellular DNA. The vesicant has an indirect rather than direct effect on cells in healthy tissue. It is eventually metabolized in the tissue and is more easily neutralized than DNA-binding vesicants (Ener, Meglathery, & Styler, 2004). Examples of non-DNA-binding vesicants include plant alkaloids (vinblastine, vincristine, vindesine, vinorelbine) and taxanes, which as a group have usually been classified as mild vesicants (Ener et al., 2004; Schrijvers, 2003; Stanford & Hardwicke, 2003).
         (1) Taxanes
            (a) Cabazitaxel (Jevtana®) infiltration had not caused skin or tissue impairment in clinical trials or postmarketing reports at the time of this writing (Sanofi-Aventis U.S. LLC, 2016); however, clinical experience with this newer drug is limited.
            (b) Docetaxel (Taxotere®) extravasation may cause hyperpigmentation, erythema, and tenderness (Sanofi-Aventis U.S. LLC, 2015b). In a case report, erythema with significant swelling and accompanying reduction of arm range of motion was noted on the day following docetaxel extravasation from an implanted port. Despite dexamethasone and chlorpheniramine treatment, the erythema progressed to 18 × 15 cm in size one week later (Chang, Wang, Chen, Chen, & Wang, 2014). Recall dermatitis at a previous docetaxel extravasation site, occurring during subsequent docetaxel administration in another location, also has been reported (Kramer, Schippert, Rinnau, Hillemanns, & Park-Simon, 2011).
            (c) Paclitaxel (Taxol®) injection site reactions, including reactions secondary to extravasation, are usually mild and consist of erythema, tenderness, skin hyperpigmentation, or swelling at the injec-

tion site. These reactions have been observed more frequently with 24-hour infusions than with 3-hour infusions. Recurrence of skin reactions at a site of previous extravasation following administration of paclitaxel injection at a different site (recall reactions) has been reported. More severe events, such as phlebitis, cellulitis, induration, skin exfoliation, necrosis, and fibrosis, have been reported, and in some cases, onset occurred during a prolonged infusion or was delayed by a week to 10 days (Teva Pharmaceuticals USA, Inc., 2015). Most clinical reports of paclitaxel extravasation were published in the first few years following its U.S. Food and Drug Administration approval and were reviewed by Stanford and Hardwicke (2003), who concluded that paclitaxel was a "mild vesicant" (p. 276). Data suggest that the potential for tissue damage is dependent on paclitaxel concentration and infusion duration (Barbee, Owonikoko, & Harvey, 2014).

(*d*) Docetaxel and paclitaxel have also been classified as *exfoliants*, or drugs that may cause inflammation and peeling of skin without causing the underlying tissue death that typically occurs with "true" vesicants (Kreidieh et al., 2016).

(*e*) Phlebitis, cellulitis, induration, fibrosis, and necrosis following extravasation of paclitaxel protein-bound particles for injectable suspension (Abraxane®) have been identified during postapproval use and reported to the manufacturer. In some cases, onset of symptoms occurred during a prolonged infusion or was delayed by 7–10 days. Recurrence of skin reactions at a site of previous extravasation following administration of paclitaxel at a different site (recall reactions) also has been reported. The manufacturer advises monitoring the infusion site closely for possible infiltration during administration (Celgene Corp., 2015).

(*f*) The available published literature supports the safety of IV administration of taxanes at recommended concentrations and duration using peripheral venous access (Barbee et al., 2014). However, some patients may require central venous access device (VAD) insertion for taxane administration. In some institutions, paclitaxel may be administered over longer than 60 minutes through a peripheral line on an infusion pump. Institutions should establish monitoring procedures to minimize the risk of extravasation.

2. Factors affecting tissue damage severity following a vesicant extravasation (Schulmeister, 2011)
   - *a)* Type of vesicant extravasated (DNA-binding vesicants cause greater tissue damage than non-DNA-binding vesicants)
   - *b)* Concentration and amount of vesicant in the tissue (higher concentration or greater amount causes more damage)
   - *c)* Location of extravasation (areas with little subcutaneous tissue and those overlying veins, arteries, and nerves are more likely to have greater damage)
   - *d)* Patient factors, such as older age, comorbidity (e.g., diabetes), and impaired immunocompetence
3. Risk factors for peripheral extravasation (Goolsby & Lombardo, 2006; Sauerland, Engelking, Wickham, & Corbi, 2006)
   - *a)* Small, fragile veins
   - *b)* Previous multiple venipunctures
   - *c)* Sensory deficits
   - *d)* Application of topical skin numbing agents prior to venipuncture, which decrease sensation at and around the venipuncture site
   - *e)* Limited vein selection because of lymph node dissection, lymphedema, or limb removal
   - *f)* Impaired cognition, altered mental status (impairs ability to detect administration site sensation changes), or somnolence
   - *g)* Probing during IV catheter insertion
   - *h)* Inadequately secured IV catheter
   - *i)* Administration site in areas prone to movement (e.g., wrist, antecubital area)
   - *j)* Use of rigid IV devices (e.g., steel winged "butterfly" needles)

k) Prior treatment with irritating or sclerosing drugs, such as chemotherapy
l) Administration of a vesicant peripherally when the manufacturer stipulates it should be administered via a central line, such as trabectedin (Yondelis®, Janssen Pharmaceutical Companies, 2015). Data suggest that trabectedin can be safely administered via a central venous catheter such as a peripherally inserted central catheter or other central VADs, such as an implanted port (Martella et al., 2015).

4. Possible etiologies of peripheral extravasations (Sauerland et al., 2006)
a) Vein wall puncture, piercing, or trauma
b) Dislodgment of the catheter from the vein
c) Administration of a vesicant in a vein below a recent (less than 24 hours) venipuncture site
d) Administration of a vesicant in a vein below a recent or nonhealed vesicant extravasation site
e) Inadvertent intramuscular or subcutaneous vesicant administration

5. Risk factors for extravasation from central VADs (Sauerland et al., 2006)
a) Difficulty encountered during device insertion (e.g., probing during venipuncture, inability to advance guidewire or catheter)
b) Inadvertent slicing, piercing, or nicking of catheter prior to or during insertion
c) Device misplacement with catheter tip outside of the venous system
d) Insufficient length of noncoring needle (implanted port)
e) Inadequately secured noncoring needle (implanted port)
f) Presence of a fibrin sheath or thrombus at the catheter tip
g) Catheter migration
h) Long dwell time of catheters inserted using a subclavian approach, in which the catheter is placed between the clavicle and first rib (increases risk of catheter fracture secondary to compression or "pinch-off")

6. Possible etiologies of extravasations from central VADs (Gibson & Bodenham, 2013; Goossens, Stas, Jérôme, & Moons, 2011; Sauerland et al., 2006)
a) Inadvertent misplacement of catheter tip outside of the venous system (e.g., pleural space) during insertion procedure
b) Vein perforation during insertion
c) Postinsertion vein erosion
d) Catheter leakage, rupture, or fracture
e) Separation of the catheter from a portal body (implanted ports)
f) Incomplete insertion of a noncoring needle into an implanted port
g) Noncoring needle dislodgment from an implanted port
h) Backflow of vesicant along the catheter to the venotomy site secondary to fibrin sheath or thrombus at the catheter tip

7. Signs and symptoms of vesicant extravasation (see Appendix H)
a) Vein irritation and flare reactions may mimic some of the signs and symptoms of vesicant extravasation (see Table 13-1).
b) Vein irritation and flare reactions are unique to peripheral chemotherapy administration; they do not occur when chemotherapy is administered via central VADs because the chemotherapy is rapidly diluted in large veins (Wickham, Engelking, Sauerland, & Corbi, 2006). However, vesicant extravasation can occur from a central VAD due to inadvertent catheter tip placement outside of the venous system or erosion of the vein wall and may cause chest pain, shortness of breath, and shock secondary to blood loss (Gibson & Bodenham, 2013). Common terminology criteria for the adverse event of infusion site extravasation are found in Table 13-2.
c) Additional signs and symptoms of vesicant extravasation (Ener et al., 2004; Pérez Fidalgo et al., 2012)
(1) IV flow rate that slows or stops
(2) Resistance during IV bolus (push) vesicant administration
(3) Leaking around the IV catheter or implanted port needle

8. Possible consequences of untreated vesicant extravasation (Goolsby & Lombardo, 2006; Pérez Fidalgo et al., 2012)
a) Blistering (usually begins within three to five days)
b) Peeling and sloughing of skin (usually begins within two weeks after extravasation)
c) Tissue necrosis (usually evident two to three weeks after extravasation)
(1) DNA-binding vesicants remain in the tissue for long periods of time. The area of tissue necrosis becomes progressively larger and deeper over time.
(2) Non-DNA-binding vesicants are more easily metabolized in the tissue. Tissue necrosis is generally localized and improves over time.
d) Damage to tendons, nerves, and joints
e) Functional and sensory impairment of the affected area

Table 13-1. Signs and Symptoms Associated With Vesicant Extravasation, Venous Irritation, and Flare Reaction

Sign/Symptom	Vesicant Extravasation	Venous Irritation	Flare Reaction
Pain	Immediate: Pain typically occurs and is described as burning, stinging, or a sensation of coolness at and around the vesicant administration site. However, some patients do not experience pain when a vesicant extravasates. Delayed: Pain usually increases in intensity over time.	Aching and tightness along a peripheral vein, above the administration site, occurs as the drug infuses.	No pain occurs; the skin overlying or above the vein may itch.
Redness	Immediate: Redness in the area of the vesicant administration site commonly occurs but is not always present or may be difficult to detect if the extravasation is occurring deeper in the tissue (e.g., as a result of needle dislodgment from implanted port). Delayed: Redness generally intensifies over time.	The vein may appear reddened or darkened.	Immediate blotches or streaks develop along the vein, which usually subside within a few minutes. Wheals may appear along the vein.
Swelling	Immediate: Swelling commonly is observed and is easier to detect when extravasation is superficial (e.g., from a peripheral vein) rather than deep in the tissue (e.g., implanted ports). Delayed: Swelling typically increases over time.	Swelling does not occur.	Swelling does not occur.
Blood return	Immediate: Loss of blood return from IV device occurs.	Blood return should be present. If loss of blood return occurs, suspect infiltration of irritant.	Blood return is present.
Ulceration	Immediate: Skin integrity is intact. Delayed: If vesicant extravasation is not treated, blistering and sloughing begin within 1–2 weeks, followed by tissue necrosis that may require surgical debridement and skin grafting or flap placement.	Ulceration does not occur.	Ulceration does not occur.

Note. Based on information from Goolsby & Lombardo, 2006; Sauerland et al., 2006; Wickham et al., 2006.

f) Disfigurement

g) Loss of limb (rare)

9. Vesicant extravasation management: A suspected vesicant extravasation is best assessed and managed using a systematic and collaborative approach that involves the patient, the nurse administering the vesicant, and the prescribing physician. Vesicant extravasation management guidelines are listed in Table 13-3.

a) Initial management of extravasation: Assess the site and patient symptoms at the first sign of extravasation, during the time the IV device is assessed, and after initial management.

b) Steps to take when a vesicant extravasation occurs or is suspected (Goolsby & Lombardo, 2006; Schulmeister, 2011)

(1) Immediately stop administering the vesicant and IV fluids.

(2) Disconnect the IV tubing from the IV device. Do not remove the IV device or noncoring port needle.

Table 13-2. Common Terminology Criteria for Adverse Events Grading for Infusion Site Extravasation

	Grade				
Adverse Event	1	2	3	4	5
Infusion site extravasation	Painless edema	Erythema with associated symptoms (e.g., edema, pain, induration, phlebitis)	Ulceration or necrosis, severe tissue damage; operative intervention indicated	Life-threatening consequences; urgent intervention indicated	Death

Note. From *Common Terminology Criteria for Adverse Events* [v.5.0], by National Cancer Institute Cancer Therapy Evaluation Program, 2017. Retrieved from https://ctep.cancer.gov/protocolDevelopment/electronic_applications/ctc.htm.

(3) Attempt to aspirate residual vesicant from the IV device or port needle using a small (1–3 ml) syringe.

(4) Remove the peripheral IV device or port needle.

(5) Initiate appropriate management measures in accordance with Table 13-3 and institutional policies.

c) Vesicant extravasation antidotes and treatments

(1) Efficacy: The efficacy of extravasation antidotes and treatments is unknown, with the exception of dexrazoxane for injection, which has a 98.2% overall efficacy for treating anthracycline extravasation (Mouridsen et al., 2007). In two European studies, 53 of 54 patients with biopsy-confirmed anthracycline extravasation did not require surgical intervention after receiving dexrazoxane administered IV daily for three days. The median baseline extravasation area was 25 cm^2 (range 1–253 cm^2), and 11 patients had extravasation areas exceeding 75 cm^2. Thirteen patients had late sequelae at the extravasation site, such as pain, fibrosis, atrophy, and local sensory disturbance; all were judged to be mild (Mouridsen et al., 2007).

(2) No clinical trials have been conducted to determine the efficacy of dimethyl sulfoxide, sodium thiosulfate, hyaluronidase, growth factors, early surgical intervention, saline washout or flushing, hyperbaric oxygen, or 3% solution of boric acid in treating biopsy-confirmed vesicant extravasations from peripheral IV catheters and implanted ports. Information about these antidotes and treatments is anecdotal and based on case reports (Firat, Erbatur, & Aytekin, 2013; Goolsby & Lombardo, 2006; Schrijvers, 2003; Wickham et al., 2006).

Table 13-3. Vesicant Extravasation Management Guidelines

Classification/Drug	Immediate Topical Therapy	Antidote or Treatment	Administration, Monitoring, and Follow-Up
Alkylating agents • Mechlorethamine hydrochloride (nitrogen mustard, Mustargen®)	Apply cold pack for 6–12 hours following sodium thiosulfate antidote injection (Lundbeck LLC, 2012).	Antidote: Sodium thiosulfate Mechanism of action: Neutralizes mechlorethamine to form nontoxic thioesters that are excreted in the urine Preparation: Prepare 1/6 molar solution (4.14 g of sodium thiosulfate per 100 ml of sterile water for injection or 2.64 g of anhydrous sodium thiosulfate per 100 ml, or dilute 4 ml of sodium thiosulfate injection [10%] with 6 ml of sterile water for injection) (Lundbeck LLC, 2012). Storage: Store at room temperature between 15°C–30°C (59°F–86°F).	Inject 2 ml of the sodium thiosulfate solution for each milligram of mechlorethamine suspected to have extravasated. Inject the solution subcutaneously into the extravasation site using a 25-gauge or smaller needle (change needle with each injection). Dose may be divided into 3–4 syringes to inject around the site of extravasation. The needle should be changed with each new injection. Assess the extravasation area for pain, blister formation, and skin sloughing periodically as needed or in accordance with institutional policy. Instruct patients to monitor the extravasation site and to report fever, chills, blistering, skin sloughing, and worsening pain. Instruct patients with peripheral extravasations to report arm or hand swelling and stiffness.
• Trabectedin (Yondelis®)	Apply cold pack for 15–20 minutes at least 4 times a day for the first 24 hours.	No known antidotes or treatments exist.	Assess the extravasation area for pain, blister formation, and skin sloughing periodically as needed or in accordance with institutional policy (Janssen Pharmaceutical Companies, 2015). In collaboration with the provider, refer patients for specialized care when indicated or needed (e.g., plastic or hand surgery consult, physical therapy, pain management, rehabilitation services).

(Continued on next page)

Table 13-3. Vesicant Extravasation Management Guidelines *(Continued)*

Classification/Drug	Immediate Topical Therapy	Antidote or Treatment	Administration, Monitoring, and Follow-Up
Anthracenedione • Mitoxantrone (Novantrone®)	Apply cold pack for 15–20 minutes at least 4 times a day for the first 24 hours.	No known antidotes or treatments exist.	Extravasation typically causes blue discoloration of the infusion site area and may require debridement and skin grafting (Fresenius Kabi USA, 2013). Assess the extravasation area for pain, blister formation, and skin sloughing periodically as needed or in accordance with institutional policy. In collaboration with the provider, refer patients for specialized care when indicated or needed (e.g., plastic or hand surgery consult, physical therapy, pain management, rehabilitation services).
Antitumor antibiotics (anthracyclines) • Daunorubicin (Cerubidine®) • Doxorubicin (Adriamycin®) • Epirubicin (Ellence®) • Idarubicin (Idamycin®)	Apply cold pack but remove at least 15 minutes prior to dexrazoxane treatment.	Treatment: Dexrazoxane for injection (Langer, 2007; Schulmeister, 2007) Mechanism of action: Unknown Dose: The recommended dose of dexrazoxane is based on the patient's body surface area: • Day 1: 1,000 mg/m² • Day 2: 1,000 mg/m² • Day 3: 500 mg/m² The maximum recommended dose is 2,000 mg on days 1 and 2 and 1,000 mg on day 3. The dose should be reduced 50% in patients with creatinine clearance values < 40 ml/min. Preparation: Each 500 mg vial of dexrazoxane must be mixed with 50 ml diluent. The patient's dose is then added to a 1,000 ml normal saline infusion bag for administration. Storage: Store at room temperature between 15°C–30°C (59°F–86°F).	Initiate the first dexrazoxane infusion as soon as possible and within 6 hours of the anthracycline extravasation. Infuse dexrazoxane over 1–2 hours in a large vein in an area other than the extravasation area (e.g., opposite arm). The same arm should be used only when the patient's clinical status (e.g., lymphedema, loss of limb) precludes use of the unaffected arm, and a large vein above the extravasation site should be used for dexrazoxane administration. Dimethyl sulfoxide should not be applied to the extravasation area. Assess the extravasation area for pain, blister formation, and skin sloughing periodically as needed or in accordance with institutional policy. Instruct patients to monitor the extravasation site and to report fever, chills, blistering, skin sloughing, and worsening pain. Instruct patients with peripheral extravasations to report arm or hand swelling and stiffness. Instruct patients about treatment side effects (e.g., nausea, vomiting, diarrhea, stomatitis, bone marrow suppression, elevated liver enzyme levels, infusion site burning). Monitor patients' complete blood count and liver enzyme levels.
Antitumor antibiotics (miscellaneous) • Dactinomycin (actinomycin D, Cosmegen®) • Daunorubicin and cytarabine (Vyxeos™) • Doxorubicin hydrochloride liposome (Doxil®) • Mitomycin (Mutamycin®)	Apply cold pack for 15–20 minutes at least 4 times a day for the first 24 hours.	No known antidotes or treatments exist.	Assess the extravasation area for pain, blister formation, and skin sloughing periodically as needed or in accordance with institutional policy. In collaboration with the provider, refer patients for specialized care when indicated or needed (e.g., plastic or hand surgery consult, physical therapy, pain management, rehabilitation services).

(Continued on next page)

Table 13-3. Vesicant Extravasation Management Guidelines *(Continued)*

Classification/Drug	Immediate Topical Therapy	Antidote or Treatment	Administration, Monitoring, and Follow-Up
Plant alkaloids and microtubule inhibitors • Vinblastine (Velban®) • Vincristine (Oncovin®)	Apply warm pack for 15–20 minutes at least 4 times a day for the first 24–48 hours. Elevate extremity (peripheral extravasations).	Antidote: Hyaluronidase (Kreidieh et al., 2016) Mechanism of action: Degrades hyaluronic acid and promotes drug dispersion and absorption Preparation: Prepare per package insert. Do not dilute. Use solution as provided. Store in refrigerator at 2°C–8°C (36°F–46°F).	Administer 150 units of the hyaluronidase solution as 5 separate injections, each containing 0.2 ml of hyaluronidase, subcutaneously into the extravasation site using a 25-gauge or smaller needle (change needle with each injection). Assess the extravasation area for pain, blister formation, and skin sloughing periodically as needed or in accordance with institutional policy. Instruct patients to monitor the extravasation site and to report fever, chills, blistering, skin sloughing, and worsening pain. Instruct patients with peripheral extravasations to report arm or hand swelling and stiffness.
Taxanes • Cabazitaxel (Jevtana®) • Docetaxel (Taxotere®) • Paclitaxel (Taxol®) • Paclitaxel protein-bound particles for injectable suspension (Abraxane®)	Apply cold pack for 15–20 minutes at least 4 times a day for the first 24 hours.	No known antidotes or treatments exist.	Assess the extravasation area for pain, blister formation, and skin sloughing periodically as needed or in accordance with institutional policy. Instruct patients to monitor the extravasation site and to report fever, chills, blistering, skin sloughing, and worsening pain. Instruct patients with peripheral extravasations to report arm or hand swelling and stiffness.

(3) Anecdotal reports of treatment of peripheral and central VAD anthracycline extravasations with IV dexrazoxane administered as directed suggest efficacy in mitigating anthracycline-induced tissue damage (Araque Arroyo, Ubago Perez, Fernandez Feijoo, & Calleja Hernandez, 2010; Conde-Estévez, Saumell, Salar, & Mateu-de Antonio, 2010; Fontaine, Noens, Pierre, & De Grève, 2012; Langer, 2007, 2008; Uges, Vollaard, Wilms, & Brouwer, 2006). In a case report of IV dexrazoxane administration 72 hours after a peripheral epirubicin extravasation (and after being initially treated with topical dimethyl sulfoxide 99%), the patient had complete recovery without any sequelae (Aigner et al., 2014).

(4) Anecdotal reports of treatment of intracavitary anthracycline vesicant extravasations include saline washout of the pleural space with concurrent IV dexrazoxane administration (Chang & Murray, 2016) and video-assisted thoracoscopy (to visualize tissue damage) followed by thoracoscopic-assisted pleural lavage with periprocedural IV infusion of dexrazoxane (Aguirre, Barnett, Burdett, Joshi, & Viana, 2017).

(5) A case report described a liposomal doxorubicin extravasation initially treated conservatively with cold compresses on the affected arm. Three days later, when the patient's pain worsened and skin redness increased, she was treated with IV dexrazoxane and completely recovered (Vos, Lesterhuis, Brüggemann, & van der Graaf, 2012).

10. Documentation of vesicant extravasation and treatment: Key elements for inclusion in vesicant extravasation documentation are listed in Figure 13-1, and Appendix I shows an example of a vesicant drug extravasation record.

11. Patient follow-up: Dependent on individual patient needs and institutional policies

a) Periodically assess the patient's response to extravasation treatment.

(1) Assess patients receiving IV dexrazoxane on each day of the three-day

Figure 13-1. Key Elements of Vesicant Extravasation Documentation

- Date and time that extravasation occurred or was suspected
- Type and size of peripheral venous access device or type of central venous access device and gauge/length of noncoring needle (implanted ports)
- Location and patency of peripheral or central venous access device
- Number and location(s) of venipuncture attempts (for peripheral vesicant administration)
- Description and quality of blood return before and during vesicant administration
- Vesicant administration technique (e.g., bolus, infusion)
- Concentration and estimated amount of extravasated vesicant
- Symptoms reported by patient (e.g., burning, pain)
- Description of administration site appearance, including measurement of edema or redness if present
- Photographs of administration site that include date and time in the photograph field (follow institutional guidelines when obtaining photographs from patients)
- Assessment of extremity (if applicable) for range of motion and discomfort with movement
- Immediate nursing interventions (e.g., topical cooling or warming, authorized prescriber notification)
- Extravasation antidote or treatment administered
- Follow-up recommendations (e.g., return appointments, referral for wound care)
- Patient teaching (e.g., assessing skin, monitoring temperature, reporting pain) and patient's response to teaching

Note. Based on information from Schulmeister, 2011.

treatment and again four to seven days after completing dexrazoxane treatment.

(2) Assess patients receiving other extravasation treatments (e.g., heat/cold, hyaluronidase) on the day after the suspected extravasation and again four to seven days later.

(3) Assessments can be done in person or via phone with photographs sent electronically per institutional policy.

(4) Reinforce patient teaching to notify the provider of worsening signs and symptoms.

b) Assessment may include inspection and measurement of the extravasation area, skin integrity, presence of pain or other symptoms, arm and hand mobility (for peripheral extravasations), and sensation.

c) Obtain follow-up photographs that include or refer to the date and time they were taken per institutional policy.

d) In collaboration with the provider, refer patients for specialized care when indicated (e.g., plastic or hand surgery consultation, physical therapy, pain management, rehabilitation services).

e) Instruct patients to protect the extravasation area from sunlight, monitor the site, and report fever, chills, blistering, skin sloughing, and worsening pain.

C. Irritation

1. Irritants: Agents that may inflame and irritate peripheral veins

a) Examples include bleomycin, carboplatin, carmustine, dacarbazine, etoposide, floxuridine, gemcitabine, ifosfamide, liposomal daunorubicin, liposomal doxorubicin, streptozocin, and topotecan (Ener et al., 2004; Pérez Fidalgo et al., 2012; Sauerland et al., 2006).

b) Measures to reduce irritation during infusion

(1) Increase dilution when possible and/or infuse with concurrent fluid administration.

(2) Administer via larger rather than smaller peripheral veins for peripheral infusions.

(3) Apply a warm pack to the administration site during infusion.

(4) Assess the administration site and monitor for pain, redness, and swelling in patients receiving irritating agents.

2. Irritants with vesicant properties: Agents that may inflame and irritate peripheral veins and have the potential to cause skin and tissue damage (e.g., blistering, sloughing) when higher concentrations or specific amounts of the drug inadvertently enter the tissue. See Table 13-4 for irritant infiltration management guidelines.

a) Bendamustine hydrochloride (Bendeka®, Teva Pharmaceuticals USA, Inc., 2017; Treanda®, Cephalon, Inc., 2016): Postmarketing reports of infiltration include hospitalization for erythema, marked swelling, and pain; precautions should be taken to avoid extravasation (Cephalon, Inc., 2016; Teva Pharmaceuticals USA, Inc., 2017). A review of more than 250,000 patients treated with bendamustine worldwide identified seven reports of extravasation-induced tissue damage (Martin, Barr, James, Pathak, & Kahl, 2017). Dilution of Treanda in 500 ml normal saline and an infusion time of one to two hours reduced bendamustine-induced venous irritation in a study of 21 patients in Japan (Watanabe et al., 2013). Bendeka is prepared in 50 ml and administered over 10 minutes, and the infusion site should be monitored for redness, swelling, pain, infection, and necrosis (Teva Pharmaceuticals USA, Inc., 2017).

b) Immunotherapy agents: Although data on infiltration of these agents are limited, anti-

Table 13-4. Irritant Infiltration Management Guidelines

Drug	Description in Literature and Package Insert	Administration, Monitoring, and Follow-Up
Bendamustine hydrochloride (Bendeka®, Treanda®)	Irritant (usually) (Kreidieh et al., 2016) Vesicant (rarely) (Pérez Fidalgo et al., 2012) Infiltration may cause painful erythema (Cephalon, Inc., 2016).	Apply cold pack for 15–20 minutes at least 4 times a day for the first 24 hours. Assess the infiltrated area for pain, blister formation, and skin sloughing periodically as needed or in accordance with institutional policy. Instruct patients to monitor the infiltration site and to report fever, chills, blistering, skin sloughing, and worsening pain.
Irinotecan (Camptosar®)	Irritant (Kreidieh et al., 2016) Exfoliative dermatitis may occur (Pfizer Inc., 2016).	Flush the skin with sterile water and apply cold pack for 15–20 minutes at least 4 times a day for the first 24 hours (Pfizer Inc., 2016). Assess the infiltrated area for pain, blister formation, and skin sloughing periodically as needed or in accordance with institutional policy. Instruct patients to monitor the infiltration site and to report fever, chills, blistering, skin sloughing, and worsening pain.
Melphalan (Alkeran®)	Irritant (usually) (Ener et al., 2004; Goolsby & Lombardo, 2006) Vesicant (rarely) (Sauerland et al., 2006) Infiltration may cause local tissue damage (GlaxoSmithKline, 2010).	Apply cold pack for 15–20 minutes at least 4 times a day for the first 24 hours. Assess the infiltrated area for pain, blister formation, and skin sloughing periodically as needed or in accordance with institutional policy. Instruct patients to monitor the infiltration site and to report fever, chills, blistering, skin sloughing, and worsening pain.
Oxaliplatin (Eloxatin®)	Irritant (usually) (de Lemos & Walisser, 2005; Kennedy et al., 2003) Vesicant (rarely) (Azaïs et al., 2015) Infiltration can lead to redness, swelling, pain, and necrosis (Sanofi-Aventis U.S. LLC, 2015a).	A warm pack may reduce local pain and inflammation (Foo et al., 2003). Apply warm pack for 15–20 minutes at least 4 times a day for the first 24–48 hours. Elevate extremity (peripheral extravasations). High-dose dexamethasone (8 mg twice daily for up to 14 days) has been reported to reduce oxaliplatin infiltration–related inflammation (Kretzschmar et al., 2003). Assess the infiltrated area for pain, blister formation, and skin sloughing periodically as needed or in accordance with institutional policy. Instruct patients to monitor the infiltration site and to report fever, chills, blistering, skin sloughing, and worsening pain. Instruct patients with peripheral extravasations to report arm or hand swelling and stiffness.
Vinorelbine (Navelbine®)	Irritant (usually) (de Lemos, 2005) Vesicant (rarely) (Das & Gogia, 2016; Hadaway, 2007; Sauerland et al., 2006) Irritant; extravasation may cause local tissue necrosis (Sagent Pharmaceuticals, 2014).	Apply warm pack for 15–20 minutes at least 4 times a day for the first 24–48 hours. Elevate extremity (peripheral extravasations). Assess the infiltrated area for pain, blister formation, and skin sloughing periodically as needed or in accordance with institutional policy. Instruct patients to monitor the infiltration site and to report fever, chills, blistering, skin sloughing, and worsening pain. Instruct patients with peripheral extravasations to report arm or hand swelling and stiffness.

bodies are classified as irritants most likely because of their ability to cause local allergic reactions at the infusion site rather than direct cellular toxicity. Immune checkpoint inhibitors (e.g., ipilimumab, nivolumab, pembrolizumab) possess irritant potential and may cause thrombophlebitis (Plusching, Haslik, Bartsch, & Mader, 2016).

c) Targeted agents: Local swelling and redness have been observed with infiltration of proteasome inhibitors (e.g., carfilzomib, ixazomib) (Plusching et al., 2016).

d) Irinotecan (Camptosar®): Care should be taken to avoid extravasation of irinotecan. If infiltration occurs, topical flushing of the skin with sterile water and application of ice are recommended (Pfizer Inc., 2016).

e) Melphalan (Alkeran®)

(1) Has been classified as neither an irritant nor a vesicant (Dorr, Alberts, & Soble, 1986), as an irritant (Ener et al., 2004; Goolsby & Lombardo, 2006), and as a vesicant (Sauerland et al., 2006). Infiltration may cause local tissue damage. Administer over 15–20 minutes into a fast-running IV solution into an injection port on the IV tubing; do not administer by direct injection into a peripheral vein (GlaxoSmithKline, 2010).

(2) Care should be taken to avoid possible infiltration (e.g., monitor the IV site during a melphalan infusion), and in cases of poor peripheral venous access, use of a central venous line is recommended (GlaxoSmithKline, 2010).

f) Oxaliplatin (Eloxatin®)

(1) Has been described as both an irritant (de Lemos & Walisser, 2005; Kennedy, Donahue, Hoang, & Boland, 2003) and a vesicant (Azaïs et al., 2015). Case reports describe induration, edema, red-brown skin discoloration, hyperpigmentation, and rare instances of tissue necrosis (Azaïs et al., 2015).

(2) The manufacturer of oxaliplatin states that infiltration has, in some cases, included necrosis and injection site reactions such as redness, swelling, and pain (Sanofi-Aventis U.S. LLC, 2015a).

(3) Kretzschmar et al. (2003) retrospectively reviewed 11 cases of peripheral oxaliplatin infiltration and found that even with large-volume (40 mg or greater) extravasations of oxaliplatin, tissue necrosis did not occur.

(4) Pericay et al. (2009) published a case report of a 165 mg dose of oxaliplatin that infiltrated when a noncoring needle dislodged from an implanted port, resulting in edema and skin discoloration. They concluded that the effect was that of an irritant rather than a vesicant.

(5) In a case report, inadvertent intrathoracic infiltration of oxaliplatin caused pleural effusion and mediastinitis. Shortness of breath and chest pain resolved within a week of discontinuing the oxaliplatin infusion and initiating IV antibiotics (Leon-Ferre, Abu Hejleh, & Halfdanarson, 2012).

(6) Because cold packs cause local vasoconstriction, they may precipitate or worsen the cold neuropathy associated with oxaliplatin (Foo, Michael, Toner, & Zalcberg, 2003).

(7) A warm pack applied to an oxaliplatin infiltration site is preferable and may reduce local pain and inflammation (Foo et al., 2003).

(8) High-dose dexamethasone (8 mg twice daily for up to 14 days) has been reported to reduce oxaliplatin infiltration–related inflammation (Kretzschmar et al., 2003).

g) Vinorelbine (Navelbine®)

(1) Has been described as both an irritant (de Lemos, 2005) and a vesicant (Ener et al., 2004; Goolsby & Lombardo, 2006; Hadaway, 2007; Sauerland et al., 2006). Case reports have described skin discoloration, chemical phlebitis, localized rash, urticaria, blistering, and rarely, skin sloughing (Manganoni et al., 2012).

(2) The manufacturer of vinorelbine states that it is an irritant, and extravasation may cause local tissue necrosis or thrombophlebitis (Sagent Pharmaceuticals, 2014).

(3) A case report of vinorelbine infiltration from an implanted port described erythema and blister formation followed by ulceration, which was treated with heat, antibiotics, and subcutaneous hyaluronidase (Das & Gogia, 2016).

(4) Rapid IV infusion over 6–10 minutes followed by a flush of more than 75–125 ml of IV fluid may reduce vinorelbine-induced irritation (de Lemos, 2005).

3. Risk factors for irritation
   a) Small veins
   b) Prior treatment with irritating or sclerosing drugs, such as chemotherapy
4. Possible etiologies of venous irritation (Doellman et al., 2009)
   a) Low or high pH (less than 5 or greater than 9) of infused drugs
   b) Solutions with high osmolality
   c) Concentrated drugs or infusion solutions
5. Signs and symptoms of venous irritation: See Table 13-1.
6. Management of venous irritation
   a) Application of a warm pack may reduce local discomfort.
   b) Restarting the peripheral IV in a larger vein in another location may be indicated.
   c) Consult a pharmacist to explore further dilution of irritating medications.
   d) Instruct patients to report the development of a hard cord along the vein, pain, erythema, and temperature elevation.

D. Flare reaction

1. Characterized by transient erythema along the vein above the peripheral IV site and may be accompanied by pruritus and urticaria; blood return is present (Wickham et al., 2006).
2. May be observed during peripheral administration of anthracyclines or mechlorethamine (Wickham et al., 2006)
3. May occur during peripheral administration of doxorubicin and is thought to be caused by local release of histamine from mast cells or basophils (Curran, Luce, & Page, 1990)
4. Management of a flare reaction (Wickham et al., 2006)
   a) Verify presence of blood return. If absent, assess for signs and symptoms of extravasation.
   b) Flush the vein slowly with saline and observe for resolution of flare, usually within 45 minutes.
   c) An antihistamine may be used to treat a flare reaction and for premedication with subsequent cycles (Wilkes & Barton-Burke, 2018).
   d) If resolution does not occur, contact the provider.
   e) Do not resume the infusion through the IV site until the flare reaction resolves completely. Consider restarting the IV in another site.
   f) Document the flare reaction, including treatment and the patient's response.

E. Acute infusion reactions: Standard infusion reactions, hypersensitivity reactions, anaphylaxis, and CRS

1. Pathophysiology
   a) Infusion reactions can occur with any medication administered intravenously, and virtually all chemotherapy agents and monoclonal antibodies (mAbs) have the potential to induce these reactions (Khan, 2016). Infusion reactions are also referred to as *standard infusion reactions* by most allergists. In general, most infusion reactions are mild and may represent an irritant effect of the chemotherapy. It is prudent to differentiate between infusion reactions and hypersensitivity reactions, as the latter type of infusion reaction is characterized by an allergic component (Castells, Matulonis, & Horton, 2018).
   b) Standard infusion reactions involving mAbs may be the result of the antibody–antigen interactions that release cytokines, but the exact mechanism is unclear. The reactions with mAbs can be mild and usually occur with the first dose. Although standard infusion reactions can affect any organ system in the body, the most common signs and symptoms are flushing, itching, change in heart rate and blood pressure, dyspnea, back pain, fever, chills, rash, throat tightening, hypoxia, seizures, and dizziness or syncope (Castells et al., 2018).
   c) Hypersensitivity reactions are unexpected, mediated by the immune system, and usually allergic in nature. Immediate hypersensitivity reactions and anaphylaxis reactions are mediated by immunoglobulin E (IgE) mast cell activation or non-IgE mediated with mast cell activation and can be further divided into immediate or delayed (de las Vecillas Sánchez, Alenazy, Garcia-Neuer, & Castells, 2017). Most immediate hypersensitivity reactions are IgE mediated and are classic allergic reactions (Jakel, Carsten, Braskett, & Carino, 2016). See Table 13-5 for examples of chemotherapy agents associated with hypersensitivity reactions.
   d) Immediate hypersensitivity reactions to immunotherapy agents are IgE mediated in nature. Reactions with immunotherapy agents such as rituximab, alemtuzumab, and cetuximab are mostly standard infusion reactions in nature but have the potential to

induce anaphylaxis, as mAbs are complete allergens. Immediate hypersensitivity reaction can occur within five minutes after the start of the infusion to as late as six hours after its completion (Giavina-Bianchi, Patil, & Banerji, 2017). See Figure 13-2 for immunotherapy agents that have the potential for hypersensitivity reaction.

e) Anaphylaxis is a hypersensitivity reaction that is a systemic allergic reaction that can be life threatening. Although uncommon with most antineoplastic agents, it is well established with platinum drugs and taxanes (Giavina-Bianchi et al., 2017). Anaphylaxis with mAbs also occurs occasionally and has been reported with rituximab (5%–10%), trastuzumab (0.6%–5%), and cetuximab (1.1%–5%) (Bonamichi-Santos & Castells, 2016). Hypersensitivity reaction with platinum agents does not usually occur until the patient has received several doses of the agent (generally after six to seven cycles) (Boulanger et al., 2014).

f) Common signs and symptoms of anaphylaxis caused by IV medications

(1) Flushing, itching, angioedema (face, eyelids, or lips), cough, nasal congestion, shortness of breath, wheezing, sensation of choking, change in voice quality, tachycardia, fainting, hypo- or hypertension, loss of consciousness, nausea, vomiting, cramping/diarrhea, impending sense of doom, tunnel vision, and back, chest, or pelvic pain (Khan, 2016)

(2) An overlap exists between standard infusion reactions and anaphylaxis, but the hallmark symptoms of anaphylaxis are urticaria and angioedema (60%–90%); upper airway symptoms such as cough, wheeze, and throat tightness (50%–60%); flush (45%–55%); dizziness, syncope, and hypotension (30%–35%); and change in voice (Commins, 2017). See Table 13-6 for the National Cancer Institute Cancer Therapy Evaluation Program's grading criteria for allergic reactions, anaphylaxis, and CRS.

g) CRS is a potentially life-threatening systemic inflammatory reaction that is observed after infusion of agents targeting the immune system. CRS develops after cells are damaged and complement pathways are activated, which results in a drastic increase in systemic inflammatory cytokines and interleukins (Kroschinsky et al., 2017). This syndrome occurs with chimeric antigen receptor (CAR) T-cell therapy and agents such as rituximab and blinatumomab, and in serious cases may result in organ failure or death (Brudno & Kochenderfer, 2016). In most patients, however, the symptoms are less serious, consisting of mild, transient fevers and myalgias (Barrett, Teachey, & Grupp, 2014).

h) Symptoms of CRS

(1) Mild: Fevers (days to weeks), tachycardia, chills, nausea, anorexia, myalgia, headaches

(2) Life threatening: Capillaries leak fluid, which results in third spacing into the lungs and interstitial tissue, leading to intravascular depletion. CRS can occur

Figure 13-2. Immunotherapy Drugs Associated With Hypersensitivity Reactions and Cytokine Release Syndrome

Bispecific Monoclonal Antibody
- Blinatumomab

Chimeric Antigen Receptor T-Cell Therapies
- Axicabtagene ciloleucel
- Tisagenlecleucel

Interferons
- Interferon alfa
- Interferon beta (1A and 1B)
- Interferon gamma

Interleukins
- Aldesleukin
- Denileukin diftitox

Monoclonal Antibodies
- Murine
  - Ibritumomab tiuxetan
  - Tositumomab
- Chimeric
  - Brentuximab
  - Cetuximab
  - Rituximab
- Humanized
  - Alemtuzumab
  - Bevacizumab
  - Gemtuzumab ozogamicin
  - Trastuzumab
- Fully human
  - Ipilimumab
  - Ofatumumab
  - Panitumumab

Note. Based on information from Bavbek et al., 2016; Bristol-Myers Squibb Co., 2017; Gobel, 2007; Kite Pharma, Inc., 2017; Kroschinsky et al., 2017; Merck and Co., Inc., 2014; Novartis Pharmaceuticals Corp., 2017; Sloane et al., 2016.

Table 13-5. Chemotherapy Agents and Associated Hypersensitivity Reactions

Drug and Chance of Reaction	Description of Reaction	Prevention	Skin Test	Future Options After Reaction
Carboplatin 1%–19.5% Mostly after cycles 6–8	Urticaria or angioedema, bronchospasm, hypotension, rash, mostly after cycles 6–8	Skin test after 6th cycle is recommended and validated. Monitor later cycles and if patient is restarting therapy after an interval > 2 years.	Intradermal injection of 0.02 ml of undiluted form of the carboplatin preparation planned for infusion	Desensitization
Cisplatin 1%–5%	Mild to severe to lethal Urticaria or angioedema, bronchospasm, hypotension, rash	Skin test is not recommended or validated.	–	Possible desensitization; more experience is needed.
Docetaxel 30% during 1st or 2nd dose	Dyspnea, hypotension, bronchospasm, urticaria, rashes, edema	Premedicate with dexamethasone 16 mg/day for 3 days, starting 1 day before chemotherapy.	–	Substitution with paclitaxel if clinically appropriate
Epipodophyllotoxins • Teniposide: 4%–6%, mostly grade 1 or 2 • Etoposide: < 2%	Hypotension, dyspnea, bronchospasm	Slowly infuse for 30–60 minutes.	–	Rechallenge after premedication with antihistamines and steroids
L-Asparaginase 5%–8% but increases to 33% after 4th dose	Urticaria or angioedema, bronchospasm, hypotension Serious anaphylactic reactions occurring in less than 10% of patients	Skin test is not validated. Some experts state the skin test is of no use because of the high rate of false positives and false negatives.	Intradermal injection of 0.1 ml of a 20 IU/ml dilution of asparaginase	Desensitization or substitution with a different preparation (*Escherichia coli*, *Erwinia*, polyethylene glycol)
Oxaliplatin 0.5%–25% Reaction after several cycles	Urticaria or angioedema, bronchospasms, hypotension, rash, hemolytic anemia, cytokine release syndrome	Skin testing is reported to be 75%–80% accurate but not validated.	European Academy of Allergy and Clinical Immunology recommends a skin test at 5 mg/ml for prick test and 0.05 mg/ml and 0.5 mg/ml for intradermal test.	Desensitization
Paclitaxel 2%–4%, if proper premodications are given Develops with 1st or 2nd dose	Urticaria or angioedema, bronchospasm, hypotension	Premedicate with antihistamines, steroids, and ranitidine.	–	Desensitization with standard 12-step program if rechallenge caused a reaction; substitution with docetaxel if clinically appropriate
Procarbazine 6%–18%	Maculopapular rash, urticaria, cough, angioedema, interstitial pneumonitis	No reliable prevention exists.	–	Discontinuation of drug

Note. Based on information from Castells et al., 2018; Jakel et al., 2016; Kroschinsky et al., 2017; Lax et al., 2015.

Table 13-6. Common Terminology Criteria for Adverse Events Grading for Allergic Reaction, Anaphylaxis, and Cytokine Release Syndrome

	Grade				
Adverse Event	**1**	**2**	**3**	**4**	**5**
Allergic reaction	Systemic intervention not indicated	Oral intervention indicated	Bronchospasm; hospitalization indicated for clinical sequelae; IV intervention indicated	Life-threatening consequences; urgent intervention indicated	Death
Anaphylaxis	–	–	Symptomatic bronchospasm, with or without urticaria; parenteral intervention indicated; allergy-related edema/angioedema; hypotension	Life-threatening consequences; urgent intervention indicated	Death
Cytokine release syndrome	Fever with or without constitutional symptoms	Hypotension responding to fluids; hypoxia responding to < 40% O_2	Hypotension managed with one pressor; hypoxia requiring ≥ 40% O_2	Life-threatening consequences; urgent intervention indicated	Death

IV—intravenous; O_2—oxygen

Note. From *Common Terminology Criteria for Adverse Events* [v.5.0], by National Cancer Institute Cancer Therapy Evaluation Program, 2017. Retrieved from https://ctep.cancer.gov/protocoldevelopment/electronic_applications/ctc.htm.

as late as seven days after completion of infusion (Maude, Barrett, Teachey, & Grupp, 2014; Smith & Venella, 2016). Severe coagulopathy, with prolonged prothrombin time, partial thromboplastin time, and low fibrinogen levels, can occur with CRS, resulting in thrombocytopenia and increased risk of thrombosis. Acute kidney injury can occur with CRS as a result of changes in hemodynamics caused by a decrease in renal blood flow and glomerular filtration rate (Smith & Venella, 2017).

2. Risk factors for hypersensitivity and anaphylaxis
   a) Administration of a chemotherapy or immunotherapy agent known to cause hypersensitivity reactions (see Table 13-5)
   b) Preexisting allergies, such as to foods, drugs, and bee stings (Kashiwagi & Kakinohana, 2015)
   c) Premedication with fosaprepitant: Serious hypersensitivity reactions are rare with fosaprepitant and occur in less than 1% of infusions but can include anaphylaxis and anaphylactic shock during or soon after infusion of fosaprepitant (Pritchett & Kinsley, 2016).
   d) Previous exposure to the agent with mild symptoms (grade 1) of allergy
   e) Failure to administer known effective prophylactic premeditations
   f) First 5–15 minutes from the start of the infusion
   g) Nurses in infusion units should confirm patients' allergy history and observe patients closely for allergic reactions. Proper patient education is critical for early detection (Kashiwagi & Kakinohana, 2015).
3. Risk factors for CRS
   a) CAR T-cell therapy: CAR T-cell therapy is a form of immunotherapy using genetically modified CD19-positive T cells to produce receptors called chimeric antigens in the treatment of B-cell malignancies. The T cells are isolated and modified using a lentiviral vector to cause apoptosis of CD19-positive cells commonly expressed on B-cell lymphomas and acute lymphoblastic leukemia.
      (1) CRS is the main complication experienced after the cell infusion and is caused by release of interleukin-6 leading to systemic inflammation. It is seen within the first 12 hours to 5 days in patients with leukemia and 2–10 days in patients with lymphoma (Smith & Venella, 2017).
      (2) In clinical trials with tisagenlecleucel (Kymriah®), an approved CAR T-cell therapy, CRS occurred in more than 20% of treated patients. Tocilizumab is a mAb used to treat CRS. It targets interleukin-6 and resolves symptoms within 24–48 hours (Genentech, Inc., 2017; Novartis Pharmaceuticals Corp., 2017).

b) First infusion of rituximab: Greater than 50% incidence (LaCasce, Castells, Burstein, & Meyerhardt, 2017)
c) Chemotherapy-naïve patients receiving mAbs
d) Patients with leukemia or lymphoma, especially those with high lymphocyte counts (greater than 25,000/mm^3) (Kroschinsky et al., 2017; Maude et al., 2014; Smith & Venella, 2017)

4. Preadministration guidelines: Implement the following steps to prevent and manage hypersensitivity reactions, anaphylaxis, and infusion reactions.
   a) Obtain and record baseline vital signs.
   b) Review patients' allergy history (e.g., food, medication, environment).
   c) Administer premedications as ordered. Common premedications include histamine (H) antagonists (e.g., H_1 antagonist [diphenhydramine], H_2 antagonist [ranitidine or famotidine]), acetaminophen (for mAbs), and corticosteroids (LaCasce et al., 2017).
   d) Ensure that emergency equipment and medications are readily available.
   e) Obtain provider orders for emergency treatment before drug administration. Written standing orders for management of hypersensitivity and infusion reactions are recommended (Gobel, 2005; Lenz, 2007; Viale, 2009).
   f) Instruct patients to report symptoms of hypersensitivity and infusion reaction.
   g) Monitor for reactions with each treatment.
      (1) Hypersensitivity reactions can occur with a patient's repeated exposure to a drug and at any time during the infusion or the treatment cycle. The majority of reactions occur during the first or second exposure, so many clinicians eliminate the premedications for subsequent infusions if no reaction occurred.
      (2) However, 10%–30% of infusion reaction will occur after the second exposure. For example, the incidence of hypersensitivity reactions with platinum-containing agents increases with multiple doses and can occur after the infusion has completed (Castells et al., 2018; LaCasce et al., 2017). No data exist to support routine premedications prior to all cycles of platinum agents in the absence of prior reaction. Although it is reasonable to consider premedications or a graduated infusion rate for patients receiving cycle 5 or beyond of a platinum-containing agent, the determination is made on a case-by-case basis (Castells et al., 2018).
      (3) See Table 13-7 for emergency medications.

5. Skin testing
   a) Skin testing has limited value with most chemotherapy with the exception of platinum-containing drugs. This practice is useful because it helps to evaluate whether the patient is truly allergic to the drug or class. Skin testing for other drugs is considered investigational and not widely performed (Lax, Long, & Banerji, 2015).
   b) Only allergy/immunology specialists with special training in technique, interpretation, and management of the rare allergic reactions should perform these tests in highly sensitive patients because of the risk of dermatologic or other toxicities associated with chemotherapy skin testing (Castells et al., 2018).
   c) Very limited data are available for skin testing with immunotherapy agents, and it is currently not recommended (Khan, 2016).

6. Emergency management of anaphylaxis: Assess and treat symptoms as quickly as possible, as respiratory or cardiac arrest and death can occur within several minutes.
   a) Stop drug infusion immediately and remove the allergen.
   b) Maintain an IV line with normal saline or another appropriate solution.
   c) Stay with the patient. Request that another staff member notify the provider and emergency team, or, if outside the hospital setting, call local emergency medical services.
   d) Place the patient in a comfortable position and assess the airway. Maintain the patient in an upright position if short of breath or vomiting. Have the patient lie flat and elevate legs if hypotensive (systolic blood pressure lower than 60 mm Hg).
   e) Monitor vital signs (pulse, respirations, blood pressure, oxygen saturation) every 2 minutes until the patient is stable, then every 5 minutes for 30 minutes, then every 15 minutes. Monitor electrocardiogram for serious reactions.
   f) Maintain airway, assessing the patient for increasing respiratory tract edema. Administer oxygen if needed. Anticipate the need for cardiopulmonary resuscitation.
   g) Administer emergency medications based on symptoms (Commins, 2017; see Table 13-7). Figure 13-3 provides a guide for the treatment of infusion reactions.

Table 13-7. Emergency Drugs for Use With Hypersensitivity or Anaphylactic Reactions[a]

Indication	Drug	Dose	Comments
Bronchial constriction (dyspnea, wheezing, stridor)	Epinephrine	0.1–0.5 mg IM into thigh (0.1–0.5 ml of 1:1,000 solution or EpiPen® 0.3 mg automatic device); IV administration is indicated for patients with profound hypotension or signs or symptoms of impending shock and have not responded to IM dose.	IM administration is preferred over IV to minimize adverse cardiac effects. Anterolateral thigh is preferable to deltoid (may also be administered by inhalation or subcutaneously). Repeat every 5–10 minutes if needed.
Shortness of breath, tachypnea (rate > 20 breaths per minute), or decreased oxygen saturation	Oxygen	8–10 L/min by face mask; 100% face mask if needed	Patients who are hemodynamically unstable may also benefit from oxygen.
	Albuterol	2.5 mg/3 ml of 0.083% inhalation solution by nebulizer	Hold if heart rate is > 110 beats per minute.
Hypotension (> 30% decrease in systolic blood pressure from baseline)	Epinephrine	0.1–0.5 mg IM into thigh (0.1–0.5 ml of 1:1,000 solution or EpiPen 0.3 mg automatic device) or 50–100 mcg IV bolus (0.2 mcg/kg) for hypotension (0.5–1 ml of 1:10,000 solution)	IM administration is preferred over IV to minimize adverse cardiac effects, except in the presence of cardiovascular collapse. Cardiac monitoring is recommended.
	Normal saline IV	500 ml fluid bolus	Administer over 10 minutes × 1, then as ordered. Multiple fluid boluses may be required if patient remains hypotensive despite epinephrine. Massive fluid shifts can occur.
Hives, itching, flushing, swollen lips or tongue	Diphenhydramine	25–50 mg IVP	To counteract the multiple effects of histamine release, both H_1 and H_2 antagonists should be administered.
	Famotidine OR	20 mg IV	
	Ranitidine	50 mg IV	
To prevent delayed reaction	Methylprednisolone	30–50 mg IV	Limited evidence is available to support this recommendation, although steroids have frequently been used.
	Hydrocortisone injection	100–500 mg IV	
	Dexamethasone	10–20 mg IV	

[a] Additional emergency medications (e.g., sodium bicarbonate, furosemide, lidocaine, naloxone hydrochloride, sublingual nitroglycerine) and emergency supplies (e.g., oxygen, suction machine with catheters, bag valve mask) should be available in case of medical emergency.

IM—intramuscular; IV—intravenous; IVP—intravenous push

Note. Based on information from Campbell & Kelso, 2017; Commins, 2017; Giavina-Bianchi et al., 2017; Soar, 2009.

h) Provide emotional support to the patient and family.

i) Document all treatments and the patient's response in the medical record.

j) Symptoms of anaphylaxis may recur hours after initial intervention; therefore, patients who have experienced a grade 3 or 4 reaction (National Cancer Institute Cancer Therapy Evaluation Program, 2017) should be hospitalized and monitored closely for 24 hours (Bonamichi-Santos & Castells, 2016). See Table 13-6 for grading criteria.

k) For patients who experience a suspected anaphylactic reaction, a red top tube, drawn one to three hours after the reaction and sent for tryptase assay, should be considered.

(1) Any elevation in serum total tryptase is consistent with anaphylaxis; however, a normal value does not exclude anaphylaxis because it may be a false negative based on the timing of the draw. To reduce the risk of a false-positive result, the sample should not be drawn at the onset of the symptoms (Giavina-Bianchi et al., 2017).

(2) Avoid administering subsequent doses if the patient is considered to be sensitized to the drug. If the drug is critical to the treatment plan, refer the patient to an allergist who is qualified in drug desensitization (Bonamichi-Santos & Castells, 2016). Drug desensitization is

Figure 13-3. Infusion-Related Toxicity Algorithm

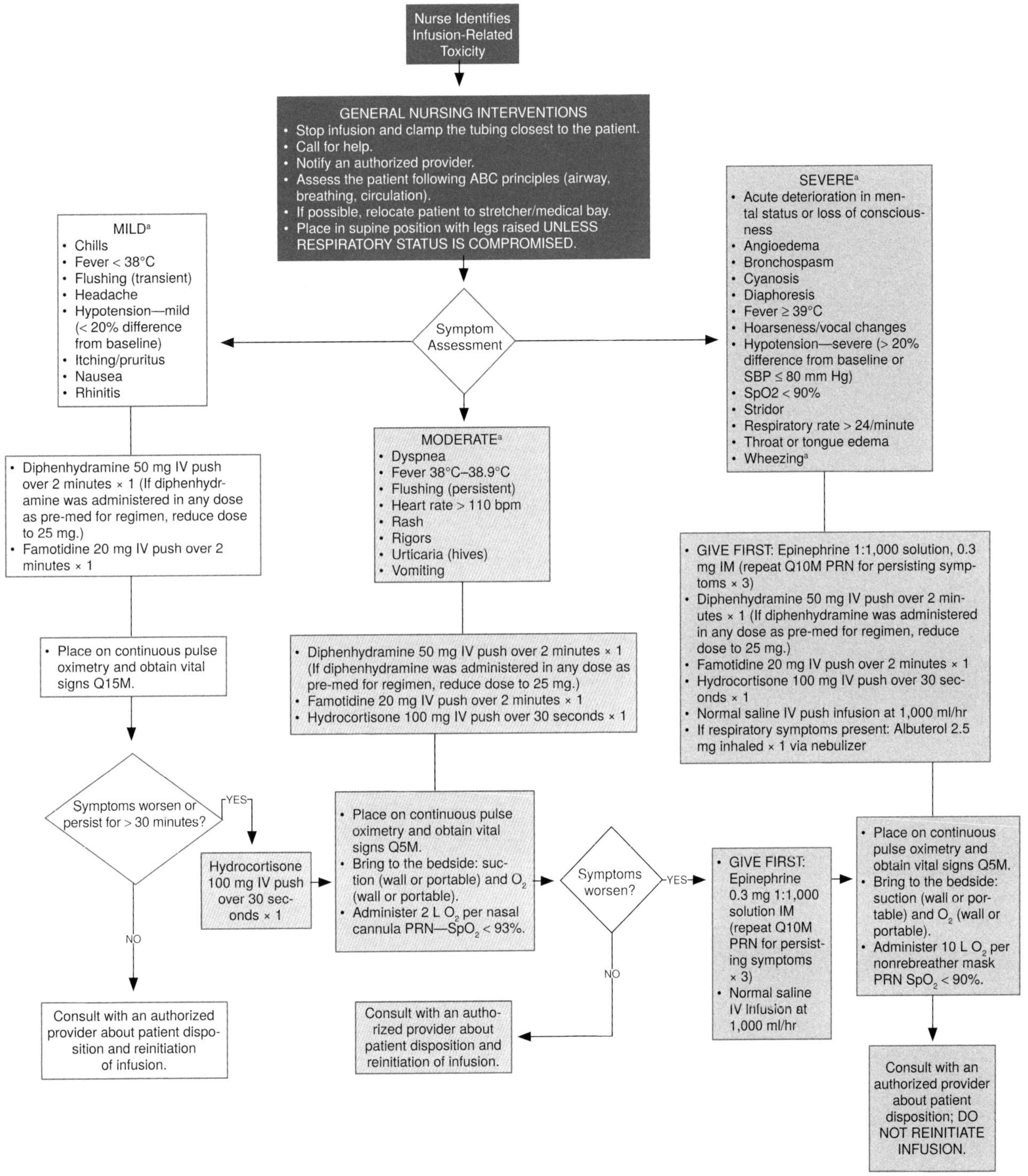
Nurse Identifies Infusion-Related Toxicity
GENERAL NURSING INTERVENTIONS
• Stop infusion and clamp the tubing closest to the patient.
• Call for help.
• Notify an authorized provider.
• Assess the patient following ABC principles (airway, breathing, circulation).
• If possible, relocate patient to stretcher/medical bay.
• Place in supine position with legs raised UNLESS RESPIRATORY STATUS IS COMPROMISED.
Symptom Assessment
MILD[a]
• Chills
• Fever < 38°C
• Flushing (transient)
• Headache
• Hypotension—mild (< 20% difference from baseline)
• Itching/pruritus
• Nausea
• Rhinitis
• Diphenhydramine 50 mg IV push over 2 minutes × 1 (If diphenhydramine was administered in any dose as pre-med for regimen, reduce dose to 25 mg.)
• Famotidine 20 mg IV push over 2 minutes × 1
• Place on continuous pulse oximetry and obtain vital signs Q15M.
Symptoms worsen or persist for > 30 minutes?
YES
Hydrocortisone 100 mg IV push over 30 seconds × 1
NO
Consult with an authorized provider about patient disposition and reinitiation of infusion.
MODERATE[a]
• Dyspnea
• Fever 38°C–38.9°C
• Flushing (persistent)
• Heart rate > 110 bpm
• Rash
• Rigors
• Urticaria (hives)
• Vomiting
• Diphenhydramine 50 mg IV push over 2 minutes × 1 (If diphenhydramine was administered in any dose as pre-med for regimen, reduce dose to 25 mg.)
• Famotidine 20 mg IV push over 2 minutes × 1
• Hydrocortisone 100 mg IV push over 30 seconds × 1
• Place on continuous pulse oximetry and obtain vital signs Q5M.
• Bring to the bedside: suction (wall or portable) and O_2 (wall or portable).
• Administer 2 L O_2 per nasal cannula PRN—SpO_2 < 93%.
Symptoms worsen?
YES
NO
Consult with an authorized provider about patient disposition and reinitiation of infusion.
SEVERE[a]
• Acute deterioration in mental status or loss of consciousness
• Angioedema
• Bronchospasm
• Cyanosis
• Diaphoresis
• Fever ≥ 39°C
• Hoarseness/vocal changes
• Hypotension—severe (> 20% difference from baseline or SBP ≤ 80 mm Hg)
• SpO2 < 90%
• Stridor
• Respiratory rate > 24/minute
• Throat or tongue edema
• Wheezing[a]
• GIVE FIRST: Epinephrine 1:1,000 solution, 0.3 mg IM (repeat Q10M PRN for persisting symptoms × 3)
• Diphenhydramine 50 mg IV push over 2 minutes × 1 (If diphenhydramine was administered in any dose as pre-med for regimen, reduce dose to 25 mg.)
• Famotidine 20 mg IV push over 2 minutes × 1
• Hydrocortisone 100 mg IV push over 30 seconds × 1
• Normal saline IV push infusion at 1,000 ml/hr
• If respiratory symptoms present: Albuterol 2.5 mg inhaled × 1 via nebulizer
• GIVE FIRST: Epinephrine 0.3 mg 1:1,000 solution IM (repeat Q10M PRN for persisting symptoms × 3)
• Normal saline IV infusion at 1,000 ml/hr
• Place on continuous pulse oximetry and obtain vital signs Q5M.
• Bring to the bedside: suction (wall or portable) and O_2 (wall or portable).
• Administer 10 L O_2 per nonrebreather mask PRN SpO_2 < 90%.
Consult with an authorized provider about patient disposition; DO NOT REINITIATE INFUSION.

[a] There may be overlap between specific factors in each category. Always choose to default to highest category for any factor.

bpm—beats per minute; IM—intramuscular; IV—intravenous; O_2—oxygen; PRN—as needed; Q5M—every 5 minutes; Q10M—every 10 minutes; Q15M—every 15 minutes; SBP—systolic blood pressure; SpO_2—blood oxygen saturation level

Note. Algorithm is to be used as a guide only.

recommended after it is shown that the benefits outweigh the risk and should be undertaken with caution by trained nurses and physicians (Giavina-Bianchi et al., 2017).

(3) Sloane et al. (2016) noted that rapid drug desensitization is cost effective and safe for allergic patients with cancer if the benefit of therapy outweighs any other risks (e.g., survival and quality of life).

7. Clinical management of CRS: Mild CRS may be indistinguishable from standard infusion reactions (Kroschinsky et al., 2017).
   a) Stop infusion, and observe the patient until symptoms resolve, which usually occurs within 30 minutes.
   b) Administer corticosteroid as ordered.
   c) Resume infusion at a slower rate (50%) after resolution of symptoms, and titrate the rate slowly.
   d) For severe reactions (see Table 13-6), administer emergency medications based on symptoms (see Table 13-7).
8. Clinical management of localized hypersensitivity (Wilkes & Barton-Burke, 2018)
   a) Observe for and evaluate symptoms (e.g., urticaria, wheals, erythema).
   b) Administer diphenhydramine, ranitidine, or corticosteroids per provider order or according to protocol.
   c) Monitor vital signs at least every 15 minutes for 1 hour or as the patient's condition requires.
   d) Document the episode, including all treatments and the patient's response, according to institutional policies.

F. Patient and caregiver education
1. Before cytotoxic therapy, inform patients and families that chemotherapy and immunotherapy agents have the potential for acute infusion reactions. Instruct them to immediately report signs and symptoms of extravasation, flare, hypersensitivity, or infusion reactions.
2. Document all patient teaching.
3. After therapy, instruct patients and families about the importance of immediately reporting symptoms of any delayed reaction.

References

Aguirre, V.J., Barnett, D., Burdett, N., Joshi, R., & Viana, F.F. (2017). Video-assisted thoracoscopy in the management of intrapleural extravasation of cytotoxic chemotherapy. *Thoracic Cancer, 8,* 363–364. https://doi.org/10.1111/1759-7714.12430

Aigner, B., Bauernhofer, T., Petru, E., Niederkorn, A., Arzberger, E.J., & Richtig, E. (2014). Complete recovery of a wide local reaction by the use of dexrazoxane 72 hours after epirubicin extravasation: Case report and review of the literature. *Dermatology, 229,* 288–292. https://doi.org/10.1159/000365391

Araque Arroyo, P., Ubago Perez, R., Fernandez Feijoo, M.A., & Calleja Hernandez, M.A. (2010). Good clinical and cost outcomes using dexrazoxane to treat accidental epirubicin extravasation. *Journal of Cancer Research and Therapeutics, 6,* 573–574. https://doi.org/10.4103/0973-1482.77081

Azaïs, H., Bresson, L., Bassil, A., Katdare, N., Merlot, B., Houpeau, J.-L., … Narducci, F. (2015). Chemotherapy drug extravasation in totally implantable venous access port systems: How effective is early surgical lavage? *Journal of Vascular Access, 16,* 31–37. https://doi.org/10.5301/jva.5000316

Barbee, M.S., Owonikoko, T.K., & Harvey, R.D. (2014). Taxanes: Vesicants, irritants, or just irritating? *Therapeutic Advances in Medical Oncology, 6,* 16–20. https://doi.org/10.1177/1758834013510546

Barrett, D.M., Teachey, D.T., & Grupp, S.A. (2014). Toxicity management for patients receiving novel T-cell engaging therapies. *Current Opinion in Pediatrics, 26,* 43–49. https://doi.org/10.1097/MOP.0000000000000043

Bavbek, S., Kendirlinan, R., Çerçi, P., Altıner, S., Soyyiğit, S., Çelebi Sözener, Z., … Gümüşburun, R. (2016). Rapid drug desensitization with biologics: A single-center experience with four biologics. *International Archives of Allergy and Immunology, 171,* 227–233. https://doi.org/10.1159/000454808

Bonamichi-Santos, R., & Castells, M. (2016). Diagnoses and management of drug hypersensitivity and anaphylaxis in cancer and chronic inflammatory diseases: Reactions to taxanes and monoclonal antibodies. *Clinical Reviews in Allergy and Immunology, 54,* 375–385. https://doi.org/10.1007/s12016-016-8556-5

Boulanger, J., Boursiquot, J.N., Cournoyer, G., Lemieux, J., Masse, M.S., Almanric, K., & Guay, M.P. (2014). Management of hypersensitivity to platinum- and taxane-based chemotherapy: CEPO review and clinical recommendations. *Current Oncology, 21,* e630–e641. https://doi.org/10.3747/co.21.1966

Bristol-Myers Squibb Co. (2017). *Yervoy® (ipilimumab)* [Package insert]. Princeton, NJ: Author.

Brudno, J.N., & Kochenderfer, J.N. (2016). Toxicities of chimeric antigen receptor T cells: Recognition and management. *Blood, 127,* 3321–3330. https://doi.org/10.1182/blood-2016-04-703751

Campbell, R.L., & Kelso, J.M. (2017). Anaphylaxis: Emergency treatment. In A.M. Feldweg (Ed.), *UpToDate.* Retrieved March 8, 2018, from https://www.uptodate.com/contents/anaphylaxis-emergency-treatment

Castells, M.C., Matulonis, U.A., & Horton, T.M. (2018). Infusion reactions to systemic chemotherapy. In D.M.F. Savarese & A.M. Feldweg (Eds.), *UpToDate.* Retrieved March 7, 2018, from https://www.uptodate.com/contents/infusion-reactions-to-systemic-chemotherapy

Celgene Corp. (2015). *Abraxane® for injectable suspension (paclitaxel protein-bound particles for injectable suspension) (albumin-bound)* [Package insert]. Summit, NJ: Author.

Cephalon, Inc. (2016). *Treanda® (bendamustine hydrochloride)* [Package insert]. Frazer, PA: Author.

Chang, P.-H., Wang, M.-T., Chen, Y.-H., Chen, Y.-Y., & Wang, C.-H. (2014). Docetaxel extravasation results in significantly delayed and relapsed skin injury: A case report. *Oncology Letters, 7,* 1497–1498. https://doi.org/10.3892/ol.2014.1921

Chang, R., & Murray, N. (2016). Management of anthracycline extravasation into the pleural space. *Oxford Medical Case Reports, 2016,* omw079. https://doi.org/10.1093/omcr/omw079

Commins, S.P. (2017). Outpatient emergencies: Anaphylaxis. *Medical Clinics of North America, 101,* 521–536. https://doi.org/10.1016/j.mcna.2016.12.003

Conde-Estévez, D., Saumell, S., Salar, A., & Mateu-de Antonio, J. (2010). Successful dexrazoxane treatment of a potentially severe extravasation of concentrated doxorubicin. *Anti-Cancer Drugs, 21,* 790–794. https://doi.org/10.1097/CAD.0b013e32833d9032

Curran, C.F., Luce, J.K., & Page, J.A. (1990). Doxorubicin-associated flare reactions. *Oncology Nursing Forum, 17,* 387–389.

Das, C.K., & Gogia, A. (2016). Vinorelbine-induced chemotherapy port extravasation. *Lancet Oncology, 17,* e568. https://doi.org/10.1016/S1470-2045(16)30556-3

de las Vecillas Sánchez, L., Alenazy, L.A., Garcia-Neuer, M., & Castells, M.C. (2017). Drug hypersensitivity and desensitizations: Mechanisms and new approaches. *International Journal of Molecular Sciences, 18,* 1316. https://doi.org/10.3390/ijms18061316

de Lemos, M.L. (2005). Vinorelbine and venous irritation: Optimal parenteral administration. *Journal of Oncology Pharmacy Practice, 11,* 79–81. https://doi.org/10.1191/1078155205jp146oa

de Lemos, M.L., & Walisser, S. (2005). Management of extravasation of oxaliplatin. *Journal of Oncology Pharmacy Practice, 11,* 159–162. https://doi.org/10.1191/1078155205jp165oa

Doellman, D., Hadaway, L., Bowe-Geddes, L.A., Franklin, M., LeDonne, J., Papke-O'Donnell, L., ... Stranz, M. (2009). Infiltration and extravasation: Update on prevention and management. *Journal of Infusion Nursing, 32,* 203–211. https://doi.org/10.1097/NAN.0b013e3181aac042

Dorr, R.T., Alberts, D.S., & Soble, M. (1986). Lack of experimental vesicant activity for the anticancer agents cisplatin, melphalan, and mitoxantrone. *Cancer Chemotherapy and Pharmacology, 16,* 91–94. https://doi.org/10.1007/BF00256155

Ener, R.A., Meglathery, S.B., & Styler, M. (2004). Extravasation of systemic hemato-oncological therapies. *Annals of Oncology, 15,* 858–862. https://doi.org/10.1093/annonc/mdh214

Firat, C., Erbatur, S., & Aytekin, A.H. (2013). Management of extravasation injuries: A retrospective study. *Journal of Plastic Surgery and Hand Surgery, 47,* 60–65. https://doi.org/10.3109/2000656X.2012.741065

Fontaine, C., Noens, L., Pierre, P., & De Grève, J. (2012). Savene® (dexrazoxane) use in clinical practice. *Supportive Care in Cancer, 20,* 1109–1112. https://doi.org/10.1007/s00520-012-1382-2

Foo, K.F., Michael, M., Toner, G., & Zalcberg, J. (2003). A case report of oxaliplatin extravasation. *Annals of Oncology, 14,* 961–962. https://doi.org/10.1093/annonc/mdg252

Fresenius Kabi USA. (2013). *Mitoxantrone injection USP* [Package insert]. Lake Zurich, IL: Author.

Genentech, Inc. (2017). *Actemra® (tocilizumab)* [Package insert]. South San Francisco, CA: Author.

Giavina-Bianchi, P., Patil, S.U., & Banerji, A. (2017). Immediate hypersensitivity reaction to chemotherapeutic agents. *Journal of Allergy and Clinical Immunology: In Practice, 5,* 593–599. https://doi.org/10.1016/j.jaip.2017.03.015

Gibson, F., & Bodenham, A. (2013). Misplaced central venous catheters: Applied anatomy and practical management. *British Journal of Anaesthesia, 110,* 333–346. https://doi.org/10.1093/bja/aes497

GlaxoSmithKline. (2010). *Alkeran® (melphalan hydrochloride)* [Package insert]. Research Triangle Park, NC: Author.

Gobel, B.H. (2005). Chemotherapy-induced hypersensitivity reactions. *Oncology Nursing Forum, 32,* 1027–1035. https://doi.org/10.1188/05.ONF.1027-1035

Gobel, B.H. (2007). Hypersensitivity reactions to biological drugs. *Seminars in Oncology Nursing, 23,* 191–200. https://doi.org/10.1016/j.soncn.2007.05.009

Goolsby, T.V., & Lombardo, F.A. (2006). Extravasation of chemotherapeutic agents: Prevention and treatment. *Seminars in Oncology, 33,* 139–143. https://doi.org/10.1053/j.seminoncol.2005.11.007

Goossens, G.A., Stas, M., Jérôme, M., & Moons, P. (2011). Systematic review: Malfunction of totally implantable venous access devices in cancer patients. *Supportive Care in Cancer, 19,* 883–898. https://doi.org/10.1007/s00520-011-1171-3

Hadaway, L. (2007). Infiltration and extravasation. *American Journal of Nursing, 107*(8), 64–72. https://doi.org/10.1097/01.NAJ.0000282299.03441.c7

Jakel, P., Carsten, C., Braskett, M., & Carino, A. (2016). Nursing care of patients undergoing chemotherapy desensitization: Part I. *Clinical Journal of Oncology Nursing, 20,* 29–32. https://doi.org/10.1188/16.CJON.29-32

Janssen Pharmaceutical Companies. (2015). *Yondelis® (trabectedin)* [Package insert]. Horsham, PA: Author.

Kashiwagi, Y., & Kakinohana, S. (2015). A retrospective analysis of oxaliplatin-related hypersensitivity reaction in colorectal cancer in patients and predictive factors. *Singapore Nursing Journal, 42*(3), 27–32.

Kennedy, J.G., Donahue, J.P., Hoang, B., & Boland, P.J. (2003). Vesicant characteristics of oxaliplatin following antecubital extravasation. *Clinical Oncology, 15,* 237–239. https://doi.org/10.1016/S09366555(02)00338-2

Khan, D.A. (2016). Hypersensitivity and immunologic reactions to biologics: Opportunities for the allergist. *Annals of Allergy, Asthma and Immunology, 117,* 115–120. https://doi.org/10.1016/j.anai.2016.05.013

Kite Pharma, Inc. (2017). *Yescarta® (axicabtagene ciloleucel)* [Package insert]. Santa Monica, CA: Author.

Kramer, F., Schippert, C., Rinnau, F., Hillemanns, P., & Park-Simon, T.-W. (2011). The first description of docetaxel-induced recall inflammatory skin reaction after previous drug extravasation. *Annals of Pharmacotherapy, 45,* e11. https://doi.org/10.1345/aph.1P440

Kreidieh, F.Y., Moukadem, H.A., & El Saghir, N.S. (2016). Overview, prevention and management of chemotherapy extravasation. *World Journal of Clinical Oncology, 7,* 87–97. https://doi.org/10.5306/wjco.v7.i1.87

Kretzschmar, A., Pink, D., Thuss-Patience, P., Dörken, B., Reichart, P., & Eckert, R. (2003). Extravasation of oxaliplatin. *Journal of Clinical Oncology, 21,* 4068–4069. https://doi.org/10.1200/JCO.2003.99.095

Kroschinsky, F., Stölzel, F., von Bonin, S., Beutel, G., Kochanek, M., Kiehl, M., & Schellongowski, P. (2017). New drugs, new toxicities: Severe side effects of modern targeted and immunotherapy of cancer and their management. *Critical Care, 21,* 89. https://doi.org/10.1186/s13054-017-1678-1

LaCasce, A.S., Castells, M.C., Burstein, H., & Meyerhardt, J.A. (2017). Infusion-related reactions to therapeutic monoclonal antibodies used for cancer therapy. In D.M.F. Savarese & A.M. Feldweg (Eds.), *UpToDate.* Retrieved March 7, 2018, from https://www.uptodate.com/contents/infusion-related-reactions-to-therapeutic-monoclonal-antibodies-used-for-cancer-therapy

Langer, S.W. (2007). Dexrazoxane for anthracycline extravasation. *Expert Review of Anticancer Therapy, 7,* 1081–1088. https://doi.org/10.1586/14737140.7.8.1081

Langer, S.W. (2008). Treatment of anthracycline extravasation from centrally inserted venous catheters. *Oncology Reviews, 2,* 114–116. https://doi.org/10.1007/s12156-008-0065-1

Lax, T., Long, A., & Banerji, A. (2015). Skin testing in the evaluation and management of carboplatin-related hypersensitivity reactions. *Journal of Allergy and Clinical Immunology: In Practice, 3,* 856–862. https://doi.org/10.1016/j.jaip.2015.07.003

Lenz, H.-J. (2007). Management and preparedness for infusion and hypersensitivity reactions. *Oncologist, 12,* 601–609. https://doi.org/10.1634/theoncologist.12-5-601

Leon-Ferre, R.A., Abu Hejleh, T.B., & Halfdanarson, T.R. (2012). Extravasation of oxaliplatin into the mediastinum: A case report and review of the literature. *Clinical Advances in Hematology and Oncology, 10,* 546–548. Retrieved from http://www.hematologyandoncology.net/archives/august-2012/extravasation-of-oxaliplatin-into-the-mediastinum-a-case-report-and-review-of-the-literature

Luedke, D.W., Kennedy, P.S., & Rietschel, R.L. (1979). Histopathogenesis of skin and subcutaneous injury induced by Adriamycin. *Plastic and Reconstructive Surgery, 63,* 463–465. https://doi.org/10.1097/00006534-197904000-00003

Lundbeck LLC. (2012). *Mustargen® (mechlorethamine hydrochloride)* [Package insert]. Deerfield, IL: Author.

Manganoni, A.M., Pavoni, L., Sereni, E., Farisoglio, C., Simoncini, E., & Calzavara-Pinton, P. (2012). Vinorelbine chemotherapy-induced blistering. *Netherlands Journal of Medicine, 70,* 294.

Martella, F., Salutari, V., Marchetti, C., Pisano, C., Di Napoli, M., Pietta, F., … Floretto, L. (2015). A retrospective analysis of trabectedin infusion by peripherally inserted central venous catheters: A multicentric Italian experience. *Anti-Cancer Drugs, 26,* 990–994. https://doi.org/10.1097/CAD.0000000000000275

Martin, P., Barr, P.M., James, L., Pathak, A., & Kahl, B. (2017). Long-term safety experience with bendamustine for injection in a real-world setting. *Expert Opinion on Drug Safety, 16,* 647–650. https://doi.org/10.1080/14740338.2017.1318125

Maude, S.L., Barrett, D., Teachey, D.T., & Grupp, S.A. (2014). Managing cytokine release syndrome associated with novel T cell-engaging therapies. *Cancer Journal, 20,* 119–122. https://doi.org/10.1097/PPO.0000000000000035

Merck and Co., Inc. (2014). *Intron® A (interferon alfa-2b, recombinant)* [Package insert]. Whitehouse Station, NJ: Author.

Mouridsen, H.T., Langer, S.W., Buter, J., Eidtmann, H., Rosti, G., de Wit, M., … Giaccone, G. (2007). Treatment of anthracycline extravasation with Savene (dexrazoxane): Results from two prospective clinical multicentre studies. *Annals of Oncology, 18,* 546–550. https://doi.org/10.1093/annonc/mdl413

National Cancer Institute Cancer Therapy Evaluation Program. (2017). *Common terminology criteria for adverse events* [v.5.0]. Retrieved from https://ctep.cancer.gov/protocoldevelopment/electronic_applications/ctc.htm

Novartis Pharmaceuticals Corp. (2017). *Kymriah® (tisagenlecleucel)* [Package insert]. East Hanover, NJ: Author.

Pérez Fidalgo, J.A., García Fabregat, L., Cervantes, A., Margulies, A., Vidall, C., & Roila, F. (2012). Management of chemotherapy extravasation: ESMO–EONS clinical practice guidelines. *Annals of Oncology, 23*(Suppl. 7), vii167–vii173. https://doi.org/10.1093/annonc/mds294

Pericay, C., López, A., Soler, J.R., Bonfill, T., Dotor, E., & Saigí, E. (2009). Extravasation of oxaliplatin: An infrequent and irritant toxicity. *Clinical and Translational Oncology, 11,* 114–116. https://doi.org/10.1007/s12094-009-0324-z

Pfizer Inc. (2016). *Camptosar® (irinotecan)* [Package insert]. New York, NY: Author.

Plusching, U., Haslik, W., Bartsch, R., & Mader, R.M. (2016). Extravasation emergencies: State-of-the-art management and progress in clinical research. *Memo—Magazine of European Medical Oncology, 9,* 226–230. https://doi.org/10.1007/s12254-016-0304-2

Pritchett, W., & Kinsley, K. (2016). Benefits and risks of fosaprepitant in patients receiving emetogenic regimens. *Clinical Journal of Oncology Nursing, 20,* 555–556. https://doi.org/10.1188/16.CJON.555-556

Sagent Pharmaceuticals. (2014). *Vinorelbine* [Package insert]. Schaumburg, IL: Author.

Sanofi-Aventis U.S. LLC. (2015a). *Eloxatin® (oxaliplatin)* [Package insert]. Bridgewater, NJ: Author.

Sanofi-Aventis U.S. LLC. (2015b). *Taxotere® (docetaxel)* [Package insert]. Bridgewater, NJ: Author.

Sanofi-Aventis U.S. LLC. (2016). *Jevtana® (cabazitaxel)* [Package insert]. Bridgewater, NJ: Author.

Sauerland, C., Engelking, C., Wickham, R., & Corbi, D. (2006). Vesicant extravasation part I: Mechanisms, pathogenesis, and nursing care to reduce risk. *Oncology Nursing Forum, 33,* 1134–1141. https://doi.org/10.1188/06.ONF.1134-1141

Schrijvers, D.L. (2003). Extravasation: A dreaded complication of chemotherapy. *Annals of Oncology, 14*(Suppl. 3), iii26–iii30. https://doi.org/10.1093/annonc/mdg744

Schulmeister, L. (2007). Totect™: A new agent for treating anthracycline extravasation. *Clinical Journal of Oncology Nursing, 11,* 387–395. https://doi.org/10.1188/07.CJON.387-395

Schulmeister, L. (2011). Extravasation management: Clinical update. *Seminars in Oncology Nursing, 27,* 82–90. https://doi.org/10.1016/j.soncn.2010.11.010

Sloane, D., Govindarajule, U., Harrow-Mortelliti, J., Barry, W., Hsu, F.I., Hong, D., … Castells, M. (2016). Safety, costs, and efficacy of rapid drug desensitizations to chemotherapy and monoclonal antibodies. *Journal of Allergy and Clinical Immunology: In Practice, 4,* 497–504. https://doi.org/10.1016/j.jaip.2015.12.019

Smith, L.T., & Venella, K. (2017). Cytokine release syndrome. *Clinical Journal of Oncology Nursing, 21*(Suppl. 2), 29–34. https://doi.org/10.1188/17.CJON.S2.29-34

Soar, J. (2009). Emergency treatment of anaphylaxis in adults: Concise guidance. *Clinical Medicine, 9,* 181–185. https://doi.org/10.7861/clinmedicine.9-2-181

Stanford, B.L., & Hardwicke, F. (2003). A review of clinical experience with paclitaxel extravasations. *Supportive Care in Cancer, 11,* 270–277. Retrieved from https://link.springer.com/article/10.1007/s00520-003-0441-0

Teva Pharmaceuticals USA, Inc. (2015). *Paclitaxel* [Package insert]. North Wales, PA: Author.

Teva Pharmaceuticals USA, Inc. (2017). *Bendeka® (bendamustine hydrochloride)* [Package insert]. North Wales, PA: Author.

Theman, T.A., Hartzell, T.L., Sinha, I., Polson, K., Morgan, J., Demetri, G.D., … George, S. (2015). Recognition of a new chemotherapeutic vesicant: Trabectedin (ecteinascidin-743) extravasation with skin and soft tissue damage. *Journal of Clinical Oncology, 27,* e198–e200. https://doi.org/10.1200/JCO.2008.21.6473

Uges, J.W.F., Vollaard, A.M., Wilms, E.B., & Brouwer, R.E. (2006). Intrapleural extravasation of epirubicin, 5-fluouracil, and cyclophosphamide, treated with dexrazoxane. *International Journal of Clinical Oncology, 11,* 467–470. https://doi.org/10.1007/s10147-006-0598-x

Viale, P.H. (2009). Management of hypersensitivity reactions: A nursing perspective. *Oncology, 23*(2, Suppl. 1), 26–30. Retrieved from http://www.cancernetwork.com/supplements/2009/infusion-reactions/display/article/10165/1382802

Vos, F.Y., Lesterhuis, W.J., Brüggemann, R.J., & van der Graaf, W.T. (2012). Recovery of symptomatic extravasation of liposomal doxorubicin after dexrazoxane treatment. *Anti-Cancer Drugs, 23,* 139–140. https://doi.org/10.1097/CAD.0b013e32834be51a

Watanabe, H., Ikesue, H., Tsujikawa, T., Nagata, K., Uchida, M., Suetsugu, K., … Oishi, R. (2013). Decrease in venous irritation by adjusting the concentration of injected bendamustine. *Biological and Pharmaceutical Bulletin, 36,* 574–578. https://doi.org/10.1248/bpb.b12-00901

Wickham, R., Engelking, C., Sauerland, C., & Corbi, D. (2006). Vesicant extravasation part II: Evidence-based management and continuing controversies. *Oncology Nursing Forum, 33,* 1143–1150. https://doi.org/10.1188/06/ONF.1143-1150

Wilkes, G.M., & Barton-Burke, M. (2018). *2018 oncology nursing drug handbook.* Burlington, MA: Jones & Bartlett Learning.

SECTION V

Treatment-Related Complications

CHAPTER 14

Myelosuppression

A. Myelosuppression: Neutropenia, anemia, and thrombocytopenia

1. *Myelosuppression* is a condition manifested by a significant decrease in the neutrophils, megakaryocytes, and erythrocytes within the bone marrow (National Cancer Institute, n.d.). It is a dose-limiting toxicity of systemic chemotherapy (Camp-Sorrell, 2018). Terms used in this section include the following.
   - *a) Neutropenia*: A significant reduction in the absolute number of circulating neutrophils in the blood. The absolute neutrophil count (ANC) is the basis for neutropenia classification and is generally defined as an ANC less than 1,500/mm^3 (Jacobson & Berliner, 2014; Noel & Jaben, 2013). The National Comprehensive Cancer Network® (NCCN®, 2017c) defines *neutropenia* as an ANC less than 500/mm^3 or less than 1,000/mm^3 with the expectation that the neutrophil count will decline to less than 500/mm^3 over 48 hours. The Common Terminology Criteria for Adverse Events stratifies grades of febrile neutropenia (National Cancer Institute Cancer Therapy Evaluation Program, 2017; see Table 14-1). Stratifying the severity of neutropenia related to relative risk for infection helps to identify those at risk following myelosuppressive therapy (Camp-Sorrell, 2018; Jacobson & Berliner, 2014; Territo, 2016).
     - (1) Mild: ANC less than the lower limit of normal (LLN) to 1,500/mm^3
     - (2) Moderate: ANC less than 1,500 to 1,000/mm^3
     - (3) Severe: ANC less than 1,000 to 500/mm^3
     - (4) Life threatening: ANC less than 500/mm^3
   - *b) Anemia*: In adults, anemia is defined as a hemoglobin (Hgb) of 11 g/dl or lower, or 2 g/dl or greater below baseline (NCCN, 2017a). Other references for adults in industrialized nations identify 14 g/dl for men and 12 g/dl for women as lower limits for normal Hgb (Means & Glader, 2014). A decrease in the hematocrit or number of red blood cells (RBCs) can be used to define anemia, but Hgb is used most often because it reflects physiologic consequences of anemia (Means & Glader, 2014). See Table 14-1 for grading of anemia.
   - *c) Thrombocytopenia*: Platelet count below the LLN, 400–140 × 10^9/L (Kuter, 2017). See Table 14-1 for grading of decreased platelet count.
   - *d) Cytopenia*: The lack of cellular elements in circulating blood
   - *e) Pancytopenia*: A depression of the normal bone marrow elements: leukocytes, platelets, and erythrocytes in the peripheral blood (Turgeon, 2018; Zack, 2018)
   - *f) Nadir*: Following cytotoxic therapy, the time or level at which the lowest blood cell count is reached (O'Leary, 2015). The nadir varies with individual agents but usually occurs 8–12 days after treatment (Camp-Sorrell, 2018).
   - *g) Hematopoiesis*
     - (1) Hematopoiesis is the process involved in the production of all blood cells from hematopoietic stem cells (HSCs). In adults, most hematopoiesis occurs in the bone marrow in myeloid tissue (see Figure 14-1).
     - (2) The process begins with HSCs, also called pluripotent stem cells (Roquiz, Al Diffalha, & Kini, 2016; Skubitz, 2014). These are the most primitive type of blood cell and the source of all hematopoietic cells. HSCs are able to self-renew and maintain their numbers because they have the ability to proliferate, differentiate, and mature into all cell lines. With each stem cell division, one daughter cell stays in the stem cell pool while the other daughter cell leaves the stem cell pool and becomes committed to a distinct cell line. These committed progenitor cells differenti-

Table 14-1. Common Terminology Criteria for Adverse Events Grading for Neutropenia, Anemia, and Thrombocytopenia

	Grade				
Adverse Event	**1**	**2**	**3**	**4**	**5**
Febrile neutropenia	–	–	ANC < 1,000/mm³ with a single temperature > 38.3°C (101°F) or a sustained temperature ≥ 38°C (100.4°F) for more than 1 hour	Life-threatening consequences; urgent intervention indicated	Death
Anemia	Hgb < LLN–10.0 g/dl; < LLN–6.2 mmol/L; < LLN–100 g/L	Hgb < 10.0–8.0 g/dl; < 6.2–4.9 mmol/L; < 100–80 g/L	Hgb < 8.0 g/dl; < 4.9 mmol/L; < 80 g/L; transfusion indicated	Life-threatening consequences; urgent intervention indicated	Death
Decreased platelet count	< LLN–75,000/mm³; < LLN–75.0 × 10⁹/L	< 75,000–50,000/mm³; < 75.0–50.0 × 10⁹/L	< 50,000–25,000/mm³; < 50.0–25.0 × 10⁹/L	< 25,000/mm³; < 25.0 × 10⁹/L	–

ANC—absolute neutrophil count; Hgb—hemoglobin; LLN—lower limit of normal

Note. From *Common Terminology Criteria for Adverse Events* [v.5.0], by National Cancer Institute Cancer Therapy Evaluation Program, 2017. Retrieved from https://ctep.cancer.gov/protocoldevelopment/electronic_applications/docs/CTCAE_v5_Quick_Reference_5x7.pdf.

ate and mature in the bone marrow. Whether HSCs proliferate or differentiate is determined by the body's needs in response to exogenous (e.g., high altitude) or endogenous (e.g., stress, infection, hemorrhage, drug therapy) influences. Once released into the bloodstream, mature cells have a varied life span (see Table 14-2).

2. Most chemotherapy agents cause some degree of myelosuppression (Zack, 2018). The degree and duration of chemotherapy-related myelosuppression are related to the agent's mechanism of action (e.g., cell cycle–specific drugs are associated with rapid cytopenias).
3. Neutropenia: Chemotherapy-induced neutropenia (CIN) is the primary dose-limiting toxicity associated with systemic chemotherapy (Zack, 2018). It has significant negative clinical consequences for patients with cancer, including life-threatening infections, prolonged hospital stays, dose reductions, and dose delays.
   a) Normal physiology of neutrophils (see Figure 14-1)
      (1) Neutrophils and monocytes stem from the colony-forming unit–granulocyte-macrophage progenitor cell. The earliest identifiable cell of the neutrophil lineage is the myeloblast. Differentiation from a myeloblast to a segmented neutrophil takes 7–11 days. Normal adult bone marrow produces approximately 1×10^{11} cells/kg neutrophils each day (Roquiz et al., 2016).
      (2) Major steps of development (Roquiz et al., 2016; Skubitz, 2014)
         (a) The HSC gives rise to the myeloblast, the earliest form of the neutrophil. During this phase, the nucleus is round. At the end of this phase, granules are evident as the cell transitions to a promyelocyte.
         (b) Promyelocytes have a large nucleus, averaging three to five times larger than the cytoplasm of the cell. During this phase, the granules begin to fade.
         (c) During the myelocyte phase, the number of primary granules decreases, and secondary neutrophilic granules appear. Myelocytes may have nuclei that are round, oval, or flattened on one side.
         (d) Metamyelocytes are observed with indented nuclei that make them appear bean-shaped.
         (e) Band neutrophils, derived from metamyelocytes, evolve when the indentation of the nucleus is more than half the width of the nucleus. At this point, the cell is approximately 24 hours from maturation into a segmented neutrophil. In the presence of acute infection or inflammation, bands are released early from the marrow and complete maturation in circulation.

Figure 14-1. Hematopoiesis and Cytokine Delineation

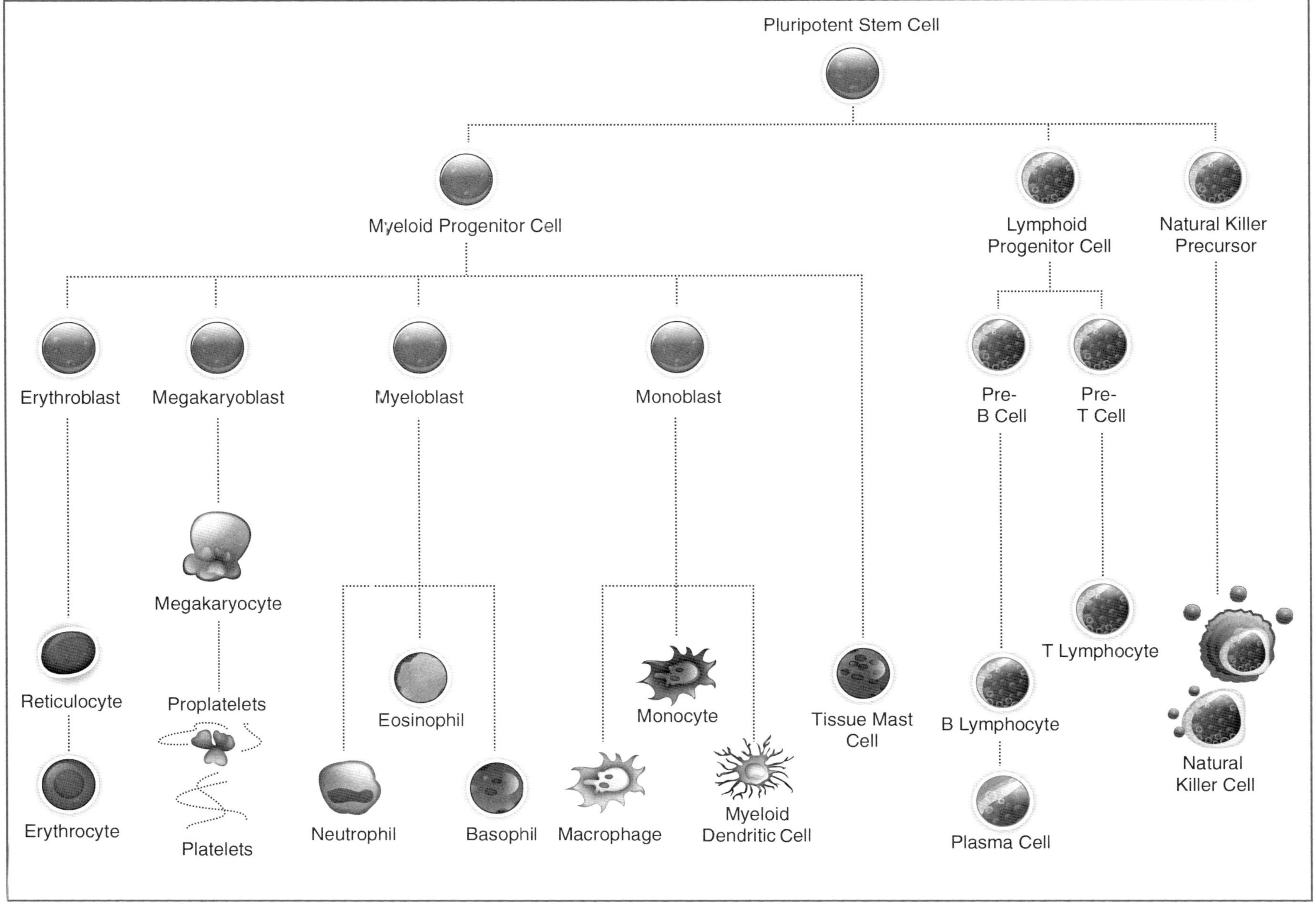

Table 14-2. Life Spans of Blood Components

Blood Component	Typical Life Span
Red blood cell	90–120 days
Platelet	8–10 days
Neutrophil	< 48 hours
Monocyte	5 days, but dependent on many factors
Macrophage	Dependent on many factors
Eosinophil	8–18 hours in blood and 2–5 days in tissue
Basophil	1–2 days
Tissue mast cell	Cutaneous: 1 year; mucosal: 1–2 weeks
B lymphocyte	Depends on type and subtype
T lymphocyte	Depends on type and subtype
Natural killer cell	Approximately 10 days

Note. Based on information from Kitamura, 1989; Milot & Filep, 2011; Min et al., 2012; Nayak et al., 2013; Park & Bochner, 2010; Pillay et al., 2010; Whitelaw, 1966; Zhang et al., 2007.

(*f*) In the segmented neutrophil phase, the nucleus has two to five lobes connected to each other by fine strands.

(3) Locations of neutrophils (Roquiz et al., 2016, Skubitz, 2014)

(*a*) The bone marrow of a healthy adult contains both mature segmented neutrophils and immature neutrophils in various stages of development. Neutrophils leave the bone marrow for the blood through pores that form between the marrow parenchyma and venous blood vessels.

(*b*) Once in the bloodstream, these cells join the functional pool by circulating or lining blood vessel walls as marginated cells, meaning they adhere to endothelial cells lining the blood vessel. Neutrophils exist in the bloodstream as mature and immature cells. These cells perform a critical role in the body's defense by generating chemotactic agents (e.g., endotoxin-activated serum [Skubitz, 2014]) in response to infection. The result is activation of neutrophil defense and movement of neutrophils to the site of infection.

(*c*) Neutrophils leave the blood for tissue by migrating through endothelial cells, a process called *diapedesis.* After neutrophils enter the tissue, they do not return to circulation or the bone marrow.

(4) Pathophysiology

(*a*) The bone marrow must constantly produce neutrophils because the life span of a neutrophil is estimated to be less than 48 hours (see Table 14-2). Chemotherapy agents suppress bone marrow activity and damage stem cells, preventing them from continuing the maturation process. Therefore, chemotherapy decreases the neutrophil count as mature neutrophils die and are not replaced (Camp-Sorrell, 2018).

(*b*) The white blood cell (WBC) nadir depends on the specific drugs and dosages used. A prolonged nadir may occur if stem cells fail to repopulate quickly following high-dose chemotherapy (O'Leary, 2015). Neutropenia occurs 8–12 days following administration of chemotherapy and resolves 21–28 days after completion of therapy.

i. Cell cycle–specific agents (e.g., antimetabolites) are generally less damaging because they primarily affect cells in a specific phase of the cell cycle. Severe neutropenia can develop when cell cycle–specific drugs are used in dose-intensification and combination chemotherapy regimens (Tortorice, 2018).

ii. Cell cycle–nonspecific agents (e.g., alkylating agents, nitrosoureas) are damaging to cells in all phases of the cell cycle, thereby causing more damage to stem cells. The extent of neutropenia with these agents is dependent on dose, schedule, and agent. For example, oxaliplatin as a single agent is expected to cause mild neutropenia, but in regimens with 5-fluorouracil and leucovorin, toxicity can be much higher (Tortorice, 2018).

iii. Some cell cycle–nonspecific agents (e.g., nitrosoureas) produce a delayed and prolonged neutropenia. In adults, nadir occurs at three to five weeks, with recovery ranging from one to two weeks to up to five to six weeks (Wilkes & Barton-Burke, 2018).

(5) Risk factors for developing neutropenia: Risk assessment for CIN should be done prior to each cycle of therapy, including initial therapy (NCCN, 2018b; O'Leary, 2015; see Figure 14-2).

(*a*) Older than 65 years old

(*b*) History of severe neutropenia with similar chemotherapy

(*c*) Previous or current chemotherapy or radiation therapy

(*d*) Chemotherapy relative dose intensity > 80%

(*e*) Dose-dense chemotherapy

(*f*) Chemotherapy regimen (e.g., high-dose cyclophosphamide or anthracyclines, etoposide)

(*g*) Hematologic malignancy, uncontrolled or advanced cancer, lung cancer

(6) Fever and febrile neutropenia: Fever is defined as a onetime oral temperature greater than 101°F (38.3°C) or oral temperature of 100.4°F (38°C) lasting one hour. Febrile neutropenia occurs when the ANC is less than 500/mm^3 or less than 1,000/mm^3 with anticipated decline to 500/mm^3 or less over the next 48 hours and fever as defined previously (NCCN, 2017c).

(7) Risk assessment

(*a*) Assess for febrile neutropenia risk prior to each treatment cycle (NCCN, 2017c; Wilson et al., 2017). Increased infection risk is present in patients with fever in the presence of neutropenia.

(*b*) Risk factors for developing febrile neutropenia (NCCN, 2017b, 2017c)

i. Advanced age

ii. Low neutrophil count at the beginning of chemotherapy cycle

iii. Tumor involvement of bone marrow

iv. Poor performance status

v. Renal dysfunction

vi. Liver dysfunction, especially elevated bilirubin

vii. Previous myelosuppressive chemotherapy or radiation

viii. Preexisting infection, open wounds, or recent surgery

ix. Chemotherapy regimen

x. Use of specific medications including but not limited to phenothiazines, diuretics, and immunosuppressive drugs

(8) Clinical manifestations of infection in patients with neutropenia (NCCN, 2017c; O'Leary, 2015)

Figure 14-2. Risk Factors for Developing Febrile Neutropenia

Patient Related
- Age > 65 years
- Female
- Poor performance status
- Poor nutritional status
- Low neutrophil count at the beginning of a treatment cycle
- Renal dysfunction
- Liver dysfunction, especially elevated bilirubin
- Cardiovascular disease
- Recent surgery
- Preexisting infection
- Open wounds

Disease Related
- Advanced disease stage
- Tumor involvement of the bone marrow
- Type of malignancy: Hematologic (leukemia, myelodysplastic syndromes), breast, lung, colorectal, ovarian, and lymphoma
- Preexisting, prolonged, or previous episode of neutropenia

Treatment Related
- Previous myelosuppressive chemotherapy or radiation
- Treatment intent (curative intent rather than palliative)
- Planned relative dose intensity (≥ 85%)
- Use of specific medications (e.g., immunosuppressive drugs)
- Chemotherapy intensity (i.e., dose dense, high dose, myeloablative)

Note. Based on information from Aapro et al., 2011; Freifeld et al., 2011; National Comprehensive Cancer Network, 2017c.

From *Putting Evidence Into Practice: Improving Oncology Patient Outcomes; Prevention of Infection* (p. 7), by M. Irwin, C. Erb, C. Williams, B.J. Wilson, and L.J. Zitella, 2013, Pittsburgh, PA: Oncology Nursing Society. Copyright 2013 by Oncology Nursing Society. Adapted with permission.

(a) A fever greater than 100.4°F (38°C) is the most reliable, and often the only, sign of infection in patients with neutropenia. Normally, WBCs cause the classic signs of infection (e.g., redness, edema, pus). Extremely neutropenic patients, however, may not be able to manifest the usual signs of infection (NCCN, 2017c).

(b) Common sites of infection and corresponding signs and symptoms in neutropenic patients (Camp-Sorrell, 2018)

i. Gastrointestinal tract: Fever, abdominal pain, alimentary mucositis (mucositis at any level of the digestive tract), diarrhea

ii. Respiratory tract: Fever, cough, dyspnea on exertion, adventitious breath sounds, chest discomfort, asymmetric chest wall movement, nasal flaring

iii. Genitourinary tract: Fever, dysuria, frequency, urgency, hematuria, cloudy urine, flank pain, perineal itching, vaginal discharge

iv. Head and neck: Swelling, itching, eye redness or drainage, ear pain or discharge, nasal congestion or drainage, oral ulcerations, difficulty swallowing, fever

v. Indwelling devices (e.g., venous access devices [VADs], ventricular peritoneal shunts): Fever, erythema, pain or tenderness, edema, drainage, induration at site

vi. Dermatologic and mucous membranes: Erythema, tenderness, warm skin, edema (especially in axilla, mouth, sinuses, perineal, or rectal areas), rashes, itching, skin lesions, fever, draining open wounds

vii. Central nervous system: Change in mental status, headache, seizure, vision changes, photosensitivity, fever, nausea, lethargy

viii. Hematologic/immunologic: Decrease in diastolic blood pressure, headache, oliguria, fever, flushed appearance

(c) Septic shock associated with neutropenia has a high mortality rate (O'Leary, 2018).

(9) ANC calculation: Use laboratory data to assess neutropenia by calculating the ANC. Note that neutropenia can occur when the total WBC count is within the normal range of 4,000–10,000/mm^3 (Camp-Sorrell, 2018; Marionneaux, 2016). Consequently, calculating the ANC is essential to achieving a correct assessment of neutrophil status. To calculate ANC, ANC = % neutrophils (polys + bands) × WBCs.

(a) Obtain complete WBC count including differential. The differential will include mature neutrophils, also referred to as *segs* for segmented neutrophils or *PMNs/polys* for polymorphonuclear neutrophils. In addition, less mature neutrophils will be present; these are known as *bands*.

(b) Add the total number of mature polys and less mature neutrophil bands.

(c) Convert sum from *(b)* to a percentage.

(d) Multiply total WBC count by total neutrophil percentage (polys + bands). ANC calculation example: WBCs = 1,500, polys = 30, bands = 5.

i. Add polys and bands: 30 + 5 = 35.

ii. Convert sum to percentage: 35 ÷ 100 = 0.35.

iii. Multiply WBC count by percentage to find ANC: 1,500 × 0.35 = 525/mm^3.

(10) Collaborative management

(a) Nurses play an important role in preventing infection in patients with neutropenia and cancer through evidence-based nursing practice, research, and patient education (Wilson et al., 2017).

i. Hand hygiene: Proper hand hygiene is the most effective measure to prevent the spread of infection. It reduces the risk of healthcare-associated infections by decreasing person-to-person transmission of pathogens (Camp-Sorrell, 2018; Centers for Disease Control and Prevention, 2017; Wilson et al., 2017).

ii. Diet: No recent studies have linked neutropenic diets (restricting fresh fruits and vegetables) with a lower risk of infection for neutropenic patients with cancer. Dietary precautions regarding the omission of fresh fruits and vegetables remain unsupported (Gardner et al., 2008). Uncooked fruits and vegetables should be thoroughly washed (Wilson et al., 2017). Basic safe food handling practices, such as avoiding uncooked and undercooked meats, seafood, and eggs and unwashed fruits and vegetables, should be employed (Camp-Sorrell, 2018).

iii. Environment: Protective or strict isolation studies reveal no significant differences in documented infections, febrile episodes, or antibiotic use for patients with CIN. Protective isolation has no effect on the host's endogenous flora and no impact on organisms transmitted by water or food (Camp-Sorrell, 2018).
- In general, patients with CIN do not require specific room ventilation.
- Allogeneic hematopoietic stem cell transplant recipients are recommended to be placed in rooms with HEPA filtration with more than 12 air exchanges per hour. Air pressure in these rooms should be positive when compared to surrounding areas, such as hallways, toilets, and anterooms (Anderson-Reitz, 2018; Stoll, da Rocha Silla, Cola, Splitt, & Moreira, 2013; Zack, 2018).

iv. Plants and flowers: No research studies are available that evaluate the potential harm of plants and flowers to patients with CIN (Wilson et al., 2017).
- Because fresh or dried flowers could expose patients with cancer to *Aspergillus* and *Fusarium*, they should be kept out of patient rooms (Freifeld et al., 2011).
- If plants must be present, plant care should be done by staff not directly caring for patients (Sehulster & Chinn, 2003).
- If patient caregivers are unable to avoid plant care, they should wear gloves and perform hand hygiene after removing gloves.

v. Treatment with colony-stimulating factors (see Table 14-3)
- Granulocyte macrophage–colony-stimulating factor (sargramostim) (Genzyme Corp., 2013)
- Granulocyte–colony-stimulating factor (G-CSF; filgrastim, pegfilgrastim) (Amgen Inc., 2015, 2016). NCCN (2018b) recommends use of these drugs when the risk of febrile neutropenia is greater than 20%.
- The manufacturer recommends initiation of G-CSF no earlier than 24 hours following chemotherapy (Amgen Inc., 2015, 2016).
- The manufacturer of G-CSF warns that safety of administration simultaneously with chemotherapy has not been established. The rationale is the potential sensitivity of rapidly

Table 14-3. Growth Factors

Classification	Mechanism of Action	Drug	Route	Indications	Side Effects	Nursing Considerations
Colony-stimulating factor	Stimulates erythropoiesis via the same mechanism as endogenous erythropoietin	Darbepoetin (Aranesp®)	IV, SC	Treatment of anemia associated with chronic renal failure whether or not the patient is receiving dialysis Treatment of anemia caused by concomitantly administered chemotherapy in patients who, upon initiation of darbepoetin, have ≥ 2 additional months of planned chemotherapy	Shortness of breath, cough, low blood pressure during dialysis, abdominal pain, edema of arms and legs, hypertension, rash, urticaria, pure red cell aplasia, myalgia, infection, fatigue, diarrhea, thrombotic events	Increased risk of death and serious cardiovascular events exists when administered if hemoglobin is > 12 g/dl. Ensure adequate iron stores in patients prior to and during use. Agent may be administered every 1, 2, or 3 weeks, but dosing schedule should be consistent. Use lowest effective dose. Do not shake vials or syringes containing the drug. Store in refrigerator. Do not freeze. (Amgen Inc., 2017a)
		Epoetin alfa (Procrit®, Epogen®)	SC	Treatment of anemia associated with renal failure whether or not the patient is receiving dialysis Treatment of anemia associated with treatment using zidovudine in HIV-infected patients Treatment of anemia in patients with nonmyeloid malignancies where anemia is caused by concomitant use of chemotherapy for ≥ 2 months. Treatment of anemia in patients scheduled to undergo elective noncardiac, nonvascular surgery to reduce the need for allogeneic red blood cell transfusions Contraindicated when goal of chemotherapy is curative	Hypertension, rash, urticaria, pure red cell aplasia, myalgia, infection, fatigue, edema, diarrhea, thrombotic events	Increased risk of death and serious cardiovascular events exists when administered if hemoglobin is > 12 g/dl. Ensure adequate iron stores in patients prior to and during use. Agent may be given three times weekly or once weekly. Use lowest effective dose. Do not shake vials or syringes containing the drug. Store in refrigerator. Do not freeze. (Amgen Inc., 2017b; Janssen Products, LP, 2017)

(Continued on next page)

Table 14-3. Growth Factors *(Continued)*

Classification	Mechanism of Action	Drug	Route	Indications	Side Effects	Nursing Considerations
Colony-stimulating factor *(cont.)*	Regulates the production of neutrophils within the bone marrow	Filgrastim (G-CSF, Neupogen®)	IV, SC	To decrease the incidence of infection in patients with nonmyeloid malignancies who are receiving myelosuppressive cancer therapies associated with severe neutropenic fever To reduce the time to neutrophil recovery and duration of fever following induction or consolidation chemotherapy in patients with AML To reduce the duration of neutropenia and associated sequelae in patients receiving myeloablative chemotherapy prior to HSCT To mobilize hematopoietic progenitor cells into peripheral blood for collection via leukapheresis For chronic administration to reduce the incidence and duration of sequelae of neutropenia in patients with congenital, cyclic, or idiopathic neutropenia	Allergic reactions, including urticaria, rash, and facial edema; acute respiratory distress syndrome, nausea, vomiting, bone pain secondary to rapid growth of myeloid cells in the bone marrow, fever, severe sickle cell crisis in patients with sickle cell disorder; risk of rare splenic rupture	Store in refrigerator. Do not freeze. Agent may be diluted with 5% dextrose in water. Do not dilute with saline solutions. Do not shake. Filgrastim is not to be administered in the 24 hours prior to chemotherapy through 24 hours after chemotherapy completion. SC dosing continues daily up to 14 days, until postnadir absolute neutrophil count > 10,000/mm³ is achieved. (Amgen Inc., 2015)
		Pegfilgrastim (Neulasta®)	SC	To decrease the incidence of infection related to neutropenia in patients with nonmyeloid malignancies receiving myelosuppressive chemotherapy	Allergic reactions, including urticaria, rash, and facial edema; acute respiratory distress syndrome, nausea, vomiting, bone pain secondary to rapid growth of myeloid cells in the bone marrow, fever, sickle cell crisis in patients with sickle cell disorder; injection site reaction; risk of rare splenic rupture	Pegfilgrastim is cleared by neutrophil receptor binding, with serum clearance directly related to number of neutrophils. Do not administer in the period beginning 14 days before and until 24 hours after administration of cytotoxic chemotherapy. Administer as a single 6 mg injection once per chemotherapy cycle. The 6 mg fixed dose should not be administered to children or adolescents weighing less than 45 kg. Store in refrigerator. Do not freeze. Do not shake. (Amgen Inc., 2016)

(Continued on next page)

Table 14-3. Growth Factors *(Continued)*

Classification	Mechanism of Action	Drug	Route	Indications	Side Effects	Nursing Considerations
Hematopoietic stem cell mobilizer	When combined with G-CSF, mobilizes hematopoietic stem cells to the peripheral blood where they can be collected for transplant	Plerixafor (Mozobil®)	SC approximately 11 hours prior to apheresis	Following 4 days of once-daily G-CSF, plerixafor is administered up to 4 consecutive days for patients with multiple myeloma and non-Hodgkin lymphoma undergoing subsequent autologous HSCT.	Diarrhea, nausea, vomiting, fatigue, headache, arthralgia, dizziness, injection site reactions Potential for splenic rupture, tumor cell mobilization, and embryo-fetal toxicity	Monitor patients during and following administration for anaphylactic shock and serious hypersensitivity reactions. Plerixafor is not indicated for patients with leukemia. For creatinine clearance < 50 ml/min, decrease dose by one-third to 0.16 mg/kg. Monitor blood counts, as an increase in circulating leukocytes and decrease in platelets have been reported. (Genzyme Corp., 2015)
	Induces committed progenitor cells to divide and differentiate in the granulocyte-macrophage pathways, including neutrophils, monocytes/macrophages, and myeloid-derived dendritic cells	Sargramostim (GM-CSF, Leukine®)	IV, SC	To shorten neutrophil recovery and reduce incidence of infection following induction chemotherapy in patients with AML To cause mobilization of hematopoietic progenitor cells for collection via leukapheresis and to speed engraftment following autologous transplantation of progenitor cells To accelerate myeloid recovery following allogeneic HSCT To prolong survival in patients with delayed or failed engraftment following HSCT	Edema, capillary leak syndrome, pleural or pericardial effusions, dyspnea, fever, abdominal pain, headache, chills, diarrhea, occasional transient supraventricular arrhythmia, bone pain secondary to rapid growth of myeloid cells in the bone marrow	Dilute in normal saline solution for IV use. Store in refrigerator. Do not freeze. Do not shake. Do not administer through in-line filter. Monitor complete blood count for elevated white blood cell and platelet count. Safety and effectiveness have not been established for pediatric patients. (Genzyme Corp., 2013)
Leukocyte growth factor (short acting)	Binds to G-CSF receptors and stimulates proliferation of neutrophils	Tbo-filgrastim (Granix®)	SC	To reduce duration of severe neutropenia in patients with nonmyeloid malignancies receiving myelosuppressive anticancer drugs associated with a clinically significant incidence of febrile neutropenia	Bone pain; allergic reactions, including angioneurotic edema, dermatitis, drug hypersensitivity, hypersensitivity reaction, rash, pruritic rash, and urticaria; sickle cell crisis; acute respiratory distress syndrome; splenic rupture	Safety and effectiveness have not been established in patients younger than age 18. Administer first dose no sooner than 24 hours following chemotherapy or within 24 hours prior to chemotherapy. (Teva Pharmaceuticals USA, Inc. 2012)

(Continued on next page)

Table 14-3. Growth Factors *(Continued)*

Classification	Mechanism of Action	Drug	Route	Indications	Side Effects	Nursing Considerations
Leukocyte growth factor	G-CSF analog used to stimulate the proliferation and differentiation of neutrophils	Filgrastim-sndz (Zarxio®)	SC	To decrease incidence of infection in patients with cancer receiving myelosuppressive chemotherapy To reduce time to neutrophil recovery and duration of fever following induction or consolidation chemotherapy for AML To reduce duration of neutropenia and neutropenia-related sequelae in patients with cancer undergoing HSCT To mobilize autologous hematopoietic progenitor cells for collection by leukapheresis To reduce incidence and duration of neutropenia-related sequelae in symptomatic patients with congenital neutropenia, cyclic neutropenia, or idiopathic neutropenia	Splenic rupture, acute respiratory distress syndrome, glomerulonephritis, alveolar hemorrhage, capillary leak syndrome, serious allergic reactions, sickle cell crisis in patients with sickle cell trait or sickle cell disease	For patients receiving myelosuppressive chemotherapy or induction/consolidation chemotherapy for AML: Recommended starting dose is 5 mcg/kg/day by SC injection, short IV infusion (15–30 minutes), or continuous IV infusion. For patients undergoing HSCT: Recommended dose is 10 mcg/kg/day given as IV infusion no longer than 24 hours. Do not inject a dose < 0.3 ml (180 mcg) from a Zarxio prefilled syringe. A dose < 0.3 ml cannot be accurately measured using the prefilled syringe. Administer drug at least 24 hours after cytotoxic chemotherapy. (Sandoz Inc., 2017)
Thrombopoietic growth factor	Stimulates megakaryocytopoiesis and thrombopoiesis	Oprelvekin (interleukin-11, Neumega®)	SC	To prevent severe thrombocytopenia and reduce the need for platelet transfusions in patients with nonmyeloid malignancies receiving chemotherapy with high risk of severe thrombocytopenia	Anaphylaxis, dilutional anemia, diarrhea, dizziness, fever, fluid retention (which can result in peripheral edema, pulmonary edema, dyspnea, capillary leak syndrome, atrial arrhythmias, and exacerbation of preexisting pulmonary effusions), headache, nausea, vomiting, insomnia, rhinitis, cough, injection site reactions	Store in refrigerator. Do not freeze. Reconstitute with sterile water. Oprelvekin should be used within 3 hours of reconstitution. Do not shake or freeze following reconstitution. Protect from light. Dosing should begin 6–24 hours after completion of chemotherapy. Discontinue when post-chemotherapy platelet nadir is > 50,000/mm³ and 2 days before next chemotherapy cycle. (Wyeth Pharmaceuticals Inc., 2015)

AML—acute myeloid leukemia; G-CSF—granulocyte–colony-stimulating factor; GM-CSF—granulocyte macrophage–colony-stimulating factor; HSCT—hematopoietic stem cell transplantation; IV—intravenous; SC—subcutaneous

dividing myeloid cells to cytotoxic agents (Amgen Inc., 2015, 2016).

vi. Prevention of trauma to the patient's skin and mucous membranes (O'Leary, 2015; Wilson et al., 2017)
- Provide meticulous care for all indwelling devices.
- Prevent pressure sores and constipation.
- Change water in pitchers, denture cups, and nebulizers at least daily.
- Consider risk–benefit ratio for invasive procedures (e.g., thoracentesis, paracentesis, VAD placement).
- Use only an electric razor to shave unwanted hair.
- Protect skin from cuts and burns. Immediately cleanse and treat any wound that breaks the skin.
- Use a soft toothbrush for frequent (minimum of three to four times daily) oral care. Allow toothbrush to dry before storing (Brown, 2015).

vii. Patient education on protective measures for neutropenic patients (Brown, 2015; Camp-Sorrell, 2018; O'Leary, 2015)
- Report fever, chills, and other signs and symptoms of infection at onset.
- Maintain personal hygiene.
- Wash hands frequently with soap and water or an antiseptic hand rub. Hands may remain colonized with microorganisms if they are not dried properly after washing.
- Bathe daily.
- Avoid activities that may compromise skin integrity.
- Wear gloves when working in the garden.
- Perform frequent (three to four times per day) oral assessment and care.
- Cleanse the perineal area from front to back after toileting.
- Avoid exposure to pathogens or people who are experiencing signs and symptoms of contagious conditions.

viii. Protective measures
- Do not share food utensils.
- Do not eat any food that has not been either cooked or washed.
- Adhere to safe food handling practices, and avoid consuming food when safety of preparation, storage, or serving is not guaranteed.
- Do not provide direct care for pets or farm animals; avoid contact with animal excreta.
- Refrain from direct or indirect contact with reptiles, fish, and birds.
- Avoid exposure to fresh or dried plants and flowers because of risk of *Aspergillus* infection. Plant care may be done by staff not directly providing care to the patient.
- Do not enter, travel through, or stay in an area of construction or renovation or where construction material or debris has been placed or where fields have recently been plowed.
- Consider vaccination for influenza and pneumonia (Centers for Disease Control and Prevention, 2015).
- Avoid contact with people who have been vaccinated with a live vaccine within the past 30 days.

(b) Management of neutropenic fever

i. Use of colony-stimulating factors after a patient is diagnosed with febrile neutropenia is not recommended (Moore, Vu, & Strickland, 2014).

ii. Obtain cultures (NCCN, 2017c).
- Urine: If symptomatic, with catheter, or if urinalysis is abnormal
- Blood: Two sets (one set includes two bottles). If patient has a central VAD and it is thought to be the cause of the infection, options include the following:
  - One peripheral and one central VAD. The lab can study time to positivity to determine if the central line is the source of the bloodstream infection.
  - Both peripheral
  - Both from central VAD
- Stool: For diarrhea, follow institutional guidelines for *Clostridium difficile* assay and enteric pathogen screen.
- Skin: Aspirate or biopsy skin lesions. Vesicular or ulcerated skin lesions require viral cultures.
- VAD cutaneous site: Consider routine fungal/*Mycobacterium* culture if inflammation is present.
- Throat/nasopharynx: When respiratory viral symptoms are present, especially during seasonal outbreaks

iii. Conduct site-specific history and physical examination with attention to identifying the source of infection (NCCN, 2017c).
- Assess VADs, skin, lungs, sinuses, mouth, pharynx, esophagus, bowel, rectum, and perivaginal and perirectal areas for signs and symptoms of infection.
- Obtain historical data, including comorbidities, date and regimen of last chemotherapy, previous infections, recent antibiotic therapy or prophylaxis, medications, and HIV status. Explore exposure risks, including anyone at home with similar symptoms, pets, travel, recent blood product transfusion, or exposure to tuberculosis.

iv. Obtain a chest x-ray if respiratory symptoms are present.

v. Once initial cultures have been obtained, administer empiric broad-spectrum antibiotics as ordered until organism source is identified.

vi. Monitor blood culture reports daily and anticipate antibiotic therapy based on findings.

4. Anemia

a) Erythropoiesis: The process of erythrocyte (RBC) production in the bone marrow (Doig, 2016)

(1) The kidneys are the primary producers of erythropoietin (EPO), the growth factor that stimulates HSCs to produce RBCs.

(2) RBC production is regulated by oxygen levels. When oxygen levels are low, the kidney releases EPO to stimulate HSCs to produce more RBCs.

b) Normal physiology of erythrocytes (Doig, 2016; Turgeon, 2018; see Figure 14-1): In the bone marrow, the HSC becomes an erythrocyte via a series of maturation phases that takes about five days.

(1) The earliest identifiable stage is the pronormoblast (rubricyte). These cells take about 12 hours to divide into basophilic normoblast daughter cells.

(2) In approximately 20 hours, the normoblast cells continue maturation marked by accumulation of more RNA and hemoglobin. When they divide, they become polychromatophilic normoblasts.

(3) Polychromatophilic normoblasts are smaller than their precursor cells, and nucleoli are no longer visible. Proliferation is apparent in this phase (about 30 hours), as polychromatophilic normoblasts outnumber cells in earlier development by 3:1. Under normal cir-

cumstances, polychromatophilic normoblasts are absent in adult peripheral blood. Small numbers are normal in the peripheral blood of newborns.

(4) Orthochromatic normoblasts are derived in about 48 hours from polychromatophilic normoblasts. In this phase, the nucleus is unable to synthesize DNA, thereby ending cell division.

(5) In the polychromatophilic erythrocyte (reticulocyte) phase, the nucleus is phagocytized after being pushed out of the cell. The reticulocyte either remains in the bone marrow for several days to mature or is released and matures in the spleen for one to two days. At this point, the erythrocyte holds approximately two-thirds of its Hgb content.

c) Without a nucleus, mature erythrocytes cannot synthesize Hgb. They are able to transport oxygen from the lungs to tissue and, because of their flexible form, move easily through microcirculation to do so.

d) Iron is essential for RBC production. Iron reaches the precursor cells bound to transferrin, where it is used for heme synthesis and stored as ferritin in bone marrow reticuloendothelial cells, the liver, and the spleen. Dietary sources provide and maintain iron stores.

e) EPO is a hormone primarily (90%) produced by the peritubular cells of the kidneys and to a lesser extent in the liver. The plasma half-life of EPO is six to nine hours. Levels vary as they respond to internal (e.g., decreased Hgb level) and external (e.g., high altitude) signals of low oxygen tension within kidney tissue. During anemia or hypoxemia, EPO is secreted into the plasma and stimulates activity of erythrocyte precursor cells. As a result, the reticulocyte count is elevated by an early and increased number of polychromatophilic cells released from the bone marrow.

f) RBC mass and volume: Homeostasis of erythropoiesis is a continuous process driven by oxygen levels and EPO response. The average number of circulating RBCs in adults is five million RBCs per microliter (Fritsma, 2016a).

g) RBC life span: A typical RBC has a life span of approximately 120 days in peripheral circulation (Manchanda, 2016; see Table 14-2). The turnover is generally 1% per day (Manchanda, 2016). The RBC life span, time for maturation in the bone marrow, and low turnover explain why anemia occurs later than neutropenia and thrombocytopenia following myelosuppressive therapy (Camp-Sorrell, 2018).

h) Pathophysiology

(1) Many causes for anemia exist in patients with cancer. Myelosuppressive therapy, bone marrow involvement, inadequate EPO levels, and RBC destruction all may contribute to the development of anemia (Camp-Sorrell, 2018; Pace, 2015).

(2) Classification of anemia based on RBC size: Mean corpuscular volume, which reflects the size of RBCs, is used in the differential diagnosis of microcytic, normocytic, or macrocytic anemia (Means & Glader, 2014; Pace, 2015; see Table 14-4).

i) Incidence

(1) Many patients (30%–90%) experience some degree of anemia associated with the diagnosis and treatment of cancer (NCCN, 2017a). Severity may increase with comorbidities, concurrent radiation therapy, and insufficient nutritional intake. The incidence of anemia in patients with hematologic malignancies has been reported as three times higher than in those with solid tumors (Camp-Sorrell, 2018).

(2) The cancer diagnosis, frequency of treatments, regimen, and dosing schedule contribute to the onset, severity, and duration of anemia (Means, 2014).

j) Risk factors

(1) Medications that suppress bone marrow function, interfere with erythrocyte development and function, or suppress EPO production

(a) Platinum drugs, due to combined renal and bone marrow toxicity (NCCN, 2017a)

(b) Immunotherapies (e.g., alemtuzumab [Genzyme Corp., 2014])

(c) Pharmacologic agents: Dapsone, methylphenylethylhydantoin, phenylbutazone, primaquine, tetracycline, and trimethadione (Keohane, 2016)

(d) High-dose chemotherapy for hematopoietic stem cell transplantation

Table 14-4. Classifications of Common Cancer-Related Anemias

Anemia Type	Description	Differential Diagnosis
Microcytic	Decreased mean corpuscular volume (MCV) (< 80 femtoliters [fl]) Red blood cells (RBCs) small in size	Iron deficiency Anemia of chronic disease Thalassemia minor Sideroblastic anemia
Normocytic	Normal MCV (80–100 fl) RBCs normal in size	Anemia of chronic disease Hemolytic anemia Aplastic anemia Renal failure
Macrocytic	Increased MCV (> 100 fl) RBCs large in size	B_{12} deficiency Folate deficiency Myelodysplastic syndromes
Low reticulocyte count	Decreased RBC production < 0.5%–1.5% of erythrocytes	Anemia of chronic disease Aplastic anemia Iron deficiency Vitamin B_{12} deficiency Folate deficiency Bone marrow suppression or infiltration
High reticulocyte count	Increased RBC destruction > 0.5%–1.5% of erythrocytes	Hemolysis Chemotherapy induced Autoimmune

Note. Based on information from Loney & Chernecky, 2000; Lynch, 2006.

From "Cancer-Related Anemia: Clinical Review and Management Update," by B. Hurter and N.J. Bush, 2007, *Clinical Journal of Oncology Nursing, 11,* p. 350. Copyright 2007 by Oncology Nursing Society. Reprinted with permission.

(2) Malignancies that originate or metastasize to the bone marrow and suppress RBC precursors

(3) Radiation therapy to areas of the skeleton involved with hematopoiesis (Camp-Sorrell, 2018; NCCN, 2017a)

(4) Acute or chronic blood loss directly related to tumor invasion

(5) Advanced age, which places patients at risk for anemia of malignancy (Means & Glader, 2014)

(6) Poor nutrition: Anorexia, nausea, vomiting, stomatitis, early satiety, and diarrhea may contribute to decreased oral intake and absorption of nutrients. Lack of calorie, protein, vitamin, and mineral intake, reflected in weight loss or weakness, compromises cellular functions, including erythrocyte production (Pace, 2015).

(7) Comorbidities

(a) Renal insufficiency: Chemotherapy agents known to have nephrotoxic properties (e.g., cisplatin) place patients at risk because kidney function is essential for EPO production. When EPO levels are low, more hypoxia is required to stimulate EPO response (Camp-Sorrell, 2018; NCCN, 2017a).

(b) Alcohol abuse and liver dysfunction (Means & Glader, 2014)

(c) Cardiopulmonary disease (Means & Glader, 2014; NCCN, 2017a)

(8) Female gender (Means & Glader, 2014)

k) Clinical manifestations (Means & Glader, 2014)

(1) Cardiopulmonary

(a) Dyspnea, hypoxia

(b) Tachycardia, heart murmurs

(c) Orthostatic hypotension

(2) Integumentary

(a) Pallor of oral mucous membranes, conjunctivae, lips, nail beds, and palms of hands or soles of feet

(b) Hair loss, thinning, and early graying

(c) Brittle fingernails and toenails

(d) Cyanosis

(e) Hypothermia

(3) Neuromuscular

(a) Headache, dizziness

(b) Drowsiness, restlessness, inability to concentrate

(c) Paresthesias

(d) Fatigue, weakness

(4) Decreased urine output

l) Adverse outcomes (Gosselin, 2018)

(1) Because low tissue oxygenation is related to reduced sensitivity of tumors to radiation therapy and some chemotherapy, hypoxia may adversely affect treatment outcomes.

(2) Low oxygen levels are directly associated with fatigue and weakness and may adversely affect quality of life.

(3) Hypoxic tissue promotes angiogenic factors that may contribute to tumor growth.

(4) Postoperative mortality is increased in the presence of anemia.

(5) Survival times of anemic patients are shorter compared to those without anemia for most tumor types.

m) Management (NCCN, 2017a, 2018a)

(1) Fatigue is an early and frequent symptom of anemia with significant negative impact on quality of life. Interventions should be aimed at identifying and managing fatigue.

(a) Encourage frequent rest periods to conserve energy.

(b) Use exercise when benefits outweigh risks.

(c) Explore complementary therapies (e.g., relaxation, massage, yoga) with potential to minimize fatigue (NCCN, 2018a).

(d) Assess nutritional intake for adequate content and quantity.

(e) Teach patients and family members/caregivers the importance of hydration.

(2) Monitor laboratory results related to anemia (see Table 14-5) and take appropriate action when abnormal (e.g., B_{12} and iron deficiencies).

(3) Interventions for hypoxia

(a) Provide supplemental oxygen.

(b) Teach energy conservation.

(c) Consider measures to increase Hgb (Camp-Sorrell, 2018; NCCN, 2017a).

i. Blood transfusions

ii. Erythropoiesis-stimulating agents (see Table 14-3)

iii. The manufacturer's (Amgen Inc., 2017a, 2017b) black box warning is supported by eight randomized studies that each demonstrated decreased overall survival and locoregional control when erythropoiesis-stimulating agents were used in patients diagnosed with advanced breast, cervical, head and neck, lymphoid, and non-small cell lung cancer.

Table 14-5. Laboratory Assessment of Anemia: Normal Values (Adults)

Laboratory Test	Normal Value
Red blood cell count	Male: 4.7–6 million cells/mcl; female: 4.2–5.4 million cells/mcl
Hemoglobin	Male: 13.5–18 g/dl; female: 12–16 g/dl
Hematocrit	Male: 42%–52%; female: 37%–47%
Mean corpuscular volume	78–100 fl
Mean corpuscular hemoglobin	27–31 pg/cell
Red cell distribution width	11.5%–14%
Reticulocyte count	0.5%–1.85% of erythrocytes
Ferritin	Male: 20–300 ng/ml; female: 15–120 ng/ml
Serum iron	Male: 75–175 mcg/dl; female: 65–165 mcg/dl
Total iron-binding capacity	250–450 mcg/dl
Serum erythropoietin level	Male: 17.2 mU/ml; female: 18.8 mU/ml
Coombs test (direct and indirect)	Negative
Serum B_{12}	190–900 pg/ml
Serum folate	> 3.5 mcg/L

Note. Based on information from Cullis, 2011; Knovich et al., 2009; Van Vranken, 2010.

From "Anemia of Chronic Disease" (p. 957), by B. Faiman in D. Camp-Sorrell and R.A. Hawkins (Eds.), *Clinical Manual for the Oncology Advanced Practice Nurse* (3rd ed.), Pittsburgh, PA: Oncology Nursing Society. Copyright 2013 by Oncology Nursing Society. Reprinted with permission.

5. Thrombocytopenia

a) Normal physiology of platelets (Fritsma, 2016b; Geddis, 2014; see Figure 14-1)

(1) The thrombocyte (platelet) precursor megakaryocyte is the largest hematopoietic cell descending from the HSC. The goal of thrombopoiesis is to produce and release mature platelets so that a normal amount (150,000–400,000/mm^3) is circulating at any given time.

(2) The major steps in thrombopoiesis

(a) Maturation begins with megakaryoblasts that increase in amounts of cytoplasm and nuclear components as they become promegakaryocytes.

(b) During the promegakaryocyte phase, the nucleus continues to enlarge and becomes lobulated in preparation for the megakaryocyte phase.

(c) When the cell reaches the megakaryocyte phase, invagination of the cytoplasm occurs, beginning delineation of individual platelets.

(d) When the megakaryocyte completes maturation, its membrane ruptures and the cytoplasm separates into platelets. One megakaryocyte is able to release thousands of platelets.

(e) Platelets are released into the circulation as the cytoplasm extends through a basement membrane of the bone marrow. Continued separation of the platelet-forming cytoplasm may occur after the cells reach the sinuses. The life span of circulating platelets is seven to eight days (see Table 14-2). There is no reserve in the bone marrow.

(3) When blood vessel wall integrity is damaged, platelets are incorporated into the vessel wall and assist the endothelial cells in regaining vessel integrity by releasing platelet-derived growth factor (Smyth, 2014).

(4) Platelet plug formation involves adhesion and aggregation of platelets in response to vascular damage. Platelets are able to fulfill this vital role in hemostasis only when normal in number and function.

(5) Aggregation is a platelet-to-platelet interaction usually occurring 10–20 seconds after loss of vascular integrity and platelet adhesion.

(6) Secondary hemostasis is accomplished by fibrin clot formation. If this process is flawed, decreased fibrin production and instability of the formed clot result.

b) Pathophysiology (Rodriguez, 2018)

(1) Thrombocytopenia after chemotherapy is evident in approximately 8–14 days and is directly related to bone marrow suppression.

(2) Severity varies with drug, dose, and schedule.

(3) For some agents (e.g., carmustine, carboplatin, dactinomycin, daunorubicin, lomustine, mitomycin C), it is a dose-limiting toxicity (Rodriguez, 2018).

c) Risk factors (Brace, 2016; Fritsma, 2016b)

(1) Myelosuppressive chemotherapy or radiation therapy to marrow-producing skeletal sites

(2) Immunotherapy (e.g., interferon)

(3) Comorbidities (e.g., liver disease)

(4) Destruction of platelets in the presence of autoimmune disease (e.g., immune thrombocytopenic purpura) or disseminated intravascular coagulation

(5) Bone marrow infiltration of primary or metastatic malignancies

(6) Drug therapy affecting platelet function (Brace, 2016; Camp-Sorrell, 2018)

(a) Aspirin

(b) Nonsteroidal anti-inflammatory drugs

(c) Quinine and quinidine

(d) Thiazide diuretics (e.g., furosemide)

(e) Benzene and benzene derivatives

(f) Tricyclic antidepressants

(g) Antimicrobials (e.g., chloramphenicol, zidovudine)

(h) Heparin

(7) Herbal agents (e.g., ginkgo, garlic, ginger, turmeric)

d) Clinical manifestations (Brace, 2016; Rodriguez, 2018)

(1) Cardiopulmonary

(a) Adverse changes in peripheral pulses, tachycardia, hypotension, orthopnea

(b) Dyspnea, tachypnea, adventitious breath sounds, hemoptysis

(2) Head and neck

(a) Petechiae of oral or nasal membranes

(b) Epistaxis

(c) Periorbital edema, subconjunctival hemorrhage, eye pain, blurred or double vision

(3) Integumentary system

(a) Petechiae, bruising, pallor, or acrocyanosis anywhere on skin or mucous membranes

(b) Bleeding from surgical, device, or wound sites

(4) Neurologic

(a) Change in mental status, confusion, restlessness, lethargy

(b) Widening pulse pressure, abnormal change in pupil size, diminished reflexes, loss of motor strength or coordination

(c) Headache, seizures

(5) Gastrointestinal

(a) Abdominal pain or distension

(b) Rectal bleeding, tarry stools, hematemesis

(c) Enlarged, palpable spleen

(6) Genitourinary

(a) Menorrhagia

(b) Hematuria, dysuria, low urine output

e) Management

(1) Monitor laboratory findings and take appropriate action.

(a) Obtain platelet count, prothrombin time, partial thromboplastin time, Hgb, hematocrit, D-dimer, fibrinogen, and fibrin.

(b) Test stool, urine, and emesis for occult blood.

(2) Maintain safe environment.

(a) Instruct patients to avoid activities that may cause injury.

(b) Assess the home environment and promote the use of nonskid rugs, night-lights, and ambulatory assistive devices to prevent falls.

(3) Educate patients and families on ways to maintain skin integrity through the following (Rodriguez, 2018):

(a) Using a soft toothbrush

(b) Blowing nose gently

(c) Using an electric razor versus a straight razor

(d) Using an emery board versus a metal nail file

(e) Using water-soluble lubricants for sexual intercourse

(f) Avoiding any sexual activity that may compromise skin or mucous membrane integrity

(g) Avoiding use of tampons

(h) Using laxatives or stool softeners to avoid constipation

(i) Refraining from using mechanical, oral irrigation, or aggressive dental flossing

(j) Avoiding dental and other invasive procedures

(4) Medications and treatments (Rodriguez, 2018)

(a) Administer platelet transfusions.

(b) Consider administering interleukin-11 (oprelvekin; see Table 14-3).

B. Biosimilars: A new product in cancer care

1. Oncology nurses must become familiar with biosimilars, as more are being developed and released over time. The U.S. Food and Drug Administration (U.S. FDA, 2017a) defines *biosimilars* as a biologic product that is "highly similar to, and has no clinically meaningful differences in safety, purity, and potency (safety and effectiveness) from, an existing FDA-approved reference product" (para. 5).

a) FDA approved the first biosimilar drug, filgrastim-sndz (Zarxio®), in the United States in 2015 (Sandoz Inc., 2017; U.S. FDA, 2017b). It can be prescribed for the same indications as filgrastim.

b) It is important to note that these are not chemically identical to the reference product, which would make them a generic version.

c) Biosimilars are produced from living systems that may cause minor structural and chemical differences, however, none of these changes result in any differences in efficacy. Biosimilars are not exact duplicates but must be chemically, functionally, and clinically similar to the reference product (U.S. FDA, 2017a).

2. Two major factors contribute to the role of biosimilars in cancer care.

a) Many drugs used for cancer treatment or supportive care are nearing the end of their patent, meaning the drug company that manufactures the agent will no longer have exclusive rights to drug production (Griffith, McBride, Stevenson, & Green, 2014).

b) Costs associated with cancer care are higher than any other area in medicine today. This is greatly due, in part, to the rising age of the baby boomers and the high cost of developing chemotherapy and other anticancer agents (Furlow, 2013).

References

Aapro, M.S., Bohlius, J., Cameron, D.A., Dal Lago, L., Donnelly, J.P., Kearney, N., ... Zielinski, C. (2011). 2010 update of EORTC guidelines for the use of granulocyte-colony stimulating factor to reduce the incidence of chemotherapy-induced febrile neutropenia in adult patients with lymphoproliferative disorders and solid tumours. *European Journal of Cancer, 47,* 8–32. https://doi.org/10.1016/j.ejca.2010.10.013

Amgen Inc. (2015). *Neupogen® (filgrastim)* [Package insert]. Thousand Oaks, CA: Author.

Amgen Inc. (2016). *Neulasta® (pegfilgrastim)* [Package insert]. Thousand Oaks, CA: Author.

Amgen Inc. (2017a). *Aranesp® (darbepoetin alfa)* [Package insert]. Thousand Oaks, CA: Author.

Amgen Inc. (2017b). *Epogen® (epoetin alfa)* [Package insert]. Thousand Oaks, CA: Author.

Anderson-Reitz, L. (2018). Complications of hematopoietic cell transplantation. In C.H. Yarbro, D. Wujcik, & B.H. Gobel (Eds.), *Cancer nursing: Principles and practice* (8th ed., pp. 591–610). Burlington, MA: Jones & Bartlett Learning.

Brace, L.D. (2016). Thrombocytopenia and thrombocytosis. In E.M. Keohane, J.L. Smith, & J.M. Walenga (Eds.), *Rodak's hematology: Clinical principles and applications* (5th ed., pp. 713–738). St. Louis, MO: Elsevier Saunders.

Brown, C.G. (2015). Oral mucositis. In C.G. Brown (Ed.), *A guide to oncology symptom management* (2nd ed., pp. 469–482). Pittsburgh, PA: Oncology Nursing Society.

Camp-Sorrell, D. (2018). Chemotherapy toxicities and management. In C.H. Yarbro, D. Wujcik, & B.H. Gobel (Eds.), *Cancer nursing: Principles and practice* (8th ed., pp. 497–554). Burlington, MA: Jones & Bartlett Learning.

Centers for Disease Control and Prevention. (2015). Vaccination of persons with primary and secondary immune deficiencies. In *Epidemiology and prevention of vaccine-preventable diseases* (13th ed., pp. A26–A27). Retrieved from https://www.cdc.gov/vaccines/pubs/pinkbook/appendix/appdx-a.html

Centers for Disease Control and Prevention. (2017). Preventing infections in cancer patients. Retrieved from https://www.cdc.gov/cancer/preventinfections

Cullis, J.O. (2011). Diagnosis and management of anaemia of chronic disease: Current status. *British Journal of Haematology, 154,* 289–300. https://doi.org/10.1111/j.1365-2141.2011.08741.x

Doig, K. (2016). Erythrocyte production and destruction. In E.M. Keohane, L.J. Smith, & J.M. Walenga (Eds.), *Rodak's hematology: Clinical principles and applications* (5th ed., pp. 95–111). St. Louis, MO: Elsevier Saunders.

Freifeld, A.G., Bow, E.J., Sepkowitz, K.A., Boeckh, M.J., Ito, J.I., Mullen, C.A., ... Wingard, J.R. (2011). Clinical practice guideline for the use of antimicrobial agents in neutropenic patients with cancer: 2010 update by the Infectious Diseases Society of America. *Clinical Infectious Diseases, 52,* e56–e93. https://doi.org/10.1093/cid/cir073

Fritsma, G.A. (2016a). Erythrocyte metabolism and membrane structure and function. In E.M. Keohane, J.L. Smith, & J.M. Walenga (Eds.), *Rodak's hematology: Clinical principles and applications* (5th ed., pp. 112–123). St. Louis, MO: Elsevier Saunders.

Fritsma, G.A. (2016b). Platelet production, structure, and function. In E.M. Keohane, J.L. Smith, & J.M. Walenga (Eds.), *Rodak's hematology: Clinical principles and applications* (5th ed., pp. 167–186). St. Louis, MO: Elsevier Saunders.

Furlow, B. (2013, May 30). Biotherapy: Entering a new era in chemotherapy. Retrieved from http://cancertherapyadvisor.com/oncology-features/biosimilars-entering-a-new-era-in-chemotherapy/article/295456

Gardner, A., Mattiuzzi, G., Faderl, S., Borthakur, G., Garcia-Manero, G., Pierce, S., ... Estey, E. (2008). Randomized comparison of cooked and noncooked diets in patients undergoing remission induction therapy for acute myeloid leukemia. *Journal of Clinical Oncology, 26,* 5684–5688. https://doi.org/10.1200/JCO.2008.16.4681

Geddis, A.E. (2014). Megakaryocytes. In J.P. Greer, D.A. Arber, B. Glader, A.F. List, R.T. Means Jr., F. Paraskevas, & G.M. Rodgers (Eds.), *Wintrobe's clinical hematology* (13th ed., pp. 371–388). Philadelphia, PA: Lippincott Williams & Wilkins.

Genzyme Corp. (2013). *Leukine® (sargramostim)* [Package insert]. Cambridge, MA: Author.

Genzyme Corp. (2014). *Campath® (alemtuzumab)* [Package insert]. Cambridge, MA: Author.

Genzyme Corp. (2015). *Mozobil® (plerixafor)* [Package insert]. Cambridge, MA: Author.

Gosselin, T.K. (2018). Principles of radiation therapy. In C.H. Yarbro, D. Wujcik, & B.H. Gobel (Eds.), *Cancer nursing: Principles and practice* (8th ed., pp. 267–284). Burlington, MA: Jones & Bartlett Learning.

Griffith, N., McBride, A., Stevenson, J.G., & Green, L. (2014). Formulary selection criteria for biosimilars: Considerations for US health-system pharmacists. *Hospital Pharmacy, 49,* 813–825. https://doi.org/10.1310/hpj4909-813

Jacobson, C.A., & Berliner, N. (2014). Neutropenia. In J.P. Greer, D.A. Arber, B. Glader, A.F. List, R.T. Means Jr., F. Paraskevas, & G.M. Rodgers (Eds.), *Wintrobe's clinical hematology* (13th ed., pp. 1279–1289). Philadelphia, PA: Lippincott Williams & Wilkins.

Janssen Products, LP. (2017). *Procrit® (epoetin alfa)* [Package insert]. Horsham, PA: Author.

Keohane, E.M. (2016). Extrinsic defects leading to increased erythrocyte destruction—nonimmune causes. In E.M. Keohane, L.J. Smith, & J.M. Walenga (Eds.), *Rodak's hematology: Clinical principles and applications* (5th ed., pp. 394–410). St. Louis, MO: Elsevier Saunders.

Kitamura, Y. (1989). Heterogeneity of mast cells and phenotypic change between subpopulations. *Annual Review of Immunology, 7,* 59–76.

Knovich, M.A., Storey, J.A., Coffman, L.G., Torti, S.V., & Torti, F.M. (2009). Ferritin for the clinician. *Blood Reviews, 23,* 95–104. https://doi.org/10.1016/j.blre.2008.08.001

Kuter, D.J. (2017). Thrombocytopenia and platelet dysfunction. In R.S. Porter (Eds.), *Merck manual* [Professional version]. Retrieved from https://www.merckmanuals.com/professional/hematology-and-oncology/thrombocytopenia-and-platelet-dysfunction

Loney, M., & Chernecky, C. (2000). Anemia. *Oncology Nursing Forum, 27,* 951–962.

Lynch, M.P. (2006). Overview of anemia. In D. Camp-Sorrell & R.A. Hawkins (Eds.), *Clinical manual for the oncology advanced practice nurse* (2nd ed., pp. 787–788). Pittsburgh, PA: Oncology Nursing Society.

Manchanda, N. (2016). Anemias: Red blood cell morphology and approach to diagnosis. In E.M. Keohane, J.L. Smith, & J.M. Walenga (Eds.), *Rodak's hematology: Clinical principles and applications* (5th ed., pp. 284–296). St. Louis, MO: Elsevier Saunders.

Marionneaux, S. (2016). Nonmalignant leukocyte disorders. In E.M. Keohane, J.L. Smith, & J.M. Walenga (Eds.), *Rodak's hematology: Clinical principles and applications* (5th ed., pp. 475–497). St. Louis, MO: Elsevier Saunders.

Means, R.T., Jr. (2014). Anemias secondary to chronic disease and systemic disorders. In J.P. Greer, D.A. Arber, B. Glader, A.F. List, R.T. Means Jr., F. Paraskevas, & G.M. Rodgers (Eds.), *Wintrobe's clinical hematology* (13th ed., pp. 998–1011). Philadelphia, PA: Lippincott Williams & Wilkins.

Means, R.T., Jr., & Glader, B. (2014). Anemia: General considerations. In J.P. Greer, D.A. Arber, B. Glader, A.F. List, R.T. Means Jr., F. Paraskevas, & G.M. Rodgers (Eds.), *Wintrobe's clinical hematology* (13th ed., pp. 587–616). Philadelphia, PA: Lippincott Williams & Wilkins.

Milot, E., & Filep, J.G. (2011). Regulation of neutrophil survival/apoptosis by Mcl-1. *Scientific World Journal, 11,* 1948–1962. https://doi.org/10.1100/2011/131539

Min, B., Brown, M.A., & LeGros, G. (2012). Understanding the roles of basophils: Breaking dawn. *Immunology, 135,* 192–197. https://doi.org/10.1111/j.1365-2567.2011.03530.x

Moore, A.J., Vu, M.A., & Strickland, S.A. (2014). Supportive care in hematologic malignancies. In J.P. Greer, D.A. Arber, B. Glader, A.F. List, R.T. Means Jr., F. Paraskevas, & G.M. Rodgers (Eds.),

Wintrobe's clinical hematology (13th ed., pp. 1426–1466). Philadelphia, PA: Lippincott Williams & Wilkins.

National Cancer Institute. (n.d.). Myelosuppression. In *NCI dictionary of cancer terms.* Retrieved from https://www.cancer.gov/publications/dictionaries/cancer-terms?cdrid=44173

National Cancer Institute Cancer Therapy Evaluation Program. (2017). *Common terminology criteria for adverse events* [v.5.0]. Retrieved from https://ctep.cancer.gov/protocolDevelopment/electronic_applications/docs/CTCAE_v5_Quick_Reference_5x7.pdf

National Comprehensive Cancer Network. (2017a). *NCCN Clinical Practice Guidelines in Oncology (NCCN Guidelines®): Cancer- and chemotherapy-induced anemia* [v.2.2018]. Retrieved from http://www.nccn.org/professionals/physician_gls/pdf/anemia.pdf

National Comprehensive Cancer Network. (2017b). *NCCN Clinical Practice Guidelines in Oncology (NCCN Guidelines®): Older adult oncology* [v.2.2017]. Retrieved from https://www.nccn.org/professionals/phuysician_gls/pdf/senior.pdf

National Comprehensive Cancer Network. (2017c). *NCCN Clinical Practice Guidelines in Oncology (NCCN Guidelines®): Prevention and treatment of cancer-related infections* [v.1.2018]. Retrieved from http://www.nccn.org/professionals/physician_gls/pdf/infections.pdf

National Comprehensive Cancer Network. (2018a). *NCCN Clinical Practice Guidelines in Oncology (NCCN Guidelines®): Cancer-related fatigue* [v.2.2018]. Retrieved from https://www.nccn.org/professionals/physician_gls/pdf/fatigue.pdf

National Comprehensive Cancer Network. (2018b). *NCCN Clinical Practice Guidelines in Oncology (NCCN Guidelines®): Myeloid growth factors* [v.1.2018]. Retrieved from http://www.nccn.org/professionals/physician_gls/PDF/myeloid_growth.pdf

Nayak, M.K., Kulkarni, P.P., & Dash, D. (2013). Regulatory role of proteasome in determination of platelet life span. *Journal of Biological Chemistry, 288,* 6826–6834. https://doi.org/10.1074/jbc.M112.403154

Noel, P., & Jaben, E.A. (2013). Consultative hematology. In G.P. Rodgers & N.S. Young (Eds.), *The Bethesda handbook of clinical hematology* (3rd ed., pp. 389–404). Philadelphia, PA: Lippincott Williams & Wilkins.

O'Leary, C. (2015). Neutropenia and infection. In C.G. Brown (Ed.), *A guide to oncology symptom management* (2nd ed., pp. 483–504). Pittsburgh, PA: Oncology Nursing Society.

O'Leary, C. (2018). Septic shock. In C.H. Yarbro, D. Wujcik, & B.H. Gobel (Eds.), *Cancer nursing: Principles and practice* (8th ed., pp. 1135–1151). Burlington, MA: Jones & Bartlett Learning.

Pace, A.F. (2015). Anemia. In C.G. Brown (Ed.), *A guide to oncology symptom management* (2nd ed., pp. 35–54). Pittsburgh, PA: Oncology Nursing Society.

Park, Y.M., & Bochner, B.S. (2010). Eosinophil survival and apoptosis in health and disease. *Allergy, Asthma and Immunology Research, 2,* 87–101. https://doi.org/10.4168/aair.2010.2.2.87

Pillay, J., den Braber, I., Vrisekoop, N., Kwast, L.M., de Boer, R.J., Borghans, J.A., ... Koenderman, L. (2010). In vivo labeling with 2H2O reveals a human neutrophil lifespan of 5.4 days. *Blood, 116,* 625–627. https://doi.org/10.1182/blood-2010-01-259028

Rodriguez, A.L. (2018). Bleeding. In C.H. Yarbro, D. Wujcik, & B.H. Gobel (Eds.), *Cancer nursing: Principles and practice* (8th ed., pp. 851–881). Burlington, MA: Jones & Bartlett Learning.

Roquiz, W., Al Diffalha, S., & Kini, A.R. (2016). Leukocyte development, kinetics, and function. In E.M. Keohane, J.L. Smith, & J.M. Walenga (Eds.), *Rodak's hematology: Clinical principles and applications* (5th ed., pp. 149–166). St. Louis, MO: Elsevier Saunders.

Sandoz Inc. (2017). *Zarxio® (filgrastim-sndz)* [Package insert]. Princeton, NJ: Author.

Sehulster, L., & Chinn, R.Y.W. (2003). Guidelines for environmental infection control in health-care facilities: Recommendations of CDC and the Healthcare Infection Control Practices Advisory Committee (HICPAC). *MMWR Recommendations and Reports, 52*(RR-10), 1–42. Retrieved from https://www.cdc.gov/mmwr/preview/mmwrhtml/rr5210a1.htm

Skubitz, K.M. (2014). Neutrophilic leukocytes. In J.P. Greer, D.A. Arber, B. Glader, A.F. List, R.T. Means Jr., F. Paraskevas, & G.M. Rodgers (Eds.), *Wintrobe's clinical hematology* (13th ed., pp. 125–159). Philadelphia, PA: Lippincott Williams & Wilkins.

Smyth, S. (2014). Platelet structure and function in hemostasis and thrombosis. In J.P. Greer, D.A. Arber, B. Glader, A.F. List, R.T. Means Jr., F. Paraskevas, & G.M. Rodgers (Eds.), *Wintrobe's clinical hematology* (13th ed., pp. 389–410). Philadelphia, PA: Lippincott Williams & Wilkins.

Stoll, P., da Rocha Silla, L.M., Cola, C.M.M., Splitt, B.I., & Moreira, L.B. (2013). Effectiveness of a protective environment implementation for cancer patients with chemotherapy-induced neutropenia on fever and mortality incidence. *Journal of Infection Control, 41,* 357–359. https://doi.org/10.1016/j.ajic.2012.05.018

Territo, M. (2016, November). Neutropenia. In R.S. Porter (Ed.), *Merck manual* [Professional version]. Retrieved from https://www.merckmanuals.com/professional/hematology-and-oncology/leukopenias/neutropenia

Teva Pharmaceuticals USA, Inc. (2012). *Granix® (tbo-filgrastim)* [Package insert]. North Wales, PA: Author.

Tortorice, P.V. (2018). Cytotoxic chemotherapy: Principles of therapy. In C.H. Yarbro, D. Wujcik, & B.H. Gobel (Eds.), *Cancer nursing: Principles and practice* (8th ed., pp. 375–416). Burlington, MA: Jones & Bartlett Learning.

Turgeon, M.L. (2018). *Clinical hematology: Theory and practice* (6th ed.). Philadelphia, PA: Wolters Kluwer.

U.S. Food and Drug Administration. (2017a, October 23). Biosimilar development, review, and approval. Retrieved from https://www.fda.gov/Drugs/DevelopmentApprovalProcess/HowDrugsareDevelopedandApproved/ApprovalApplications/TherapeuticBiologicApplications/Biosimilars/ucm580429.htm

U.S. Food and Drug Administration. (2017b, December 13). Biosimilar product information. Retrieved from https://www.fda.gov/Drugs/DevelopmentApprovalProcess/HowDrugsareDevelopedandApproved/ApprovalApplications/TherapeuticBiologicApplications/Biosimilars/ucm580432.htm

Van Vranken, M. (2010). Evaluation of microcytosis. *American Family Physician, 82,* 1117–1122. Retrieved from http://www.aafp.org/afp/2010/1101/p1117.html

Whitelaw, D.M. (1966). The intravascular lifespan of monocytes. *Blood, 28,* 455–464. Retrieved from http://www.bloodjournal.org/content/28/3/455.long?sso-checked=true

Wilkes, G.M., & Barton-Burke, M. (2018). *2018 oncology nursing drug handbook.* Burlington, MA: Jones & Bartlett Learning.

Wilson, B.J., Ahmed, F., Crannell, C.E., Crego, W., Erb, C.H., Foster, J., ... Zitella, L. (2017, April 20). ONS Putting Evidence Into Practice: Prevention of infection. Retrieved from https://www.ons.org/practice-resources/pep/prevention-infection

Wyeth Pharmaceuticals Inc. (2015). *Neumega® (oprelvekin)* [Package insert]. Philadelphia, PA: Author.

Zack, E. (2018). Principles and techniques of bone marrow transplantation. In C.H. Yarbro, D. Wujcik, & B.H. Gobel (Eds.), *Cancer nursing: Principles and practice* (8th ed., pp. 555–590). Burlington, MA: Jones & Bartlett Learning.

Zhang, Y., Wallace, D.L., de Lara, C.M., Ghattas, H., Asquith, B., Worth, A., ... Macallan, D.C. (2007). In vivo kinetics of human natural killer cells: The effects of ageing and acute and chronic viral infection. *Immunology, 121,* 258–265. https://doi.org/10.1111/j.1365-2567.2007.02573.x

CHAPTER 15

Gastrointestinal and Mucosal Toxicities

A. Nausea and vomiting

1. Overview: Nausea and vomiting may be experienced by up to 80% of patients with cancer and can be the most distressing side effects of cancer treatment (J. Lee et al., 2017; National Cancer Institute [NCI], 2017e). Adherence to antiemetic guidelines has been shown to decrease the incidence of chemotherapy-induced nausea and vomiting (CINV) in patients receiving highly or moderately emetogenic chemotherapy (Abunahlah, Sancar, Dane, & Özyavuz, 2016; Gilmore et al., 2014). Advances in modern antiemetics have led to improvements, and now approximately 13%–35% of patients receiving highly or moderately emetogenic chemotherapy will experience acute CINV (Grunberg et al., 2004). Oncology nurses must be knowledgeable and proactive when managing CINV.
2. Definitions
   a) *Nausea* is an unpleasant subjective experience that is described as a "wavelike" feeling occurring in the stomach or back of the throat that may be accompanied by vomiting (NCI, 2017b).
   b) *Retching* is a rhythmic contraction involving the esophagus, diaphragm, and abdominal muscles in an attempt to eject stomach contents (NCI, 2017b).
   c) *Vomiting* is the forceful expulsion of gastric contents through the mouth (NCI, 2017b).
3. Pathophysiology
   a) Nausea, retching, and vomiting are independent phenomena that can occur sequentially or as separate entities. The subjective nature of nausea prevents a clear understanding of it; however, mechanisms of vomiting related to chemotherapy administration are becoming better understood.
   b) Vomiting results from the stimulation of a complex process that involves the activation of various pathways and neurotransmitter receptors (see Figures 15-1 and 15-2).
   c) The vomiting center (VC) is a cluster of neurons located in the medulla. Stimulation of the VC results in efferent impulses from the central nervous system to the salivation center, cranial nerves, respiratory center, and abdominal muscles. This leads to the initiation of emesis (National Comprehensive Cancer Network® [NCCN®], 2018b; Navari & Aapro, 2016). In other words, the VC receives input or stimuli from a variety of sources and then sends signals to different organs and tissues, resulting in vomiting.
   d) The VC may be stimulated through peripheral or central pathways.
      (1) Vagal afferents (gastrointestinal [GI] and pharyngeal)
         (a) The GI vagal afferent is thought to be the primary cause of acute chemotherapy-induced vomiting (Hesketh, 2008).
         (b) Chemotherapy stimulates enterochromaffin cells in the GI tract, causing them to release serotonin (5-hydroxytryptamine-3 [5-HT_3]) (Hesketh, 2008).
         (c) Serotonin release causes the activation of the vagus nerve, which stimulates vomiting through the VC (Hesketh, 2008; Navari & Aapro, 2016).
         (d) 5-HT_3 receptors along the vagus nerve may also be involved in acute nausea and vomiting related to abdominal distension, radiation to the abdomen or chest, and pharyngeal irritation (Tipton, 2014).

Figure 15-1. Mechanisms of Emesis

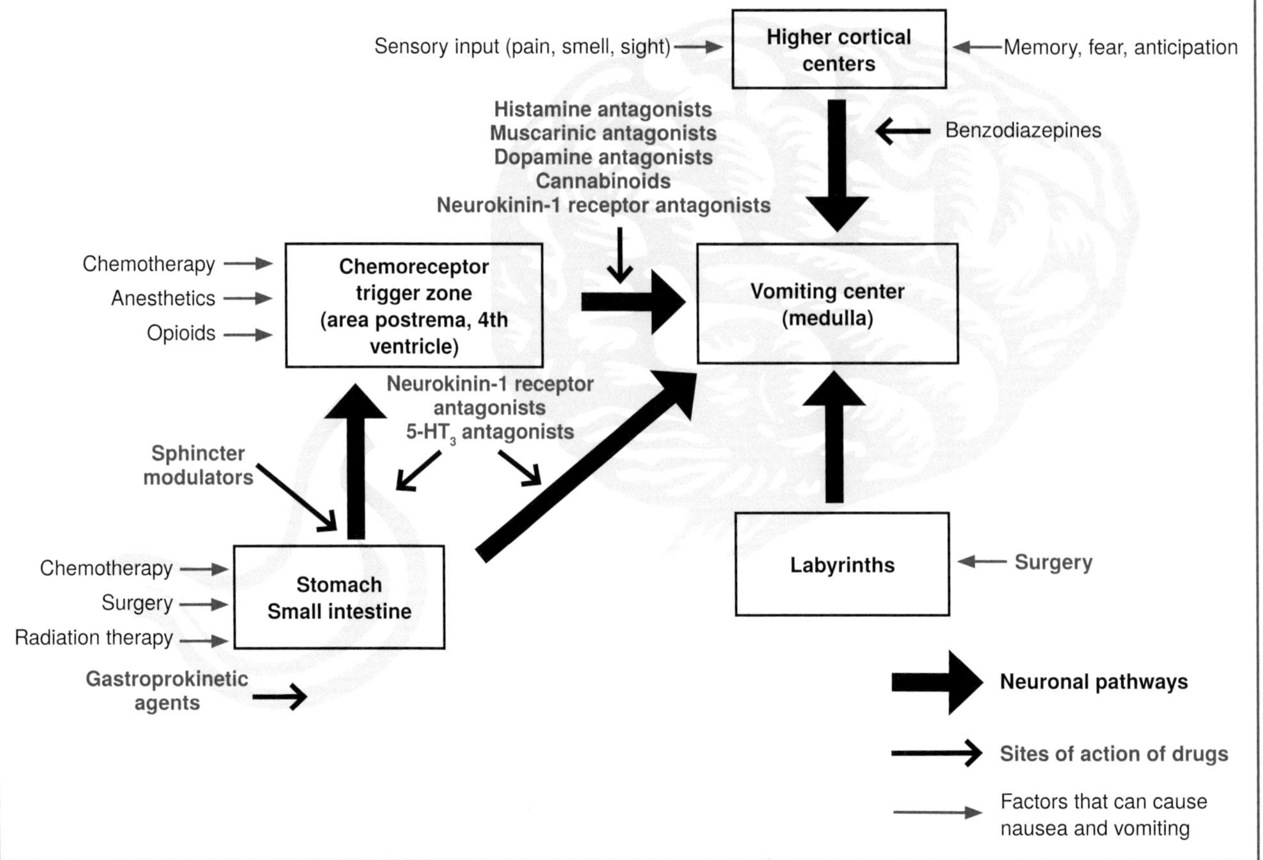

(e) Additional receptors involved in this process may include neurokinin-1 (NK_1) and cholecystokinin-1 (Hesketh, 2008).

(2) Chemoreceptor trigger zone (CTZ)

(a) The CTZ is found in the area postrema in the fourth ventricle of the brain (Hesketh, 2008; Navari & Aapro, 2016).

(b) The CTZ is an area of the brain where the blood–brain barrier is less restrictive. As a result, the CTZ may be stimulated by emetogens in the blood or cerebrospinal fluid (Hesketh, 2008).

(c) Opioids, dopaminergic agonists, chemotherapy, and toxins may all stimulate the CTZ and result in vomiting (Hesketh, 2008).

(3) Higher cortical centers: Nausea and vomiting may be a result of anxiety, memory, fear, pain, or a conditioned response to sights or smells.

(4) Vestibular apparatus

(a) Labyrinthitis and motion sickness may result in nausea and vomiting (Tipton, 2014).

(b) Surgery can also induce vomiting through stimulation of the vestibular system.

(5) Other potential causes of nausea and vomiting (NCCN, 2018b)

(a) Brain metastases
(b) Side effect of other medications
(c) Excessive secretions
(d) Gastroparesis
(e) Electrolyte imbalance
(f) Uremia
(g) Anxiety
(h) Vestibular dysfunction
(i) Malignant ascites

4. Types of CINV

a) Anticipatory CINV: Occurs before chemotherapy administration; is likely a conditioned response and therefore occurs after a previous experience with CINV (NCCN, 2018b)

(1) It may be triggered by a particular smell, taste, or sight.

Figure 15-2. Neuroreceptors

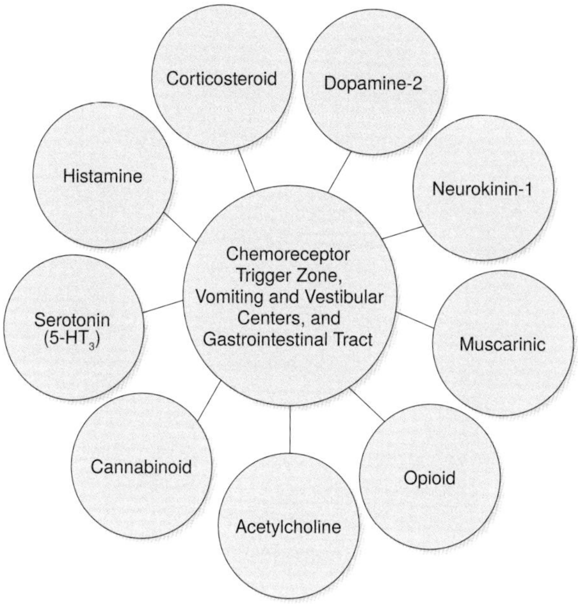

Note. Based on information from National Comprehensive Cancer Network, 2018b.

(2) Incidence: Anticipatory CINV occurs in 18%–57% of patients, with nausea being more common than vomiting (NCCN, 2018b).

(3) Risk factors (Molassiotis et al., 2016; NCI, 2017e)

(a) Anxiety prior to chemotherapy cycle

(b) History of poorly controlled CINV with previous encounters

(c) Young or middle-aged (e.g., patients younger than age 50)

(d) Female gender

(e) Feeling warm, hot, dizzy, or sweaty after chemotherapy

(f) Susceptibility to motion sickness

(g) History of pregnancy-induced nausea and vomiting

(4) To minimize the risk of anticipatory CINV, adequate antiemetic control and prevention of acute and delayed CINV is essential.

b) Acute-onset CINV: May occur within a few minutes of chemotherapy administration and normally peaks after 5–6 hours and resolves within 24 hours (NCCN, 2018b)

(1) Incidence: The incidence of acute CINV is related to the emetogenic potential of the antineoplastic medication.

(a) Grunberg et al. (2005) developed categories for the emetogenic potential of IV chemotherapy. These categories are based on the number of people who experience acute emesis without the use of antiemetic prophylaxis. Current treatment guidelines published by NCCN, the American Society of Clinical Oncology (ASCO), and the Multinational Association of Supportive Care in Cancer/European Society for Medical Oncology are based on these categories (Hesketh et al., 2017; NCCN, 2018b; Roila et al., 2016).

i. High: Emesis occurs in greater than 90% of patients.

ii. Moderate: Emesis occurs in 30%–90% of patients.

iii. Low: Emesis occurs in 10%–30% of patients.

iv. Minimal: Emesis occurs in fewer than 10% of patients.

(b) The use of antiemetic prophylaxis also affects the incidence of acute CINV (Gilmore et al., 2014).

(2) Risk factors (NCI, 2017e; NCCN, 2018b; Warr, Street, & Carides, 2011)

(a) Female gender

(b) Young or middle-aged (e.g., patients younger than age 50)

(c) Alcohol use: Patients who have a history of low or no alcohol consumption have more nausea and vomiting than patients with a history of high alcohol consumption.

(d) History of motion sickness

(e) History of pregnancy-induced nausea and vomiting

(3) Prevention of acute CINV (NCCN, 2018b)

(a) Prophylactic medications should be administered before chemotherapy.

(b) If the patient is receiving chemotherapy from multiple emetogenic risk categories, antiemetic prophylactic therapy should be based on the highest emetogenic risk medication (Hesketh et al., 2017; NCCN, 2018b).

c) Delayed-onset CINV: Occurs more than 24 hours after chemotherapy administration and may last for several days (NCI, 2017b; NCCN, 2018b)

(1) Occurs commonly with carboplatin, cisplatin, cyclophosphamide, and doxorubicin

(2) More common in patients who have experienced acute emesis

(3) Risk factors for delayed CINV are similar to risk factors for acute CINV.

(4) The time frame of delayed emesis may depend on the regimen and the emetogenic potential of the chemotherapy medication(s) administered on the last day of treatment.

d) Breakthrough CINV: Occurs despite prophylactic treatment and may require rescue antiemetics (Navari, 2015)

e) Refractory CINV: Occurs when antiemetic prophylaxis has not been effective in previous cycles, and antiemetic prophylaxis is not effective in the subsequent cycle (Navari, 2015)

5. Assessment: Determine the potential causes of nausea and vomiting, the specific type or types of nausea and vomiting, and the level of emetogenicity (see Tables 15-1 and 15-2). See Table 15-3 for NCI's nausea and vomiting grading scale.

a) Chemotherapy (NCCN, 2018b)

(1) Evaluate the emetogenic potential of all chemotherapy agents the patient will be taking, and ensure that the patient has prescriptions for antiemetics.

(2) Also consider the emetogenic potential of oral antineoplastic therapies.

b) Immunotherapy

(1) Patients receiving immunotherapy agents may experience nausea and vomiting as part of a flu-like syndrome.

(2) Monoclonal antibodies may be associated with nausea and vomiting during the infusion.

(3) Cytokine release syndrome, a possible toxicity related to chimeric antigen receptor T cells, monoclonal antibodies, and other immunotherapies, may result in nausea and vomiting (Bonifant, Jackson, Brentjens, & Curran, 2016; Kroschinsky et al., 2017)

c) Targeted therapy (Navari & Aapro, 2016; Roila et al., 2016)

(1) New targeted therapies have varying schedules and combinations, as well as different doses.

(2) Because of the lack of prospective trials regarding nausea and vomiting related to targeted therapies, evidence regarding antiemetic therapy for these medications is lacking.

(3) The incidence and severity of nausea and vomiting with targeted therapies are not well studied.

(4) Some newer targeted therapies have low or minimal emetogenic potential (see Table 15-2).

d) Physical causes

(1) Tumor obstruction

(2) Gastroparesis

(3) Constipation

(4) Increased intracranial pressure

(5) Brain metastasis

(6) Vestibular dysfunction

(7) Uncontrolled pain

(8) Fluid volume status

e) Metabolic causes

(1) Hypercalcemia

(2) Hyponatremia

(3) Hyperglycemia

(4) Uremia

(5) Increased creatinine

f) Other medications (e.g., opioids, antibiotics)

g) Psychological causes

(1) Anxiety

(2) Fear

(3) Emotional distress

6. Potential complications of nausea and vomiting (NCI, 2017e; Tipton, 2014)

a) Discomfort

b) Treatment delay or withdrawal from treatment

c) Interference with quality of life (e.g., impaired mobility, fatigue)

d) Dehydration

e) Metabolic disturbances

f) Anorexia, weight loss, and nutritional depletion

g) Physical and mental deterioration

h) Increased intracranial pressure

i) Aspiration

j) Decreased ability to perform self-care

k) Costs associated with treatment

l) Family/caregiver strain

m) Lost productivity and missed work

7. Collaborative management: Pharmacologic interventions (see Table 15-4)

a) The goal of antiemetic therapy is prevention of nausea and vomiting (NCCN, 2018b).

(1) Consider the level of emetogenicity based on the medication, route of administration, and dose administered. Choose the prophylactic antiemetic regimen based on the drug with the highest emetogenicity. Also

Table 15-1. Emetogenic Potential of Intravenous Antineoplastic Drugs

Incidence	Medication	Onset (hours)	Duration (hours)
High (90%–100%)	AC combination (doxorubicin or epirubicin + cyclophosphamide)[a]	–	–
	Carboplatin (AUC ≥ 4 mg/ml × min)[b]	–	–
	Carmustine (> 250 mg/m²)	–	–
	Cisplatin	1–6	24–48
	Cyclophosphamide (≥ 1,500 mg/m²)	–	–
	Dacarbazine	1–3	1–12
	Doxorubicin (≥ 60 mg/m²)[b]	–	–
	Epirubicin (> 90 mg/m²)[b]	–	–
	Ifosfamide (≥ 2 g/m² per dose)[b]	–	–
	Mechlorethamine	0.5–2	8–24
	Streptozocin	1–6	12–24
Moderate (30%–90%)	Aldesleukin (> 12–15 MIU/m²)	–	–
	Amifostine (> 300 mg/m²)	–	–
	Arsenic trioxide	–	–
	Azacitidine	–	–
	Bendamustine	–	–
	Busulfan[b]	–	–
	Carboplatin (AUC < 4 mg/ml × min)	–	–
	Carmustine (≤ 250 mg/m²)[b]	–	–
	Clofarabine	–	–
	Cyclophosphamide (< 1,500 mg/m²)	–	–
	Cytarabine (> 200 mg/m²)	–	–
	Dactinomycin	2–5	24
	Daunorubicin	2–6	24
	Dinutuximab	–	–
	Doxorubicin (< 60 mg/m²)	–	–
	Epirubicin (≤ 90 mg/m²)	–	–
	Idarubicin	6–12	24+
	Ifosfamide (< 2 g/m² per dose)[b]	3–6	24+
	Interferon alfa (≥ 10 MIU/m²)	–	–
	Irinotecan	–	–
	Irinotecan liposomal injection	–	–
	Melphalan[b]	–	–
	Methotrexate (≥ 250 mg/m²)[b]	1–12	12–72
	Oxaliplatin	1–6	24
	Temozolomide[b]	–	–
	Trabectedin	–	–
Low (10%–30%)	Aldesleukin (≤ 12 MIU/m²)	–	–
	Amifostine (≤ 300 mg/m²)	–	–

(Continued on next page)

Table 15-1. Emetogenic Potential of Intravenous Antineoplastic Drugs *(Continued)*

Incidence	Medication	Onset (hours)	Duration (hours)
Low (10%–30%) *(cont.)*	Atezolizumab	–	–
	Belinostat	–	–
	Blinatumomab	–	–
	Brentuximab	–	–
	Cabazitaxel	–	–
	Carfilzomib	–	–
	Cytarabine (100–200 mg/m²)[b]	–	–
	Docetaxel[b]	–	–
	Doxorubicin (liposomal)	–	–
	Eribulin	–	–
	Etoposide	3–8	–
	5-Fluorouracil[b]	3–6	24+
	Floxuridine	–	–
	Gemcitabine	–	–
	Interferon alfa (> 5–10 MIU/m²)	–	–
	Ixabepilone	–	–
	Methotrexate (> 50 mg/m² but < 250 mg/m²)[b]	–	–
	Mitomycin[b]	1–4	48–72
	Mitoxantrone	4–6	6+
	Necitumumab	–	–
	Olaratumab	–	–
	Omacetaxine	–	–
	Paclitaxel[b]	4–8	–
	Paclitaxel, albumin bound	–	–
	Pemetrexed	–	–
	Pentostatin	–	–
	Pralatrexate[b]	–	–
	Romidepsin	–	–
	Talimogene laherparepvec	–	–
	Thiotepa[b]	–	–
	Topotecan	6–12	24–72
	Ziv-aflibercept	–	–
Minimal (< 10%)	Alemtuzumab[b]	–	–
	Asparaginase	–	–
	Avelumab	–	–
	Bevacizumab	–	–
	Bleomycin[b]	3–6	–
	Bortezomib[b]	–	–
	Cetuximab[b]	–	–

(Continued on next page)

Table 15-1. Emetogenic Potential of Intravenous Antineoplastic Drugs *(Continued)*

Incidence	Medication	Onset (hours)	Duration (hours)
Minimal (< 10%) *(cont.)*	Cladribine (2-chlorodeoxyadenosine)	–	–
	Cytarabine (< 100 mg/m²)[b]	6–12	3–12
	Daratumumab	–	–
	Decitabine	–	–
	Denileukin diftitox	–	–
	Dexrazoxane	–	–
	Elotuzumab[b]	–	–
	Fludarabine[b]	–	–
	Interferon alfa (≤ 5 MIU/m²)	–	–
	Ipilimumab[b]	–	–
	Methotrexate (< 50 mg/m²)[b]	4–12	3–12
	Nelarabine	–	–
	Nivolumab	–	–
	Obinutuzumab	–	–
	Ofatumumab	–	–
	Panitumumab[b]	–	–
	Pegaspargase	–	–
	Peginterferon	–	–
	Pembrolizumab	–	–
	Pertuzumab[b]	–	–
	Ramucirumab	–	–
	Rituximab	–	–
	Siltuximab	–	–
	Temsirolimus[b]	–	–
	Trastuzumab[b]	–	–
	Valrubicin	–	–
	Vinblastine[b]	4–8	–
	Vincristine	4–8	–
	Vincristine (liposomal)	–	–
	Vinorelbine[b]	–	–

[a] Any regimen that includes an anthracycline and cyclophosphamide (e.g., regimen consisting of cyclophosphamide, doxorubicin, vincristine, and prednisone)

[b] Discrepancies noted in the references

AC—anthracycline plus cyclophosphamide; AUC—area under the plasma concentration versus time curve; MIU—million international units

Note. Based on information from Grunberg et al., 2011; National Comprehensive Cancer Network, 2018b; Roila et al., 2016.

From "Chemotherapy Toxicities and Management" (pp. 518–519), by D. Camp-Sorrell in C.H. Yarbro, D. Wujcik, and B.H. Gobel (Eds.), *Cancer Nursing: Principles and Practice* (8th ed.), 2018, Burlington, MA: Jones & Bartlett Learning. Copyright 2018 by Jones & Bartlett Learning. Adapted with permission.

consider patient-specific risk factors (Hesketh et al., 2017; Roila et al., 2016).

(2) Patient response to pharmacologic interventions for nausea and vomiting requires frequent assessment, with treatment modification as appropriate (NCCN, 2018b).

(3) Steroids are not recommended to be used as antiemetic prophylaxis for immunotherapies and cellular therapies (NCCN, 2018b).

Table 15-2. Emetogenic Potential of Oral Antineoplastic Drugs

Incidence	Medication
Moderate to high (≥ 30%)	Altretamine Busulfan (≥ 4 mg/dl) Ceritinib Crizotinib Cyclophosphamide (≥ 100 mg/m²/day) Enasidenib Estramustine Etoposide[a] Hexamethylmelamine Lenatinib Lomustine (single day) Midostaurin Mitotane Niraparib Olaparib[a] Panobinostat Procarbazine Rucaparib Temozolomide (> 75 mg/m²/day)[a] Trifluiridine/tipiracil Vinorelbine
Minimal to low (< 30%)	Abemaciclib Afatinib Alectinib Axitinib Bexarotene Bosutinib[a] Brigatinib Busulfan (< 4 mg/day)[a] Cabozantinib[a] Capecitbine Chlorambucil Cobimetinib Cyclophosphamide (< 100 mg/m²/day)[a] Dabrafenib Dasatinib Erlotinib Everolimus Fludarabine Gefitinib Hydroxyurea Ibrutinib Idelalisib Imatinib[a] Ixazomib Lapatinib Lenalidomide L-Phenylalanine mustard Melphalan Mercaptopurine Methotrexate Neratinib Nilotinib Osimertinib Palbociclib Pazopanib Pomalidomide

(Continued in next column)

Table 15-2. Emetogenic Potential of Oral Antineoplastic Drugs *(Continued)*

Incidence	Medication
Minimal to low (< 30%) *(cont.)*	Ponatinib Regorafenib Ribociclib Ruxolitinib Sonidegib Sorafenib Sunitinib Tegafur-uracil Temozolomide (≤ 75 mg/m²/day)[a] Thalidomide Thioguanine Topotecan Trametinib Tretinoin Vandetanib Vemurafenib Venetoclax Vismodegib Vorinostat

[a] Discrepancies noted in the references

Note. Based on information from Grunberg et al., 2011; National Comprehensive Cancer Network, 2018b; Roila et al., 2016.

b) Prevention and management of anticipatory CINV: Benzodiazepines may reduce the occurrence of anticipatory CINV. They should be administered beginning the night before treatment and may be repeated one to two hours before chemotherapy administration (NCCN, 2018b; Roila et al., 2016).

c) Prevention and management of acute and delayed CINV related to IV antineoplastic administration

(1) ASCO and NCCN have published antiemetic guidelines (Hesketh et al., 2017; NCCN, 2018b). Although the guidelines are similar, there are some differences.

(2) For patients receiving IV agents categorized as high emetogenic risk

(a) NCCN recommends use of a three-drug combination of a 5-HT_3 receptor antagonist, a NK_1 receptor antagonist, and dexamethasone prior to chemotherapy administration (NCCN, 2018b).

i. Olanzapine may be added to the three-drug combination (NCCN, 2018b).

ii. Alternatively, an olanzapine-containing regimen consisting of olanzapine, palonosetron, and dexamethasone may be used (NCCN, 2018b).

Table 15-3. Common Terminology Criteria for Adverse Events Grading for Nausea and Vomiting

	Grade				
Adverse Event	**1**	**2**	**3**	**4**	**5**
Nausea	Loss of appetite without alteration in eating habits	Oral intake decreased without significant weight loss, dehydration, or malnutrition	Inadequate oral caloric or fluid intake; tube feeding, total parenteral nutrition, or hospitalization indicated	–	–
Vomiting	Intervention not indicated	Outpatient IV hydration; medical intervention indicated	Tube feeding, total parenteral nutrition, or hospitalization indicated	Life-threatening consequences	Death

Note. From *Common Terminology Criteria for Adverse Events* [v.5.0], by National Cancer Institute Cancer Therapy Evaluation Program, 2017. Retrieved from https://ctep.cancer.gov/protocoldevelopment/electronic_applications/docs/CTCAE_v5_Quick_Reference_5x7.pdf.

iii. Lorazepam may be used in combination with the aforementioned antiemetics to improve control in high-risk regimens (NCCN, 2018b).

iv. Consider adding an H_2 antagonist or proton pump inhibitor (NCCN, 2018b).

v. Antiemesis prophylaxis consisting of dexamethasone; olanzapine; aprepitant and dexamethasone; or a combination of aprepitant, dexamethasone, and olanzapine should be given on days 2–4. This varies depending on what prophylaxis was given day 1 (NCCN, 2018b).

(b) ASCO recommends use of a four-drug combination consisting of a 5-HT_3 receptor antagonist, an NK_1 receptor antagonist, dexamethasone, and olanzapine prior to chemotherapy administration (Hesketh et al., 2017).

i. Dexamethasone and olanzapine should be administered on days 2–4. Exception: Patients receiving an anthracycline and cyclophosphamide should only receive olanzapine on days 2–4.

ii. If aprepitant was administered on day 1, it will be administered on day 2–3 also (Hesketh et al., 2017).

(c) Anthracycline plus cyclophosphamide regimens are classified as highly emetogenic and should be treated as such (Hesketh et al., 2017; Roila et al., 2016).

(d) Pediatric patients should receive a three-drug combination consisting of a 5-HT_3 receptor antagonist, aprepitant, and dexamethasone (Hesketh et al., 2017).

i. If the patient cannot receive aprepitant, a 5-HT_3 receptor antagonist and dexamethasone should be administered (Hesketh et al., 2017).

ii. If the patient cannot receive dexamethasone, palonosetron and aprepitant should be administered (Hesketh et al., 2017).

(3) For patients receiving IV agents categorized as moderate emetogenic risk

(a) NCCN recommends use of a two-drug combination of a 5-HT_3 receptor antagonist and dexamethasone prior to chemotherapy administration (NCCN, 2018b).

i. An NK_1 receptor antagonist or olanzapine may be added to the regimen (NCCN, 2018b).

ii. Alternatively, an olanzapine-containing regimen consisting of olanzapine, palonosetron, and dexamethasone may be used (NCCN, 2018b).

iii. Lorazepam may be used in combination with the aforementioned antiemetics to improve control (NCCN, 2018b).

iv. Addition of an H_2 antagonist or proton pump inhibitor

Table 15-4. Commonly Used Agents for Prevention and Treatment of Chemotherapy-Induced Nausea and Vomiting

Classification	Mechanism of Action	Drug	Route, Dose, and Schedule for Adult Patients	Indications	Side Effects	Nursing Considerations
Atypical antipsychotic	Acts on multiple receptor sites, including dopamine, histamine, serotonin, and acetylcholine-muscarine	Olanzapine	2.5–10 mg PO daily	Prevention of acute and delayed n/v	Dizziness, sedation, weight gain, altered cardiac conduction (prolonged QTc), anticholinergic effects (e.g., constipation, dry mouth, blurry vision, urinary retention)	Drug is contraindicated in patients with dementia. Risk of extrapyramidal symptoms is increased in patients receiving metoclopramide or haloperidol.
Benzodiazepine	Acts as CNS depressant; interferes with afferent nerves from cerebral cortex by gamma-aminobutyric acid inhibition, causing sedation	Alprazolam	0.5–1 mg PO given the night before treatment and repeated 1–2 hours before chemotherapy administration	Prevention of anticipatory n/v	Sedation, confusion, hyperactivity, agitation, dizziness, lightheadedness, hallucinations	Use starting dose of 0.5 mg PO in older adult patients, patients with advanced liver disease, or patients with other pertinent comorbidities.
		Lorazepam	0.5–2 mg PO, sublingual, or IV every 6 hours For anticipatory n/v: 0.5–2 mg PO beginning the night before treatment and repeated 1–2 hours before chemotherapy administration	In combination with other antiemetics as needed for acute or delayed n/v Prevention of anticipatory n/v	Sedation, confusion, hyperactivity, agitation, dizziness, lightheadedness, hallucinations	Use with caution in older adult patients and those with hepatic or renal dysfunction.
Cannabinoid	Activates cannabinoid receptors	Dronabinol	5–10 mg PO every 4–6 hours	Treatment of breakthrough or refractory n/v	Sedation, vertigo, euphoria, dysphoria, dry mouth, tachycardia, orthostasis	Incidence of paranoid reactions or abnormal thinking increases with maximum doses.
		Nabilone	1–2 mg PO BID Maximum recommended dose is 6 mg given in divided doses TID.	Treatment of breakthrough or refractory n/v	Sedation, vertigo, euphoria, dysphoria, dry mouth, tachycardia, orthostasis	Incidence of paranoid reactions or abnormal thinking increases with maximum doses.

(Continued on next page)

Table 15-4. Commonly Used Agents for Prevention and Treatment of Chemotherapy-Induced Nausea and Vomiting *(Continued)*

Classification	Mechanism of Action	Drug	Route, Dose, and Schedule for Adult Patients	Indications	Side Effects	Nursing Considerations
Corticosteroid	Antiprostaglandin synthesis activity; mechanism of antiemetic activity unknown	Dexamethasone	12 mg IV or PO day 1 of chemotherapy, then 8 mg IV or PO days 2–4 of chemotherapy	Prevention of acute and delayed n/v	Insomnia, anxiety, acne, hyperglycemia, dyspepsia	Dexamethasone metabolism may be affected by administration of fosaprepitant, aprepitant, and netupitant, and the dosage of dexamethasone may require adjustment. Administer slowly over at least 10 minutes to prevent perianal or vaginal burning or itching.
Dopamine antagonist	Blocks dopamine receptors	Haloperidol	0.5–2 mg PO or IV every 4–6 hours	Treatment of breakthrough n/v	Sedation, extrapyramidal symptoms, dystonia, dizziness, orthostasis, prolonged QT interval	Extrapyramidal symptoms are more common in younger patients. Drug is highly sedating.
		Metoclopramide	10–40 mg PO or IV every 4–6 hours	Prevention of acute or delayed n/v Treatment of breakthrough n/v	Sedation, extrapyramidal symptoms, dystonia, dizziness, orthostasis, diarrhea	Drug increases gut motility and may be given to manage gastroparesis. Risk of tardive dyskinesia increases with duration of treatment and increasing cumulative dose.
		Prochlorperazine	Doses vary; 10 mg PO or IV every 6 hours. Also available as 25 mg suppositories every 12 hours	Prevention of acute and delayed n/v Treatment of breakthrough n/v	Sedation, extrapyramidal symptoms, dystonia, dizziness, orthostasis	Drug is highly sedating.
$5\text{-}HT_3$ antagonist	$5\text{-}HT_3$ receptor antagonist	Dolasetron	100 mg PO on day 1; may also be given on days 2 and 3 or daily	Prevention of acute and delayed n/v	Headache, diarrhea, dizziness, fatigue, prolonged QT interval, cardiac arrhythmia	IV dolasetron is not recommended because it is associated with increased risk of cardiac arrhythmias.
Neurokinin-1 antagonist	Neurokinin-1 receptor antagonist	Aprepitant	125 mg PO day 1 of chemotherapy, then 80 mg PO days 2 and 3	Prevention of acute and delayed n/v	Fatigue, headache, dyspepsia, decreased appetite, hiccups	When administered with dexamethasone, aprepitant causes an increase in dexamethasone serum levels. Consider decreasing dose of dexamethasone by 50%.
		Fosaprepitant	150 mg IV once on day 1	Prevention of acute and delayed n/v	Fatigue, infusion site reactions, infusion-related hypersensitivity reactions, diarrhea, hiccups, lack of appetite, headache	When administered with dexamethasone, fosaprepitant causes an increase in dexamethasone serum levels. Consider decreasing dose of dexamethasone by 50%.

(Continued on next page)

Table 15-4. Commonly Used Agents for Prevention and Treatment of Chemotherapy-Induced Nausea and Vomiting *(Continued)*

Classification	Mechanism of Action	Drug	Route, Dose, and Schedule for Adult Patients	Indications	Side Effects	Nursing Considerations
Neurokinin-1 antagonist *(cont.)*		Granisetron	10 mg SC, 2 mg PO, or 0.01 mg/kg (max 1 mg) IV once prior to chemotherapy IV or PO dose may be repeated on days 2 and 3.	Prevention of acute and delayed n/v	Headache, nausea, constipation, vomiting, weakness, prolonged QT interval	The SC formulation should not be given more frequently than 1-week intervals.
		Granisetron transdermal	Transdermal patch containing 34.3 mg of granisetron One patch delivers 3.1 mg per 24 hours. Apply a single patch to the upper outer arm a minimum of 24–48 hours before chemotherapy. Patch can be worn for up to 7 days (depending upon the duration of the regimen). Remove patch a minimum of 24 hours after completion of chemotherapy.	Prevention of acute and delayed n/v	Headache, nausea, constipation, vomiting, weakness	Remove patch if severe skin reactions occur (allergic, erythematous, macular, or papular rash or pruritus). Instruct patients to avoid direct exposure of application site to natural and artificial light while wearing the patch and for 10 days after removal.
		Ondansetron	16–24 mg PO or 8–16 mg IV (maximum 32 mg/day) Orally disintegrating tablet formulation: 8 mg	Prevention of acute and delayed n/v	Headache, fatigue, malaise, constipation, drowsiness, sedation, QT prolongation	PO ondansetron has a lower risk of cardiac arrhythmia than IV ondansetron. A single dose larger than 16 mg of ondansetron is not recommended because of increased risk of prolonged QT interval.
		Palonosetron	0.25 mg IV on day 1 or 0.5 mg PO given once, 30 minutes prior to chemotherapy on day 1	Prevention of acute and delayed n/v	Headache, constipation	Mean terminal elimination half-life is approximately 40 hours. IV palonosetron is more effective for the prevention of delayed nausea than other 5-HT_3 receptor antagonists.
Combination	Neurokinin-1 receptor antagonist/5-HT_3 receptor antagonist	Netupitant/palonosetron	Netupitant 300 mg plus palonosetron 0.5 mg PO given once on day 1	Prevention of acute and delayed n/v	Headache, fatigue, weakness	Monitor patients for hypersensitivity reaction. Avoid use in patients with severe hepatic impairment or end-stage renal disease.

BID—twice daily; CNS—central nervous system; 5-HT_3—5-hydroxytryptamine-3; IV—intravenous; n/v—nausea and vomiting; PO—by mouth; QTc—QT interval corrected; SC—subcutaneous; TID—three times daily

Note. Based on information from Camp-Sorrell, 2018; National Comprehensive Cancer Network, 2018b; Wolters Kluwer Health, 2017.

may be considered (NCCN, 2018b).

v. Antiemesis prophylaxis consisting of dexamethasone; olanzapine; aprepitant with or without dexamethasone; or a 5-HT_3 receptor antagonist may be given on days 2 and 3. This will depend on what prophylaxis was given day 1 (NCCN, 2018b).

(*b*) ASCO recommends use of a two-drug combination of a 5-HT_3 receptor antagonist and dexamethasone prior to chemotherapy administration (Hesketh et al., 2017).

i. For patients receiving carboplatin area under the plasma concentration versus time curve greater than or equal to 4 mg/ml × min, an NK_1 receptor antagonist should be added (Hesketh et al., 2017).

ii. Dexamethasone should be administered on days 2 and 3 if the patient is receiving chemotherapy associated with delayed nausea and vomiting (Hesketh et al., 2017).

iii. Pediatric patients should receive a 5-HT_3 receptor antagonist and dexametha sone (Hesketh et al., 2017). If dexamethasone cannot be administered, the patient should receive a 5-HT_3 receptor antagonist and aprepitant (Hesketh et al., 2017).

(4) For patients receiving IV agents categorized as low emetogenic risk

(*a*) NCCN recommends a single dose of dexamethasone, metoclopramide, prochlorperazine, or a 5-HT_3 receptor antagonist (NCCN, 2018b).

i. Lorazepam may be used in combination with the aforementioned antiemetics to improve control (NCCN, 2018b).

ii. Addition of an H_2 antagonist or proton pump inhibitor may be considered (NCCN, 2018b).

(*b*) ASCO recommends a single dose of dexamethasone or a 5-HT_3 receptor antagonist (Hesketh et al., 2017).

(*c*) Pediatric patients should receive ondansetron or granisetron (Hesketh et al., 2017).

(5) For patients receiving IV agents categorized as minimal emetogenic risk: No routine prophylaxis is recommended for adults or pediatric patients (Hesketh et al., 2017; NCCN, 2018b).

d) Prevention and management of acute and delayed CINV related to oral antineoplastic administration (NCCN, 2018b)

(1) For patients receiving oral agents categorized as high to moderate emetogenic risk

(*a*) Administer a 5-HT_3 receptor antagonist prior to chemotherapy and continue daily (NCCN, 2018b).

(*b*) Lorazepam may be used in combination with the aforementioned antiemetics to improve control (NCCN, 2018b).

(*c*) Consider adding an H_2 antagonist or proton pump inhibitor (NCCN, 2018b).

(2) For patients receiving oral agents categorized as low to minimal emetogenic risk

(*a*) No routine prophylaxis is recommended, but antiemetics may be prescribed as needed. If the patient experiences nausea and vomiting, consider metoclopramide, prochlorperazine, or a 5-HT_3 receptor antagonist (NCCN, 2018b).

(*b*) Lorazepam may be used in combination with the aforementioned antiemetics to improve control (NCCN, 2018b).

(*c*) Addition of an H_2 antagonist or proton pump inhibitor may be considered (NCCN, 2018b).

e) Treatment of delayed CINV

(1) Delayed nausea is often more common and severe than acute nausea and is more difficult to treat (NCCN, 2018b).

(2) 5-HT_3 receptor antagonists, although effective for the prevention of acute vomiting, are not as effective for delayed vomiting.

(3) For patients receiving moderately or highly emetogenic chemotherapy,

dexamethasone should be administered daily during chemotherapy and for two to three days after chemotherapy administration to help prevent delayed CINV (NCCN, 2018b). ASCO recommends dexamethasone and olanzapine on days 2–4 for patients receiving highly emetogenic chemotherapy, unless the patient receives an anthracycline and cyclophosphamide. In this case, ASCO recommends olanzapine only for days 2–4 (Hesketh et al., 2017).

(4) To prevent delayed CINV in patients receiving carboplatin, an NK_1 receptor antagonist should be given in combination with a 5-HT_3 receptor antagonist and dexamethasone (Roila et al., 2016).

f) Management of breakthrough CINV

(1) Consider adding other antiemetic agents from different drug classifications, using caution to avoid overlapping side effects (Hesketh et al., 2017).

(2) Around-the-clock antiemetic dosing should be strongly considered for patients with breakthrough CINV (NCCN, 2018b).

(3) Consider an H_2 antagonist or proton pump inhibitor for patients with dyspepsia (NCCN, 2018b).

(4) Monitor the patient's hydration and electrolytes, and correct as needed (NCCN, 2018b).

(5) Olanzapine may be an effective option for breakthrough CINV (Chiu et al., 2016; Roila et al., 2016) and should be included in the prophylactic antiemesis regimen for patients with breakthrough nausea and vomiting (Hesketh et al., 2017).

(6) Consider using nonpharmacologic interventions in conjunction with antiemetics.

8. Collaborative management: Nonpharmacologic interventions

a) Behavioral interventions, including hypnosis, progressive muscle relaxation, biofeedback, yoga, and systematic desensitization; music therapy; and acupuncture or acupressure may be used as adjunct therapies to manage anticipatory CINV (NCCN, 2018b; Roila et al., 2016).

b) Management of patient expectations may be one approach to help prevent chemotherapy-induced nausea (J. Lee et al., 2017).

c) Several nonpharmacologic interventions have been studied for the prevention and management of CINV; however, their effectiveness is not established. These interventions may be considered for use in conjunction with antiemetics and include acupuncture, acupressure, aromatherapy, exercise, ginger, massage, therapeutic touch, and yoga (J. Lee et al., 2017; Marx et al., 2017).

9. Dietary interventions (American Cancer Society, 2017; NCCN, 2018b)

a) Encourage patients to eat small, frequent meals and food that is cold or room temperature.

b) Encourage patients to eat bland food.

c) Encourage patients to drink clear liquids (e.g., fruit juice, broth).

d) Encourage patients to avoid food that is fried, spicy, fatty, or very sweet and to avoid food with strong odors.

e) Ensure that patients are eating enough protein and calories. A liquid replacement meal (protein shake) may be used.

f) Encourage patients to avoid overeating.

g) Encourage patients to use plastic forks and spoons if metal silverware causes a bitter taste.

h) Consider a dietary consult.

10. Patient and family education

a) Instruct patients to take antiemetics as prescribed and to notify the provider if they are unable to take medications as prescribed.

b) Remind patients as necessary to take antiemetics before arriving for treatment. Ensure that antiemetics have been taken prior to administration of chemotherapy.

c) Instruct patients to notify providers if nausea and vomiting persists for longer than 24 hours or if they are unable to maintain fluid intake. Ensure that parents of pediatric patients notify providers if vomiting persists for more than two hours.

d) Refer patients to educational materials such as NCI's *Eating Hints: Before, During and After Cancer Treatment* (NCI, 2018a).

B. Anorexia

1. Definitions

a) Anorexia: Loss of a desire to eat (NCI, 2017c).

b) Cachexia: *Cancer cachexia* is "a multifactorial syndrome characterised by an ongoing loss of skeletal muscle mass (with or without loss of fat mass) that cannot be fully reversed by conventional nutritional support and leads to progressive functional impairment" (Fearon et al., 2011, p. 490; see Figure 15-3). This is

Figure 15-3. Cancer Cachexia

Diagnostic Criteria
- Weight loss > 5% over the past 6 months; or
- Body mass index < 20 kg/m² and any degree of weight loss > 2%; or
- Appendicular skeletal muscle index consistent with sarcopenia (another wasting syndrome) and weight loss of > 2%

Stages of Cancer Cachexia
- Precachexia: Weight loss of ≤ 5%, along with other symptoms such as impaired glucose tolerance or anorexia
- Cachexia: Weight loss > 5% or other symptoms and conditions consistent with the diagnostic criteria for cachexia
- Refractory cachexia: Patients experiencing cachexia who are no longer responsive to cancer treatment, have a low performance score, and have a life expectancy of < 3 months

Note. Based on information from Fearon et al., 2011.

the most complete international definition of cancer cachexia at this time (Bruggeman et al., 2016).

2. Pathophysiology
   a) Anorexia and cachexia result from a complicated process involving numerous physiologic and psychological factors.
      (1) Tumor effects (Aapro et al., 2014)
         (a) May be present at diagnosis in some malignancies (e.g., pancreatic, upper GI, lung)
         (b) Obstruction of the esophageal or GI tract can lead to nutrient malabsorption, nausea, vomiting, and pain (e.g., tumors causing dysphagia or affecting GI function).
         (c) Proinflammatory cytokines such as interleukin-1, interleukin-6, tumor necrosis factor-alpha, and interferon alfa may be released by the tumor or malignant inflammation, which can lead to satiety and metabolic abnormalities (Aoyagi, Terracina, Raza, Matsubara, & Takabe, 2015; Mattox, 2017).
         (d) Metabolic abnormalities may lead to increased hepatic glucose and lipolysis production of glycerol and free fatty acids (Mattox, 2017).
         (e) Hypercalcemia secondary to bony involvement or paraneoplastic syndrome may lead to nausea, vomiting, and anorexia.
         (f) Decreased hypothalamic response signals lead to reduced appetite (Mattox, 2017).
         (g) Low levels of protein and albumin lead to more extracellular water, and less intracellular water causes low oncotic pressure and increases weight loss (Schwarz et al., 2017).
      (2) Treatment effects (Suzuki, Asakawa, Amitani, Nakamura, & Inui, 2013)
         (a) Surgery may result in malabsorption, obstruction, and fluid and electrolyte abnormalities.
         (b) Chemotherapy and radiation therapy side effects include nausea, vomiting, mucositis, taste changes, xerostomia, constipation, and diarrhea.
         (c) Combination therapy results in a greater number of adverse effects.
         (d) Body composition can predict toxicity, as noted with sarcopenic obesity. *Sarcopenia* is the degenerative loss of skeletal muscle mass. High body mass index can mask sarcopenia (Bruggeman et al., 2016).
      (3) Psychosocial effects (Weber & O'Brien, 2017)
         (a) Cancer-related depression often coexists with anorexia and cachexia, especially in patients with late-stage disease or multiple symptoms. The prevalence of depression among patients with cancer is estimated to be 15%–25% (Weber & O'Brien, 2017).
         (b) Anxiety, fear, grief, fatigue, pain, and the patient's reaction to body image changes may contribute to anorexia.
         (c) Cachexia results in decreased survival and poor response to treatment (Aoyagi et al., 2015; NCI, 2017c).
3. Incidence: Historical data have demonstrated a 50% overall incidence of anorexia and cachexia in patients with cancer, increasing to 86% in the last week or two before death (Aoyagi et al., 2015).
4. Risk factors (Aapro et al., 2014; Aoyagi et al., 2015)
   a) Advanced cancer
   b) Solid tumor, with head and neck, GI, and lung as most common types
   c) Chronic illness such as pulmonary disease and congestive heart failure
   d) Increased prevalence in the very young and older adults
   e) Surgery, radiation, chemotherapy, immunotherapy, and targeted therapy

f) Data suggest that certain targeted therapy agents (e.g., sorafenib) may increase muscle wasting (Aapro et al., 2014).
g) Biomarkers: Researchers are in the early stages of using genotype to identify predisposition to cachexia (Aapro et al., 2014).

5. Clinical manifestations: Patients have reduced ability to tolerate treatment based on the following, especially if they present with pretreatment cachexia (Aapro et al., 2014).
a) Involuntary weight loss of more than 5% of usual weight
b) Changes in appetite
(1) Changes in taste and smell
(2) Early satiety
c) Changes in GI tract function
(1) Dysmotility
(2) Inactivation of bile salts or pancreatic enzymes
(3) Partial or complete obstruction
d) Loss of muscle mass
e) Loss of adipose tissue
f) Fatigue and weakness
g) Immune system impairment
h) Metabolic dysfunction
i) Hypoalbuminemia

6. Assessment (Dev, Wong, Hui, & Bruera, 2017; Schwarz et al., 2017)
a) Perform a nutritional assessment.
b) Grading: See Table 15-5 for NCI's anorexia grading scale.
c) Monitor weight: Compare with pretreatment weight.
d) Obtain a diet history or have the patient complete a food diary for several days.
e) Measure body composition.
(1) Triceps skinfold thickness estimates body fat.
(2) Mid-arm muscle circumference estimates muscle mass.
f) Assess laboratory results (Aapro et al., 2014).
(1) Evaluate plasma markers for inflammation.
(2) Assess for endocrine abnormalities (e.g., thyroid dysfunction, metabolic abnormalities, hypogonadism).
g) Assess functional status (LeBlanc et al., 2015; Wheelwright et al., 2013).
(1) The Functional Assessment of Anorexia/Cachexia Therapy (FAACT) is used to assess patients' status.
(2) Functional status tools include symptom distress and quality-of-life questions.
(3) Incorporate early initiatives for high-risk disease processes.

7. Collaborative management and impact on clinical outcomes: The extent of nutritional intervention depends on the cause of weight loss and overall goals of the patient, family, and healthcare team. Early consultation of a palliative care team has proved to be effective for improving outcomes (Aapro et al., 2014; Dev et al., 2017; Schwarz et al., 2017).
a) Treatment of the cancer is the primary objective.
b) Symptom management: Management of symptoms such as nausea and vomiting, mucositis, oral candidiasis, diarrhea, constipation, taste changes, dysphagia, xerostomia, fatigue, pain, and depression may improve anorexia. See the discussion of management in the specific sections of this publication.
c) Pharmacologic intervention: Progestins and corticosteroids are the only two classes of drugs to have demonstrated effectiveness as appetite stimulants (NCCN, 2017a; Zhan, Wang, Qian, & Yu, 2013).
(1) Progestins (Zhan et al., 2013)
(a) Megestrol acetate is most commonly used.

Table 15-5. Common Terminology Criteria for Adverse Events Grading for Anorexia

	Grade				
Adverse Event	**1**	**2**	**3**	**4**	**5**
Anorexia	Loss of appetite without alteration in eating habits	Oral intake altered without significant weight loss or malnutrition; oral nutritional supplements indicated	Associated with significant weight loss or malnutrition (e.g., inadequate oral caloric and/or fluid intake); tube feeding or total parenteral nutrition indicated	Life-threatening consequences; urgent intervention indicated	Death

Note. From *Common Terminology Criteria for Adverse Events* [v.5.0], by National Cancer Institute Cancer Therapy Evaluation Program, 2017. Retrieved from https://ctep.cancer.gov/protocoldevelopment/electronic_applications/docs/CTCAE_v5_Quick_Reference_5x7.pdf.

(b) It improves appetite and weight gain in patients with cancer; however, it does not improve quality of life.
(c) Mechanism of action is not well established.
(d) Optimal dose is not defined but ranges from 100–1,600 mg/day.
(e) Side effects include deep vein thrombosis, edema, impotence in men, and GI disturbances.
(2) Corticosteroids (Matsuo et al., 2017)
(a) Mechanism of action is unknown but may be related to euphoric and anti-inflammatory effects.
(b) Effects are short lived.
(c) Many side effects, both short and long term, can occur, including immunosuppression, hyperglycemia, and muscle wasting.

d) Nonpharmacologic interventions (Dev et al., 2017; NCCN, 2017a)
(1) Interventions may not increase weight or length of survival but may improve quality of life.
(2) Refer to a dietitian for early nutritional counseling. Strong evidence supports early nutritional counseling as beneficial for prevention and reduction of cachexia (J.L.C. Lee, Leong, & Lim, 2016).
(3) Provide high-calorie/high-protein oral supplements as needed and tolerated.
(4) Consider enteral or parenteral nutrition if the disease or treatment interferes with the patient's ability to eat or to absorb nutrients (J.L.C. Lee et al., 2016; NCCN, 2017a).
(a) Enteral: Patients must have a functioning bowel. Complications include aspiration pneumonia, electrolyte abnormalities, diarrhea, and infection.
(b) Parenteral: Types include central parenteral nutrition, which requires a central venous access device, and peripheral parenteral nutrition. Complications include high infection rate.
(5) Integrative medicine (NCI, 2017d): Complementary and alternative medicine may be helpful, including Reiki, music therapy, prayer, and spiritual uplifting.
(6) Improved outcomes result when an interprofessional team is involved (Scott, Reid, Hudson, Martin, & Porter, 2016).

8. Patient and family education
a) Provide written handouts, stressing high-calorie/high-protein foods.
b) Monitor and record weight weekly, using the same scale at the same time of the day.
c) Encourage patients to eat small, frequent meals.
d) Provide an attractive setting for meals.
e) Encourage patients to engage in physical activity.
f) Use measures to control nausea and vomiting, mucositis, dry mouth, taste changes, and other side effects of treatment.
g) Include patients in family activities to avoid isolation, even if patients have no appetite. Do not force patients to eat.
h) Remind families that patients' lack of appetite is caused by the effects of the disease and treatment and is not their fault.
i) Refer to community resources as needed, such as home care and Meals on Wheels.
j) Loss of muscle and weight is an overt symptom and can cause both patient and family distress (Aapro et al., 2014). Refer for psychosocial and emotional support.

C. Diarrhea
1. Overview
a) Definition: *Diarrhea* is defined as loose or watery stools three or more times daily that may be acute, chronic, or persistent in nature (National Institute of Diabetes and Digestive and Kidney Diseases, 2016). Diagnostic criteria include greater than 75% water content, increase in daily stool weight, and frequency (Pessi et al., 2014).
(1) Classification based on duration (National Institute of Diabetes and Digestive and Kidney Diseases, 2016)
(a) Acute: Diarrhea lasting one to two days that typically resolves on its own
(b) Persistent: Diarrhea lasting two to four weeks
(c) Chronic: Diarrhea that lasts at least four weeks with potentially transient symptoms
(2) Classification based on intensity (Shaw & Taylor, 2012; see Figure 15-4)
(a) Uncomplicated: Grade 1 or 2 toxicity without additional signs or symptoms
(b) Complicated: Grade 3 or 4 diarrhea OR grade 1 or 2 diarrhea with one or more of the follow-

Figure 15-4. Evidence-Based Recommendations for the Management of Cancer Treatment–Induced Diarrhea

ASSESSMENT AND EVALUATION

History
- Physiologic history of GI disturbances (baseline, treatment, and disease related)
- Current treatment type
- Duration, volume, consistency, and frequency of diarrhea
- Presence of nocturnal diarrhea
- Confounding factors (fever, orthostatic hypotension, abdominal pain or cramping, weakness)
- Symptom interference with QOL and function

Physical assessment: Abdominal assessment (visual assessment, auscultation for bowel sounds, palpation, percussion as appropriate)

Laboratory assessment: CBC, electrolytes, stool workup (presence of blood, fecal leukocytes, infectious sources), lactoferrin, and fecal calprotectin testing may be indicated at baseline and every 3 weeks during treatment with anti–PD-1 checkpoint inhibitors.

CTCAE GRADING

Grade 1	Grade 2	Grade 3	Grade 4	Grade 5
Increase of < 4 stools daily from baseline; mild increase in ostomy output compared to base ine	Increase of 4–6 stools daily from baseline; moderate increase in ostomy output compared to baseline; diarrhea interferes with or limits instrumental ADL	Increase of ≥ 7 stools daily from baseline; severe increase in ostomy output compared to baseline; limitations in self-care ADL; hospitalization indicated for management	Life-threatening consequences with urgent intervention indicated	Death

CLASSIFICATION

Uncomplicated	Complicated
• Grade 1 or 2 toxicity • No additional signs or symptoms • May be managed with nonpharmacologic approaches including dietary changes and increased oral hydration to 3–4 L of water daily • May also introduce pharmacologic measures	• Grade 3 or 4 toxicity • Grade 1 or 2 toxicity with ≥ 1 complicating symptoms (e.g., cramping, nausea, vomiting, fever, bleeding, dehydration, sepsis, neutropenia, decreased performance status) • The patient should be managed in the hospital with IV fluids, electrolyte replacement, and pharmacologic measures.

MANAGEMENT BY TREATMENT TYPE

Chemotherapy

Grade 1	Grade 2	Grades 3–4
• Decrease or delay chemotherapy; oral hydration and electrolyte replacement, if indicated, are recommended. • Initiate loperamide.[a] • Consider dietary modifications.[b]	• Decrease or delay chemotherapy dosing. • Initiate IV fluids if the patient is unable to tolerate oral fluids. • Initiate or continue loperamide.[a] • Diphenoxylate/atropine may also be used if the patient is not on opioids. • For *Clostridium difficile*–related diarrhea, initiate metronidazole (500 mg PO/IV QID × 10–14 days) or vancomycin 125–500 mg PO QID × 10–14 days; probiotics may also be used to stabilize and restore the gut flora. • For non-*Clostridium difficile* infection, treat according to culture findings.	• Discontinuation (temporarily or permanently) of causative agent may be necessary. • Provide IV fluids. • Manage with antidiarrheal and anticholinergic agents. • Transition to or escalate dosing of octreotide.[a] • Continue or initiate antibiotics as outlined for grade 2 management.

Radiation Therapy[c]

Grade 1	Grade 2	Grades 3–4
• Initiate loperamide.[a] • Consider dietary modifications;[b] psyllium fiber may be effective.	• Initiate loperamide.[a] • Progress to octreotide[a] if diarrhea is unresponsive to loperamide.	• IV fluids are recommended though may not need to be administered in the hospital setting. • Octreotide may be indicated with complicating symptoms.[a] • In grade 3–4 diarrhea, octreotide is indicated in the presence of complicating symptoms but may not be required in uncomplicated cases. IV antibiotics may worsen symptoms in some cases. Carefully assess workup results to determine if the indication for IV antibiotics outweighs the risk.

(Continued on next page)

Figure 15-4. Evidence-Based Recommendations for the Management of Cancer Treatment–Induced Diarrhea *(Continued)*

Hormone Therapy[d]	
Grade 1	**Grade 2**
• Consider dietary modifications.[b] • Initiate loperamide.[a]	• Consider octreotide;[a] escalate dose if diarrhea persists of worsens. • Tincture of opium at 10–15 drops every 3–4 hours has also been recommended.

Targeted Therapy		
Grade 1	**Grade 2**	**Grades 3–4**
• Dose reduce or hold targeted therapy. • Initiate loperamide; discontinue and progress to octreotide if diarrhea is unresponsive to loperamide.[a] • Oral hydration and electrolyte replacement, if indicated, are recommended. • Consider dietary modifications.[b]	• Decrease or delay targeted therapy. • Consider IV fluids if patient is unable to tolerate PO; continue antidiarrheal with loperamide; discontinue and progress to octreotide if diarrhea is unresponsive to loperamide.[a] • Consider anticholinergics, corticosteroids, infliximab, and probiotics.	• Discontinuation (temporarily until symptoms resolve or possibly permanently) of causative targeted agent may be necessary. • Hospitalization may be required for supportive care. • Manage with antidiarrheal and anticholinergic agents. • IV fluids may be indicated.

Immunotherapy			
Grade 1	**Grade 2**	**Grade 3**	**Grade 4**
• Consider holding immunotherapy per NCCN guidelines. • Initiate loperamide,[a] oral hydration, and close monitoring.	• Hold immunotherapy. • Administer IV methylprednisolone (1 mg/kg/day). • If no response in 2–3 days: – Increase dose to 2 mg/kg/day. – Consider infliximab. – If refractory to infliximab, consider vedolizumab.	• Discontinue anti–CTLA-4 agents. • Anti–PD-1/PD-L1 therapy may be reinstated after toxicity resolution. • Hospitalization may be required for supportive care. • Administer IV methylprednisolone (2 mg/kg/day). • If no response in 2 days: – Consider infliximab (5 mg/kg/day). – If refractory to infliximab, consider vedolizumab.	• Permanently discontinue immunotherapy. • Hospitalization may be required for supportive care. • Administer IV methylprednisolone (2 mg/kg/day). • If no response in 2 days: – Consider infliximab (5–10 mg/kg). – If refractory to infliximab, consider vedolizumab.

ASSESSMENT FOR SYMPTOM RESOLUTION

- **Chemotherapy, hormone therapy, and targeted therapy:** Assess diarrhea every 12–24 hours and escalate care as required in the presence of increased grading or persistent diarrhea; discontinue loperamide after 12 hours without diarrhea.
- **Radiation therapy:** Assess diarrhea every 12–24 hours and escalate care as required in the presence of increased grading or persistent diarrhea; continue loperamide throughout radiation therapy.
- **Immunotherapy:** Assess diarrhea every 12–24 hours; taper corticosteroids over 4–6 weeks before resuming. When symptoms improve to grade 1 or better, may be able to restart treatment in the presence of low-dose steroids after evaluation of risks and benefits.
- Regardless of treatment, consider use of a patient journal to document stool frequency and characteristics in the ambulatory setting.

[a] Loperamide dosing is 4 mg starting dose followed by 2 mg every 4 hours or after every unformed stool (maximum daily dose of 16 mg). Octreotide is generally dosed at 100–150 mcg TID up to 500 mcg TID.

[b] Dietary modifications include eliminating all lactose-containing products, alcohol, caffeine, foods containing sugar alcohols (e.g., sorbitol), foods high in insoluble fiber (e.g., raw fruits and vegetables), and high-fat foods.

[c] Many cases can be managed in the outpatient setting; evaluate patients for complicating conditions (e.g., fever, sepsis, neutropenia), which may require hospitalization for management.

[d] Diarrhea is a less frequent but possible side effect of hormone therapy.

ADL—activities of daily living; CBC—complete blood count; CTCAE—Common Terminology Criteria for Adverse Events; CTLA-4—cytotoxic T-lymphocyte antigen 4; GI—gastrointestinal; IV—intravenous; NCCN—National Comprehensive Cancer Network; PD-1—programmed cell death protein 1; PD-L1—programmed cell death-ligand 1; PO—by mouth; QID—four times daily; QOL—quality of life; TID—three times daily

Note. Based on information from Benson et al., 2004; Kottschade et al., 2016; Lui et al., 2017; National Cancer Institute Cancer Therapy Evaluation Program, 2017; National Comprehensive Cancer Network, 2017a, 2018c; Pessi et al., 2014; Shaw & Taylor, 2012; Thorpe, Byar, Conley, Drapek, et al., 2017.

ing: cramping, nausea, vomiting, fever, bleeding, dehydration, sepsis, neutropenia, or decreased performance status

b) Antineoplastic treatment–induced diarrhea

(1) Diarrhea in patients with cancer is associated with both the disease and its treatments, including radiation therapy, chemotherapy, targeted therapy, and immunotherapies, as well as graft-versus-host disease (Koselke & Kraft, 2012).

(2) Chemotherapy-induced diarrhea contributes to treatment alterations (60%), interference in daily activities (30%), dose delays (28%), treatment discontinuation (15%), and death related to dehydration (5%) (McQuade, Stojanovska, Abalo, Bornstein, & Nurgali, 2016).

2. Pathophysiology: The pathophysiology and etiology of diarrhea in patients with cancer can be multifaceted. All possible causes of diarrhea need to be considered to treat the patient appropriately.

a) Classifications of diarrhea

(1) Osmotic diarrhea: Osmotic diarrhea usually is related to injury to the gut, dietary factors, or problems with digestion. Water is drawn into the intestinal lumen, resulting in increased stool volume and weight. Lactose intolerance is an example of this type of diarrhea. New-onset lactose intolerance can occur in patients undergoing cancer treatment (Andreyev, Davidson, Gillespie, Allum, & Swarbrick, 2012). Osmotic diarrhea is associated with large stool volumes and sometimes is improved with fasting or elimination of the causative factor (e.g., lactose, sorbitol).

(2) Secretory diarrhea: The small and large intestines secrete more fluids and electrolytes than can be absorbed. Infection and inflammation of the gut; damage to the gut caused by chemotherapy, radiation therapy, or graft-versus-host disease; and certain endocrine tumors can cause secretory diarrhea. The imbalance between absorption and secretion leads to production of a large volume of fluid and electrolytes in the small bowel. This type of diarrhea is associated with large volumes and may require a period of bowel rest with parenteral nutrition followed by slow diet progression as tolerated (Muehlbauer, 2014).

(3) Exudative diarrhea: This type is caused by alterations in mucosal integrity, epithelial loss, enzyme destruction, and defective absorption of the colon. Mucosal inflammation and ulceration caused by inflammatory diseases, cancers, and cancer treatment may result in the outpouring of plasma, proteins, mucus, and blood into the stool, all of which can result in exudative diarrhea (Deshpande, Lever, & Soffer, 2013).

(4) Inflammatory diarrhea: Inflammatory diarrhea develops from invasive or toxin-producing bacteria causing impaired mucosal integrity that may result in tissue damage (Barr & Smith, 2014).

(5) Dysentery: Dysentery is diarrhea characterized by blood in the stool (Schmidt-Hieber et al., 2017).

b) Pathophysiologic mechanisms by antineoplastic agent category

(1) Chemotherapy (Koselke & Kraft, 2012): Direct mucosal damage and toxicity can be caused by the metabolic by-products of agents (e.g., SN-38G from irinotecan), mitotic arrest of cells in the GI tract resulting in alterations to the osmotic gradient (e.g., with 5-fluorouracil), or stimulation of inflammatory cytokines, tumor necrosis factor-alpha, and prostaglandins.

(2) Targeted therapy (Pessi et al., 2014)

(a) Secretive diarrhea is believed to be associated with excessive chloride secretion associated with many of the anti–epidermal growth factor receptor agents; this toxicity also may be amplified by combination with radiation therapy.

(b) Ischemic mucosal damage may result from agents such as sorafenib.

(3) Immunotherapy (Spain, Diem, & Larkin, 2016): Immune-mediated colitis, as well as resulting diarrhea, is a primary immune-related adverse event associated with immunotherapies, specifically checkpoint inhibitors, and may present as acute or delayed (often five to seven weeks after therapy).

c) Differential diagnosis for diarrhea in patients with cancer (Schmidt-Hieber et al., 2017)

(1) Paraneoplastic diarrhea: Rare and triggered by secretion of vasoactive intestinal polypeptide leading to watery diarrhea and electrolyte alterations

(2) Infection-related diarrhea (see section D on colitis)

(a) Neutropenic enterocolitis: Observed in patients with chemotherapy-associated neutropenia resulting from penetration of the bowel wall by various pathogens

(b) Bacterial infections: Nontyphoidal *Salmonella, Shigella, Yersinia, Clostridium* enterocolitis, and *Campylobacter*

(c) Viral infections: Norovirus, rotavirus, adenovirus, cytomegalovirus

(d) Parasitic infections: *Blastocystis, Cryptosporidium, Cyclospora cayetanensis, Entamoeba histolytica, Giardia lamblia, Cystoisospora belli, Sarcocystis hominis, Sarcocystis suihominis, Strongyloides stercoralis*

3. Incidence

a) The incidence of diarrhea varies greatly depending on the agent(s) used. The specific agent, dose, schedule, and combination with other cancer therapies influence the severity of chemotherapy-induced diarrhea (McQuade et al., 2016).

(1) Chemotherapy: Overall incidence may be as high as 80%; incidence of post-chemotherapy chronic diarrhea may be as high as 49%. Regimens containing either irinotecan or 5-fluorouracil account for up to 80% of the incidence of chemotherapy-induced diarrhea and for one-third of patients experiencing grade 3 or 4 diarrhea (McQuade et al., 2016).

(2) Targeted therapy: Overall incidence is approximately 60% and primarily associated with tyrosine kinase inhibitors (Pessi et al., 2014).

(a) Erlotinib: Up to 18%

(b) Gefitinib: 25.9%–51.6%

(c) Lapatinib: Up to 64%; increased toxicity in combination with trastuzumab (up to 60%)

(d) Afatinib: 14.4% (grade 3–4) to 95% (grade 1–2)

(e) Regorafenib: 34%–40% (grade 3–4: 5%–8%)

(f) Cabozantinib: 64% (12% reported as severe)

(g) Imatinib: 20%–26% (1% reported as severe)

(h) Pazopanib: 52% (grade 3 or 4: less than 4%)

(i) Sunitinib: 44% (grade 3 or 4: 5%)

(j) Sorafenib: 43%–55.3% (grade 3 or 4: 2%–7.8%)

(k) Ziv-aflibercept: 69.2% (grade 3 or 4: 19%)

(l) Axitinib: 11% (grade 3 or higher)

(m) Vandetanib: 74% (10% reported as severe and leading to dose reduction)

(n) Everolimus: 1%–3% (grade 3 or 4)

(o) Vemurafenib: 5%–6%

(p) Dabrafenib: 1%

(q) Trametinib and selumetinib: 45%–50% (grade 3 or 4: 4%)

(r) Crizotinib: 50%–60%

(3) Immunotherapy (Pessi et al., 2014)

(a) Monoclonal antibodies: Associated with 1%–2% (grade 3) to 21% (grade 2) incidence of diarrhea (Pessi et al., 2014)

i. Trastuzumab: Up to 7%; increased in combination with other therapies (e.g., hormone therapy, 19%; chemotherapy, up to 47%)

ii. Pertuzumab: 3% as monotherapy; up to 7.9% in combination with trastuzumab and docetaxel

iii. Cetuximab: 13%–28% as monotherapy (2% reported as severe); incidence of 80% in combination therapy with chemotherapy (grade 3 or 4: 6%–28%)

iv. Panitumumab: 21% as monotherapy (2% reported as severe); incidence of 70% in combination therapy with chemotherapy (grade 3 or 4: 8%–20%)

v. Bevacizumab: 69.2% (grade 3 or 4: 19%)

(b) Checkpoint inhibitors (Spain et al., 2016)

i. Ipilimumab: 22%–33%

ii. Anti–programmed cell death protein 1 antibodies: 8%–19%

iii. Combination ipilimumab and nivolumab: 44%

4. Clinical manifestations: Diarrhea can contribute to numerous sequelae, including dehydration, fever, malnutrition, sepsis, frank bleeding, moderate to severe cramping, renal insufficiency, cardiac dysfunction, and severe electrolyte imbalance, that can contribute to impaired quality of life and treatment delays, dose reductions and discontinuation, and even death (Andreyev et al., 2014; Koselke & Kraft, 2012).
   a) Additional sequelae may include perianal skin breakdown, discomfort, or infection; reduced absorption of oral medications; anxiety; and exhaustion.
   b) Immune-mediated colitis is characterized by abdominal pain, rectal or mucosal bleeding, and inflammation of the large bowel. In severe cases, it can progress to intestinal colitis and possibly death (Spain et al., 2016).
5. Risk factors
   a) Disease related (NCI, 2017a)
      (1) Carcinoid syndrome
      (2) Colon cancer
      (3) Lymphoma
      (4) Medullary carcinoma of the thyroid
      (5) Pancreatic cancer
      (6) Pheochromocytoma
   b) Treatment related
      (1) Chemotherapy: Capecitabine, cisplatin, cytosine arabinoside, cyclophosphamide, daunorubicin, docetaxel, doxorubicin, 5-fluorouracil, interferon, irinotecan, leucovorin, methotrexate, oxaliplatin, paclitaxel, topotecan (NCI, 2017a)
      (2) Targeted therapy: Tyrosine kinase inhibitors, epidermal growth factor receptor–targeted therapies (Pessi et al., 2014)
      (3) Immunotherapy: Checkpoint inhibitors (Pessi et al., 2014)
      (4) Radiation therapy: Monotherapy or combination radiation therapy, particularly to the pelvis, abdomen, or lower thoracic and lumbar spine, can lead to destruction of the cells of the lumen of the bowel and can be an acute or chronic toxicity (NCI, 2017a).
      (5) Surgery: Celiac plexus block, cholecystectomy, esophagogastrectomy, gastrectomy, pancreatic duodenectomy, intestinal resection, vagotomy (NCI, 2017a). Manipulation of the bowel during surgery may cause diarrhea or ileus.
      (6) Other pharmacologic agents: Antibiotics, magnesium-containing antacids, antihypertensives, colchicine, digoxin, iron, lactulose, laxatives, methyldopa, metoclopramide, misoprostol, potassium supplements, propranolol, theophylline (NCI, 2017a)
   c) Acute or chronic conditions (NCI, 2017a)
      (1) Immunosuppression
      (2) Infection related to mucositis and neutropenia (e.g., infection with rotavirus, *Escherichia coli*, *Shigella*, *Salmonella*, *Giardia*, or *Clostridium difficile*)
      (3) Graft-versus-host disease
      (4) Diabetes, hyperthyroidism, inflammatory bowel disease (Crohn disease, diverticulitis, gastroenteritis, HIV/AIDS, ulcerative colitis), obstruction (tumor related)
      (5) Malabsorption, partial bowel obstruction, bowel edema, motility disruption
   d) Behavioral and psychosocial (NCI, 2017a)
      (1) Anxiety and stress
      (2) Dietary causes (e.g., lactose intolerance; ingestion of caffeine, alcohol, or spicy or fatty foods; use of hyperosmotic dietary supplements)
6. Assessment: Timely and accurate assessment is critical to the management of diarrhea and prevention of severe sequelae, including death (NCI, 2017a).
   a) Assessment (Andreyev et al., 2014)
      (1) History
         (a) Assess patients for concerning symptoms, which include abdominal cramps or nausea not responsive to pharmacologic management, inability to eat, increased fatigue, chest pain, vomiting, reduced urine output secondary to dehydration, fever (higher than 38.5°C), GI bleed, and previous admission for diarrhea.
         (b) Include a diet history to evaluate for items that could contribute to diarrhea (e.g., irritating foods, alcohol, coffee, fiber, fruit, lactose-containing foods or fluids, sorbitol-based gum, candy, herbal teas that may contain laxatives), as well as history or new onset of food or lactose intolerance or allergies.
         (c) Assess stool quality and characteristics, including continence and changes in bowel patterns,

frequency, consistency, volume, odor, and visible presence of blood in stool.

(*d*) Evaluate current or recent medications, including antacids (especially those containing magnesium), antiarrhythmics, antibiotics, antihypertensives, caffeine, diuretics, laxatives or stool softeners, magnesium oxide, nonsteroidal anti-inflammatory drugs, potassium or calcium supplements, promotility agents (metoclopramide), and theophylline.

(*e*) Evaluate other confounding factors, including travel history (outside the United States), use of alternative therapies (e.g., dietary supplements, herbal remedies), and opioid withdrawal.

(2) Physical assessment

(*a*) Vital signs

(*b*) Weight (with attention to significant weight gain or loss)

(*c*) Peripheral perfusion

(*d*) Physical examination, with particular attention to the GI system (e.g., visual inspection; palpation and auscultation of the abdomen with particular attention to guarding and rebound tenderness; assessment for fecal impaction, including in patients with neutropenia, unless such an examination would cause severe rectal pain)

(*e*) Alterations in skin integrity, particularly focused on the perianal area

(*f*) Evaluation for signs and symptoms of dehydration, including delayed capillary refill and reduced skin turgor

(3) Laboratory assessment

(*a*) Stool sample for consistency, presence of blood, and infectious sources. Conduct *Clostridium difficile* testing and consider testing for rotavirus and norovirus in the winter and bacterial and parasite cultures if travel would put the patient at risk (NCCN, 2017a).

(*b*) Serum chemistries for electrolyte imbalance, specifically potassium

(*c*) Albumin levels, which may be decreased with diarrhea

(*d*) Complete blood count to determine if neutropenia or infection is present

(*e*) Acid–base balance and lactate concentrations in presence of hypotension and tachycardia

(*f*) Urinalysis

(*g*) Biopsy of ulcerations to evaluate for viral infection, particularly cytomegalovirus

(4) Radiographic assessment

(*a*) Computed tomography scan of the abdomen to evaluate for enterocolitis, perforation, abscess, and pancreatitis

(*b*) Endoscopy and flexible sigmoidoscopy

b) Assessment tools: The Common Terminology Criteria for Adverse Events is the current standard for assessment and grading of treatment-related toxicities, including diarrhea (NCI Cancer Therapy Evaluation Program [CTEP], 2017; see Figure 15-4).

7. Collaborative management (see Figure 15-4)

a) Fluid resuscitation

(1) Oral: Daily fluid intake of 3–4 L of water is recommended, in some cases with the addition of salt and sugar (Pessi et al., 2014).

(2) IV: Fluid bolus, preferably using normal saline (never hypotonic solutions such as 5% dextrose), should be implemented to evaluate for blood plasma volume increases. If hemodynamic stability is not achieved, further evaluation from an intensivist or nephrologist should be sought (Andreyev et al., 2014).

b) Electrolyte repletion

(1) Hypokalemia: Potassium less than 3.5 mEq/L

(2) Magnesium: Less than 0.4 mmol/L or, in symptomatic patients, less than 0.4–0.7 mmol/L

(3) Calcium: Adjusted calcium concentration less than 2.2 mmol/L

(4) Phosphates: If severe (less than 0.3 mmol/L) or moderate (0.3–0.6 mmol/L), consider repletion; hypomagnesemia and hypocalcemia might predispose patients to hypophosphatemia.

c) Pharmacologic management

(1) Chemotherapy- and targeted therapy–induced diarrhea

(a) Loperamide: Nonanalgesic agonist that decreases intestinal motility through activity on the mu-opioid receptor in the mesenteric plexus (McQuade et al., 2016). Dosing: Starting dose is 4 mg, followed by 2 mg every two hours, taken 30 minutes before food if possible (Andreyev et al., 2014; Shaw & Taylor, 2012; Thorpe, Byar, Conley, Drapek, et al., 2017).

(b) Octreotide: Synthetic somatostatin analog that increases intestinal transit time through inhibition of gut hormones (McQuade et al., 2016). Dosing: 500 mcg twice daily is currently recommended and may be administered via IV or subcutaneous administration. Octreotide may be effective in patients who are refractory to loperamide (Andreyev et al., 2014; Thorpe, Byar, Conley, Drapek, et al., 2017).

(c) Tincture of opium: Decreases intestinal motility through activity on the mu-opioid receptors; contains 10 mg/ml of morphine (McQuade et al., 2016)

i. Dosing: 10–15 drops per 3–4 hours. Evidence is limited, specifically in the presence of chemotherapy- and targeted therapy–induced diarrhea; however, it may be used as second-line therapy (Koselke & Kraft, 2012).

ii. Monitor for side effects, which may include nausea and vomiting (most common), painful urination, allergic reaction, seizure, abdominal pain, constipation, and potential for respiratory depression (McQuade et al., 2016).

(d) Evidence is mixed regarding the use of steroids alone or in combination with loperamide (Pessi et al., 2014).

(e) Antibiotics should be introduced in diarrhea lasting greater than 24 hours to reduce the risk of sepsis (Koselke & Kraft, 2012).

(f) Irinotecan is a chemotherapy drug that can cause acute diarrhea (during or immediately after drug administration) or delayed diarrhea. Immediate-onset diarrhea is caused by acute cholinergic properties and often is accompanied by other symptoms including abdominal cramping, rhinitis, lacrimation, and salivation. The mean duration of symptoms is 30 minutes, and they usually respond rapidly to atropine. *Delayed diarrhea* is defined as diarrhea occurring greater than 24 hours after administration of irinotecan and commonly is treated with loperamide (Stein, Voigt, & Jordan, 2010). Prophylactic atropine may be considered (unless clinically contraindicated) for patients who experience cholinergic symptoms (Pfizer Inc., 2016; see Table 15-6).

(2) Immune-mediated diarrhea (Spain et al., 2016): Refer to section D for a full review of the management of colitis.

(a) Implement supportive care measures and introduction of loperamide in grade 1 cases, as outlined below.

(b) Prednisolone 0.5–1 mg/kg/day should be initiated in the presence of grade 2 diarrhea or grade 1 diarrhea with no improvement in or worsening symptoms; increase to 1–2 mg/kg/day at grade 3 diarrhea.

(c) Introduce infliximab 5 mg/kg and continue steroid use in the presence of grade 3 diarrhea (except in patients with sepsis or perforation, for whom infliximab is contraindicated).

(d) Include additional use of immunosuppressants, including tacrolimus or mycophenolate mofetil, if the diarrhea is refractory to first-line therapy.

d) Other management strategies

(1) In the presence of severe immune-mediated colitis with resulting diarrhea, colectomy may be appropriate in select cases (Spain et al., 2016).

(2) Dietary modifications, including bland diet, may be implemented (Schmidt-Hieber et al., 2017; Thorpe, Byar, Conley, Drapek, et al., 2017).

Table 15-6. Common Antidiarrheal Medications

Classification	Mechanism of Action	Drug	Route, Dose, and Schedule for Adult Patients[a]	Side Effects[a]	Nursing Considerations[a]
Antimotility agents	Slows GI transit time and promotes reabsorption of water from bowel; antiperistaltic	Diphenoxylate hydrochloride with atropine sulfate (Lomotil®)	Individualize dosage. Initial dose is 10 mg followed by 5 mg PO QID; maximum dose is 20 mg/day.	Dry mouth, urinary retention, confusion, sedation, restlessness	Bacterial diarrhea should also be managed with the appropriate antimicrobial therapy. Lomotil is contraindicated for the treatment of diarrhea secondary to pseudomembranous colitis. In patients with advanced liver disease, drug may precipitate hepatic coma. Do not use in children younger than age 2.
		Loperamide (Imodium® A-D)	4 mg PO initially, followed by 2 mg PO after each unformed stool; do not exceed 16 mg/day. Exception: Doses are higher for late-onset irinotecan-induced diarrhea (2 mg every 2 hours).	Constipation, fatigue, urinary retention, drowsiness, dizziness	Bacterial diarrhea should also be managed with the appropriate antimicrobial therapy. Do not use in children younger than age 2.
Somatostatin analogs	Inhibits growth hormone, glucagon, and insulin; prolongs intestinal transit time; increases sodium and water absorption	Octreotide (Sandostatin®)	100–150 mcg SC or IV TID. Doses may be escalated to 500 mcg SC or IV TID or by continuous IV infusion 25–50 mcg/hr.	Abdominal discomfort, flatulence, constipation, diarrhea, nausea, dizziness, headache, cardiac dysrhythmias, bradycardia	Drug may interact with insulin, oral hypoglycemic medications, beta-blockers, and calcium channel blockers. Insulin requirements may be decreased. Observe for hyperglycemia and hypoglycemia. Drug may decrease levels of cyclosporine when given concurrently. Drug may increase risk of developing gallstones. Drug is recommended after failure of loperamide or in patients with complicated diarrhea. Complicated diarrhea is defined as involving abdominal cramping, nausea and vomiting, fever, sepsis, neutropenia, or bleeding. Sandostatin LAR Depot is under investigation for the treatment of chemotherapy-induced diarrhea.
Anticholinergics	Antagonist of acetylcholine	Atropine	Used for early-onset cholinergic diarrhea (e.g., irinotecan induced), 0.25–1 mg IV or SC	Dry mouth, blurred vision, photophobia, constipation, xerostomia, tachyarrhythmia	Antacids interfere with absorption of atropine. Drug is contraindicated in patients with closed-angle glaucoma.

[a] Consult product information for complete list of contraindications, drug interactions, and dosage ranges.

GI—gastrointestinal; IV—intravenous; PO—oral; QID—four times daily; SC—subcutaneous; TID—three times daily

Note. Based on information from Benson et al., 2004; Engelking, 2008; Gibson & Stringer, 2009; Stein et al., 2010; and manufacturers' prescribing information.

(3) Evidence suggests the potential efficacy of probiotics in reducing antibiotic-associated diarrhea; however, more studies are needed to evaluate safety (Schmidt-Hieber et al., 2017).

e) Interventions by grade (NCCN, 2017a)

(1) Grade 1

(a) Oral hydration and electrolyte replacement

(b) Antidiarrheal medication: Administer antidiarrheal medication as appropriate once infection has been ruled out. This will reduce stool frequency, volume, and peristalsis. Mistakenly using an antidiarrheal to treat diarrhea caused by infection can intensify diarrhea severity and infectious complications.

(c) Dose reduction or discontinuation of chemotherapy if diarrhea is chemotherapy induced

(d) Bland diet or clear liquids

(2) Grade 2

(a) IV fluids if patient cannot tolerate oral hydration

(b) Initiation or continuation of antidiarrheal medication

(c) Introduction or continuation of bland diet or clear liquids

(d) Consideration of anticholinergic agents

(e) Treatment with antibiotics if diarrhea is infection related

(f) Delay or discontinuation of chemotherapy if diarrhea is chemotherapy induced

(g) Withholding of immunotherapy agent if diarrhea is immune mediated

(h) Consideration of corticosteroids, infliximab, and probiotics for immune-related diarrhea

(3) Grade 3 or 4

(a) Inpatient hospitalization, including intensive care for grade 4

(b) For graft-versus-host disease–related diarrhea, dietary limitations, steroids, and consideration of IV nutrition

(c) IV fluids

(d) Antidiarrheal and anticholinergic agents

(e) Consideration of somatostatin

(f) Permanent discontinuation of causative immunotherapy agent (Spain et al., 2016)

8. Patient and family education (Muehlbauer et al., 2009)

a) Discuss treatment-related risks and diarrhea manifestations with patients and caregivers at the outset of treatment, using visual aids, such as the Bristol stool chart, as appropriate (Andreyev et al., 2014).

b) Educate patients to be aware of their baseline bowel functioning, monitor for changes in bowel habits, and report changes to their provider.

c) Start antidiarrheal medications at the specified time. With certain chemotherapy agents, antidiarrheal medication should be provided so that patients can self-administer at the onset.

d) Instruct patients on dietary recommendations and fluid intake.

(1) Avoid foods high in insoluble fiber (e.g., raw fruits and vegetables), greasy or fried foods, lactose, skins, seeds, legumes, caffeine, alcohol, and hyperosmotic liquids. These may be stimulating or irritating to the GI tract.

(2) Include foods high in soluble fiber or pectin in their diets and low insoluble fiber foods such as rice noodles, bananas, white toast, skinned turkey or chicken, fish, and mashed potatoes.

(3) Maintain fluid intake by drinking 8–10 large glasses each day of clear fluids (e.g., bouillon; weak, tepid decaffeinated tea; gelatin; sports drinks). Water alone lacks the needed electrolytes and vitamins. Carbonated and caffeinated drinks contain relatively few electrolytes and may worsen diarrhea. Fluids with glucose are useful because glucose absorption drives sodium and water back into the body.

(4) Limit the use of sugar-free candies or gum made with sugar alcohol (sorbitol), which can cause diarrhea (NCI, 2017a).

(5) Eat food at room temperature if not tolerated otherwise. Hot and cold foods may aggravate diarrhea.

(6) Limit or avoid milk and other dairy products.

(7) Avoid hyperosmotic supplements (e.g., Ensure®), which can contribute to the production of loose, high-volume stools.

e) Instruct patients and families on skin care.

(1) Clean the rectal area with mild soap and water after each bowel movement, rinsing well and patting dry with a soft towel. Cleansing decreases the risk of infection and skin irritation.

(2) Apply moisture-barrier ointment to protect perianal skin.

(3) Take warm sitz baths to relieve pain related to perianal inflammation. Anesthetic creams or sprays may help to relieve pain related to inflammation.

f) Educate patients and families on symptoms to report.

(1) Understand when diarrhea can be self-managed and when to seek help.

(2) Report excessive thirst, fever, dizziness or light-headedness, palpitations, rectal spasms, excessive cramping, watery or bloody stools, and continued diarrhea despite antidiarrheal treatment. These symptoms can be life threatening.

D. Colitis

1. Definitions and pathophysiology: *Colitis* is a general term for a disorder characterized by the inflammation of the colon (NCI CTEP, 2017). Colitis has multiple causes and, therefore, slightly different definitions based on the causative agent.

a) *Neutropenic enterocolitis*, also called *typhlitis*, results from the combination of neutropenia and damage to the bowel mucosa from chemotherapy (Palmore, Parta, Cuellar-Rodriguez, & Gea-Banancloche, 2015). Neutropenic enterocolitis can be life threatening (Nesher & Rolston, 2012).

(1) Severe neutropenia (absolute neutrophil count [ANC] less than 500/mm^3) decreases the immune response against the invasion of local tissue by intestinal microbes.

(2) Mucosal injury predisposes the colon to distension and necrosis (Rodrigues, Dasilva, & Wexner, 2017).

(3) Mucosal motility can be altered, allowing for the colon to become more vulnerable to bacterial invasion and overgrowth (Rodrigues et al., 2017).

(4) Multiple proinflammatory mediators inside the intestinal lumen cause increased mucosal permeability (Nesher & Rolston, 2012).

(5) The cause is frequently polymicrobial and includes bacterial and fungal species, such as *Clostridium difficile* (*C. difficile*) or *Candida albicans* (Nesher & Rolston, 2012; Palmore et al., 2015).

b) *C. difficile* colitis (Anand & Glatt, 1993)

(1) This type of colitis is a superficial necrosis causing exudative plaque of mucosa in the colon caused by *C. difficile* and its toxin.

(2) Chemotherapy agents and antibiotics alter the normal gut flora, causing overgrowth of *C. difficile* and its toxin.

(3) Following chemotherapy administration, the colon may undergo desquamation and necrosis, secondarily providing an anaerobic environment, which in turn allows for overgrowth of *C. difficile* and its toxin.

(4) The bacteria and toxin are unable to be degraded or passed because the colon accumulates protein-rich fluids, such as albumin, in the intraluminal layer.

(5) Decreased degradation of the toxin and increased overgrowth of the *C. difficile* bacteria occur.

(6) This cycle of normal mucosa being destroyed, creating a seemingly perfect environment for *C. difficile* and its toxin to overgrow, is repeated with future cycles of chemotherapy and likely affects the body's ability to reestablish normal flora.

c) Immune-mediated colitis

(1) Cytotoxic T-lymphocyte antigen 4 (CTLA-4) monoclonal antibody (e.g., ipilimumab)

(a) Fully humanized monoclonal antibody (immunoglobulin G1) against CTLA-4 that promotes antitumor T-cell immunity

(b) Causes apoptosis of activated T cells, which negatively regulates T-cell activation

(c) Mechanism of action (Barina et al., 2016)

i. Suppresses CTLA-4, which causes activation of T cells

ii. Activated T cells cause tissue damage inside the colon, which destroys mucosal immunity, disrupting the enteric flora and antibody levels.

iii. Causes inflammation in the GI mucosa and is manifested in diarrhea and immune-mediated colitis

(2) Programmed cell death-protein 1 (PD-1) inhibitor monoclonal antibodies (e.g., nivolumab, pembrolizumab)
  (a) Nivolumab and pembrolizumab are human immunoglobulin G4 monoclonal antibodies that bind to the PD-1 receptor and block its interaction with programmed cell death-ligand 1 and 2 (PD-L1 and PD-L2)
  (b) Mechanism of action (Chen, Pezhouh, Lauwers, & Masia, 2017)
    i. Signaling limits effector function on the activated T cells in the periphery.
    ii. Depletion of regulatory T cells causes inhibition or block of anti-inflammatory mechanisms.
    iii. Inhibited cytokine production and widespread immune dysregulation result.
  (c) PD-1 inhibitors can cause collagenous colitis (Baroudjian et al., 2016).
    i. Characterized by subepithelial collagen band (more than 10 mcm) with increased intraepithelial lymphocytes
    ii. Blocking the PD-1 pathway may trigger mucosal T lymphocytes.
    iii. Diagnosed from colonoscopy with pathologic interpretation
(3) PD-L1 inhibitors (e.g., atezolizumab, avelumab, durvalumab)
  (a) Mechanism of action: Blockade of the PD-L1 pathway causes an increase in T-cell activation, which ultimately leads to decreased tumor size.
  (b) When the PD-L1 pathway is blocked, immune responses are inhibited without causing antibody-dependent cell-mediated cytotoxicity.
  (c) Diarrhea and colitis with PD-L1 agents have a similar presentation as with PD-1 agents.
  (d) The combination of checkpoint inhibitors such as ipilimumab and nivolumab further increases risk and toxicity (Kroschinsky et al., 2017).
  (e) The combination of checkpoint inhibitors and radiation therapy to the abdomen also increases risk of toxicity, most frequently, diarrhea and colitis.
(4) PI3K inhibitors (e.g., idelalisib): Mechanism of action
  (a) Inhibits PI3K pathway to induce apoptosis of malignant B cells
  (b) Causes tissue damage in the colon and mucosal lining, which manifests as diarrhea and immune-mediated colitis (Louie et al., 2015)

2. Incidence
  a) Neutropenic enterocolitis: Incidence is 0.8%–26%, but it is frequently underreported (Nesher & Rolston, 2012).
  b) *C. difficile* colitis
    (1) Incidence of positive *C. difficile* blood cultures is 18%–44% (Nesher & Rolston, 2012).
    (2) Relapse can occur with each subsequent cycle of chemotherapy in as many as 43% of patients (Anand & Glatt, 1993).
  c) Invasive fungal–induced colitis: The incidence of invasive fungal–induced colitis is approximately 5% (Nesher & Rolston, 2012).
  d) Immune-mediated colitis (see Table 15-7)
    (1) CTLA-4 monoclonal antibodies—ipilimumab
      (a) 14% of patients developed symptoms, 33% developed diffuse colitis (Barina et al., 2016).
      (b) 8%–22% of patients developed colitis (Gupta, De Felice, Loftus, & Khanna, 2015).
      (c) 17% of patients developed segmental colitis with diverticulosis (Barina et al., 2016).
      (d) 50% of patients developed isolated rectosigmoid colitis without diverticulosis (Barina et al., 2016).
      (e) The median onset of ipilimumab-induced colitis was 34 days or following three treatments (Cramer & Bresalier, 2017).
      (f) Ipilimumab 3 mg/kg—7% of patients experienced diarrhea with up to six stools above baseline, with only 5% of patients experiencing colitis (Bristol-Myers Squibb Co., 2017).
        i. The median onset to grade 2 colitis was 1.4 months.

Table 15-7. Drug Classes and Associated Colitis and Diarrhea Risk

Drug	Target	Indication	Route	Toxicity Incidence	Median Time to Onset
Tyrosine Kinase Inhibitor					
Idelalisib (Zydelig®)	PI3K	Relapsed CLL/SLL Relapsed follicular lymphoma	PO	Grade 3–4 diarrhea or colitis: 14%	1 week to 1 month
Checkpoint Inhibitors					
Atezolizumab (Tecentriq®)	PD-L1	NSCLC Urothelial carcinoma	IV	Diarrhea or colitis: 19.7%	21 days
Avelumab (Bavencio®)	PD-L1	Merkel cell carcinoma Urothelial carcinoma	IV	Diarrhea: 1.5% Colitis: 0.4%	2.1 months; median duration 6 weeks
Durvalumab (Imfinzi®)	PD-L1	Urothelial carcinoma	IV	Any diarrhea or colitis: 12.6% Grade 3–4 diarrhea or colitis: 1.1%	73 days
Ipilimumab (Yervoy®)	CTLA-4	Melanoma	IV	Diarrhea: 7% Colitis: 5%	1.4–1.7 months
Nivolumab (Opdivo®)	PD-1	Melanoma NSCLC RCC Hodgkin lymphoma Urothelial carcinoma Head and neck cancer	IV	Grade 3–4 diarrhea: 1.6% Colitis: 2.9%	5.3 months
Pembrolizumab (Keytruda®)	PD-1	Melanoma NSCLC HNSCC Hodgkin lymphoma	IV	Grade 3–4 diarrhea: 0.8% Colitis: 1.7%	6–18 weeks

CLL/SLL—chronic lymphocytic leukemia/small lymphocytic lymphoma; CTLA-4—cytotoxic T-lymphocyte antigen 4; HNSCC—head and neck squamous cell carcinoma; IV—intravenous; NSCLC—non-small cell lung cancer; PD-L1—programmed cell death-ligand 1; PD-1—programmed cell death protein 1; PI3K—phosphoinositide 3-kinase; PO—oral; RCC—renal cell carcinoma

Note. Based on information from AstraZeneca Pharmaceuticals LP, 2017; Barina et al., 2016; Baroudjian et al., 2016; Bristol-Myers Squibb Co., 2017, 2018; Cramer & Bresalier, 2017; EMD Serono, Inc., 2017; Genentech, Inc., 2017; Gilead Sciences, Inc., 2018; Gupta et al., 2015; Merck and Co., Inc., 2017; Weidner et al., 2015.

ii. The median onset to grade 3–5 colitis was 1.7 months.

(2) PD-1 inhibitor monoclonal antibodies—nivolumab and pembrolizumab

(*a*) Up to 61% of patients experience immune-related adverse events, including GI, dermatologic, and hepatic toxicities (Cramer & Bresalier, 2017; Gupta et al., 2015).

(*b*) 27% of patients present with mild to severe diarrhea (Cramer & Bresalier, 2017).

(*c*) Up to 12% of patients may develop enterocolitis (Cramer & Bresalier, 2017).

(*d*) Nivolumab (Bristol-Myers Squibb Co., 2018)

i. 2.9% of patients receiving nivolumab as a single agent across clinical trials experienced immune-mediated colitis.

ii. Median time to onset was 5.3 months.

iii. 1% of patients required drug hold.

iv. 0.7% of patients required permanent discontinuation of drug.

(*e*) Pembrolizumab (Merck and Co., Inc., 2017)

i. In the trials that led to U.S. Food and Drug Administration approval, 1.7% of patients experienced colitis.

ii. Median time to onset was 3.5 months, and median duration was 1.3 months.

(3) PD-L1 inhibitor monoclonal antibodies—atezolizumab, avelumab, durvalumab

(a) 9% of patients receiving PD-L1 agents on clinical trials reported diarrhea of all grades (including disease types of melanoma, non-small cell lung cancer, colorectal cancer, ovarian cancer, renal cell carcinoma, pancreatic carcinoma, gastric cancer, and breast cancer) (Brahmer et al., 2012).

(b) Avelumab (EMD Serono, Inc., 2017)

i. 1.5% of patients developed colitis with 0.4% grade 3 colitis.

ii. Median time to onset was 2.1 months, and median duration was six weeks.

(c) Atezolizumab (Genentech, Inc., 2017)

i. 19.7% of patients across clinical trials developed colitis or diarrhea.

ii. 0.8% of patients with urothelial carcinoma and 0.5% of patients with non-small cell lung cancer developed immune-mediated colitis.

iii. Median time to onset was 21 days.

(d) Durvalumab (AstraZeneca Pharmaceuticals LP, 2017)

i. 12.6% of patients in clinical trials developed colitis or diarrhea.

ii. 1.1% developed grade 3–4 colitis or diarrhea.

iii. Median time to onset was 73 days.

(4) PI3K inhibitor—idelalisib

(a) According to a study by Weidner et al. (2015), 30%–45% of patients will develop severe diarrhea with more than seven stools above baseline. Approximately 71% of patients with severe diarrhea will develop colitis.

(b) According to clinical trials leading to U.S. Food and Drug Administration approval of idelalisib, 14% of patients experienced grade 3–4 diarrhea or colitis with median time to onset ranging from one week to one month (Gilead Sciences, Inc., 2018).

3. Risk factors

a) Currently receiving an immunotherapy agent that induces colitis

b) History of colitis, whether chemotherapy induced or from previous immunotherapy agents. Patients who received anti-CTLA-4 therapy and had associated colitis had a higher incidence of colitis when exposed to other immunotherapy agents such as PD-1 inhibitors (Chen et al., 2017).

c) Preexisting bowel abnormalities such as autoimmune diseases (Crohn disease or ulcerative colitis), diverticulitis, history of bowel surgery, and extensive tumor infiltration (Nesher & Rolston, 2012)

d) Neutropenic enterocolitis can occur in patients receiving high-dose chemotherapy and chemotherapy given for acute leukemia treatment (Palmore et al., 2015).

e) Neutropenia, as it reduces the body's immune response and allows for overgrowth of the intestinal microbes (Nesher & Rolston, 2012)

f) Radiation therapy, as it increases risk of mucosal damage and causes injury and destruction to the normal mucosa (Nesher & Rolston, 2012)

4. Clinical manifestations (see Table 15-8)

a) Neutropenic enterocolitis (Palmore et al., 2015)

(1) Febrile and neutropenic (ANC less than $500/mm^3$)

(2) Bowel wall thickening of greater than 4 mm

(3) Right lower quadrant inflammatory mass and mucosal edema; extensive involvement of the large bowel and terminal ileum may occur.

(4) Abdominal pain, cramping, distension, diarrhea, and possibly bloody stool (hematochezia)

b) Immune-mediated colitis

(1) Diarrhea: The hallmark symptom of ipilimumab-associated colitis is 3–20 loose bowel movements per day with possible associated hematochezia (Barina et al., 2016).

(2) Nausea

(3) Abdominal pain

(4) Possible fever or chills

(5) PD-1 inhibitor–induced colitis

Table 15-8. Comparison of Chemotherapy-Induced and Immune-Mediated Colitis

Characteristic	Chemotherapy Induced	Immune Related
Distribution	Superficial	Continuous, superficial
Primary location of inflammation	Diffuse pancolitis	Left colon Distal colon and rectum Diffuse pancolitis
Suspected etiology	Predisposition due to neutropenia *C. difficile* and associated toxin Fungal etiologies Cytomegalovirus	CTLA-4, PD-1, or PI3K inhibition T-cell activation Regulatory T-cell depletion PI3K inhibitor
Histologic findings	Bowel wall thickening > 4 mm Various degrees of hemorrhage, ulcerations, and ecchymosis Exudates have fibrin and cellular debris on severely ulcerated areas Microscopic findings: Mucosal and submucosal edema with associated necrosis	Cryptitis and granulomas Lymphoplasmacytic expansion of lamina propria Apoptotic bodies Neutropenia
Management	Drug hold or discontinuation Bowel rest Antidiarrheal contraindicated Testing to rule out microbial source Consideration of G-CSF until resolution or ANC > 1,000/mm^3 Initiation of empiric antimicrobials Supportive care: Fluids/electrolyte replacement; maintaining hemoglobin > 7 g/dl, platelets > 50,000/mm^3	Drug hold or discontinuation Corticosteroids Use of infliximab in corticosteroid-resistant colitis Surgical intervention as last resort

ANC—absolute neutrophil count; CTLA-4—cytotoxic T-lymphocyte antigen 4; G-CSF—granulocyte–colony-stimulating factor; PD-1—programmed cell death protein 1; PI3K—phosphoinositide 3-kinase

Note. Based on information from Anand & Glatt, 1993; Barina et al., 2016; Baroudjian et al., 2016; Bavi et al., 2017; Cramer & Bresalier, 2017; Gupta et al., 2015; Nesher & Rolston, 2012; Palmore et al., 2015; Rodrigues et al., 2017; Weidner et al., 2015; Yanai et al., 2017.

(*a*) Grade 3 diarrhea

(*b*) Abdominal pain, cramping, discomfort

(*c*) Pembrolizumab (Baroudjian et al., 2016)

i. 16% of patients have diarrhea of any grade, while 1% of patients will have grade 3–4 diarrhea.

ii. Nonbloody diarrhea that can be severe, causing hypokalemia and weight loss as well as other electrolyte imbalances

5. Assessment

a) Neutropenic enterocolitis

(1) Plain radiographic films (x-rays) demonstrate lack of bowel gas, usually in the right lower quadrant with a dilated fluid-filled ascending colon and gaseous dilation in the cecum (Nesher & Rolston, 2012).

(2) Occasionally, a small bowel obstruction is demonstrated. Plain films typically are of limited value and have nonspecific findings, unless a patient has a suspected bowel perforation, in which the presence of free air is demonstrated (Nesher & Rolston, 2012).

(3) Ultrasonography may be used to measure the thickness of the bowel wall and may be useful to measure the clinical course of colitis (Nesher & Rolston, 2012).

(4) Computed tomography (CT) scans can differentiate from other sources of abdominal pain, such as appendicitis and cholecystitis.

(5) CT will demonstrate greater than 4 mm thickening in any segment of the bowel (Nesher & Rolston, 2012).

(6) Colonoscopy is rarely indicated because of the risk of perforation and neutropenia (Rodrigues et al., 2017).

(7) On surgery or autopsy, the bowel appears to be edematous and thickened. It has various degrees of hemorrhage, ulcerations, and ecchymosis.

(8) Exudates have fibrin and cellular debris on severely ulcerated areas (Nesher & Rolston, 2012).

(9) Microscopic findings show mucosal and submucosal edema with associated necrosis (Nesher & Rolston, 2012).

b) Immune-mediated colitis

(1) Ipilimumab-associated colitis

(a) Assessment is based on symptom recognition because of the high incidence.

(b) Most patients do not require colonoscopy (Barina et al., 2016).

(c) CT of the abdomen/pelvis reveals mesenteric vessel engorgement (75%), pericolonic inflammation, hyper-enhancement of colonic mucosa (83%), thickening of the colon wall (75%), distension of the colon with fluid infiltration (25%), pneumatosis, and diverticulosis in the inflamed colon segment. Positron-emission tomography images reveal increased fluorodeoxyglucose avidity in the areas of the colon affected (86%) (Barina et al., 2016)

(d) Colonoscopic findings include distal and diffuse inflammatory colitis with neutrophilic infiltration and ulceration of the mucosal surface (Barina et al., 2016).

(2) PD-1 inhibitor–induced colitis

(a) Colonoscopy reveals inflammatory changes in the GI tract: ulcerations, granularity, exudates, and loss of vascularity (Cramer & Bresalier, 2017; Gupta et al., 2015). Biopsies demonstrate neutrophilic cryptitis and erosions of the mucosal surface (Cramer & Bresalier, 2017).

(b) Three types of colitis seen with colonoscopy via pathologic features (Chen et al., 2017)

i. Active colitis with increased apoptosis and crypt atrophy

ii. Lymphocytic colitis with increased intraepithelial lymphocytes and surface epithelial damage

iii. Recurrent PD-1 inhibitor–induced colitis with features mimicking inflammatory bowel disease due to chronicity

(c) Collagenous colitis induced by pembrolizumab (Baroudjian et al., 2016)

i. Colonoscopy with macroscopic and microscopic evaluation

ii. Colonoscopy reveals predominance of intraepithelial lymphocytes both in surface mucosa and within the tubules in the lamina propria, showing similar presentations between PD-1 and PD-L1 therapies as described previously (Bavi, Butler, Serra, & Chetty, 2017).

(3) PI3K inhibitor–induced colitis: Colonoscopy reveals mild to severe pancolitis with intraepithelial lymphocytosis (86%), crypt epithelial apoptosis (79%), and neutrophilic cryptitis (79%) (Weidner et al., 2015).

6. Collaborative management and prevention

a) Preventing diarrhea includes early recognition of symptoms.

(1) Grading of diarrhea: Proper grading of diarrhea is essential for proper management.

(2) NCI CTEP's (2017) grading criteria are used to assess symptoms of diarrhea or colitis and implement a treatment management strategy (see Table 15-9).

b) Interprofessional collaboration (Mistry, Forbes, & Fowler, 2017)

(1) Educate and inform clinicians on how to identify, grade, and manage diarrhea and colitis.

(2) Early intervention can improve patient outcomes.

(3) Minimize the likelihood of permanent or severe side effects.

c) Rule out infectious colitis.

(1) Perform stool tests for enteric pathogens and *C. difficile* (by polymerase chain reaction, or PCR) (Gupta et al., 2015).

(2) Rule out cytomegalovirus infection by performing immunohistochemical staining on biopsy samples from colonoscopy (Gupta et al., 2015).

Table 15-9. Common Terminology Criteria for Adverse Events Grading for Colitis

	Grade				
Adverse Event	**1**	**2**	**3**	**4**	**5**
Colitis	Asymptomatic; clinical or diagnostic observations only; intervention not indicated	Abdominal pain; mucus or blood in stool	Severe abdominal pain; peritoneal signs	Life-threatening consequences; urgent intervention indicated	Death

Note. From *Common Terminology Criteria for Adverse Events* [v.5.0], by National Cancer Institute Cancer Therapy Evaluation Program, 2017. Retrieved from https://ctep.cancer.gov/protocoldevelopment/electronic_applications/docs/CTCAE_v5_Quick_Reference_5x7.pdf.

(3) Rule out fungal causes of colitis.

d) Perform colonoscopy in any patient with grade 2 or higher diarrhea (Cramer & Bresalier, 2017).

e) Neutropenic enterocolitis

(1) Hold chemotherapy

(2) Bowel rest

(3) IV fluid replacement

(4) Maintenance of hemoglobin greater than 7 g/dl

(5) Maintenance of platelet count greater than 50,000/mm^3

(6) Initiation of broad-spectrum antibiotics with consideration of antifungal agents

(7) Consideration of granulocyte–colony-stimulating factor until resolution or ANC is greater than 1,000/mm^3

(8) Initiation of empiric antimicrobial therapy (Rodrigues et al., 2017)

(9) Testing to rule out infectious etiologies—perform stool cultures for fungal, cytomegalovirus sources, and PCR assay for *C. difficile*.

(10) Delay of chemotherapy until full resolution and consideration of dose modification for subsequent cycles (Nesher & Rolston, 2012)

f) *C. difficile* colitis

(1) Management with oral vancomycin and/or metronidazole

(2) Antidiarrheals are contraindicated because they decrease motility, allowing for the *C. difficile* bacteria and toxin to fester and overgrow (Anand & Glatt, 1993).

g) Immune-mediated colitis (see example case report in Figure 15-5)

(1) Regardless of the immunotherapy agent used, effective colitis and diarrhea management is accomplished by early intervention.

(2) Colitis-related mortality with immunotherapy agents has been associated with

Figure 15-5. Case Report

- **Age:** 61
- **Sex:** Female
- **Diagnosis:** Relapsed stage IV, grade 2 follicular lymphoma
- **Treatment:** Oral PI3K inhibitor
- **Risk factors:** None
  - No history of irritable bowel syndrome, malabsorption disorders, or malignancy in GI tract
  - No recent travel
  - No dietary changes
  - No increased stressors in life
  - No recent oral antibiotics
- **Symptoms:** Abdominal pain, tenderness, and distension with associated diarrhea, reported 8 times per day
  - Loose, watery, and unformed stools
  - Afebrile
  - Mild associated nausea
- **Grade of diarrhea:** 3
- **Timeline to occur:** 5 cycles
- **Management**
  - Drug hold
  - Supportive care—oral fluids and electrolyte replacement
  - Patient tested negative for *C. difficile* and had negative stool cultures.
  - PET-CT demonstrated FDG-avid colon.
- **Symptoms:** Symptoms worsened
  - Reported grade 4 diarrhea—12 episodes of diarrhea daily
  - Concerns for colitis
- **Assessment:** Colonoscopy
  - Diffuse pancolitis
  - Diffuse erythema with ulcerations
  - Intraepithelial lymphocytosis
  - Neutrophilic cryptitis
- **Management:** Initiated oral corticosteroids with improvement in symptoms
  - Steroid taper over 6–12 weeks
  - Continued drug hold, with discontinuation in drug due to grade 4 toxicity

FDG—fluorodeoxyglucose; GI—gastrointestinal; PET-CT—positron-emission tomography–computed tomography; PI3K—phosphoinositide 3-kinase

delayed reporting, nonadherence with antidiarrheal regimen, and failure to hold the immunotherapy agent (Naidoo et al., 2015).

(3) Early identification and diagnosis with timely implementation of therapy is critical (Gondal, Patel, Gallan, Hart, & Bissonnette, 2016).

(4) With early intervention, colitis is reversible.

h) Interventions by grade

(1) Grade 1 bowel symptoms (see Table 15-9)

(a) Treat symptomatically using antidiarrheals (Cramer & Bresalier, 2017).

(b) Institute fluid and electrolyte replacement (Gupta et al., 2015).

(2) Grade 2 bowel symptoms

(a) Hold checkpoint inhibitor therapy, and continue treatment with antidiarrheal (Cramer & Bresalier, 2017).

(b) If symptoms persist up to one week, it is recommended to initiate corticosteroids (Cramer & Bresalier, 2017).

(c) Initiate at a dosage of 0.5–1 mg/kg/day of prednisone or equivalent for five to seven days. If no improvement occurs, increase dosage and manage as grade 3–4 (Bristol-Myers Squibb Co., 2018).

(d) Once symptoms decrease to grade 1, resume therapy, and continue a one-month steroid taper. Rapid tapering of steroids may result in recurrent colitis (Cramer & Bresalier, 2017).

(e) Use of infliximab, a monoclonal antibody against inflammatory cytokine tumor necrosis factor-alpha, for corticosteroid-resistant colitis (Gupta et al., 2015; Yanai, Nakamura, & Matsumoto, 2017)

i. 17% of patients with ipilimumab-related colitis are treated with infliximab after corticosteroid failure of symptom reduction (Barina et al., 2016).

ii. Infliximab is contraindicated in patients with perforation or sepsis (Yang, Yu, Dong, Zhong, & Hu, 2017).

(3) Grade 3–4 bowel symptoms

(a) Permanently discontinue checkpoint inhibitor therapy, and initiate corticosteroids (Cramer & Bresalier, 2017).

(b) Initiate at a dosage of 1–2 mg/kg/day of prednisone or equivalent followed by one-month steroid taper (Bristol-Myers Squibb Co., 2017, 2018).

(c) If grade 3–4 symptoms persist with corticosteroids after three to five days, initiate infliximab (Cramer & Bresalier, 2017).

i) Use of corticosteroids

(1) Of patients with ipilimumab-related colitis, 67% were treated with corticosteroid taper, and 25% were treated with IV corticosteroids (Barina et al., 2016).

(2) Prednisone therapy 0.5–1 mg/kg/day or equivalent is recommended for grade 2 symptoms that persist up to one week (Cramer & Bresalier, 2017; Gupta et al., 2015).

j) Total colectomy

(1) Colectomy was used as definitive treatment in 8% of patients with ipilimumab-related colitis after failure of medical therapy (Barina et al., 2016).

(2) Surgery is reserved for patients in whom medical therapy has failed or those who have bowel perforation (Gupta et al., 2015).

k) Management of PD-1 inhibitor–induced colitis (Baroudjian et al., 2016)

(1) Pembrolizumab-induced collagenous colitis

(a) It is recommended to perform colonoscopy with biopsies.

(b) If a diagnosis of collagenous colitis is made with pathology, it is recommended to continue with PD-1 inhibitor therapy while initiating corticosteroid therapy, such as budesonide 9 mg/day, along with symptomatic management.

(2) General early intervention includes withdrawal of PD-1 inhibitor therapy and initiation of steroids.

7. Patient and family education

a) Educate patients and caregivers on definition of diarrhea and importance of reporting bowel movements.

(1) Underreporting of diarrheal episodes may cause a delay in therapy.

(2) Patients should report to the treatment team any changes in bowel patterns, increase in stools over baseline, or other symptoms such as cramping, blood in stool, or increased gas or bloating.

b) Although the median onset of colitis and diarrhea has been outlined previously, symptoms of colitis or diarrhea can occur any time after a patient has received an immunotherapy or chemotherapy agent.

(1) Drink fluids to maintain clear or pale yellow–colored urine.

(2) Eat a well-balanced diet. Patients with mild grade 1 diarrhea or colitis can follow the colitis diet from the Academy of Nutrition and Dietetics (Naidoo et al., 2015).

(3) Work with a dietitian to determine foods that cause flares and avoid those foods.

E. Pancreatitis

1. Definition and pathophysiology

a) Acute inflammatory process of the pancreas

b) Classification (Vege, 2017)

(1) Mild acute: Absence of organ failure or local or systemic complication

(2) Moderately severe: Transient organ failure (resolves within 48 hours) or local or systemic complications without persistent organ failure (greater than 48 hours)

(3) Severe: Persistent organ failure that may involve one or multiple organs

c) The International Association of Pancreatology/American Pancreatic Association (IAP/APA) defined the diagnosis of acute pancreatitis as the presence of at least two of the following three features: upper abdominal pain, serum amylase or lipase more than three times the upper limit of normal, and/or imaging, such as CT, magnetic resonance imaging, or ultrasonography (Working Group IAP/APA Acute Pancreatitis Guidelines, 2013).

2. Incidence and risk factors

a) L-Asparaginase and PEG-asparaginase: Prevalence of pancreatitis is 2%–16% (Ngo, Jia, Green, Gulati, & Lall, 2015) and usually occurs with the first three to five doses.

b) Other chemotherapy agents: Carboplatin, cisplatin, cytarabine, ifosfamide, paclitaxel, and vinorelbine. Onset is variable and may range from hours to one month after administration (Ngo et al., 2015).

c) Immune checkpoint inhibitors: Ipilimumab, nivolumab, pembrolizumab, atezolizumab (Davies, 2016). Pancreatitis can occur during treatment or weeks to months after treatment is discontinued.

d) Targeted therapies: Pancreatic effects can range from asymptomatic pancreatic enzyme elevation to acute pancreatitis.

(1) Frequency of acute pancreatitis in clinical trials is 0%–4.3%.

(2) Amylase and lipase elevation frequently is reported with tyrosine kinase inhibitors.

(3) A meta-analysis evaluating pancreatitis with vascular endothelial growth factor receptor tyrosine kinase inhibitors (sunitinib, sorafenib, pazopanib, axitinib, vandetanib, cabozantinib, ponatinib, regorafenib) observed a 1.95-fold increase in risk of all grades of pancreatitis; however, the risk of severe (grade 3 or higher) was not significant (Ghatalia et al., 2105).

e) Obstructions of the duct system, including periampullary neoplasms, cholelithiasis, and congenital alterations in the ductal system, such as pancreas divisum

f) Hypertriglyceridemia, hypercalcemia

g) Diabetes

h) Tumor lysis syndrome

i) Post–endoscopic retrograde cholangiopancreatography: Pancreatitis is the most common postprocedure complication. Risk is increased with chronic pancreatitis and after inadvertent cannulation of the pancreatic duct (Phillip, Schwab, Haf, & Algül, 2017).

j) Alcohol abuse

k) Illicit drug use

l) Pediatrics: Hematopoietic stem cell transplantation (HSCT)

m) Infection

3. Clinical manifestations (Vege, 2017)

a) Three main manifestations

(1) Acute onset of persistent, severe epigastric abdominal pain, which may be right upper quadrant or, rarely, confined to the left side. Approximately 50% radiates to the back. Pain may be partially relieved by sitting up or bending forward.

(2) Pancreatic enzyme elevations

(a) Serum amylase: Rises within 6–12 hours. Elevation greater than

three times the upper limit of normal has sensitivity for diagnosis of acute pancreatitis; if uncomplicated, amylase returns to normal three to five days.

(*b*) Serum lipase: Rises 4–8 hours after onset of symptoms, peaks at 24 hours, and returns to normal within 8–14 days. These elevations occur earlier, last longer compared to amylase elevations, and are more sensitive in patients with pancreatitis secondary to alcohol abuse.

(*c*) Trypsinogen activation peptide: Is elevated early and may be useful in detection of early acute pancreatitis and as a predictor of severity (Vege, 2017).

(3) CT positive for signs of pancreatic inflammation

b) Other clinical findings (Vege, 2017)

(1) Fever

(2) Tachycardia and hypovolemia

(3) Hypoxemia

(4) Dyspnea due to diaphragmatic inflammation

(5) Nausea and vomiting (incidence of approximately 90%)

(6) Jaundice, elevated liver function tests

(7) Hypoactive bowel sounds, ileus

(8) Leukocytosis, elevated hematocrit from hemoconcentration due to extravasation of intravascular fluid into third space

(9) Elevated blood urea nitrogen, hypocalcemia, hyperglycemia, hypoglycemia

(10) Hemorrhagic pancreatitis is manifested by ecchymotic discoloration around the umbilicus (Cullen sign) or along the flank (Grey Turner sign). These suggest possible retroperitoneal bleeding in the setting of pancreatic necrosis.

(11) Later complications include hemorrhage, sepsis, and multisystem organ failure.

4. Assessment

a) Perform a physical examination to find and document the preceding clinical manifestations.

b) The epigastrium may be minimally tender to palpation. With severe pancreatitis, patients may have significant tenderness to palpation, abdominal distention, and hypoactive bowel sounds due to ileus from inflammation (Vege, 2017).

5. Collaborative management: Treatment and follow-up will depend on the etiology of the pancreatitis (Working Group IAP/APA Acute Pancreatitis Guidelines, 2013). Holding or discontinuing any agent that may be the cause of the condition is the primary treatment.

a) Pancreatitis associated with checkpoint inhibitors may require immunosuppression with corticosteroids (Davies, 2016).

b) Pancreatitis associated with L-asparaginase tends to respond after the drug is discontinued and aggressive treatment is initiated and will most likely recur if the drug is used again (Kearney et al., 2009; Stock et al., 2011; Tokimasa & Yamato, 2012; Treepongkaruna et al., 2009). Because reduced L-asparaginase exposure is related to a decreased cure rate in acute lymphoblastic leukemia, the drug should not be stopped unless pancreatitis is diagnosed. L-Asparaginase is contraindicated in patients with a history of severe pancreatitis (Jazz Pharmaceuticals, 2016).

c) Insert a nasogastric tube if patients have nausea and vomiting or ileus to rest the gut and pancreas during the acute phase (Working Group IAP/APA Acute Pancreatitis Guidelines, 2013).

d) Fluids: Use Ringer's lactate for initial fluid resuscitation (Working Group IAP/APA Acute Pancreatitis Guidelines, 2013).

e) Implement nutritional support (Working Group IAP/APA Acute Pancreatitis Guidelines, 2013).

(1) Restart oral feeding if pancreatitis is mild, abdominal pain is decreasing, and inflammatory markers are improving.

(2) Provide enteral tube feeding if pancreatitis is predicted to be severe. Either the nasojejunal or nasogastric route can be used.

(3) Parenteral nutrition is a second-line therapy if tube feeding is not tolerated and nutritional support is required.

f) Monitor serum lipase, amylase, glucose, electrolytes, and liver function tests.

g) Treat hyperglycemia as indicated.

h) Provide effective pain control and monitor for increasing pain, which may indicate progression of pancreatitis.

i) Prevent infectious complications.

(1) IV antibiotic therapy is not recommended for the prevention of infectious complications in acute pancre-

atitis (Working Group IAP/APA Acute Pancreatitis Guidelines, 2013). IV antibiotics should be given in the case of suspected infection with necrotizing pancreatitis (Working Group IAP/APA Acute Pancreatitis Guidelines, 2013).

(2) Probiotic prophylaxis is not recommended.

(3) Selective gut decontamination has shown some benefits, but further studies are needed (Working Group IAP/APA Acute Pancreatitis Guidelines, 2013).

j) Monitor patients' vital signs, oxygen saturation, level of consciousness, and condition carefully for signs of hypovolemic shock. Hypotension occurs because of sequestration of protein-rich fluids in the pancreas, retroperitoneal space, and abdominal cavity in severe acute pancreatitis.

6. Patient and family education

a) Instruct patients to use analgesics for pain control.

b) Implement oral and nasal care while patients are NPO (nothing by mouth) with a nasogastric tube.

c) Ensure that patients know the importance of adherence to dietary, pharmacologic, and lifestyle recommendations.

d) Ensure that patients and significant others can recognize the early symptoms of pancreatitis, such as abdominal pain, especially associated with vomiting, and instruct them to seek medical intervention when these occur.

F. Mucositis

1. Definitions: Mucositis is a potential complication of systemic cytotoxic therapy, epidermal growth factor receptor (EGFR) inhibitors, tyrosine kinase inhibitors, and radiation therapy (Eilers, Harris, Henry, & Johnson, 2014). Severe mucositis can contribute to hospitalization, need for narcotic analgesic or total parenteral nutrition, suboptimal delivery of antineoplastic treatment, and morbidity and mortality (Mercadante et al., 2015). *Mucositis* and *stomatitis* are often used interchangeably, but they do not reflect identical processes (Peterson, Srivastava, & Lalla, 2015).

a) *Mucositis:* Refers to inflammatory or ulcerative lesions of the oral or GI tract resulting from chemotherapy agents or ionizing radiation (Peterson et al., 2015)

b) *Stomatitis:* Refers to an array of symptoms in the oral cavity, including mucosal inflammation, ulcers, chelates or dry lips, and oral pain (Hartl et al., 2017)

c) *Alimentary tract mucositis*: Refers to mucosal injury across the continuum of the oral and GI mucosa from the mouth to the anus (Peterson et al., 2015)

2. Pathophysiology

a) Historically, oral mucositis was attributed to the direct effects of cytotoxic drugs or radiation therapy on the epithelial stem cells. It is now known to be a result of a complex, sequential series of biologic events that culminates in the destruction of epithelial stem cells and interruption of epithelial renewal, a critical process by which tissue health is maintained (Yuan & Sonis, 2014). It is a complex interaction between epithelial and connective tissue compartments (Stringer & Logan, 2015).

b) Based on observations of oral mucositis in animal models, researchers developed a five-phase model that describes the sequence of genetic and histopathologic events following cytotoxic treatment (Al-Dasooqi et al., 2013).

c) The five phases are initiation, upregulation/activation, signaling and amplification, ulceration, and healing (Sonis, 2011).

(1) Initiation: Radiation and chemotherapy adversely affect the cells and strands of DNA in the basal epithelium and submucosa. Free radicals (reactive oxygen species) also are generated and play an interfering role in the biologic events of the later stages (Moslemi et al., 2016).

(2) Upregulation and generation of messenger signals: The negative effect on the cells and DNA and the reactive oxygen species activate a cascade of reactions that bring about the production of proinflammatory cytokines. These compounds stimulate several pathways leading to lesions or the death of basal cells by apoptosis (Moslemi et al., 2016). Nuclear factor-κB results in upregulation of many genes and the release of proinflammatory cytokines, such as tumor necrosis-alpha, interleukin (IL)-1 beta (IL-1β), and IL-6.

(3) Signaling and amplification: In addition to causing direct tissue damage, proinflammatory cytokines activate the production of tissue-damaging tumor necrosis-alpha, IL-1β, and IL-6, as well as other cytokines that alter mucosal

tissues. The release of proinflammatory cytokines not only damages the cells but also provides a positive feedback that amplifies the lesions caused directly by the radiation or chemotherapy (Moslemi et al., 2016).

(4) Ulceration: Tissue injury in the GI mucosa appears as ulcers that penetrate through the epithelium to the submucosa. Bacteria penetrate the submucosa and stimulate macrophage activity, which increases the release of proinflammatory cytokines. Angiogenesis also is stimulated.

(5) Healing: Signals from extracellular tissues stimulate epithelial proliferation until the mucosa returns to its normal thickness. Neutropenia may prolong the healing process.

3. Incidence of oral mucositis
   a) Prevalence and incidence are inconsistent because of the lack of standardized scoring criteria, tumor location, and different treatment regimens, as well as underreporting (Villa & Sonis, 2015). Incidence varies depending on the type of cancer treatment, dose, and frequency (Fulton, 2018).
   b) Incidence in HSCT recipients varies between 47% and 100%. Intensity of the conditioning regimen, transplant type, and total body irradiation (TBI) can influence incidence as well as severity (Chaudhry et al., 2015).
   c) Incidence in patients undergoing head and neck radiation therapy is 65%–90% (Sonis, 2011).
      (1) It occurs in almost all patients who are treated for cancers of the mouth, oropharynx, and nasopharynx and about two-thirds of patients treated for cancers of the hypopharynx or larynx (Moslemi et al., 2016).
      (2) The use of concomitant chemotherapy and/or targeted therapy agents increases the risk (Villa & Sonis, 2015).
   d) Both stomatitis and diarrhea have been reported with targeted therapies.
      (1) The term *stomatitis* has been used for oral lesions secondary to targeted therapy agents to distinguish from mucositis due to conventional chemotherapy and radiation therapy (Al-Dasooqi et al., 2013).
      (2) Certain mammalian target of rapamycin (mTOR) inhibitors have reported rates of 66% (Al-Dasooqi et al., 2013).
      (3) Lesions secondary to targeted therapy agents are often accompanied by a skin rash (Al-Dasooqi et al., 2013).
4. Risk factors
   a) Development of mucositis depends on both therapy- and patient-related factors (Villa & Sonis, 2016).
   b) Treatment-related factors
      (1) Chemotherapy agents (Chaveli-López & Bagán-Sebastián, 2016; Epstein et al., 2012)
         (a) Antimetabolites
            i. Increased risk with bolus 5-fluorouracil
            ii. Methotrexate for prophylaxis of graft-versus-host disease following HSCT (Brennan, von Bültzingslöwen, Schubert, & Keefe, 2006; Cutler et al., 2005)
         (b) Antitumor antibiotics
         (c) Alkylating agents: High-dose melphalan
         (d) Plant alkaloids
      (2) Targeted therapy
         (a) mTOR inhibitors (Martins et al., 2013)
         (b) Tyrosine kinase inhibitors (Califano et al., 2015)
      (3) Immunotherapy agents: PD-1/PD-L1 inhibitor therapy may induce or accelerate oral complications by aberrant cell activation, such as what has been seen in graft-versus-host disease or autoimmune conditions (Jackson, Johnson, Sosman, Murphy, & Epstein, 2015).
      (4) Leukemia, lymphoma, and HSCT put patients at risk because treatment involves drugs with a great potential to produce oral mucositis and cause prolonged neutropenia.
      (5) Radiation therapy
         (a) Radiation therapy following surgical resection in patients with head and neck cancer
         (b) Combined chemotherapy and radiation (Eilers & Million, 2011)
         (c) TBI or radiation therapy to the head or neck (Maria, Eliopoulos, & Muanza, 2017)
         (d) Greater incidence when EGFR inhibitor treatment added to radiation therapy (De Sanctis et al., 2016)

(6) Drugs or therapies that alter mucous membranes (Wujcik, 2014)
   (a) Oxygen therapy: Dries out the mucosal lining
   (b) Anticholinergics: Decrease salivary flow
   (c) Phenytoin: Causes gingival hyperplasia
   (d) Steroids: Can result in fungal overgrowth

c) Patient-related risk factors
(1) Ill-fitting dentures, as they can irritate the mucosa and break integrity
(2) Poor oral hygiene, periodontal disease: Periodontitis-associated bacteria have been related to onset and worsening of ulcerative mucositis (De Sanctis et al., 2016).
(3) Persistent alcohol or tobacco use
   (a) Alcohol and tobacco irritate the mucosa. Tobacco affects microcirculation, which may delay healing (Eilers & Million, 2011).
   (b) Chronic alcohol use is associated with mucosal atrophy and hyper-regeneration of the basal layer cells, thereby increasing susceptibility of the mucosa, as well as predisposing patients to malnutrition (De Sanctis et al., 2016).
(4) Xerostomia or hyposalivation
(5) Dehydration, as it alters mucosal integrity
(6) Nutrition
   (a) Poor nutrition can lead to delayed healing and increase risk of breakdown (Maria et al., 2017).
   (b) Unintentional weight loss before therapy (i.e., more than 5% weight loss over one month or more than 10% in the last six months) (De Sanctis et al., 2016).
   (c) Low body mass index (less than 18.5 kg/m^2) (Maria et al., 2017)
   (d) Irritating foods: Acidic, spicy foods may inflame and traumatize mucosa (Wujcik, 2014).
(7) Immunosuppression due to comorbidities
(8) Neutropenia
(9) Hepatic or renal impairment: Inadequate metabolism or excretion of drugs
(10) Age (Fulton, 2018)
   (a) Older patients, because of age-related decline in kidney function and decreased creatinine clearance rates, which can affect excretion of chemotherapy and lead to drugs remaining longer in the circulation, causing more damage
   (b) Younger patients (20 years and younger), because of increased epithelial mitotic rates and increased EGFR in epithelial tissue (Treister & Sankar, 2017)
(11) Genetic factors may play a major role. Animal studies have shown that a variety of gene expression–related changes occur after chemotherapy or radiation therapy (Villa & Sonis, 2016).

5. Clinical manifestations
a) Presentation of oral mucositis depends on the modality (chemotherapy, targeted therapy, immunotherapy, radiation therapy, or combined therapy), the type of drugs administered, the dosage or intensity, and the schedule of administration (Villa & Sonis, 2016).
(1) First signs of mucositis usually begin about three to four days after the infusion of chemotherapy, and patients complain of mucosal irritation. Ulcer formation develops, peaks days 7–14, and resolves in about a week after peaking (Villa & Sonis, 2016).
(2) HSCT recipients experience mucositis three to five days following the conditioning regimen.
(3) Patients receiving radiation to the head and neck complain of oral soreness and develop erythema at the end of the first week of treatment, when cumulative doses reach 10 Gy. By 12–14 days, when cumulative doses reach 30 Gy, multiple ulcerations develop, and as radiation accumulates, ulcerative lesions become more diffuse and painful. These lesions are then present throughout the duration of therapy (usually 60–70 Gy). Ulcerations remain at peak for at least two weeks following completion of therapy. They usually begin to resolve over two to four weeks but can persist for up to eight weeks (Moslemi et al., 2016; Villa & Sonis, 2015).

b) Intensity increases with higher doses of cytotoxic drugs. Drugs that are not usually stomatotoxic at standard doses (e.g., cyclophosphamide) can cause cellular damage to the mucosa at high doses (Keefe et al., 2007).

c) Signs and symptoms
   (1) Oral mucosal changes (e.g., erythema, pallor, white patches, discolored lesion, ulcers), edematous oral mucosa and tongue
   (2) Mucosal ulcerations: Irregularly shaped lesions that typically lack peripheral erythema (Pilotte, Hohos, Polson, Hutalen, & Treister, 2011)
   (3) Mouth lesions with mTOR inhibitors: Clinically mimic aphthous stomatitis (commonly called canker sores) (Pilotte et al., 2011)
   (4) Difficulty talking, changes in voice strength, pain when talking
   (5) Pain on swallowing or inability to swallow
   (6) Saliva: Changes in amount or consistency, watery or thick and ropy

6. Assessment
   a) Use a standardized assessment tool or scale when performing a physical examination. Scales designed for clinical use consider the symptoms, signs, and functional disturbances associated with oral mucositis and assign an overall score. The following are some common tools.
      (1) Oral Assessment Guide: This tool contains eight categories that reflect oral health and function (Eilers, Berger, & Peterson, 1988). It has been identified as the only validated tool consistently judged to be user-friendly and appropriate for both children and adults (Peters, 2016; see Table 15-10).
      (2) The World Health Organization (1979) Oral Toxicity Scale combines mucosal changes, pain, and functionality into

Table 15-10. Oral Assessment Guide

Category	Tools for Assessment	Methods of Measurement	Numeric and Descriptive Ratings		
			1	2	3
Voice	Auditory	Converse with patient.	Normal	Deeper or raspy	Difficulty talking or painful
Swallow	Observation	Ask patient to swallow. To test gag reflex, gently place blade on back of tongue and depress. Observe result.	Normal swallow	Some pain on swallowing	Unable to swallow
Lips	Visual/palpatory	Observe and feel tissue.	Smooth and pink and moist	Dry or cracked	Ulcerated or bleeding
Tongue	Visual and/or palpatory	Feel and observe appearance of tissue.	Pink and moist and papillae present	Coated or loss of papillae with a shiny appearance with or without redness	Blistered or cracked
Saliva	Tongue blade	Insert blade into mouth, touching the center of the tongue and the floor of the mouth.	Watery	Thick or ropy	Absent
Mucous membranes	Visual	Observe appearance of tissue.	Pink and moist	Reddened or coated (increased whiteness) without ulcerations	Ulcerations with or without bleeding
Gingiva	Tongue blade and visual	Gently press tissue with tip of blade.	Pink, stippled, and firm	Edematous with or without redness	Spontaneous bleeding or bleeding with pressure
Teeth or dentures (or denture-bearing area)	Visual	Observe appearance of teeth or denture-bearing area.	Clean and no debris	Plaque or debris in localized areas (between teeth if present)	Plaque or debris generalized along gum line or denture-bearing area

Note. Table courtesy of June Eilers, PhD, APRN-CNS, BC, Nebraska Medical Center. Used with permission.

a single composite score (Epstein et al., 2012).
- *(a)* Grade 0: No changes
- *(b)* Grade 1: Soreness, erythema
- *(c)* Grade 2: Soreness, erythema, ulceration, and can eat solid food
- *(d)* Grade 3: Soreness, erythema, ulceration, and can consume a liquid diet only
- *(e)* Grade 4: Soreness, erythema, ulceration, and oral alimentation is not possible

(3) The World Health Organization tool grades the severity of mucositis, whereas the Oral Assessment Guide addresses overall changes in the oral cavity (Peters, 2016).

(4) NCI CTEP's (2017) Common Terminology Criteria for Adverse Events consists of a 1–5 grading scale that is associated with descriptions of oral mucosal changes.
- *(a)* Grade 1: Asymptomatic or mild symptoms; intervention not indicated
- *(b)* Grade 2: Moderate pain or ulcer that does not interfere with oral intake; modified diet indicated
- *(c)* Grade 3: Severe pain; interfering with oral intake
- *(d)* Grade 4: Life-threatening consequences; urgent intervention indicated
- *(e)* Grade 5: Death

(5) Patient-reported outcome measures are questionnaires completed by patients to assess symptom burden and functionality (Epstein et al., 2012). These may be helpful and a feasible substitute for clinical situations where patients cannot endure an oral examination (Gussgard, Hope, Jokstad, Tenenbaum, & Wood, 2014).
- *(a)* Patient-Reported Oral Mucositis Symptom scale (Kushner et al., 2008; see Figure 15-6)
- *(b)* Oral Mucositis Weekly Questionnaire (Epstein et al., 2007)

(6) Whichever tool is used, it should be used as standard practice for all relevant patients in the health service (Peters, 2016).

7. Collaborative management and prevention

a) Several agents and interventions have been studied for the prevention and treatment of mucositis (Van Sebille et al., 2015). The Multinational Association of Supportive Care in Cancer and International Society of Oral Oncology provides evidence-based guidelines that have been endorsed by the American Society of Clinical Oncology, the European Society for Medical Oncology, and the Oncology Nursing Society (Epstein et al., 2012). The Oncology Nursing Society Putting Evidence Into Practice resources provide evidence-based interventions for patient care (Eilers et al., 2017).

b) Good oral hygiene practices and oral care protocols are beneficial and may reduce the risk, duration, and severity of oral mucositis (McGuire et al., 2013).
- (1) The single most important aspect of any oral care protocol is consistency of use; oral care has a positive effect on mucositis prevention and management (Eilers et al., 2017).
- (2) The protocol should include brushing with a soft toothbrush and flossing at least two times per day (Eilers et al., 2014).
- (3) Microorganism colonization of oral ulcerations may prolong healing, so it is important to reduce the oral bacterial load with daily tooth brushing and flossing (Villa & Sonis, 2015).

c) Orthodontic appliances or poorly fitting dentures may traumatize the oral mucosa and should be removed or adjusted (Villa & Sonis, 2016). Braces may need to be removed if patients are to undergo transplantation or if prolonged periods of neutropenia are anticipated.

d) Patient education may improve adherence with oral care, frequency, and ability to cope with mucositis.

e) Conduct a pretreatment dental evaluation with attention to potentially irritating teeth surfaces, underlying gingivitis, periodontal infection, and ill-fitting dentures. Crucial dental work should be done before chemotherapy begins.

f) Emphasize intake of high-protein foods and increased fluid intake (greater than 1,500 ml/day).

g) Prevention of oral mucositis
- (1) Oral cryotherapy is recommended for patients receiving bolus 5-fluorouracil or high-dose melphalan with or without TBI, a conditioning regimen for HSCT (Lalla et al., 2014).

Figure 15-6. Patient-Reported Oral Mucositis Symptom (PROMS) Scale

This questionnaire asks you to evaluate some situations you may have experienced in the past week. All of the situations refer to the condition of your mouth. You can indicate the severity of the situation by placing a vertical mark along the lines below.

Mouth pain

No pain ________________________________ worst possible pain

Difficulty speaking because of mouth sores

No trouble speaking ________________________________ impossible to speak

Restriction of speech because of mouth sores

No restriction of speech ________________________________ complete restriction of speech

Difficulty eating hard foods (hard bread, potato chips, etc.) because of mouth sores

No trouble eating hard foods ________________________________ impossible to eat hard foods

Difficulty eating soft foods (Jello, pudding, etc.) because of mouth sores

No trouble eating soft foods ________________________________ impossible to eat soft foods

Restriction of eating because of mouth sores

No restriction of eating ________________________________ complete restriction of eating

Difficulty drinking because of mouth sores

No trouble drinking ________________________________ impossible to drink

Restriction of drinking because of mouth sores

No restriction of drinking ________________________________ complete restriction of drinking

Difficulty swallowing because of mouth sores

Not difficult to swallow ________________________________ impossible to swallow

Change in taste

No change in taste ________________________________ complete change in taste

Note. Figure courtesy of Howard C. Tenenbaum, DDS, Dipl Perio, PhD, FRCD(C). Used with permission.

(2) Recombinant human keratinocyte growth factor-1 (palifermin) at a dose of 60 mcg/kg/day for three days prior to conditioning treatment and for three days after treatment is recommended in patients receiving high-dose chemotherapy and TBI followed by autologous HSCT for a hematologic malignancy (Lalla et al., 2014).

(3) Low-level laser therapy is recommended for patients receiving HSCT conditioned with high-dose chemotherapy with or without TBI and patients receiving radiation therapy without concomitant chemotherapy for head and neck cancer (Lalla et al., 2014).

(4) Benzydamine mouthwash is recommended for patients with head and neck cancer receiving moderate-dose radiation therapy (up to 50 Gy) without concomitant chemotherapy.

(5) Zinc supplements may be of benefit to prevent mucositis in patients with oral

cancer receiving radiation or chemoradiation (Jensen & Peterson, 2013).

(6) *Lactobacillus* lozenges may be effective in patients with head and neck cancer undergoing chemoradiation (Sharma et al., 2012).

h) Prevention of GI mucositis (Lalla et al., 2014)

(1) Amifostine greater than 340 mg/m^2 IV is recommended to prevent proctitis in patients receiving radiation therapy.

(2) Octreotide greater than 100 mcg subcutaneously twice daily is recommended to treat diarrhea induced by standard- or high-dose chemotherapy associated with HSCT, if loperamide is ineffective.

(3) The following recommendations have been suggested; however, evidence is weaker:

(a) Amifostine IV to prevent esophagitis induced by chemoradiation in patients with non-small cell lung cancer

(b) Sucralfate enemas to treat chronic radiation-induced proctitis in patients with rectal bleeding who are not neutropenic or thrombocytopenic

(c) Sulfasalazine 500 mg twice daily to prevent radiation-induced enteropathy in patients receiving radiation therapy to the pelvis

(d) Probiotics containing *Lactobacillus* species to prevent diarrhea in patients receiving chemotherapy or radiation therapy for a pelvic malignancy

(e) Hyperbaric oxygen to treat radiation-induced proctitis in patients receiving radiation therapy for a solid tumor

i) Symptom control: Pain reduction

(1) Oral agents to promote cleansing, moisture, and comfort (see Table 15-11)

(2) Patient-controlled analgesia for patients undergoing HSCT

(3) Use of 2% morphine mouthwash for patients receiving chemoradiation for head and neck cancer

(4) Use of 0.5% doxepin mouthwash for all patients with oral mucositis–induced pain

(5) Transdermal fentanyl for patients receiving conventional or high-dose chemotherapy, with or without TBI

j) Colonization of damaged mucosa by bacteria, fungi, and viruses is thought to occur during the ulceration phase (Vanhoecke, De Ryck, Stringer, Van de Wiele, & Keefe, 2015). Culture mucosal lesions so that appropriate antimicrobial agents can be prescribed. *Candida* lesions look like whitish or cream-colored plaques on the mucosa and often are treated while cultures are pending.

8. Patient and family education: Teach oral cavity self-management techniques.

a) Perform a daily oral self-examination, and report signs and symptoms of mucositis.

b) Comply with an oral hygiene program. Oral hygiene should be performed after every meal and at bedtime. If mild to moderate dysfunction is present, the frequency of oral hygiene should be increased to every two to four hours. If the condition progresses to a more severe dysfunction, hourly care may be indicated. The program should include the following:

(1) Floss the teeth with dental tape at least once daily or as advised by the clinician (Harris, Eilers, Harriman, Cashavelly, & Maxwell, 2008). However, patients who do not regularly floss should not do so while immunosuppressed (Eilers & Million, 2011).

(2) Brush all tooth surfaces with a soft toothbrush for at least 90 seconds at least twice daily. Allow toothbrush to air dry before storing, and replace toothbrush frequently (Harris et al., 2008). Sponge swabs are not as effective as toothbrushes and should be avoided when cleaning the teeth except in patients who cannot tolerate a toothbrush because of severe pain with mucositis. However, sponge swabs may be beneficial for cleaning the mucous membranes of the oral cavity (Eilers & Million, 2011).

(3) Cleanse the oral cavity after meals, at bedtime, and at other times by vigorously swishing the mouth with a non-alcohol-based bland rinse (see Table 15-11). Oral rinsing should be done to remove excess debris, hydrate the oral mucosa, and aid in the removal of organisms (Eilers & Million, 2011; Harris et al., 2008).

(4) Apply water-based moisturizers to lips.

(5) Maintain hydration.

Table 15-11. Mucositis Management: MASCC/ISOO and ONS PEP Recommendations

Agent	Efficacy	Comments
Amifostine	Strong evidence supports use of amifostine for prevention of radiation-induced proctitis. Weaker evidence supports use to prevent esophagitis induced by chemoradiation in patients with non-small cell lung cancer.	Dose of 340 mg/m² IV
Benzydamine mouthwash	Strong evidence supports effectiveness in patients with HNC receiving moderate-dose radiation therapy (up to 50 Gy).	Nonsteroidal anti-inflammatory analgesic Inhibits production of proinflammatory cytokines
Chlorhexidine	Chlorhexidine is not recommended for prevention, but may have other indications, such as treatment of gingivitis.	Contains alcohol Reports of rinse-induced discomfort and taste alteration Can turn teeth brown
Cryotherapy (ice chips)	Cryotherapy demonstrates consistent reduction in incidence and severity of oral mucositis among patients receiving bolus 5-FU. Weaker evidence supports use for patients receiving high-dose melphalan with or without TBI followed by autologous HSCT.	Ice chips applied to mouth 5 minutes before bolus 5-FU therapy and continued for 30 minutes after Not recommended in patients receiving capecitabine or oxaliplatin because of potential discomfort with exposure to coldness
Dexamethasone mouthwash (0.1 mg/ml)	Dexamethasone mouthwash is recommended for patients receiving mTOR inhibitors.	Relieves aphthous-like ulcers, which differ from chemotherapy-induced ulcers, which are irregularly shaped and typically lack peripheral erythema
0.5% doxepin mouthwash	Evidence is weaker but supports benefit to treat pain.	Tricyclic antidepressant
Keratinocyte growth factor-1: Palifermin	Palifermin is approved for prevention of oral mucositis in patients undergoing autologous HSCT receiving high-dose chemotherapy or TBI.	60 mcg/kg/day IV for 3 days prior to the preparatory regimen and for 3 days post-transplant Can cause tongue discoloration and unpleasant aftertaste
Low-level laser therapy	Low-level laser therapy to reduce incidence of oral mucositis is recommended in patients receiving high-dose chemotherapy with or without TBI before HSCT and suggested in patients with HNC receiving radiation therapy without concomitant chemotherapy.	Requires expensive equipment and specialized operator training; limited to centers capable of supporting this technology
Mixed rinses, which may include lidocaine, diphenhydramine, milk of magnesia, Mylanta®	Data demonstrating efficacy are lacking for prevention and treatment of mucositis.	Agents potentially useful for pain or discomfort only Alcohol-based elixirs to be avoided May adhere to mucous membranes and build up residue, making oral care difficult or uncomfortable Potential of some preparations to contribute to tooth decay due to sugar content
2% morphine mouthwash	Evidence is weaker but supports effectiveness.	For patients receiving chemoradiation for HNC Limited utility with topical morphine Potential for burning with oral alcohol-based formulations
Mucosal coating agents	Evidence from randomized trials is lacking to support benefit.	Variety of agents: Gelclair®, Orabase®, sucralfate suspension
Non-alcohol-based bland rinses	Evidence may be insufficient or lacking; however, bland rinses are harmless and can be helpful for oral hygiene maintenance and patient comfort.	0.9% saline, sodium bicarbonate, or 0.9% saline plus sodium bicarbonate Sodium bicarbonate recommended by ONS PEP

(Continued on next page)

Table 15-11. Mucositis Management: MASCC/ISOO and ONS PEP Recommendations *(Continued)*

Agent	Efficacy	Comments
Octreotide	Strong evidence supports effectiveness.	Dose of ≥ 100 mcg subcutaneously twice daily to treat diarrhea induced by standard- or high-dose chemotherapy associated with HSCT, if loperamide is ineffective
Oral zinc supplements	Evidence is weaker but supports effectiveness in patients receiving radiation therapy or chemoradiation for HNC.	Essential trace element needed for tissue repair; has antioxidant effect
Patient-controlled analgesia	Strong evidence supports effectiveness to treat pain.	Recommended for patients undergoing HSCT
Probiotics: *Lactobacillus* species	Evidence is weaker but supports effectiveness.	To prevent diarrhea in patients receiving chemotherapy or radiation therapy for a solid tumor
Sucralfate enemas	Weaker evidence supports effectiveness.	For chronic radiation-induced proctitis in patients with rectal bleeding
Topical capsaicin	Pilot data demonstrated marked reduction in oral pain.	Clinical potential possibly linked to epithelialization and elevation of pain threshold Further study warranted
Topical lidocaine	Limited data exist; use may provide significant relief of limited duration.	Requires frequent application; may lead to decreased sensitivity and additional trauma and impair taste perception Prophylaxis not recommended

5-FU—5-fluorouracil; HNC—head and neck cancer; HSCT—hematopoietic stem cell transplantation; MASCC/ISOO—Multinational Association of Supportive Care in Cancer and International Society of Oral Oncology; mTOR—mammalian target of rapamycin; ONS PEP—Oncology Nursing Society Putting Evidence Into Practice; TBI—total body irradiation

Note. Based on information from Eilers et al., 2014; Gibson et al., 2013; Harris et al., 2008; Lalla et al., 2014; Maria et al., 2017; McGuire et al., 2013; Peterson et al., 2015; Pilotte et al., 2011; Van Sebille et al., 2015; Wardill et al., 2014.

(6) Consider the use of oral moisturizers to promote comfort if xerostomia exists (Eilers & Million, 2011).

(7) Avoid irritating agents, including commercial mouthwashes containing phenol, astringents, or alcohol; highly abrasive toothpastes; acidic, hot, or spicy foods and beverages; rough foods; alcohol; tobacco; poorly fitting dentures; braces; and lemon-glycerin swabs and solutions (Harris et al., 2008).

(8) Recommendations for patients with dentures (NCI, 2016)

(*a*) Remove dentures and other oral devices when cleaning the mouth. If mouth sores are present, or if the mouth is inflamed or painful, avoid using removable oral devices to prevent further irritation.

(*b*) Brush and rinse dentures daily.

(*c*) Clean dentures twice a day with a denture cleaner, and rinse well.

(*d*) Report pain associated with mucositis.

G. Perirectal cellulitis

1. Definition: Inflammation and edema of the perineal and rectal area
2. Pathophysiology

a) Tears of the anorectal mucosa allow infection. The most common anaerobic organisms include *Bacteroides fragilis*, *Peptostreptococcus*, *Prevotella*, *Fusobacterium*, *Porphyromonas*, and *Clostridium*. The most common aerobic bacteria include *Staphylococcus aureus*, *Streptococcus*, and *Escherichia coli*. Community-acquired methicillin-resistant *Staphylococcus aureus* (known as MRSA) has been implicated in rectal abscess infections (Hebra, 2017).

b) A perianal abscess is a simple anorectal abscess.

c) Perirectal abscesses are more complex and can involve different planes in the anorectum (Bleday, 2018).

d) Infection starting as a local abscess can lead to systemic sepsis.

3. Incidence: Overall incidence has decreased in the past decade, presumably because of the early use of empiric antibiotics in febrile neutropenic

patients. Perirectal abscesses are more common in patients with anorectal cancer or hematologic malignancies and may be present at initial diagnosis (Hebra, 2017).

4. Risk factors
   a) Chronic neutropenia or thrombocytopenia
   b) Constipation: The passage of hard stool causes trauma to the rectal mucosa.
   c) Diarrhea: Caustic fluid irritates and breaks down perirectal tissue.
   d) Perirectal mucositis caused by chemotherapy or radiation therapy
   e) Any rectal trauma, such as rectal stimulation or the use of rectal thermometers, enemas, or suppositories
   f) Hemorrhoids or anal fissures/abscesses
5. Assessment
   a) Ask patients if they are experiencing perineal or rectal discomfort.
      (1) Patients with an anorectal abscess often present with severe pain in anal or rectal area. Pain is constant and not necessarily associated with a bowel movement (Bleday, 2018). Pain may be described as dull, aching, or throbbing, which may worsen when sitting or before defecation.
      (2) Fear of defecation related to pain may not be reported and may increase the risk of constipation.
   b) Monitor for the presence of fever.
   c) Perform a physical examination of the perineal area. The entrance site for the infective agent may be a small tear that shows minimal irritation.
      (1) An area of fluctuance or patch of erythematous indurated skin overlying perianal skin may be seen with a superficial perianal abscess (Bleday, 2018).
      (2) Localized tenderness, gross swelling, fluctuance, erythema, and drainage may be observed if an abscess is present. An abscess of the perirectal area may produce bloody, purulent, or mucoid drainage.
      (3) Deeper abscesses may not have findings on physical examination and may only be discovered via digital rectal examination or by imaging (Bleday, 2018).
      (4) Obtain a culture, if possible, for identification of infectious organisms (Hebra, 2017).
   d) Consider abdominal or pelvic CT if an abscess is suspected. Magnetic resonance imaging and transperitoneal or endorectal ultrasound can confirm diagnosis when a deep abscess is suspected (Bleday, 2018).
6. Collaborative management
   a) Ensure that antibiotic coverage includes a specific anaerobic agent in addition to broad-spectrum aerobic coverage. Consider *Enterococcus* or *Candida* coverage if appropriate (NCCN, 2017b).
   b) The primary treatment for anorectal abscess is surgical drainage. Any undrained abscess can expand and progress to systemic infection (Bleday, 2018).
   c) Administer antipyretic medications to relieve fever.
   d) Teach and encourage patients to take sitz baths or use gentle external perineal irrigation.
   e) Administer stool softeners, and encourage patients to eat a low-bulk diet. Consult a dietitian as needed.
   f) Inspect the perirectal mucosa frequently for any signs of irritation or skin breakdown.
7. Patient and family education
   a) Instructions for patients and significant others
      (1) Maintain meticulous perineal hygiene, especially in the presence of neutropenia.
      (2) Apply appropriate barrier creams.
      (3) Monitor carefully for any signs of infection or worsening of tissue integrity.
   b) Ensure that patients and significant others can perform the following:
      (1) Identify the risk factors for perirectal cellulitis.
      (2) Implement measures that minimize the risk of developing perirectal cellulitis.
      (3) Identify situations that require prompt professional intervention.
         (a) Pain, redness, or swelling in the affected area
         (b) Body temperature greater than 100.4°F (38°C)

H. Constipation

1. Definition: The decreased passage of stool characterized by infrequent bowel movements, hard stool, sensation of abdominal bloating or cramping, straining with bowel movements, and feeling of incomplete evacuation (Thorpe, Byar, Conley, Held-Warmkessel, & Ramsdell, 2017). Constipation commonly is associated with decreased frequency in defecation of less than three bowel movements in a week and often is accompanied by discomfort (Rangwala, Zafar, & Abernathy, 2012). Constipation may be a pre-

senting symptom of the cancer diagnosis, a side effect of therapy, the result of tumor progression, or unrelated to the cancer or therapy. The cause is usually multifactorial; the most common are decrease in bowel motility due to decrease in fiber intake, dehydration, immobility, and use of pain medications (Connolly & Larkin, 2012; Dzierżanowski & Ciałkowska-Rysz, 2015; Nelson, 2016).

2. Pathophysiology: Decrease in intestinal motility by one of the following mechanisms (Nelson, 2016):
   a) Primary: Intrinsic factors that slow peristalsis, such as decreased physical activity, lack of time or privacy for defecation, decreased fiber in the diet
   b) Secondary: Pathologic processes such as autonomic nervous system dysfunction, obstruction, spinal cord compression from tumor, hypercalcemia, hypokalemia, and hypothyroidism
   c) Iatrogenic: Use of pharmacologic agents such as opioids, chemotherapy, anticonvulsants, and psychotropic medications (Ahmedzai & Boland, 2010; Connolly & Larkin, 2012; Rangwala et al., 2012; Woolery et al., 2008)
3. Incidence: Clinically, constipation is a common problem for patients with cancer but is not well defined. In the palliative care population, constipation is reported to occur in 40%–60% of patients (Candy et al., 2015). In hospitalized patients with cancer, incidence can be as high as 70%–100% (Thorpe, Byar, Conley, Held-Warmkessel, et al., 2017). In 85%–95% of cases, constipation is shown to decrease quality of life, even though two-thirds may be mild to moderate in degree (Dzierżanowski & Ciałkowska-Rysz, 2015).
4. Clinical manifestations
   a) Abdominal or rectal discomfort or pain
   b) Nausea and/or vomiting
   c) Anorexia
   d) Impaction/obstruction
   e) Ileus
   f) Anal fissures
   g) Hemorrhoids
   h) Ruptured bowel and life-threatening sepsis
5. Risk factors
   a) Disease related: Mesenteric and omental masses or malignant adhesions, internal or external obstruction of bowel by tumor
   b) Mechanical pressure on the bowel (e.g., bowel obstruction secondary to tumor in the GI tract, pressure from ascites)
   c) Damage to the spinal cord from T8 to L3, which causes compression of nerves that innervate the bowel
   d) Pressure from ascites
   e) Neurologic disorders: Stroke, Parkinson disease, multiple sclerosis
   f) Systemic disorders: Lupus, amyloidosis, scleroderma
   g) Decreased mobility
   h) Anorexia causing poor nutritional intake
   i) Metabolic and endocrine disorders
      (1) Hypothyroidism
      (2) Hyperthyroidism
      (3) Diabetes mellitus
   j) Electrolyte disturbances
      (1) Hypokalemia
      (2) Hypercalcemia
   k) Treatment related
      (1) Neurotoxic effect of cancer chemotherapy, targeted therapy, or immunotherapy agents
      (2) Surgical: Manipulation of intestines, surgical trauma to neurogenic pathways of intestines or rectum
      (3) Nutritional deficiencies: Decreased intake of fiber, roughage, and fluids
      (4) Side effect of pharmacologic agents (see Table 15-12)
         (a) Antineoplastics
         (b) Anticholinergics
         (c) Diuretics
         (d) Opioids
         (e) Aluminum- and calcium-based antacids
         (f) Calcium and iron supplements
         (g) Tricyclic antidepressants
         (h) Antihypertensives
         (i) Antispasmodics
         (j) 5-HT_3 antagonists
         (k) Nonsteroidal anti-inflammatory drugs
         (l) Barbiturates
      (5) Personal factors (Dzierżanowski & Ciałkowska-Rysz, 2015)
         (a) Interference with usual bowel movement routine
         (b) Lack of privacy
         (c) Lack of response to the defecation reflex: Pain, fatigue, social circumstances
         (d) Depression, anxiety
         (e) Decreased physical activity/exercise
         (f) Overuse of laxatives
6. Assessment
   a) Assess presence of risk factors.

Table 15-12. Common Antineoplastic Regimens and Other Treatments With High Risk for Constipation

Causative Agent	Agents	Mechanism of Action
Highly emetogenic chemotherapy	AC (doxorubicin and cyclophosphamide) combination Carmustine Cisplatin Cyclophosphamide Cytarabine Dacarbazine Doxorubicin Epirubicin Ifosfamide Mechlorethamine Melphalan Streptozocin	Nausea and vomiting Decreased oral intake Slowed peristaltic movement in gastrointestinal tract Decreased intake that leads to fewer stools, increased transit time, hard stools, and difficulty eliminating (Camp-Sorrell, 2017; Chu & DeVita, 2017; Truven Health Analytics, 2017)
Chemotherapy	Taxanes (docetaxel, paclitaxel) Vinca alkaloids (vinblastine, vincristine, vinorelbine) (Camp-Sorrell, 2017)	Decreased motility and peristalsis due to autonomic nervous system dysfunction; may result in colon impaction, colicky abdominal pain, and paralytic ileus Rectal emptying decreased when nonfunctional afferent and efferent pathways from the sacral cord are interrupted (Camp-Sorrell, 2017; Chu & DeVita, 2017; Truven Health Analytics, 2017)
Opioids	Opioid analgesics: Fentanyl, hydrocodone, hydromorphone, morphine, oxycodone (Brant et al., 2016)	Affect the colon's ability to maintain motility and peristalsis Primary agents causing medication-induced constipation (Siemens et al., 2015; Truven Health Analytics, 2017)
Immunotherapy	Ado-trastuzumab emtansine Blinatumomab Lenalidomide Thalidomide	Decreased bowel peristalsis Conjugated monoclonal antibodies and bispecific immunotherapies have 36% incidence of constipation (Camp-Sorrell, 2017; Truven Health Analytics, 2017; Villadolid & Amin, 2015)
Targeted therapy	Antiangiogenesis agents: Axitinib, crizotinib, ibrutinib, nilotinib, vorinostat	Decreased bowel peristalsis
Surgery	Colon, ovarian, and abdominal surgeries	Impaired defecation resulting from muscle weakness, surgical pain, and bowel impairment from manipulation of the bowel during surgery (Camp-Sorrell, 2017; Nelson, 2016; Truven Health Analytics, 2017)
Radiation	Radiation to the bowel or abdominal field	Small bowel obstruction and stricture (Russell, 2017; Truven Health Analytics, 2017)

b) Assess patterns of elimination, including the amount and frequency of elimination and the urge to defecate, the character and volume of stool, and the use of laxatives, stool softeners, or other measures to enhance bowel function. Note that small amounts of loose stool may indicate constipation, as the liquid stool passes around a stool mass. Small, pellet-like stool indicates slow colonic transit time, and long, thin pieces of stool may indicate stenosis or hemorrhoids (McQuade et al., 2016; Nelson, 2016).

c) Assess usual dietary patterns, focusing on fluid and fiber intake.

d) Assess mobility, activity level, and functional status.

e) Assess for abdominal pain, distension, and presence or absence of bowel sounds.

f) Assess for the presence of straining, rectal pressure, excessive flatulence, or cramping.

g) Determine facts about the patient's last bowel movement (e.g., when it occurred, amount, consistency, color, presence of blood). Structured self-rating tools can be useful for more accurate assessment of constipation. Available tools are the Bristol Stool Form Scale, the Constipation Assessment Scale, and the Common Terminology Criteria for

Adverse Events (Camp-Sorrell, 2017; NCI CTEP, 2017).

h) Determine current medication usage.

i) Use laboratory results to assist in metabolic evaluation.

j) Perform abdominal palpation and rectal examination if appropriate. A rectal examination is not routinely performed in pediatric patients. Rectal or stoma manipulation for examinations, enemas, or suppositories should be avoided in myelosuppressed patients because of the risk for bleeding, fissures, or abscesses (NCI, 2018b; NCCN, 2018a; Woolery et al., 2008).

k) Use radiographic imaging to differentiate between mechanical obstruction and decreased motility from an ileus.

7. Collaborative management: The cause of the constipation should be considered prior to beginning treatment. The preponderance of the literature on constipation management in patients with cancer is directed at palliative care and opioid-related constipation. Optimal pharmacologic management of constipation requires further investigation (Brick, 2013; Candy et al., 2015; Ishihara et al., 2012; Tarumi, Wilson, Szafran, & Spooner, 2013; Thorpe, Byar, Conley, Held-Warmkessel, et al., 2017). NCCN (2017a) palliative care guidelines offer guidance for the treatment of constipation. The Oncology Nursing Society Putting Evidence Into Practice (PEP) resource on constipation provides the most recent evidence for management. Nurses must have knowledge of the GI side effects of patients' medications. Prevention of constipation is a priority in patients with cancer. All patients on opioids require a prophylactic bowel regimen prior to initiation of opioid therapy (Camilleri, 2011).

a) Pharmacologic interventions (see Table 15-13)

(1) Opioid receptor agonists are used to treat constipation caused by opioid pain medication. Methylnaltrexone injection works by protecting the bowel from the effects of the opioid at the receptor sites in the bowel. Methylnaltrexone is recommended for practice (Thorpe, Byar, Conley, Held-Warmkessel, et al., 2017).

(2) Opioid agonist and opioid receptor antagonist combination drugs cause a local inhibitory effect on opioid action in the GI tract. The combination of oxycodone and naloxone has been shown to reduce constipation in patients on opioids. This combination is recommended for practice (Thorpe, Byar, Conley, Held-Warmkessel, et al., 2017).

(3) Mu-opioid receptor antagonists counteract the effects of opioids on GI motility and secretion. Alvimopan, a gut motility stimulator, is categorized as likely to be effective (Thorpe, Byar, Conley, Held-Warmkessel, et al., 2017).

(4) Osmotic laxatives increase the bulk of stools by attracting and retaining water in the bowel, resulting in softer stool.

(a) Lactulose

(b) Sorbitol

(5) Stimulant laxatives chemically stimulate the smooth muscles of the bowel to increase contractions (Shoemaker, Estfan, Induru, & Walsh, 2011).

(a) Bisacodyl (Dulcolax®)

(b) Senna (Senokot®)

(6) Emollient and lubricant laxatives soften hardened feces and facilitate the passage through the lower intestine.

(a) Docusate

(b) Mineral oil

(c) Glycerin suppository

(d) Enema

b) Nonpharmacologic management to prevent constipation

(1) Include increased physical activity or passive exercise as appropriate in a bowel retraining regimen. This promotes the urge to defecate by helping to move feces into the rectum.

(2) Help patients to maintain usual bowel habits during hospitalization. Baseline bowel habits are important to determine adequate bowel function. The change from baseline is more important than the number of bowel movements (Rangwala et al., 2012).

(3) Provide privacy and comfort. Inadequate conditions of privacy and dependence on a caregiver are directly correlated to risk for constipation (Dzierżanowski & Ciałkowska-Rysz, 2015; Shoemaker et al., 2011). Avoid use of a bedpan when constipation exists.

(4) Increase fluid intake to 3,000 ml/day unless contraindicated.

(5) Modify diet, as tolerated, to include high-fiber foods, as fiber adds bulk to the stool and assists food in passing more quickly through the stomach and intestines. Insoluble fiber includes wheat bran, fruit and root vegetable

Table 15-13. Pharmacologic Management of Constipation in Adult Patients

Classification	Mechanism of Action	Drug	Route, Dose, and Schedule	Side Effects	Nursing Considerations
Treatment of Opioid-Induced Constipation					
Opioid receptor agonist	Peripherally acting mu-opioid antagonist that reverses or prevents opioid-induced constipation without diminishing pain, palliating symptoms, or precipitating opioid withdrawal (Thorpe, Byar, Conley, Held-Warmkessel, et al., 2017)	Methylnaltrexone	Subcutaneous; 0.15 mg/kg every other day, no more than once a day	Flatulence, abdominal pain, dizziness, diarrhea, nausea, hyperhidrosis	Methylnaltrexone is recommended for patients on opioids and contraindicated in those with known or suspected mechanical gastrointestinal obstruction. Median time to laxation is approximately 6 hours. (Brick, 2013; Bull et al., 2015; Dunphy & Walker, 2017; Truven Health Analytics, 2017)
Opioid agonist and opioid receptor antagonist	Combination opioid that exerts a local inhibitory effect on the opioid action in the gastrointestinal tract (Thorpe, Byar, Conley, Held-Warmkessel, et al., 2017)	Oxycodone/naloxone	Oral prolonged-release tablets; initial dose oxycodone 10 mg/naloxone 5 mg	Nausea, vomiting, respiratory depression	The combination of oxycodone/naloxone improves bowel function by reducing constipation without compromising pain relief. (Ahmedzai et al., 2012; Koopmans-Klein et al., 2016; Truven Health Analytics, 2017)
Mu-opioid receptor antagonist	Counteracts the effects of opioids on gastrointestinal motility and secretion by acting on the peripheral opioid receptors in the gastrointestinal tract, increasing the frequency of spontaneous bowel movement (Thorpe, Byar, Conley, Held-Warmkessel, et al., 2017)	Alvimopan	Oral capsule; 12 mg twice daily; maximum 12 doses	Abdominal pain, indigestion, nausea, diarrhea	Alvimopan is approved for short-term hospital use only and is available only through a Risk Evaluation and Mitigation Strategy program. Drug is used in patients on opioids. It does not cross the blood–brain barrier and therefore blocks constipation without compromising pain relief. (Siemens et al., 2015; Truven Health Analytics, 2017; Webster et al., 2008)
Osmotic laxative	Hyperosmolar water-soluble radiology contrast medium that functions as an osmotic laxative retaining water in the bowel, resulting in softer stool (Thorpe, Byar, Conley, Held-Warmkessel, et al., 2017)	Amidotrizoate	Oral; in palliative care: 50 ml daily; may repeat once the following day (Mercadante et al., 2011)	Diarrhea	Studies in palliative care demonstrated that osmotic laxatives are an effective and well-tolerated alternative therapy for patients with advanced cancer and constipation after surgery. (Mercadante et al., 2011; Truven Health Analytics, 2017)

(Continued on next page)

Table 15-13. Pharmacologic Management of Constipation in Adult Patients *(Continued)*

Classification	Mechanism of Action	Drug	Route, Dose, and Schedule	Side Effects	Nursing Considerations
Bowel Regimen Agents					
Hyperosmotic laxative	Increases water content and bulk of stool by attracting and retaining water in the bowel (Nelson, 2016)	Polyethylene glycol (Golytely® or Colyte®)	Oral; 17 g (1 tbsp) dissolved in 8 oz of water, juice, soda, or other beverage, 2 times per day (NCCN, 2018a)	Diarrhea, flatulence, nausea, stomach cramps, bloating	NCCN (2018a) recommends polyethylene glycol for persistent constipation. Do not administer electrolytes with polyethylene glycol when kidney function is compromised. (Truven Health Analytics, 2017; Wirz et al., 2012)
Rectal preparations	Have a direct action on the intestine, allowing water and fats to penetrate dry stool; suppositories stimulate the intestinal nerve plexus and cause rectal emptying (Polovich et al., 2014)	Arachis oil enema Glycerol suppository Phosphate enema Sodium citrate enema	Once daily for suppositories and enemas (NCCN, 2018a)	Electrolyte imbalance	Avoid rectal manipulation in neutropenic patients. Effectiveness is unknown in constipation in patients with cancer.
Large bowel stimulants	Act directly on the colon to stimulate motility and are activated by bacterial degradation in the intestine	Senna	Oral; not to exceed 34 mg/day	Electrolyte or fluid imbalance with excess catharsis or excess use	Initiate senna 2 days prior to opioid therapy. It is recommended prophylactically for patients on vinca alkaloids. No evidence shows that adding docusate with senna has any added benefit. Senna can cause gastric irritation. It is contraindicated in patients with suspected intestinal obstruction or severe dehydration. (Feudtner et al., 2014; Tarumi et al., 2013; Truven Health Analytics, 2017)
Stimulant laxative	Act directly on the colon to stimulate motility and are activated by bacterial degradation in the intestine	Bisacodyl (Dulcolax®)	Oral; 5–15 mg daily, up to 30 mg daily	Abdominal cramps or discomfort, diarrhea, proctitis	Stimulant laxatives chemically stimulate bowel smooth muscles to increase contractions. (Shoemaker et al., 2011; Truven Health Analytics, 2017)

(Continued on next page)

Table 15-13. Pharmacologic Management of Constipation in Adult Patients *(Continued)*

Classification	Mechanism of Action	Drug	Route, Dose, and Schedule	Side Effects	Nursing Considerations
Bowel Regimen Agents *(Cont.)*					
Bulk-forming laxatives	Nondigestible substances that pass through the stomach, causing water to be retained, thus increasing the bulk of the stool (Nelson, 2016; Polovich et al., 2014)	Psyllium Calcium polycarbophil Methylcellulose	Psyllium: Oral; 1–2 tsp 1–3 times a day Calcium polycarbophil: Oral; up to 1 tbsp (2 g fiber) or 4 caplets (500 mg fiber/caplet) 3 times a day Methylcellulose: Oral; 1 tbsp in 8 oz of water daily or every 8 hours, or 2 caplets up to 6 times daily (NCCN, 2018a)	Flatulence, abdominal distention, bloating, mechanical obstruction, anaphylactic reaction	Bulk-forming laxatives must be taken with 200–300 ml of water to avoid intestinal obstruction and are not an option for patients with poor tolerance of fluids. (Dzierżanowski & Ciałkowska-Rysz, 2015; Truven Health Analytics, 2017)
Prokinetic agents	Promotes motility in the upper gastrointestinal tract and increases gastric emptying and intestinal transit time (Polovich et al., 2014)	Metoclopramide	Oral; 10–20 mg every 6 hours	–	Prokinetic agents should be reserved for use in individuals with severe constipation and those resistant to bowel programs.
Osmotic laxatives	Increase gastric secretion and motor activity and exert an osmotic effect in the small and large intestines, improving stool consistency (Camp-Sorrell, 2017)	Lactulose Sorbitol Magnesium hydroxide (milk of magnesia) Magnesium citrate Sodium phosphate	Lactulose: Oral; 15–30 ml (10–20 g) daily, up to 60 ml/day Sorbitol: Oral; 30–150 ml every day Magnesium hydroxide: Oral; 30–60 ml Magnesium citrate: Oral; 240 ml Sodium phosphate: • Oral: 15–45 ml/day • Enema: 1/day	Bloating, diarrhea, flatulence, nausea, vomiting, epigastric pain	Administer as a single dose. Oral formulations may be mixed in fruit juice, water, or milk to improve taste. Onset of action may require 48 hours. Adding conventional laxatives may be necessary. Watch for dehydration. Sodium phosphate: Use caution in patients with renal insufficiency. (Lee-Robichaud et al., 2010; Truven Health Analytics, 2017)
Detergent laxatives and surfactants (softeners)	Direct action on the intestine allowing water and fats to penetrate into dry stool and decreasing electrolyte and water absorption from the colon (Polovich et al., 2014)	Docusate sodium Docusate calcium	Docusate sodium: Oral; 50–400 mg daily Docusate calcium: Oral; 240 mg daily	Abnormal, bitter taste in mouth; cramps, diarrhea, nausea	Increase fluid intake and take with a full glass of fluid with each dose. These agents are used prophylactically in combination with an oral laxative for patients on vinca alkaloids. (Tarumi et al., 2013; Truven Health Analytics, 2017)

(Continued on next page)

Table 15-13. Pharmacologic Management of Constipation in Adult Patients *(Continued)*

Classification	Mechanism of Action	Drug	Route, Dose, and Schedule	Side Effects	Nursing Considerations
Bowel Regimen Agents *(Cont.)*					
Lubricants	Coat the stool and reduce friction (Polovich et al., 2014)	Glycerol suppositories Mineral oil Mineral oil enema	Glycerol suppositories: Rectal; 2–3 g suppository for 15 minutes once daily Mineral oil: Oral; 10–30 ml daily Mineral oil enema: 1/day	–	Excessive doses can lead to malabsorption of fat-soluble vitamins. (Truven Health Analytics, 2017)
Milk and molasses enema	Sugar in the milk and molasses irritates the intestinal lining and produces gas, causing pressure, peristalsis, and evacuation. (Hansen et al., 2011; Woolery et al., 2008)	–	3 oz of powdered milk in 6 oz of warm water, mix with 4 oz molasses Insert enema tube 12 in. or until resistance is met. Administer less than 300 ml and allow to dwell 20 minutes with patient on right side. (Woolery et al., 2008)	–	Use caution with hypertonic solutions; assess intravascular volume status. Enema may be repeated up to 4 times/day until impaction is relieved. (Hansen et al., 2011; Truven Health Analytics, 2017; Woolery et al., 2008)

GI—gastrointestinal; NCCN—National Comprehensive Cancer Network

skins, whole wheat and whole grains, beans, berries, and seeds and nuts. Soluble fiber absorbs liquid to form a gel that eases stool movement. Sources include fruits, vegetables, beans, barley, and oat bran. Studies have not established the effectiveness of fiber for constipation (Thorpe, Byar, Conley, Held-Warmkessel, et al., 2017). Obtain a nutritional consult to individualize diet modifications.

c) Complementary and alternative medicine: Probiotics have been used for the treatment of diarrhea and constipation. Probiotics such as *Bifidobacterium* or *Lactobacillus* are live microorganisms capable of colonizing the intestinal tract, altering the microflora, and exerting a positive effect on the host. Probiotics can be found in some yogurts, some cheeses, dairy products such as *Lactobacillus* milk or kefir, sauerkraut, and kimchi. Not all probiotics are the same, and not all have beneficial effects. The positive effects can support the immune system, aid in weight management, and prevent diarrhea and constipation. Effectiveness is not established (Thorpe, Byar, Conley, Held-Warmkessel, et al., 2017).

8. Patient and family education

a) Encourage patients to exercise regularly. Regular exercise stimulates GI motility.

b) Instruct patients to report constipation and to be aware of the complications associated with constipation, such as fecal impaction.

c) Stress that patients should call a physician to initiate a bowel program if three days pass without a bowel movement.

d) Ensure that all patients who are prescribed opioids are started on pharmacologic and nonpharmacologic interventions to prevent constipation and maintain the bowel program until opioids are discontinued (Ahmedzai & Boland, 2010; Bohnenkamp & LeBaron, 2010; Dzierżanowski & Ciałkowska-Rysz, 2015; Thorpe, Byar, Conley, Held-Warmkessel, et al., 2017; Wirz, Nadstawek, Elsen, Junker, & Wartenberg, 2012).

References

Aapro, M., Arends, J., Bozzetti, F., Fearon, K., Grunberg, S.M., Herrstedt, J., … Strasser, F. (2014). Early recognition of malnutrition and cachexia in the cancer patient: A position paper of a European School of Oncology Task Force. *Annals of Oncology, 25,* 1492–1499. https://doi.org/10.1093/annonc/mdu085

Abunahlah, N., Sancar, M., Dane, F., & Özyavuz, M.K. (2016). Impact of adherence to antiemetic guidelines on the incidence of chemotherapy-induced nausea and vomiting and quality of life. *International Journal of Clinical Pharmacy, 38,* 1464–1476. https://doi.org/10.1007/s11096-016-0393-3

Ahmedzai, S.H., & Boland, J. (2010). Constipation in people prescribed opioids. *BMJ Clinical Evidence, 2010,* 2407. Retrieved from https://www.ncbi.nlm.nih.gov/pmc/articles/PMC2907601

Ahmedzai, S.H., Nauck, F., Bar-Sela, G., Bosse, B., Leyendecker, P., & Hopp, M. (2012). A randomized, double-blind, active-controlled, double-dummy, parallel-group study to determine the safety and efficacy of oxycodone/naloxone prolonged-release tablets in patients with moderate/severe, chronic cancer pain. *Palliative Medicine, 26,* 50–60. https://doi.org/10.1177/0269216311418869

Al-Dasooqi, N., Sonis, S.T., Bowen, J.M., Bateman, E., Blijlevens, N., Gibson, R.J., … Lalla, R.V. (2013). Emerging evidence on the pathobiology of mucositis. *Supportive Care in Cancer, 21,* 3233–3241. https://doi.org/10.1007/s00520-013-1900-x

American Cancer Society. (2017). Managing nausea and vomiting at home. Retrieved from https://www.cancer.org/treatment/treatments-and-side-effects/physical-side-effects/nausea-and-vomiting/nausea-and-vomiting.html

Anand, A., & Glatt, A.E. (1993). *Clostridium difficile* infection associated with antineoplastic chemotherapy: A review. *Clinical Infectious Diseases, 17,* 109–113. https://doi.org/10.1093/clinids/17.1.109

Andreyev, H.J.N., Davidson, S.E., Gillespie, C., Allum, W.H., & Swarbrick, E. (2012). Practice guidance on the management of acute and chronic gastrointestinal problems arising as a result of treatment for cancer. *Gut, 61,* 179–192. https://doi.org/10.1136/gutjnl-2011-300563

Andreyev, J., Ross, P., Donnellan, C., Lennan, E., Leonard, P., Waters, C., … Ferry, D. (2014). Guidance on the management of diarrhoea during cancer chemotherapy. *Lancet Oncology, 15,* e447–e460. https://doi.org/10.1016/S1470-2045(14)70006-3

Aoyagi, T., Terracina, A.P., Raza, A., Matsubara, H., & Takabe, K. (2015). Cancer cachexia, mechanism and treatment. *World Journal of Gastrointestinal Oncology, 7,* 17–29. https://doi.org/10.4251/wjgo.v7.i4.17

AstraZeneca Pharmaceuticals LP. (2017). *Imfinzi® (durvalumab)* [Package insert]. Wilmington, DE: Author.

Barina, A.R., Bashir, M.R., Howard, B.A., Hanks, B.A., Salama, A.K., & Jaffe, T.A. (2016). Isolated recto-sigmoid colitis: A new imaging pattern of ipilimumab-associated colitis. *Abdominal Radiology, 41,* 207–214. https://doi.org/10.1007/s00261-015-0560-3

Baroudjian, B., Lourenco, N., Pagès, C., Chami, I., Maillet, M., Bertheau, P., … Allez, M. (2016). Anti-PD1-induced collagenous colitis in a melanoma patient. *Melanoma Research, 26,* 308–311. https://doi.org/10.1097/CMR.0000000000000252

Barr, W., & Smith, A. (2014). Acute diarrhea in adults. *American Family Physician, 89,* 180–189.

Bavi, P., Butler, M., Serra, S., & Chetty, R. (2017). Immune modulator-induced changes in the gastrointestinal tract. *Histopathology, 71,* 494–496. https://doi.org/10.1111/his.13224

Benson, A.B., III, Ajani, J.A., Catalano, R.B., Engelking, C., Kornblau, S.M., Martensen, J.A., Jr., … Wadler, S. (2004). Recommended guidelines for the treatment of cancer treatment-induced diarrhea. *Journal of Clinical Oncology, 22,* 2918–2926. https://doi.org/10.1200/JCO.2004.04.132

Bleday, R. (2018). Perianal and perirectal abscess. In W. Chen (Ed.), *UpToDate.* Retrieved April 13, 2018, from https://www.uptodate.com/contents/perianal-and-perirectal-abscess

Bohnenkamp, S., & LeBaron, V.T. (2010). Management of constipation in patients with cancer? *Journal of the Advanced Practitioner in Oncology, 1,* 211–217.

Bonifant, C.L., Jackson, H.J., Brentjens, R.J., & Curran, K.J. (2016). Toxicity and management in CAR T-cell therapy. *Molecular Therapy Oncolytics, 3,* 16011. https://doi.org/10.1038/mto.2016.11

Brahmer, J.R., Tykodi, S.S., Chow, L.Q.M., Hwu, W.-J., Topalian, S.L., Hwu, P., … Wigginton, J.M. (2012). Safety and activity of anti–PD-L1 antibody in patients with advanced cancer. *New England Journal of Medicine, 366,* 2455–2465. https://doi.org/10.1056/NEJMoa1200694

Brant, J.M., Walton, A., & Dyk, L. (2016). Comfort. In J.K. Itano (Ed.), *Core curriculum for oncology nursing* (5th ed., pp. 418–434). St. Louis, MO: Elsevier.

Brennan, M.T., von Bültzingslöwen, I., Schubert, M.M., & Keefe, D. (2006). Alimentary mucositis: Putting the guidelines into practice. *Supportive Care in Cancer, 14,* 573–579. https://doi.org/10.1007/s00520-006-0054-5

Brick, N. (2013). Laxatives or methylnaltrexone for the management of constipation in palliative care patients. *Clinical Journal of Oncology Nursing, 17,* 91–92. https://doi.org/10.1188/13.CJON.91-92

Bristol-Myers Squibb Co. (2017). *Yervoy® (ipilimumab)* [Package insert]. Princeton, NJ: Author.

Bristol-Myers Squibb Co. (2018). *Opdivo® (nivolumab)* [Package insert]. Princeton, NJ: Author.

Bruggeman, A.R., Kamal, A.H., LeBlanc, T.W., Ma, J.D., Baracos, V.E., & Roeland, E.J. (2016). Cancer cachexia: Beyond weight loss. *Journal of Oncology Practice, 12,* 1163–1171. https://doi.org/10.1200/JOP.2016.016832

Bull, J., Wellman, C.V., Israel, R.J., Barrett, A.C., Paterson, C., & Forbes, W.P. (2015). Fixed-dose subcutaneous methylnaltrexone in patients with advanced illness and opioid-induced constipation: Results of a randomized, placebo-controlled study and open-label extension. *Journal of Palliative Medicine, 18,* 593–600. https://doi.org/10.1089/jpm.2014.0362

Califano, R., Tariq, N., Compton, S., Fitzgerald, D.A., Harwood, C.A., Lal, R., … Nicolson, M. (2015). Expert consensus on the management of adverse events from EGFR tyrosine kinase inhibitors in the UK. *Drugs, 75,* 1335–1348. https://doi.org/10.1007/s40265-015-0434-6

Camilleri, M. (2011). Opioid-induced constipation: Challenges and therapeutic opportunities. *American Journal of Gastroenterology, 106,* 835–842. https://doi.org/10.1038/ajg.2011.30

Camp-Sorrell, D. (2017). Constipation and diarrhea management for patients with cancer. In D. Cope (Ed.), *InPractice.* Retrieved from https://www.inpractice.com/Textbooks/Oncology-Nursing/Symptom-Management/Diarrhea-and-Constipation/Chapter-Pages/Page-3/Subpage-6/Subsubpage-2.aspx

Camp-Sorrell, D. (2018). Chemotherapy toxicities and management. In C.H. Yarbro, D. Wujcik, & B.H. Gobel (Eds.), *Cancer nursing: Principles and practice* (8th ed., pp. 497–554). Burlington, MA: Jones & Bartlett Learning.

Candy, B., Jones, L., Larkin, P.J., Vickerstaff, V., Tookman, A., & Stone, P. (2015). Laxatives for the management of constipation in people receiving palliative care. *Cochrane Database of Systematic Reviews, 2015*(5). https://doi.org/10.1002/14651858.CD003448.pub4

Chaudhry, H.M., Bruce, A.J., Wolf, R.C., Litzow, M.R., Hogan, W.J., Patnaik, M.S., … Hashmi, S.K. (2015). The incidence and severity of oral mucositis among allogeneic hematopoietic stem cell transplantation patients: A systematic review. *Biology of Blood and Marrow Transplantation, 22,* 605–616. https://doi.org/10.1016/j.bbmt.2015.09.014

Chaveli-López, B., & Bagán-Sebastián, J.V. (2016). Treatment of oral mucositis due to chemotherapy. *Journal of Clinical and Experimental Dentistry, 8,* e201–e209. https://doi.org/10.4317/jced.52917

Chen, J.H., Pezhouh, M.K., Lauwers, G.Y., & Masia, R. (2017). Histopathologic features of colitis due to immunotherapy with anti-PD-1 antibodies. *American Journal of Surgical Pathology, 41,* 643–654. https://doi.org/10.1097/PAS.0000000000000829

Chiu, L., Chow, R., Popovic, M., Navari, R.M., Shumway, N.M., Chiu, N., … DeAngelis, C. (2016). Efficacy of olanzapine for the prophylaxis and rescue to chemotherapy-induced nausea and vomiting (CINV): A systematic review and meta-analysis. *Supportive Care in Cancer, 24,* 2381–2392. https://doi.org/10.1007/s00520-016-3075-8

Chu, E., & DeVita, V.T., Jr. (2017). *Physician's cancer chemotherapy drug manual 2017.* Burlington, MA: Jones & Bartlett Learning.

Connolly, M., & Larkin, P. (2012). Managing constipation: A focus on care and treatment in the palliative setting. *British Journal of Community Nursing, 17,* 60–67.

Cramer, P., & Bresalier, R.S. (2017). Gastrointestinal and hepatic complications of immune checkpoint inhibitors. *Current Gastroenterology Reports, 19,* 3. https://doi.org/10.1007/s11894-017-0540-6

Cutler, C., Li, S., Kim, H.T., Laglenne, P., Szeto, K.C., Hoffmeister, L., … Antin, J.H. (2005). Mucositis after allogeneic hematopoietic stem cell transplantation: A cohort study of methotrexate and non-methotrexate-containing graft-versus-host disease prophylaxis regimens. *Biology of Blood and Marrow Transplantation, 11,* 383–388. https://doi.org/10.1016/j.bbmt.2005.02.006

Davies, M. (2016). How checkpoint inhibitors are changing the treatment paradigm in solid tumors: What advanced practitioners in oncology need to know. *Journal of the Advanced Practitioner in Oncology, 7,* 498–509. https://doi.org/10.6004/jadpro.2016.7.5.3

De Sanctis, V., Bossi, P., Sanguineti, G., Trippa, F., Ferrari, D., Bacigalupo, A., … Lalla, R.V. (2016). Mucositis in head and neck cancer patients treated with radiotherapy and systemic therapies: Literature review and consensus statements. *Critical Reviews in Oncology/Hematology, 100,* 147–166. https://doi.org/10.1016/j.critrevonc.2016.01.010

Deshpande, A., Lever, D.S., & Soffer, E. (2013). Acute diarrhea. Retrieved from http://www.clevelandclinicmeded.com/medicalpubs/diseasemanagement/gastroenterology/acute-diarrhea

Dev, R., Wong, A., Hui, D., & Bruera, E. (2017). The evolving approach to management of cancer cachexia. *Oncology, 31,* 23–32.

Dunphy, E.P., & Walker, S. (2017). Gastrointestinal symptoms. In J. Eggert (Ed.), *Cancer basics* (2nd ed., pp. 431–473). Pittsburgh, PA: Oncology Nursing Society.

Dzierżanowski, T., & Ciałkowska-Rysz, A. (2015). Behavioral risk factors in constipation in palliative care patients. *Supportive Care in Cancer, 23,* 1787–1793. https://doi.org/10.1007/s00520-014-2495-6

Eilers, J.G., Asakura, Y., Blecher, C.S., Burgoon, D., Chiffelle, R., Ciccolini, K., … Valinski, S. (2017, May 10). Putting evidence into practice: Mucositis. Retrieved from https://www.ons.org/practice-resources/pep/mucositis

Eilers, J., Berger, A.M., & Peterson, M.C. (1988). Development, testing and application of the oral assessment guide. *Oncology Nursing Forum, 15,* 325–330.

Eilers, J., Harris, D., Henry, K., & Johnson, L.A. (2014). Evidence-based interventions for cancer treatment-related mucositis: Putting evidence into practice. *Clinical Journal of Oncology Nursing, 18*(Suppl. 6), 80–96. https://doi.org/10.1188/14.CJON.S3.80-96

Eilers, J., & Million, R. (2011). Clinical update: Prevention and management of oral mucositis in patients with cancer. *Seminars in Oncology Nursing, 27,* e1–e16. https://doi.org/10.1016/j.soncn.2011.08.001

EMD Serono, Inc. (2017). *Bavencio® (avelumab)* [Package insert]. Rockland, MA: Author.

Engelking, C. (2008). Diarrhea and constipation. In R.A. Gates & R.M. Fink (Eds.), *Oncology nursing secrets* (3rd ed., pp. 372–397). St. Louis, MO: Elsevier Mosby.

Epstein, J.B., Beaumont, J.L., Gwede, C.K., Murphy, B., Garden, A.S., Meredith, R., ... Cella, D. (2007). Longitudinal evaluation of the oral mucositis weekly questionnaire-head and neck cancer, a patient-reported outcomes questionnaire. *Cancer, 109,* 1914–1922. https://doi.org/10.1002/cncr.22620

Epstein, J.B., Thariat, J., Bensadoun, R.-J., Barasch, A., Murphy, B.A., Kolnick, L., ... Maghami, E. (2012). Oral complications of cancer and cancer therapy: From cancer treatment to survivorship. *CA: A Cancer Journal for Clinicians, 62,* 400–422. https://doi.org/10.3322/caac.21157

Fearon, K., Strasser, F., Anker, S.D., Bosaeus, I., Bruera, E., Fainsinger, R.L., ... Baracos, V.E. (2011). Definition and classification of cancer cachexia: An international consensus. *Lancet Oncology, 12,* 489–495. https://doi.org/10.1016/S1470-2045(10)70218-7

Feudtner, C., Freedman, J., Kang, T., Womer, J.W., Dai, D., & Faerber, J. (2014). Comparative effectiveness of senna to prevent problematic constipation in pediatric oncology patients receiving opioids: A multicenter study of clinically detailed administrative data. *Journal of Pain and Symptom Management, 48,* 272–280. https://doi.org/10.1016/j.jpainsymman.2013.09.009

Fulton, J. (2018). Oral mucositis. In C.H. Yarbro, D. Wujcik, & B.H. Gobel (Eds.), *Cancer nursing: Principles and practice* (8th ed., pp. 922–938). Burlington, MA: Jones & Bartlett Learning.

Genentech, Inc. (2017). *Tecentriq® (atezolizumab)* [Package insert]. South San Francisco, CA: Author.

Ghatalia, P., Morgan, C.J., Choueiri, T.K., Rocha, P., Naik, G., & Sonpavde, G. (2015). Pancreatitis with vascular endothelial growth factor receptor tyrosine kinase inhibitors. *Critical Reviews in Oncology/Hematology, 94,* 136–145. https://doi.org/10.1016/j.critrevonc.2014.11.008

Gibson, R.J., Keefe, D.M.K., Lalla, R.V., Bateman, E., Blijlevens, N., Fijlstra, M., ... Bowen, J.M. (2013). Systematic review of agents for the management of gastrointestinal mucositis in cancer patients. *Supportive Care in Cancer, 21,* 313–326. https://doi.org/10.1007/s00520-012-1644-z

Gibson, R.J., & Stringer, A.M. (2009). Chemotherapy-induced diarrhoea. *Current Opinion in Supportive and Palliative Care, 3,* 31–35. https://doi.org/10.1097/SPC.0b013e32832531bb

Gilead Sciences, Inc. (2018). *Zydelig ® (idelalisib)* [Package insert]. Foster City, CA: Author.

Gilmore, J.W., Peacock, N.W., Gu, A., Szabo, S., Rammage, M., Sharpe, J., ... Burke, T.A. (2014). Antiemetic guideline consistency and incidence of chemotherapy-induced nausea and vomiting in US community oncology practice: INSPIRE study. *Journal of Oncology Practice, 10,* 68–74. https://doi.org/10.1200/JOP.2012.000816

Gondal, B., Patel, P., Gallan, A., Hart, J., & Bissonnette, M. (2016). Immune-mediated colitis with novel immunotherapy: PD-1 inhibitor associated gastrointestinal toxicity. *Acta Gastro-Enterologica Belgica, 79,* 379–381.

Grunberg, S.M., Deuson, R.R., Mavros, P., Geling, O., Hansen, M., Cruciani, G., ... Daugaard, G. (2004). Incidence of chemotherapy-induced nausea and emesis after modern antiemetics: Perception versus reality. *Cancer, 100,* 2261–2668. https://doi.org/10.1002/cncr.20230

Grunberg, S.M., Osoba, D., Hesketh, P.J., Gralla, R.J., Borjeson, S., Rapoport, B.L., ... Tonato, M. (2005). Evaluation of new antiemetic agents and definition of antineoplastic agent emetogenicity—An update. *Supportive Care in Cancer, 13,* 80–84. https://doi.org/10.1007/s00520-004-0718-y

Grunberg, S.M., Warr, D., Gralla, R.J., Rapoport, B.L., Hesketh, P.J., Jordan, K., & Espersen, B.T. (2011). Evaluation of new antiemetic agents and definition of antineoplastic agent emetogenicity—State of the art. *Supportive Care in Cancer, 19*(Suppl. 1), S43–S47. https://doi.org/10.1007/s00520-010-1003-x

Gupta, A., De Felice, K.M., Loftus, E.V., Jr., & Khanna, S. (2015). Systematic review: Colitis associated with anti-CTLA-4 therapy. *Alimentary Pharmacology and Therapeutics, 42,* 406–417. https://doi.org/10.1111/apt.13281

Gussgard, A.M., Hope, A.J., Jokstad, A., Tenenbaum, H., & Wood, R. (2014). Assessment of cancer therapy-induced oral mucositis using a patient-reported oral mucositis experience questionnaire. *PLOS ONE, 9,* e91733. https://doi.org/10.1371/journal.pone.0091733

Hansen, S.E., Whitehill, J.L., Goto, C.S., Quintero, C.A., Darling, B.E., & Davis, J. (2011). Safety and efficacy of milk and molasses enemas compared with sodium phosphate enemas for the treatment of constipation in a pediatric emergency department. *Pediatric Emergency Care, 27,* 1118–1120. https://doi.org/10.1097/PEC.0b013e31823b0088

Harris, D.J., Eilers, J., Harriman, A., Cashavelly, B.J., & Maxwell, C. (2008). Putting Evidence Into Practice®: Evidence-based interventions for the management of oral mucositis. *Clinical Journal of Oncology Nursing, 12,* 141–152. https://doi.org/10.1188/08.CJON.141-152

Hartl, D.M., Morel, D., Saavedra, E., Massard, C., Rinaldo, A., Saba, N.F., ... Soria, J.-C. (2017). Otorhinolaryngological toxicities of new drugs in oncology. *Advances in Therapy, 34,* 866–894. https://doi.org/10.1007/s12325-017-0512-0

Hebra, A. (2017). Anorectal abscess. Retrieved from https://emedicine.medscape.com/article/191975-overview

Hesketh, P.J. (2008). Chemotherapy-induced nausea and vomiting. *New England Journal of Medicine, 358,* 2482–2494. https://doi.org/10.1056/NEJMra0706547

Hesketh, P.J., Kris, M.G., Basch, E., Bohlke, K., Barbour, S.Y., Clark-Snow, R.A., ... Lyman, G.H. (2017). Antiemetics: American Society of Clinical Oncology clinical practice guideline update. *Journal of Clinical Oncology, 35,* 3240–3261. https://doi.org/10.1200/JCO.2017.74.4789

Ishihara, M., Ikesue, H., Matsunaga, H., Suemaru, K., Kitaichi, K., Suetsugu, K., ... Itoh, Y. (2012). A multi-institutional study analyzing effect of prophylactic medication for prevention of opioid-induced gastrointestinal dysfunction. *Clinical Journal of Pain, 28,* 373–381. https://doi.org/10.1097/AJP.0b013e318237d626

Jackson, L.K., Johnson, D.B., Sosman, J.A., Murphy, B.A., & Epstein, J.B. (2015). Oral health in oncology: Impact of immunotherapy. *Supportive Care in Cancer, 23,* 1–3. https://doi.org/10.1007/s00520-014-2434-6

Jazz Pharmaceuticals. (2016). *Erwinaze® (asparaginase* Erwinia chrysanthemi*)* [Package insert]. Palo Alto, CA: Author.

Jensen, S.B., & Peterson, D.E. (2013). Oral mucosal injury caused by cancer therapies: Current management and new frontiers in research. *Journal of Oral Pathology and Medicine, 43,* 81–90. https://doi.org/10.1111/jop.12135

Kearney, S.L., Dahlberg, S.E., Levy, D.E., Voss, S.D., Sallan, S.E., & Silverman, L.B. (2009). Clinical course and outcome in children with acute lymphoblastic leukemia and asparaginase-associated pancreatitis. *Pediatric Blood and Cancer, 53,* 162–167. https://doi.org/10.1002/pbc.22076

Keefe, D.M., Schubert, M.M., Elting, L.S., Sonis, S.T., Epstein, J.B., Raber-Durlacher, J.E., ... Peterson, D.E. (2007). Updated clinical practice guidelines for the prevention and treatment of mucositis. *Cancer, 109,* 820–831. https://doi.org/10.1002/cncr.22484

Koopmans-Klein, G., Wagemans, M.F.M., Wartenberg, H.C.H, Van Megen, Y.J.B., & Huygen, F.J.P.M. (2016). The efficacy of standard laxative use for the prevention and treatment of opioid induced constipation during oxycodone use: A small Dutch observational pilot study. *Expert Review of Gastroenterology and Hepatology, 10,* 547–553. https://doi.org/10.1586/17474124.2016.1129275

Koselke, E.A., & Kraft, S. (2012). Chemotherapy-induced diarrhea: Options for treatment and prevention. *Journal of Hematology Oncology Pharmacy, 2,* 143–151. Retrieved from http://jhoponline.com/jhop-issue-archive/2012-issues/december-2012-vol-3-no-4/15408-chemotherapy-unduced-diarrhea-options

Kottschade, L., Brys, A., Peikert, T., Ryder, M., Raffals, L., Brewer, J., ... Markovic, S. (2016). A multidisciplinary approach to toxicity management of modern immune checkpoint inhibitors in cancer therapy. *Melanoma Research, 26,* 469–480. https://doi.org/10.1097/CMR.0000000000000273

Kroschinsky, F., Stölzel, F., von Bonin, S., Beutel, G., Kochanek, M., Kiehl, M., & Schellongowski, P. (2017). New drugs, new toxicities: Severe side effects of modern targeted and immunotherapy of cancer and their management. *Critical Care, 21,* 89. https://doi.org/10.1186/s13054-017-1678-1

Kushner, J.A., Lawrence, H.P., Shoval, I., Kiss, T.L., Devins, G.M., Lee, L., & Tenenbaum, H.C. (2008). Development and validation of a patient-reported oral mucositis symptom (PROMS) scale. *Journal of the Canadian Dental Association, 74,* 59. Retrieved from http://www.cda-adc.ca/jcda/vol-74/issue-1/59.html

Lalla, R.V., Bowen, J., Barasch, A., Elting, L., Epstein, J., Keefe, D.M., ... Elad, S. (2014). MASCC/ISOO clinical practice guidelines for the management of mucositis secondary to cancer therapy. *Cancer, 120,* 1453–1461. https://doi.org/10.1002/cncr.28592

LeBlanc, T.W., Samsa, G.P., Wolf, S.P., Locke, S.C., Cella, D.F., & Abernethy, A.P. (2015). Validation and real-world assessment of the Functional Assessment of Anorexia-Cachexia Therapy (FAACT) scale in patients with advanced non-small cell lung cancer and the cancer anorexia-cachexia syndrome (CACS). *Supportive Care in Cancer, 23,* 2341–2347. https://doi.org/10.1007/s00520-015-2606-z

Lee, J., Cherwin, C., Czaplewski, L.M., Dabbour, R., Doumit, M., Lewis, C., ... Whiteside, S. (2017, April 14). Putting evidence into practice: Chemotherapy-induced nausea and vomiting. Retrieved from https://www.ons.org/practice-resources/pep/chemotherapy-induced-nausea-and-vomiting

Lee, J.L.C., Leong, L.P., & Lim, S.L. (2016). Nutrition intervention approaches to reduce malnutrition in oncology patients: A systematic review. *Supportive Care in Cancer, 24,* 469–480. https://doi.org/10.1007/s00520-015-2958-4

Lee-Robichaud, H., Thomas, K., Morgan, J., & Nelson, R.L. (2010). Lactulose versus polyethylene glycol for chronic constipation. *Cochrane Database of Systematic Reviews, 2010*(7). https://doi.org/10.1002/14651858.CD007570.pub2

Louie, C.Y., DiMaio, M.A., Matsukuma, K.E., Coutre, S.E., Berry, G.J., & Longacre, T.A. (2015). Idelalisib-associated enterocolitis: Clinicopathologic features and distinction from other enterocolitides. *American Journal of Surgical Pathology, 39,* 1653–1660. https://doi.org/10.1097/PAS.0000000000000525

Lui, M., Gallo-Hershberg, D., & DeAngelis, C. (2017). Development and validation of a patient-reported questionnaire assessing systemic therapy induced diarrhea in oncology patients. *Health and Quality of Life Outcomes, 15,* 249. https://doi.org/10.1186/s12955-017-0794-6

Maria, O.M., Eliopoulos, N., & Muanza, T. (2017). Radiation-induced oral mucositis. *Frontiers in Oncology, 7,* 89. https://doi.org/10.3389/fonc.2017.00089

Martins, F., de Oliveira, M.A., Wang, Q., Sonis, S., Gallottini, M., George, S., & Treister, N. (2013). A review of oral toxicity associated with mTOR inhibitor therapy in cancer patients. *Oral Oncology, 49,* 293–298. http://doi.org/10.1016/j.oraloncology.2012.11.008

Marx, W., McCarthy, A.L., Ried, K., McKavanagh, D., Vitetta, L., Sali, A., ... Isenring, E. (2017). The effect of a standardized ginger extract on chemotherapy-induced nausea-related quality of life in patients undergoing moderately or highly emetogenic chemotherapy: A double-blind, randomized, placebo controlled trial. *Nutrients, 9,* 867. https://doi.org/10.3390/nu9080867

Matsuo, N., Morita, T., Matsuda, Y., Okamoto, K., Matsumoto, Y., Kaneishi, K., Odagiri, T., ... Iwase, S. (2017). Predictors of responses to corticosteroids for anorexia in advanced cancer patients: A multicenter prospective observational study. *Supportive Care in Cancer, 25,* 41–50. https://doi.org/10.1007/s00520-016-3383-z

Mattox, T.W. (2017). Cancer cachexia: Cause, diagnosis, and treatment. *Nutrition in Clinical Practice, 32,* 599–606. https://doi.org/10.1177/0884533617722986

McGuire, D.B., Fulton, J.S., Park, J., Brown, C.G., Correa, M.E.P., Eilers, J., ... Lalla, R.V. (2013). Systematic review of basic oral care for the management of oral mucositis in cancer patients. *Supportive Care in Cancer, 21,* 3165–3177. https://doi.org/10.1007/s00520-013-1942-0

McQuade, R.M., Stojanovska, V., Abalo, R., Bornstein, J.C., & Nurgali, K. (2016). Chemotherapy induced constipation and diarrhea: Pathophysiology, current and emerging treatments. *Frontiers in Pharmacology, 7,* 414. https://doi.org/10.3389/fphar.2016.00414

Mercadante, S., Aielli, F., Adile, C., Ferrera, P., Valle, A., Fusco, F., ... Porzio, G. (2015). Prevalence of oral mucositis, dry mouth, and dysphagia in advanced cancer patients. *Supportive Care in Cancer, 23,* 3249–3255. https://doi.org/10.1007/s00520-015-2720-y

Mercadante, S., Ferrera, P., & Casuccio, A. (2011). Effectiveness and tolerability of amidotrizoate for the treatment of constipation resistant to laxatives in advanced cancer patients. *Journal of Pain and Symptom Management, 41,* 421–425. https://doi.org/10.1016/j.jpainsymman.2010.04.022

Merck and Co., Inc. (2017). *Keytruda® (pembrolizumab)* [Package insert]. Whitehouse Station, NJ: Author.

Mistry, H.E., Forbes, S.G., & Fowler, N. (2017). Toxicity management: Development of a novel and immune-mediated adverse events algorithm. *Clinical Journal of Oncology Nursing, 21*(Suppl. 2), 53–59. https://doi.org/10.1188/17.CJON.S2.53-59

Molassiotis, A., Lee, P.H., Burke, T.A., Dicato, M., Gascon, P., Roila, F., & Aapro, M. (2016). Anticipatory nausea, risk factors, and its impact on chemotherapy-induced nausea and vomiting: Results from the Pan European Emesis Registry Study. *Journal of Pain and Symptom Management, 51,* 987–993. https://doi.org/10.1016/j.jpainsymman.2015.12.317

Moslemi, D., Nokhandani, A.M., Otaghsaraei, M.T., Moghadamnia, Y., Kazemi, S., & Moghadamnia, A.A. (2016). Management of chemo/radiation-induced oral mucositis in patients with head and neck cancer: A review of the literature. *Radiotherapy and Oncology, 120,* 13–20. https://doi.org/10.1016/j.radonc.2016.04.001

Muehlbauer, P.M. (2014). Diarrhea. In C.H. Yarbro, D. Wujcik, & B.H. Gobel (Eds.), *Cancer symptom management* (4th ed., pp. 185–212). Burlington, MA: Jones & Bartlett Learning.

Muehlbauer, P.M., Thorpe, D., Davis, A., Drabot, R., Rawlings, B.L., & Kiker, E. (2009). Putting evidence into practice: Evidence-based interventions to prevent, manage, and treat chemotherapy- and radiotherapy-induced diarrhea. *Clinical Journal of Oncology Nursing, 13,* 336–341. https://doi.org/10.1188/09.CJON.336-341

Naidoo, J., Page, D.B., Li, B.T., Connell, L.C., Schindler, K., Lacouture, M.E., ... Wolchok, J.D. (2015). Toxicities of the anti-PD-1 and anti-PD-L1 immune checkpoint antibodies. *Annals of Oncology, 26,* 2375–2391. https://doi.org/10.1093/annonc/mdv383

National Cancer Institute. (2016). Oral complications of chemotherapy and head/neck radiation (PDQ®) [Patient version]. Retrieved from https://www.cancer.gov/about-cancer/treatment/side-effects/mouth-throat/oral-complications-pdq

National Cancer Institute. (2017a). Gastrointestinal complications (PDQ®) [Health professional version]. Retrieved from https://www.cancer.gov/about-cancer/treatment/side-effects/constipation/GI-complications-hp-pdq

National Cancer Institute. (2017b). Nausea and vomiting (PDQ®) [Patient version]. Retrieved from https://www.cancer.gov/about-cancer/treatment/side-effects/nausea/nausea-pdq

National Cancer Institute. (2017c). Nutrition in health care (PDQ®) [Health professional version]. Retrieved from https://www.cancer.gov/about-cancer/treatment/side-effects/appetite-loss/nutrition-hp-pdq

National Cancer Institute. (2017d). Topics of integrative, complementary and alternative therapies (PDQ®) [Health professional version]. Retrieved from https://www.cancer.gov/about-cancer/treatment/cam/hp/cam-topics-pdq

National Cancer Institute. (2017e). Treatment-related nausea and vomiting (PDQ®) [Health professional version]. Retrieved from https://www.cancer.gov/about-cancer/treatment/side-effects/nausea/nausea-hp-pdq

National Cancer Institute. (2018a). *Eating hints: Before, during, and after cancer treatment* (NIH Publication No. 18-7157). Retrieved from https://www.cancer.gov/publications/patient-education/eatinghints.pdf

National Cancer Institute. (2018b). Gastrointestinal complications (PDQ®) [Health professional version]. Retrieved from http://www.cancer.gov/cancertopics/pdq/supportivecare/gastrointestinalcomplications/HealthProfessional

National Cancer Institute Cancer Therapy Evaluation Program. (2017). *Common terminology criteria for adverse events* [v.5.0]. Retrieved from https://ctep.cancer.gov/protocoldevelopment/electronic_applications/docs/CTCAE_v5_Quick_Reference_5x7.pdf

National Comprehensive Cancer Network. (2017a). *NCCN Clinical Practice Guidelines in Oncology (NCCN Guidelines®): Palliative care* [v.1.2018]. Retrieved from https://www.nccn.org/professionals/physician_gls/PDF/palliative.pdf

National Comprehensive Cancer Network. (2017b). *NCCN Clinical Practice Guidelines in Oncology (NCCN Guidelines®): Prevention and treatment of cancer-related infections* [v.1.2018]. Retrieved from http://www.nccn.org/professionals/physician_gls/pdf/infections.pdf

National Comprehensive Cancer Network. (2018a). *NCCN Clinical Practice Guidelines in Oncology (NCCN Guidelines®): Adult cancer pain* [v.1.2018]. Retrieved from https://www.nccn.org/professionals/physician_gls/pdf/pain.pdf

National Comprehensive Cancer Network. (2018b). *NCCN Clinical Practice Guidelines in Oncology (NCCN Guidelines®): Antiemesis* [v.1.2018]. Retrieved from https://www.nccn.org/professionals/physician_gls/pdf/antiemesis.pdf

National Comprehensive Cancer Network. (2018c). *NCCN Clinical Practice Guidelines in Oncology (NCCN Guidelines®) in partnership with the American Society of Clinical Oncology (ASCO): Management of immunotherapy-related toxicities (immune checkpoint inhibitor-related toxicities)* [v.1.2018]. Retrieved from https://www.nccn.org/professionals/physician_gls/pdf/immunotherapy.pdf

National Institute of Diabetes and Digestive and Kidney Diseases. (2016). Definition and facts for diarrhea. Retrieved from https://www.niddk.nih.gov/health-information/digestive-diseases/diarrhea/definition-facts

Navari, R.M. (2015). Treatment of breakthrough and refractory chemotherapy-induced nausea and vomiting. *BioMed Research International, 2015,* 595894. https://doi.org/10.1155/2015/595894

Navari, R.M., & Aapro, M. (2016). Antiemetic prophylaxis for chemotherapy-induced nausea and vomiting. *New England Journal of Medicine, 374,* 1356–1367. https://doi.org/10.1056/NEJMra1515442

Nelson, L. (2016). Alterations in gastrointestinal function. In J.K. Itano (Ed.), *Core curriculum for oncology nursing* (5th ed., pp. 340–362). St. Louis, MO: Elsevier.

Nesher, L., & Rolston, K.V.I. (2012). Neutropenic enterocolitis, a growing concern in the era of widespread use of aggressive chemotherapy. *Clinical Infectious Diseases, 56,* 711–717. https://doi.org/10.1093/cid/cis998

Ngo, D., Jia, J.B., Green, C.S., Gulati, A.T., & Lall, C. (2015). Cancer therapy related complications in the liver, pancreas, and biliary system: An imaging perspective. *Insights Into Imaging, 6,* 665–677. https://doi.org/10.1007/s13244-015-0436-7

Palmore, T.N., Parta, M., Cuellar-Rodriguez, J., & Gea-Banancloche, J.C. (2015). Infections in the cancer patient. In V.T. DeVita Jr., T.S. Lawrence, & S.A. Rosenberg (Eds.), *DeVita, Hellman, and Rosenberg's cancer: Principles and practice of oncology* (10th ed., pp. 1931–1959). Philadelphia, PA: Wolters Kluwer Health.

Pessi, M.A., Zilembo, N., Haspinger, E.R., Molino, L., Di Cosimo, S., Garassino, M., & Ripamonti, C.I. (2014). Targeted therapy-induced diarrhea: A review of the literature. *Critical Reviews in Oncology/Hematology, 90,* 165–179. https://doi.org/10.1016/j.critrevonc.2013.11.008

Peters, M.D.J. (2016, January 20). Oral mucositis: Assessment [Evidence summary]. Retrieved June 12, 2017, from Joanna Briggs Institute Library Database: http://connect.jbiconnectplus.org

Peterson, D.E., Srivastava, R., & Lalla, R.V. (2015). Oral mucosal injury in oncology patients: Perspectives on maturation of a field. *Oral Diseases, 21,* 133–141. https://doi.org/10.1111/odi.12167

Pfizer Inc. (2016). *Camptosar® (irinotecan)* [Package insert]. New York, NY: Author.

Phillip, V., Schwab, M., Haf, D., & Algül, H. (2017). Identification of risk factors for post-endoscopic retrograde cholangiopancreatography pancreatitis in a high-volume center. *PLOS ONE, 12,* e0177874. https://doi.org/10.1371/journal.pone.0177874

Pilotte, A.P., Hohos, M.B., Polson, K.M.O., Hutalen, T.M., & Treister, N. (2011). Managing stomatitis in patients treated with mammalian target of rapamycin inhibitors [Online exclusive]. *Clinical Journal of Oncology Nursing, 15,* E83–E89. https://doi.org/10.1188/11.CJON.E83-E89

Polovich, M., Olsen, M., & LeFebvre, K.B. (Eds.). (2014). *Chemotherapy and biotherapy guidelines and recommendations for practice* (4th ed.). Pittsburgh, PA: Oncology Nursing Society.

Rangwala, F., Zafar, S.Y., & Abernathy, A.P. (2012). Gastrointestinal symptoms in cancer patients with advanced disease: New methodologies, insights and a proposed approach. *Current Opinion in Supportive and Palliative Care, 6,* 69–75. https://doi.org/10.1097/SPC.0b013e32834f689d

Rodrigues, F.G., Dasilva, G., & Wexner, S.D. (2017). Neutropenic enterocolitis. *World Journal of Gastroenterology, 23,* 42–47. https://doi.org/10.3748/wjg.v23.i1.42

Roila, F., Molassiotis, A., Herrstedt, J., Aapro, M., Gralla, R.J., Bruera, E., … van der Wetering, M. (2016). 2016 MASCC and ESMO guideline update for the prevention of chemotherapy- and radiotherapy-induced nausea and vomiting and of nausea and vomiting in advanced cancer patients. *Annals of Oncology, 27*(Suppl. 5), v119–v133. https://doi.org/10.1093/annonc/mdw270

Russell, M.L. (2016). Nursing implications of radiation therapy. In J.K. Itano (Ed.), *Core curriculum for oncology nursing* (5th ed., pp. 226–236). St. Louis, MO: Elsevier.

Schmidt-Hieber, M., Bierwirth, J., Buchheidt, D., Cornely, O.A., Hentrich, M., Maschmeyer, G., ... Vehreschild, M.J.G.T. (2017). Diagnosis and management of gastrointestinal complications in adult cancer patients: 2017 updated evidence-based guidelines of the Infectious Diseases Working Party (AGIHO) of the German Society of Hematology and Medical Oncology (DGHO). *Annals of Hematology, 97,* 31–49. https://doi.org/10.1007/s00277-017-3183-7

Schwarz, S., Prokopchuk, O., Esefeld, K., Gröschel, S., Bachmann, J., Lorenzen, S., ... Martignoni, M.E. (2017). The clinical picture of cachexia: A mosaic of different parameters (experience of 503 patients). *BMC Cancer, 17,* 130. https://doi.org/10.1186/s12885-017-3116-9

Scott, D., Reid, J., Hudson, P., Martin, P., & Porter, S. (2016). Health care professionals' experience, understanding and perception of need of advanced cancer patients with cachexia and their families: The benefits of a dedicated clinic. *BMC Palliative Care, 15,* 100. https://doi.org/10.1186/s12904-016-0171-y

Sharma, A., Rath, G.K., Chaudhary, S.P., Thakar, A., Mohanti, B.K., & Bahadur, S. (2012). *Lactobacillus brevis* CD2 lozenges reduce radiation- and chemotherapy-induced mucositis in patients with head and neck cancer: A randomized double-blind placebo-controlled study. *European Journal of Cancer, 48,* 875–881. https://doi.org/10.1016/j.ejca.2011.06.010

Shaw, C., & Taylor, L. (2012). Treatment-related diarrhea in patients with cancer. *Clinical Journal of Oncology Nursing, 16,* 413–417. https://doi.org/10.1188/12.CJON.413-417

Shoemaker, L.K., Estfan, B., Induru, R., & Walsh, T.D. (2011). Symptom management: An important part of cancer care. *Cleveland Clinic Journal of Medicine, 78,* 25–34. https://doi.org/10.3949/ccjm.78a.10053

Siemens, W., Gaertner, J., & Becker, G. (2015). Advances in pharmacotherapy for opioid-induced constipation—A systematic review. *Expert Opinion on Pharmacotherapy, 16,* 515–532. https://doi.org/10.1517/14656566.2015.995625

Sonis, S.T. (2011). Oral mucositis. *Anti-Cancer Drugs, 22,* 607–612. https://doi.org/10.1097/CAD.0b013e3283462086

Spain, L., Diem, S., & Larkin, J. (2016). Management of toxicities of immune checkpoint inhibitors. *Cancer Treatment Reviews, 44,* 51–60. https://doi.org/10.1016/j.ctrv.2016.02.001

Stein, A., Voigt, W., & Jordan, K. (2010). Chemotherapy-induced diarrhea: Pathophysiology, frequency and guideline-based management. *Therapeutic Advances in Medical Oncology, 2,* 51–63. https://doi.org/10.1177/1758834009355164

Stock, W., Douer, D., DeAngelo, D.J., Arellano, M., Advani, A., Damon, L., ... Bleyer, A. (2011). Prevention and management of asparaginase/pegasparaginase-associated toxicities in adults and older adolescents: Recommendations of an expert panel. *Leukemia and Lymphoma, 52,* 2237–2253. https://doi.org/10.3109/10428194.2011.596963

Stringer, A.M., & Logan, R.M. (2015). The role of oral flora in the development of chemotherapy-induced oral mucositis. *Journal of Oral Pathology and Medicine, 44,* 81–87. https://doi.org/10.1111/jop.12152

Suzuki, H., Asakawa, A., Amitani, H., Nakamura, N., & Inui, A. (2013). Cancer cachexia—Pathophysiology and management. *Journal of Gastroenterology, 48,* 574–594. https://doi.org/10.1007/s00535-013-0787-0

Tarumi, Y., Wilson, M.P., Szafran, O., & Spooner, G.R. (2013). Randomized, double-blind, placebo-controlled trial of oral docusate in the management of constipation in hospice patients. *Journal of Pain and Symptom Management, 45,* 2–13. https://doi.org/10.1016/j.jpainsymman.2012.02.008

Thorpe, D.M., Byar, K.L., Conley, S., Drapek, L., Held-Warmkessel, J., Ramsdell, M.J., ... Wolles, B. (2017, February 27). Putting evidence into practice: Diarrhea. Retrieved from https://www.ons.org/practice-resources/pep/diarrhea

Thorpe, D.M., Byar, K.L., Conley, S., Held-Warmkessel, J., & Ramsdell, M.J. (2017, February 27). Putting evidence into practice: Constipation. Retrieved from https://www.ons.org/practice-resources/pep/constipation

Tipton, J. (2014). Nausea and vomiting. In C.H. Yarbro, D. Wujcik, & B.H. Gobel (Eds.), *Cancer symptom management* (4th ed., pp. 213–239). Burlington, MA: Jones & Bartlett Learning.

Tokimasa, S., & Yamato, K. (2012). Does octreotide prevent L-asparaginase-associated pancreatitis in children with acute lymphoblastic leukaemia? *British Journal of Haematology, 157,* 381–382. https://doi.org/10.1111/j.1365-2141.2011.08971.x

Treepongkaruna, S., Thongpak, N., Pakakasama, S., Pienvichit, P., Sirachaninan, N., & Hongeng, S. (2009). Acute pancreatitis in children with acute lymphoblastic leukemia after chemotherapy. *Journal of Pediatric Hematology/Oncology, 31,* 812–815. https://doi.org/10.1097/MPH.0b013e3181b87035

Treister, N.S., & Sankar, V. (2017). Chemotherapy-induced oral mucositis. Retrieved from http://www.emedicine.com/derm/topic682.htm

Truven Health Analytics. (2017). Micromedex® Solutions [Web application]. Retrieved from http://www.micromedexsolutions.com/micromedex2/librarian

Van Sebille, Y.Z.A., Stansborough, R., Wardill, H.R., Bateman, E., Gibson, R.J., & Keefe, D.M. (2015). Management of mucositis during chemotherapy: From pathophysiology to pragmatic therapeutics. *Current Oncology Reports, 17,* 50. https://doi.org/10.1007/s11912-015-0474-9

Vanhoecke, B., De Ryck, T., Stringer, A., Van de Wiele, T., & Keefe, D. (2015). Microbiota and their role in the pathogenesis of oral mucositis. *Oral Diseases, 21,* 17–30. https://doi.org/10.1111/odi.12224

Vege, S.S. (2017). Clinical manifestations and diagnosis of acute pancreatitis. In S. Grover (Ed.), *UpToDate.* Retrieved July 7, 2017, from https://www.uptodate.com/contents/clinical-manifestations-and-diagnosis-of-acute-pancreatitis

Villa, A., & Sonis, S.T. (2015). Mucositis: Pathobiology and management. *Current Opinion in Oncology, 27,* 159–164. https://doi.org/10.1097/CCO.0000000000000180

Villa, A., & Sonis, S.T. (2016). Pharmacotherapy for the management of cancer regimen-related oral mucositis. *Expert Opinion on Pharmacotherapy, 17,* 1801–1807. https://doi.org/10.1080/14656566.2016.1217993

Villadolid, J., & Amin, A. (2015). Immune checkpoint inhibitors in clinical practice: Update on management of immune-related toxicities. *Translational Lung Cancer Research, 4,* 560–575. https://doi.org/10.3978/j.issn.2218-6751.2015.06.06

Wardill, H.R., Bowen, J.M., & Gibson, R.J. (2014). New pharmacotherapy options for chemotherapy-induced alimentary mucositis. *Expert Opinion on Biological Therapy, 14,* 347–354. https://doi.org/10.1517/14712598.2014.874412

Warr, D.G., Street, J.C., & Carides, A.D. (2011). Evaluation of risk factors predictive of nausea and vomiting with current standard-of-care antiemetic treatment: Analysis of phase 3 trial of aprepitant in patients receiving adriamycin–cyclophosphamide-based chemotherapy. *Supportive Care in Cancer, 19,* 807–813. https://doi.org/10.1007/s00520-010-0899-5

Weber, D., & O'Brien, K. (2017). Cancer and cancer-related fatigue and the interrelationships with depression, stress, and inflammation. *Journal of Evidence-Based Complementary and Alternative Medicine, 22,* 502–512. https://doi.org/10.1177/2156587216676122

Webster, L., Jansen, J.P., Peppin, J., Lasko, B., Irving, G., Morlion, B., ... Carter, E. (2008). Alvimopan, a peripherally acting mu-opioid receptor (PAM-OR) antagonist for the treatment of opioid-induced bowel dysfunction: Results from a randomized, double-blind, placebo-controlled, dose-finding study in subjects taking opioids for chronic non-cancer pain. *Pain, 137,* 428–440. https://doi.org/10.1016/j.pain.2007.11.008

Weidner, A.-S., Panarelli, N.C., Geyer, J.T., Bhavsar, E.B., Furman, R.R., Leonard, J.P., … Yantiss, R.K. (2015). Idelalisib-associated colitis: Histologic findings in 14 patients. *American Journal of Surgical Pathology, 39,* 1661–1667. https://doi.org/10.1097/PAS.0000000000000522

Wheelwright, S., Darlington, A.-S., Hopkinson, J.B., Fitzsimmons, D., White, A., & Johnson, C.D. (2013). A systematic review of health-related quality of life instruments in patients with cancer cachexia. *Supportive Care in Cancer, 21,* 2625–2636. https://doi.org/10.1007/s00520-013-1881-9

Wirz, S., Nadstawek, J., Elsen, C., Junker, U., & Wartenberg, H.C. (2012). Laxative management in ambulatory cancer patients on opioid therapy: A prospective, open-label investigation of polyethylene glycol, sodium picosulphate and lactulose. *European Journal of Cancer Care, 21,* 131–140. https://doi.org/10.1111/j.1365-2354.2011.01286.x

Wolters Kluwer Health. (2017). Lexicomp Online. Retrieved from https://online.lexi.com

Woolery, M., Bisanz, A., Lyons, H.F., Gaido, L., Yenulevich, M., Fulton, S., & McMillan, S.C. (2008). Putting Evidence Into Practice®: Evidence-based interventions for the prevention and management of constipation in patients with cancer. *Clinical Journal of Oncology Nursing, 12,* 317–337. https://doi.org/10.1188/08.CJON.317-337

Working Group IAP/APA Acute Pancreatitis Guidelines. (2013). IAP/APA evidence-based guidelines for the management of acute pancreatitis. *Pancreatology, 13,* e1–e15. https://doi.org/10.1016/j.pan.2013.07.063

World Health Organization. (1979). *WHO handbook for reporting of cancer treatment.* Geneva, Switzerland: Author.

Wujcik, D. (2014). Mucositis. In C.H. Yarbro, D. Wujcik, & B.H. Gobel (Eds.), *Cancer symptom management* (4th ed., pp. 403–419). Burlington, MA: Jones & Bartlett Learning.

Yanai, S., Nakamura, S., & Matsumoto, T. (2017). Nivolumab-induced colitis treated by infliximab. *Clinical Gastroenterology and Hepatology, 15,* e80–e81. https://doi.org/10.1016/j.cgh.2016.09.017

Yang, L., Yu, H., Dong, S., Zhong, Y., & Hu, S. (2017). Recognizing and managing on toxicities in cancer immunotherapy. *Tumor Biology, 39.* https://doi.org/10.1177/1010428317694542

Yuan, A., & Sonis, S. (2014). Emerging therapies for prevention and treatment or oral mucositis. *Expert Opinion on Emerging Drugs, 19,* 343–351. https://doi.org/10.1517/14728214.2014.946403

Zhan, P., Wang, Q., Qian, Q., & Yu, L.-K. (2013). Megestrol acetate in cancer patients with anorexia-cachexia syndrome: A meta-analysis. *Translational Cancer Research, 2,* 74–79. https://doi.org/10.3978/j.issn.2218-676X.2013.04.13

CHAPTER 16

Cardiovascular Toxicities

A. Overview

1. Cardiovascular toxicity is a potential complication of cancer therapy that may result from the direct effects of cancer treatment on heart function and structure or may be due to accelerated development of cardiovascular disease, especially in the presence of traditional cardiovascular risk factors (Armstrong et al., 2013).
2. Although novel targeted therapies are considered to be less toxic and better tolerated by patients compared with classic chemotherapy agents, rare but serious cardiovascular complications have been described. For cancer survivors, the risk of death from cardiovascular causes exceeds that of tumor recurrence for many forms of cancer (Carver et al., 2007; Silber et al., 2004).
3. Cardiovascular toxicity encompasses a broad range of cardiovascular side effects related to cancer therapy, including alterations in conduction pathways (dysrhythmias), vasculature (hypertension), coronary arteries (myocardial ischemia), cardiac myocytes (left ventricular dysfunction and heart failure), pericardial fluid accumulation (pericardial effusion), and valvular disease (Rowinsky et al., 1991; Sorrentino, Kim, Foderaro, & Truesdell, 2012; Yeh & Bickford, 2009).
4. This chapter will discuss the common cardiovascular toxicities associated with cancer therapy (see Table 16-1 at the end of this chapter) and provide a concise review of the pathophysiology, risk factors, clinical manifestations, and recommendations for effective management.

B. Conduction pathway disorders

1. Definition: Disturbance in the regular excitation of the heart (Chummun, 2009; Mottram & Svenson, 2011). Conduction disturbances are classified according to their origin (e.g., atrial, ventricular) or their degree of life-threatening symptoms. Sinus dysrhythmias associated with antineoplastic agents usually are transient dysrhythmias, are of short duration, and often are asymptomatic and do not necessitate alteration of the chemotherapy regimen. The most commonly observed dysrhythmias associated with cancer treatment include atrial fibrillation as well as cardiac repolarization abnormalities manifested as QT prolongation and ventricular arrhythmias (torsades de pointes) (Tamargo, Caballero, & Delpon, 2015).
   a) Atrial fibrillation is the most common of the atrial dysrhythmias and is characterized by an absence of discrete P waves and an "irregularly irregular" ventricular rate that may be caused by factors such as heart disease, hypertension, thyroid problems, and viral infection.
   b) QT prolongation
      (1) The QT interval represents the duration of electrical depolarization and repolarization of the ventricles (Strevel, Ing, & Siu, 2007), beginning at the initiation of the QRS complex and ending where the T wave returns to isoelectric baseline. The approximate duration of a normal QT interval is 350–460 ms. The QT interval is inversely correlated with heart rate; therefore, it is shorter with more rapid heart rates and longer with slower rates. Because of this inverse relationship, the QT interval is routinely transformed (normalized) by means of various formulas into a heart rate–dependent "corrected" value known as the QTc interval. The QTc interval is intended to represent the QT interval at a standardized heart rate of 60 bpm. Several correction formulas have been developed to improve the accuracy of QT measurement with corrected QT (QTc) values (Desai, Li, Desta, Malik, & Flockhart, 2003; Fridericia, 2003; Sagie, Larson, Goldberg, Bengtson, & Levy, 1992; Strevel et al., 2007). QTc intervals at the upper limit of normal

have been proposed for males (greater than 450 ms) and females (greater than 460 ms). A QTc greater than 500 ms or a QT change from baseline of greater than 60 ms (Strevel et al., 2007) should be of particular concern because it can predispose patients to torsades de pointes (TdP), a polymorphic ventricular tachyarrhythmia that appears on electrocardiogram (ECG) as a continuous twisting of the vector of the QRS complex around the isoelectric baseline. TdP may degenerate into ventricular fibrillation leading to sudden cardiac death (Haverkamp et al., 2000). A feature of TdP is pronounced prolongation of the QT interval in the supraventricular beat preceding the arrhythmia.

2. Pathophysiology
   a) Atrial fibrillation: The exact mechanism leading to increased rates of atrial fibrillation in patients with cancer remains unclear; however, it has been suggested that atrial fibrillation may actually represent an inflammatory complication of cancer (Farmakis, Parissis, & Filippatos, 2014; Guo, Lip, & Apostolakis, 2012).
   b) QT prolongation: The arrhythmogenic mechanisms underlying cardiac dysrhythmias (QT prolongation) in patients with cancer is not well established. Dysrhythmias may be caused by the tumor, cancer treatment, metabolic abnormalities (e.g., abnormal electrolytes), or underlying cardiac disease (myocardial ischemia and heart failure), which create an arrhythmogenic substrate (Tamargo et al., 2015). The most commonly identified chemotherapy agents that affect cardiac repolarization include histone deacetylase inhibitors, tyrosine kinase inhibitors (TKIs), the BRAF inhibitor vemurafenib, and arsenic trioxide (Bello et al., 2009; Burris et al., 2009; Deremer, Ustun, & Natarajan, 2008; Hazarika et al., 2008; Johnson et al., 2010; Soignet et al., 2001; Westervelt et al., 2001).
3. Incidence: The incidence of dysrhythmias specifically associated with cancer treatments is largely underestimated because of the probable attribution to other causes (Fadol & Lech, 2011; Guglin, Aljayeh, Saiyad, Ali, & Curtis, 2009; Sereno et al., 2008). Incidence rates have been reported with specific therapies.
   a) Asymptomatic bradycardia occurs in 3%–30% of patients receiving paclitaxel. More profound cardiac events (e.g., ventricular tachycardia, left bundle branch block) have been observed in rare instances (Fadol & Lech, 2011; Yeh & Bickford, 2009).
   b) Bradycardia from thalidomide has been reported with a variable frequency from less than 1% to up to 55% of patients treated. The proposed mechanisms include therapy-related hypothyroidism, sedative effects, and increased vagal sensitivity (Fadol & Lech, 2011; Guglin et al., 2009).
   c) Atrial fibrillation is the most common supraventricular dysrhythmia in patients with cancer, particularly following lung resection, which carries a 13%–20% chance of developing postoperative atrial fibrillation (Murphy & Salire, 2013; Onaitis, D'Amico, Zhao, O'Brien, & Harpole, 2010). Surgical patients with esophageal cancer have a 20%–25% chance of developing postoperative atrial fibrillation (Murphy & Salire, 2013; Murthy et al., 2003). Atrial fibrillation may occur acutely; during or after chemotherapy and/or radiation therapy; or following a surgical intervention (Erichsen et al., 2012; Guzzetti, Costantino, & Fundaro, 2002; Guzzetti, Costantino, Vernocchi, Sada, & Fundaro, 2008; Onaitis et al., 2010).
4. Risk factors (Fadol & Lech, 2011; Guzzetti et al., 2002)
   a) Atrial fibrillation (Camm et al., 2012)
      (1) Older age
      (2) Preexisting cardiovascular disease
      (3) Hypertension
      (4) Heart failure
      (5) Sleep apnea
      (6) Pericardial disease
      (7) Pulmonary embolism
      (8) Valvular disease
      (9) Chronic obstructive pulmonary disease
      (10) Electrolyte abnormalities
      (11) Thyroid disorders
      (12) Chronic kidney disease
   b) QT prolongation
      (1) Medications known to prolong the QTc, including arsenic trioxide, dasatinib, 5-fluorouracil, lapatinib, nilotinib, pazopanib, sunitinib, tamoxifen, temsirolimus, and vorinostat (Al-Khatib, LaPointe, Kramer, & Califf, 2003; Cahoon, 2009; Drew et al., 2004, 2010; Fadol & Lech, 2011; Guglin et al., 2009; Kim & Ewer, 2014; Kubota, Shimizu, Kamakura, & Horie, 2000; Kulkarni, Bhattacharya, & Petros, 1992; Lenihan & Kowey, 2013)

(2) Presence of multiple comorbidities (e.g., preexisting cardiac disease)
(3) Polypharmacy with concomitant QT-prolonging agents (e.g., antiemetics, antidepressants, antibiotics)
(4) Electrolyte disturbances (particularly hypokalemia and hypomagnesemia) and other metabolic abnormalities
(5) Diurnal effects
(6) Autonomic tone

5. Clinical manifestations
   a) Some patients with dysrhythmias may be asymptomatic; however, most patients with dysrhythmias report subjective symptoms such as palpitations, chest discomfort, dyspnea, or dizziness (Carey & Pelter, 2009). Syncope as the first presenting symptom is more common with ventricular dysrhythmias (Hazinski, Samson, & Schexnayder, 2010).
   b) Atrial fibrillation (Bontempo & Goralnick, 2011; Carey & Pelter, 2009)
      (1) Palpitations
      (2) Chest discomfort
      (3) Dyspnea and fatigue may result from decreased cardiac output due to loss of "atrial kick" (approximately one-third of cardiac output), which leads to worsening of all other cardiac disease symptoms.
      (4) Dizziness
   c) QT prolongation (Ederhy et al., 2009; Lech, 2013)
      (1) Palpitations
      (2) Syncope
      (3) Presyncope
6. Assessment
   a) Assess patients' history for known medical conditions or medications that may precipitate dysrhythmias. Elimination of preventable risks may reduce incidence or severity (Jolobe, 2010).
   b) Obtain a baseline ECG.
   c) Maintain ongoing monitoring (continuous or intermittent) of ECG rhythm.
   d) Compare apical and peripheral heart rate (Carey & Pelter, 2009).
   e) Perform follow-up assessments of vital signs and for symptoms of dyspnea, hypoxemia (shown as low oxygen saturation), hypotension, or chest discomfort (Hazinski et al., 2010).
   f) Replace electrolytes and maintain within normal ranges.
   g) Identify the etiology of the QT prolongation—toxic substances, other metabolic abnormalities, or primary or structural abnormalities of the heart itself.
7. Collaborative management
   a) Correct contributing factors such as hypoxemia, anemia, fluid imbalance, and electrolyte abnormalities. Administer electrolyte replacement to a goal potassium value greater than 4 mEq/L and magnesium value greater than 2 mEq/L (Hinkle, 2011; Pepin & Shields, 2012). Optimal calcium levels are not established, but ionized calcium levels greater than 1.1 mEq/L are the usual goal.
   b) Prior to starting medications with potential for QT prolongation, obtain a baseline ECG with QT measurement, with subsequent ECG monitoring for QT intervals as indicated by the drug's prescribing information.
   c) In patients with excessive corrected QT interval prolongation (greater than 500 ms), QT-prolonging cancer drugs should not be started, and potential causes or contributing factors should be evaluated and corrected.
   d) Concomitant treatment with QT-prolonging drugs (e.g., certain antiarrhythmic, antibiotic, and antifungal agents) should be avoided.
   e) Monitor electrolytes, particularly potassium and magnesium levels, and supplement as needed.
8. Patient and family education (Chopra, 2011)
   a) Teach patients and families the symptoms of dysrhythmia and the potential urgency of treatment.
   b) Once dysrhythmias have been identified in a patient, teach preventive strategies, such as hydration or electrolyte replacement. Emphasize that vomiting or diarrhea may disrupt fluid or electrolyte balance.
   c) If supraventricular tachycardia has occurred, teach patients to induce vagal maneuvers via coughing or bearing down as if defecating.
   d) Patients with ventricular dysrhythmias are at risk for sudden death, and if indicated, family members may be advised to learn basic life support skills.
   e) Emphasize the importance of periodic evaluation of laboratory values and ECG in patients at risk for dysrhythmias.
   f) Atrial fibrillation
      (1) Patients with truly "lone" atrial fibrillation need to be aware that their risk of stroke is extremely low, approximately 1.3% over a 15-year period (Lane, Barker, & Lip, 2015; Potpara & Lip, 2011). However, regular clinical

reassessment of their stroke risk using the CHA2DS2-VASc score (Lane et al., 2015; Lip, Nieuwlaat, Pisters, Lane, & Crijns, 2010) is essential, particularly as age increases and the prospect of developing comorbidities becomes more likely (Lane et al., 2015; Olesen, Torp-Pedersen, Hansen, & Lip, 2012; Potpara & Lip, 2011; Potpara et al., 2012).

(2) All patients with atrial fibrillation should be aware of the risk factors that can increase their risk of stroke.

(3) Patients need to be aware of the potential harms of medications used to treat atrial fibrillation (beta-blockers, antidysrhythmics), which can include life-threatening ventricular arrhythmias (and lead to death in rare cases), deterioration of left ventricular systolic function, and organ toxicity (particularly with long-term use).

(4) Patients need to be aware that late recurrences of atrial fibrillation after cardioversion or catheter ablation are a possibility and that more than one procedure may be required.

(5) Patients need to know what has caused their atrial fibrillation, how it will affect their life (consequences), and what the therapeutic options are.

(6) Patients need to know what they have been prescribed and why they are taking it, how to take the medication (e.g., dose; frequency; timings; with, before, or after food; with other tablets), what will happen if they fail to adhere as prescribed, any factors that may modify drug efficacy, any possible side effects (Dickinson & Raynor, 2003; Lane et al., 2015), and the likelihood of treatment success or failure, to enable realistic treatment expectations.

g) QT prolongation

(1) Patients need to know the importance of maintaining magnesium levels within normal limits.

(2) Patients need to be aware if they are on medications that can result in QT prolongation.

C. Vascular abnormalities

1. Hypertension is defined as a systolic blood pressure of 140 mm Hg or greater or a diastolic blood pressure of 90 mm Hg or greater (Lenihan & Kowey, 2013; Maitland et al., 2010).

a) Hypertension is the most frequent comorbid condition reported in patients with cancer and is associated with increased risk of cardiovascular complications, including stroke, myocardial infarction, and heart failure (Lenihan & Kowey, 2013; Maitland et al., 2010).

b) It is particularly increased in patients treated with angiogenesis inhibitors, commonly known as vascular signaling pathway (VSP) inhibitors, including the vascular endothelial growth factor (VEGF) inhibitors and other small molecule TKIs (Lankhorst, Saleh, Danser, & van den Meiracker, 2015). Drug-related hypertension can occur from initiation until one year after treatment onset (Zamorano et al., 2016).

2. Pathophysiology

a) The exact mechanism underlying the development of hypertension related to cancer therapy is unknown. Proposed mechanisms include abnormalities in endothelial function and angiogenesis, nitric oxide pathway inhibition, decrease in vascular wall compliance and flexibility, oxidative stress, and glomerular injury developing from loss of VEGF effect, as well as renal thrombotic microangiopathy (Izzedine et al., 2009; Mancia et al., 2013; Priori et al., 2015; Ranpura, Pulipati, Chu, Zhu, & Wu, 2010; Zamorano et al., 2016).

b) Multikinase inhibition results in antiangiogenesis by blocking the *BCR-ABL* receptor and the actions of VEGF, which decreases cellular nitric oxide (Force, Krause, & Van Etten, 2007; Yusuf, Razeghi, & Yeh, 2008). Hypertension is thought to be related to the loss of VEGF effect on the vascular endothelial wall, leading to diminished nitric oxide synthase and loss of the vasodilatory effects of nitric oxide (Kamba & McDonald, 2007; Kurtin, 2009; Subbiah, Lenihan, & Tsimberidou, 2011; Yusuf et al., 2008).

c) Lower nitric oxide levels are associated with sodium and water retention (Chen, 2009; Kajdaniuk, Marek, Borgiel-Marek, & Kos-Kudla, 2011; Kamba & McDonald, 2007; Zeb, Ali, & Rohra, 2007).

d) Vasoconstriction (Mourad, des Guetz, Debbabi, & Levy, 2008; Sereno et al., 2008; Zeb et al., 2007)

3. Incidence

a) Hypertension incidence has increased to 80% in patients with cancer treated with VEGF inhibitors (Lankhorst et al., 2015).

b) Hypertension associated with antiangiogenic therapies and multikinase inhibitors occurs with high frequency, ranging from 4%–67% of cases (Chu et al., 2007; Fadol & Lech, 2011; Force et al., 2007; Kamba & McDonald, 2007; Mourad et al., 2008; Patel et al., 2008; Viale & Yamamoto, 2008; Yusuf et al., 2008). Approximately 11%–16% of patients receiving bevacizumab have significant hypertension that requires addition or adjustment of antihypertensive medications (Subbiah et al., 2011; Yusuf et al., 2008).

4. Risk factors
   a) Advancing age
   b) Preexisting hypertension or cardiovascular disease (Kajdaniuk et al., 2011; Steingart et al., 2012; Subbiah et al., 2011)
   c) Treatment with bevacizumab, pazopanib, sorafenib, sunitinib, or vandetanib (Fadol & Lech, 2011). Proteinuria usually precedes hypertension with bevacizumab therapy (Gerber, 2008; Patel et al., 2011).
   d) Renal insufficiency, hyperthyroidism, Cushing syndrome, increased intracranial pressure, and hypomagnesemia independent of chemotherapy toxicity (Costa, Tejpar, Prenen, & Van Cutsem, 2011; Houston, 2011)
   e) Medications such as antidepressants, including tricyclic antidepressants and selective serotonin reuptake inhibitors
   f) Race: Hypertension tends to be more common, be more severe, occur earlier in life, and be associated with greater target-organ damage in African Americans.
5. Clinical manifestations
   a) Most patients with high blood pressure have no signs or symptoms, even if blood pressure readings reach dangerously high levels.
   b) A few people with high blood pressure may have headaches, shortness of breath, or nosebleeds, but these signs and symptoms are not specific and usually do not occur until blood pressure has reached a severe or life-threatening stage.
   c) Increases in blood pressure with multikinase inhibitors and antiangiogenic agents may be asymptomatic or accompanied by headache, visual disturbances, fatigue, tachycardia, or heart failure.
6. Assessment (Lenihan & Kowey, 2013; Maitland et al., 2010)
   a) Obtain a comprehensive patient history to establish baseline. Assess for medications (e.g., sinus or cold remedies) or clinical conditions that may contribute to altered blood pressure.
   b) Evaluate laboratory values to determine specific cardiovascular risk factors prior to starting VSP inhibitors.
   c) Blood pressure assessment should have a minimum of two standardized measurements and set a goal of less than 140/90 mm Hg for most patients, in accordance with recommendations for all adults.
   d) Higher-risk patients, including those with diabetes or chronic kidney disease, should achieve a lower goal (e.g., 130/80 mm Hg).
   e) Evaluate pain control, as pain may contribute to hypertension.
   f) Assess for stress management and other medications used in these patients (e.g., steroids, nonsteroidal anti-inflammatory drugs, erythropoietin) that can cause hypertension to obtain an adequate estimation of blood pressure.
7. Collaborative management of hypertension (Maitland et al., 2010)
   a) Early diagnosis and control of blood pressure to the recommended guideline parameters allow for effective antiangiogenic therapy for optimal cancer treatment (Ranpura et al., 2010).
   b) A baseline blood pressure measurement and regular monitoring are recommended while patients are receiving VEGF inhibitors, especially during the first cycle of chemotherapy when most patients experience an elevation in blood pressure.
   c) Blood pressure should be actively monitored weekly during the first cycle of VSP inhibitor therapy and then at least every two to three weeks for the duration of treatment.
   d) Patients with preexisting hypertension and on multiple antihypertensive agents should be evaluated for renal function and proteinuria.
   e) The choice of antihypertensive therapy must be individualized to patients according to their medical history and the specific properties of different classes of antihypertensive agents (Lenihan & Kowey, 2013; Mancia et al., 2013).
   f) Antihypertensive agent classes that have been specifically prescribed to control hypertension associated with VSP inhibitor therapy include thiazide diuretics, beta-blockers, dihydropyridine calcium channel blockers, angiotensin-converting enzyme inhibitors, and angiotensin receptor blockers (Lenihan & Kowey, 2013; Maitland et al., 2010).
   g) Some agents may be preferable (e.g., renin-angiotensin or sympathetic system

inhibitors) over others (e.g., thiazide diuretics) to minimize the risk of electrolyte depletion.

h) Hypertension associated with TKIs is typically quite manageable with appropriate therapy. Early intervention is key to minimizing additional cardiovascular adverse effects such as heart failure (Lenihan & Kowey, 2013).

i) Patients should keep a blood pressure measurement log, especially during the first week of treatment because the magnitude of elevation is unpredictable.

j) Target blood pressure should be based on the Eighth Joint National Committee classification and guidelines (James et al., 2014).

k) Antihypertensive therapy should be adjusted accordingly based on associated comorbidities (e.g., less than 140/90 mm Hg) in patients with diabetes or chronic kidney disease.

8. Patient and family education

a) Hypertension can be life threatening and cause stroke, so patients should be prepared to recognize signs of a hypertensive crisis or stroke.

(1) Memory lapses

(2) Blackouts or near-syncope

(3) Visual abnormalities

(4) Persistent headache

(5) Slurred words

(6) Numbness or tingling of an extremity

(7) Facial droop

b) Patients may require guidance with self-administration of antihypertensive agents.

c) Many antihypertensive agents can cause immediate orthostasis, dizziness, nausea, and risk of falling.

d) Patients should be instructed to use a validated, automated oscillometric device that measures blood pressure in the brachial artery (upper arm) and to perform measurements in a quiet room after five minutes of rest in the seated position with the back and arm supported.

e) Blood pressure generally should be checked in both arms to determine if a difference exists. It is important to use an appropriately sized arm cuff.

f) Adherence to taking the medications as prescribed should be emphasized to patients.

g) Patients should be aware of the potential side effects of their medications and when to report them to their healthcare provider.

h) Before starting TKIs, patients need to have a baseline blood pressure measurement and be aware of what the target blood pressure should be.

D. Venous thromboembolism (VTE)

1. VTE is a serious, life-threatening disorder and the second leading cause of death in hospitalized patients with cancer (Lyman et al., 2007). VTE consists of deep vein thrombosis, which typically involves the deep veins of the legs or pelvis, and its complication, pulmonary embolism.

2. Pathophysiology: Endothelial wall damage is thought to have a direct relationship to atherosclerotic events such as VTE, supported by the fact that VTE occurs with higher incidence in patients treated with VEGF inhibitors (Force et al., 2007; Kamba & McDonald, 2007).

3. Incidence: The risk of VTE in patients with cancer is 1.9%–11% based on a variety of factors. The addition of thalidomide increases this risk to as high as 30%, and antiangiogenic agents increase the risk up to 30%, even in lower-risk individuals (Yusuf et al., 2008).

4. Risk factors

a) Treatment with chemotherapy and immunotherapy agents, including bevacizumab, cisplatin, erlotinib, lenalidomide, tamoxifen, thalidomide, and vorinostat (Fadol & Lech, 2011; Zangari, Berno, Zhan, Tricot, & Fink, 2012)

b) Edema, immobility, dehydration, congestive heart failure, and erythropoiesis-stimulating agents (Connolly, Dalal, Lin, & Khorana, 2012)

5. Clinical manifestations: Unilateral pain, redness, and swelling of affected extremity

6. Assessment: Obtain a health history at every clinic or hospital visit. Assess patients for signs and symptoms of VTE, such as pain, redness, and swelling of extremities, especially unilaterally.

7. Collaborative management: Refer patients for diagnostic testing (e.g., venous Doppler study). Initiate anticoagulant therapy when indicated, and monitor therapeutic levels when necessary. Discontinue medications thought to contribute to VTE.

8. Patient and family education (Viale & Yamamoto, 2008)

a) Teach patients the signs and symptoms of vascular complications.

b) Teach lifestyle changes, such as smoking cessation, low-fat diet, moderate exercise, and stress management, that may reduce the incidence and severity of vascular complications.

c) Advise patients to report symptoms to healthcare providers so that assessment and preventive strategies can be implemented early.

E. Coronary artery disease
   1. Myocardial ischemia: Several cancer treatments, including cytotoxic drugs, radiation therapy, and targeted therapies, are associated with an increased risk of coronary artery disease with or without acute coronary syndromes. The most common cancer therapies associated with myocardial infarction and myocardial ischemia are angiogenesis inhibitors (e.g., lenalidomide, thalidomide), antimetabolites (e.g., capecitabine; 5-fluorouracil), antimicrotubule agents (e.g., docetaxel, ixabepilone, paclitaxel), monoclonal antibody TKIs (e.g., bevacizumab), proteasome inhibitors (e.g., carfilzomib), and small molecule TKIs (e.g., erlotinib, imatinib, nilotinib, pazopanib, ponatinib, ramucirumab, regorafenib, sorafenib, ziv-aflibercept).
   2. Pathophysiology
      a) The exact mechanism of cardiotoxicity resulting in myocardial ischemia associated with these agents is not entirely understood. Potential mechanisms include coronary artery thrombosis, coronary arteritis, coronary vasospasm, direct toxic effects, interaction with the coagulation system, autoimmune responses, and apoptosis of the myocardial cells and endothelium, mimicking toxic myocarditis (Yeh & Bickford, 2009).
      b) Myocarditis-induced edema of myocytes creates increased automaticity and impaired perfusion. Increased workload and myocardial stress is thought to be the mechanism for myocardial ischemia and infarction. Thromboses occurring as a result of increased propensity for clotting may involve coronary arteries (Kusama et al., 2011).
   3. Incidence
      a) 5-Fluorouracil: Incidence of myocardial ischemia varies from 1%–68%. It occurs within two to five days after the start of treatment and presents as angina-like chest pains; however, myocardial infarction, arrhythmias, heart failure, cardiogenic shock, and sudden death have been reported (Bonita & Pradhan, 2013; Fadol & Lech, 2011). Cardiac mortality rate with 5-fluorouracil is 2.2%–13%.
      b) Capecitabine: Incidence of cardiotoxicity is 3%–9%. The onset of anginal symptoms ranges from three hours to four days after therapy (Yeh & Bickford, 2009).
      c) Antimicrotubule agents: Incidence of myocardial ischemia is 0.5%–5% with paclitaxel and 1.7% with docetaxel (Yeh & Bickford, 2009).
      d) Monoclonal antibody TKIs (e.g., bevacizumab): Incidence of high-grade ischemia is 0.6%–1.5% (Fadol & Lech, 2011; Ranpura et al., 2010).
      e) Small molecule TKIs (e.g., erlotinib, sorafenib): Incidence of myocardial infarction and ischemia was 2.3% when erlotinib was combined with gemcitabine (Fadol & Lech, 2011). Sorafenib is associated with myocardial infarction in 2.7%–3% of patients (Fadol & Lech, 2011; Porto et al., 2010).
   4. Risk factors
      a) Cancer therapies associated with myocardial ischemia, which include bevacizumab, bortezomib, capecitabine, docetaxel, doxorubicin, erlotinib, 5-fluorouracil, hydroxyurea, paclitaxel, pazopanib, rituximab, and sorafenib (Arima et al., 2009; Kalsch, Wieneke, & Erbel, 2010; Molteni et al., 2010; Saif, Shah, & Shah, 2009; Subbiah et al., 2011; Takamatsu et al., 2010; Tunio, Hashmi, & Shoaib, 2012; Winchester & Bavry, 2010)
      b) Androgen deprivation (Saylor & Smith, 2009)
      c) Cetuximab used for locally advanced squamous cell head and neck cancer. Similar events were not observed with cetuximab when used for treatment of metastatic colorectal cancer (ImClone LLC, 2016).
      d) Interleukin-2 resulting in capillary permeability with myocarditis (Jones & Ewer, 2006; Muehlbauer, Callahan, Zlott, & Dahl, 2018)
      e) Taxane therapy (Londhey & Parikh, 2009): Few patients suffer coronary artery disease with now-established drug monitoring and dose attenuation plans.
      f) Agents enhancing hypercoagulability, although no relationship to any specific chemotherapy or immunotherapy agent has been demonstrated (Yusuf et al., 2008)
      g) High-dose chemotherapy: Rare unexplained chest pain with ischemic ECG changes that spontaneously resolve (Fadol & Lech, 2011; Yusuf et al., 2008)
      h) Aromatase inhibitors (Bird & Swain, 2008; Towns, Bedard, & Verma, 2008)
      i) Transarterial chemoembolization, with unclear etiology (Lai et al., 2010)
   5. Clinical manifestations
      a) General signs and symptoms: Anxiety, generalized fatigue and weakness, restlessness, agitation
      b) Cardiovascular: Retrosternal chest discomfort, tachycardia, new murmur or S_2 or S_3, congestive heart failure symptoms, hypertension or hypotension
      c) Gastrointestinal: Nausea, abdominal pain, indigestion, vomiting

d) Neurologic: Light-headedness, near-syncope, syncope
e) Pulmonary: Dyspnea, wheezing, tachypnea, pulmonary rales
f) Integumentary: Diaphoresis; cool, clammy skin; pallor
g) Elevated cardiac enzymes indicative of a myocardial infarction (Curigliano et al., 2012)
h) Ischemic ECG changes are seen in up to 68% of patients (Bonita & Pradhan, 2013).

6. Assessment
   a) Dysrhythmias are common in patients with cancer; life-threatening ventricular tachycardia or ventricular fibrillation is most common in the first two hours.
   b) Cardiac enzymes (creatine phosphokinase-MB, troponin I, or troponin T) measured in the serum are elevated when myocardial injury occurs (Gaze, 2011).
   c) Echocardiogram or multigated acquisition scan
   d) Diagnostic right heart catheterization
7. Collaborative management (Daga, Kaul, & Mansoor, 2011; Hazinski et al., 2010; Jugdutt, 2012)
   a) Initiate medical treatment as appropriate (e.g., supplemental oxygen; morphine 2–4 mg IV as needed for analgesia; nitroglycerin sublingually as needed for chest pains).
   b) Administer oxygen at a rate sufficient to maintain oxygen saturation above 90% unless otherwise contraindicated.
   c) Implement cardiac monitoring: Observe for dysrhythmias and ischemic changes, low oxygen saturation, or extremes in blood pressure.
   d) Obtain an order for aspirin 325 mg to be chewed as soon as a 12-lead ECG is performed and ST changes are present. Administer with caution in patients with low platelet counts and brain metastases.
   e) Consider patient candidacy for reperfusion strategies, such as cardiac catheterization with angioplasty, stent placement, or intracoronary/IV thrombolysis (Iyengar & Godbole, 2011).
   f) Consider ischemia-reducing or myocardial preservation strategies, such as administration of nitrates, beta-blockers, or statins (Ferreira & Mochly-Rosen, 2012; Gerczuk & Kloner, 2012).
   g) Maintain potassium greater than 4 mEq/L, magnesium greater than 2 mEq/L, and ionized calcium greater than 1 mEq/L (Akhtar, Ullah, & Hamid, 2011).
   h) Consider discontinuation of antineoplastic agents that are thought to cause cardiac ischemia or infarction, such as fluoropyrimidines, oxaliplatin, sorafenib, or tamoxifen (Basselin et al., 2011; Chang, Hung, Yeh, Yang, & Wang, 2011; Shah, Shah, & Rather, 2012).
   i) Determine the need for follow-up assessment of coronary arteries and myocardial function with exercise stress testing, cardiac catheterization, echocardiogram, or multigated acquisition scan (Al-Zaiti, Pelter, & Carey, 2011; Arrighi & Dilsizian, 2012).
   j) Aggressively manage cardiac risk factors (e.g., hypertension, hyperlipidemia).
8. Patient and family education
   a) Explain the disease process, diagnostic tests, and medications to patients and families.
   b) Provide emotional support to patients and families to lower patients' level of anxiety, which can reduce heart rate and myocardial oxygen demand.
   c) Provide instruction regarding risk factor modification (Anderson et al., 2017; Crumlish & Magel, 2011).
   d) Educate patients and families regarding reportable symptoms, such as chest discomfort, left arm or neck pain, and dyspnea.
   e) Educate patients and families regarding management of risks for cardiac ischemia that are specific to oncology (e.g., anemia, cardiac demands of infection, electrolyte disturbances).
   f) Include patient teaching on cardiac medications and unique considerations in oncology care (e.g., risk for low blood pressure increased when febrile; electrolyte disturbances with nausea and vomiting may contribute to cardiac dysrhythmias).
   g) Provide referral and education regarding cardiac rehabilitation programs (Anderson et al., 2016).

F. Left ventricular dysfunction/heart failure
1. Definition: Heart failure is defined as inadequate contractile force to eject the required amount of blood for perfusion of the body (Hunt et al., 2009; Lindenfeld et al., 2010).
   a) It is classified as primary or secondary based on the primary etiology and has three types: acute, early-onset progressive, or chronic late progressive (Gianni, Salvatorelli, & Minotti, 2007).
   b) A consensus definition for cardiotoxicity-induced cardiomyopathy and heart failure is still lacking. Multiple definitions are listed below.

(1) The National Cancer Institute (NCI) broadly defines *cardiotoxicity* as "toxicity that affects the heart" (NCI, n.d.).

(2) The Common Terminology Criteria for Adverse Events (version 5.0) defines left ventricular dysfunction and heart failure based on severity (grades 1–5), with a decrease in left ventricular ejection fraction (LVEF) of 10% or greater from baseline or LVEF less than 50% (NCI Cancer Therapy Evaluation Program, 2017).

(3) The Cardiac Review and Evaluation Committee supervising trastuzumab clinical trials defined drug-related cardiotoxicity as one or more of the following (Bloom et al., 2016; Raschi & De Ponti, 2012; Seidman et al., 2002):

(a) Cardiomyopathy characterized by a decrease in LVEF, either global or more severe in the septum

(b) Symptoms associated with congestive heart failure

(c) Signs associated with congestive heart failure (e.g., S_3 gallop, tachycardia, or both)

(d) Reduction in LVEF from baseline of at least 5% to less than 55% with accompanying signs or symptoms of congestive heart failure, or a reduction in LVEF of at least 10% to less than 55% without accompanying signs or symptoms

(4) The U.S. Food and Drug Administration defined anthracycline-induced cardiotoxicity as greater than 20% decrease in LVEF when baseline is normal or greater than 10% decrease when baseline is not normal (Bloom et al., 2016).

(5) The American Society of Echocardiography and European Association of Cardiovascular Imaging defined cancer therapeutics–related cardiac dysfunction as a decrease in the LVEF of more than 10% to a value less than 53% confirmed by repeat imaging (Bloom et al., 2016; Plana et al., 2014).

2. Pathophysiology

a) Anthracycline-induced cardiotoxicity: The exact mechanism is not fully understood, although multiple pathways have been implicated (Wouters, Kremer, Miller, Herman, & Lipshultz, 2005). The most commonly accepted pathophysiologic mechanism is the oxidative stress hypothesis, which suggests that the generation of reactive oxygen species and lipid peroxidation of the cell membrane damage cardiomyocytes. Other proposed mechanisms include intercalation into nuclear DNA to impair protein synthesis and inhibition of topoisomerase II to inhibit DNA repair (Doroshow, 1983; Drafts et al., 2013; Franco & Lipshultz, 2015; Lim et al., 2004; Steinherz, Steinherz, Tan, Heller, & Murphy, 1991; Tewey, Rowe, Yang, Halligan, & Liu, 1984; Zhang et al., 2012).

(1) Several agents have been identified as potentially effective prophylaxis for anthracycline-induced cardiotoxicity, including beta-blockers, statins, angiotensin antagonists, and dexrazoxane (Kalam & Marwick, 2013).

(2) Dexrazoxane is a topoisomerase IIβ inhibitor that converts an active ion-binding form to prevent toxic radical injury. The recommended dosing ratio of dexrazoxane to doxorubicin is 10:1 (Kalam & Marwick, 2013; Pfizer Inc., 2012).

(3) Dexrazoxane is reconstituted with sterile water and may be further diluted with lactated Ringer's solution for rapid IV infusion; it should not be administered via IV push (Pfizer Inc., 2012).

b) TKI-associated toxicity: The mechanisms of action proposed for TKI-associated toxicity (e.g., trastuzumab) are typically related to their individual targets of action for cancer therapy, either on- or off-target adverse reactions, such as left ventricular dysfunction or heart failure.

(1) On-target toxicity occurs when the specific kinase targeted by the therapy provides an important physiologic function in addition to the target tumor tissue (Cheng & Force, 2010; Lenihan & Kowey, 2013). An example of on-target toxicity is cardiotoxicity that may occur with trastuzumab. It is believed that trastuzumab interferes with HER2 functioning in cardiac tissue, which manifests as left ventricular systolic dysfunction (Cheng & Force, 2010; Fabian et al., 2005; Force et al., 2007; Kerkela et al., 2006; Lenihan & Kowey, 2013; Mann, 2006).

(2) Off-target toxicity is observed when a nonselective TKI modulates the function of a kinase involved in normal vas-

cular physiology and is not the target in cancer cells (Mouhayar, Durand, & Cortes, 2013). A typical example is the unintended inhibition of the AMP-activated protein kinase (known as AMPK) by sunitinib, a mechanism that may be partially responsible for cardiomyopathy.

3. Incidence (Chen, 2009; Ewer & Ewer, 2008; Steinherz et al., 1991; Von Hoff et al., 1979; Yeh & Bickford, 2009; Yusuf et al., 2008; Zamorano et al., 2016)
   a) Cardiotoxicities resulting in left ventricular dysfunction or cardiomyopathy and heart failure are relatively common and serious side effects of cancer treatment (Carver et al., 2007). Heart failure due to cancer therapy has been linked to a 3.5-fold increased mortality risk compared with idiopathic cardiomyopathy (Bloom et al., 2016; Felker et al., 2000).
   b) Anthracyclines produce some degree of cardiac dysfunction in 50% of patients over a 10–20-year period after exposure. Approximately 3%–5% develop overt heart failure (Fadol & Lech, 2011). Anthracycline-induced left ventricular dysfunction or heart failure may be classified as the following:
      (1) Acute-onset anthracycline-induced toxicity, which develops in 1% of patients, presents immediately after infusion, and is manifested as supraventricular arrhythmia, ECG changes, and transient decline in myocardial contractility, which is usually reversible.
      (2) Early-onset chronic progressive anthracycline-induced cardiotoxicity, which occurs during therapy or within the first year after treatment in 1.6%–2.1% of patients (Gianni et al., 2008)
      (3) Late-onset chronic progressive anthracycline-induced cardiotoxicity, which occurs one year or later after completion of therapy in 1.6%–5% of patients. Late-occurring cardiotoxicity may not be clinically evident until 10–20 years after the first dose of treatment (Bloom et al., 2016; Curigliano et al., 2012; Volkova & Russell, 2011), with a median of 7 years after treatment (Steinherz et al., 1991; Von Hoff et al., 1979; Zamorano et al., 2016).
   c) Trastuzumab-induced cardiotoxicity does not appear to be cumulative dose dependent and is associated with reversible cardiomyocyte dysfunction, which typically recovers after treatment discontinuation of the targeted agent and initiation of heart failure therapy (Ewer & Lippman, 2005; Le, Cao, & Yang, 2014).
      (1) Patients who received the combination therapy of trastuzumab with anthracyclines have a higher chance of developing left ventricular dysfunction or heart failure (Piccart-Gebhart et al., 2005; Slamon et al., 2001, 2011). A meta-analysis on the use of trastuzumab reported an incidence of left ventricular dysfunction of 3%–7% (trastuzumab alone) but increased to 27% when administered with anthracyclines (Lazzari, De Paolis, Bovelli, & Boschetti, 2013; Piccart-Gebhart et al., 2005; Seidman et al., 2002).
      (2) Adjuvant trastuzumab after anthracyclines and paclitaxel is associated with an incidence of 4%–18.6% for left ventricular dysfunction and 1.6%–3.3% for heart failure (Bria et al., 2008; Lazzari et al., 2013; Perez et al., 2008; Slamon et al., 2011).
   d) Bevacizumab, another humanized monoclonal antibody against VEGF, has an adverse complication of heart failure, with an incidence of 1.7%–3% (Lazzari et al., 2013; Yeh & Bickford, 2009).
4. Risk factors
   a) Anthracycline-induced cardiotoxicity
      (1) Lifetime cumulative dose (Camp-Sorrell, 2018)
      (2) Infusion regimen (Fadol & Lech, 2011)
      (3) Preexisting cardiac disease (Fadol & Lech, 2011)
      (4) Preexisting hypertension
      (5) Concomitant use of other chemotherapy agents known to cause cardiotoxicity (e.g., cyclophosphamide, trastuzumab, paclitaxel) (Bird & Swain, 2008; Ewer & O'Shaughnessy, 2007; Mackey et al., 2008; Perez et al., 2008)
      (6) History of prior mediastinal radiation therapy (Yeh & Bickford, 2009; Yusuf et al., 2008)
      (7) Female gender (Fulbright, Huh, Anderson, & Chandra, 2010)
      (8) Age (young and elderly) (Fulbright et al., 2010)
      (9) Increased length of time since completion of chemotherapy
      (10) Increase in biomarkers (e.g., troponins, natriuretic peptides) during and after

administration (Braverman, Antin, Plappert, Cook, & Lee, 1991; Cardinale et al., 2002, 2004; Curigliano et al., 2012; Herrmann et al., 2014; Pichon et al., 2005; Volkova & Russell, 2011; Zamorano et al., 2016)

b) Trastuzumab-induced cardiotoxicity
  (1) Age greater than 50 years
  (2) Borderline LVEF before treatment
  (3) History of cardiovascular disease
  (4) Presence of cardiovascular risk factors (e.g., diabetes, dyslipidemia, elevated body mass index greater than 30 kg/m^2)
  (5) Prior treatment with anthracyclines (de Azambuja, Bedard, Suter, & Piccart-Gebhart, 2009; Hayes & Picard, 2006; Lazzari et al., 2013; Telli, Hunt, Carlson, & Guardino, 2007)
  (6) Genetic predisposition and immune status (Force et al., 2007; Lazzari et al., 2013)

5. Clinical manifestation
  a) Signs
    (1) Edema (lower-extremity swelling, abdominal ascites)
    (2) Jugular venous distension
    (3) Hepatomegaly (enlarged liver)
    (4) Abnormal heart sounds (S_3 gallop, murmurs)
    (5) Tachycardia
    (6) Hypotension
    (7) Tachypnea
    (8) Abnormal lung sounds (crackles)
  b) Symptoms
    (1) Fatigue, weakness, exercise intolerance
    (2) Dyspnea
    (3) Orthopnea
    (4) Paroxysmal nocturnal dyspnea
    (5) Increased abdominal girth
    (6) Frequent coughing, especially at night when lying flat
    (7) Sudden weight gain

6. Assessment
  a) Perform a comprehensive history and physical assessment.
  b) Obtain history of treatments received for cancer therapy.
  c) Determine the etiology of heart failure (e.g., ischemic versus nonischemic).
  d) Classify the presenting syndrome (e.g., acute vs. chronic; systolic vs. diastolic).
  e) Identify concomitant disease relevant to heart failure (e.g., amyloidosis, hemochromatosis).
  f) Evaluate for presence of coronary artery disease and valvular problems.
  g) Assess severity of symptoms.
  h) Perform diagnostic and interventional procedures as needed (e.g., cardiac catheterization).

7. Collaborative management and prevention (Fares, 2008; Yusuf et al., 2008)
  a) Identify precipitating factors for acute decompensated heart failure.
    (1) Patient-related factors (Fadol, 2013)
      (a) Nonadherence to medications
      (b) Excessive salt intake
      (c) Physical and environmental stressors
    (2) Cardiac-related factors
      (a) Cardiac arrhythmias (e.g., atrial fibrillation, ventricular fibrillation, bradyarrhythmias)
      (b) Uncontrolled hypertension
      (c) Acute myocardial infarction
      (d) Valvular disease, worsening mitral regurgitation
    (3) Adverse effects of anticancer agents
      (a) Steroids
      (b) Chemotherapy (e.g., doxorubicin, cyclophosphamide)
      (c) Nonsteroidal anti-inflammatory drugs
      (d) Thiazolidinediones
  b) Establish diagnosis of left ventricular dysfunction or heart failure.
    (1) Echocardiography to assess left ventricular function
    (2) Chest x-ray to evaluate for pulmonary edema, pleural effusion, and cardiomegaly
    (3) Nuclear imaging to detect location and severity of coronary artery disease
    (4) Coronary angiography to evaluate coronary artery disease
    (5) Endomyocardial biopsy to diagnose anthracycline-induced cardiomyopathy
    (6) Thyroid profile to evaluate for hypothyroidism or hyperthyroidism as heart failure etiology
    (7) Viral titers to evaluate causes of myocarditis, endocarditis, and pericarditis
    (8) Iron studies to evaluate for hemochromatosis resulting in heart failure
  c) Initiate recommended pharmacologic therapies for heart failure.
    (1) Angiotensin-converting enzyme inhibitors

(2) Angiotensin receptor blocker
(3) Aldosterone antagonists
(4) Cardiac glycosides
(5) Direct-acting vasodilator

8. Patient and family education
   a) Dietary modifications: Instruct patients on sodium restriction to 2,000 mg/day to prevent volume overload (Fadol, 2013).
   b) Physical activity: Encourage physical activity, except during periods of acute exacerbation when physical rest is recommended.
   c) Weight monitoring: Patients should be advised to perform daily weight monitoring and notify their healthcare provider in case of a sudden unexpected weight gain (more than 2 lbs per day for two consecutive days or more than 5 lbs per week) for possible adjustment of diuretic dose.
   d) Alcohol intake: Moderate intake (one drink per day for women and two drinks per day for men) is permitted except in cases of alcoholic cardiomyopathy.
   e) Encourage smoking cessation.

Table 16-1. Cardiotoxicity of Cancer Therapy

Classification	Drug	Side Effects	Nursing Considerations
Chemotherapy Agents			
Alkylating agents	Busulfan (IV: Busulfex®; oral: Myleran®)	When used in combination with cyclophosphamide • Atrial fibrillation • Cardiac dysrhythmia • Complete atrioventricular block • Hypertension (36% with IV formulation) • Left heart failure (with IV formulation) • Pericardial effusion (with IV formulation) • Tachycardia (44% with IV formulation) • Vasodilation (25% with IV formulation) • Ventricular premature heart beats Cardiac tamponade (2% with high doses of oral formulation) Chest pain (26% with IV formulation) Pericardial fibrosis (with oral formulation)	Monitor for nausea and vomiting, which often preceded fatal cardiac tamponade. Monitor pediatric patients with thalassemia, as they may be prone to cardiac tamponade, particularly during concurrent treatment with cyclophosphamide. (Truven Health Analytics, 2017)
	Cisplatin	Bradyarrhythmia Cardiomyopathy (22% with prior chest wall radiation; 5.1% without) Hypertension MI Orthostatic hypotension	Monitor for serum electrolyte disturbances, including hypomagnesemia, hypocalcemia, hyponatremia, hypokalemia, and hypophosphatemia. Monitor levels of magnesium, calcium, sodium, and potassium before first and subsequent cisplatin therapy. Monitor serum creatinine and blood urea nitrogen levels, which may be elevated in individuals experiencing orthostatic hypotension. Monitor for bradyarrhythmia within 2 hours of starting infusion and for up to 3 hours after. Maintain normal serum electrolyte levels by supplementation as appropriate. Hypertension is associated with combination therapy containing cisplatin, etoposide, vinblastine, and bleomycin. (Truven Health Analytics, 2017)

(Continued on next page)

Table 16-1. Cardiotoxicity of Cancer Therapy *(Continued)*

Classification	Drug	Side Effects	Nursing Considerations
Chemotherapy Agents *(Cont.)*			
Alkylating agents *(cont.)*	Cyclophosphamide (high-dose)	Atrial fibrillation Cardiac tamponade Cardiogenic shock Cardiomyopathy Cardiotoxicity (27%; grade 3–4: 3%) CHF Heart failure (7%–28%) Myocardial hemorrhage Left ventricular systolic dysfunction MI Myocardial necrosis Myocarditis Acute myopericarditis Pericardial effusion (33%) Pericarditis Prolonged QT interval Supraventricular arrhythmia Ventricular fibrillation Ventricular tachycardia	Monitor ECG for QT (QTc) prolongation in patients treated with high-dose cyclophosphamide-containing chemotherapy. ECG may show diminished QRS complex. Monitor cardiac biomarker (BNP) in patients on high-dose cyclophosphamide as an indicator of acute heart failure because it is elevated within the first 24 hours of therapy and remains persistently elevated for up to 1 week after the clinical presentation of acute heart failure. Monitor for cardiotoxicity, including myocarditis, myopericarditis, pericardial effusion, including cardiac tamponade, and CHF, which have been reported and may be fatal. Risk for cardiotoxicity increases with high doses, older patients, history of radiation to the chest wall, and previous or current treatment with cardiotoxic agents. Monitor for supraventricular (atrial fibrillation and flutter) and ventricular (tachyarrhythmia associated with severe QT prolongation) arrhythmias. Monitor patients with risk factors and preexisting cardiac disease for cardiotoxicities. Diuretics, ACE inhibitors, and beta-blockers should be instituted early if no contraindications exist. The spectrum of clinical manifestations from cyclophosphamide-induced cardiotoxicity is variable in presentation and severity. Common manifestations include tachyarrhythmias, hypotension, heart failure, myocarditis, and pericardial disease. These typically present within the first 48 hours of drug administration but may be seen up to 10 days after initiation. Hemorrhagic myocarditis is a rare complication that is uniformly and rapidly fatal. Mild to moderate heart failure and small pericardial effusions generally resolve within a few days to weeks after discontinuation of cyclophosphamide. The risk of cardiotoxicity appears to be dose related (150 mg/kg and 1.5 g/m^2/day) and occurs 1–10 days after the administration of the first dose of cyclophosphamide. Higher doses of this drug may produce significant cardiotoxicity, including fatal hemorrhagic myocarditis. Pediatric patients with thalassemia have been shown to have a potential for cardiac tamponade when cyclophosphamide is given with busulfan. Myocardial necrosis may result in rare circumstances. (Dhesi et al., 2013; Shaikh & Shih, 2012; Truven Health Analytics, 2017)
	Dacarbazine	Orthostatic hypotension ECG abnormalities	Monitor blood pressure and observe for ECG abnormalities for patients receiving this therapy. Educate patients about signs and symptoms of hypotension. (Truven Health Analytics, 2017)
	Estramustine (estradiol and nitrogen mustard)	CHF MI Edema	Monitor for signs and symptoms of CHF (e.g., shortness of breath, lower-extremity edema) and acute MI (e.g., chest pain, shortness of breath, palpitation). Because hypertension may occur, monitor blood pressure periodically. Use estramustine with caution in patients with a history of cerebral vascular or coronary artery disease. (Truven Health Analytics, 2017)

(Continued on next page)

Classification	Drug	Side Effects	Nursing Considerations
Chemotherapy Agents *(Cont.)*			
Alkylating agents *(cont.)*	Ifosfamide (Ifex®)	Cardiotoxicity (0.5%) Hypotension (0.3%) MI Myocarditis	Monitor electrolyte levels. Establish baseline cardiac status and monitor for acute changes. Risk is dose dependent and increased with previous treatment with cardiotoxic agents and regimens, preexisting cardiac disease, and renal impairment. Cardiotoxicity includes supraventricular or ventricular arrhythmias, decreased QRS voltage and changes in ST segment or T-wave, toxic cardiomyopathy leading to heart failure, and pericardial effusion, some of which have caused fatalities. (Truven Health Analytics, 2017)
	Melphalan (Alkeran®, Evomela®)	Atrial fibrillation or flutter (11%) Peripheral edema (33%) Supraventricular tachycardia (11%)	Monitor for signs and symptoms of cardiotoxicity, including ECG changes. This drug includes a black box warning for hypersensitivity reaction that may include cardiac arrest. Paroxysmal atrial fibrillation was observed in 5 patients undergoing stem cell transplantation. Supraventricular tachycardia has been associated with longer hospital stays. (Truven Health Analytics, 2017)
	Trabectedin (Yondelis®)	Cardiomyopathy (all grades: 6%; grade 3–4: 4%) Peripheral edema (all grades: 28%; grade 3–4: 0.8%)	Assess neutrophil count, creatine phosphokinase levels, and liver function tests prior to each dose. Assess LVEF by ECG or MUGA scan prior to initiation of therapy. Assess for cardiomyopathy, which may be fatal. Delay next dose for up to 3 weeks in the presence of LVEF < LLN or clinical evidence of cardiomyopathy. Reduce next dose by 1 dose level for adverse event during the prior cycle in the presence of absolute decrease of ≥ 10% from baseline to < LLN, or clinical evidence of cardiomyopathy. Once dosage has been reduced, it should not be increased in subsequent cycles. Permanently discontinue trabectedin for symptomatic cardiomyopathy or persistent left ventricular dysfunction that does not recover to LLN within 3 weeks. (Truven Health Analytics, 2017)
Antimetabolites	Azacitidine	Atrial fibrillation (< 5%) Cardiorespiratory arrest (< 5%) Chest pain (16.4%) CHF (< 5%) Dilated cardiomyopathy (< 5%) Heart failure (< 5%) Hypertension (8.6%) Hypotension (6.8%) Pericarditis	Monitor coadministration with other cardiotoxic medications. Toxicity usually is self-limiting and responds to a drug holiday. (Celgene Corp., 2012; Truven Health Analytics, 2017)

Table 16-1. Cardiotoxicity of Cancer Therapy *(Continued)*

(Continued on next page)

Table 16-1. Cardiotoxicity of Cancer Therapy *(Continued)*

Classification	Drug	Side Effects	Nursing Considerations
Chemotherapy Agents *(Cont.)*			
Antimetabolites *(cont.)*	Capecitabine (Xeloda®)	Cardiotoxicity Chest pain Edema (33%) Takotsubo cardiomyopathy Vasospasm	Monitor for MI, ischemia, angina, dysrhythmias, cardiac arrest, cardiac failure, sudden death, ECG changes, and cardiomyopathy, all of which have been observed with use of this agent. Assess for chest pain, even in patients with no prior history, as it has been observed in patients within the first few doses of capecitabine in combination with other chemotherapy, radiation therapy, or both. Patients may have elevated ST intervals but may also show no signs of ischemia on ECG or stress echo. These adverse events may be more common in patients with a prior history of coronary artery disease. Assess for edema, particularly in patients undergoing combination therapy with docetaxel, for whom rates were highest. Interrupt drug if grade 2–3 adverse reactions occur; discontinue drug for grade 4 toxicity. Takotsubo cardiomyopathy is a reversible condition characterized by transient apical and midventricular wall motion; patients may present with radiating chest pain, nausea and vomiting, and shortness of breath. (Truven Health Analytics, 2017)
	Clofarabine (Clolar®)	Edema (12.2%) Hypertension (13%) Hypotension (29%) Pericardial effusion (7.8%) Tachycardia (35%)	Monitor for hypotension and tachycardia, which may be indicative of cytokine release syndrome or systematic inflammatory response syndrome. Monitor cardiac function during the 5 days of clofarabine administration. Evaluate for signs and symptoms of cytokine release and systemic inflammatory response syndrome (e.g., tachypnea, tachycardia, hypotension, pulmonary edema) that can lead to systemic inflammatory response syndrome, capillary leak syndrome, and organ failure. Discontinue drug if hypotension occurs during infusion. Cardiotoxicities were most commonly observed among pediatric patients with relapsed or refractory acute lymphoblastic leukemia or acute myeloid leukemia. (Truven Health Analytics, 2017)
	5-Fluorouracil (5-FU; Adrucil®)	Cardiotoxicity (1.2%–18%) • Acute coronary syndrome • Angina pectoris • Cardiogenic shock • Cardiomyopathy • Heart failure • MI • ST-T abnormalities on ECG	Assess for signs and symptoms of acute coronary syndrome, which may include radiating chest pain, diarrhea, and vomiting. Assess for nausea, vomiting, diaphoresis, and signs of ECG changes that may occur with angina; angina pain may occur within hours of receiving a second or third dose but may be associated with the first dose. Assess for angina attacks with rechallenge of the drug. Assess for cardiotoxicities during continuous infusion of the drug. Monitor for ST segment changes on ECG. Withhold treatment if cardiotoxicity occurs. Perform an ECG prior to each administration. Treatment-induced cardiotoxicity may be treated prophylactically or therapeutically with long-acting nitrates or calcium channel blockers. Patients at higher risk for developing cardiotoxicity include those with heart disease, electrolyte disturbances, or radiation exposure to the heart. Incidence of 5-FU cardiotoxicity is dependent on dose and schedule. Incidence of 10% has been associated with doses > 800 mg/m^2/day. (Fadol & Lech, 2011; Truven Health Analytics, 2017)

(Continued on next page)

Table 16-1. Cardiotoxicity of Cancer Therapy *(Continued)*

Classification	Drug	Side Effects	Nursing Considerations
Chemotherapy Agents *(Cont.)*			
Antimetabolites *(cont.)*	Gemcitabine hydrochloride	Atrial fibrillation Capillary leak syndrome Cardiac dysrhythmia CHF MI Pericardial effusion Peripheral edema (20%) Vasculitis	Monitor for hypotension, particularly in patients with an infusion time of > 60 minutes or more than once per week. Assess for tachypnea, pulmonary crackles, and arterial hypoxemia, which may occur in the presence of atrial fibrillation. Assess for dyspnea, diffuse swelling, weight gain, and hypotension, which may occur in the presence of capillary leak syndrome. Discontinue treatment in the presence of capillary leak syndrome, which may occur in monotherapy or combination therapy. Radiation therapy is not recommended during or within 7 days of infusion. (Truven Health Analytics, 2017)
	Pemetrexed (Alimta®)	Chest pain (up to 5%)	Monitor patients for and educate patients and families about signs and symptoms of chest pain, which have been observed in combination with cisplatin. (Truven Health Analytics, 2017)
	Pentostatin (Nipent™)	Chest pain (3%–10%) Hypotension (3%–10%) Peripheral edema (3%–10%)	Monitor patients for and educate patients and families about signs and symptoms of cardiac complications, which have been observed in patients treated with pentostatin for hairy cell leukemia. (Truven Health Analytics, 2017)
Anthracyclines	Daunorubicin	CHF (50%–80% mortality rate) Tachycardia Supraventricular arrhythmias Heart block ECG abnormalities (e.g., ST-T changes)	Assess for pericarditis and myocarditis, which have been reported with treatment. Monitor cardiac function via ECG or ejection fraction prior to each treatment course and following treatment to assess for acute and late effects. Cardiac monitoring in children should include echo and radionuclide angiocardiography, with at least 1 of these tests consistently performed throughout treatment. The Cardiology Committee of the Children's Cancer Study Group suggests the following monitoring schedule during and after treatment: • During therapy – Perform baseline cardiac assessment with an ECG, echo, and, when available, a radionuclide angiography (MUGA). – Obtain an echo (or a radionuclide angiocardiogram) before every other subsequent course of therapy with a cumulative dose < 300 mg/m². – Obtain an echo (or a radionuclide angiocardiogram) before each subsequent course of therapy above a cumulative dose of 300 mg/m² with mediastinal irradiation < 1,000 cGy. – Obtain an echo and radionuclide angiocardiogram before each subsequent course of therapy above a cumulative dose of 300 mg/m² with mediastinal irradiation > 1,000 cGy. – Obtain an echo and radionuclide angiocardiogram before each subsequent course of therapy above a cumulative dose of 400 mg/m² in the absence of mediastinal irradiation. • After therapy – Obtain an echo at 3–6 months and 12 months after therapy completion. An ECG and radionuclide angiocardiogram should be performed at 1 year following therapy completion. – For patients with normal cardiac function in the 1-year post-treatment period, follow-up ECG and echo should be performed every 2–3 years, with a radionuclide angiocardiogram and 24-hour continuous taped ECG performed every 5 years post-treatment. – For patients with abnormal cardiac function in the 1-year post-treatment period, follow-up ECG and echo should be performed yearly, with a radionuclide angiocardiogram and 24-hour continuous taped ECG performed every 5 years post-treatment.

(Continued on next page)

Table 16-1. Cardiotoxicity of Cancer Therapy *(Continued)*

Classification	Drug	Side Effects	Nursing Considerations
Chemotherapy Agents *(Cont.)*			
Anthracyclines *(cont.)*	Daunorubicin *(cont.)*		Treatment with anthracycline-based therapy should be avoided for up to 7 months after completing trastuzumab. Cardiotoxicity risk is associated with cumulative doses > 400–550 mg/m^2 in adults, 300 mg/m^2 in children older than 2 years, and 10 mg/kg in children younger than 2 years. Acute or subacute toxicity may occur within 1–23 days after treatment and is not related to cumulative dose, with delayed toxicity occurring months to years after treatment. CHF may be irreversible and resistant to treatment with digitalis. Cardiotoxicity risk increases with history of radiation to the chest wall, age > 70 years, underlying heart disease or hypertension, and history of or concurrent administration with other anthracyclines or cardiotoxic agents (e.g., trastuzumab). Infants or young children appear to be at higher risk for cardiotoxicity than adults. (Truven Health Analytics, 2017)
	Daunorubicin and cytarabine liposome (Vyxeos™)	Cardiac dysrhythmia (30%) Cardiotoxicity (non-conduction related; 20%) Edema (51%) Hypertension (18%) Hypotension (20%)	Assess cardiac function prior to starting drug and each treatment cycle using an ECG, echo, or MUGA scan. Monitor more frequently if patients are receiving concomitant therapy with other cardiotoxic drugs. Discontinue use of drug in the presence of impaired cardiac function unless benefit outweighs the risk. Drug is not recommended for use in patients with LVEF below normal limits. Cardiotoxicity risk is increased with prior anthracycline-based therapy, chest wall irradiation, and history of cardiac disease or concomitant use of cardiotoxic drugs. CHF risk is increased with total cumulative nonliposomal daunorubicin doses > 550 mg/m^2. Avoid use of this drug in patients who have reached a lifetime cumulative limit of anthracyclines. Periodic monitoring with an echo or MUGA scans is recommended. (Truven Health Analytics, 2017)
	Doxorubicin liposomal (Doxil®)	Cardiomyopathy (Kaposi sarcoma; < 1%) CHF (up to 2%)	Assess for a history of cardiovascular disease, which increases risk for cardiac complications. Assess left ventricular cardiac function via MUGA or ECG at baseline, during therapy, and after discontinuation to assess for acute and delayed toxicities. Cardiotoxicity risk has been observed with cumulative anthracycline doses of 450–550 mg/m^2. Cardiotoxicity at lower doses may occur in patients who received mediastinal irradiation or patients with preexisting heart disease. Chronic effects seen with cumulative doses approaching 550 mg/m^2 may result in CHF. (Truven Health Analytics, 2017)

(Continued on next page)

Table 16-1. Cardiotoxicity of Cancer Therapy *(Continued)*

Classification	Drug	Side Effects	Nursing Considerations
Chemotherapy Agents *(Cont.)*			
Anthracyclines *(cont.)*	Doxorubicin (Adriamycin®)	Cardiogenic shock Cardiomyopathy (1%–20%) CHF (1%–20%) ECG abnormality Heart failure Left ventricular failure (1%–20%) MI Myocarditis Pericarditis Sinus tachycardia Tachyarrhythmia	Assess for arrhythmia, which may occur within hours of therapy and can be life threatening. Assess cardiac function via ECG and evaluate for ST-T wave changes and atrioventricular and bundle branch block. Assess for myocarditis or pericarditis, both of which may occur during or after therapy. Assess for tachyarrhythmias, including sinus tachycardia, premature ventricular contractions, and ventricular tachycardia. Periodic monitoring with an echo or MUGA scans is recommended. Protect against cardiotoxicity with dexrazoxane in 10:1 ratio of dexrazoxane to doxorubicin. Protective agent is administered by rapid infusion 30 minutes prior to doxorubicin. The National Institute for Occupational Safety and Health recommends the use of double gloves and a protective gown in the preparation and administration of injections. Prepare in a biosafety cabinet or a compounding aseptic containment isolator; eye/face and respiratory protection may be needed. Prepare compounds in a closed-system drug-transfer device. During administration, if there is a potential that the substance could splash or if the patient may resist, use eye/face protection. Dexrazoxane as a cardioprotectant is not recommended during doxorubicin administration. Avoid use of CYP3A4, CYP2D6, and P-glycoprotein inhibitors and inducers and trastuzumab, which may increase risk of cardiac dysfunction. This drug is contraindicated in patients with a recent MI (within 4–6 weeks). Cardiotoxicity risk factors include prior or concomitant radiation therapy to the chest wall, previous therapy with other anthracyclines or anthracenediones, and concomitant use of other cardiotoxic drugs. Cardiotoxicity risk is dose dependent. Cumulative doses > 550 mg/m² are associated with an increased risk of cardiomyopathy. The maximum recommended cumulative doxorubicin dose in combination with paclitaxel is 340–380 mg/m². Fatal cases of cardiotoxicity have occurred at doses < 400 mg/m² (all in combination with concurrent administration of cardio- or hepatotoxic agents); therefore, cardiac monitoring is imperative regardless of dosing. Continuous infusion administration may allow for higher cumulative dosing of > 450 mg/m², which have been administered with no observed cardiac abnormalities. Administration using a weekly schedule of 20 mg/m² was associated with less cardiac damage than an every-3-week schedule of 60 mg/m². Prior doses of other anthracyclines or anthracenediones should be included when calculating total cumulative doses of doxorubicin. Delayed-onset, dose-related cardiomyopathy is the most common and well-known cardiotoxicity and is likely to be irreversible and unresponsive to treatment. (Truven Health Analytics, 2017)

(Continued on next page)

Table 16-1. Cardiotoxicity of Cancer Therapy *(Continued)*

Classification	Drug	Side Effects	Nursing Considerations
Chemotherapy Agents *(Cont.)*			
Anthracyclines *(cont.)*	Epirubicin (Ellence®)	Atrioventricular block Bradyarrhythmia Bundle branch block Cardiotoxicity CHF (0.4%–3.3%) Left ventricular cardiac dysfunction (1.4%–2.1%) Phlebitis (3%–10%) Thrombophlebitis Ventricular tachycardia	Monitor for dysrhythmias, including premature ventricular contractions, sinus tachycardia, bradycardia, and heart block. Obtain LVEF at baseline and during treatment with ECG and MUGA scan or echo, especially in patients with risk factors for increased cardiotoxicity. Continued LVEF evaluation is recommended in patients with previous anthracycline or anthracenedione exposure. Avoid concomitant use of cardiotoxic agents unless cardiac function is closely monitored. Active or dormant cardiovascular disease, prior or concomitant radiation to the mediastinal or pericardial area, previous therapy with other anthracyclines or anthracenediones, or concomitant use of other cardiotoxic drugs may increase cardiotoxicity risk. In the adjuvant treatment of breast cancer, the maximum cumulative dose used in clinical trials was 720 mg/m². Cardiotoxicity may occur at lower cumulative doses regardless of whether cardiac risk factors are present. The probability of developing clinically evident CHF is estimated at approximately 0.9% with a cumulative dose of 550 mg/m², 1.6% with 700 mg/m², and 3.3% with 900 mg/m². CHF risk rises rapidly with increasing total cumulative doses > 900 mg/m²; cumulative dose should be exceeded only with extreme caution. High single doses have been associated with acute myocardial ischemia. Myocardial toxicity, manifested in its most severe form by potentially fatal CHF, may occur either during therapy with epirubicin or months to years after termination of therapy. Cardiomyopathy is notably late in onset, occurring 6 months to years after therapy. (Shaikh & Shih, 2012; Truven Health Analytics, 2017)
	Idarubicin (Idamycin®)	Cardiovascular findings • Acute MI • Bundle branch block • CHF • Conduction defects • Heart failure • LVEF abnormalities • Supraventricular extrasystoles • T-wave flattening	Monitor cardiac function closely while on treatment. Manifestations include ECG changes such as ventricular and supraventricular extrasystoles, bundle branch block, T-wave flattening, and conduction defects. Evaluate for anemia and infection prior to and during treatment, which may increase cardiotoxicity risk. Patients receiving concurrent therapy with cardiotoxic agents, including trastuzumab, cyclophosphamide, or paclitaxel, should have cardiac function closely monitored. Hold other cardiotoxic agents during treatment unless benefit outweighs risk. Anthracycline use (e.g., trastuzumab, cyclophosphamide, paclitaxel) should be held for at least 5 half-lives following treatment with idarubicin, and, if used, cardiac function should be closely monitored. Cardiotoxicities may be worsened by previous treatment with doxorubicin. Cardiotoxicity risk may increase with history of preexisting heart disease or previous therapy with anthracyclines, anthracenediones, or other cardiotoxic agents, as well as concomitant or previous treatment with chest wall irradiation or drugs that suppress cardiac contractility. Drug may be less cardiotoxic than other agents. CHF has been reported with IV idarubicin when given alone or with cytarabine. (Truven Health Analytics, 2017)

(Continued on next page)

Table 16-1. Cardiotoxicity of Cancer Therapy *(Continued)*

Classification	Drug	Side Effects	Nursing Considerations
Chemotherapy Agents *(Cont.)*			
Anthracyclines *(cont.)*	Mitoxantrone	Bradyarrhythmia Cardiovascular abnormalities (4%–15%) CHF (2.6%)	Monitor patients for bradyarrhythmia, which has been reported as low as 38 bpm on day 2 of therapy. Establish baseline cardiac function. Monitor cardiac status with ECG. Monitor for cardiac arrhythmias, including decreased LVEF, CHF, tachycardia, ECG changes, and MI (rare). Assess cardiac function and LVEF by physical examination, history, and ECG prior to the start of therapy in all patients and consistently after treatment initiation in patients at elevated risk (e.g., history of anthracycline therapy or mediastinal irradiation, preexisting cardiovascular disease). Cardiotoxicity is observed with prolonged administration and at doses > 80–100mg/m^2. Previous treatment with doxorubicin, radiation therapy, or a history of cardiac disease increases risk. Cardiac dysfunction may be observed in both adult and pediatric patients undergoing treatment with mitoxantrone. Monitor for cardiotoxicity beyond doses of 100 mg/m^2. Maximum dose is considered 160 mg/m^2; cardiotoxicity risk increases with cumulative dose. (Truven Health Analytics, 2017)
Antitumor antibiotics	Bleomycin	Acute chest pain Arterial thrombosis Cerebrovascular accident Coronary arteriosclerosis Edema (50%) MI Raynaud phenomenon	Monitor for signs and symptoms of arterial thrombosis, including coronary artery disease and arterial thrombosis, which have been observed in patients receiving combination therapy with vinblastine and cisplatin. Assess for acute chest pain during infusion, as it may indicate pleuropericarditis. Assess for edema, particularly in the hands and feet. Cerebrovascular accident has been noted in combination regimens with bleomycin. Maximum lifetime dose is 400 units, but lower doses are recommended when administered with other cardiotoxic agents or chest irradiation involving the heart. Perform routine monitoring with echocardiography as maximum tolerated dose is approached. Raynaud phenomenon is observed in monotherapy or combination therapy with vinblastine with or without cisplatin. Combination therapy with cisplatin, vinblastine, and etoposide for germ cell tumors is associated with severe myocardial complications. (Truven Health Analytics, 2017)

(Continued on next page)

Table 16-1. Cardiotoxicity of Cancer Therapy *(Continued)*

Classification	Drug	Side Effects	Nursing Considerations
Chemotherapy Agents *(Cont.)*			
Miscellaneous	Arsenic trioxide	Chest pain (25%) Complete atrioventricular block CHF Edema (40%) Hypertension (10%) Hypotension (25%) Palpitations (10%) Prolonged QT interval (2%–40%) Tachycardia (55%) Torsades de pointes (2.5%) Ventricular arrhythmia	Assess for QT prolongation, torsades de pointes, and complete atrioventricular block, which may be fatal. Assess for a history of QT-prolonging drugs, torsades de pointes, QT-interval prolongation, CHF, current use of potassium-wasting diuretics, conditions resulting in hypokalemia or hypomagnesemia, or current use of drugs that can cause electrolyte abnormalities, as these can worsen QT prolongation. Perform an ECG and assess electrolyte levels prior to treatment. Check 12-lead ECG prior to therapy and hold if QTc is > 500 ms. Check all electrolytes prior to administration of medication and replenish prior to therapy. Potassium should be kept > 4 mEq/L and magnesium > 1.8 mEq/L. Discontinue QT-prolonging agents if possible, and perform frequent cardiac monitoring if not possible. Consider dose adjustment prior to restarting therapy after QTc prolongation occurs. Drug should not be administered unless the QTc is < 500 ms. Therapy can be resumed once the QTc returns to < 460 ms. QT prolongation with dysrhythmias: Usual onset of QT prolongation > 0.50 ms was 1–4 weeks after treatment. QT prolongation effects may persist up to 8 weeks after therapy. Complete atrioventricular block has been reported with arsenic trioxide. Assess for other causes of dysrhythmias prior to administering drug. (Truven Health Analytics, 2017)
	Eribulin (Halaven®)	Hypotension (5%–10% in adult patients with liposarcoma) Peripheral edema (12%) QTc prolongation	Monitor for QT prolongation (via ECG) in high-risk patients, including those with CHF, bradyarrhythmias, and electrolyte abnormalities and those using QT-prolonging medications. Monitor for electrolyte abnormalities, and correct hypokalemia or hypomagnesemia prior to starting the drug and during its use. Use with caution in patients with congenital long QT syndrome. (Truven Health Analytics, 2017)
Plant alkaloids: Taxanes	Docetaxel	Cardiac dysrhythmia (2%–8%) Cardiotoxicity, including left ventricular diastolic dysfunction CHF (2.3% reported in combination therapy with doxorubicin and cyclophosphamide) Fluid retention (6.5%–67%) Hypotension (2% observed in hypersensitivity reactions) Myocardial ischemia (1%–2%) Peripheral edema (18%–34%) Syncope (2%) Vasodilation (27% observed in combination with doxorubicin and cyclophosphamide)	Monitor patients for signs and symptoms of fluid retention, particularly those with preexisting history. Assess cardiac function by ECG and serum concentration of the cardiac neurohormone BNP in patients preparing to undergo therapy with this drug. Premedicate with corticosteroids for 3 days starting 1 day prior to each dose; in patients with prostate cancer, oral dexamethasone is recommended at 12 hours, 3 hours, and 1 hour before drug administration. Black box warning for fluid retention with a median weight gain of 2 kg, with up to 15 kg reported in the presence of multiple courses of the drug; may require drug discontinuation. (Truven Health Analytics, 2017)

(Continued on next page)

Table 16-1. Cardiotoxicity of Cancer Therapy *(Continued)*			
Classification	**Drug**	**Side Effects**	**Nursing Considerations**
Chemotherapy Agents *(Cont.)*			
Plant alkaloids: Taxanes *(cont.)*	Paclitaxel	Atrial fibrillation (< 1% with severe conduction abnormalities) Atrioventricular block (< 1%) Bradyarrhythmia (3%) Cardiac dysrhythmia (< 1%) Cardiotoxicity (1%–13% in combination with trastuzumab and as monotherapy, respectively) CHF, including cardiac dysfunction and reduction of LVEF Edema (21%) Hypotension (9%–17%) Left ventricular diastolic dysfunction MI Supraventricular tachycardia (< 1%) Ventricular arrhythmia (< 1%)	Obtain a baseline ECG, history and physical, and cardiac assessment before treatment. Monitor vital signs frequently, especially during the first hour of infusion. Perform continuous cardiac monitoring during infusion in patients with history of serious cardiac conduction abnormalities. Cardiac dysrhythmia may require pacemaker placement. Premedication with corticosteroids plus diphenhydramine and an H_2 antagonist (e.g., ranitidine) is recommended, with dosing and route of administration varying based on drug administration. Drug has a black box warning for hypersensitivity reactions, including hypotension, which may be fatal. Asymptomatic bradycardia has been observed during infusion even in patients with no known cardiac history or risk factors. Patients who have undergone treatment with other anthracyclines may be at increased risk for cardiotoxicity. Ventricular tachycardia and ventricular ectopy have been observed in combination therapy with paclitaxel. (Truven Health Analytics, 2017)
Plant alkaloids: Vinca alkaloids	Vinblastine	Angina pectoris (rare) Cardiovascular autonomic neuropathy, including abnormal variations in heart rate and blood pressure ECG abnormalities, potentially associated with coronary ischemia Hypertension MI Raynaud phenomenon	Most presentations are rare, but patients should be monitored for signs and symptoms of cardiac dysfunction, including ECG changes and variations in blood pressure and heart rate. (Truven Health Analytics, 2017)
	Vincristine	Angina pectoris (rare) Cardiovascular autonomic neuropathy, including abnormal variations in heart rate and blood pressure Hypertension Hypotension MI	Most presentations are rare, but patients should be monitored for signs and symptoms of cardiac dysfunction, including ECG changes and variations in blood pressure and heart rate. (Truven Health Analytics, 2017)
	Vinorelbine (Navelbine®)	MI (rare)	Most presentations are rare, but patients should be monitored for signs and symptoms of cardiac dysfunction. (Truven Health Analytics, 2017)

(Continued on next page)

Table 16-1. Cardiotoxicity of Cancer Therapy *(Continued)*

Classification	Drug	Side Effects	Nursing Considerations
Targeted Therapy Agents			
Small molecule inhibitors	Afatinib (Gilotrif®)	Diastolic dysfunction, including left ventricular dysfunction, and ventricular dilation (2.2% in afatinib-treated patients vs. 0.9% in chemotherapy-treated patients)	Most presentations are rare, but patients should be monitored for signs and symptoms of cardiac dysfunction. Discontinue drug in the presence of symptomatic diastolic dysfunction. (Truven Health Analytics, 2017)
	Alectinib (Alecensa®)	Bradyarrhythmia (8.6%–11%) Fatal cardiac arrest reported in 1 patient in clinical trials Fatal endocarditis (0.4%)	Monitor patients for signs and symptoms of cardiac dysfunction, particularly bradycardia, which may require dose reduction, pause in therapy, or discontinuation. Monitor heart rate and blood pressure regularly. Advise patients to report any changes in heart or blood pressure medication. Dosing may be reinstated with recovery to asymptomatic bradycardia or to a heart rate of at least 60 bpm. Discontinue drug in the presence of recurrent bradycardia. (Truven Health Analytics, 2017)
	Axitinib (Inlyta®)	Heart failure (2%; grade 3–4: 1%) Hypertension (40%; grade 3–4: 16%) Hypertensive crisis (< 1%)	Monitor patients for signs and symptoms of cardiac dysfunction, particularly heart failure and hypertension, including hypertensive crisis, which may require dose reduction, pause in therapy, or discontinuation. Monitor for hypertension (> 150 mm Hg systolic; > 100 mm Hg diastolic), which has been reported, particularly in patients with renal cell carcinoma. Onset of hypertension occurred at a median of 1 month after treatment initiation, although blood pressure increases have occurred as early as 4 days after initiation. Blood pressure should be well controlled prior to starting this drug; monitor blood pressure regularly during therapy. (Truven Health Analytics, 2017)
	Bortezomib (Velcade®)	Heart disease (15%) Heart failure (5%) Hypertension (6%) Hypotension (12%–15%) Peripheral edema (7%)	Closely monitor patients with existing heart disease or risk factors for heart disease during therapy. Assess for cardiac dysfunction, including development or exacerbation of CHF and new-onset decreased LVEF, which have been observed, even in patients with no prior history of cardiac abnormalities. Hypotension, including orthostatic and postural hypotension, has been reported; risk is increased with concurrent use of medications that can cause hypotension, a history of syncope, and dehydration. Management may include adjustment of antihypertensive medications, hydration, and administration of mineralocorticoids (e.g., fludrocortisone) and/or adrenergic agents (e.g., epinephrine). (Truven Health Analytics, 2017)
	Bosutinib (Bosulif®)	Chest pain (7%–12%) Edema (17%–20%) Hypertension (1% to < 10%) Pericardial effusion (1% to < 10%) Pericarditis (0.1% to < 1%) Prolonged QT interval (1% to < 10%)	Monitor for signs of fluid retention, which may present as pericardial effusion, pleural effusion, pulmonary edema, or peripheral edema. Consider dose reductions or temporary interruptions of therapy for symptomatic pericardial effusions. (Truven Health Analytics, 2017)

(Continued on next page)

Table 16-1. Cardiotoxicity of Cancer Therapy *(Continued)*			
Classification	**Drug**	**Side Effects**	**Nursing Considerations**
Targeted Therapy Agents *(Cont.)*			
Small molecule inhibitors *(cont.)*	Brigatinib (Alunbrig®)	Bradyarrhythmia (5.7%–7.6%) Hypertension (11%–21%)	Assess and control blood pressure prior to start of therapy; monitoring is recommended, and therapy interruption, dosage reduction, or discontinuation may be required. Measure blood pressure 2 weeks after initiation and at least monthly thereafter during use. Measure heart rate regularly throughout treatment and more frequently in patients requiring concomitant therapy known to cause bradycardia. For patients with symptomatic bradycardia (heart rate < 60 bpm), hold drug until the patient is asymptomatic with resting heart rate of ≥ 60 bpm. If drug is anticipated to be the primary or monotherapeutic source of bradycardia, resume dosing at the next lowest efficacious level. Permanently discontinue drug if no contributing concomitant medication is identified or if bradycardia is recurrent or unresponsive to therapy. For patients with grade 3 hypertension (SBP ≥ 160 mm Hg or DBP ≥ 100 mm Hg), initiate antihypertensive therapy. Withhold drug until hypertension has recovered to grade 1 or less (SBP < 140 mm Hg and DBP < 90 mm Hg), then restart with next lower dose. If grade 3 hypertension recurs, withhold therapy until recovery to grade 1 or less and resume at next lower dose. Permanently discontinue drug in presence of recurrent grade 3 or higher hypertension. (Truven Health Analytics, 2017)
	Cabozantinib (capsules: Cometriq®; tablets: Cabometyx®)	Hypertension (33%–39%) Hypotension (7%)	Monitor blood pressure before treatment initiation and regularly during therapy. Discontinue drug in the presence of malignant hypertension, hypertensive crisis, or persistent uncontrolled hypertension despite medical management. Hypertension may require drug pause, dose reduction, or discontinuation. Hypertension is one of the most common adverse events leading to dose reduction in patients with renal cell carcinoma. (Truven Health Analytics, 2017)

(Continued on next page)

Table 16-1. Cardiotoxicity of Cancer Therapy *(Continued)*			
Classification	**Drug**	**Side Effects**	**Nursing Considerations**
Targeted Therapy Agents *(Cont.)*			
Small molecule inhibitors *(cont.)*	Carfilzomib (Kyprolis®)	Cardiac arrest (> 10% combination therapy; > 20% monotherapy) Chest wall pain (11.4%) CHF (> 10% combination therapy; > 20% monotherapy) Heart failure (> 10% combination therapy; > 20% monotherapy) MI (> 10% combination therapy; > 20% monotherapy) Myocardial ischemia (> 10% combination therapy; > 20% monotherapy) Peripheral edema (16%–20%) Restrictive cardiomyopathy Venous thrombosis (9%–13% combination therapy; 2% monotherapy)	Monitor patients for signs and symptoms of cardiac dysfunction, especially those that may require dose reduction, pause in therapy, or discontinuation. Monitor for volume overload, particularly in patients with risk factors for cardiac failure. Monitor for signs or symptoms of cardiac failure or cardiac ischemia, and evaluate promptly. Hypertension, hypertensive crisis, and hypertensive emergency have been reported and included fatalities; monitoring is recommended, and dosage interruption or discontinuation may be required. Adjust total fluid intake as appropriate in patients with baseline cardiac failure or risk factors for cardiac failure. Withhold treatment for grade 3–4 cardiac adverse events, and consider restarting at a reduced dose after resolution, if appropriate. Risk of cardiac complications is increased in individuals aged 75 years or older, with NYHA class III or IV heart failure, recent MI, or uncontrolled conduction abnormalities. New or worsening cardiac failure (e.g., CHF, pulmonary edema, decreased LVEF), restrictive cardiomyopathy, myocardial ischemia, and MI have been reported, with potential for fatality. Fatal cardiac arrest within 1 day of carfilzomib administration has been reported. (Truven Health Analytics, 2017)
	Ceritinib (Zykadia®)	Bradyarrhythmia (1%) Cardiac tamponade (rare but can be fatal) Prolonged QT interval (12%)	Monitor ECGs and electrolytes in patients treated with QT-prolonging drugs or with concurrent electrolyte abnormalities, bradyarrhythmias, or CHF. Perform periodic ECGs in patients at risk for QT interval prolongation (i.e., CHF, bradyarrhythmias, electrolyte abnormalities, or concomitant QT-prolonging drugs). Advise patients to report any changes in heart or blood pressure medication. Withhold drug in presence of prolonged QT interval until recovery to baseline, then resume with a reduced dose; may require permanent discontinuation if condition persists. Permanently discontinue if QTc interval prolongation occurs with torsades de pointes, polymorphic ventricular tachycardia, or serious arrhythmia. Drug may cause concentration-dependent increases in the QTc interval, resulting in increased risk for ventricular tachyarrhythmias (e.g., torsades de pointes) or sudden death. Drug should not be used in patients with congenital long QT syndrome. Monitor heart rate and blood pressure regularly during treatment. (Truven Health Analytics, 2017)

(Continued on next page)

Table 16-1. Cardiotoxicity of Cancer Therapy *(Continued)*			
Classification	**Drug**	**Side Effects**	**Nursing Considerations**
Targeted Therapy Agents *(Cont.)*			
Small molecule inhibitors *(cont.)*	Cobimetinib (Cotellic®)	Cardiomyopathy, including decreased symptomatic or asymptomatic cardiac ejection fraction Hypertension (15%)	Evaluate LVEF prior to initiation of treatment, 1 month after initiation, and every 3 months thereafter. Drug may require pause, dose reduction, or discontinuation based on recovery of ejection fraction. When resuming treatment after interruption or dose reduction, monitor LVEF after 2 weeks, 4 weeks, 10 weeks, and 16 weeks, and as clinically indicated. Median time to onset was 4 months, and median time to resolution was 3 months for decreased ejection fraction; resolution often is to above the LLN or within 10% of baseline. (Truven Health Analytics, 2017)
	Crizotinib (Xalkori®)	Bradyarrhythmia (5%–14%) Edema (31%–49%) Prolonged QT interval (2.1%–6%)	Regularly monitor heart rate and blood pressure. Consider periodic monitoring with ECG and electrolytes in patients with risk factors for QT prolongation. Perform baseline and periodic monitoring of electrolytes with a potassium goal of 4 mEq/L and magnesium goal of 2 mEq/L. Withhold treatment if symptomatic bradycardia occurs; treatment may be resumed when heart rate is ≥ 60 bpm. Permanently discontinue drug in the presence of life-threatening bradycardia. Use with caution in patients with higher risk of developing prolonged QT interval or with baseline cardiac disease, including congenital long QT syndrome. Interrupt treatment for QTc > 500 ms on at least 2 separate ECGs. May resume at a reduced dose following recovery to QTc ≤ 480 ms. Discontinue use if QTc > 500 ms develops (or a 60 ms or more increase from baseline) with torsades de pointes or polymorphic ventricular tachycardia or signs and symptoms of serious arrhythmia. Edema can intensify with combination treatment with pemetrexed plus cisplatin. (Truven Health Analytics, 2017)
	Dabrafenib (Tafinlar®)	Cardiomyopathy (2.9%–6%) Deep vein thrombosis (up to 7%) Peripheral edema (17%–31%) Prolonged QT interval (2%–13%)	Assess LVEF by ECG or MUGA scan prior to treatment, 1 month after initiation of treatment, and every 2–3 months following. Monitor for QT prolongation of > 500 ms, which has been reported. Cardiomyopathy may require dose interruption (reported in 2.4% of patients on monotherapy and 4.4% on combination therapy), dose reduction, or discontinuation (reported in 1% of patients). Withhold treatment for symptomatic cardiomyopathy or asymptomatic left ventricular dysfunction of > 20% from baseline and below LLN. Resume treatment at same dose level. Median time to onset of cardiomyopathy was 4.4 months (monotherapy) and 8.2 months (combination therapy with dabrafenib plus trametinib). Incidence of deep vein thrombosis and pulmonary embolism is increased when dabrafenib is used in combination with trametinib. (Truven Health Analytics, 2017)

(Continued on next page)

Table 16-1. Cardiotoxicity of Cancer Therapy *(Continued)*

Classification	Drug	Side Effects	Nursing Considerations
Targeted Therapy Agents *(Cont.)*			
Small molecule inhibitors *(cont.)*	Dasatinib (Sprycel®)	CHF or cardiac dysfunction, including acute cardiac failure, cardiomyopathy, diastolic and left ventricular dysfunction, ventricular failure, and decreases in ejection fraction (2%–4%) Edema (generalized: 1%–4%; localized/superficial: 3%–22%) Palpitations (1%–10%) Pericardial effusion (3%–4%) Prolonged QT interval (1%) Tachyarrhythmia (1%–10%) Ventricular arrhythmia (< 1%)	Monitor patients for signs and symptoms of cardiac dysfunction, which may require dose reduction, pause in therapy, or discontinuation. Assess for signs and symptoms of fluid retention, which is one of the most commonly reported adverse events but appears less frequently with once daily dosing. Use with caution in patients who have or may develop QTc prolongation (maximum mean change in QTcF from baseline ranged 7–13.4 ms), including patients with hypokalemia or hypomagnesemia, those who are receiving antiarrhythmic medications or other medications that prolong the QT interval, or those who have had high cumulative doses of anthracyclines. Correct hypokalemia and hypomagnesemia prior to therapy initiation. (Truven Health Analytics, 2017)
	Ibrutinib (Imbruvica®)	Atrial fibrillation and flutter (6%–9%) Hypertension (6%–17%) Peripheral edema (12%–25%)	Monitor patients for signs and symptoms of cardiac dysfunction, which may require dose reduction, pause in therapy, or discontinuation. Perform ECG in patients who develop arrhythmic symptoms (e.g., palpitations, light-headedness) or new-onset dyspnea. Conduct periodic clinical monitoring for atrial fibrillation, especially in older adult patients. Monitor for uncontrolled or new-onset hypertension. Atrial fibrillation was one of the most common grade 3–4 nonhematologic adverse reactions in mantle cell lymphoma trials. Incidence of atrial fibrillation is increased in patients with cardiac risk factors, hypertension, acute infections, and a previous history of atrial fibrillation. (Truven Health Analytics, 2017)
	Imatinib mesylate (Gleevec®)	Cardiac tamponade Cardiogenic shock Chest pain (7%–11%) CHF (up to 1%) Edema Heart failure Hypotension (11%) Palpitations (up to 5.2%) Pericardial effusion Pericarditis Peripheral edema (up to 33%) Tachycardia (up to 1%)	Weigh patients regularly, and monitor for signs and symptoms of fluid volume overload. Monitor for signs and symptoms of cardiac dysfunction, which may require dose reduction, pause in therapy, or discontinuation. Monitor ECG and serum troponin levels for signs and symptoms of hypereosinophilic syndrome and cardiac involvement, which have been associated with cardiogenic shock and left ventricular dysfunction. Assess for CHF in older adult patients and those with a history of coronary disease. Assess for edema, including potential for pleural effusion, pericardial effusion, pulmonary edema, and ascites, with superficial edema most prominent in the lower extremities. In patients with chronic myeloid leukemia, edema risk is increased in those receiving high-dose therapy and those older than age 65. Manage edema with a pause in therapy and diuretic agents. Cardiogenic shock can be reversible when managed with systemic steroids, circulatory support, and interruption of imatinib treatment. Prophylactic concurrent use of systemic steroids 1–2 mg/kg for 1–2 weeks may be indicated if either ECG or troponin is abnormal at the initiation of imatinib therapy. (Truven Health Analytics, 2017)

(Continued on next page)

Table 16-1. Cardiotoxicity of Cancer Therapy *(Continued)*			
Classification	**Drug**	**Side Effects**	**Nursing Considerations**
Targeted Therapy Agents *(Cont.)*			
Small molecule inhibitors *(cont.)*	Lapatinib (Tykerb®)	Depression of left ventricular systolic function (1.52%–3.98%; grade 3–4: < 1%) Heart failure Prolonged QT interval Torsades de pointes Variant angina (< 1%) Ventricular arrhythmia	Monitor for signs and symptoms of cardiac dysfunction, particularly QT interval prolongation, and decreased LVEF, which may require dose reduction, pause in therapy, or discontinuation. Confirm normal LVEF before beginning drug. Obtain baseline cardiac evaluation with echo or MUGA scan. Assess for prolonged QT interval in patients with hypokalemia or hypomagnesemia, congenital long QT syndrome, concomitant use of antiarrhythmic agents or other agents that lead to QT prolongation, or cumulative high-dose anthracycline therapy. Discontinue treatment in patients with a decreased LVEF that is grade 2 or greater and in patients with an LVEF that drops below LLN. May rechallenge at a reduced dose if after 2 weeks the LVEF has recovered to normal and the patient is asymptomatic. Monitor and correct for hypomagnesemia and hypokalemia to reduce risk of QT prolongation. Evaluate and correct electrolyte abnormalities prior to the start of and during treatment, specifically hypokalemia and hypomagnesemia, to reduce risk for prolonged QT interval. (Truven Health Analytics, 2017)
	Lenvatinib (Lenvima®)	Hypertension (42%–73%) Hypotension (9%) Myocardial dysfunction (7%–10%) Peripheral edema (21%–42%) Prolonged QT interval (9%–11%)	Monitor for signs and symptoms of cardiac dysfunction, particularly QT interval prolongation, hypertension, and decreased ventricular function, which may require dose reduction, pause in therapy, or discontinuation. Monitor blood pressure and correct at baseline, prior to treatment initiation, and monitor after 1 week, then every 2 weeks for the first 2 months, and then at least monthly thereafter during treatment. Monitor ECG in patients with congenital long QT syndrome, CHF, bradyarrhythmias, and concomitant use of drugs that prolong the QT interval (including class Ia and III antiarrhythmics). Monitor for and correct electrolyte abnormalities in all patients. Hold treatment for grade 3 hypertension despite optimal antihypertensive therapy, grade 3 cardiac dysfunction, and QT prolongation > 500 ms. Treatment may be resumed at a reduced dose when hypertension is controlled at grade 2 or lower; cardiac dysfunction improves to grade 0, 1, or baseline; or when QT prolongation improves to < 480 ms or baseline. Discontinue treatment in the presence of life-threatening hypertension or grade 4 cardiac dysfunction. (Truven Health Analytics, 2017)

(Continued on next page)

Table 16-1. Cardiotoxicity of Cancer Therapy *(Continued)*

Classification	Drug	Side Effects	Nursing Considerations
Targeted Therapy Agents *(Cont.)*			
Small molecule inhibitors *(cont.)*	Nilotinib (Tasigna®)	Hypertension (10%–11%) Ischemic heart disease (5%–9.4%) MI (< 1%) Pericardial effusion (< 1%) Peripheral arterial occlusive disease (2.9%–3.6%) Peripheral edema (9%–15%) Prolonged QT interval (< 10%) Sudden death due to cardiotoxicity (0.3%; likely due to ventricular repolarization)	Monitor for signs and symptoms of cardiac dysfunction, particularly QT interval prolongation, which may require dose reduction, pause in therapy, or discontinuation. Assess ECG at baseline, 7 days after treatment initiation, with dose adjustments, and periodically thereafter. Assess lipid profiles and glucose periodically during the first year of treatment and at least once a year with long-term therapy. Evaluate potential for drug interactions if statin treatment is warranted. Evaluate cardiovascular status at baseline, and monitor risk factors during therapy. Avoid concomitant use with CYP34A inhibitors because of risk for prolonged QT intervals. Instruct patients to avoid eating 2 hours before and 1 hour after administration because of risk for prolonged QT intervals. Dose reduction may be necessary if inhibitors must be given, and the QTc should be monitored closely. Avoid concomitant use of drugs known to prolong QT interval. Dose modifications are required based on the severity of the adverse reaction. Monitor for and correct hypomagnesemia and hypokalemia to reduce risk of QT prolongation. Drug has a black box warning for QT interval prolongation that may progress to torsades de pointes; it should be avoided in patients with long QT syndrome, hypokalemia, hypomagnesemia, and QT prolongation, which may be fatal. (Truven Health Analytics, 2017)
	Niraparib (Zejula®)	Hypertension (20%) Palpitations (10%) Peripheral edema (1%–10%) Tachycardia (1%–10%)	Monitor for signs and symptoms of cardiac dysfunction, particularly hypertension, which may require dose reduction, pause in therapy, or discontinuation. Monitor blood pressure and heart rate monthly for the first year and periodically thereafter, especially in patients with cardiovascular disorders (e.g., coronary insufficiency, cardiac arrhythmias, hypertension). Administer antihypertensives, which may require dose adjustment of niraparib. (Truven Health Analytics, 2017)
	Osimertinib (Tagrisso®)	Cardiomyopathy (1.9%) Decreased cardiac ejection fraction (4%) Prolonged QT interval (0.7%)	Monitor for signs and symptoms of cardiac dysfunction, particularly QTc prolongation and cardiomyopathy, which may require dose reduction, pause in therapy, or discontinuation. Assess for cardiomyopathies, including cardiac failure, CHF, decreased LVEF, or pulmonary edema, which may be fatal. Closely monitor patients with congenital long QT syndrome, CHF, electrolyte abnormalities, or concomitant use of medications that can prolong the QTc interval, and discontinue therapy in the presence of life-threatening arrhythmia. Permanently discontinue therapy in patients with symptomatic CHF or persistent, asymptomatic left ventricular dysfunction that does not resolve within 4 weeks. Assess LVEF at baseline and every 3 months following with ECG or MUGA. (Truven Health Analytics, 2017)

(Continued on next page)

Table 16-1. Cardiotoxicity of Cancer Therapy *(Continued)*			
Classification	**Drug**	**Side Effects**	**Nursing Considerations**
Targeted Therapy Agents *(Cont.)*			
Small molecule inhibitors *(cont.)*	Panobinostat (Farydak®)	Cardiac dysrhythmia (12%) ECG T-wave abnormalities (40%) Hemorrhage (grade 3–4: 4%) Hypertension (< 10%) Hypotension (< 10%) MI (< 4%) Orthostatic hypotension (< 10%) Palpitations (< 10%) Peripheral edema (29%) ST segment depression (22%)	Monitor for signs and symptoms of cardiac dysfunction, particularly cardiac dysrhythmias, which may require dose reduction, pause in therapy, or discontinuation. Monitor electrolytes during treatment, and correct abnormalities as clinically indicated. Assess for ECG changes, which may include ST segment depression and T-wave abnormalities and prolongation of cardiac ventricular repolarization (QT interval). Do not initiate therapy in patients with recent MI or unstable angina or in patients with a QTcF > 450 ms or clinically significant baseline ST segment or T-wave abnormalities. Avoid concomitant use with antiarrhythmics (e.g., amiodarone, disopyramide, procainamide, quinidine, sotalol) or drugs known to prolong the QT interval (e.g., bepridil, chloroquine, clarithromycin, halofantrine, methadone, moxifloxacin, pimozide). Obtain an ECG at baseline and periodically to monitor for abnormalities. Drug has a black box warning for severe and fatal cardiac ischemic events, including severe arrhythmias, and ECG changes that may be exacerbated by electrolyte abnormalities. (Truven Health Analytics, 2017)
	Pazopanib (Votrient®)	Bradyarrhythmia (2%–19%) Chest pain (5%–10%) CHF (1%) Heart failure Hypertension (40%; grade 3–4: 4%–7%) Left ventricular cardiac dysfunction (0.6%–8%) MI (2%) Peripheral edema (14%; grade 3: 2%) Prolonged QT interval (0.2%–2%) Torsades de pointes (< 1%)	Perform baseline and periodic monitoring of electrolytes with a potassium goal of 4 mEq/L and magnesium goal of 2 mEq/L. Control preexisting hypertension before beginning pazopanib therapy. Monitor for cardiac dysfunction, including signs and symptoms of CHF and decreased LVEF, as well as QT prolongation. Consider periodic monitoring with ECG in patients with risk factors for QT prolongation. Use with caution in patients with higher risk of developing prolonged QT interval or with baseline cardiac disease. Dose reduction is permitted if hypertension persists despite supportive antihypertensive therapies; persistent or severe hypertension may require discontinuation of therapy. Avoid use of pazopanib in patients with a recent (within 6 months) arterial thromboembolic event. (GlaxoSmithKline, 2013; Nguyen & Shayahi, 2012; Truven Health Analytics, 2017)

(Continued on next page)

Table 16-1. Cardiotoxicity of Cancer Therapy *(Continued)*

Classification	Drug	Side Effects	Nursing Considerations
Targeted Therapy Agents *(Cont.)*			
Small molecule inhibitors *(cont.)*	Ponatinib (Iclusig®)	Arterial ischemia (11%–42%) Atrial fibrillation (7%) Bradyarrhythmia (1%) Cardiac dysrhythmia (19%) Heart failure (6%–15%) Hypertension (53%–71%) Myocardial ischemia (21%) Peripheral artery occlusive disease (12%) Peripheral edema (13%–22%)	Monitor for signs and symptoms of cardiac dysfunction, particularly cardiac ischemia, infarction, or hypertension, which may require dose reduction, pause in therapy, or discontinuation. Assess patients with hypertension for confusion, headache, chest pain, or shortness of breath, which may require urgent clinical intervention. Frequently assess and manage blood pressure prior to and during treatment. Hold therapy to evaluate patients with signs and symptoms of abnormal heart rate, including rapid heart rate in the presence of atrial fibrillation and slow heart rate in the presence of bradyarrhythmia. Interrupt treatment and consider evaluating for renal artery stenosis if significant worsening, labile, or treatment-resistant hypertension occurs. Cardiac vascular occlusions requiring revascularization procedures have occurred, including life-threatening and fatal MI and coronary artery occlusion. Interrupt or discontinue treatment immediately if arterial occlusion is suspected. Consider risks versus benefits before restarting therapy. Drug has a black box warning for arterial occlusion (i.e., MI, stroke, stenosis of large arteries of the brain, severe peripheral vascular disease), venous occlusive events, and life-threatening or fatal heart failure and left ventricular dysfunction. Arterial ischemia includes cardiovascular, cerebrovascular, and peripheral vascular ischemia. Atrial fibrillation was the most common arrhythmia reported during clinical trials, and approximately 50% of cases were grade 3–4. Additional grade 3–4 arrhythmia events included syncope, tachycardia, bradycardia, QT prolongation, atrial flutter, supraventricular tachycardia, ventricular tachycardia, atrial tachycardia, complete atrioventricular block, cardiorespiratory arrest, loss of consciousness, and sinus node dysfunction, with some patients requiring hospitalization. Fatal and life-threatening arterial occlusions may occur within 2 weeks of initiation and at dosages as low as 15 mg/day; median time to first onset is 193 days, so monitoring should be long term for these patients. Risk factors include hypertension, hyperlipidemia, and preexisting cardiac disease, and event frequency increased with age. Occlusions also occurred in patients without cardiovascular risk factors and in patients aged 50 years or younger. Peripheral arterial occlusive events requiring revascularization procedures have occurred, including fatal mesenteric artery occlusion and life-threatening peripheral arterial disease. Digital or distal extremity necrosis requiring amputation has also occurred. The median time to onset of the first peripheral vascular arterial occlusive event was 478 days. (Truven Health Analytics, 2017)

(Continued on next page)

Table 16-1. Cardiotoxicity of Cancer Therapy *(Continued)*

Classification	Drug	Side Effects	Nursing Considerations
Targeted Therapy Agents *(Cont.)*			
Small molecule inhibitors *(cont.)*	Regorafenib (Stivarga®)	Hypertension (30%–59%; grade 3–4: 8%–28%) Hypertensive crisis (0.25%) MI (1.2%) Myocardial ischemia (1.2%)	Patients should be monitored for signs and symptoms of cardiac dysfunction, particularly cardiac ischemia, infarction, or hypertension, which may require dose reduction, pause in therapy, or discontinuation. Blood pressure should be adequately controlled prior to initiation of drug and monitored weekly for the first 6 weeks during therapy, then at least every cycle. Drug should be temporarily withheld or permanently discontinued in patients with severe or uncontrolled hypertension. (Truven Health Analytics, 2017)
	Ribociclib (Kisqali®)	Peripheral edema (12%) Prolonged QT interval (3%) Sudden cardiac death (0.3%) Syncope (2.7%)	Monitor for signs and symptoms of cardiac dysfunction, particularly prolongation of QT interval, electrolyte imbalances, and syncope, which may require dose reduction, pause in therapy, or discontinuation. Assess ECG prior to initiation, during therapy, and as clinically indicated, as ECG changes have been observed within first 4 weeks of treatment and were reversible with dose interruption. Monitor serum potassium, calcium, phosphorus, and magnesium prior to initiation, during therapy, and as clinically indicated. Prolongation of the QT interval, which is drug concentration dependent, can result in sudden death. Avoid use of ribociclib in patients with preexisting QT prolongation or those at risk (e.g., long QT syndrome, recent MI, CHF, unstable angina, bradyarrhythmias). Avoid concomitant use of drugs known to prolong the QT interval. Correct any electrolyte abnormalities prior to starting therapy to avoid QT prolongation. (Truven Health Analytics, 2017)
	Romidepsin (Istodax®)	ECG changes (QT prolongation) ECG ST segment changes (2%–63%) Hypotension (7%–23%) QTc prolongation (at least 2%) Supraventricular arrhythmia (6%) Ventricular arrhythmia (4%)	Monitor INR more frequently in patients receiving concurrent warfarin therapy. ECG changes, including T-wave and ST segment changes, have been reported; prior to administration, confirm that potassium and magnesium levels are within normal limits. Monitor for ECG changes in patients with congenital long QT syndrome, a history of significant cardiovascular disease, or concomitant use of antiarrhythmic or QT-prolonging agents, for whom these risks are elevated. Obtain baseline and periodic ECGs. Monitor for and correct electrolyte abnormalities. (Truven Health Analytics, 2017)
	Sorafenib (Nexavar®)	Cardiac dysrhythmia (< 1%) CHF (1.9%) Edema Heart failure exacerbation Hypertension (19.1%; grade 3–4: 4.3%) Hypertensive crisis (< 1%) MI (1.9%–2.9%) Myocardial ischemia (1.9%–2.9%) Prolonged QT interval (< 0.1%)	Monitor for signs and symptoms of cardiac dysfunction, particularly cardiac ischemia, hypertension, and MI, which may require dose reduction, pause in therapy, or discontinuation. Monitor for QT interval prolongation in patients with CHF, bradyarrhythmias, electrolyte abnormalities, and concomitant use of other drugs known to prolong the QT interval. Monitor blood pressure weekly for the first 6 weeks of treatment, then every 2–3 weeks for the duration of treatment. Avoid use in patients with congenital long QT syndrome. Hypertension can be severe and potentially persistent. Treat preexisting hypertension with standard hypertensive agents before treatment initiation. In the presence of prolonged QT interval, monitor ECGs and electrolytes (i.e., magnesium, calcium, potassium) in at-risk patients, and interrupt treatment with QTc interval > 500 ms or increases from baseline ≥ 60 ms. (Truven Health Analytics, 2017)

(Continued on next page)

Table 16-1. Cardiotoxicity of Cancer Therapy *(Continued)*

Classification	Drug	Side Effects	Nursing Considerations
Targeted Therapy Agents *(Cont.)*			
Small molecule inhibitors *(cont.)*	Sunitinib (Sutent®)	Aortic dissection (rare but potentially fatal) Heart failure (up to 2%) Hypertension (15%–39%) Left ventricular cardiac dysfunction (11%–27%) Peripheral edema (10%–24%) Prolonged QT interval Thromboembolic disorder Torsades de pointes (< 0.1%)	Monitor for signs and symptoms of cardiac dysfunction, particularly CHF and hypertension, which may require dose reduction, pause in therapy, or discontinuation. Monitor for cardiotoxicity (e.g., myocardial disorders, cardiomyopathy), especially in patients with a history of cardiac events, pulmonary embolism, cerebrovascular accident, or transient ischemic attack. Monitor for LVEF changes 20%–50% of baseline, which may occur without clinical evidence of CHF; monitoring is recommended. Patients with a history of QT interval prolongation, relevant preexisting cardiac disease, bradycardia, electrolyte disturbances, or concomitant use of antiarrhythmics or strong CYP3A4 inhibitors may experience QT interval prolongation and torsades de pointes. Obtain baseline LVEF prior to initiation of drug, especially in patients with cardiac risk factors. Monitor for and correct hypomagnesemia and hypokalemia to reduce risk of QT prolongation. Monitor blood pressure weekly for the first 6 weeks, then periodically throughout therapy. Standard antihypertensive agents are recommended for management of hypertension. Therapy breaks have been effective for resolution of hypertension. Hypertension seems to be related to presence of proteinuria, and both usually are present prior to cardiac failure. Halt all therapy if symptomatic myocardial ischemia or manifestations of CHF occur temporally related to drug administration. (Truven Health Analytics, 2017)
	Temsirolimus (Torisel®)	Chest pain (16%) Edema (35%) Hypertension (7%) Venous thromboembolism (2%)	Assess for angioedema, which has been reported in combination with ACE inhibitors or calcium channel blockers. Monitor for signs and symptoms of angioedema and for elevations in blood pressure. Treatment-induced or intensified hypertension may require management with one or more antihypertensive agents. (Hall et al., 2013; Truven Health Analytics, 2017)
	Trametinib (Mekinist®)	Bradyarrhythmia (up to 10%) Cardiomyopathy (6%–9%) Hypertension (15%–26%) Peripheral edema	Monitor for signs and symptoms of cardiac dysfunction, which may require dose reduction, pause in therapy, or discontinuation. Assess LVEF by echo or MUGA scan before initiating treatment, 1 month after initiation, and at 2–3-month intervals thereafter during therapy. Monitor for cardiomyopathy, defined as a decrease in LVEF below the institutional LLN with an absolute decrease in LVEF > 10% below baseline, which has occurred with the use of this drug as both monotherapy and in combination regimens. Median time to onset of cardiomyopathy was 2.1 months with monotherapy and 6.7–8.2 months with combination therapy; therefore, patients should have long-term monitoring for this toxicity. Withhold treatment in patients with LVEF > 10% below baseline; however, treatment may be resumed at a lower dosing level if LVEF improves to normal value. Permanently discontinue treatment for symptomatic cardiomyopathy or persistent, asymptomatic LVEF dysfunction (> 20% from baseline and is < LLN) that does not resolve within 4 weeks. (Truven Health Analytics, 2017)

(Continued on next page)

Table 16-1. Cardiotoxicity of Cancer Therapy *(Continued)*			
Classification	**Drug**	**Side Effects**	**Nursing Considerations**
Targeted Therapy Agents *(Cont.)*			
Small molecule inhibitors *(cont.)*	Vandetanib (Caprelsa®)	Heart failure (0.9%) Hypertension (all grades: 33%; grades 3–4: 5%) Prolonged QT interval (all grades: 14%; grades 3–4: 8%)	Monitor for and correct hypocalcemia, hypomagnesemia, and hypokalemia to reduce risk of QT prolongation. Correct these electrolyte abnormalities prior to treatment initiation. Monitor for QT prolongation, torsades de pointes, ventricular tachycardia, and sudden death at baseline, during initiation of treatment, and at dose escalation. Therapy is contingent on QTc; treatment should not be initiated if > 450 ms. If QTcF interval > 500 ms during therapy, temporarily discontinue therapy, and resume at reduced dose. Hold drug in the presence of Common Terminology Criteria for Adverse Events (National Cancer Institute Cancer Therapy Evaluation Program, 2017) grade 3 or greater toxicity; resume at reduced dose. Heart failure and hypertension, including hypertensive crisis, has been reported, which may require holding, dose modifying, or discontinuing the drug. Do not use in patients with history of or active torsades de pointes, bradyarrhythmias, or uncompensated heart failure. Use is contraindicated in patients with congenital long QT syndrome. Avoid concomitant use of drugs that prolong QT interval (e.g., clarithromycin, chloroquine, dolasetron, granisetron, haloperidol, methadone, moxifloxacin, pimozide), or perform more frequent ECG monitoring if use is necessary. (Truven Health Analytics, 2017)
	Vemurafenib (Zelboraf®)	Atrial fibrillation (< 10%) Cardiac tamponade Hypertension (36%) Peripheral edema (17%–23%) Prolonged QT interval (55%) Vasculitis (< 10%)	To reduce risk of QT prolongation, monitor for and correct hypocalcemia, hypomagnesemia, and hypokalemia. Obtain ECGs at baseline, 15 days after the start of treatment, monthly during the first 3 months of treatment, and then at least every 3 months. Assess for QT prolongation, which may increase the risk of torsades de pointes and other ventricular arrhythmias. Hold treatment in patients with uncorrectable electrolyte abnormalities, corrected QT interval of > 500 ms, congenital long QT syndrome, or concomitant use of products known to prolong the QT interval. Withhold treatment in patients who develop grade 3 corrected QT interval prolongation (i.e., more than 500 ms). May restart at a reduced dose in patients who improve to corrected QT interval prolongation of grade 2 or better (i.e., ≤ 500 ms). Permanently discontinue treatment if QTc remains above 500 ms and more than 60 ms higher than baseline values (after controlling for electrolyte abnormalities, CHF, bradyarrhythmias, or other cardiac risk factors). (Truven Health Analytics, 2017)
	Vorinostat (Zolinza®)	MI Peripheral edema (12.8%) Prolonged QT interval Syncope	Monitor electrolytes, including potassium, magnesium, and calcium, every 2 weeks during the first 2 months of therapy and then monthly, and more frequently in symptomatic patients (e.g., with nausea, vomiting, diarrhea, fluid imbalance, or cardiac symptoms). Use in combination with warfarin may lead to elevated INR. Monitor INR frequently. Teach patients methods to reduce risk of venous thromboembolism: drink fluids and maintain mobility. Consider thromboprophylaxis for patients with additional risks for venous thromboembolism. (Truven Health Analytics, 2017)

(Continued on next page)

Table 16-1. Cardiotoxicity of Cancer Therapy *(Continued)*

Classification	Drug	Side Effects	Nursing Considerations
Targeted Therapy Agents *(Cont.)*			
Small molecule inhibitors *(cont.)*	Ziv-aflibercept (Zaltrap®)	Angina pectoris Decreased ejection fraction Heart failure Hypertension (41%; grade 3: 19%; grade 4: 0.2%)	Monitor for signs and symptoms of cardiac dysfunction, which may require dose reduction, pause in therapy, or discontinuation. Monitor blood pressure every 2 weeks or more frequently as indicated. Treat with appropriate antihypertensive therapy (Regeneron Pharmaceuticals, Inc., 2013). Hold dosing if recurrent or severe hypertension occurs, and restart at a lower dose once blood pressure is controlled. (Truven Health Analytics, 2017)
Immunotherapy Agents			
Checkpoint inhibitors (CTLA-4)	Ipilimumab (Yervoy®)	Heart failure with reduced ejection fraction Immune-mediated myocarditis (severe or fatal: 0.2%) Immune-mediated pericarditis (severe or fatal: 0.2%–1%)	Monitor for signs and symptoms of heart failure, including reduced ejection fraction. Steroid therapy (1–2 mg/kg/day) may be used in the presence of immune-mediated myocarditis and pericarditis; however, severe presentation may require drug discontinuation. (Truven Health Analytics, 2017)
Chimeric antigen receptor T-cell immunotherapy	Tisagenlecleucel (Kymriah®)	Hypertension (19%) Hypotension (31%) Tachycardia (26%)	Establish baseline cardiac status and monitor for acute changes. (Truven Health Analytics, 2017)
Cytokines: Cell signaling molecules	Epoetin alfa (Procrit®)	Cardiovascular events (14%–18%), including MI, stroke, and CHF CHF (6.6%–9%) Edema (1%–3%) MI (0.8%–2.8%) Hypertension (incidence varies based on indication; surgery: 3%–6%; chronic kidney disease: 13.7%–27.7%)	Monitor for hemoglobin rate increase of > 1 g/dl over a 2-week period, which may increase risk for death, MI, stroke, and CHF. Use the lowest dose sufficient to reduce need for blood transfusions. Reduce or withhold dosing if blood pressure cannot be therapeutically controlled. Drug has a black box warning that it may increase risk of serious cardiovascular and thromboembolic events. (Truven Health Analytics, 2017)
	Filgrastim (G-CSF; Neupogen®)	Capillary leak syndrome Chest pain (13%) Syncope (resulting in loss of consciousness: 15%)	Assess for signs and symptoms of capillary leak syndrome, including hypotension, hypoalbuminemia, edema, and hemoconcentration, as this presentation may be life threatening. In the presence of capillary leak syndrome, which may be life threatening, discontinue the drug and initiate methylprednisolone. Capillary leak syndrome may require management in the intensive care setting. (Truven Health Analytics, 2017)
	Pegfilgrastim (PEG-G-CSF)	Capillary leak syndrome	Assess for signs and symptoms of capillary leak syndrome, including hypotension, hypoalbuminemia, edema, and hemoconcentration, as this presentation may be life threatening. In the presence of capillary leak syndrome, which may be life threatening, discontinue the drug and initiate methylprednisolone. Capillary leak syndrome may require management in the intensive care setting. (Truven Health Analytics, 2017)

(Continued on next page)

Table 16-1. Cardiotoxicity of Cancer Therapy *(Continued)*

Classification	Drug	Side Effects	Nursing Considerations
Immunotherapy Agents *(Cont.)*			
Cytokines: Cell signaling molecules *(cont.)*	Sargramostim (GM-CSF; Leukine®)	Capillary leak syndrome (< 1%) Cardiac dysrhythmia Chest pain (15%) Edema (bone marrow transplant: 15%; acute myeloid leukemia: 25%) Hypertension (34%) Hypotension Left bundle branch block (rarely observed) Pericardial effusion (4%–25%) Pericarditis Supraventricular arrhythmia Tachycardia (11%)	Assess for signs and symptoms of capillary leak syndrome, including hypotension, hypoalbuminemia, edema, and hemoconcentration. Establish baseline cardiac status and monitor for acute changes. Use with caution in patients with history of fluid retention, pulmonary infiltrates, or CHF. Discontinue drug in presence of arrhythmias. Diuretic therapy may be indicated for fluid retention/edema. (Truven Health Analytics, 2017)
Cytokines: Interferons	Interferon alfa-2b (Intron-A®)	Cardiac dysrhythmia (< 5%) Cardiomegaly (< 5%) Cardiomyopathy (< 5%) Chest pain (1%–28%, varies by diagnosis) Coronary artery disorder (< 5%) Heart failure (< 5%) Hypotension (< 5%) MI Raynaud disease (< 5%) Supraventricular arrhythmia Tachycardia (< 5%) Vasculitis	Monitor closely for signs and symptoms of cardiac complications. Obtain ECGs prior to and during therapy for patients with preexisting cardiac abnormalities and patients who are in advanced stages of cancer. Discontinue drug in the presence of severe or life-threatening symptoms. Use with caution in patients with a history of cardiovascular disease. (Truven Health Analytics, 2017)
	Interferon alfa-2b (pegylated; Sylatron™)	Angina pectoris Bundle branch block (4%) Cardiac dysrhythmia Cardiomyopathy Chest pain (6%–8%) Heart failure Hypotension MI (4%) Pericarditis Supraventricular arrhythmia (4%) Tachycardia Ventricular tachycardia (4%)	Assess for history of cardiovascular disease, including MI or arrhythmic disorder, which is associated with an increased risk for cardiovascular adverse events. Monitor for signs and symptoms of cardiotoxicity. In patients with a history of significant or unstable cardiac disease, do not treat with combination peginterferon/ribavirin. Permanently discontinue drug if new onset of ventricular arrhythmia or cardiovascular decompensation occurs. Use with caution in patients with history of cardiac dysfunction. (Truven Health Analytics, 2017)
	Interferon-gamma (IFN-gamma; Actimmune®)	Cardiac dysrhythmia Heart failure Hypotension MI Syncope	Assess for signs and symptoms of cardiac dysrhythmia, including supraventricular tachycardia, atrial flutter, sinus tachycardia, premature ventricular contractions, heart block, and ventricular tachycardia. Monitor for signs and symptoms of cardiotoxicity and adjust dosage or discontinue drug as indicated. Preexisting cardiac conditions, including ischemia, CHF, or arrhythmia, may be exacerbated by flu-like symptoms (e.g., fever, chills) from higher-than-recommended doses. Cardiotoxicity generally is reported in the presence of doses > 100 mcg/m² administered 3 times weekly. (Truven Health Analytics, 2017)

(Continued on next page)

Table 16-1. Cardiotoxicity of Cancer Therapy *(Continued)*

Classification	Drug	Side Effects	Nursing Considerations
Immunotherapy Agents *(Cont.)*			
Cytokines: Interleukins	Aldesleukin (IL-2; Proleukin®)	Atrial arrhythmia (grade 4: < 1%) Blood pressure alteration (11%) Bradyarrhythmia (< 1%) Capillary leak syndrome Cardiac arrest (1%) Cardiac dysrhythmia (10%) CHF (11%) Coronary artery thrombosis Disorder of cardiovascular system (11%) ECG waveform abnormalities (11%) Edema (15%) Endocarditis (fatal) Hypotension (71%; grade 4: 3%) MI (1%) Myocardial ischemia (grade 4: 1%) Myocarditis Peripheral edema (28%) Second-degree atrioventricular block (< 1%) Supraventricular tachycardia (12%; grade 4: 1%) Tachycardia (23%) Vasodilation (13%) Ventricular premature beats (1%) Ventricular tachycardia (1%)	Monitor for signs and symptoms of capillary leak syndrome, which may occur immediately following initiation of treatment and is characterized by the following, as observed in clinical trials: extravasation of plasma proteins and fluids into the extravascular space, severe hypotension, cardiac arrhythmias, angina, MI, respiratory insufficiency requiring intubation, gastrointestinal bleeding or infarction, renal insufficiency, edema, and mental status changes. Capillary leak syndrome–associated hypotension is characterized by a drop in mean arterial blood pressure within 2–12 hours; reduced organ perfusion may result in death. Assess for hypovolemia by catheterization and central pressure monitoring. Monitor serum electrolytes at baseline and daily during treatment. Monitor vital signs (temperature, pulse, blood pressure, and respiration rate), weight, and fluid intake and output daily. Monitor cardiac function daily through vital signs monitoring and physical assessment. Discontinue treatment in the event of reduced organ perfusion, including altered mental status, decreased urine output, and SBP decreases to < 90 mm Hg. Administer IV fluids with careful monitoring of fluid status. Initiate dopamine (1–5 mcg/kg/min) prior to the onset of hypotension; phenylephrine hydrochloride (1–5 mcg/kg/min) has also been used to stabilize blood pressure. Pressor therapy may be needed to maintain blood pressure and renal output during treatment. Withhold IL-2 in patients developing ventricular dysrhythmias until cardiac ischemia and wall motion can be assessed. If adverse events occur, drug should be withheld, not dose reduced. Side effects appear to be dose related (Shelton, 2012). Risk increases with doses > 100,000 IU/kg (Shelton, 2012). Average dose is 600,000 IU/kg (Prometheus Laboratories Inc., 2012). Most adverse reactions are self-limiting and usually, but not invariably, reverse or improve within 2–3 days of discontinuing therapy. Electrical changes caused by cytokine immunotherapy usually relate to cellular swelling or inflammatory cytokine release causing disruption of conduction pathways. Capillary permeability and hypovolemia enhance the risk of supraventricular tachycardia. Patients should have normal cardiac, pulmonary, hepatic, and central nervous system function at the start of therapy. Electrical changes associated with immunotherapy agents generally necessitate temporary discontinuation of the drug. Once inflammatory effects have resolved, rechallenge is possible. (Shelton, 2012; Truven Health Analytics, 2017)
	Oprelvekin (IL-11; Neumega®)	Cardiomegaly (21%) Edema (59%) Increased plasma volume Palpitations (14%) Syncope (13%) Tachyarrhythmia (20%) Ventricular arrhythmia	Monitor for signs and symptoms of cardiotoxicity, and adjust dosage or discontinue drug as indicated. Monitor heart rate, blood pressure, and ECG. Use with caution in patients with history of atrial arrhythmias, thromboembolic disorders, and left ventricular dysfunction or CHF. (Truven Health Analytics, 2017)

(Continued on next page)

Table 16-1. Cardiotoxicity of Cancer Therapy *(Continued)*

Classification	Drug	Side Effects	Nursing Considerations
Immunotherapy Agents *(Cont.)*			
Miscellaneous: Autologous cellular immunotherapy	Sipuleucel-T (Provenge®)	Hypertension (7.5%)	Monitor for signs and symptoms of hypertension, and manage as indicated. Observe patients for at least 30 minutes after each infusion for acute infusion reactions, especially those with cardiac or pulmonary conditions.
Miscellaneous: Immunomodulators	Lenalidomide (Revlimid®)	Atrial fibrillation (grade 3–4: 3.7%) Cerebrovascular accident (1.4%–2.3%) CHF (grade 3–4: 1.4%) Edema (10.1%) Heart failure (1%–10%) Hypotension (7.1%) MI (< 5%) Peripheral edema (20.3%–26.3%) Syncope (1.4%–2.8%) Tachycardia (1.7%)	Establish baseline blood pressure, heart rate and regularity, and ECG findings to identify drug-related changes. Monitor heart rate, rhythm, and blood pressure frequently during therapy or with new cardiac symptoms. Assess for atrial fibrillation and CHF, which may be fatal in patients receiving lenalidomide in combination with dexamethasone, as observed in patients treated for multiple myeloma. Assess for cerebrovascular accident and MI in patients with multiple myeloma who have an increased risk of stroke while being treated with lenalidomide; risk factors for thrombosis include use of erythropoiesis-stimulating agents and estrogen agents. Assess for thrombosis, which may occur at least 2.7 months after treatment, particularly in patients who have not undergone prophylaxis. Assess for hypotension, edema, syncope, and tachycardia, which have been observed in patients treated in combination with dexamethasone. Thromboprophylaxis is recommended during treatment, especially for those at elevated risk for stroke; patients should be assessed and managed for risk factors for stroke, including hyperlipidemia, hypertension, and smoking. Cardiac failure was observed in patients treated for chronic lymphocytic leukemia. (Celgene Corp., 2013; Truven Health Analytics, 2017)
	Thalidomide (Thalomid®)	Atrial fibrillation (grade 3–4: 5%) Bradyarrhythmia (3%) Cardiac dysrhythmia Edema (13%–56%; grade 3: 6%) Heart failure Hypotension (3%) Ischemic heart disease (11.1%) MI (1.3%) Orthostatic hypotension (3%) Peripheral edema (34%)	Assess for ischemic heart disease, MI, and stroke. Assess for bradycardia, particularly in patients taking drugs that may reduce heart rate, who are at an increased risk for this toxicity. Monitor for hypotensive reaction, including dizziness or orthostatic hypotension. Monitor for signs and symptoms of thromboembolism, which may include upper- and lower-extremity swelling, shortness of breath, or chest pain. Assess patients for dizziness, palpitations, or other symptoms of dysrhythmias. Assess for cardiac arrhythmias, including ECG abnormalities, atrial fibrillation, bradycardia, tachycardia, sick sinus syndrome, and MI. Treatment may need to be held or discontinued in the presence of bradycardia. Initiate thromboprophylaxis when not contraindicated. Evaluate for and use drugs that increase risk of thromboembolism cautiously. Cardiotoxicity often is observed in combination with dexamethasone. Bradyarrhythmia and hypotension may result from activation of the vasovagal pathway. (Truven Health Analytics, 2017)

(Continued on next page)

Table 16-1. Cardiotoxicity of Cancer Therapy *(Continued)*			
Classification	**Drug**	**Side Effects**	**Nursing Considerations**
Immunotherapy Agents *(Cont.)*			
Monoclonal antibodies: Chimeric	Cetuximab (anti-EGFR antibody; Erbitux®)	Cardiorespiratory event (2%–3%) Sudden cardiac death (2%–3%)	Monitor electrolytes, particularly magnesium, calcium, and potassium levels, throughout treatment and up to 8 weeks after conclusion of therapy, and maintain within normal limits. Monitor for infusion reaction up to 1 hour after infusion; in the presence of reaction, monitor until reaction is resolved. Concomitant use of this drug with radiation (and cisplatin) increases the risk of life-threatening events, including cardiac events and electrolyte abnormalities. MI has been observed in patients receiving cetuximab for head and neck cancer but was not evident in patients receiving the drug for metastatic colorectal cancer. (Truven Health Analytics, 2017)
	Dinutuximab (anti-GD2 antibody; Unituxin®)	Capillary leak syndrome (40%), including fatal cases Edema (17%) Hypertension (14%) Hypotension (60%) Tachycardia (19%)	Monitor blood pressure during infusion. In moderate to severe cases, hold drug until supportive management resolves capillary leak syndrome, after which the drug may be restarted at a reduced rate. In life-threatening cases, withhold drug until next cycle or permanently discontinue if capillary leak syndrome recurs or persists. In the presence of symptomatic hypotension (SBP < LLN for age or decreased by > 15% from baseline), stop therapy and implement supportive management. Infusion may be reinstated at reduced rate 2 hours after symptoms resolve. Administer IV hydration prior to each infusion. (Truven Health Analytics, 2017)
	Ramucirumab (anti-VEGFR2 antibody; Cyramza®)	Hypertension (11%–36%) Hypertension (grade 3 or higher: 3% in monotherapy; 6%–15% in combination therapy) Peripheral edema (16%–25% in combination therapy)	Monitor blood pressure every 2 weeks or more frequently during therapy. Control hypertension before treatment initiation. Pause treatment until severe hypertension is controlled. Permanently discontinue therapy for hypertension uncontrolled by antihypertensives, hypertensive crisis, or hypertensive encephalopathy. (Truven Health Analytics, 2017)
	Rituximab (anti-CD20 antibody; Rituxan®)	Cardiac complications (29%) Heart failure Hypotension (10%) Peripheral edema (16%) Supraventricular arrhythmia (4.5%) Vasculitis	Monitor older patients for signs and symptoms of cardiac complications, including supraventricular arrhythmias, for whom these events are more common. Monitor for changes in blood pressure; however, hypertension has primarily been reported in patients with rheumatoid arthritis who are being treated with this agent. Monitor patients with a history of arrhythmia and angina for new-onset or exacerbated arrhythmia. Monitor patients with a history of cardiac abnormalities or cardiac reactions for infusion reaction, as risk is increased. Assess for inflammatory skin lesions, which may appear on the abdomen and lower extremities and become purpuric, as these have been observed in the presence of vasculitis in patients treated for B-cell chronic lymphoid leukemia. Monitor for hypotension, which may be a sign of infusion reaction and is most commonly observed during the first infusion or in patients with active or history of cardiac or pulmonary conditions or adverse events. Perform cardiac monitoring during infusion for patients with a cardiac history of arrhythmia or angina or in those who develop significant arrhythmia during treatment. Discontinue drug in the presence of life-threatening cardiac arrhythmias.

(Continued on next page)

Table 16-1. Cardiotoxicity of Cancer Therapy *(Continued)*

Classification	Drug	Side Effects	Nursing Considerations
Immunotherapy Agents *(Cont.)*			
Monoclonal antibodies: Chimeric *(cont.)*	Rituximab (anti-CD20 antibody; Rituxan®) *(cont.)*		After symptoms resolve, resume treatment by reducing the infusion rate by 50%. Risk of potentially fatal cardiac arrhythmia is increased in patients with current arrhythmia or history of arrhythmia and angina. Infusion-related deaths have occurred within 24 hours of infusion. Infusion-related complications include MI, ventricular fibrillation, and cardiogenic shock. (Biogen Inc. & Genentech, Inc., 2016; Truven Health Analytics, 2017)
Monoclonal antibodies: Human	Ado-trastuzumab emtansine (anti-HER2 antibody conjugated with emtansine; Kadcyla®)	Hypertension (5.1%) Left ventricular cardiac dysfunction (1.8%) Pulmonary arterial hypertension	Evaluate LVEF prior to treatment initiation and at regular intervals (e.g., every 3 months) during treatment and within 3 weeks if LVEF is ≤ 45%. Drug has a black box warning that reduction of LVEF may occur; assess LVEF before, during, and after treatment. Drug may need to be held or discontinued if LVEF does not resolve. (Truven Health Analytics, 2017)
	Elotuzumab (anti-SLAMF7 antibody; Empliciti™)	Bradycardia (66%) Decreased systolic arterial pressure (28.9%) Increased diastolic arterial pressure (17.3%) Increased systolic arterial pressure (33.3%) Tachycardia (47.8%)	Monitor for signs and symptoms of cardiotoxicity, and manage symptoms as indicated. Monitor vital signs for changes in blood pressure (increase or decrease). Assess for cardiac abnormalities, particularly in patients receiving combination therapy with lenalidomide and dexamethasone, with which their presentations have been observed. (Truven Health Analytics, 2017)
Monoclonal antibodies: Humanized	Alemtuzumab (anti-CD52 antibody; Campath®)	Cardiomyopathy Chest discomfort (7%) CHF Decreased cardiac ejection fraction Peripheral edema (5%) Tachycardia (8%)	Monitor vital signs before and during infusions. Monitor for infusion reactions during and for a minimum of 2 hours after each infusion, with additional monitoring as indicated for patients with conditions that have a higher risk of cardiovascular or pulmonary complications. (Truven Health Analytics, 2017)
	Bevacizumab (anti-VEGF antibody; Avastin®)	Hypertension (19%–42%; grade 3–5: 5%–18%) CHF (1.6%–4%) Hypertensive encephalopathy Hypotension (7%–15%) Ischemic heart disease (1%) Left ventricular cardiac dysfunction (10%) Peripheral edema (15%)	Monitor for severe hypertension (grade 3–4), for which holding or stopping the drug may be necessary. Monitor for mild or moderate blood pressure elevations, which also may be a sign of infusion reaction or posterior reversible encephalopathy syndrome. Monitor for left ventricular dysfunction and CHF for up to 6 months following therapy. Monitor for hypertensive crisis, particularly in patients with metastatic renal cell carcinoma receiving combination therapy with interferon alfa. Continue to monitor blood pressure even after discontinuation of bevacizumab in patients with hypertension. Check baseline vital signs, particularly blood pressure, with each clinic visit or at least every 2–3 weeks during therapy, with routine monitoring after treatment. Discontinue therapy in the presence of CHF. Initiate antihypertensive therapy with elevated blood pressure, as this has been demonstrated to control treatment-related elevations in blood pressure in most cases. Hold treatment in the presence of uncontrolled hypertension, and discontinue in the presence of hypertensive crisis or encephalopathy. Temporarily suspend treatment if urine shows 3+ urine dipstick reading, particularly if accompanied by hypertension; perform 24-hour urine collection and analysis in patients with a dipstick reading of 2+.

(Continued on next page)

Table 16-1. Cardiotoxicity of Cancer Therapy *(Continued)*

Classification	Drug	Side Effects	Nursing Considerations
Immunotherapy Agents *(Cont.)*			
Monoclonal antibodies: Humanized *(cont.)*	Bevacizumab (anti-VEGF antibody; Avastin®) *(cont.)*		Risk of severe hypertension or hypotension is increased in patients aged 65 and older with metastatic colorectal cancer. Hypertension may persist for several weeks after discontinuation of bevacizumab. CHF occurs more frequently in patients who have received prior anthracyclines or left chest wall irradiation. Hypertensive encephalopathy was observed in a patient with breast cancer receiving dosing of 3 mg/kg every 2 weeks. (Truven Health Analytics, 2017)
	Pertuzumab (anti-HER2 antibody; Perjeta®)	CHF (0.9%–4%) Left ventricular dysfunction (3%–7%)	Assess LVEF prior to initiation of pertuzumab and at regular intervals (e.g., every 3 months) during therapy to ensure that ventricular function is not impaired. Monitored for hypersensitivity reactions for 60 minutes after first infusion and 30 minutes after subsequent infusions. Withhold pertuzumab if significant decrease in LVEF occurs, then reassess within 3 weeks. If it continues to be decreased, discontinue pertuzumab. LVEF and CHF have been reported and may require therapy interruption or discontinuation; cardiotoxicity risk is increased with prior anthracycline therapy or chest wall irradiation. (Truven Health Analytics, 2017)
	Trastuzumab (anti-HER2 antibody; Herceptin®)	Cardiac dysrhythmia (3%) Edema (4.7%) Heart failure (0.4%–3.2% with adjuvant therapy; 7%–28% in metastatic breast cancer) Palpitations (3%) Peripheral edema (5%–22%)	Perform assessment including cardiac history, physical examination, and LVEF evaluation by MUGA scan or echo at baseline immediately prior to therapy, every 3 months during treatment, and every 6 months following treatment, and every 4 weeks if drug is held for significant LVEF dysfunction. Frequently monitor for deteriorating cardiac function. Assess for asymptomatic decreases in LVEF and symptomatic myocardial dysfunction, arrhythmias, hypertension, disabling cardiac failure, and cardiomyopathy, which have been observed during treatment. LVEF monitoring is of critical importance for patients with the following risks for CHF: • Baseline LVEF < 54% • Age > 50 years • Receiving antihypertensive treatment • BMI > 25 kg/m² Evaluate LVEF before, during, and for at least 2 years after treatment. Decreases in LVEF may necessitate holding or discontinuing treatment. Cardiotoxicity contributed to treatment discontinuation in 2.6%–15% of patients receiving adjuvant therapy with IV trastuzumab. Cardiac dysfunction risk is increased in patients receiving anthracycline-based therapy during or after treatment with trastuzumab. Advanced age may increase the probability of cardiac dysfunction. Cardiotoxicity risk is increased in older patients with breast cancer. Treatment has been associated with cardiac death. Symptomatic myocardial dysfunction increases 4–6-fold with monotherapy or combination therapy, as compared to treatment without trastuzumab. Hold anthracycline-based treatment for at least 7 months after discontinuation of trastuzumab. (Truven Health Analytics, 2017)

(Continued on next page)

Table 16-1. Cardiotoxicity of Cancer Therapy *(Continued)*

Classification	Drug	Side Effects	Nursing Considerations
Immunotherapy Agents *(Cont.)*			
Monoclonal antibodies: Murine	Blinatumomab (anti-CD19/ CD3 antibody; Blincyto®)	Cardiac dysrhythmia, including atrial fibrillation, atrial flutter, bradycardia, sinus bradycardia, sinus tachycardia, supraventricular tachycardia, and tachycardia (14%) Edema (18%)	Monitor for signs and symptoms of cardiotoxicity, including capillary leak syndrome, which may result from cytokine release syndrome. (Truven Health Analytics, 2017)
Hormone Therapy Agents			
Androgen inhibitor	Abiraterone acetate (Zytiga®)	Cardiac dysrhythmia (7.2%) Cardiorespiratory arrest (0.5%) Chest discomfort/pain (3.8%; grade 3–4: 0.5%) Edema (25.1%–26.7%) Heart failure (2.3%–2.6%) Hypertension (8.5%–37%) MI (rare, but may be fatal) Torsades de pointes	Monitor blood pressure and fluid balance/retention at least monthly during therapy. Monitor serum potassium monthly. Use with caution in patients who are sensitive to increased blood pressure, hypokalemia, or fluid retention. Corticosteroids may be coadministered to reduce incidence and severity of edema. Use with caution in patients with known heart or vascular disease known to be compromised by hypertension, hypokalemia, or fluid retention. Heart failure may lead to treatment discontinuation. (Truven Health Analytics, 2017)

ACE—angiotensin-converting enzyme; BMI—body mass index; BNP—B-type (brain) natriuretic peptide; bpm—beats per minute; CHF—congestive heart failure; CTLA-4—cytotoxic T-lymphocyte antigen 4; DBP—diastolic blood pressure; ECG—electrocardiogram; echo—echocardiography; EGFR—epidermal growth factor receptor; 5-FU—5-fluorouracil; G-CSF—granulocyte–colony-stimulating factor; GM-CSF—granulocyte macrophage–colony-stimulating factor; HER2—human epidermal growth factor receptor 2; IFN—interferon; IL—interleukin; INR—international normalized ratio; IV—intravenous; LLN—lower limit of normal; LVEF—left ventricular ejection fraction; MI—myocardial infarction; ms—milliseconds; MUGA—multigated acquisition; NYHA—New York Heart Association; PEG-G-CSF—pegylated granulocyte–colony-stimulating factor; QTc—corrected QT interval; QTcF—corrected QT interval using Fridericia's calculation; SBP—systolic blood pressure; VEGFR2—vascular endothelial growth factor receptor 2

References

Akhtar, M.I., Ullah, H., & Hamid, M. (2011). Magnesium, a drug of diverse use. *Journal of the Pakistan Medical Association, 61,* 1220–1225. Retrieved from http://jpma.org.pk/full_article_text.php?article_id=3191

Al-Khatib, S.M., LaPointe, N.M.A., Kramer, J.M., & Califf, R.M. (2003). What clinicians should know about the QT interval. *JAMA, 289,* 2120–2127. https://doi.org/10.1001/jama.289.16.2120

Al-Zaiti, S.S., Pelter, M.M., & Carey, M.G. (2011). Exercise stress treadmill testing. *American Journal of Critical Care, 20,* 259–260. https://doi.org/10.4037/ajcc2011492

Anderson, L., Brown, J.P.R., Clark, A.M., Dalal, H., Rossau, H.K., Bridges, C., & Taylor, R.S. (2017). Patient education in the management of coronary heart disease. *Cochrane Database of Systematic Reviews, 2017*(6). https://doi.org/10.1002/14651858.CD008895.pub3

Anderson, L., Thompson, D.R., Oldridge, N., Zwisler, A.D., Rees, K., Martin, N., & Taylor RS. (2016). Exercise-based cardiac rehabilitation for coronary heart disease. *Cochrane Database of Systematic Reviews, 2016*(1). https://doi.org/10.1002/14651858.CD001800.pub3

Arima, Y., Oshima, S., Noda, K., Fukushima, H., Taniguchi, I., Nakamura, S., ... Ogawa, H. (2009). Sorafenib-induced acute myocardial infarction due to coronary artery spasm. *Journal of Cardiology, 54,* 512–515. https://doi.org/10.1016/j.jjcc.2009.03.009

Armstrong, G.T., Oeffinger, K.C., Chen, Y., Kawashima, T., Yasui, Y., Leisenring, W., ... Meacham, L.R. (2013). Modifiable risk factors and major cardiac events among adult survivors of childhood cancer. *Journal of Clinical Oncology, 31,* 3673–3680. https://doi.org/10.1200/JCO.2013.49.3205

Arrighi, J.A., & Dilsizian, V. (2012). Multimodality imaging for assessment of myocardial viability: Nuclear, echocardiography, MR, and CT. *Current Cardiology Reports, 14,* 234–243. https://doi.org/10.1007/s11886-011-0242-x

Basselin, C., Fontanges, T., Descotes, J., Chevalier, P., Bui-Xuan, B., Feinard, G., & Timour, Q. (2011). 5-Fluorouracil–induced Tako-Tsubo–like syndrome. *Pharmacotherapy, 31,* 226. https://doi.org/10.1592/phco.31.2.226

Bello, C.L., Mulay, M., Huang, X., Patyna, S., Dinolfo, M., Levine, S., ... Rosen, L. (2009). Electrocardiographic characterization of the QTc interval in patients with advanced solid tumors: Pharmacokinetic-pharmacodynamic evaluation of sunitinib. *Clinical Cancer Research, 15,* 7045–7052. https://doi.org/10.1158/1078-0432.CCR-09-1521

Biogen Inc. & Genentech, Inc. (2016). *Rituxan®* (rituximab) [Package insert]. South San Francisco, CA: Genentech, Inc.

Bird, B.R., & Swain, S.M. (2008). Cardiac toxicity in breast cancer survivors: Review of potential cardiac problems. *Clinical Can-*

cer Research, 14, 14–24. https://doi.org/10.1158/1078-0432.CCR-07-1033

Bloom, M.W., Hamo, C.E., Cardinale, D., Ky, B., Nohria, A., Baer, L., … Butler, J. (2016). Cancer therapy–related cardiac dysfunction and heart failure: Part 1: Definitions, pathophysiology, risk factors, and imaging. *Circulation: Heart Failure, 9,* e002661. https://doi.org/10.1161/CIRCHEARTFAILURE.115.002661

Bonita, R., & Pradhan, R. (2013). Cardiovascular toxicities of cancer chemotherapy. *Seminars in Oncology, 40,* 156–167. https://doi.org/10.1053/j.seminoncol.2013.01.004

Bontempo, L.J., & Goralnick, E. (2011). Atrial fibrillation. *Emergency Medicine Clinics of North America, 29,* 747–758. https://doi.org/10.1016/j.emc.2011.08.008

Braverman, A.C., Antin, J.H., Plappert, M.T., Cook, E.F., & Lee, R.T. (1991). Cyclophosphamide cardiotoxicity in bone marrow transplantation: A prospective evaluation of new dosing regimens. *Journal of Clinical Oncology, 9,* 1215–1223. https://doi.org/10.1200/JCO.1991.9.7.1215

Bria, E., Cuppone, F., Fornier, M., Nistico, C., Carlini, P., Milella, M., … Giannarelli, D. (2008). Cardiotoxicity and incidence of brain metastases after adjuvant trastuzumab for early breast cancer: The dark side of the moon? A meta-analysis of the randomized trials. *Breast Cancer Research and Treatment, 109,* 231–239. https://doi.org/10.1007/s10549-007-9663-z

Burris, H.A., III, Taylor, C.W., Jones, S.F., Koch, K.M., Versola, M.J., Arya, N., … Wilding, G. (2009). A phase I and pharmacokinetic study of oral lapatinib administered once or twice daily in patients with solid malignancies. *Clinical Cancer Research, 15,* 6702–6708. https://doi.org/10.1158/1078-0432.CCR-09-0369

Cahoon, W.D., Jr. (2009). Acquired QT prolongation. *Progress in Cardiovascular Nursing, 24,* 30–33. https://doi.org/10.1111/j.1751-7117.2009.00021.x

Camm, A.J., Lip, G.Y.H., De Caterina, R., Savelieva, I., Atar, D., Hohnloser, S.H., … Kirchhof, P. (2012). 2012 focused update of the ESC guidelines for the management of atrial fibrillation: An update of the 2010 ESC guidelines for the management of atrial fibrillation. Developed with the special contribution of the European Heart Rhythm Association. *European Heart Journal, 33,* 2719–2747. https://doi.org/10.1093/eurheartj/ehs253

Camp-Sorrell, D. (2018). Chemotherapies toxicities and management. In C.H. Yarbro, D. Wujcik, & B.H. Gobel (Eds.), *Cancer nursing: Principles and practice* (8th ed., pp. 497–554). Burlington, MA: Jones & Bartlett Learning.

Cardinale, D., Sandri, M.T., Colombo, A., Colombo, N., Boeri, M., Lamantia, G., … Cipolla, C.M. (2004). Prognostic value of troponin I in cardiac risk stratification of cancer patients undergoing high-dose chemotherapy. *Circulation, 109,* 2749–2754. https://doi.org/10.1161/01.CIR.0000130926.51766.CC

Cardinale, D., Sandri, M.T., Martinoni, A., Borghini, E., Civelli, M., Lamantia, G., … Cipolla, C.M. (2002). Myocardial injury revealed by plasma troponin I in breast cancer treated with high-dose chemotherapy. *Annals of Oncology, 13,* 710–715. https://doi.org/10.1093/annonc/mdf170

Carey, M.G., & Pelter, M.M. (2009). Complaints of skipped beats. *American Journal of Critical Care, 18,* 483–484. https://doi.org/10.4037/ajcc2009882

Carver, J.R., Shapiro, C.L., Ng, A., Jacobs, L., Schwartz, C., Virgo, K.S., … Vaughn, D.J. (2007). American Society of Clinical Oncology clinical evidence review on the ongoing care of adult cancer survivors: Cardiac and pulmonary late effects. *Journal of Clinical Oncology, 25,* 3991–4008. https://doi.org/10.1200/JCO.2007.10.9777

Celgene Corp. (2012). *Vidaza® (azacitidine)* [Package insert]. Summit, NJ: Author.

Celgene Corp. (2013). *Revlimid® (lenalidomide)* [Package insert]. Summit, NJ: Author.

Chang, P.-H., Hung, M.-J., Yeh, K.-Y., Yang, S.-Y., & Wang, C.-H. (2011). Oxaliplatin-induced coronary vasospasm manifesting as Kounis syndrome: A case report. *Journal of Clinical Oncology, 29,* e776–e778. https://doi.org/10.1200/JCO.2011.36.4265

Chen, M.H. (2009). Cardiac dysfunction induced by novel targeted anticancer therapy: An emerging issue. *Current Cardiology Reports, 11,* 167–174. https://doi.org/10.1007/s11886-009-0025-9

Cheng, H., & Force, T. (2010). Why do kinase inhibitors cause cardiotoxicity and what can be done about it? *Progress in Cardiovascular Disease, 53,* 114–120. https://doi.org/10.1016/j.pcad.2010.06.006

Chopra, H.K. (2011). Arrhythmia management: Current perspectives. *Indian Heart Journal, 63,* 304.

Chu, T.F., Rupnick, M.A., Kerkela, R., Dallabrida, S.M., Zurakowski, D., Nguyen, L., … Chen, M.H. (2007). Cardiotoxicity associated with tyrosine kinase inhibitor sunitinib. *Lancet, 370,* 2011–2019. https://doi.org/10.1016/S0140-6736(07)61865-0

Chummun, H. (2009). Understanding changes in cardiovascular pathophysiology. *British Journal of Nursing, 18,* 359–364. https://doi.org/10.12968/bjon.2009.18.6.40768

Connolly, G.C., Dalal, M., Lin, J., & Khorana, A.A. (2012). Incidence and predictors of venous thromboembolism (VTE) among ambulatory patients with lung cancer. *Lung Cancer, 78,* 253–258. https://doi.org/10.1016/j.lungcan.2012.09.007

Costa, A., Tejpar, S., Prenen, H., & Van Cutsem, E. (2011). Hypomagnesaemia and targeted anti-epidermal growth factor receptor (EGFR) agents. *Targeted Oncology, 6,* 227–233. https://doi.org/10.1007/s11523-011-0200-y

Crumlish, C.M., & Magel, C.T. (2011). Patient education on heart attack response: Is rehearsal the critical factor in knowledge retention? *Medsurg Nursing, 20,* 310–317.

Curigliano, G., Cardinale, D., Suter, T., Plataniotis, G., de Azambuja, E., Sandri, M.T., … Roila, F. (2012). Cardiovascular toxicity induced by chemotherapy, targeted agents and radiotherapy: ESMO clinical practice guidelines. *Annals of Oncology, 23*(Suppl. 7), vii155–vii166. https://doi.org/10.1093/annonc/mds293

Daga, L.C., Kaul, U., & Mansoor, A. (2011). Approach to STEMI and NSTEMI. *Journal of the Association of Physicians of India, 59*(Suppl.), 19–25.

de Azambuja, E., Bedard, P.L., Suter, T., & Piccart-Gebhart, M. (2009). Cardiac toxicity with anti-HER-2 therapies—What have we learned so far? *Targeted Oncology, 4,* 77–88. https://doi.org/10.1007/s11523-009-0112-2

Deremer, D.L., Ustun, C., & Natarajan, K. (2008). Nilotinib: A second-generation tyrosine kinase inhibitor for the treatment of chronic myelogenous leukemia. *Clinical Therapeutics, 30,* 1956–1975. https://doi.org/10.1016/j.clinthera.2008.11.014

Desai, M., Li, L., Desta, Z., Malik, M., & Flockhart, D. (2003). Variability of heart rate correction methods for the QT interval. *British Journal of Clinical Pharmacology, 55,* 511–517. https://doi.org/10.1046/j.1365-2125.2003.01791.x

Dhesi, S., Chu, M.P., Blevins, G., Paterson, I., Larratt, L., Oudit, G.Y., & Kim, D.H. (2013). Cyclophosphamide-induced cardiomyopathy: A case report, review, and recommendations for management. *Journal of Investigative Medicine High Impact Case Reports, 1*(1). https://doi.org/10.1177/2324709613480346

Dickinson, D., & Raynor, D.K. (2003). What information do patients need about medicines? Ask the patients—they may want to know more than you think. *BMJ, 327,* 861. https://doi.org/10.1136/bmj.327.7419.861-a

Doroshow, J.H. (1983). Anthracycline antibiotic-stimulated superoxide, hydrogen peroxide, and hydroxyl radical production by NADH dehydrogenase. *Cancer Research, 43,* 4543–4551.

Drafts, B.C., Twomley, K.M., D'Agostino, R., Jr., Lawrence, J., Avis, N., Ellis, L.R., ... Hundley, W.G. (2013). Low to moderate dose anthracycline-based chemotherapy is associated with early non-invasive imaging evidence of subclinical cardiovascular disease. *JACC: Cardiovascular Imaging, 6,* 877–885. https://doi.org/10.1016/j.jcmg.2012.11.017

Drew, B.J., Ackerman, M.J., Funk, M., Gibler, W.B., Kligfield, P., Menon, V., ... Zareba, W. (2010). Prevention of torsade de pointes in hospital settings: A scientific statement from the American Heart Association and the American College of Cardiology Foundation. *Circulation, 121,* 1047–1060. https://doi.org/10.1161/CIRCULATIONAHA.109.192704

Drew, B.J., Califf, R.M., Funk, M., Kaufman, E.S., Krucoff, M.W., Laks, M.M., ... Van Hare, G.F. (2004). Practice standards for electrocardiographic monitoring in hospital settings: An American Heart Association scientific statement from the Councils on Cardiovascular Nursing, Clinical Cardiology, and Cardiovascular Disease in the Young: Endorsed by the International Society of Computerized Electrocardiology and the American Association of Critical-Care Nurses. *Circulation, 110,* 2721–2746. https://doi.org/10.1161/01.CIR.0000145144.56673.59

Ederhy, S., Cohen, A., Dufaitre, G., Izzedine, H., Massard, C., Meuleman, C., ... Soria, J.C. (2009). QT interval prolongation among patients treated with angiogenesis inhibitors. *Targeted Oncology, 4,* 89–97. https://doi.org/10.1007/s11523-009-0111-3

Erichsen, R., Christiansen, C.F., Mehnert, F., Weiss, N.S., Baron, J.A., & Sorensen, H.T. (2012). Colorectal cancer and risk of atrial fibrillation and flutter: A population-based case-control study. *Internal and Emergency Medicine, 7,* 431–438. https://doi.org/10.1007/s11739-011-0701-9

Ewer, M.S., & Lippman, S.M. (2005). Type II chemotherapy-related cardiac dysfunction: Time to recognize a new entity. *Journal of Clinical Oncology, 23,* 2900–2902. https://doi.org/10.1200/JCO.2005.05.827

Ewer, M.S., & O'Shaughnessy, J.A. (2007). Cardiac toxicity of trastuzumab-related regimens in HER2-overexpressing breast cancer. *Clinical Breast Cancer, 7,* 600–607. https://doi.org/10.3816/CBC.2007.n.017

Ewer, S.M., & Ewer, M.S. (2008). Cardiotoxicity profile of trastuzumab. *Drug Safety, 31,* 459–467. https://doi.org/10.2165/00002018-200831060-00002

Fabian, M.A., Biggs, W.H., III, Treiber, D.K., Atteridge, C.E., Azimioara, M.D., Benedetti, M.G., ... Lockhart, D.J. (2005). A small molecule-kinase interaction map for clinical kinase inhibitors. *Nature Biotechnology, 23,* 329–336. https://doi.org/10.1038/nbt1068

Fadol, A.P. (2013). Heart failure in patients with cancer. In A.P. Fadol (Ed.), *Cardiac complications of cancer therapy* (pp. 159–194). Pittsburgh, PA: Oncology Nursing Society.

Fadol, A.P., & Lech, T. (2011). Cardiovascular adverse events associated with cancer therapy. *Journal of the Advanced Practitioner in Oncology, 2,* 229–242. https://doi.org/10.6004/jadpro.2011.2.4.2

Fares, W.H. (2008). Management of acute decompensated heart failure in an evidence-based era: What is the evidence behind the current standard of care? *Heart and Lung, 37,* 173–178. https://doi.org/10.1016/j.hrtlng.2007.05.001

Farmakis, D., Parissis, J., & Filippatos, G. (2014). Insights into onco-cardiology: Atrial fibrillation in cancer. *Journal of the American College of Cardiology, 63,* 945–953. https://doi.org/10.1016/j.jacc.2013.11.026

Felker, G.M., Thompson, R.E., Hare, J.M., Hruban, R.H., Clemetson, D.E., Howard, D.L., ... Kasper, E.K. (2000). Underlying causes and long-term survival in patients with initially unexplained cardiomyopathy. *New England Journal of Medicine, 342,* 1077–1084. https://doi.org/10.1056/NEJM200004133421502

Ferreira, J.C., & Mochly-Rosen, D. (2012). Nitroglycerin use in myocardial infarction patients. *Circulation Journal, 76,* 15–21. https://doi.org/10.1253/circj.CJ-11-1133

Force, T., Krause, D.S., & Van Etten, R.A. (2007). Molecular mechanisms of cardiotoxicity of tyrosine kinase inhibition. *Nature Reviews Cancer, 7,* 332–344. https://doi.org/10.1038/nrc2106

Franco, V.I., & Lipshultz, S.E. (2015). Cardiac complications in childhood cancer survivors treated with anthracyclines. *Cardiology in the Young, 25*(Suppl. 2), 107–116. https://doi.org/10.1017/S1047951115000906

Fridericia, L.S. (2003). The duration of systole in an electrocardiogram in normal humans and in patients with heart disease. 1920. *Annals of Noninvasive Electrocardiology, 8,* 343–351. https://doi.org/10.1046/j.1542-474X.2003.08413.x

Fulbright, J.M., Huh, W., Anderson, P., & Chandra, J. (2010). Can anthracycline therapy for pediatric malignancies be less cardiotoxic? *Current Oncology Reports, 12,* 411–419. https://doi.org/10.1007/s11912-010-0129-9

Gaze, D.C. (2011). The perils, pitfalls and opportunities of using high sensitivity cardiac troponin. *Current Medicinal Chemistry, 18,* 3442–3445. https://doi.org/10.2174/092986711796642571

Gerber, D.E. (2008). Targeted therapies: A new generation of cancer treatments. *American Family Physician, 77,* 311–319.

Gerczuk, P.Z., & Kloner, R.A. (2012). An update on cardioprotection: A review of the latest adjunctive therapies to limit myocardial infarction size in clinical trials. *Journal of the American College of Cardiology, 59,* 969–978. https://doi.org/10.1016/j.jacc.2011.07.054

Gianni, L., Herman, E.H., Lipshultz, S.E., Minotti, G., Sarvazyan, N., & Sawyer, D.B. (2008). Anthracycline cardiotoxicity: From bench to bedside. *Journal of Clinical Oncology, 26,* 3777–3784. https://doi.org/10.1200/JCO.2007.14.9401

Gianni, L., Salvatorelli, E., & Minotti, G. (2007). Anthracycline cardiotoxicity in breast cancer patients: Synergism with trastuzumab and taxanes. *Cardiovascular Toxicology, 7,* 67–71. https://doi.org/10.1007/s12012-007-0013-5

GlaxoSmithKline. (2013). *Votrient® (pazopanib)* [Package insert]. Research Triangle Park, NC: Author.

Guglin, M., Aljayeh, M., Saiyad, S., Ali, R., & Curtis, A.B. (2009). Introducing a new entity: Chemotherapy-induced arrhythmia. *Europace, 11,* 1579–1586. https://doi.org/10.1093/europace/eup300

Guo, Y., Lip, G.Y., & Apostolakis, S. (2012). Inflammation in atrial fibrillation. *Journal of the American College of Cardiology, 60,* 2263–2270. https://doi.org/10.1016/j.jacc.2012.04.063

Guzzetti, S., Costantino, G., & Fundaro, C. (2002). Systemic inflammation, atrial fibrillation, and cancer. *Circulation, 106,* e40. https://doi.org/10.1161/01.CIR.0000028399.42411.13

Guzzetti, S., Costantino, G., Vernocchi, A., Sada, S., & Fundaro, C. (2008). First diagnosis of colorectal or breast cancer and prevalence of atrial fibrillation. *Internal Emergency Medicine, 3,* 227–231. https://doi.org/10.1007/s11739-008-0124-4

Hall, P.S., Harshman, L.C., Srinivas, S., & Witteles, R.M. (2013). The frequency and severity of cardiovascular toxicity from targeted therapy in advanced renal cell carcinoma patients. *JACC: Heart Failure, 1,* 72–78. https://doi.org/10.1016/j.jchf.2012.09.001

Haverkamp, W., Breithardt, G., Camm, A.J., Janse, M.J., Rosen, M.R., Antzelevitch, C., ... Shah, R. (2000). The potential for QT prolongation and pro-arrhythmia by non-anti-arrhythmic drugs: Clinical and regulatory implications. Report on a policy conference of the European Society of Cardiology. *Cardiovascular Research, 47,* 219–233. https://doi.org/10.1016/S0008-6363(00)00119-X

Hayes, D.F., & Picard, M.H. (2006). Heart of darkness: The downside of trastuzumab. *Journal of Clinical Oncology, 24,* 4056–4058. https://doi.org/10.1200/JCO.2006.07.5143

Hazarika, M., Jiang, X., Liu, Q., Lee, S.L., Ramchandani, R., Garnett, C., … Pazdur, R. (2008). Tasigna for chronic and accelerated phase Philadelphia chromosome–positive chronic myelogenous leukemia resistant to or intolerant of imatinib. *Clinical Cancer Research, 14,* 5325–5331. https://doi.org/10.1158/1078-0432.CCR-08-0308

Hazinski, M., Samson, R., & Schexnayder, S. (2010). *2010 handbook of emergency cardiovascular care for healthcare providers.* Dallas, TX: American Heart Association.

Herrmann, J., Lerman, A., Sandhu, N.P., Villarraga, H.R., Mulvagh, S.L., & Kohli, M. (2014). Evaluation and management of patients with heart disease and cancer: Cardio-oncology. *Mayo Clinic Proceedings, 89,* 1287–1306. https://doi.org/10.1016/j.mayocp.2014.05.013

Hinkle, C. (2011). Electrolyte disorders in the cardiac patient. *Critical Care Nursing Clinics of North America, 23,* 635–643. https://doi.org/10.1016/j.ccell.2011.08.008

Houston, M. (2011). The role of magnesium in hypertension and cardiovascular disease. *Journal of Clinical Hypertension, 13,* 843–847. https://doi.org/10.1111/j.1751-7176.2011.00538.x

Hunt, S.A., Abraham, W.T., Chin, M.H., Feldman, A.M., Francis, G.S., Ganiats, T.G., … Yancy, C.W. (2009). 2009 focused update incorporated into the ACC/AHA 2005 guidelines for the diagnosis and management of heart failure in adults: A report of the American College of Cardiology Foundation/American Heart Association Task Force on Practice Guidelines developed in collaboration with the International Society for Heart and Lung Transplantation. *Journal of the American College of Cardiology, 53,* e1–e90. https://doi.org/10.1016/j.jacc.2008.11.013

ImClone LLC. (2016). *Erbitux® (cetuximab)* [Package insert]. Branchburg, NJ: Author.

Iyengar, S.S., & Godbole, G.S. (2011). Thrombolysis in the era of intervention. *Journal of the Association of Physicians of India, 59*(Suppl.), 26–30.

Izzedine, H., Ederhy, S., Goldwasser, F., Soria, J.C., Milano, G., Cohen, A., … Spano, J.P. (2009). Management of hypertension in angiogenesis inhibitor-treated patients. *Annals of Oncology, 20,* 807–815. https://doi.org/10.1093/annonc/mdn713

James, P.A., Oparil, S., Carter, B.L., Cushman, W.C., Dennison-Himmelfarb, C., Handler, J., … Ortiz, E. (2014). 2014 evidence-based guideline for the management of high blood pressure in adults: Report from the panel members appointed to the Eighth Joint National Committee (JNC 8). *JAMA, 311,* 507–520. https://doi.org/10.1001/jama.2013.284427

Johnson, F.M., Agrawal, S., Burris, H., Rosen, L., Dhillon, N., Hong, D., … Chiappori, A.A. (2010). Phase 1 pharmacokinetic and drug-interaction study of dasatinib in patients with advanced solid tumors. *Cancer, 116,* 1582–1591. https://doi.org/10.1002/cncr.24927

Jolobe, O.M. (2010). Baseline drug history is also important for interpretation of the electrocardiogram. *American Journal of Emergency Medicine, 28,* 637–638. https://doi.org/10.1016/j.ajem.2010.04.009

Jones, R.L., & Ewer, M.S. (2006). Cardiac and cardiovascular toxicity of nonanthracycline anticancer drugs. *Expert Review of Anticancer Therapy, 6,* 1249–1269. https://doi.org/10.1586/14737140.6.9.1249

Jugdutt, B.I. (2012). Ischemia/infarction. *Heart Failure Clinics, 8,* 43–51. https://doi.org/10.1016/j.hfc.2011.08.006

Kajdaniuk, D., Marek, B., Borgiel-Marek, H., & Kos-Kudla, B. (2011). Vascular endothelial growth factor (VEGF)—part 1: In physiology and pathophysiology. *Endokrynologia Polska, 62,* 444–455.

Kalam, K., & Marwick, T.H. (2013). Role of cardioprotective therapy for prevention of cardiotoxicity with chemotherapy: A systematic review and meta-analysis. *European Journal of Cancer, 49,* 2900–2909. https://doi.org/10.1016/j.ejca.2013.04.030

Kalsch, H., Wieneke, H., & Erbel, R. (2010). Acute myocardial infarction in a patient with chronic myelocytic leukemia during chemotherapy with hydroxyurea. *Herz, 35,* 420–422. https://doi.org/10.1007/s00059-010-3367-6

Kamba, T., & McDonald, D.M. (2007). Mechanisms of adverse effects of anti-VEGF therapy for cancer. *British Journal of Cancer, 96,* 1788–1795. https://doi.org/10.1038/sj.bjc.6603813

Kerkela, R., Grazette, L., Yacobi, R., Iliescu, C., Patten, R., Beahm, C., … Force, T. (2006). Cardiotoxicity of the cancer therapeutic agent imatinib mesylate. *Nature Medicine, 12,* 908–916. https://doi.org/10.1038/nm1446

Kim, P.Y., & Ewer, M.S. (2014). Chemotherapy and QT prolongation: Overview with clinical perspective. *Current Treatment Options in Cardiovascular Medicine, 16,* 303. https://doi.org/10.1007/s11936-014-0303-8

Kubota, T., Shimizu, W., Kamakura, S., & Horie, M. (2000). Hypokalemia-induced long QT syndrome with an underlying novel missense mutation in S4–S5 linker of KCNQ1. *Journal of Cardiovascular Electrophysiology, 11,* 1048–1054. https://doi.org/10.1111/j.1540-8167.2000.tb00178.x

Kulkarni, P., Bhattacharya, S., & Petros, A.J. (1992). Torsade de pointes and long QT syndrome following major blood transfusion. *Anaesthesia, 47,* 125–127. https://doi.org/10.1111/j.1365-2044.1992.tb02008.x

Kurtin, S.E. (2009). Hypertension management in the era of targeted therapies for cancer. *Oncology, 23*(4, Suppl. Nurse Ed.), 41–45.

Kusama, Y., Kodani, E., Nakagomi, A., Otsuka, T., Atarashi, H., Kishida, H., & Mizuno, K. (2011). Variant angina and coronary artery spasm: The clinical spectrum, pathophysiology, and management. *Journal of Nippon Medical School, 78,* 4–12. https://doi.org/10.1272/jnms.78.4

Lai, Y.L., Chang, W.C., Kuo, W.H., Huang, T.Y., Chu, H.C., Hsieh, T.Y., & Chang, W.K. (2010). An unusual complication following transarterial chemoembolization: Acute myocardial infarction. *Cardiovascular and Interventional Radiology, 33,* 196–200. https://doi.org/10.1007/s00270-009-9683-7

Lane, D.A., Barker, R.V., & Lip, G.Y.H. (2015). Best practice for atrial fibrillation patient education. *Current Pharmaceutical Design, 21,* 533–543. https://doi.org/10.2174/1381612820666140825125715

Lankhorst, S., Saleh, L., Danser, A.J., & van den Meiracker, A.H. (2015). Etiology of angiogenesis inhibition-related hypertension. *Current Opinion in Pharmacology, 21,* 7–13. https://doi.org/10.1016/j.coph.2014.11.010

Lazzari, L., De Paolis, M., Bovelli, D., & Boschetti, E. (2013). Target therapies-induced cardiotoxicity. *European Oncology and Haematology, 9,* 56–60. https://doi.org/10.17925/EOH.2013.09.1.56

Le, D.L., Cao, H., & Yang, L.-X. (2014). Cardiotoxicity of molecular-targeted drug therapy. *Anticancer Research, 34,* 3243–3249. Retrieved from http://ar.iiarjournals.org/content/34/7/3243.long

Lech, T. (2013). QT prolongation and antineoplastic agents. In A.P. Fadol (Ed.), *Cardiac complications of cancer therapy* (pp. 217–225). Pittsburgh, PA: Oncology Nursing Society.

Lenihan, D.J., & Kowey, P.R. (2013). Overview and management of cardiac adverse events associated with tyrosine kinase inhibitors. *Oncologist, 18,* 900–908. https://doi.org/10.1634/theoncologist.2012-0466

Lim, C.C., Zuppinger, C., Guo, X., Kuster, G.M., Helmes, M., Eppenberger, H.M., … Sawyer, D.B. (2004). Anthracyclines induce calpain-dependent titin proteolysis and necrosis in cardiomyocytes. *Journal of Biological Chemistry, 279,* 8290–8299. https://doi.org/10.1074/jbc.M308033200

Lindenfeld, J., Albert, N.M., Boehmer, J.P., Collins, S.P., Ezekowitz, J.A., Givertz, M.M., ... Walsh, M.N. (2010). HFSA 2010 comprehensive heart failure practice guideline. *Journal of Cardiac Failure, 16,* e1–e194. https://doi.org/10.1016/j.cardfail.2010.04.004

Lip, G.Y.H., Nieuwlaat, R., Pisters, R., Lane, D.A., & Crijns, H.J.G.M. (2010). Refining clinical risk stratification for predicting stroke and thromboembolism in atrial fibrillation using a novel risk factor-based approach: The Euro Heart Survey on Atrial Fibrillation. *Chest, 137,* 263–272. https://doi.org/10.1378/chest.09-1584

Londhey, V.A., & Parikh, F.S. (2009). Paclitaxel-induced myocardial infarction in a case of carcinoma ovary. *Journal of the Association of Physicians of India, 57,* 342–343.

Lyman, G.H., Khorana, A.A., Falanga, A., Clarke-Pearson, D., Flowers, C., Jahanzeb, M., ... Francis, C.W. (2007). American Society of Clinical Oncology guideline: Recommendations for venous thromboembolism prophylaxis and treatment in patients with cancer. *Journal of Clinical Oncology, 25,* 5490–5505. https://doi.org/10.1200/JCO.2007.14.1283

Mackey, J.R., Clemons, M., Côté, M.A., Delgado, D., Dent, S., Paterson, A., ... Verma, S. (2008). Cardiac management during adjuvant trastuzumab therapy: Recommendations of the Canadian Trastuzumab Working Group. *Current Oncology, 15,* 24–35. https://doi.org/10.3747/co.2008.199

Maitland, M.L., Bakris, G.L., Black, H.R., Chen, H.X., Durand, J.-B., Elliott, W.J., ... Tang, W.H.W. (2010). Initial assessment, surveillance, and management of blood pressure in patients receiving vascular endothelial growth factor signaling pathway inhibitors. *Journal of the National Cancer Institute, 102,* 596–604. https://doi.org/10.1093/jnci/djq091

Mancia, G., Fagard, R., Narkiewicz, K., Redon, J., Zanchetti, A., Bohm, M., ... Wood, D.A. (2013). 2013 ESH/ESC guidelines for the management of arterial hypertension: The Task Force for the Management of Arterial Hypertension of the European Society of Hypertension (ESH) and of the European Society of Cardiology (ESC). *European Heart Journal, 34,* 2159–2219. https://doi.org/10.1093/eurheartj/eht151

Mann, D.L. (2006). Targeted cancer therapeutics: The heartbreak of success. *Nature Medicine, 12,* 881–882. https://doi.org/10.1038/nm0806-881

Molteni, L.P., Rampinelli, I., Cergnul, M., Scaglietti, U., Paino, A.M., Noonan, D.M., ... Albini, A. (2010). Capecitabine in breast cancer: The issue of cardiotoxicity during fluoropyrimidine treatment. *Breast Journal, 16*(Suppl. 1), S45–S48. https://doi.org/10.1111/j.1524-4741.2010.01004.x

Mottram, A.R., & Svenson, J.E. (2011). Rhythm disturbances. *Emergency Medicine Clinics of North America, 29,* 729–746. https://doi.org/10.1016/j.emc.2011.08.007

Mouhayar, E., Durand, J.-B., & Cortes, J. (2013). Cardiovascular toxicity of tyrosine kinase inhibitors. *Expert Opinion on Drug Safety, 12,* 687–696. https://doi.org/10.1517/14740338.2013.788642

Mourad, J.J., des Guetz, G., Debbabi, H., & Levy, B.I. (2008). Blood pressure rise following angiogenesis inhibition by bevacizumab. A crucial role for microcirculation. *Annals of Oncology, 19,* 927–934. https://doi.org/10.1093/annonc/mdm550

Muehlbauer, P.M., Callahan, A., Zlott, D., & Dahl, B.J. (2018). Biotherapy. In C.H. Yarbro, D. Wujcik, & B.H. Gobel (Eds.), *Cancer nursing: Principles and practice* (8th ed., pp. 611–652). Burlington, MA: Jones & Bartlett Learning.

Murphy, S.W., & Salire, E.C. (2013). Atrial dysrhythmias and atrioventricular blocks. In A.P. Fadol (Ed.), *Cardiac complications of cancer therapy* (pp. 195–215). Pittsburgh, PA: Oncology Nursing Society.

Murthy, S.C., Law, S., Whooley, B.P., Alexandrou, A., Chu, K.M., & Wong, J. (2003). Atrial fibrillation after esophagectomy is a marker for postoperative morbidity and mortality. *Journal of Thoracic and Cardiovascular Surgery, 126,* 1162–1167. https://doi.org/10.1016/S0022-5223(03)00974-7

National Cancer Institute. (n.d.). Cardiotoxicity. In *NCI Dictionary of cancer terms.* Retrieved from https://www.cancer.gov/publications/dictionaries/cancer-terms/def/cardiotoxicity

National Cancer Institute Cancer Therapy Evaluation Program. (2017). *Common terminology criteria for adverse events* [v.5.0]. Retrieved from https://ctep.cancer.gov/protocoldevelopment/electronic_applications/docs/CTCAE_v5_Quick_Reference_5x7.pdf

Nguyen, D.T., & Shayahi, S. (2012). Pazopanib: Approval for soft-tissue sarcoma. *Journal of the Advanced Practitioner in Oncology, 4,* 53–57.

Olesen, J.B., Torp-Pedersen, C., Hansen, M.L., & Lip, G.Y.H. (2012). The value of the CHA_2DS_2-VASc score for refining stroke risk stratification in patients with atrial fibrillation with a $CHADS_2$ score 0–1: A nationwide cohort study. *Thrombosis and Haemostasis, 107,* 1172–1179. https://doi.org/10.1160/TH12-03-0175

Onaitis, M., D'Amico, T., Zhao, Y., O'Brien, S., & Harpole, D. (2010). Risk factors for atrial fibrillation after lung cancer surgery: Analysis of the Society of Thoracic Surgeons General Thoracic Surgery Database. *Annals of Thoracic Surgery, 90,* 368–374. https://doi.org/10.1016/j.athoracsur.2010.03.100

Patel, M.R., Mahaffey, K.W., Garg, J., Pan, G., Singer, D.E., Hacke, W., ... Califf, R.M. (2011). Rivaroxaban versus warfarin in nonvalvular atrial fibrillation. *New England Journal of Medicine, 365,* 883–891. https://doi.org/10.1056/NEJMoa1009638

Patel, T.V., Morgan, J.A., Demetri, G.D., George, S., Maki, R.G., Quigley, M., & Humphreys, B.D. (2008). A preeclampsia-like syndrome characterized by reversible hypertension and proteinuria induced by the multitargeted kinase inhibitors sunitinib and sorafenib. *Journal of the National Cancer Institute, 100,* 282–284. https://doi.org/10.1093/jnci/djm311

Pepin, J., & Shields, C. (2012). Advances in diagnosis and management of hypokalemic and hyperkalemic emergencies. *Emergency Medicine Practice, 14,* 1–17.

Perez, E.A., Suman, V.J., Davidson, N.E., Sledge, G.W., Kaufman, P.A., Hudis, C.A., ... Rodeheffer, R.J. (2008). Cardiac safety analysis of doxorubicin and cyclophosphamide followed by paclitaxel with or without trastuzumab in the North Central Cancer Treatment Group N9831 adjuvant breast cancer trial. *Journal of Clinical Oncology, 26,* 1231–1238. https://doi.org/10.1200/JCO.2007.13.5467

Pfizer Inc. (2012). *Zinecard® (dexrazoxane)* [Package insert]. New York, NY: Author.

Piccart-Gebhart, M.J., Procter, M., Leyland-Jones, B., Goldhirsch, A., Untch, M., Smith, I., ... Gelber, R.D. (2005). Trastuzumab after adjuvant chemotherapy in HER2-positive breast cancer. *New England Journal of Medicine, 353,* 1659–1672. https://doi.org/10.1056/NEJMoa052306

Pichon, M.F., Cvitkovic, F., Hacene, K., Delaunay, J., Lokiec, F., Collignon, M.A., & Pecking, A.P. (2005). Drug-induced cardiotoxicity studied by longitudinal B-type natriuretic peptide assays and radionuclide ventriculography. *In Vivo, 19,* 567–576.

Plana, J.C., Galderisi, M., Barac, A., Ewer, M.S., Ky, B., Scherrer-Crosbie, M., ... Lancellotti, P. (2014). Expert consensus for multimodality imaging evaluation of adult patients during and after cancer therapy: A report from the American Society of Echocardiography and the European Association of Cardiovascular Imaging. *Journal of the American Society of Echocardiography, 27,* 911–939. https://doi.org/10.1016/j.echo.2014.07.012

Porto, I., Leo, A., Miele, L., Pompili, M., Landolfi, R., & Crea, F. (2010). A case of variant angina in a patient under chronic treatment with sorafenib. *Nature Reviews Clinical Oncology, 7,* 476–480. https://doi.org/10.1038/nrclinonc.2010.67

Potpara, T.S., & Lip, G.Y.H. (2011). Lone atrial fibrillation: What is known and what is to come. *International Journal of Clinical Practice, 65,* 446–457. https://doi.org/10.1111/j.1742-1241.2010.02618.x

Potpara, T.S., Polovina, M.M., Licina, M.M., Marinkovic, J.M., Prostran, M.S., & Lip, G.Y.H. (2012). Reliable identification of "truly low" thromboembolic risk in patients initially diagnosed with "lone" atrial fibrillation: The Belgrade Atrial Fibrillation Study. *Circulation: Arrhythmia and Electrophysiology, 5,* 319–326. https://doi.org/10.1161/CIRCEP.111.966713

Priori, S.G., Blomström-Lundqvist, C., Mazzanti, A., Blom, N., Borggrefe, M., Camm, J., … Van Veldhuisen, D.J. (2015). 2015 ESC guidelines for the management of patients with ventricular arrhythmias and the prevention of sudden cardiac death: The Task Force for the Management of Patients with Ventricular Arrhythmias and the Prevention of Sudden Cardiac Death of the European Society of Cardiology (ESC). Endorsed by: Association for European Paediatric and Congenital Cardiology (AEPC). *European Heart Journal, 36,* 2793–2867. https://doi.org/10.1093/eurheartj/ehv316

Prometheus Laboratories Inc. (2012). *Proleukin® (aldesleukin)* [Package insert]. San Diego, CA: Author.

Ranpura, V., Pulipati, B., Chu, D., Zhu, X., & Wu, S. (2010). Increased risk of high-grade hypertension with bevacizumab in cancer patients: A meta-analysis. *American Journal of Hypertension, 23,* 460–468. https://doi.org/10.1038/ajh.2010.25

Raschi, E., & De Ponti, F. (2012). Cardiovascular toxicity of anticancer-targeted therapy: Emerging issues in the era of cardio-oncology. *Internal and Emergency Medicine, 7,* 113–131. https://doi.org/10.1007/s11739-011-0744-y

Regeneron Pharmaceuticals, Inc. (2013). *Zaltrap® (ziv-aflibercept)* [Package insert]. Bridgewater, NJ: Author.

Rowinsky, E.K., McGuire, W.P., Guarnieri, T., Fisherman, J.S., Christian, M.C., & Donehower, R.C. (1991). Cardiac disturbances during the administration of taxol. *Journal of Clinical Oncology, 9,* 1704–1712. https://doi.org/10.1200/JCO.1991.9.9.1704

Sagie, A., Larson, M.G., Goldberg, R.J., Bengtson, J.R., & Levy, D. (1992). An improved method for adjusting the QT interval for heart rate (the Framingham Heart Study). *American Journal of Cardiology, 70,* 797–801. https://doi.org/10.1016/0002-9149(92)90562-D

Saif, M.W., Shah, M.M., & Shah, A.R. (2009). Fluoropyrimidine-associated cardiotoxicity: Revisited. *Expert Opinion on Drug Safety, 8,* 191–202. https://doi.org/10.1517/14740330902733961

Saylor, P.J., & Smith, M.R. (2009). Metabolic complications of androgen deprivation therapy for prostate cancer. *Journal of Urology, 181,* 1998–2006. https://doi.org/10.1016/j.juro.2009.01.047

Seidman, A., Hudis, C., Pierri, M.K., Shak, S., Paton, V., Ashby, M., … Keefe, D. (2002). Cardiac dysfunction in the trastuzumab clinical trials experience. *Journal of Clinical Oncology, 20,* 1215–1221. https://doi.org/10.1200/JCO.2002.20.5.1215

Sereno, M., Brunello, A., Chiappori, A., Barriuso, J., Casado, E., Belda, C., … Gonzalez-Baron, M. (2008). Cardiac toxicity: Old and new issues in anti-cancer drugs. *Clinical and Translational Oncology, 10,* 35–46. https://doi.org/10.1007/s12094-008-0150-8

Shah, N.R., Shah, A., & Rather, A. (2012). Ventricular fibrillation as a likely consequence of capecitabine-induced coronary vasospasm. *Journal of Oncology Pharmacy Practice, 18,* 132–135. https://doi.org/10.1177/1078155211399164

Shaikh, A.Y., & Shih, J.A. (2012). Chemotherapy-induced cardiotoxicity. *Current Heart Failure Reports, 9,* 117–127. https://doi.org/10.1007/s11897-012-0083-y

Shelton, B.K. (2012). Biological agents. In D.S. Aschenbrenner & S.J. Venable (Eds.), *Drug therapy in nursing* (4th ed., pp. 644–668). Philadelphia, PA: Lippincott Williams & Wilkins.

Silber, J.H., Cnaan, A., Clark, B.J., Paridon, S.M., Chin, A.J., Rychik, J., … Zhao, H. (2004). Enalapril to prevent cardiac function decline in long-term survivors of pediatric cancer exposed to anthracyclines. *Journal of Clinical Oncology, 22,* 820–828. https://doi.org/10.1200/JCO.2004.06.022

Slamon, D., Eiermann, W., Robert, N., Pienkowski, T., Martin, M., Press, M., … Crown, J. (2011). Adjuvant trastuzumab in HER2-positive breast cancer. *New England Journal of Medicine, 365,* 1273–1283. https://doi.org/10.1056/NEJMoa0910383

Slamon, D.J., Leyland-Jones, B., Shak, S., Fuchs, H., Paton, V., Bajamonde, A., … Norton, L. (2001). Use of chemotherapy plus a monoclonal antibody against HER2 for metastatic breast cancer that overexpresses HER2. *New England Journal of Medicine, 344,* 783–792. https://doi.org/10.1056/NEJM200103153441101

Soignet, S.L., Frankel, S.R., Douer, D., Tallman, M.S., Kantarjian, H., Calleja, E., … Warrell, R.P., Jr. (2001). United States multicenter study of arsenic trioxide in relapsed acute promyelocytic leukemia. *Journal of Clinical Oncology, 19,* 3852–3860. https://doi.org/10.1200/JCO.2001.19.18.3852

Sorrentino, M.F., Kim, J., Foderaro, A.E., & Truesdell, A.G. (2012). 5-Fluorouracil induced cardiotoxicity: Review of the literature. *Cardiology Journal, 19,* 453–457. https://doi.org/10.5603/CJ.2012.0084

Steingart, R.M., Bakris, G.L., Chen, H.X., Chen, M.-H., Force, T., Ivy, S.P., … Tang, W.H. (2012). Management of cardiac toxicity in patients receiving vascular endothelial growth factor signaling pathway inhibitors. *American Heart Journal, 163,* 156–163. https://doi.org/10.1016/j.ahj.2011.10.018

Steinherz, L.J., Steinherz, P.G., Tan, C.T., Heller, G., & Murphy, M.L. (1991). Cardiac toxicity 4 to 20 years after completing anthracycline therapy. *JAMA, 266,* 1672–1677. https://doi.org/10.1001/jama.1991.03470120074036

Strevel, E.L., Ing, D.J., & Siu, L.L. (2007). Molecularly targeted oncology therapeutics and prolongation of the QT interval. *Journal of Clinical Oncology, 25,* 3362–3371. https://doi.org/10.1200/JCO.2006.09.6925

Subbiah, I.M., Lenihan, D.J., & Tsimberidou, A.M. (2011). Cardiovascular toxicity profiles of vascular-disrupting agents. *Oncologist, 16,* 1120–1130. https://doi.org/10.1634/theoncologist.2010-0432

Takamatsu, H., Yamashita, T., Kotani, T., Sawazaki, A., Okumura, H., & Nakao, S. (2010). Ischemic heart disease associated with bortezomib treatment combined with dexamethasone in a patient with multiple myeloma. *International Journal of Hematology, 91,* 903–906. https://doi.org/10.1007/s12185-010-0586-9

Tamargo, J., Caballero, R., & Delpon, E. (2015). Cancer chemotherapy and cardiac arrhythmias: A review. *Drug Safety, 38,* 129–152. https://doi.org/10.1007/s40264-014-0258-4

Telli, M.L., Hunt, S.A., Carlson, R.W., & Guardino, A.E. (2007). Trastuzumab-related cardiotoxicity: Calling into question the concept of reversibility. *Journal of Clinical Oncology, 25,* 3525–3533. https://doi.org/10.1200/JCO.2007.11.0106

Tewey, K.M., Rowe, T.C., Yang, L., Halligan, B.D., & Liu, L.F. (1984). Adriamycin-induced DNA damage mediated by mammalian DNA topoisomerase II. *Science, 226,* 466–468. https://doi.org/10.1126/science.6093249

Towns, K., Bedard, P.L., & Verma, S. (2008). Matters of the heart: Cardiac toxicity of adjuvant systemic therapy for early-stage breast cancer. *Current Oncology, 15*(Suppl. 1), S16–S29. https://doi.org/10.3747/co.2008.173

Truven Health Analytics. (2017). Micromedex® Solutions [Web application]. Retrieved from http://www.micromedexsolutions.com/micromedex2/librarian

Tunio, M.A., Hashmi, A., & Shoaib, M. (2012). Capecitabine induced cardiotoxicity: A case report and review of literature. *Pakistan Journal of Pharmaceutical Sciences, 25,* 277–281.

Viale, P.H., & Yamamoto, D.S. (2008). Cardiovascular toxicity associated with cancer treatment. *Clinical Journal of Oncology Nursing, 12,* 627–638. https://doi.org/10.1188/08.CJON.627-638

Volkova, M., & Russell, R., III. (2011). Anthracycline cardiotoxicity: Prevalence, pathogenesis and treatment. *Current Cardiology Reviews, 7,* 214–220. https://doi.org/10.2174/157340311799960645

Von Hoff, D.D., Layard, M.W., Basa, P., Davis, H.L., Jr., Von Hoff, A.L., Rozencweig, M., & Muggia, F.M. (1979). Risk factors for doxorubicin-induced congestive heart failure. *Annals of Internal Medicine, 91,* 710–717. https://doi.org/10.7326/0003-4819-91-5-710

Westervelt, P., Brown, R.A., Adkins, D.R., Khoury, H., Curtin, P., Hurd, D., ... DiPersio, J.F. (2001). Sudden death among patients with acute promyelocytic leukemia treated with arsenic trioxide. *Blood, 98,* 266–271. https://doi.org/10.1182/blood.V98.2.266

Winchester, D.E., & Bavry, A.A. (2010). Acute myocardial infarction during infusion of liposomal doxorubicin for recurrent breast cancer. *Breast Journal, 16,* 313–314. https://doi.org/10.1111/j.1524-4741.2009.00898.x

Wouters, K.A., Kremer, L.C., Miller, T.L., Herman, E.H., & Lipshultz, S.E. (2005). Protecting against anthracycline-induced myocardial damage: A review of the most promising strategies. *British Journal of Haematology, 131,* 561–578. https://doi.org/10.1111/j.1365-2141.2005.05759.x

Yeh, E.T.H., & Bickford, C.L. (2009). Cardiovascular complications of cancer therapy: Incidence, pathogenesis, diagnosis, and management. *Journal of the American College of Cardiology, 53,* 2231–2247. https://doi.org/10.1016/j.jacc.2009.02.050

Yusuf, S.W., Razeghi, P., & Yeh, E.T. (2008). The diagnosis and management of cardiovascular disease in cancer patients. *Current Problems in Cardiology, 33,* 163–196. https://doi.org/10.1016/j.cpcardiol.2008.01.002

Zamorano, J.L., Lancellotti, P., Rodriguez Muñoz, D., Aboyans, V., Asteggiano, R., Galderisi, M., ... Suter, T.M. (2016). 2016 ESC position paper on cancer treatments and cardiovascular toxicity developed under the auspices of the ESC Committee for Practice Guidelines: The Task Force for cancer treatments and cardiovascular toxicity of the European Society of Cardiology (ESC). *European Heart Journal, 37,* 2768–2801. https://doi.org/10.1093/eurheartj/ehw211

Zangari, M., Berno, T., Zhan, F., Tricot, G., & Fink, L. (2012). Mechanisms of thrombosis in paraproteinemias: The effects of immunomodulatory drugs. *Seminars in Thrombosis and Hemostasis, 38,* 768–779. https://doi.org/10.1055/s-0032-1328888

Zeb, A., Ali, S.R., & Rohra, D.K. (2007). Mechanism underlying hypertension and proteinuria caused by bevacizumab. *Journal of the College of Physicians and Surgeons—Pakistan, 17,* 448–449.

Zhang, S., Liu, X., Bawa-Khalfe, T., Lu, L.S., Lyu, Y.L., Liu, L.F., & Yeh, E.T. (2012). Identification of the molecular basis of doxorubicin-induced cardiotoxicity. *Nature Medicine, 18,* 1639–1642. https://doi.org/10.1038/nm.2919

CHAPTER 17

Pulmonary Toxicities

A. Overview

1. Pulmonary toxicity ranges from reversible short-term reactive airway disease to diffuse permanent fibrosis and structural destruction.
   a) Most side effects are rare, occurring in less than 1% of low-risk patients and up to 33% in high-risk groups (Balk, 2017; Maldonado & Limper, 2018; Schwaiblmair et al., 2012). On rare occasions, these toxicities are fatal (Abdel-Rahman & Elhalawani, 2015; Chatterjee, Pilaka, Mukhopadhyay, Shrinali, & Ahmed, 2015; Feldman & Vander Els, 2017; Osawa et al., 2015; Qi, Sun, Shen, & Yao, 2015; Specks, 2017; Vahid & Marik, 2008).
   b) As patients survive increasingly aggressive and multimodal therapy and the use of multitargeted therapies becomes more commonplace, additional pulmonary toxicities are emerging.
   c) Interstitial pneumonitis related to immune checkpoint inhibitors may also demonstrate a unique physiologic mechanism (Shannon, 2017; Teuwen, Van den Mooter, & Dirix, 2015).
2. Chemotherapy-induced pulmonary toxicities are divided into acute, chronic, and indeterminate (undefined) disorders (Schwaiblmair et al., 2012; Travis et al., 2013).
   a) Acute disorders occur within minutes to a few months after exposure to the offending agent. Toxicities usually have a direct effect on the lungs. Many are believed to be at least partially reversible yet may still be fatal in their most acute forms. Examples of acute disorders include bronchospasm, hypersensitivity pneumonitis, alveolar hemorrhage, differentiation/retinoic acid syndrome, noncardiogenic pulmonary edema, pulmonary alveolar proteinosis, and interstitial pneumonitis.
   b) Chronic disorders occur months to years after exposure. Most chronic disorders cause irreversible lung injury and may be progressive in nature, leading to severe disability or death. Examples of chronic lung toxicities include progressive interstitial pneumonitis, organizing pneumonia, pulmonary veno-occlusive disease (VOD), and pulmonary fibrosis.
   c) Indeterminate lung toxicities are those conditions that are undefined or have an unclear trajectory. They may begin with features of both acute and chronic disorders and are ultimately defined when the degree of alveolar damage is identified.
3. Determining the etiology of pulmonary signs and symptoms in patients with cancer can be challenging because toxicity can mimic a broad spectrum of pathogenic causes, including infectious and neoplastic (Kaner & Zappetti, 2017, 2018; Maldonado & Limper, 2018; Schwaiblmair et al., 2012; Sverzellati et al., 2015; Travis et al., 2013). Consequently, it is imperative to understand the potential for toxicity and to detect pulmonary toxicity as early as possible.
   a) Common symptoms of pulmonary toxicities include dyspnea, tachypnea, exercise intolerance, and increased work of breathing. Some disorders also cause fever, substernal discomfort, and hypoxemia (Parshall et al., 2012; Schwaiblmair et al., 2012; Travis et al., 2013).
   b) The primary diagnostic test used to differentiate specific conditions is the computed tomography (CT) scan. Although unique findings indicate some disorders, histologic sampling may be necessary to determine the precise pathology (Diederich, 2016; Sverzellati et al., 2015; Torrisi et al., 2011; Travis et al., 2013).

B. Interstitial lung disease (ILD)

1. ILD is a heterogeneous group of lung disorders involving damage to the alveoli and surrounding interstitium. ILD includes acute chemotherapy-induced pneumonitis, pulmonary capillary permeability syndrome, chemotherapy-related acute respiratory distress syndrome, hypersensitivity/eosinophilic pneumonitis, cryptogenic (of unknown cause) organizing pneumonia, pulmonary fibrosis, and pul-

monary alveolar proteinosis (King, 2017a, 2017b; National Cancer Institute Cancer Therapy Evaluation Program, 2017; Vande Vusse & Madtes, 2017; Yakabe et al., 2013).

2. Pathophysiology
   a) Postulated pathologic changes (Ryu et al., 2014; Schwaiblmair et al., 2012; Specks, 2017; Travis et al., 2013; Vahid & Marik, 2008)
      (1) Injury to lung parenchyma
      (2) Inflammation of alveoli, alveolar cell walls, interstitial spaces, and terminal bronchioles
      (3) Release of interleukins and transforming growth factors
      (4) Destruction of the alveolar-capillary endothelium leading to changes in interstitial fibroblasts
      (5) Activation of fibroblasts and microfibroblasts, which cause collagen deposition in the alveolar interstitium
      (6) Pulmonary alveolar proteinosis–like changes, which may occur with long-term interstitial pneumonitis and may be linked to severity of disease (Nunomura et al., 2016)
   b) Disease results predominantly from inflammatory features.
      (1) Fluid or bloody exudates in alveoli
      (2) Fluid between alveoli (interstitial spaces) from degradation of the alveolar wall
      (3) Fibrosis and stiffening of vascular, airway, and alveolar walls
   c) Immune checkpoint inhibitors create a T-cell hyperexpansion with immune hyperactivity (Possick, 2017; Shannon, 2017).
      (1) Direct interaction of T cells with normal tissues
      (2) High levels of CD4 T-helper cytokines and increased migration of cytolytic CD8 T cells and organ damage.
      (3) Programmed cell death-ligand 2 (PD-L2) localized to antigen-presenting cells (e.g., macrophages) with lung toxic effects
      (4) Direct lung injury caused by cytokines
   d) Resolution results in scarring and fibrosis of tissue, beginning in the interstitium and later involving the alveolar sacs. Pulmonary fibrosis is the chronic continuation of some acute pneumonitis syndromes (Travis et al., 2013).
   e) Stiff, noncompliant lungs have poor elasticity and cause increased work of breathing.
   f) Chronic exposure to chemotherapy agents may result in changes in lung connective tissue, obliteration of alveoli, and dilation of air spaces, leading to a honeycomb appearance on x-rays and scans (Diederich, 2016; Torrisi et al., 2011).
   g) Increased pulmonary pressure from connective tissue and fibrotic banding leads to pulmonary hypertension, cor pulmonale, and heart failure.
   h) Cellular mechanisms of injury (Ryu et al., 2014; Travis et al., 2013)
      (1) Direct damage: Some chemotherapy agents cause direct damage to the alveoli and capillary endothelium (e.g., high-dose cytarabine or mitomycin C) (Chan & King, 2016; Maldonado & Limper, 2018; Nucci, Nouér, & Annaisie, 2015).
      (2) Metabolic damage: Cyclophosphamide metabolism in the lung leads to the formation of alkylating metabolites and acrolein, which may cause toxicity (Specks, 2017; Vahid & Marik, 2008).
      (3) Multikinase inhibitors (e.g., sorafenib), including tyrosine kinase inhibitors (e.g., imatinib, dasatinib), and epidermal growth factor receptor inhibitors (e.g., cetuximab, panitumumab) can cause injury (Achermann et al., 2012; Maldonado & Limper, 2018; Vahid & Marik, 2008). Inhibition of the tyrosine kinase pathway may affect the alveoli and pneumocytes.
      (4) Immune checkpoint inhibitors may produce a unique physiologic autoimmune response that results in interstitial pneumonitis, but exact mechanisms of pathology remain unclear (Possick, 2017; Shannon, 2017; Teuwen et al., 2015).
      (5) Acute onset of pulmonary edema (noncardiogenic) is related to cytokine-induced capillary leak syndrome (Binder, Hübner, Temmesfeld-Wollbrück, & Schlattmann, 2011; Goebeler & Bargou, 2016; Maldonado & Limper, 2017a, 2018; Nucci et al., 2015).
      (6) Hemorrhagic pneumonitis is parenchymal injury and microvascular bleeding similar to alveolar hemorrhage but occurs in both alveolar and interstitial spaces (Balk, 2017; Vion, Pautou, Durand, Boulanger, & Valla, 2015).
      (7) Hypersensitivity pneumonitis is characterized by an acute, rapid-onset immu-

nologic alveolar reaction that leads to capillary permeability, fluid extravasation, and lymphocytic or eosinophilic infiltration of the alveoli and interstitium, impeding gas exchange (Balk, 2017; Y.-J. Kim, Song, & Ryu, 2009; King, 2017c; Maldonado & Limper, 2017a, 2018; Mankikian et al., 2014; Yakabe et al., 2013).

(8) Cryptogenic organizing pneumonia, previously called bronchiolitis obliterans organizing pneumonia, is characterized by development of fibrous connective tissue between and involving alveolar and bronchiolar spaces, inflammatory activation of autoimmune collagen deposition, and obstruction of the ventilating airways. This disorder may be associated with immune disorders (e.g., autoimmune diseases, post-transplant), infectious diseases, hematologic malignancies, and some antineoplastic medications (Bellanger et al., 2015; Kaner & Zappetti, 2017, 2018; Vande Vusse & Madtes, 2017). It has been reported in patients with breast and lung cancer receiving chemoradiation (Falcinelli et al., 2015; Murofushi, Oguchi, Gosho, Kozuka, & Sakurai, 2015).

(9) Pulmonary alveolar proteinosis is a syndrome of phospholipidosis and frothy exudates of the distal airways. Although the triggering mechanisms are not well understood, autoimmune activation is suspected. It is characterized by granulocyte macrophage–colony-stimulating factor (GM-CSF) deficiency. It has most commonly been reported after hematopoietic stem cell transplantation (HSCT), but it is unclear if it is triggered by medication exposure or immune deficits (Bonella & Campo, 2014; Chan & King, 2017a; Suzuki & Trapnell, 2016).

3. Incidence: ILD incidence varies based on individual patient and medication-related factors. Pneumonitis syndromes are infrequent.
   a) Incidence increases when pulmonary toxic agents are administered concomitantly with thoracic radiation (Maldonado & Limper, 2018; Olivier & Peikert, 2017).
   b) Incidence is influenced by cumulative dose with some agents.
   c) Combination of agents with similar pulmonary toxicities may enhance the risk for adverse effects (Teuwen et al., 2015).
   d) Incidence of pneumonitis is higher in specific populations, even when equivalent drug exposure has been experienced. Immune checkpoint inhibitor therapy–induced pneumonitis is more common among patients with lung cancer and renal cell cancer than those with melanoma (Possick, 2017; Shannon, 2017).
4. Risk factors (Maldonado & Limper, 2017a, 2017b, 2018; Vahid & Marik, 2008)
   a) The anticancer drugs most commonly associated with pulmonary toxicity are all-trans-retinoic acid (ATRA), bleomycin, busulfan, carmustine, cyclophosphamide, cytosine arabinoside, everolimus, gemcitabine, methotrexate, mitomycin C, oxaliplatin, rituximab, and tamoxifen (Maldonado & Limper, 2017a; Mizuno et al., 2012; Specks, 2017).

(1) Agents associated with bronchospasm include asparaginase, cetuximab, etoposide, gemcitabine, oxaliplatin, rituximab, taxanes, trastuzumab, and vinorelbine (Hospira, Inc., 2017; Maldonado & Limper, 2017a; Syrigou et al., 2011).

(2) Agents associated with noncardiogenic pulmonary edema include blinatumomab, cytarabine, gemcitabine, interleukins, and vinca alkaloids (Binder et al., 2011; Dhupkar & Gordon, 2017; Goebeler & Bargou, 2015; Maldonado & Limper, 2017a, 2018; Nucci et al., 2015).

(3) Agents associated with hypersensitivity pneumonitis include bortezomib, docetaxel, gemcitabine, imatinib, lenalidomide, methotrexate, oxaliplatin, paclitaxel, procarbazine, and thalidomide (Balk, 2017; Gurram, Pulivarthi, & McGary, 2013; King, 2017c; Maldonado & Limper, 2017a, 2018; Mankikian et al., 2014; Toma, Rapoport, Burke, & Sachdeva, 2017).

(4) Antineoplastic therapies associated with cryptogenic organizing pneumonia include radiofrequency ablation, radiation therapy, bleomycin, busulfan, everolimus, interferon alfa-1, platinum agents, rituximab, sirolimus, tacrolimus, temozolomide, thalidomide, and trastuzumab (Bräunlich, Seyfarth, Frille, & Wirtz, 2015; Maldonado

& Limper, 2017a, 2018; Olivier & Peikert, 2017; Vande Vusse & Madtes, 2017).

b) Agents associated with nonspecific dyspnea include ATRA, azathioprine, cetuximab, chlorambucil, chlorozotocin, crizotinib, dasatinib, docetaxel, doxorubicin, erlotinib, etoposide, fludarabine, gemcitabine, ifosfamide, imatinib, irinotecan, lenalidomide, lomustine, melphalan, mercaptopurine, mitoxantrone, nilotinib, panitumumab, pemetrexed, procarbazine, semustine, temozolomide, temsirolimus, thalidomide, trastuzumab, vinblastine, and vindesine (Maldonado & Limper, 2017a, 2018).

c) General patient-specific risk factors for ILD (King, 2017a; Maldonado & Limper, 2017a; Olivier & Peikert, 2017; Takeda et al., 2012)

(1) Age: Because the effectiveness of the antioxidant defense system decreases with age, susceptibility to pulmonary toxicity from certain cytotoxic drugs increases significantly after age 70 (Maldonado & Limper, 2017a).

(2) Tobacco smoking (Keldsen, Jöhnk, & Ejlersen, 2016; Margaritopoulos, Vasarmidi, Jacob, Wells, & Antoniou, 2015; Shannon, 2017)

(3) Deteriorating creatinine clearance affecting drug clearance has been implicated in increased risk for pneumonitis and pulmonary fibrosis (Balk, 2017).

(4) High oxygen concentrations (above 60% fraction of inspired oxygen), such as those used during administration of general anesthesia, can enhance the pulmonary toxicity of bleomycin (Olivier & Peikert, 2017).

(5) Prior lung disease (e.g., chronic obstructive pulmonary disease) or reduced lung reserve (King, 2017a; Willemsen et al., 2016; Xu et al., 2012)

(6) Autoimmune disease enhances release of inflammatory mediators that increase drug-related pulmonary toxicity (King, 2017a; Teuwen et al., 2015).

(7) Graft-versus-host disease (Abugideiri et al., 2016)

d) Treatment-related factors (see Table 17-1)

(1) Thoracic radiation therapy (Abugideiri et al., 2016; Maldonado & Limper, 2018; Olivier & Peikert, 2017)

(2) Multidrug regimens such as those including bleomycin, busulfan, carmustine, melphalan, mitomycin, cyclophosphamide, or methotrexate (Binder et al., 2011; Desai et al., 2016; Maldonado & Limper, 2017a, 2018; Specks, 2017). It has not been determined whether any single drug is the causative agent or if the interaction of these antineoplastics results in enhanced toxicity.

(3) Concurrent chemotherapy and radiation therapy, especially with transplant therapies, bleomycin, carmustine, cyclophosphamide, or doxorubicin, has been associated with interstitial pulmonary pneumonitis (Desai et al., 2016; Maldonado & Limper, 2018; Olivier & Peikert, 2017; Specks, 2017).

(4) Cumulative dose: Increasing toxicity with increasing dose is believed to be a result of drug accumulation in the lung itself. Two patterns of dose-related pulmonary toxicity are clinically observed.

(a) A threshold effect: A definite increase in risk for pulmonary toxicity occurs when a cumulative dose is reached.

i. Total lifetime dose of bleomycin exceeding 400 units (Feldman & Vander Els, 2017; Fresenius Kabi USA, LLC, 2016a): Recent studies suggest that toxicity may occur as early as 180–240 units in patients treated for germ cell malignancies (Stein, Zidan, Charas, Gershuny, & Ben-Yosef, 2015).

ii. Busulfan, in the absence of other predisposing factors, total dose greater than 500 mg (Aspen Global Inc., 2011)

iii. Mitomycin maximum dose of 30 mg/m^2 (Chan & King, 2016)

iv. Lomustine dose greater than 1,100 mg/m^2 (NextSource Biotechnology, LLC, 2013)

(b) A linear effect: Risk for the development of pulmonary toxicity constantly increases as more drug is administered (e.g., carmustine [Heritage Pharmaceuticals, 2017]).

(5) Long-term treatment (e.g., busulfan, imatinib treatment)

e) Risk factors for direct injury

Table 17-1. Pulmonary Toxicities of Antineoplastic and Supportive Agents

Classification	Drug	Incidence	Side Effects	Nursing Considerations
Chemotherapy Agents				
Alkylating agents	Busulfan (IV: Busulfex®; oral: Myleran®)	Incidence is rare but serious. Busulfan is associated with pulmonary damage and pneumonitis. Toxicity occurs in 2.5%–11.5% of patients, usually those on long-term treatment, although it can occur more acutely. Mean time from exposure to interstitial pneumonitis toxicity is 4 years (range = 8 months to 10 years). Risk increases with total doses > 500 mg, concurrent pulmonary toxic medications, and preexisting lung disease. (Aspen Global Inc., 2011; Ranchoux et al., 2015; Russi & Negrin, 2018)	Interstitial pneumonitis, pulmonary fibrosis, organizing pneumonia, pulmonary VOD; insidious-onset cough, dyspnea, and low-grade fever; bronchopulmonary dysplasia progressing to interstitial pulmonary fibrosis ("busulfan lung") Bronchopulmonary dysplasia with pulmonary fibrosis is a rare but serious complication following chronic busulfan therapy. Chest x-rays show diffuse linear densities, sometimes with reticular nodular or nodular infiltrates or consolidation. Pleural effusions have occurred. (Aspen Global Inc., 2011; Maldonado & Limper, 2017a; Russi & Negrin, 2018)	Establish baseline pulmonary function. Assess x-rays, PFTs, and CT scans as indicated.
	Chlorambucil (Leukeran®)	Incidence is low. Respiratory dysfunction is usually reported at high doses but occurs at total doses of 540–834 mg. Onset is 6 months to 3 years after initiation of therapy. (Aspen Global Inc., 2016; Dweik, 2017)	Interstitial pneumonitis, organizing pneumonia, pulmonary fibrosis Pulmonary fibrosis and bronchopulmonary dysplasia in patients receiving long-term therapy Biopsy findings may include T-cell infiltration and alveolitis. Periodic monitoring of PFTs shows decreased lung volumes and reduced DLCO before clinical symptoms. Toxicity is steroid responsive in < 10% of cases. (Aspen Global Inc., 2016; Dweik, 2017; Maldonado & Limper, 2017a)	Establish baseline pulmonary function.
	Cyclophosphamide (Cytoxan®)	Incidence is rare. Diffuse alveolar damage is the most common manifestation of cyclophosphamide-induced lung disease. In early-onset toxicity occurring within the first 48 days, no relationship exists among development of lung injury, dose, and duration of administration. Incidence of pulmonary toxicity is reportedly increased in patients who have received concomitant methotrexate or amiodarone and in chronic graft-versus-host disease. (Specks, 2017)	Interstitial pneumonitis, pulmonary fibrosis, alveolar hemorrhage Edema, fibrosis, alveolar hemorrhage, and fibrin deposition are thought to be due to accumulation of the alkylating agent metabolite acrolein. The metabolite causes lipid peroxidation normally cleared by pulmonary antioxidant mechanisms, but when accumulated, it erodes the lipid layer and causes microvascular damage. Onset of chronic fibrosis can be 15 weeks to 6 years after medication administration. Interstitial pulmonary fibrosis has been reported in patients receiving high doses of cyclophosphamide over a prolonged period. Anaphylactic reactions are associated with death. Possible cross-sensitivity with other alkylating agents has been reported.	Concomitant oxygen delivery > 60% FiO_2 may exacerbate incidence and severity. Treatment involves discontinuing the agent and administering steroids, which have good to variable response in early-onset toxicity. Delayed-onset interstitial fibrosis with pleural thickening is less responsive to corticosteroids. (Baxter Healthcare Corp., 2013; Specks, 2017)

(Continued on next page)

Table 17-1. Pulmonary Toxicities of Antineoplastic and Supportive Agents *(Continued)*

Classification	Drug	Incidence	Side Effects	Nursing Considerations
Chemotherapy Agents *(Cont.)*				
Alkylating agents *(cont.)*	Cyclophosphamide (Cytoxan®) *(cont.)*		One clinical change in PFTs that has been proved significantly predictive for cyclophosphamide-induced pulmonary toxicity is reduction of DLCO. (Baxter Healthcare Corp., 2013; McCormack, 2017; Specks, 2017)	
	Ifosfamide (Ifex®)	Interstitial pneumonitis with pulmonary fibrosis occurs with variable incidence, with the highest incidence of 6% in non-small cell lung cancer. Acute dyspnea with hypoxemia due to transient methemoglobinemia may occur in some patients. (Maldonado & Limper, 2017a; Vahid & Marik, 2008)	Interstitial pneumonitis Dyspnea, tachypnea, and cough warrant investigation of possible pulmonary toxicity. (Fresenius Kabi USA, LLC, 2016b)	Methemoglobinemia occurs because of reactions between 4-thioifosfamide and glutathione to deplete antioxidant reserves. (Maldonado & Limper, 2017a, 2018; Vahid & Marik, 2008)
	Melphalan (Alkeran®, Evomela®)	Reports of bronchopulmonary dysplasia Acute hypersensitivity reactions including anaphylaxis: 2.4% of 425 patients receiving the injected drug for myeloma (GlaxoSmithKline, 2011)	Bronchospasm, interstitial pneumonitis Pulmonary fibrosis, interstitial pneumonia, bronchospasm, and dyspnea can signal rare hypersensitivity reaction, not pulmonary toxicity. These patients responded to antihistamine and corticosteroid therapy. (GlaxoSmithKline, 2011; Maldonado & Limper, 2017a)	If a hypersensitivity reaction occurs, IV or PO melphalan should not be readministered because hypersensitivity reactions have been reported with PO melphalan. (GlaxoSmithKline, 2011)
	Oxaliplatin (Eloxatin®)	Pulmonary fibrosis: < 1% of study patients; may be fatal Peak incidence of ILD is > 3–6 months after start of therapy but is not clearly cumulative dose related. Incidence of events increases with combined therapy. An acute syndrome of grade 3–4 pharyngolaryngeal dysesthesia is seen in 1%–2% of patients with previously untreated advanced colorectal cancer. Combined incidence of cough, dyspnea, and hypoxia was 43% (any grade) and 7% (grades 3–4) in the oxaliplatin plus 5-FU/LV arm compared to 32% (any grade) and 5% (grades 3–4) in the irinotecan plus 5-FU/LV arm for patients with previously untreated colorectal cancer. (Maldonado & Limper, 2017a; Sanofi-Aventis U.S. LLC, 2015a)	Dyspnea of uncertain significance, bronchospasm, hypersensitivity pneumonitis, interstitial pneumonitis, pulmonary fibrosis, diffuse alveolar hemorrhage, organizing pneumonia Anaphylactic-like reactions, thought to be related to eosinophilic infiltration of the lungs, are treatable with epinephrine, corticosteroids, and antihistamines. Corticosteroids are of uncertain benefit for interstitial pneumonitis, pulmonary fibrosis, or organizing pneumonia. Rare cases of diffuse alveolar hemorrhage have been fatal. Previously treated patients experienced subjective sensations of dysphagia or dyspnea, without laryngospasm or bronchospasm (no stridor or wheezing). (Bellanger et al., 2015; Falcinelli et al., 2015; Sanofi-Aventis U.S. LLC, 2015a; Shogbon et al., 2013; Vahid & Marik, 2008)	In cases of unexplained respiratory symptoms such as nonproductive cough, dyspnea, crackles, or radiologic pulmonary infiltrates, oxaliplatin should be discontinued until further pulmonary investigation excludes ILD or pulmonary fibrosis. (Sanofi-Aventis U.S. LLC, 2015a)

(Continued on next page)

Table 17-1. Pulmonary Toxicities of Antineoplastic and Supportive Agents *(Continued)*

Classification	Drug	Incidence	Side Effects	Nursing Considerations
Chemotherapy Agents *(Cont.)*				
Alkylating agents *(cont.)*	Temozolomide (Temodar®)	Dyspnea: 5%–8%; sinusitis: 6%; cough: 5% Interstitial pneumonitis: Up to 4.8% in patients receiving doses > 150–200 mg/m^2 (Sun Pharmaceutical Industries, Inc., 2017; Vahid & Marik, 2008)	Dyspnea of uncertain significance, bronchospasm, interstitial pneumonitis, organizing pneumonia Toxicity may be enhanced by pneumocystis prophylaxis with trimethoprim-sulfamethoxazole, as incidence seems to have increased since introduction of this practice. Allergic reactions, including rare cases of anaphylaxis, have occurred when temozolomide was used with nitrosoureas and procarbazine. Pneumonitis may occur with high doses. Organizing pneumonia has been treated with methylprednisolone 1 mg/kg/day with moderate success. (Balzarini et al., 2014; T.-O. Kim et al., 2012; Sun Pharmaceutical Industries, Inc., 2017)	Establish baseline pulmonary function and reassess with any respiratory symptoms.
Antimetabolites	Capecitabine (Xeloda®)	Dyspnea: 14% Pulmonary effects are not considered a major toxicity but these side effects have occurred: dyspnea, cough: 0.1%; epistaxis, hemoptysis, and respiratory distress: 0.1%; and asthma: 0.2%. Most reported cases have been in combination with another pulmonary toxic agent, such as oxaliplatin. (Bellanger et al., 2015; Genentech, Inc., 2016c)	Interstitial pneumonitis, dyspnea, cough, respiratory distress	Manage toxicities with symptomatic treatment, dose interruptions, and dose adjustment. Once dose has been adjusted, it should not be increased later. (Genentech, Inc., 2016c)
	Cytarabine (Cytosar®)	Noncardiogenic pulmonary edema in doses > 5 g/m^2 (6–12 hours after dose) Incidence is approximately 14% of patients, with most (approximately 75%) reversible. Cytarabine liposomal: No pulmonary data exist. (Breccia et al., 2012; Mayne Pharma Inc., 2011; Sigma-Tau Pharmaceuticals, Inc., 2014; Villa et al., 2014)	Noncardiogenic pulmonary edema (previously known as cytarabine syndrome)—a syndrome of sudden respiratory distress, rapidly progressing to pulmonary edema, capillary leak syndrome, respiratory failure, and ARDS (Nucci et al., 2015; Sanz & Montesinos, 2014)	High-resolution CT will show diffuse bilateral patchy infiltrates. Symptoms may be reduced with fluid restrictions. (Nucci et al., 2015)

(Continued on next page)

Table 17-1. Pulmonary Toxicities of Antineoplastic and Supportive Agents *(Continued)*

Classification	Drug	Incidence	Side Effects	Nursing Considerations
Chemotherapy Agents *(Cont.)*				
Antimetabolites *(cont.)*	Fludarabine phosphate	Cough: 10%–44%; pneumonia: 16%–22%; dyspnea: 9%–22%; allergic pneumonitis: 0%–6% Rare cases of progression to debilitating or fatal pulmonary fibrosis have occurred. (Hospira, Inc., 2013; Maldonado & Limper, 2018)	Alveolitis, noncardiogenic pulmonary edema, hypersensitivity pneumonitis, pulmonary fibrosis Pulmonary hypersensitivity reactions such as dyspnea, cough, and interstitial pulmonary infiltrate have been observed. A clinical investigation using fludarabine phosphate injection in combination with pentostatin for the treatment of refractory chronic lymphocytic leukemia in adults showed an unacceptably high incidence of fatal pulmonary toxicity. Therefore, this combination is not recommended. Corticosteroids are of uncertain benefit. (Hospira, Inc., 2013; Maldonado & Limper, 2018)	Rechallenge after suspected toxicity is contraindicated.
	Gemcitabine hydrochloride (Gemzar®)	Pulmonary toxicity: 0.2%–13% Dyspnea: 23% (severe dyspnea in 3%) Bronchospasm: 0.6% Parenchymal lung toxicity, including interstitial pneumonitis, pulmonary fibrosis, pulmonary edema, and ARDS, has been reported rarely. Severe pulmonary toxicities likely to be related to bronchospastic events, capillary permeability-induced pulmonary edema, or diffuse alveolar hemorrhage have been reported. These have led to death in approximately 0.3% of cases. Late pulmonary fibrosis has been reported in < 1% of patients. Incidence increased to 2.7% when gemcitabine was administered with other pulmonary toxic agents. Pulmonary hemorrhage has been associated with a 20% mortality rate. Radiation recall after thoracic irradiation has been reported rarely in patients with lung cancer. (Abdel-Rahman & Elhalawani, 2015; Binder et al., 2011; Eli Lilly and Co., 2017; Maldonado & Limper, 2017a; Olivier & Peikert, 2017; Vahid & Marik, 2008)	Dyspnea of uncertain significance, bronchospasm, eosinophilic pneumonitis, noncardiogenic pulmonary edema, ILD, pulmonary fibrosis, alveolar hemorrhage, pleural effusion, pulmonary VOD, radiation recall Dyspnea, cough, bronchospasm, and parenchymal lung toxicity (rare) may occur. If such effects develop, gemcitabine should be discontinued. Early use of supportive care measures may help to ameliorate these conditions. Respiratory failure and death occurred very rarely in some patients despite discontinuation of therapy. Some patients experienced onset of pulmonary symptoms up to two weeks after the last dose. (Abdel-Rahman & Elhalawani, 2015; Eli Lilly and Co., 2017; Kido et al., 2012; Maldonado & Limper, 2018; Qi et al., 2015; Yakabe et al., 2013)	Prolonged infusion time beyond 60 minutes and doses more than once weekly increase toxicities. Risk is increased when gemcitabine is administered with other pulmonary toxic medications. Bronchospasm can be treated and resolved with corticosteroids. Rechallenge may require premedication with corticosteroids. Hypersensitivity skin testing has been useful in identification of reactions. (Kuo et al., 2015; Vahid & Marik, 2008)

(Continued on next page)

Table 17-1. Pulmonary Toxicities of Antineoplastic and Supportive Agents *(Continued)*

Classification	Drug	Incidence	Side Effects	Nursing Considerations
Chemotherapy Agents *(Cont.)*				
Antimetabolites *(cont.)*	Methotrexate	Allergic pneumonitis: 1%–33% Toxicity is not dose related, but patients who receive treatment more frequently may be more susceptible to lung injury. (Balk, 2017)	Hypersensitivity pneumonitis, pulmonary fibrosis, organizing pneumonia; fever, dyspnea, cough (especially dry nonproductive), nonspecific pneumonitis, or chronic interstitial obstructive pulmonary disease (deaths have been reported); pulmonary infiltrates Higher risk for complications is associated with older age, previous use of disease-modifying immunosuppressive drugs, preexisting lung disease, abnormal baseline PFTs, daily dosing rather than weekly administration, and decreased elimination of methotrexate (e.g., renal insufficiency). (Balk, 2017; West-Ward Pharmaceuticals Corp., 2017)	Readministration with a desensitization protocol has been successfully implemented. (Balk, 2017)
	Pemetrexed (Alimta®)	Postmarketing data show low incidence of ILD with variable severity.	Alveolar hemorrhage (rare), ILD, and pleural effusions have been reported. ILD presents initially as dyspnea without pulmonary infiltrates and is reported within the first through fifth courses of therapy. Pulmonary infiltrates are diffuse with ground-glass opacities. Pleural effusions occur in 7%–12% of patients and are more common if premedication with corticosteroids is not administered. (Adhikari et al., 2016; Breuer & Nechushtan, 2012; Hochstrasser et al., 2012; Tomii et al., 2017)	Establish baseline pulmonary function and imaging to have for comparison if respiratory symptoms develop. Discontinue medication with respiratory symptoms until etiology can be established. Corticosteroids have been used with anecdotal evidence of benefit.
Antitumor antibiotics	Bleomycin sulfate (Blenoxane®)	Average incidence: 10% of treated patients Dose-related incidence: • < 270 units: 0%–2% • > 360 units: 6%–18% Nonspecific pneumonitis progresses to pulmonary fibrosis and death in approximately 1% of patients. More common in patients older than age 70 receiving a total dose > 400 units, concomitant pulmonary toxic agents, renal dysfunction, concomitant radiation therapy, or oxygen therapy. Toxicity may be lower if drug is not given as IV bolus. (Feldman & Vander Els, 2017; Fresenius Kabi USA, LLC, 2016a; Specks, 2017; Stein et al., 2015)	Hypersensitivity pneumonitis, pulmonary fibrosis, pulmonary VOD, organizing pneumonia, spontaneous pneumothorax Characteristics of bleomycin-induced pneumonitis include dyspnea and fine rales. Bleomycin-induced pneumonitis produces patchy x-ray opacities usually of the lower lung fields that look the same as infectious bronchopneumonia or even lung metastases in some patients. DLCO may be abnormal before other symptoms appear. (Feldman & Vander Els, 2017; McCormack, 2017; Stein et al., 2015)	Early toxicity may be self-resolving. Monitor for early warning signs of toxicity to avoid irreversible pulmonary damage. Chest x-rays should be taken every 1–2 weeks. If pulmonary changes are noted, treatment should be discontinued. Exposure to increasing concentrations of oxygen—increasing toxicity warrants prudently maintaining oxygen levels at room air (25%). (Feldman & Vander Els, 2017; Fresenius Kabi USA, LLC, 2016a; Stein et al., 2015)

(Continued on next page)

Table 17-1. Pulmonary Toxicities of Antineoplastic and Supportive Agents *(Continued)*

Classification	Drug	Incidence	Side Effects	Nursing Considerations
Chemotherapy Agents *(Cont.)*				
Antitumor antibiotics *(cont.)*	Mitomycin (Mitosol®)	Pulmonary toxicity (3%–36%) has been reported with single-agent therapy and combination chemotherapy 6–12 months after therapy. Prior treatment with mitomycin C, cumulative doses > 30 mg/m², and other anticancer drugs may increase risk of toxicity. (Accord Healthcare Inc., 2013; Chan & King, 2016)	Bronchospasm, noncardiogenic pulmonary edema, ILD, pulmonary VOD Dyspnea, nonproductive cough, crackles, and capillary leak with progressive respiratory dysfunction are indicative of ILD. Severe bronchospasm has been reported following administration of vinca alkaloids in patients who previously or simultaneously received mitomycin C. Acute respiratory distress occurred within minutes to hours after the vinca alkaloid injection. The total doses for each drug varied considerably. Pulmonary VOD occurs later after exposure (up to 10 years) and leads to symptoms of pulmonary hypertension. (Accord Healthcare Inc., 2013; Chan & King, 2016)	Signs and symptoms of pneumonitis may be reversed if therapy is instituted early. Drug may be discontinued if dyspnea occurs even with normal chest radiograph. Caution should be exercised when using oxygen because oxygen toxic injury occurs even in the absence of other medication-related etiologic precipitators. Pay careful attention to fluid balance, and avoid overhydration. (Accord Healthcare Inc., 2013; Schwaiblmair et al., 2012)
	Mitoxantrone (Novantrone®)	Hypersensitivity-like acute pneumonitis occurs variably when given in combination with other chemotherapy agents. (Vahid & Marik, 2008)	Hypersensitivity pneumonitis, ILD, organizing pneumonia; sudden-onset dyspnea and tachypnea with hypoxemia; patchy infiltrates on x-ray or CT scan Toxicity usually only occurs when drug is given with other potentially pulmonary toxic medications. (Chan & King, 2017a)	Organizing pneumonia detectable on bronchial biopsy or open lung biopsy usually is responsive to corticosteroid treatment. (Vahid & Marik, 2008)
Camptothecins	Topotecan hydrochloride (Hycamtin®)	Dyspnea, all grades: 20% Dyspnea, grade 3–4: 4% in patients with ovarian cancer; 12% in patients with small cell lung cancer Pulmonary fibrosis (rare): < 1%; higher incidence with combination chemotherapy or radiation therapy (Maldonado & Limper, 2017a; Novartis Pharmaceuticals Corp., 2015)	Dyspnea, coughing, and pneumonitis are the main pulmonary side effects. Pulmonary infections are more common than interstitial pneumonitis syndromes. (Maldonado & Limper, 2017a; Novartis Pharmaceuticals Corp., 2015)	Establish baseline pulmonary function.

(Continued on next page)

Table 17-1. Pulmonary Toxicities of Antineoplastic and Supportive Agents *(Continued)*

Classification	Drug	Incidence	Side Effects	Nursing Considerations
Chemotherapy Agents *(Cont.)*				
Differentiating agents	All-trans-retinoic acid (ATRA; tretinoin; Vesanoid®)	Acute differentiation syndrome in patients receiving ATRA: 14%–25%, with an associated mortality of approximately 2%. Severe and moderate disease occur with equal frequency. (Weinberger & Larson, 2017)	Retinoic acid differentiation syndrome Pulmonary infiltration of differentiating leukemic cells and their associated chemokines cause inflammatory capillary permeability with sudden and severe hypoxemia. Differentiation syndrome is present with ATRA or arsenic individually or in combination therapies. It occurs in a bimodal pattern, with 46% developing symptoms in the first week of therapy and an additional 36% having symptoms between the third and fourth weeks. Characteristic features of this syndrome include fever, myalgias, arthralgias, weight gain, peripheral edema, respiratory distress with pulmonary infiltrates, hypotension, hepatic and renal dysfunction, rash, and effusions. Respiratory findings usually include an increased cardiothoracic ratio, peribronchial cuffing, and ground-glass opacities. Consolidation and pleural effusions are common. Approximately 40% may have a clear radiograph, although this is uncommon in severe disease. Pulmonary hemorrhage has occurred in severe cases of differentiation syndrome but may be difficult to differentiate from coagulopathies common in acute progranulocytic leukemia. (Elemam & Abdelmoety, 2013; Nucci et al., 2015; Sanz & Montesinos, 2014; Villa et al., 2014; Weinberger & Larson, 2017)	Close monitoring of intake and output, weight, vital signs, and breath sounds may assist early detection. Monitor oxygen saturation for early signs of hypoxemia on exertion. Monitor chest x-ray for pulmonary infiltrates that may precede clinical symptoms. Monitor labs for evidence of renal dysfunction.
Miscellaneous	Arsenic trioxide (Trisenox®)	Respiratory events (all grades, N = 40): • Cough: 65% • Dyspnea: 53% • Hypoxia: 23% • Pleural effusion: 20% • Wheezing: 13% Grades 3–4: • Dyspnea: 10% • Hypoxia: 10% • Pleural effusion: 3% (Teva Pharmaceuticals USA, Inc., 2016)	Differentiation syndrome These adverse effects usually are not permanent or irreversible and usually do not require interruption of therapy. Risk increases with high WBC count, high percentage of blasts, and preexisting lung disease. (Leblejian et al., 2013; Sanz & Montesinos, 2014; Teva Pharmaceuticals USA, Inc., 2016; Weinberger & Larson, 2017)	Establish baseline pulmonary function. Monitor WBC counts and blast percentages.

(Continued on next page)

Table 17-1. Pulmonary Toxicities of Antineoplastic and Supportive Agents *(Continued)*

Classification	Drug	Incidence	Side Effects	Nursing Considerations
Chemotherapy Agents *(Cont.)*				
Nitrosoureas	Carmustine (BiCNU®)	Although rare, cases of fatal pulmonary toxicity have been reported. Most of these patients were receiving prolonged therapy with total doses > 1,400 mg/m². However, reports exist of pulmonary fibrosis in patients receiving lower total doses. In a long-term study of carmustine, all participants initially treated before age 5 died of delayed pulmonary fibrosis. In another report, 40% of those experiencing delayed toxicity after childhood treatment died of pulmonary fibrosis. (Heritage Pharmaceuticals, 2017; Versluys & Bresters, 2016)	ILD, pulmonary VOD Pulmonary infiltrates and fibrosis have been reported to occur from 9 days to 43 months after treatment and appear to be dose related. Fibrosis may be slowly progressive. When carmustine is used in high doses (300–600 mg/m²) prior to HSCT, pulmonary toxicity may occur and may be dose limiting. The pulmonary toxicity of high-dose carmustine may manifest as severe interstitial pneumonitis, which occurs most frequently in patients who have had recent mediastinal irradiation. A linear relationship exists between total dose and pulmonary toxicity at doses > 1,000 mg/m², with 50% of patients developing pulmonary toxicity at total cumulative doses of 1,500 mg/m². Risk factors include preexisting lung disease, smoking, cyclophosphamide therapy, and recent (within months) thoracic irradiation. Patients with baseline forced vital capacity and/or DLCO < 70% of the predicted value are at high risk. Delayed toxicity after childhood treatment has increased mortality compared to toxicities from other causes. Other risks for increased pulmonary toxicity with carmustine include history of lung disease and treatment duration. (Heritage Pharmaceuticals, 2017; Maldonado & Limper, 2017a; Versluys & Bresters, 2016)	Perform baseline and regular PFTs, especially in patients with risk factors or those who have received > 800 mg/m². CT abnormalities with carmustine occur in the upper zones of the lungs. (Heritage Pharmaceuticals, 2017; Versluys & Bresters, 2016)
	Lomustine (Gleostine®)	Pulmonary toxicity is rare; it usually occurs with doses > 1,100 mg/m² (one reported case at a dose of 600 mg/m²). There appeared to be some late reduction of pulmonary function in all long-term survivors. This form of lung fibrosis may be slowly progressive and has resulted in death in some cases. Incidence is increased in childhood survivors treated before age 5. (NextSource Biotechnology, LLC, 2013)	ILD, pulmonary fibrosis Pulmonary toxicity onset is characterized by an interval of 6 months or longer from the start of therapy with cumulative doses of lomustine usually > 1,100 mg/m². Delayed-onset pulmonary fibrosis occurring up to 17 years after treatment has been reported in patients who received nitrosoureas in childhood and early adolescence (1–16 years) combined with cranial irradiation for intracranial tumors. (NextSource Biotechnology, LLC, 2013)	Establish baseline pulmonary function. Monitor high-risk patients with PFTs.

(Continued on next page)

Table 17-1. Pulmonary Toxicities of Antineoplastic and Supportive Agents *(Continued)*

Classification	Drug	Incidence	Side Effects	Nursing Considerations
Chemotherapy Agents *(Cont.)*				
Plant alkaloids: Epipodophyllotoxins	Etoposide (Toposar®) Etoposide phosphate (Etopophos®)	Cases of pulmonary events have been reported infrequently: pneumonitis, pulmonary fibrosis, and pulmonary hypertension in < 1% of patients. Anaphylactic-like reactions characterized by chills, fever, tachycardia, bronchospasm, dyspnea, and/or hypotension: 0.7%–4% of patients receiving IV etoposide and < 1% of patients treated with oral capsules Incidence of ILD is as high as 24% when drug is given with methotrexate and cyclophosphamide. (Bristol-Myers Squibb Co., 2016)	Bronchospasm, interstitial pneumonitis, pulmonary fibrosis, pulmonary hypertension Anaphylactic-like reactions have occurred during the initial infusion of etoposide. Facial/tongue swelling, coughing, diaphoresis, cyanosis, tightness in throat, laryngospasm, back pain, and/or loss of consciousness have occurred with aforementioned reactions. An apparent hypersensitivity-associated apnea has been reported rarely. Toxicity is increased with low serum albumin and impaired renal function. Increased methotrexate blood levels occurred when drugs were given concomitantly, but it is unclear whether this is due to etoposide interaction or decreased clearance. Chronic lung disease is difficult to identify, as this agent is usually administered with other pulmonary toxic agents. PET scintigraphy may demonstrate clear ventilation abnormalities with etoposide pulmonary toxicity. Rechallenge with agent has been done with premedications without repeat of bronchospasm. (Bristol-Myers Squibb Co., 2016; Maldonado & Limper, 2017a)	Higher rates of anaphylactic-like reactions have been reported in children who received infusions at concentrations higher than those recommended. The role of infusion concentration (or infusion rate) in the development of anaphylactic-like reactions is uncertain. Treatment is symptomatic. (Bristol-Myers Squibb Co., 2016)
Plant alkaloids: Taxanes	Docetaxel (Taxotere®)	Non-dose-related interstitial pneumonitis with pulmonary fibrosis: Approximately 3%–5% of cases, most often manifesting 4–8 weeks after exposure Progression to pulmonary fibrosis: < 1% of patients Incidence of ILD is higher (up to 47%) when drug is given with gemcitabine. Pleural effusion is more common after cumulative dose of 400 mg/m^2 if no steroid premedications were given. Incidence is reduced from 20% to 6% with steroid premedications. (Binder et al., 2011; Genestreti et al., 2015; King, 2017c; Sanofi-Aventis U.S. LLC, 2015b; Tamiya et al., 2012)	Bronchospasm, hypersensitivity pneumonitis, ILD, pleural effusion, noncardiogenic pulmonary edema Usual steroid dose to prevent pleural effusions is dexamethasone 4–8 mg the day prior or same day as docetaxel administration. Bronchoalveolar lavage in early lung toxicity showed lymphocytosis in cases of reported hypersensitivity pneumonitis. (Gurram et al., 2013; King, 2017c; Syrigou et al., 2011)	Pleural effusions may be reversible with diuretics. Pulmonary fibrosis is not consistently responsive to corticosteroids. Hypersensitivity skin testing has been useful in identification of reactions. (Kuo et al., 2015; Sanofi-Aventis U.S. LLC, 2015b)

(Continued on next page)

Table 17-1. Pulmonary Toxicities of Antineoplastic and Supportive Agents *(Continued)*

Classification	Drug	Incidence	Side Effects	Nursing Considerations
Chemotherapy Agents *(Cont.)*				
Plant alkaloids: Taxanes *(cont.)*	Paclitaxel	Dyspnea (rare for single agent): 2% Rare reports of interstitial pneumonia, lung fibrosis, and pulmonary embolism: 8.5%–9% with combined therapy Events usually occur with high doses or in combined therapy. (Hospira, Inc., 2017)	Bronchospasm, hypersensitivity pneumonitis, pulmonary fibrosis, radiation recall Rare reports exist of radiation pneumonitis recall phenomenon in patients receiving concurrent radiation. Incidence may be higher in weekly rather than every-three-week dosing. Incidence is higher when administered with gemcitabine or radiation. Bronchoalveolar lavage in early lung toxicity showed lymphocytosis in cases of reported hypersensitivity pneumonitis. (Hospira, Inc., 2017; King, 2017c; Syrigou et al., 2011)	Toxicity is rarely severe or fatal and often responds to corticosteroids. (King, 2017c)
Plant alkaloids: Vinca alkaloids	Vinorelbine tartrate (Navelbine®)	Shortness of breath: 3%; severe: 2% Rare but severe cases of ILD, most of which were fatal, occurred in patients treated with single-agent vinorelbine. (Pierre Fabre Pharmaceuticals, Inc., 2014)	Bronchospasm, ILD Acute shortness of breath and severe bronchospasm occurred, most commonly when vinorelbine was used in combination with mitomycin; these adverse events may require treatment with supplemental oxygen, bronchodilators, or corticosteroids, particularly with preexisting pulmonary dysfunction. The mean time to onset of these symptoms after vinorelbine administration was 1 week (range = 3–8 days). (Pierre Fabre Pharmaceuticals, Inc., 2014)	Patients with alterations in their baseline pulmonary function or with new onset of dyspnea, cough, hypoxia, or other symptoms should be evaluated promptly. (Pierre Fabre Pharmaceuticals, Inc., 2014)
Targeted Therapy Agents				
Small molecule inhibitors	Afatinib (Gilotrif®)	All toxicities are rare (< 1%) but present with monotherapy, so are likely drug related. (Teuwen et al., 2015)	Dyspnea, cough, interstitial pneumonitis, respiratory infection. (Teuwen et al., 2015)	–
	Bortezomib (Velcade®)	Acute pneumonitis syndrome and diffuse alveolar hemorrhage have been reported rarely in case reports. (Sugita et al., 2015; Wirk, 2012)	Differentiation syndrome, hypersensitivity pneumonitis; sudden respiratory distress with accompanying pulmonary infiltrates Proposed pathophysiology is acute vasculitis. Toxicities have inconsistent reversibility or responsiveness to corticosteroids. (Dy & Adjei, 2013; Maldonado & Limper, 2017a; Oudart et al., 2012)	Immediate discontinuation of this drug is recommended when pulmonary symptoms occur. (Millennium Pharmaceuticals, Inc., 2017)

(Continued on next page)

Table 17-1. Pulmonary Toxicities of Antineoplastic and Supportive Agents *(Continued)*

Classification	Drug	Incidence	Side Effects	Nursing Considerations
Targeted Therapy Agents *(Cont.)*				
Small molecule inhibitors *(cont.)*	Brigatinib (Alunbrig®)	Incidence varies by dosage. ILD/pneumonitis: 3.7% of patients who received 90 mg once-daily dosage; 9.1% of patients whose dosage was advanced from 90 mg to 180 mg once daily (Ariad Pharmaceuticals, Inc., 2017)	ILD/pneumonitis Usually occurs early, within 9 days of initiation of medication Adverse reactions of ILD/pneumonitis can occur in varying grades of severity. (Ariad Pharmaceuticals, Inc., 2017)	Unlike similar kinase inhibitors, brigatinib has the potential for tolerization and continued dosing after pulmonary toxicity. Therefore, brigatinib is started at a low dose and ramped up to higher doses if tolerated without adverse effects in first 7 days. Monitor for new or worsening respiratory symptoms such as dyspnea or cough during the first week of initiating treatment. If new or worsening respiratory symptoms occur, discontinue brigatinib and evaluate for ILD/pneumonitis. If ILD/pneumonitis is present, follow grade-specific dosage instructions: • Grade 1: If symptoms occur <u>during</u> first 7 days of treatment, withhold brigatinib until recovery to baseline. Resume at same dose and do not escalate to 180 mg. If symptoms occur <u>after</u> the first 7 days of treatment, withhold brigatinib until recovery to baseline, then resume at same dose. If ILD/pneumonitis recurs, permanently discontinue brigatinib. • Grade 2: If symptoms occur <u>during</u> first 7 days of treatment, withhold brigatinib until recovery to baseline.

(Continued on next page)

Table 17-1. Pulmonary Toxicities of Antineoplastic and Supportive Agents *(Continued)*

Classification	Drug	Incidence	Side Effects	Nursing Considerations
Targeted Therapy Agents *(Cont.)*				
Small molecule inhibitors *(cont.)*	Brigatinib (Alunbrig®) *(cont.)*			Resume at next lower dose and do not escalate if ILD/pneumonitis is suspected (90 mg then 60 mg then discontinue; or 180 mg then 120 mg then 90 mg then 60 mg). If symptoms occur <u>after</u> the first 7 days of treatment, withhold brigatinib until recovery to baseline. If ILD/pneumonitis is suspected resume at next lower dose; otherwise, resume at same dose. If ILD/pneumonitis recurs, permanently discontinue brigatinib. • Grade 3–4: Permanently discontinue brigatinib. (D.-W. Kim et al., 2017)
	Carfilzomib (Kyprolis®)	All toxicities are rare (< 1%) but present with monotherapy, so are likely drug related. (Dy & Adjei, 2013)	Cough, dyspnea, pulmonary arterial hypertension (Dy & Adjei, 2013)	Withhold therapy until symptoms resolve for grades 1–2; permanently discontinue therapy for grades 3–4. (Dy & Adjei, 2013)
	Crizotinib (Xalkori®)	ILD (rare): Approximately 1.6% during registration trials, but is potentially life threatening Alveolar hemorrhage (rare; case reports) (Ono et al., 2013; Pfizer Inc., 2017)	Dyspnea of uncertain significance, ILD, respiratory tract infections, ARDS ILD presents as dyspnea with pulmonary infiltrates. All cases of ILD presented within the first 2 months of crizotinib therapy. Reports of dyspnea warrant temporary discontinuation of agent until ILD can be ruled out. (Kwon & Meagher, 2012; Pfizer Inc., 2017)	Coadministration of other pulmonary toxic agents or lung irradiation warrants frequent physical assessment and diagnostic tests such as imaging or PFTs. If treatment-related ILD is strongly suspected, permanent discontinuation of crizotinib is recommended.

(Continued on next page)

Table 17-1. Pulmonary Toxicities of Antineoplastic and Supportive Agents *(Continued)*

Classification	Drug	Incidence	Side Effects	Nursing Considerations
Targeted Therapy Agents *(Cont.)*				
Small molecule inhibitors *(cont.)*	Dasatinib (Sprycel®)	Pleural effusion: Approximately 10%–35% of patients across multiple studies ILD and pulmonary VOD: Rare but can be fatal Pleural effusions: Onset is 1–55 days, average 36 days. Incidence is increased with twice-daily dosing and higher daily dose (> 100 mg/day), or dose concentration > 2.5 ng/ml. Incidence is also increased when lymphocytosis is present. (Bristol-Myers Squibb Co., 2015; Eskazan et al., 2014; Miura, 2015; Montani et al., 2012; Schiffer et al., 2016)	ILD, pleural effusion, pulmonary VOD Most effusions are exudative and characterized by lymphocytic infiltration of the pleura. Lymphocytic effusion is associated with tumor response rates. Most patients who develop grade 3–4 pleural effusions have accelerated- or blast-phase chronic myeloid leukemia. Symptoms include dyspnea, cough, and chest pain. (Bristol-Myers Squibb Co., 2015; Eskazan et al., 2014; Maldonado & Limper, 2017b; Montani et al., 2012; Schiffer et al., 2016)	Most pleural effusions are reversible but may recur with future treatment (48%). Lymphocytosis during dasatinib therapy has been associated with improved tumor response rates. Treatment may include interruption of medication and administration of diuretics or corticosteroids. (Eskazan et al., 2014; Kaifi et al., 2012; Latagliata et al., 2013; Paydas, 2014; Schiffer et al., 2016)
	Erlotinib (Tarceva®)	Incidence is rare (< 1%) except when the drug is given in combination with gemcitabine, where incidence is approximately 2.5%. (Genentech, Inc., & Astellas Pharma US, Inc., 2016)	ILD, pulmonary fibrosis, organizing pneumonia, radiation recall pneumonitis Fatal ILD has been associated with oral erlotinib therapy for lung cancer. Toxicities can occur days to months after exposure. (Awad & Nott, 2016; Maldonado & Limper, 2017b; Qi et al., 2015)	Some patients have shown clinical improvement with corticosteroid treatment. Strong suspicion of erlotinib-induced lung injury warrants discontinuation of the drug. (Genentech, Inc., & Astellas Pharma US, Inc., 2016; Maldonado & Limper, 2017b)
	Everolimus (Afinitor®; Afinitor Disperz® tablets for oral suspension)	Cough of unknown clinical significance while receiving everolimus: Up to 20% of patients ILD (most common significant respiratory toxicity): 14%–45% of patients within 6 months of starting therapy. Incidence is higher when including radiologic evaluation for asymptomatic pulmonary changes. Pleural effusions: 7% Alveolar hemorrhage associated with everolimus therapy (rare): < 0.2% (Maldonado & Limper, 2018; Mizuno et al., 2012; Nishino et al., 2016; Novartis Pharmaceuticals Corp., 2016; Willemsen et al., 2016)	Cough, dyspnea, ILD, hypersensitivity pneumonitis, diffuse alveolar hemorrhage, organizing pneumonia, pleural effusion (Nishino et al., 2016; Willemsen et al., 2016)	Acute onset of respiratory distress warrants immediate discontinuation of medication with diagnostic testing.

(Continued on next page)

Table 17-1. Pulmonary Toxicities of Antineoplastic and Supportive Agents *(Continued)*

Classification	Drug	Incidence	Side Effects	Nursing Considerations
Targeted Therapy Agents *(Cont.)*				
Small molecule inhibitors *(cont.)*	Gefitinib (Iressa®)	Overall incidence of cases of ILD: 1%–3%, the highest incidence of all tyrosine kinase inhibitors Approximately one-third of the ILD cases have been fatal. ILD has occurred in patients who have received prior radiation therapy (31%), prior chemotherapy (57%), and no previous therapy (12%). Incidence of ILD with gefitinib is increased among smokers, older adults, and those with chronic lung disease, poor performance status, or concurrent cardiac disease. (AstraZeneca Pharmaceuticals LP, 2015; Maldonado & Limper, 2017b; Teuwen et al., 2015)	ILD, diffuse alveolar hemorrhage, pulmonary fibrosis, organizing pneumonia Patients often present with acute-onset dyspnea, sometimes associated with cough or low-grade fever and often becoming severe quickly and requiring hospitalization. Increased mortality has been observed in patients with concurrent idiopathic pulmonary fibrosis whose condition worsens while receiving gefitinib. Alveolar hemorrhage presents within 24–42 days after administration. (AstraZeneca Pharmaceuticals LP, 2015; Qi et al., 2015)	If acute onset or worsening of pulmonary symptoms (dyspnea, cough, and fever) occurs, therapy should be interrupted and symptoms promptly investigated. If ILD is confirmed, discontinue drug. Corticosteroids are of uncertain benefit with ILD but are routinely administered. (AstraZeneca Pharmaceuticals LP, 2015)
	Imatinib mesylate (Gleevec®)	Severe superficial edema and severe fluid retention (pleural effusion, pulmonary edema, and ascites): 2%–6% of patients taking imatinib for gastrointestinal stromal tumors Dyspnea: 14%–15% Interstitial pneumonitis and pulmonary fibrosis: Rare (Giannou et al., 2015; Kantarjian et al., 2012; K.W. Kim et al., 2015; Lindauer & Hochhaus, 2014; Novartis Pharmaceuticals Corp., 2017a)	Dyspnea of uncertain significance, hypersensitivity pneumonitis, noncardiogenic pulmonary edema, ILD, pulmonary alveolar proteinosis, pleural effusions Fluid retention events include pleural effusion, ascites, pulmonary edema, pericardial effusion, and anasarca. Differentiation of these as complications of disease or therapy was difficult to ascertain. Fluid extravasation and pleural effusions appear to be dose related, were more common in the blast crisis and accelerated-phase studies (where the dose was 600 mg/day), and were more common in older adults. However, a few of these events may be serious or life threatening, and 1 patient with blast crisis died with pleural effusion, congestive heart failure, and renal failure. (Novartis Pharmaceuticals Corp., 2017a; Vahid & Marik, 2008)	These events usually were managed by interrupting imatinib mesylate treatment and using diuretics or other appropriate supportive care measures. Symptoms often resurface when rechallenging with this agent. The overall safety profile in pediatric patients (39 children studied) was similar to that found in studies of adult patients treated with imatinib; however, no peripheral edema has been reported in children. (Novartis Pharmaceuticals Corp., 2017a; Vahid & Marik, 2008)
	Pazopanib (Votrient®)	ILD: 0.1% (Novartis Pharmaceuticals Corp., 2017b)	Pneumothorax and bronchopleural fistulae in patients with metastatic sarcoma (Teuwen et al., 2015)	–

(Continued on next page)

Table 17-1. Pulmonary Toxicities of Antineoplastic and Supportive Agents *(Continued)*

Classification	Drug	Incidence	Side Effects	Nursing Considerations
Targeted Therapy Agents *(Cont.)*				
Small molecule inhibitors *(cont.)*	Sorafenib (Nexavar®)	Incidence is very low (< 1%). (Teuwen et al., 2015)	Interstitial pneumonitis	–
	Sunitinib (Sutent®)	Pleural effusions (most common): 1%–13% Other toxicities are uncommon and usually only case reports. (Miura et al., 2014; Teuwen et al., 2015)	Interstitial pneumonitis, recall pneumonitis, cryptogenic organizing pneumonia (Teuwen et al., 2015)	Temporary discontinuation followed by dose reduction improved symptoms. High-dose corticosteroids are recommended. (Teuwen et al., 2015)
	Temsirolimus (Torisel®)	Incidence is 3%–54% of patients treated for renal cell cancer. (Dy & Adjei, 2013; Willemsen et al., 2016)	Cases of ILD, some resulting in death, have occurred. Some patients with ILD were asymptomatic, and others presented with symptoms. (Willemsen et al., 2016; Wyeth Pharmaceuticals, 2017)	Some patients with ILD required discontinuation of temsirolimus and treatment with corticosteroids or antibiotics.
Immunotherapy Agents				
Checkpoint inhibitors: CTLA-4	Ipilimumab (Yervoy®)	Toxicities are rare (< 1.5%) but potentially severe. Effects occur during induction (first 12 weeks), but risk persists for months following therapy discontinuation. Peak incidence is 2.8 months after start of therapy. Infusion reactions: 2%–4% Granulomatous pneumonitis with lymphadenopathy occurs in 5%–7% of patients with thoracic disease. Hypoxia at rest may signal early detectable toxicity. Risk is increased when combination immune therapies are administered. Incidence is less with CTLA-4 inhibitors (e.g., ipilimumab) than with PD-1 and PD-L1 inhibitors. (Shannon, 2017; Teuwen et al., 2015)	Infusion reactions, interstitial pneumonitis, sarcoid-like granulomatous pneumonitis, pulmonary edema	Treatment is corticosteroids. Permanent discontinuation of the agent is indicated in grade 3–4 toxicity. Corticosteroids continued approximately 1 month before a gradual taper. Refractory symptoms may be treated with additional immunosuppressive medications (e.g., infliximab, mycophenolate mofetil). COPD exacerbations after treatment are common. (Dy & Adjei, 2013; Shannon, 2017)

(Continued on next page)

Table 17-1. Pulmonary Toxicities of Antineoplastic and Supportive Agents *(Continued)*

Classification	Drug	Incidence	Side Effects	Nursing Considerations
Immunotherapy Agents *(Cont.)*				
Checkpoint inhibitors: PD-1	Nivolumab (Opdivo®)	Cough: 22%–35% Dyspnea: 10%–16% Interstitial pneumonitis: 1%–12%, with higher incidence in patients with nonmelanoma cancers, patients receiving combination therapy, smokers, and patients with prior lung disease. Onset is usually in first 3 months of therapy. (Bristol-Myers Squibb Co., 2017; Shannon, 2017)	Cough, dyspnea, infusion reactions, interstitial pneumonitis	Corticosteroids are used for treatment of ILD in 89% of cases for an average of 26 days, and complete resolution occurred in 67% following steroid taper. Withhold drug for grade 2 (moderate ILD) and permanently discontinue for grades 3–4 (severe ILD). Recurrent pneumonitis occurred in 8% with ILD after reinitiation of nivolumab. (Bristol-Myers Squibb Co., 2017)
	Pembrolizumab (Keytruda®)	Cough: 17% Dyspnea: 11% ILD: 3.4% Toxicities have a later onset than with nivolumab. ILD occurred more frequently in patients with prior thoracic radiation (6.9%). (Merck and Co., Inc., 2017)	Cough, dyspnea, infusion reactions, interstitial pneumonitis	Recommend 2–7 weeks of steroid therapy. Registration trials showed 67% of patients were given steroids, and symptoms resolved in 59%. Refractory symptoms may be treated with additional immunosuppressive medications (e.g., infliximab, mycophenolate mofetil). Rechallenge with agent often has been successful without recurrence of toxicity. (Merck and Co., Inc., 2017; Shannon, 2017)
Checkpoint inhibitors: PD-L1	Atezolizumab (Tecentriq®)	Dyspnea and cough: 12%–16% during registration trials ILD: 1%–2.6% (Genentech, Inc., 2017b)	Cough, dyspnea, infusion reactions, hypoxia, ILD (Shannon, 2017)	Recommend 2–7 weeks of steroid therapy (Shannon, 2017). Refractory symptoms may be treated with additional immunosuppressive medications (e.g., infliximab, mycophenolate mofetil). (Shannon, 2017)

(Continued on next page)

Table 17-1. Pulmonary Toxicities of Antineoplastic and Supportive Agents *(Continued)*

Classification	Drug	Incidence	Side Effects	Nursing Considerations
Immunotherapy Agents *(Cont.)*				
Checkpoint inhibitors: PD-L1	Durvalumab (Imfinzi®)	Cough and dyspnea: 2%–10% during registration trials (AstraZeneca Pharmaceuticals LP, 2017)	Cough, dyspnea, ILD, infusion reactions (Shannon, 2017)	Recommend 2–7 weeks of steroid therapy. Refractory symptoms may be treated with additional immunosuppressive medications (e.g., infliximab, mycophenolate mofetil). (Shannon, 2017)
Cytokines: Interferons	Interferon alfa-2b (Intron-A®)	Rare (Merck and Co., Inc., 2016)	Fever, cough, dyspnea, nonspecific pulmonary infiltrates, pneumonitis, pulmonary alveolar proteinosis, organizing pneumonia, pleural effusions, pulmonary hypertension (Bräunlich et al., 2015; Merck and Co., Inc., 2016; Papani et al., 2017)	Consider holding drug while evaluating symptoms.
Cytokines: Interleukins	Aldesleukin (IL-2; Proleukin®)	Life-threatening grade 4 respiratory disorders: 3% (ARDS, respiratory failure, intubation); apnea: 1% Adverse events occurred in 10% of patients (N = 525). Dyspnea: 43% Lung disorder: 24% (physical findings associated with pulmonary congestion, rales, rhonchi) Respiratory disorder: 11% (ARDS, chest x-ray infiltrates, unspecified pulmonary changes) Increased cough: 11% (Prometheus Laboratories Inc., 2012)	Noncardiogenic pulmonary edema, dyspnea, respiratory failure, tachypnea, pleural effusion, wheezing, apnea, pneumothorax, hemoptysis Toxicities may worsen with continued exposure or occur more quickly with each subsequent therapy cycle. (Dhupkar & Gordon, 2017; Kai-Feng et al., 2011; Prometheus Laboratories Inc., 2012; Shelton, 2012)	Establish baseline pulmonary function with PFTs, and assess abnormalities that indicate ineligibility for high-dose aldesleukin. Consider fluid limitations with respiratory symptoms if blood pressure tolerates. Consider holding or discontinuing dose with refractory symptoms. (Dhupkar & Gordon, 2017; Prometheus Laboratories Inc., 2012)
	Oprelvekin (IL-11; Neumega®)	Dyspnea: 48%; increased cough: 29%; pleural effusions: 10% (Kai-Feng et al., 2011; Wyeth Pharmaceuticals, 2011)	Noncardiogenic pulmonary edema, pleural effusions, dyspnea of uncertain significance Peripheral edema, dyspnea, and preexisting fluid collections, including pleural and pericardial effusions or ascites, should be monitored. Patients should be advised to immediately seek medical attention if any of the following signs or symptoms develop: swelling of the face, tongue, or throat; difficulty breathing, swallowing, or talking; shortness of breath; or wheezing. (Wyeth Pharmaceuticals, 2011)	Fluid retention is reversible within several days of discontinuing Oprelvekin. Fluid balance should be monitored, and appropriate medical management is advised. Closely monitor fluid and electrolyte status in patients receiving chronic diuretic therapy. (Kai-Feng et al., 2011; Vahid & Marik, 2008; Wyeth Pharmaceuticals, 2011)

(Continued on next page)

Table 17-1. Pulmonary Toxicities of Antineoplastic and Supportive Agents *(Continued)*

Classification	Drug	Incidence	Side Effects	Nursing Considerations
Immunotherapy Agents *(Cont.)*				
Immunomodulators	Lenalidomide (Revlimid®)	Dyspnea of uncertain significance: 15%–23%, but only 4% severe Hypersensitivity reactions (rare): < 1%, but can be severe and progress to irreversible pulmonary fibrosis (Maldonado & Limper, 2018; Mankikian et al., 2014)	Dyspnea of uncertain significance, hypersensitivity pneumonitis, interstitial pneumonitis, organizing pneumonia (Mankikian et al., 2014; Toma et al., 2017)	Immediately discontinue medication if pulmonary toxicity is suspected. Rechallenge with the agent after resolution of toxicity has been successful in select cases. (Celgene Corp., 2017a; Sakai et al., 2015)
	Thalidomide (Thalomid®)	Dyspnea of uncertain significance: 50%, but only 4% severe Other acute pulmonary toxicities are rare and have no reported incidence rate. (Celgene Corp., 2017b; Maldonado & Limper, 2018)	Dyspnea of uncertain significance, hypersensitivity pneumonitis, alveolar hemorrhage, pulmonary fibrosis, organizing pneumonitis, pulmonary VOD with pulmonary hypertension Sudden-onset ground-glass opacities have been noted with thalidomide. Case reports reflect multiple different etiologies: infection, interstitial lung toxicity, organizing pneumonia, and alveolar hemorrhage. It is believed that antiangiogenic properties have been temporally associated with alveolar hemorrhage in patients receiving thalidomide. (Schwaiblmair et al., 2012)	Consider infectious etiology as higher risk for pulmonary symptoms than drug toxicity. Other bleeding symptoms may support suspicion for alveolar hemorrhage in patients with respiratory distress temporally related to thalidomide administration.
Monoclonal antibodies: Chimeric	Brentuximab vedotin (anti-CD30 antibody; Adcetris®)	–	–	Concomitant use with bleomycin is contraindicated because of pulmonary toxicity. In a clinical trial that studied brentuximab with bleomycin as part of a combination regimen, noninfectious pulmonary toxicity was greater than with ABVD (doxorubicin, bleomycin, vinblastine, and dacarbazine). Cough and dyspnea were reported, and imaging showed interstitial infiltration and inflammation. Most patients responded to corticosteroids. (Seattle Genetics, Inc., 2016)

(Continued on next page)

Table 17-1. Pulmonary Toxicities of Antineoplastic and Supportive Agents *(Continued)*

Classification	Drug	Incidence	Side Effects	Nursing Considerations
Immunotherapy Agents *(Cont.)*				
Monoclonal antibodies: Chimeric *(cont.)*	Cetuximab (anti-EGFR antibody; Erbitux®)	Bronchospasm with hypersensitivity reaction: Generally uncommon (3%), but frequent severe reactions (20%) have a geographic propensity (southeast United States through southern Midwest states such as Oklahoma, Arkansas, and Texas). Most reactions (> 90%) occur during the first infusion. ILD: < 1%, idiosyncratic in nature (ImClone, LLC, 2016; Maldonado & Limper, 2017b; Teuwen et al., 2015)	Bronchospasm, interstitial pneumonitis, organizing pneumonia ILD has been reported as serious and potentially fatal. Pneumonitis syndromes have an onset of 2–6 months after start of drug and may worsen after discontinuation of medication. Toxicities are characterized by dyspnea, tachypnea, and activity intolerance. Symptoms can progressively worsen even after initial discontinuation of medication. (Achermann et al., 2012; ImClone, LLC, 2016; Maldonado & Limper, 2017b)	All dyspnea noted between cycles warrants evaluation of PFTs. Hold medication until ILD is ruled out. If drug is resumed, administer at 50% of previous rate. Recurrence of toxicity has been reported. (ImClone, LLC, 2016; Teuwen et al., 2015)
	Rituximab (anti-CD20 antibody; Rituxan®)	Pulmonary events: 38% (N = 135) in clinical trials. Infusion-related deaths involving pulmonary function occurred in 0.04%–0.07%. Bronchospasm: 8% ILD: Approximately 2%, but up to 4.8% with low lymphocyte counts (Genentech, Inc., 2016b; Maldonado & Limper, 2017b)	Bronchospasm, hypersensitivity pneumonitis, ILD, alveolar hemorrhage, pulmonary alveolar proteinosis, organizing pneumonia Most common adverse events were increased cough, rhinitis, bronchospasm, dyspnea, and sinusitis. Infusion-related symptom complex includes pulmonary effects: hypoxia, bronchospasm, dyspnea, pulmonary infiltrates, and ARDS. Increased pulmonary toxicities are seen in patients with low absolute lymphocyte count. Pulmonary toxicities are more frequent in patients with cancer than in patients with autoimmune disease. Hypersensitivity pneumonitis has an onset of days to weeks after exposure and shows eosinophilic infiltration on bronchoscopy. Alveolar hemorrhage can be acute in onset and fatal. Pulmonary alveolar proteinosis occurs more often in patients with immature lymphocyte cell types and has not been reported in patients with multiple myeloma treated with rituximab. Reports exist of organizing pneumonia presenting up to 6 months after infusion and a limited number of reports of pneumonitis (including interstitial pneumonitis) presenting up to 3 months after infusion, some of which resulted in fatal outcomes. Treatment with corticosteroids is standard for most toxicity but is not clearly helpful. It is most substantiated with alveolar hemorrhage and organizing pneumonia. (Bonella & Campo, 2014; Genentech, Inc., 2016b; Ikpeama & Bailes, 2012; King, 2017a; Maldonado & Limper, 2017b; Teuwen et al., 2015; Urun et al., 2012	Interrupt treatment for severe reactions and resume at 50% reduced infusion rate when symptoms resolve. The safety of resuming or continuing administration of rituximab in patients with ILD or organizing pneumonitis is unknown. (Genentech, Inc., 2016b)

(Continued on next page)

Table 17-1. Pulmonary Toxicities of Antineoplastic and Supportive Agents *(Continued)*

Classification	Drug	Incidence	Side Effects	Nursing Considerations
Immunotherapy Agents *(Cont.)*				
Monoclonal antibodies: Human	Panitumumab (anti-EGFR; Vectibix®)	Bronchospasm: Infusion reactions occur in 4% of patients, but severe reactions with bronchospasm occur in 1%–2%. ILD: < 1% (Amgen Inc., 2015; Osawa et al., 2015)	Bronchospasm, ILD ILD is characterized by dyspnea, cough, and pulmonary infiltrates that occur 2–4 months into therapy and worsen even after drug discontinuation. (Amgen Inc., 2015)	Monitor for infusion reactions. Evidence of interstitial pneumonitis via PFTs and high-resolution CT scan prompts permanent discontinuation of drug.
Monoclonal antibodies: Humanized	Alemtuzumab (anti-CD52 antibody; Campath®)	Infusion rate–related dyspnea: 17% Acute infusion-related events were most common during the first week of therapy. Incidence (N = 149): • Dyspnea: 26% • Cough: 25% • Bronchitis/pneumonitis: 21% • Pneumonia: 16% • Bronchospasm: 9% (Genzyme Corp, 2014)	Dyspnea of uncertain significance, bronchospasm, interstitial pneumonitis Alemtuzumab has been associated with infusion-related events including hypotension, rigors, fever, shortness of breath, bronchospasm, chills, and rash. Side effects include asthma, bronchitis, COPD, hemoptysis, hypoxia, pleural effusion, pleurisy, pulmonary edema, pulmonary fibrosis, pulmonary infiltration, respiratory depression, respiratory insufficiency, sinusitis, stridor, and throat tightness. (Genzyme Corp, 2014)	To ameliorate or avoid infusion-related events, premedicate patients with an oral antihistamine and acetaminophen prior to dosing, and monitor closely for infusion-related adverse events.
	Bevacizumab (Avastin®)	Hemoptysis: More common with squamous cell lung cancer (31%) than with nonsquamous cell lung cancer (2%–3%). Interstitial pneumonitis and organizing pneumonia: Incidence is difficult to quantify because it usually is associated with thoracic radiation. Alveolar hemorrhage: 4.4% of patients, of which 1.3% were fatal. Incidence of all-grade toxicity is lower in nonsquamous lung cancer. (Genentech, Inc. 2016a; Teuwen et al., 2015)	Hemoptysis, interstitial pneumonia, pleural effusion, organizing pneumonia All toxicities are more common in patients with squamous cell carcinoma of the lung. Most common clinical presentation is hemoptysis. Use of bevacizumab clearly increases risk of radiation pneumonitis syndromes. Mechanism of toxicity is unclear but thought to be related to blocking of VEGF. (Hollebecque et al., 2012; Lind et al., 2012; Maldonado & Limper, 2017b; Teuwen et al., 2015)	This medication is always discontinued when pulmonary bleeding of any type is noted. (Genentech, Inc., 2016a)
	Pertuzumab (Perjeta®)	All toxicities are rare (< 1%) but present with monotherapy, so are likely drug related, and may be serious in some cases. Cough of uncertain significance occurs in a larger number of patients. (Teuwen et al., 2015)	Cough, interstitial pneumonitis, pleural effusions, ARDS (Teuwen et al., 2015)	–

(Continued on next page)

Table 17-1. Pulmonary Toxicities of Antineoplastic and Supportive Agents *(Continued)*

Classification	Drug	Incidence	Side Effects	Nursing Considerations
Immunotherapy Agents *(Cont.)*				
Monoclonal antibodies: Humanized *(cont.)*	Trastuzumab (anti-HER2 antibody; Herceptin®)	As a single agent: • Increased cough: 26% • Dyspnea: 22% In the postmarketing setting, severe hypersensitivity reactions (including anaphylaxis), infusion reactions, and pulmonary adverse events have been reported. Severe pulmonary events leading to death have been reported rarely. Interstitial pneumonitis: 1%–2%, but severe in only 0.3% Chronic organizing pneumonia: < 1% Pulmonary toxicities rarely reported with trastuzumab emtansine as compared to trastuzumab regular formulation. Cough was noted in 2%–3% of patients. (Genentech, Inc., 2017a; Maldonado & Limper, 2017b; Teuwen et al., 2015; Vahid & Marik, 2008)	Dyspnea of uncertain significance, bronchospasm, interstitial pneumonitis, organizing pneumonia, increased cough, dyspnea, rhinitis, pharyngitis, pulmonary infiltrates, pleural effusions, noncardiac edema, pulmonary insufficiency, hypoxia, ARDS Other severe events reported rarely in the postmarketing setting include pneumonitis and pulmonary fibrosis. Bronchospasm in conjunction with hypersensitivity reactions have occurred. (Genentech, Inc., 2017a; Teuwen et al., 2015)	Patients with symptomatic intrinsic lung disease or extensive tumor involvement of the lungs, resulting in dyspnea at rest, may be at greater risk for severe reactions. Adverse effects increase with combined drug therapy. Corticosteroids may be helpful. Rechallenge with this agent is not recommended. (Genentech, Inc., 2017a; Vahid & Marik, 2008)

ARDS—acute respiratory distress syndrome; ATRA—all-trans-retinoic acid; COPD—chronic obstructive pulmonary disease; CTLA-4—cytotoxic T-lymphocyte antigen 4; CT—computed tomography; DLCO—diffusing capacity of the lung for carbon monoxide; EGFR—epidermal growth factor receptor; FiO_2—fraction of inspired oxygen; 5-FU/LV—5-fluorouracil/leucovorin; HER2—human epidermal growth factor receptor 2; HSCT—hematopoietic stem cell transplantation; IL—interleukin; ILD—interstitial lung disease; IV—intravenous; PD-1—programmed cell death protein 1; PD-L1—programmed cell death-ligand 1; PET—positron-emission tomography; PFTs—pulmonary function tests; PO—by mouth; VEGF—vascular endothelial growth factor; VOD—veno-occlusive disease; WBC—white blood cell

(1) Rare reports of interstitial pulmonary infiltrates and acute alveolitis with hydroxyurea

(2) Metabolic injury

(a) Metabolites of cyclophosphamide cause acute pneumonitis that may be hemorrhagic in nature. The mortality rate associated with this syndrome is approximately 50% (Specks, 2017).

(b) Renal dysfunction may cause delayed drug excretion and increase the pulmonary toxicity of bleomycin, cyclophosphamide, and methotrexate (Balk, 2017; Specks, 2017).

(3) Disruption of intracellular kinases

(a) Tyrosine kinase inhibitors (e.g., erlotinib, gefitinib) (Maldonado & Limper, 2017b; Teuwen et al., 2015)

(b) Epidermal growth factor receptor inhibitors (e.g., cetuximab) (Achermann et al., 2012)

(c) Mammalian target of rapamycin (mTOR) inhibitors (e.g., everolimus, temsirolimus) (Maldonado & Limper, 2017b; Nishino et al., 2016; Novartis Pharmaceuticals Corp, n.d.; Willemsen et al., 2016): Genetic risks may be activated by these agents (Willemsen et al., 2016).

(4) Pulmonary edema

(a) Biologic agents cause this toxicity (Bräunlich et al., 2015; Shelton, 2012). Interleukin-2 is associated with a high incidence of capillary leak syndrome. Pulmonary edema is a dose-limiting toxicity of high-dose interleukin-2 therapy (Prometheus Laboratories Inc., 2012). Severity depends on the route, dose, and administration schedule (Dhupkar & Gordon, 2017; Shelton, 2012). It resolves quickly after therapy ends and diuresis begins.

(b) Docetaxel is associated with fluid retention, alveolar permeability, and pulmonary infiltrates. These may be prevented with corticosteroid premedication and are treated with diuretics (King, 2017c).

(c) Cytosine arabinoside (Nucci et al., 2015)

(d) Blinatumomab (Goebeler & Bargou, 2016)

(e) Leuprolide acetate (Tan & Lake, 2016)

(f) Tyrosine kinase inhibitors (e.g., bortezomib, dasatinib, gefitinib, imatinib mesylate) cause capillary permeability, pulmonary edema, and effusions (Teuwen et al., 2015; Vahid & Marik, 2008).

(5) Hypersensitivity pneumonitis

(a) Paclitaxel can cause acute pneumonitis, which no longer appears to be a hypersensitivity reaction to the drug's emulsification agents (polyoxyl 40 hydrogenated castor oil [Kolliphor® EL, formerly Cremophor® EL]) as originally postulated (Maldonado & Limper, 2017a).

(b) Docetaxel: Hypersensitivity pneumonitis occurs in 7%–47% of patients depending on total dose, chemotherapy schedule, and concurrent administration with gemcitabine or radiation (Genestreti et al., 2015; Olivier & Peikert, 2017).

(c) Gemcitabine-induced eosinophilic pneumonitis suggests that hypersensitivity may be an element of this drug reaction (Yakabe et al., 2013).

(d) Acute methotrexate reaction is likely allergic in origin (Balk, 2017).

(e) Pathologically confirmed hypersensitivity pneumonitis has occurred with bortezomib, imatinib, lenalidomide, mTOR inhibitors, oxaliplatin, procarbazine, and thalidomide, but no clear etiologic mechanisms have been identified (Maldonado & Limper, 2017b; Toma et al., 2017).

(f) Hypersensitivity skin testing may be used to differentiate the etiology when multiple agents are implicated (Kuo, Hawkins, & Yip, 2015).

5. Clinical manifestations: May be difficult to detect when subtle

a) Signs and symptoms (King, 2017a)

(1) Dyspnea
(2) Tachypnea
(3) Increased work of breathing
(4) Dry, nonproductive cough
(5) Fever with some types of ILD
(6) Hypoxemia: Cyanosis, low oxygen saturation
(7) Anxiety, uneasiness
(8) Weight loss
(9) Fatigue

b) Timing of signs and symptoms
(1) Hypersensitivity reactions may occur as early as hours after exposure or up to weeks after discontinuation.
(2) Hypersensitivity pneumonitis occurs 7–10 days after exposure, although it may not always present on the first cycle of therapy, as would normally be expected (Yakabe et al., 2013).
(3) Methotrexate hypersensitivity reactions occur 12–18 hours after the first dose (Balk, 2017).
(4) Delayed toxicity may occur 8 months to 10 years after therapy.

6. Assessment
a) Past medical history
(1) Chemotherapy and immunotherapy drug exposure
(2) Other medications known to cause pulmonary toxicity (e.g., amiodarone, nitrofurantoin, penicillamine, phenytoin, procainamide, propranolol, statins, sulfonamides) (Olivier & Peikert, 2017; Vahid & Marik, 2008; Xu et al., 2012)
(3) Recent or chronic pulmonary conditions (Maldonado & Limper, 2017b)
(4) Recent viral illnesses that predispose to hemorrhagic airway disease
(5) Autoimmune or connective tissue diseases (King, 2017a)
(6) Occupational exposures such as silica, dusts, coal, and cotton (King, 2017a)
(7) Environmental exposures such as asbestos, gases, and dusts (King, 2017a)

b) Physical examination
(1) Vital signs: Tachypnea, tachycardia
(2) Crackles on auscultation
(3) Cough and sputum production; hemoptysis
(4) Pleuritic pain may accompany some disorders (e.g., erlotinib-induced reactions).
(5) Accessory muscle use for breathing
(6) Evidence of poor tissue oxygenation: Cyanosis, oliguria, decreased bowel sounds, altered mentation

c) Diagnostic tests (Sverzellati et al., 2015)
(1) Arterial blood gases usually show hypoxemia with respiratory alkalosis.
(2) Changes suggesting pulmonary edema were observed in radiographs of patients receiving high-dose interleukin-2 during initial registration trials, but the incidence of this toxicity has been minimized with careful assessment and management of hypotension and cardiac dysfunction (Prometheus Laboratories Inc., 2012; Shelton, 2012).
(3) Chest x-rays show ground-glass opacities/infiltrates and interstitial or alveolar thickening of interlobular septum (Matsuno, 2012; Stark, 2017). Nodular patterns indicate fibrosis (Stark, 2017).
(4) Chest CT is highly sensitive and able to differentiate pneumonitis from pulmonary embolism or fibrosis that may occur in patients with cancer experiencing respiratory distress. Immune checkpoint inhibitor toxicity has a more peripheral distribution, although many CT changes are similar to those with other toxicities (Diederich, 2016; Matsuno, 2012; Nucci et al., 2015; Shannon, 2017; Tamura et al., 2013). A sensitive test of pulmonary function is the carbon monoxide diffusing capacity, which is reduced prior to symptoms in many patients (McCormack, 2017).
(5) Serum markers KL-6, SP-A, and SP-D have been used as indicators of ILD for some agents (e.g., gefitinib) (King, 2017b; Matsuno, 2012).
(6) Positron-emission tomography scintigraphy has been helpful for early diagnosis of pulmonary fibrosis related to etoposide (Maldonado & Limper, 2017a).
(7) Bronchoscopy with lavage may provide definitive diagnostic findings with toxicities such as alveolar hemorrhage, pulmonary alveolar proteinosis, and hypersensitivity pneumonitis. Immune checkpoint inhibitor pneumonitis produces lymphocyte-predominant bronchoalveolar lavage specimens (Shannon, 2017).
(8) Open lung biopsy provides definitive diagnosis.

7. Collaborative management
   a) Pulmonary function testing is a prerequisite for the following patients being evaluated for therapy:
      (1) Heavy smokers (Margaritopoulos et al., 2015)
      (2) Patients with extensive pulmonary disease
      (3) Patients with symptoms suggesting decreased pulmonary reserve, such as exercise intolerance, new cough, or tachypnea
   b) Avoid exceeding maximum recommended doses.
      (1) Bleomycin: 400 units total lifetime dose (Fresenius Kabi USA, LLC, 2016a; Feldman & Vander Els, 2017)
      (2) Mitomycin C: 30 mg/m^2 (Chan & King, 2016)
   c) If pulmonary toxicity is suspected, hold chemotherapy and notify prescriber. Rechallenge with the offending agent varies with toxicity severity, timing, probable mechanism of injury, and specific agent.
   d) Administer oxygen cautiously and only if patient is hypoxemic (Stein et al., 2015).
      (1) Some lung-toxic medications have produced increased toxicity (diffuse alveolar damage) with oxygen therapy (e.g., bleomycin).
      (2) Oxygen can cause absorption atelectasis and loss of surfactant, which may exacerbate toxicity risk.
   e) Establish fluid balance goals.
      (1) Carefully record intake and output.
      (2) Determine if fluid boluses or fluid restrictions are warranted.
      (3) Consider using goal "dry" weight to target diuretic therapy. Weigh patients on a regular basis.
      (4) Diuretics decrease parenchymal edema, drawing fluid from interstitial spaces. This is not always effective when capillary permeability is impaired and cell and vessel boundaries have been compromised.
   f) Supportive care
      (1) Oxygen therapy: When using bleomycin, be alert for oxygen-induced lung damage (Feldman & Vander Els, 2017; Stein et al., 2015).
      (2) Bronchodilators: A metered dose inhaler provides better delivery than a nebulizer.
      (3) Position for best breathing: Head of bed elevated, tripod position (arms elevated and extended, with knees separated while leaning forward), legs over side of bed
   g) Treatment of possible etiologies of ILD
      (1) Administer corticosteroids as ordered. Corticosteroids usually are contraindicated for patients receiving lymphokines, such as aldesleukin (Dhupkar & Gordon, 2017).
         (a) Corticosteroids are dosed as low dose, moderate dose, or high dose.
         (b) Risks and benefits of corticosteroids should be considered when choosing to treat pulmonary toxicities.
         (c) Exact dosages remain controversial, but specific recommendations based on the toxicity grade have been established for immune checkpoint inhibitors (Teuwen et al., 2015).
      (2) Initiate antimicrobial therapy when infection superimposed on other lung toxicity is suspected.
   h) Unproven/investigational treatments
      (1) Pirfenidone 1,800 mg/day has been used with steroid-refractory bleomycin toxicity (Sakamoto, Ito, Hashimoto, & Hasegawa, 2017).
      (2) Inhaled lecithinized superoxide dismutase catalyzes with pirfenidone in bleomycin toxicity (Tanaka, Azuma, Miyazaki, Sato, & Mizushima, 2012).
      (3) Rituximab has been effective in cases of refractory hypersensitivity pneumonitis (Keir et al., 2014).
   i) Follow-up evaluation of patients at risk
      (1) Monitor x-rays and CT scans routinely with disorders that can produce hypersensitivity, idiopathic, or non-dose-related toxicities.
         (a) For targeted and immunotherapies (e.g., cetuximab, erlotinib, rituximab), imaging at least monthly is recommended (Achermann et al., 2012; Qi et al., 2015).
         (b) Frequency is based on risk for ILD and may increase with cumulative dose or added risk factors.
         (c) A chest x-ray may be recommended every one to two weeks to monitor for bleomycin toxicity (Fresenius Kabi USA, LLC, 2016a).
      (2) Perform periodic monitoring of pulmonary function tests for patients at

risk for ILD (at baseline and every three months during active therapy; often performed years after HSCT) (Keldsen et al., 2016; King, 2017b; McCormack, 2017; Willemsen et al., 2016). Most ILD produces restrictive disease. The ratio of forced expiratory volume in one second to forced vital capacity is most sensitive to detect restrictive disease. Ratios that are normal to only slightly elevated indicate restrictive lung disease. Low forced vital capacity with normal forced expiratory volume in one second and total lung capacity below the lower limit of normal suggests restrictive lung disease.

(3) Low diffusing capacity of the lung for carbon monoxide (DLCO) corrected for hemoglobin (Hgb) and lung volume indicates parenchymal restrictive disease. DLCO may differentiate parenchymal restrictive disease associated with chemotherapy agents from other physical causes (e.g., obesity, pleural effusions). It is used more frequently to detect pulmonary fibrosis (McCormack, 2017; Willemsen et al., 2016). The use of threshold values to trigger therapy breaks in bleomycin has been questioned, given the number of patients with 20% reduction in DLCO who did not develop progressive respiratory dysfunction. The negative impact of bleomycin on dose-dependent responses may not be equivalent to the incidence of pulmonary toxicity (Roncolato et al., 2016).

(4) In patients with acute-onset symptomatic disorders such as alveolar hemorrhage or acute hypersensitivity reaction, screening is not performed, because of the usual acute presentation.

(5) Late or delayed onset of lung toxicity may occur and be related to treatment and host factors, but plans for follow-up care are not clearly defined (Versluys & Bresters, 2016).

C. Alveolar hemorrhage

1. Pathophysiology

a) Unlike tumor invasion of the upper airways, alveolar hemorrhage as a toxicity of antineoplastic therapy occurs in the microvasculature of small airways. Three types exist (Ikpeama & Bailes, 2012; Schwarz, 2017).

(1) *Bland pulmonary hemorrhage* occurs due to hydrostatic pressure changes and is most common with coagulopathies, anticoagulant therapy, heart failure, or renal failure.

(2) *Diffuse alveolar hemorrhage* occurs as a result of direct lung injury causing alveolar edema and development of hyaline membranes. Toxic metabolites from cyclophosphamide and gemcitabine produce lung toxicity by this mechanism.

(3) *Pulmonary/capillary vasculitis* is an autoimmune process resulting in the fibrinous destruction of alveolar basement membranes. It is caused by agents that trigger immunologic mechanisms (e.g., rituximab).

b) Vascular endothelial wall destruction by chemotherapy or chemoradiation causes microcapillary bleeding (Ueda et al., 2014). Repeated episodes of alveolar hemorrhage may lead to pulmonary fibrosis.

2. Incidence

a) Alveolar hemorrhage incidence rates are 1.9% in patients receiving nonmyeloablative transplant regimens, as high as 10.3% in those undergoing myeloablative HSCT, and lower in pediatric transplant recipients. Incidence may also be related to severe systemic viral infection in high-risk groups (Kaner & Zappetti, 2018; X.-D. Mo et al., 2013).

b) Incidence is rare with other antineoplastic therapies.

3. Risk factors

a) Alveolar hemorrhage is best documented in the setting of HSCT, although some acute pneumonitis syndromes may be hemorrhagic in nature (Kaner & Zappetti, 2018; Schwarz, 2017; Vande Vusse & Madtes, 2017).

b) Alveolar hemorrhage has been rarely associated with normal doses of bevacizumab, bortezomib, crizotinib, cyclophosphamide, docetaxel, etoposide, everolimus, gefitinib, gemcitabine, lenalidomide, nilotinib, oxaliplatin, pemetrexed, rituximab, and sirolimus (Chatterjee et al., 2015; Donatelli, Chongnarungsin, & Ashton, 2014; Kurimoto et al., 2015; Maldonado & Limper, 2018; Mankikian et al., 2014; Ono et al., 2013; Sakai et al., 2015; Saleem, Ammannagari, Winans, & Leonardo, 2015; Schwarz, 2017; Specks, 2017; Sugita et al., 2015; Toma et al., 2017; Wirk, 2012; Willemsen et al., 2016).

c) Concomitant pulmonary infection may be present with adenovirus, cytomegalovirus, dengue fever, Epstein-Barr virus, *Stenotrophomonas maltophilia*, and *Strongyloides* (parasite) (Mori et al., 2014; Schwarz, 2017).

d) Non-oncologic drugs can cause alveolar hemorrhage (e.g., amiodarone, crack cocaine, nitrofurantoin, propylthiouracil, valproate) (Ikpeama & Bailes, 2012).

e) Unlike other bleeding syndromes, pulmonary hemorrhage is not always related to platelet counts or coagulation values (Nanjappa et al., 2016).

4. Clinical manifestations (Ikpeama & Bailes, 2012)
   a) Onset of bleeding often is sudden, over a single day. It usually begins within the first two weeks after the preparative regimen for HSCT.
   b) Symptoms include dyspnea, fever, cough, chest discomfort, and profound hypoxemia.
   c) Hemoptysis occurs in up to one-third of patients. Pink, frothy sputum and blood in bronchoalveolar specimens may be found (Schwarz, 2017).
   d) Hypoxemia-related symptoms include agitation, confusion, air hunger, cyanosis, tachycardia, and bradycardia.
5. Assessment
   a) Breath sounds (early crackles and diminished breath sounds as the airways become filled with bloody exudate)
   b) Oxygen saturation (decreased)
   c) Sputum (increase in quantity and change in quality)
   d) Hgb, platelet count, and coagulation parameters: Hgb may not fall until bleeding is life threatening.
   e) Nonspecific findings of inflammation: Increased erythrocyte sedimentation rate, leukocytosis (if not marrow suppressed)
   f) Pulmonary function tests (increased DLCO with hypoxemia) if patient is able to participate (Keldsen et al., 2016; McCormack, 2017)
   g) Chest x-ray or CT scan: Bilateral patchy, irregular interstitial infiltrates (Nucci et al., 2015; Torrisi et al., 2011)
   h) Bronchoalveolar lavage: Bloody returns, higher yield than instilled, and positive hemosiderin-laden macrophages in the sputum (Escuissato, Warszawiak, & Marchiori, 2015; Gilbert, Lerner, Baram, & Awsare, 2013)
6. Collaborative management
   a) Corticosteroids are standard treatment, although they have not been proved effective in treatment of medication-induced alveolar hemorrhage (Rathi et al., 2015; Schwarz, 2017; Sugita et al., 2015).
      (1) Methylprednisolone at doses of 500–2,000 mg IV daily for approximately five days
      (2) No standard tapering regimen is recommended. Close observation for rebleeding during steroid tapering is recommended to guide practice.
   b) Coagulation factors can be administered, although no one therapy has been proved effective. Unproven coagulation therapies include IV aminocaproic acid and coagulation factor VII (Heslet, Nielson, & Nepper-Christensen, 2012; Larcombe, Kapur, Fraser, Coulthard, & Schlapbach, 2014).
   c) Consider noninvasive or invasive mechanical ventilation with positive pressure to produce intra-alveolar pressure and reduce bleeding (Ikpeama & Bailes, 2012; Spira et al., 2013).
   d) Experimental therapies are based on suspected etiologic factor and include plasma exchange and IV immunoglobulin (Schwarz, 2017).
   e) Ensure adequate airway clearance with bronchodilator therapy, adequate hydration, and deep endotracheal suctioning as needed. Retained blood can cause secondary infection and worsened hypoxemia (Ikpeama & Bailes, 2012).
   f) Provide supportive management of dyspnea.
   g) When tumor involvement of pulmonary cells is implicated, such as with myeloma, rechallenge may be more successful (Sugita et al., 2015).

D. Acute promyelocytic leukemia (APL) treatment–related differentiation syndrome

1. Pathophysiology (Sanz & Montesinos, 2014; Villa et al., 2014)
   a) APL treatment–related differentiation syndrome occurs with APL (M3 leukemia). It was initially named retinoic acid syndrome because of its association with administration of ATRA, but the newer term *APL treatment–related differentiation syndrome* was introduced because it was realized that the syndrome occurs with any effective initial treatment for APL (Sanz & Montesinos, 2014).
   b) The syndrome is caused by rapid proliferation and differentiation of white blood cells (WBCs). This results in immunologic stimu-

lation by vasoactive cytokines, thus creating inflammatory capillary permeability of the lungs and a widespread erythematous rash (Leblejian et al., 2013; Villa et al., 2014; Weinberger & Larson, 2017).

c) It is more a condition of tumor responsiveness to therapy than a toxicity.

d) It is unclear whether pulmonary changes are related to the disease, rejection phenomena, chemotherapy agents, or the combined effects of chemoradiation (Nucci et al., 2015; Sanz & Montesinos, 2014).

2. Incidence

a) It occurs in approximately 27%–48% of patients with APL receiving induction therapy (Elemam & Abdelmoety, 2013; Leblejian et al., 2013; Lengfelder et al., 2015; Weinberger & Larson, 2017). It also has occurred in other settings of retinoid administration, emphasizing the need for monitoring when administering any retinoid or other differentiating agent (e.g., arsenic trioxide).

b) It has been reported to occur in 10%–15% of patients receiving combination retinoid and chemotherapy and is more prevalent in patients with high WBC counts (Watts & Tallman, 2014).

3. Risk factors (Breccia et al., 2012; Villa et al., 2014; Weinberger & Larson, 2017)

a) Increased body mass index is the only validated risk factor that predicts for presence of the syndrome (Breccia et al., 2012; Leblejian et al., 2013).

b) Induction therapy with active disease is a risk factor; the syndrome does not occur during consolidation therapy when there is no active leukemia.

c) High WBC count may or may not be associated with increased risk, but it is clear that a rapid rise of WBC count, or large percentage of immature cells, is related to the presence of APL treatment–related differentiation syndrome (Leblejian et al., 2013; Watts & Tallman, 2014; Weinberger & Larson, 2017).

d) Acute leukemia, M3 subtype, expression of CD13 on APL blast cells (Breccia et al., 2014)

(1) CD34/CD2 subgroup shows increased risk.

(2) CD56 expression with prevalent bcr3 expression shows increased risk.

e) Treatment-specific variables

(1) ATRA treatment

(2) Arsenic trioxide

(3) Bortezomib

(4) Azacitidine (Laufer & Roberts, 2015)

4. Clinical manifestations (Dhar & Barman, 2012; Weinberger & Larson, 2017)

a) Signs and symptoms include fever, dyspnea, cough, hypotension, crackles, hypoxemia, musculoskeletal pain (e.g., arthralgias, myalgias), effusions, edema, and weight gain more than 5 kg from baseline.

b) Rash can be diffuse, erythematous, and nonpruritic and is more common in severe cases (Weinberger & Larson, 2017).

c) Renal dysfunction may occur but often is slower in onset than other symptoms, so it may be noted after recognition of the syndrome.

d) Approximately one-half of patients have symptoms within one week, and the rest develop symptoms between the third and fourth week of induction therapy (Sanz & Montesinos, 2014).

e) Common Terminology Criteria for Adverse Events grading (National Cancer Institute Cancer Therapy Evaluation Program, 2017)

(1) Weight gain

(a) Grade 1: 5% to less than 10% from baseline

(b) Grade 2: 10% to less than 20% weight gain from baseline

(c) Grade 3: Greater than or equal to 20% weight gain from baseline

(2) Toxicity of differentiation syndrome is graded according to severity of symptoms.

(a) Grade 1: Fluid retention of less than 3 kg requiring intervention with fluid restriction and/or diuretics

(b) Grade 2: Moderate signs and symptoms requiring steroid administration

(c) Grade 3: Severe symptoms and hospitalization indicated

(d) Grade 4: Life-threatening consequences with mechanical ventilation indicated

(e) Grade 5: Death due to the disorder

5. Assessment

a) Breath sounds and oxygen saturation

b) Intake and output, weight; monitor for overhydration, which may worsen respiratory symptoms.

c) Laboratory studies

(1) WBC count with differential daily; assessment of blast percentage

(2) Periodic assessment of Hgb, hematocrit, and platelet count; anemia and thrombocytopenia are common.

(3) Periodic evaluation of coagulation parameters and platelet count; disseminated intravascular coagulation may be present.
(4) Renal function tests to monitor for impairment; it is unclear if dysfunction is related to hypotension or thrombosis (Weinberger & Larson, 2017).

d) Chest x-ray or CT: Nodular or ground-glass opacities with patchy bilateral distribution, consolidation, air bronchograms, prominent septal lines, and possible pleural effusions, although up to 40% of patients will have no initial x-ray findings of peribronchial cuffing or increased cardiothoracic ratio (Nucci et al., 2015; Weinberger & Larson, 2017).

6. Collaborative management
   a) Prevention
   (1) Immediate administration of chemotherapy when WBC count rises
   (2) Fluid management (strict intake and output)

   b) Although the clinical benefit is still unclear, immediate treatment with corticosteroids (Sanz & Montesinos, 2014) or conventional chemotherapy is still believed by some to improve outcomes.
   (1) Dexamethasone, which usually inhibits inflammatory chemokines, does not appear to be effective in reduction of this syndrome's clinical manifestations (Aznab & Rezaei, 2017).
   (2) If treatment with steroids is selected, the usual treatment is dexamethasone 10 mg IV twice daily for at least three days (Sanz & Montesinos, 2014).
   (3) Even with steroid treatment, the syndrome carries an approximate 10% mortality rate (Aznab & Rezaei, 2017).

   c) Noninvasive or invasive mechanical ventilation with positive pressure
   d) Removal of pleural or pericardial effusions
   e) Continuous dialysis has been used with some success to remove inflammatory cytokines (Villa et al., 2014).

E. Pleural effusions

1. Definition: Accumulation of excess fluid in the pleural space that impairs lung expansion. Four to six liters of pleural fluid usually pass daily through the potential space between the visceral and parietal pleura (Villena Garrido et al., 2014).
2. Pathophysiology: Excess fluid is retained in the pleural space, which restricts full alveolar expansion (Muzumdar, 2012; Villena Garrido et al., 2014).
   a) Major causes of pleural effusion are obstruction to fluid outflow and pleural irritation leading to exudative capillary permeability into the space (Muzumdar, 2012).
   (1) Mast cell degranulation may mediate pleural effusion and potential physiology for drug-related effusions (Giannou et al., 2015).
   (2) Pleural effusions after HSCT may be multifactorial. Engraftment syndrome resulting from the treatment and cell engraftment has been associated with pleural effusions (Brownback et al., 2014).

   b) Transudative effusions are produced by passive capillary permeability and are characteristic of fluid overload, heart failure, or hypothyroidism (Dasanu, Jen, & Skulski, 2017; Kust et al., 2016).
   c) Hydrophilic drugs with low plasma protein binding (e.g., methotrexate, pemetrexed) may accumulate in the pleural space, enhancing the incidence of pleural effusion and potentiating drug toxicity (Honoré, Joensen, Olsen, Hansen, & Mellemgaard, 2014).
3. Incidence of drug-related pleural effusions
   a) Incidence varies and is dependent on agent, dose, schedule, and comorbid conditions.
   b) Incidence can be as high as 54% with some agents (Maldonado & Limper, 2017a, 2017b, 2018).
4. Risk factors
   a) Pleural effusions are a common complication of cancer and other medical disorders, such as cirrhosis, gout, heart failure, infections, pneumonia, pulmonary embolism, renal failure, rheumatoid conditions, or hypothyroidism, and medications, such as valproate and clozapine (Findik, 2012).
   b) When associated with chemotherapy and immunotherapy agents, pleural effusions are the result of capillary permeability that is temporally related to administration of the offending agent. Most resolve with discontinuation of treatment.
   c) Chemotherapy and immunotherapy agents that have been associated with development of pleural effusions
   (1) Antimetabolites/folate inhibitors (e.g., methotrexate, pemetrexed)—eosinophilic pleural effusions (Cudzilo, Aragaki, Guitron, & Benzaquen, 2014; Honoré et al., 2014)

(2) Bacillus Calmette Guérin—lymphocyte infiltration of the pleura (Tobiume et al., 2014)
(3) Bortezomib (Oudart et al., 2012)
(4) Cytosine arabinoside when combined with daunorubicin (He et al., 2014)
(5) Cyclophosphamide (high-dose) (Nakazawa et al., 2014)
(6) Kinase *BCR-ABL* inhibitors (e.g., dasatinib, which is the most common and significant in this drug class; imatinib; nilotinib); more common in second-generation agents (Chakraborty, Bossaer, Patel, & Krishnan, 2013; Cortes et al., 2015; Eskazan et al., 2014; Schiffer et al., 2016)
(7) Docetaxel (Park et al., 2014)
(8) Fludarabine (Nakazawa et al., 2014)
(9) Gemcitabine (Kido et al., 2012)
(10) Immune checkpoint inhibitors (e.g., ipilimumab)—late onset and uncommon, but may be linked to drug-related hypothyroidism (Dasanu et al., 2017)
(11) mTOR inhibitors (e.g., everolimus, temsirolimus) (Fukushima, Saito, Sakata, & Sawa, 2013; Willemsen et al., 2016)
(12) Oprelvekin (Wyeth Pharmaceuticals, 2011)
(13) Sunitinib (Miura et al., 2014)

5. Clinical manifestations and assessment (Muzumdar, 2012; Villena Garrido et al., 2014; Willemsen et al., 2016)
   a) Patients present with tachypnea, dyspnea, increased work of breathing, abnormal chest excursion, and fatigue.
   b) Onset varies by agent and mechanism of toxicity; hypersensitivity reactions may occur sooner than direct injury (Willemsen et al., 2016).
   c) Large pleural effusions are easily documented by an upright chest x-ray; smaller effusions are seen on chest CT.
   d) Tyrosine kinase inhibitor–induced pleural effusions are characterized by exudative features and lymphocytic infiltration of the pleura.
6. Collaborative management (Kaifi et al., 2012; Villena Garrido et al., 2014)
   a) In most cases, pleural effusions are uncomplicated and spontaneously resolve upon discontinuation of the causative agent.
   b) Dose reduction has been successful at eliminating pleural effusion related to some drugs.
   c) Concomitant corticosteroids have been effective at reducing the severity of pleural effusions related to docetaxel.
   d) Other treatment strategies have included albumin supplementation, fluid restrictions, diuretics, and corticosteroids, but these interventions do not have a body of evidence to support their use (Villena Garrido et al., 2014).
   e) Medical or surgical pleurodesis is rarely required to treat drug-induced pleural effusion.
      (1) On rare occasions, thoracentesis has been performed as a temporary measure or to rule out other causes of the effusion.
      (2) Tunneled or temporary pleural catheters may be used with persistent drug-related pleural effusion.

F. Pulmonary alveolar proteinosis/pulmonary alveolar phospholipoproteinosis
1. Pathophysiology (Suzuki & Trapnell, 2016)
   a) Pulmonary alveolar proteinosis or pulmonary alveolar phospholipoproteinosis is a distal airway disorder characterized by accumulation of lipoproteinaceous exudate with surfactant components and cell fragments that stain positive for periodic acid-Schiff protein (Bonella & Campo, 2014; Chan & King, 2017a).
   b) The thick proteinaceous exudate causes bronchiolar occlusion, poor respiratory compliance, and hypoxemia (Bonella & Campo, 2014; Chan & King, 2017a).
   c) Primary pathologic mechanism is likely related to GM-CSF deficiency. In adults, it is thought to be due to anti–GM-CSF antibodies (Ben-Dov & Segal, 2014; Papiris et al., 2014).
   d) Gene mutations for normal surfactant production and clearance have been implicated in the pathophysiology and propensity to develop this disorder (Suzuki & Trapnell, 2016). These genetic variations may be inherited, acquired, or a combination of both etiologies. This suggests that more cases and etiologic agents may be identified over time (Antoon et al., 2016).
2. Incidence: Rare
3. Risk factors
   a) After HSCT (Ansari et al., 2012; Chaulagain, Pilichowska, Brinckerhoff, Tabba, & Erban, 2014; Kaner & Zappetti, 2018)
   b) Autoimmune disease or concomitant autoimmune pathologic process (e.g., autoimmune hemolytic anemia, immune thrombocytope-

nia); associated with more than 90% of cases (Boerner et al., 2016; Bonella & Campo, 2014; Chan & King, 2017a)

c) Hematologic malignancies (Chaulagain et al., 2014; Papiris et al., 2015)

d) Myelodysplastic syndromes (Ishii et al., 2014)

e) Profound neutropenia at the onset of the disorder

f) Infection with *Acinetobacter, Aspergillus, Pneumocystis, Nocardia,* or *Mycobacterium* (Arai, Inoue, Akira, Nakata, & Kitaichi, 2015; Bonella & Campo, 2014; Chan & King, 2017a; Shattuck & Bean, 2013)

g) Isolated cases with specific antineoplastic agents

(1) Unclear whether disorder is caused by antineoplastic agents, such as alkylating agents, or imatinib, or the underlying disease (Yoshimura et al., 2014)

(2) Everolimus (Darley, Malouf, & Glanville, 2016)

4. Clinical manifestations and assessment (Ben-Dov & Segal, 2014)

a) Signs and symptoms include dyspnea, mainly with exertion; tachypnea; cough; and increased work of breathing.

b) Pulmonary alveolar proteinosis/pulmonary alveolar phospholipoproteinosis occurs over a few days with progressive worsening.

c) CT scan shows widespread air-space consolidation with "crazy-paving" patterns, appearing like octagonal pavement stones pieced together, with even, bilateral distribution centrally located and sparing the apices and costophrenic angle. Pulmonary fibrosis will occur over time with long-term pathology (Akira et al., 2016; Chan & King, 2017b; Choi et al., 2015; Diederich, 2016; Nunomura et al., 2016; Shattuck & Bean, 2013).

d) DLCO is below predicted value, but this is a nonspecific finding (Bai et al., 2016).

e) Although open lung biopsy has historically been the diagnostic test of choice, today 75%–90% of cases are diagnosed by bronchoscopy (Chan & King, 2017a; Kroll, Kumar, Grossman, Price, & Srigley, 2016; Q. Mo et al., 2016).

(1) Lung biopsy specimens are positive for periodic acid-Schiff stain.

(2) Lavage specimens are cloudy, with alveolar macrophages and eosinophils.

(3) Myelin-like lamellar bodies are present (Huang et al., 2016; Yi et al., 2012).

f) High serum titer of immunoglobulin G anti–GM-CSF antibodies is an indicator of pulmonary alveolar proteinosis/pulmonary alveolar phospholipoproteinosis (Ben-Dov & Segal, 2014).

g) Other markers include increased lactate dehydrogenase, high total cholesterol and low-density lipoprotein, carcinoembryonic antigen, CA 19-9, CYFRA 21-1, neuron-specific enolase, and GATA2 deficiency (Chan & King, 2017a; Griese et al., 2015; Li et al., 2014; Q. Mo et al., 2016).

h) Induced sputum may be helpful but is not as accurate as bronchoalveolar lavage (Huang et al., 2016).

i) The syndrome usually corrects itself when patients go into remission or recover normal WBC counts.

j) It may be fatal in patients with persistent disease or those who fail to recover counts (Chaulagain et al., 2014).

5. Collaborative management (Ben-Dov & Segal, 2014; Bonella & Campo, 2014; Campo et al., 2012; Chan & King, 2017b)

a) Whole lung lavage: An operative procedure where single lung ventilation is performed during warmed saline flushing of the other lung; may require multiple procedures. Repeated whole lung lavage procedures may be necessary (Abdelmalak, Khanna, Culver, & Popovich, 2015; Zhang et al., 2016).

b) Antibiotics to treat causative organisms or prevent secondary infections (Chan & King, 2017b)

c) Chest percussion (Vymazal & Krecmerova, 2015)

d) GM-CSF subcutaneously or by inhalation over 8–12 weeks (Papiris et al., 2014; Satoh et al., 2012; Tazawa et al., 2014)

e) Rituximab (Garber, Albores, Wang, & Neville, 2015; Malur et al., 2012; Nagasawa, Kurasawa, & Hanaoka, 2016)

f) Corticosteroids have been used to treat this disorder and have a strong scientific basis validated by the inflammatory nature of this disorder. Despite their extensive use, some authors believe them to be ineffective in altering the disease course (Akasaka et al., 2015; Chan & King, 2017b).

g) Hydration, sputum expectoration, and bronchodilators (Vymazal & Krecmerova, 2015)

h) Investigational use of plasmapheresis to remove GM-CSF antibodies (Garber et al., 2015)

G. Pulmonary VOD

1. Pathophysiology (Mandel & LeVarge, 2018a; Olsson & Palazzini, 2015)

a) Subgroup of patients with pulmonary arteriolar hypertension who subsequently develop venous pathology as well. Also called obstructive disease in the pulmonary veins or isolated pulmonary venous sclerosis
b) Endothelial wall damage is the proposed mechanism of injury.
c) Post-capillary pulmonary venular obstruction occurs with fibrous tissue that becomes dense and sclerotic.
   (1) Calcium deposits in elastic fibers of venule walls
   (2) Engorgement of alveolar capillaries
   (3) Dilated lymphatics with interstitial edema
   (4) Venous fibrosis
d) It is unclear whether pulmonary changes are related to the disease, rejection phenomena, chemotherapy agents, or the combined effects of chemoradiation (Cutler, 2017).
e) Pulmonary VOD presents 40–60 days after HSCT as hypoxemia, volume-dependent hypotension, atrial arrhythmias, right bundle branch block, or hepatic congestion (Kaner & Zappetti, 2018).

2. Incidence
   a) Pulmonary VOD is an infrequent manifestation of endothelial injury, occurring in less than 2% of HSCT recipients (Tewari, Wallis, & Kebriaei, 2017).
   b) Incidence is likely underestimated because symptoms mimic other adverse effects.
   c) Pulmonary VOD possibly accounts for 5%–10% of all cases of idiopathic pulmonary hypertension (Mandel & LeVarge, 2018a; Olsson & Palazzini, 2015).
3. Risk factors (Bishop, Mauro, & Khouri, 2012; Mandel & LeVarge, 2018a)
   a) HSCT, especially matched unrelated transplant recipients and those with graft-versus-host disease (Tewari et al., 2017)
   b) High-dose alkylating agents: Busulfan, carmustine, other alkylating agents used for the preparative regimen for HSCT (Ranchoux et al., 2015)
   c) Other agents: Dasatinib, interferon alfa-2a, mitomycin (Buchelli Ramirez, Álvarez Álvarez, Rodríguez Reguero, García Clemente, & Casan Clarà, 2014; Morishita et al., 2016; Papani, Duarte, Lin, Kuo, & Sharma, 2017; Perros et al., 2015)
   d) Prior lung injury; familial pulmonary hypertension
   e) Viral illnesses (e.g., cytomegalovirus, Epstein-Barr virus)
   f) Thrombotic disorders
4. Clinical manifestations and assessment
   a) Subtle and vague symptoms: Dyspnea, fatigue
   b) Heart failure symptoms (Mandel & LeVarge, 2018a; Olsson & Palazzini, 2015)
      (1) Right heart failure early: Elevated jugular venous pressure, hepatomegaly, edema
      (2) Left heart failure later: Crackles, heart murmurs and gallops, subxiphoid retraction, oliguria
   c) Definitive diagnosis requires a right heart catheterization, but risk of bleeding is high. Elevated right heart pressures on echocardiogram may be suggestive of this disorder.
   d) CT demonstrates patchy, ground-glass, or nodular infiltrates with perihilar distribution and engorgement of major central pulmonary veins that are unique to pulmonary VOD, differentiating pulmonary hypertension from other causes (Mandel & LeVarge, 2018b; Mineo et al., 2014).
   e) Bronchoscopic examination shows hyperemia of lobar and segmental bronchi with vascular engorgement (Mandel & LeVarge, 2018b).
5. Collaborative management (Mandel & LeVarge, 2018b; Olsson & Palazzini, 2015)
   a) Correct etiologic factors (e.g., viral infections, disseminated intravascular coagulation, offending medications).
   b) Avoid calcium channel blockers and prostacyclins (usual treatments for pulmonary hypertension), which can cause pulmonary edema in pulmonary VOD (Bishop et al., 2012; Mandel & LeVarge, 2018b).
   c) Nitric oxide, prostanoids, endothelin-1 receptor antagonists, and phosphodiesterase inhibitors have been used with limited success (Bishop et al., 2012).
   d) If an autoimmune component is present (e.g., graft-versus-host disease), corticosteroids may be beneficial (Mandel & LeVarge, 2018b).
   e) Anticoagulant, antiplatelet, and fibrinolytic agents used with hepatic VOD have not been proved effective and may increase bleeding risk (Mandel & LeVarge, 2018b).
   f) Differential diagnosis between pulmonary VOD and other etiologies of pulmonary hypertension is essential to ensure appropriate treatment with minimization of adverse effects.
   g) Pulmonary VOD has a poor prognosis, even when identified early, but it has been reversible in cases of dasatinib etiology (Buchelli Ramirez et al., 2014).

H. Patient and family education (Camp-Sorrell, 2018)
   1. Provide education regarding symptoms associated with pulmonary toxicity (e.g., cough, dyspnea, chest pain, shallow breathing, chest wall discomfort). Make sure all patients know to seek medical assistance immediately if symptoms occur.
   2. Advise smoking cessation or reduction, as any reduced exposure may reverse lung changes and slow the progression of interstitial lung disease (Margaritopoulos et al., 2015).
   3. Inform patients that treatment may be delayed or held until pulmonary symptoms resolve.
   4. Explore with patients their wishes regarding intubation and resuscitation status; establish advance directives.
   5. Teach patients that raising the head of the bed may facilitate breathing.
   6. Instruct patients to conserve energy by performing daily activities when their energy level is highest.
   7. Teach patients and significant others methods to decrease symptoms of dyspnea (e.g., exercising to tolerance, practicing pursed-lip breathing, refraining from smoking, using a small fan).
   8. Teach patients to take an opioid (e.g., morphine) as prescribed by their physician to relieve discomfort caused by air hunger.
   9. Review the safety issues (e.g., flammability) related to oxygen administration.

References

Abdelmalak, B.B., Khanna, A.K., Culver, D.A., & Popovich, M.J. (2015). Therapeutic whole-lung lavage for pulmonary alveolar proteinosis: A procedural update. *Journal of Bronchology and Interventional Pulmonology, 22,* 251–258. https://doi.org/10.1097/LBR.0000000000000180

Abdel-Rahman, O., & Elhalawani, H. (2015). Risk of fatal pulmonary events in patients with advanced non-small-cell lung cancer treated with EGF receptor tyrosine kinase inhibitors: A comparative meta-analysis. *Future Oncology, 11,* 1109–1122. https://doi.org/10.2217/fon.15.16

Abugideiri, M., Nanda, R.H., Butker, C., Zhang, C., Kim, S., Chiang, K.-Y., … Esiashvilli, N. (2016). Factors influencing pulmonary toxicity in children undergoing allogeneic hematopoietic stem cell transplantation in the setting of total body irradiation-based myeloablative conditioning. *International Journal of Radiation Oncology, Biology, Physics, 94,* 349–359. https://doi.org/10.1016/j.ijrobp.2015.10.054

Accord Healthcare Inc. (2013). *Mitomycin* [Package insert]. Durham, NC: Author.

Achermann, Y., Frauenfelder, T., Obrist, S., Zaugg, K., Corti, N., & Gunthard, H.F. (2012). A rare but severe pulmonary side effect of cetuximab in two patients. *BMJ Case Reports, 2012.* https://doi.org/10.1136/bcr-03-2012-5973

Adhikari, B., Dongol, R.M., Baral, D., Hewett, Y., & Shah, B.K. (2016). Pemetrexed and interstitial lung disease. *Acta Oncologica, 55,* 521–522. https://doi.org/10.3109/0284186X.2015.1080859

Akasaka, K., Tanaka, T., Kitamura, N., Ohkouchi, S., Tazawa, R., Takada, T., … Nakata, K. (2015). Outcome of corticosteroid administration in autoimmune pulmonary alveolar proteinosis: A retrospective cohort study. *BMC Pulmonary Medicine, 15,* 88. https://doi.org/10.1186/s12890-015-0085-0

Akira, M., Inoue, Y., Arai, T., Sugimoto, C., Tokura, S., Nakata, K., & Kitaichi, M. (2016). Pulmonary fibrosis on high-resolution CT of patients with pulmonary alveolar proteinosis. *American Journal of Roentgenology, 207,* 544–551. https://doi.org/10.2214/AJR.15.14982

Amgen Inc. (2015). *Vectibix® (panitumumab)* [Package insert]. Thousand Oaks, CA: Author.

Ansari, M., Rougemont, A.-L., Le Deist, F., Ozsahin, H., Duval, M., Champagne, M.A., & Fournet, J.-C. (2012). Secondary pulmonary alveolar proteinosis after unrelated cord blood hematopoietic cell transplantation. *Pediatric Transplantation, 16,* E146–E149. https://doi.org/10.1111/j.1399-3046.2011.01487.x

Antoon, J.W., Hernandez, M.L., Roehrs, P.A., Noah, T.L., Leigh, M.W., & Byerley, J.S. (2016). Endogenous lipoid pneumonia preceding diagnosis of pulmonary alveolar proteinosis. *Clinical Respiratory Journal, 10,* 246–249. https://doi.org/10.1111/crj.12197

Arai, T., Inoue, Y., Akira, M., Nakata, K., & Kitaichi, M. (2015). Autoimmune pulmonary alveolar proteinosis following aspergillosis. *Internal Medicine, 54,* 3177–3180. https://doi.org/10.2169/internalmedicine.54.5034

Ariad Pharmaceuticals, Inc. (2017). *Alunbrig® (brigatinib)* [Package insert]. Cambridge, MA: Author.

Aspen Global Inc. (2011). *Myleran® (busulfan)* [Package insert]. Grand Bay, Mauritius: Author.

Aspen Global Inc. (2016). *Leukeran® (chlorambucil)* [Package insert]. Grand Bay, Mauritius: Author.

AstraZeneca Pharmaceuticals LP. (2015). *Iressa® (gefitinib)* [Package insert]. Wilmington, DE: Author.

AstraZeneca Pharmaceuticals LP. (2017). *Imfinzi® (durvalumab)* [Package insert]. Wilmington, DE: Author.

Awad, R., & Nott, L. (2016). Radiation recall pneumonitis induced by erlotinib after palliative thoracic radiotherapy for lung cancer: Case report and literature review. *Asia-Pacific Journal of Clinical Oncology, 12,* 91–95. https://doi.org/10.1111/ajco.12447

Aznab, M., & Rezaei, M. (2017). Induction, consolidation, and maintenance therapies with arsenic as a single agent for promyelocytic leukaemia in a 11-year follow-up. *Hematological Oncology, 35,* 113–117. https://doi.org/10.1002/hon.2253

Bai, J.W., Xu, J.F., Yang, W.L., Gao, B., Cao, W., Liang, S., & Li, H. (2016). A new scale to assess the severity and prognosis of pulmonary alveolar proteinosis. *Canadian Respiratory Journal, 2016,* 3412836. https://doi.org/10.1155/2016/3412836

Balk, R.A. (2017). Methotrexate-induced lung injury. In H. Hollingsworth & D.M.F. Savarese (Eds.), *UpToDate.* Retrieved May 4, 2018, from http://www.uptodate.com/contents/methotrexate-induced-lung-injury

Balzarini, L., Mancini, C., & Marvisi, M. (2014). A fatal case of acute interstitial pneumonia (AIP) in a woman affected by glioblastoma. *Current Drug Safety, 9,* 73–76. https://doi.org/10.2174/1574886308666140106154343

Baxter Healthcare Corp. (2013). *Cyclophosphamide* [Package insert]. Deerfield, IL: Author.

Bellanger, C., Dhooge, M., Tabouret, T., Chapron, J., Dreanic, J., Brezault, C., … Coriat, R. (2015). Incidence of organizing pneumonia induced by oxaliplatin chemotherapy for digestive cancer. *Annals of Pharmacotherapy, 49,* 494–495. https://doi.org/10.1177/1060028015569595

Ben-Dov, I., & Segal, M.J. (2014). Autoimmune pulmonary alveolar proteinosis: Clinical course and diagnostic criteria. *Autoimmune Reviews, 13,* 513–517. https://doi.org/10.1016/j.autrev.2014.01.046

Binder, D., Hübner, R.-H., Temmesfeld-Wollbrück, B., & Schlattmann, P. (2011). Pulmonary toxicity among cancer patients treated with a combination of docetaxel and gemcitabine: A meta-analysis of clinical trials. *Cancer Chemotherapy and Pharmacology, 68,* 1575–1583. https://doi.org/10.1007/s00280-011-1648-2

Bishop, B.M., Mauro, V.F., & Khouri, S.J. (2012). Practical considerations for the pharmacotherapy of pulmonary arterial hypertension. *Pharmacotherapy, 32,* 838–855. https://doi.org/10.1002/j.1875-9114.2012.01114.x

Boerner, E.B., Costabel, U., Wessendorf, T.E., Theegarten, D., Hetzel, M., Drent, M., & Bonella, F. (2016). Pulmonary alveolar proteinosis: Another autoimmune disease associated with sarcoidosis? *Sarcoidosis, Vasculitis and Diffuse Lung Diseases, 33,* 90–94.

Bonella, F., & Campo, I. (2014). Pulmonary alveolar proteinosis. *Pneumologia, 63,* 144, 147–155.

Bräunlich, J., Seyfarth, H.-J., Frille, A., & Wirtz, H. (2015). Diffuse interstitial pulmonary infiltrates in malignant melanoma. *Respiratory Care, 60,* e115–e117. https://doi.org/10.4187/respcare.03621

Breccia, M., De Propris, M.S., Stefanizzi, C., Raponi, S., Molica, M., Colafigli, G., … Foà, R. (2014). Negative prognostic value of CD34 antigen also if expressed on a small population of acute promyelocytic leukemia cells. *Annals of Hematology, 93,* 1819–1823. https://doi.org/10.1007/s00277-014-2130-0

Breccia, M., Mazzarella, L., Bagnardi, V., Disalvatore, D., Loglisci, G., Cimino, G., … Lo-Coco, F. (2012). Increased BMI correlates with higher risk of disease relapse and differentiation syndrome in patients with acute promyelocytic leukemia treated with the AIDA protocols. *Blood, 119,* 49–54. https://doi.org/10.1182/blood-2011-07-369595

Breuer, S., & Nechushtan, H. (2012). Pemetrexed-induced lung toxicity: A case report. *Clinical Oncology, 24,* 76–77. https://doi.org/10.1016/j.clon.2011.08.009

Bristol-Myers Squibb Co. (2015). *Sprycel® (dasatinib)* [Package insert]. Princeton, NJ: Author.

Bristol-Myers Squibb Co. (2016). *Etopophos® (etoposide phosphate)* [Package insert]. Princeton, NJ: Author.

Bristol-Myers Squibb Co. (2017). *Opdivo® (nivolumab)* [Package insert]. Princeton, NJ: Author.

Brownback, K.R., Simpson, S.Q., McGuirk, J.P., Lin, T.L., Abhyankar, S., Ganguly, S., & Aljitawi, O.S. (2014). Pulmonary manifestations of the pre-engraftment syndrome after umbilical cord blood transplantation. *Annals of Hematology, 95,* 847–854. https://doi.org/10.1007/s00277-013-1981-0

Buchelli Ramirez, H.L., Álvarez Álvarez, C.M., Rodríguez Reguero, J.J., García Clemente, M.M., & Casan Clarà, P. (2014). Reversible pre-capillary pulmonary hypertension due to dasatinib. *Respiratory Care, 59,* e77–e80. https://doi.org/10.4187/respcare.02692

Campo, I., Kadija, Z., Mariani, F., Paracchini, E., Rodi, G., Majoli, F., … Luisetti, M. (2012). Pulmonary alveolar proteinosis: Diagnostic and therapeutic challenges. *Multidisciplinary Respiratory Medicine, 7,* 4. https://doi.org/10.1186/2049-6958-7-4

Camp-Sorrell, D. (2018). Chemotherapy toxicities and management. In C.H. Yarbro, D. Wujcik, & B.H. Gobel (Eds.), *Cancer nursing: Principles and practice* (8th ed., pp. 497–554). Burlington, MA: Jones & Bartlett Learning.

Celgene Corp. (2017a). *Revlimid® (lenalidomide)* [Package insert]. Summit, NJ: Author.

Celgene Corp. (2017b). *Thalomid® (thalidomide)* [Package insert]. Summit, NJ: Author.

Chakraborty, K., Bossaer, J.B., Patel, R., & Krishnan, K. (2013). Successful treatment of nilotinib-induced pleural effusion with prednisone. *Journal of Oncology Pharmacy Practice, 19,* 175–177. https://doi.org/10.1177/1078155212447530

Chan, E.D., & King, T.E., Jr. (2016). Mitomycin-C pulmonary toxicity. In H. Hollingsworth & D.M.F. Savarese (Eds.), *UpToDate.* Retrieved May 4, 2018, from http://www.uptodate.com/contents/mitomycin-c-pulmonary-toxicity

Chan, E.D., & King, T.E., Jr. (2017a). Causes, clinical manifestations, and diagnosis of pulmonary alveolar proteinosis in adults. In H. Hollingsworth (Ed.), *UpToDate.* Retrieved May 4, 2018, from https://www.uptodate.com/contents/causes-clinical-manifestations-and-diagnosis-of-pulmonary-alveolar-proteinosis-in-adults

Chan, E.D., & King, T.E., Jr. (2017b). Treatment and prognosis of pulmonary alveolar proteinosis in adults. In H. Hollingsworth (Ed.), *UpToDate.* Retrieved May 4, 2018, from http://www.uptodate.com/contents/treatment-and-prognosis-of-pulmonary-alveolar-proteinosis-in-adults

Chatterjee, S., Pilaka, V.K.R., Mukhopadhyay, S., Shrinali, R.K., & Ahmed, R. (2015). Docetaxel-induced haemorrhagic interstitial pneumonitis—An acute life-threatening adverse effect. *Clinical Oncology, 27,* 483–484. https://doi.org/10.1016/j.clon.2015.03.011

Chaulagain, C.P., Pilichowska, M., Brinckerhoff, L., Tabba, M., & Erban, J.K. (2014). Secondary pulmonary alveolar proteinosis in hematologic malignancies. *Hematology/Oncology and Stem Cell Therapy, 7,* 127–135. https://doi.org/10.1016/j.hemonc.2014.09.003

Choi, Y.R., Chang, Y.-J., Kim, S.W., Choe, K.H., Lee, K.M., & An, J.-Y. (2015). Crazy paving radiography finding in asymptomatic pulmonary alveolar proteinosis. *Asian Cardiovascular and Thoracic Annals, 23,* 588–590. https://doi.org/10.1177/0218492314548232

Cortes, J., Mauro, M., Steegmann, J.L., Saglio, G., Malhotra, R., Ukropec, J.A., & Wallis, N.T. (2015). Cardiovascular and pulmonary adverse events in patients treated with *BCR-ABL* inhibitors: Data from the FDA Adverse Event Reporting System. *American Journal of Hematology, 90,* E66–E72. https://doi.org/10.1002/ajh.23938

Cudzilo, C., Aragaki, A., Guitron, J., & Benzaquen, S. (2014). Methotrexate-induced pleuropericarditis and eosinophilic pleural effusion. *Journal of Bronchology and Interventional Pulmonology, 21,* 90–92. https://doi.org/10.1097/LBR.0000000000000031

Cutler, C. (2017). The approach to hematopoietic cell transplantation survivorship. In A.G. Rosmarin (Ed.), *UpToDate.* Retrieved May 4, 2018, from https://www.uptodate.com/contents/the-approach-to-hematopoietic-cell-transplantation-survivorship

Darley, D.R., Malouf, M.A., & Glanville, A.R. (2016). A rare case of everolimus-induced pulmonary alveolar proteinosis. *Journal of Heart and Lung Transplantation, 35,* 147–148. https://doi.org/10.1016/j.healun.2015.10.001

Dasanu, C.A., Jen, T., & Skulski, R. (2017). Late-onset pericardial tamponade, bilateral pleural effusions and recurrent immune monoarthritis induced by ipilimumab use for metastatic melanoma. *Journal of Oncology Pharmacy Practice, 23,* 231–234. https://doi.org/10.1177/1078155216635853

Desai, A.V., Heneghan, M.B., Li, Y., Bunin, N.J., Grupp, S.A., Bagatell, R., & Seif, A.E. (2016). Toxicities of busulfan/melphalan versus carboplatin/etoposide/melphalan for high-dose chemotherapy with stem cell rescue for high risk neuroblastoma. *Bone Marrow Transplantation, 51,* 1204–1210. https://doi.org/10.1038/bmt.2016.84

Dhar, A.K., & Barman, P.K. (2012). Retinoic acid syndrome—Cardiac complication. *Journal of the Association of Physicians of India, 60,* 63–65.

Dhupkar, P., & Gordon, N. (2017). Interleukin-2: Old and new approaches to enhance immune-therapeutic efficacy. In A. Naing & J. Hajjar (Eds.), *Advances in Experimental Medicine and Biology: Vol. 995. Immunotherapy* (pp. 33–51). https://doi.org/10.1007/978-3-319-53156-4_2

Diederich, S. (2016). Chest CT for suspected pulmonary complications of oncologic therapies: How I review and report. *Cancer Imaging, 16,* 7. https://doi.org/10.1186/s40644-016-0066-4

Donatelli, C., Chongnarungsin, D., & Ashton, R. (2014). Acute respiratory failure from nilotinib-associated diffuse alveolar hemorrhage. *Leukemia and Lymphoma, 55,* 2408–2409. https://doi.org/10.3109/10428194.2014.887714

Dweik, R.A. (2017). Chlorambucil-induced pulmonary injury. In H. Hollingsworth (Ed.), *UpToDate.* Retrieved May 4, 2018, from http://www.uptodate.com/contents/chlorambucil-induced-pulmonary-injury

Dy, G.K., & Adjei, A.A. (2013). Understanding, recognizing, and managing toxicities of targeted anticancer therapies. *CA: A Cancer Journal for Clinicians, 63,* 249–279. https://doi.org/10.3322/caac.21184

Elemam, O., & Abdelmoety, D. (2013). Acute promyelocytic leukemia, study of predictive factors for differentiation syndrome, single center experience. *Journal of the Egyptian National Cancer Institute, 25,* 13–19. https://doi.org/10.1016/j.jnci.2012.10.004

Eli Lilly and Co. (2017). *Gemzar® (gemcitabine for injection)* [Package insert]. Indianapolis, IN: Author.

Escuissato, D.L., Warszawiak, D., & Marchiori, E. (2015). Differential diagnosis of diffuse alveolar haemorrhage in immunocompromised patients. *Current Opinion in Infectious Diseases, 28,* 337–342. https://doi.org/10.1097/QCO.0000000000000181

Eskazan, A.E., Eyice, D., Kurt, E.A., Elverdi, T., Yalniz, F.F., Salihoglu, A., ... Soysal, T. (2014). Chronic myeloid leukemia patients who develop grade I/II pleural effusion under second-line dasatinib have better responses and outcomes than patients without pleural effusion. *Leukemia Research, 38,* 781–787. https://doi.org/10.1016/j.leukres.2014.04.004

Falcinelli, L., Bellavita, R., Rebonato, A., Chiari, R., Vannucci, J., Puma, F., & Aristei, C. (2015). Bronchiolitis obliterans organizing pneumonia after radiation for lung cancer: A case report. *Tumori Journal, 101,* e88–e91. https://doi.org/10.5301/TJ.2015.14508

Feldman, D., & Vander Els, N. (2017). Bleomycin-induced lung injury. In H. Hollingsworth & D.M.F. Savarese (Eds.), *UpToDate.* Retrieved May 4, 2018, from http://www.uptodate.com/contents/bleomycin-induced-lung-injury

Findik, S. (2012). Pleural effusion in pulmonary embolism. *Current Opinion in Pulmonary Medicine, 18,* 347–354. https://doi.org/10.1097/MCP.0b013e32835395d5

Fresenius Kabi USA, LLC. (2016a). *Bleomycin sulfate* [Package insert]. Lake Zurich, IL: Author.

Fresenius Kabi USA, LLC. (2016b). *Ifosfamide* [Package insert]. Lake Zurich, IL: Author.

Fukushima, N., Saito, S., Sakata, Y., & Sawa, Y. (2013). A case of everolimus-associated chylothorax in a cardiac transplant recipient. *Transplantation Proceedings, 45,* 3144–3146. https://doi.org/10.1016/j.transproceed.2013.08.082

Garber, B., Albores, J., Wang, T., & Neville, T.H. (2015). A plasmapheresis protocol for refractory pulmonary alveolar proteinosis. *Lung, 193,* 209–211. https://doi.org/10.1007/s00408-014-9678-2

Genentech, Inc. (2016a). *Avastin® (bevacizumab)* [Package insert]. South San Francisco, CA: Author.

Genentech, Inc. (2016b). *Rituxan® (rituximab)* [Package insert]. South San Francisco, CA: Author.

Genentech, Inc. (2016c). *Xeloda® (capecitabine)* [Package insert]. South San Francisco, CA: Author.

Genentech, Inc. (2017a). *Herceptin® (trastuzumab)* [Package insert]. South San Francisco, CA: Author.

Genentech, Inc. (2017b). *Tecentriq® (atezolizumab)* [Package insert]. South San Francisco, CA: Author.

Genentech, Inc., & Astellas Pharma US, Inc. (2016). *Tarceva® (erlotinib)* [Package insert]. South San Francisco, CA, and Northbrook, IL: Authors.

Genestreti, G., Di Battista, M., Trisolini, R., Denicolo, F., Valli, M., Lazzari-Agli, L.A., ... Brandes, A.A. (2015). A commentary on interstitial pneumonitis induced by docetaxel: Clinical cases and systematic review of the literature. *Tumori Journal, 101,* e92–e95. https://doi.org/10.5301/tj.5000275

Genzyme Corp. (2014). *Campath® (alemtuzumab)* [Package insert]. Cambridge, MA: Author.

Giannou, A.D., Marazioti, A., Spella, M., Kanellakis, N.I., Apostolopoulou, H., Psallidas, I., ... Stathopoulos, G.T. (2015). Mast cells mediate malignant pleural effusion formation. *Journal of Clinical Investigation, 125,* 2317–2334. https://doi.org/10.1172/JCI79840

Gilbert, C.R., Lerner, A., Baram, M., Awsare, B.K. (2013). Utility of flexible bronchoscopy in the evaluation of pulmonary infiltrates in the hematopoietic stem cell transplant population—A single center fourteen year experience. *Archivos de Bronconeumología, 49,* 189–195. https://doi.org/10.1016/j.arbres.2012.11.012

GlaxoSmithKline. (2011). *Alkeran® (melphalan)* [Package insert]. Research Triangle Park, NC: Author.

Goebeler, M.-E., & Bargou, R. (2016). Blinatumomab: A CD19/CD3 bispecific T cell engager (BiTE) with unique anti-tumor efficacy. *Leukemia and Lymphoma, 57,* 1021–1032. https://doi.org/10.3109/10428194.2016.1161185

Griese, M., Zarbock, R., Costabel, U., Hildebrandt, J., Theegarten, D., Albert, M., ... Bonella, F. (2015). GATA2 deficiency in children and adults with severe pulmonary alveolar proteinosis and hematologic disorders. *BMC Pulmonary Medicine, 15,* 87. https://doi.org/10.1186/s12890-015-0083-2

Gurram, M.K., Pulivarthi, S., & McGary, C.T. (2013). Fatal hypersensitivity pneumonitis associated with docetaxel. *Tumori Journal, 99,* e100–e103. https://doi.org/10.1177/030089161309900325

He, Y., Li, X.D., Wang, D.N., Hu, Y., Xiao, R.Z., Wang, W.W., & Lin, D.J. (2014). Acute pleural and pericardial effusion induced by chemotherapy in treating chronic myelocytic leukemia. *Clinical Laboratory, 60,* 853–857.

Heritage Pharmaceuticals. (2017). *BiCNU® (carmustine)* [Package insert]. Eatontown, NJ: Author.

Heslet, L., Nielson, J.D., & Nepper-Christensen, S. (2012). Local pulmonary administration of factor VIIa (rFVIIa) in diffuse alveolar hemorrhage (DAH)—A review of a new treatment paradigm. *Biologics: Targets and Therapy, 6,* 37–46. https://doi.org/10.2147/BTT.S25507

Hochstrasser, A., Benz, G., Joerger, M., Templeton, A., Brutsche, M., & Früh, M. (2012). Interstitial pneumonitis after treatment with pemetrexed: A rare event? *Chemotherapy, 58,* 84–88. https://doi.org/10.1159/000336131

Hollebecque, A., Massard, C., & Soria, J.-C. (2012). Vascular disrupting agents: A delicate balance between efficacy and side effects. *Current Opinion in Oncology, 24,* 305–315. https://doi.org/10.1097/CCO.0b013e32835249de

Honoré, P.H., Joensen, S.J., Olsen, M., Hansen, S.H., & Mellemgaard, A. (2014). Third-space fluid distribution of pemetrexed in non-small cell lung cancer patients. *Cancer Chemotherapy and Pharmacology, 74,* 349–357. https://doi.org/10.1007/s00280-014-2485-x

Hospira, Inc. (2013). *Fludarabine phosphate* [Package insert]. Lake Forest, IL: Author.

Hospira, Inc. (2017). *Paclitaxel* [Package insert]. Lake Forest, IL: Author.

Huang, Z., Yi, X., Luo, B., Zhu, J., Wu, Y., Jiang, W., … Zeng, Y. (2016). Induced sputum deposition improves diagnostic yields of pulmonary alveolar proteinosis: A clinicopathological and methodological study of 17 cases. *Ultrastructural Pathology, 40,* 7–13. https://doi.org/10.3109/01913123.2015.1104404

Ikpeama, L.C., & Bailes, B.K. (2012). Diffuse alveolar hemorrhage-induced respiratory failure. *Critical Care Nursing Quarterly, 35,* 124–133. https://doi.org/10.1097/CNQ.0b013e31824566fb

ImClone LLC. (2016). *Erbitux® (cetuximab)* [Package insert]. Branchburg, NJ: Author.

Ishii, H., Seymour, J.F., Tazawa, R., Inoue, Y., Uchida, N., Nishida, A., … Nakata, K. (2014). Secondary pulmonary alveolar proteinosis complicating myelodysplastic syndrome results in worsening prognosis: A retrospective cohort study in Japan. *BMC Pulmonary Medicine, 14,* 37. https://doi.org/10.1186/1471-2466-14-37

Kai-Feng, W., Hong-Ming, P., Hai-Zhou, L., Li-Rong, S., & Xi-Yan, Z. (2011). Interleukin-11 induced capillary leak syndrome in primary hepatic carcinoma patients with thrombocytopenia. *BMC Cancer, 11,* 204. https://doi.org/10.1186/1471-2407-11-204

Kaifi, J.T., Toth, J.W., Gusani, N.J., Kimchi, E.T., Staveley-O'Carroll, K.F., Belani, C.P., & Reed, M.F. (2012). Multidisciplinary management of malignant pleural effusions. *Journal of Surgical Oncology, 105,* 731–738. https://doi.org/10.1002/jso.22100

Kaner, R.J., & Zappetti, D. (2017). Pulmonary complications after autologous hematopoietic cell transplantation. In H. Hollingsworth (Ed.), *UpToDate.* Retrieved May 4, 2018, from https://www.uptodate.com/contents/pulmonary-complications-after-autologous-hematopoietic-cell-transplantation

Kaner, R.J., & Zappetti, D. (2018). Pulmonary complications after allogeneic hematopoietic cell transplantation. In H. Hollingsworth (Ed.), *UpToDate.* Retrieved May 4, 2018, from https://www.uptodate.com/contents/pulmonary-complications-after-allogeneic-hematopoietic-cell-transplantation

Kantarjian, H.M., Shah, N.P., Cortes, J.E., Baccarani, M., Agarwal, M.B., Undurraga, M.S., … Hochhaus, A. (2012). Dasatinib or imatinib in newly diagnosed chronic-phase myeloid leukemia: 2-year follow-up from a randomized phase 3 trial (DASISION). *Blood, 119,* 1123–1129. https://doi.org/10.1182/blood-2011-08-376087

Keir, G.J., Maher, T.M., Ming, D., Abdullah, R., de Lauretis, A., Wickremasinghe, M., … Renzoni, E.A. (2014). Rituximab in severe, treatment-refractory interstitial lung disease. *Respirology, 19,* 353–359. https://doi.org/10.1111/resp.12214

Keldsen, N., Jöhnk, M.L., & Ejlersen, J.A. (2016). Impairment of lung function during adjuvant oxaliplatin treatment in patients with colorectal cancer: A prospective trial. *Current Drug Safety, 11,* 215–221. https://doi.org/10.2174/1574886311666160427104624

Kido, H., Morizane, C., Tamura, T., Hagihara, A., Kondo, S., Ueno, H., & Okusaka, T. (2012). Gemcitabine-induced pleuropericardial effusion in a patient with pancreatic cancer. *Japanese Journal of Clinical Oncology, 42,* 845–850. https://doi.org/10.1093/jjco/hys099

Kim, D.-W., Tiseo, M., Ahn, M.-J., Reckamp, K.L., Hansen, K.H., Kim, S.-W., … Camige, D.R. (2017). *Journal of Clinical Oncology, 35,* 2490–2498. https://doi.org/10.1200/JCO.2016.71.5904

Kim, K.W., Shinagare, A.B., Krajewski, K.M., Pyo, J., Tirumani, S.H., Jagannathan, J.P., & Ramaiya, N.H. (2015). Fluid retention associated with imatinib treatment in patients with gastrointestinal stromal tumor: Quantitative radiologic assessment and implications for management. *Korean Journal of Radiology, 16,* 304–313. https://doi.org/10.3348/kjr.2015.16.2.304

Kim, T.-O., Oh, I.-J., Kang, H.-W., Chi, S.-Y., Ban, H.-J., Kwon, Y.-S., … Kim, Y.-C. (2012). Temozolomide-associated bronchiolitis obliterans organizing pneumonia successfully treated with high-dose corticosteroid. *Journal of Korean Medical Science, 27,* 450–453. https://doi.org/10.3346/jkms.2012.27.4.450

Kim, Y.-J., Song, M., & Ryu, J.-C. (2009). Mechanisms underlying methotrexate-induced pulmonary toxicity. *Expert Opinion on Drug Safety, 8,* 451–458. https://doi.org/10.1517/14740330903066734

King, T.E., Jr. (2017a). Approach to the adult with interstitial lung disease: Clinical evaluation. In H. Hollingsworth (Ed.), *UpToDate.* Retrieved May 4, 2018, from http://www.uptodate.com/contents/approach-to-the-adult-with-interstitial-lung-disease-clinical-evaluation

King, T.E., Jr. (2017b). Approach to the adult with interstitial lung disease: Diagnostic testing. In H. Hollingsworth (Ed.), *UpToDate.* Retrieved May 4, 2018, from http://www.uptodate.com/contents/approach-to-the-adult-with-interstitial-lung-disease-diagnostic-testing

King, T.E., Jr. (2017c). Taxane-induced pulmonary toxicity. In D.M.F. Savarese & H. Hollingsworth (Eds.), *UpToDate.* Retrieved May 4, 2018, from http://www.uptodate.com/contents/taxane-induced-pulmonary-toxicity

Kroll, R.P., Kumar, S., Grossman, R.F., Price, C., & Srigley, J.R. (2016). Rare presentation of pulmonary alveolar proteinosis causing acute respiratory failure. *Canadian Respiratory Journal, 2016,* 4064539. https://doi.org/10.1155/2016/4064539

Kuo, J.C., Hawkins, C.A., & Yip, D. (2015). Application of hypersensitivity skin testing in chemotherapy-induced pneumonitis. *Asia Pacific Allergy, 5,* 234–236. https://doi.org/10.5415/apallergy.2015.5.4.234

Kurimoto, R., Sekine, I., Iwasawa, S., Sakaida, E., Tada, Y., Tatsumi, K., … Takiguchi, Y. (2015). Alveolar hemorrhage associated with pemetrexed administration. *Internal Medicine, 54,* 833–836. https://doi.org/10.2169/internalmedicine.54.3414

Kust, D., Kruljac, I., Peternac, A.S., Ostojić, J., Prpić, M., Čaržavec, D., & Gaćina, P. (2016). Pleural and pericardial effusions combined with ascites in a patient with severe sunitinib-induced hypothyroidism. *Acta Clinica Belgica, 71,* 175–177. https://doi.org/10.1179/2295333715Y.0000000065

Kwon, J., & Meagher, A. (2012). Crizotinib: A breakthrough for targeted therapies in lung cancer. *Journal of the Advanced Practitioner in Oncology, 3,* 267–272. https://doi.org/10.6004/jadpro.2012.3.4.8

Larcombe, P.J., Kapur, N., Fraser, C.J., Coulthard, M.G., & Schlapbach, L.J. (2014). Intrabronchial administration of activated recombinant factor VII in a young child with diffuse alveolar hemorrhage. *Pediatric Blood and Cancer, 61,* 570–571. https://doi.org/10.1002/pbc.24841

Latagliata, R., Breccia, M., Fava, C., Stagno, F., Tiribelli, M., Luciano, L., … Alimena, G. (2013). Incidence, risk factors and management of pleural effusions during dasatinib treatment in unselected elderly patients with chronic myelogenous leukaemia. *Hematological Oncology, 31,* 103–109. https://doi.org/10.1002/hon.2020

Laufer, C.B., & Roberts, O. (2015). Differentiation syndrome in acute myeloid leukemia after treatment with azacitidine. *European Journal of Haematology, 95,* 484–485. https://doi.org/10.1111/ejh.12598

Leblejian, H., DeAngelo, D.J., Skirvin, J.A., Stone, R.M., Wadleigh, M., Werner, L., … McDonnell, A.M. (2013). Predictive factors for all-trans retinoic acid-related differentiation syndrome in patients with acute promyelocytic leukemia. *Leukemia Research, 37,* 747–751. https://doi.org/10.1016/j.leukres.2013.04.011

Lengfelder, E., Lo-Coco, F., Ades, L., Montesinos, P., Grimwade, D., Kishore, B., … Sanz, M. (2015). Arsenic trioxide-based therapy of relapsed acute promyelocytic leukemia: Registry results from the European LeukemiaNet. *Leukemia, 29,* 1084–1091. https://doi.org/10.1038/leu.2015.12

Li, Y., Tian, X.-L., Gui, Y.-S., Ma, A.-P., Li, X., Zeng, N., … Xu, K.-F. (2014). Characteristics of serum lipid metabolism in patients with autoimmune pulmonary alveolar proteinosis. *Zhongguo Yi Xue Ke Xue Yuan Bao, 36,* 645–649. https://doi.org/10.3881/j.issn.1000-503X.2014.06.016

Lind, J.S.W., Senan, S., & Smit, E.F. (2012). Pulmonary toxicity after bevacizumab and concurrent thoracic radiotherapy observed in a phase I study for inoperable stage III non-small-cell lung cancer. *Journal of Clinical Oncology, 30,* e104–e108. https://doi.org/10.1200/JCO.2011.38.4552

Lindauer, M., & Hochhaus, A. (2014). Dasatinib. In U.M. Martens (Ed.), *Recent Results in Cancer Research: Vol. 201. Small molecules in oncology* (pp. 27–65). https://doi.org/10.1007/978-3-642-54490-3_2

Maldonado, F., & Limper, A.H. (2017a). Pulmonary toxicity associated with antineoplastic therapy: Cytotoxic agents. In D.M.F. Savarese & H. Hollingsworth (Eds.), *UpToDate.* Retrieved May 4, 2018, from http://www.uptodate.com/contents/pulmonary-toxicity-associated-with-antineoplastic-therapy-cytotoxic-agents

Maldonado, F., & Limper, A.H. (2017b). Pulmonary toxicity associated with antineoplastic therapy: Molecularly targeted agents. In D.M.F. Savarese & H. Hollingsworth (Eds.), *UpToDate.* Retrieved May 4, 2018, from http://www.uptodate.com/contents/pulmonary-toxicity-associated-with-antineoplastic-therapy-molecularly-targeted-agents

Maldonado, F., & Limper, A.H. (2018). Pulmonary toxicity associated with systemic antineoplastic therapy: Clinical presentation, diagnosis, and treatment. In H. Hollingsworth & D.M.F. Savarese (Eds.), *UpToDate.* Retrieved May 4, 2018, from http://www.uptodate.com/contents/pulmonary-toxicity-associated-with-systemic-antineoplastic-therapy-clinical-presentation-diagnosis-and-treatment

Malur, A., Kavuru, M.S., Marshall, I., Barna, B.P., Huizar, I., Karnekar, R., & Thomassen, M.J. (2012). Rituximab therapy in pulmonary alveolar proteinosis improves alveolar macrophage lipid homeostasis. *Respiratory Research, 13,* 46. https://doi.org/10.1186/1465-9921-13-46

Mandel, J., & LeVarge, B. (2018a). Epidemiology, pathogenesis, clinical evaluation, and diagnosis of pulmonary veno-occlusive disease in adults. In G. Finlay (Ed.), *UpToDate.* Retrieved May 4, 2018, from https://www.uptodate.com/contents/epidemiology-pathogenesis-clinical-evaluation-and-diagnosis-of-pulmonary-veno-occlusive-disease-in-adults

Mandel, J., & LeVarge, B. (2018b). Treatment and prognosis of pulmonary veno-occlusive disease in adults. In G. Finlay (Ed.), *UpToDate.* Retrieved May 4, 2018, from https://www.uptodate.com/contents/treatment-and-prognosis-of-pulmonary-veno-occlusive-disease-in-adults

Mankikian, J., Lioger, B., Diot, E., D'Halluin, P., Lissandre, S., Marchand Adam, S., … Beau Salinas, F. (2014). Pulmonary toxicity associated with the use of lenalidomide: Case report of late-onset acute respiratory distress syndrome and literature review. *Heart and Lung, 43,* 120–123. https://doi.org/10.1016/j.hrtlng.2013.11.007

Margaritopoulos, G.A., Vasarmidi, E., Jacob, J., Wells, A.U., & Antoniou, K.M. (2015). Smoking and interstitial lung disease. *European Respiratory Review, 24,* 428–435. https://doi.org/10.1183/16000617.0050-2015

Matsuno, O. (2012). Drug-induced interstitial lung disease: Mechanisms and best diagnostic approaches. *Respiratory Research, 13,* 39. https://doi.org/10.1186/1465-9921-13-39

Mayne Pharma Inc. (2011). *Cytarabine* [Package insert]. Paramus, NJ: Author.

McCormack, M.C. (2017). Diffusing capacity for carbon monoxide. In H. Hollingsworth (Ed.), *UpToDate.* Retrieved May 4, 2018, from http://www.uptodate.com/contents/diffusing-capacity-for-carbon-monoxide

Merck and Co., Inc. (2016). *Intron® A (interferon alfa-2b, recombinant)* [Package insert]. Whitehouse Station, NJ: Author.

Merck and Co., Inc. (2017). *Keytruda® A (pembrolizumab)* [Package insert]. Whitehouse Station, NJ: Author.

Millennium Pharmaceuticals, Inc. (2017). *Velcade® (bortezomib)* [Package insert]. Cambridge, MA: Author.

Mineo, G., Attinà, D., Mughetti, M., Balacchi, C., De Luca, F., Niro, F., … Zompatori, M. (2014). Pulmonary veno-occlusive disease: The role of CT. *La Radiologia Medica, 119,* 667–673. https://doi.org/10.1007/s11547-013-0363-y

Miura, M. (2015). Therapeutic drug monitoring of imatinib, nilotinib, and dasatinib for patients with chronic myeloid leukemia. *Biological and Pharmaceutical Bulletin, 38,* 645–654. https://doi.org/10.1248/bpb.b15-00103

Miura, Y., Imamura, C.K., Fukunaga, K., Katsuyama, Y., Suyama, K., Okaneya, T., … Tanigawara, Y. (2014). Sunitinib-induced severe toxicities in a Japanese patient with *ABCG2* 421 AA genotype. *BMC Cancer, 14,* 964. https://doi.org/10.1186/1471-2407-14-964

Mizuno, R., Asano, K., Mikami, S., Nagata, H., Kaneko, G., & Oya, M. (2012). Patterns of interstitial lung disease during everolimus treatment in patients with metastatic renal cell carcinoma. *Japanese Journal of Clinical Oncology, 42,* 442–446. https://doi.org/10.1093/jjco/hys033

Mo, Q., Wang, B., Dong, N., Bao, L., Su, X., Li, Y., & Chen, C. (2016). The clinical clues of pulmonary alveolar proteinosis: A report of 11 cases and literature review. *Canadian Respiratory Journal, 2016,* 4021928. https://doi.org/10.1155/2016/4021928

Mo, X.-D., Xu, L.-P., Liu, D.-H., Zhang, X.-H., Chen, H., Chen, Y.-H., … Huang, X.-J. (2013). High-dose cyclophosphamide therapy associated with diffuse alveolar hemorrhage after allogeneic hematopoietic stem cell transplantation. *Respiration, 86,* 453–461. https://doi.org/10.1159/000345592

Montani, D., Bergot, E., Günther, S., Savale, L., Bergeron, A., Bourdin, A., … Humbert, M. (2012). Pulmonary artery hypertension in patients treated with dasatinib. *Circulation, 125,* 2128–2137. https://doi.org/10.1161/CIRCULATIONAHA.111.079921

Mori, M., Tsunemine, H., Imada, K., Ito, K., Kodaka, T., & Takahashi, T. (2014). Life-threatening hemorrhagic pneumonia caused by *Stenotrophomonas maltophilia* in the treatment of hematologic diseases. *Annals of Hematology, 93,* 901–911. https://doi.org/10.1007/s00277-014-2028-x

Morishita, S., Hagihara, M., Itabashi, M., Ishii, Y., Yamamoto, W., Numata, A., … Nakajima, H. (2016). Development of pulmonary hypertension during oral dasatinib therapy for chronic myelogenous leukemia. *Rinsho Ketsueki, 57,* 999–1003. https://doi.org/10.11406/rinketsu.57.999

Murofushi, K.N., Oguchi, M., Gosho, M., Kozuka, T., & Sakurai, H. (2015). Radiation-induced bronchiolitis obliterans organizing pneumonia (BOOP) syndrome in breast cancer patients is associated with age. *Radiation Oncology, 10,* 103. https://doi.org/10.1186/s13014-015-0393-9

Muzumdar, H. (2012). Pleural effusion. *Pediatrics in Review, 33,* 45–47. https://doi.org/10.1542/pir.33-1-45

Nagasawa, J., Kurasawa, K., & Hanaoka, R. (2016). Rituximab improved systemic lupus erythematosus-associated pulmonary alveolar proteinosis without decreasing anti-GM-CSF antibody levels. *Lupus, 25,* 783–784. https://doi.org/10.1177/0961203315627204

Nakazawa, H., Nishina, S., Mimura, Y., Kawakami, T., Senoo, Y., Sakai, K., ... Kitano, K. (2014). Tumor lysis syndrome in a chronic lymphocytic leukemia patient with pleural effusion after oral fludarabine and cyclophosphamide therapy. *International Journal of Hematology, 99,* 782–785. https://doi.org/10.1007/s12185-014-1560-8

Nanjappa, S., Jeong, D.K., Muddaraju, M., Jeong, K., Hill, E.D., & Greene, J.N. (2016). Diffuse alveolar hemorrhage in acute myeloid leukemia. *Cancer Control, 23,* 272–277. https://doi.org/10.1177/107327481602300310

National Cancer Institute Cancer Therapy Evaluation Program. (2017). *Common terminology criteria for adverse events* [v.5.0]. Retrieved from https://ctep.cancer.gov/protocoldevelopment/electronic_applications/docs/CTCAE_v5_Quick_Reference_5x7.pdf

NextSource Biotechnology, LLC. (2013). *Gleostine® (lomustine)* [Package insert]. Miami, FL: Author.

Nishino, M., Brais, L.K., Brooks, N.V., Hatabu, H., Kulke, M.H., & Ramaiya, N.H. (2016). Drug-related pneumonitis during mammalian target of rapamycin inhibitor therapy in patients with neuroendocrine tumors: A radiographic pattern-based approach. *European Journal of Cancer, 53,* 163–170. https://doi.org/10.1016/j.ejca.2015.10.015

Novartis Pharmaceuticals Corp. (n.d.). Mechanism of action. Retrieved from https://www.hcp.novartis.com/products/afinitor/advanced-pancreatic-neuroendocrine-tumor-net/mechanism-of-action

Novartis Pharmaceuticals Corp. (2015). *Hycamtin® (topotecan)* [Package insert]. East Hanover, NJ: Author.

Novartis Pharmaceuticals Corp. (2016). *Afinitor® (everolimus)* [Package insert]. East Hanover, NJ: Author.

Novartis Pharmaceuticals Corp. (2017a). *Gleevec® (imatinib mesylate)* [Package insert]. East Hanover, NJ: Author.

Novartis Pharmaceuticals Corp. (2017b). *Votrient® (pazopanib)* [Package insert]. East Hanover, NJ: Author.

Nucci, M., Nouér, S.A., & Anaissie, E. (2015). Distinguishing the causes of pulmonary infiltrates in patients with acute leukemia. *Clinical Lymphoma, Myeloma and Leukemia, 15*(Suppl.), S98–S103. https://doi.org/10.1016/j.clml.2015.03.007

Nunomura, S., Tanaka, T., Nakayama, T., Otani, K., Ishii, H., Tabata, K., ... Fukuoka, J. (2016). Pulmonary alveolar proteinosis-like change: A fairly common reaction associated with the severity of idiopathic pulmonary fibrosis. *Respiratory Investigation, 54,* 272–279. https://doi.org/10.1016/j.resinv.2016.02.004

Olivier, K.R., & Peikert, T. (2017). Radiation-induced lung injury. In H. Hollingsworth (Ed.), *UpToDate.* Retrieved May 4, 2018, from https://www.uptodate.com/contents/radiation-induced-lung-injury

Olsson, K.M., & Palazzini, M. (2015). Challenges in pulmonary hypertension: Managing the unexpected. *European Respiratory Review, 24,* 674–681. https://doi.org/10.1183/16000617.0060-2015

Ono, A., Takahashi, T., Oishi, T., Sugino, T., Akamatsu, H., Shukuya, T., ... Yamamoto, N. (2013). Acute lung injury with alveolar hemorrhage as adverse drug reaction related to crizotinib. *Journal of Clinical Oncology, 31,* e417–e419. https://doi.org/10.1200/JCO.2012.47.1110

Osawa, M., Kudoh, S., Sakai, F., Endo, M., Hamaguchi, T., Ogino, Y., ... Gemma, A. (2015). Clinical features and risk factors of panitumumab-induced interstitial lung disease: A post-marketing all-case surveillance study. *International Journal of Clinical Oncology, 20,* 1063–1071. https://doi.org/10.1007/s10147-015-0834-3

Oudart, J.-B., Maquart, F.-X., Semouma, O., Lauer, M., Arthuis-Demoulin, P., & Ramont, L. (2012). Pleural effusion in a patient with multiple myeloma. *Clinical Chemistry, 58,* 672–674. https://doi.org/10.1373/clinchem.2010.160994

Papani, R., Duarte, A.G., Lin, Y.-L., Kuo, Y.-F., & Sharma, G. (2017). Pulmonary arterial hypertension associated with interferon therapy: A population-based study. *Multidisciplinary Respiratory Medicine, 12,* 1. https://doi.org/10.1186/s40248-016-0082-z

Papiris, S.A., Tsirigotis, P., Kolilekas, L., Papadaki, G., Papaioannou, A.I., Triantafillidou, C., ... Manali, E.D. (2014). Long-term inhaled granulocyte macrophage–colony-stimulating factor in autoimmune pulmonary alveolar proteinosis: Effectiveness, safety, and lowest effective dose. *Clinical Drug Investigations, 34,* 553–564. https://doi.org/10.1007/s40261-014-0208-z

Papiris, S.A., Tsirigotis, P., Kolilekas, L., Papadaki, G., Papaioannou, A.I., Triantafillidou, C., ... Manali, E.D. (2015). Pulmonary alveolar proteinosis: Time to shift? *Expert Review of Respiratory Medicine, 9,* 337–349. https://doi.org/10.1586/17476348.2015.1035259

Park, S.I., Jeon, W.H., Jeung, H.J., Kim, G.C., Kim, D.K., & Sim, Y.-J. (2014). Clinical features of docetaxel chemotherapy-related lymphedema. *Lymphatic Research and Biology, 12,* 197–202. https://doi.org/10.1089/lrb.2013.0037

Parshall, M.B., Schwartzstein, R.M., Adams, L., Banzetti, R.B., Manning, H.L., Bourbeau, J., ... O'Donnell, D.E. (2012). An official American Thoracic Society statement: Update on the mechanisms, assessment, and management of dyspnea. *American Journal of Respiratory and Critical Care Medicine, 185,* 435–452. https://doi.org/10.1164/rccm.201111-2042ST

Paydas, S. (2014). Dasatinib, large granular lymphocytosis, and pleural effusion: Useful or adverse effect? *Critical Reviews in Oncology/Hematology, 89,* 242–247. https://doi.org/10.1016/j.critrevonc.2013.10.005

Perros, F., Günther, S., Ranchoux, B., Godinas, L., Antigny, F., Chaumais, M.-C., ... Montani, D. (2015). Mitomycin-induced pulmonary veno-occlusive disease: Evidence from human disease and animal model. *Circulation, 132,* 834–847. https://doi.org/10.1161/CIRCULATIONAHA.115.014207

Pfizer Inc. (2017). *Xalkori® (crizotinib)* [Package insert]. New York, NY: Author.

Pierre Fabre Pharmaceuticals, Inc. (2014). *Navelbine® (vinorelbine tartrate)* [Package insert]. Parsippany, NJ: Author.

Possick, J.D. (2017). Pulmonary toxicities from checkpoint immunotherapy for malignancy. *Clinics in Chest Medicine, 38,* 223–232. https://doi.org/10.1016/j.ccm.2016.12.012

Prometheus Laboratories Inc. (2012). *Proleukin® (aldesleukin)* [Package insert]. San Diego, CA: Author.

Qi, W.-X., Sun, Y.-J., Shen, Z., & Yao, Y. (2015). Risk of interstitial lung disease associated with EGFR-TKIs in advanced non-small-cell lung cancer: A meta-analysis of 24 phase III clinical trials. *Journal of Chemotherapy, 27,* 40–51. https://doi.org/10.1179/1973947814Y.0000000189

Ranchoux, B., Günther, S., Quarck, R., Chaumais, M.-C., Dorfmüller, P., Antigny, F., ... Perros, F. (2015). Chemotherapy-induced pulmonary hypertension: Role of alkylating agents. *American Journal of Pathology, 18,* 356–371. https://doi.org/10.1016/j.ajpath.2014.10.021

Rathi, N.K., Tanner, A.R., Dinh, A., Dong, W., Feng, L., Ensor, J., ... Nates, J.L. (2015). Low-, medium- and high-dose steroids with or without aminocaproic acid in adult hematopoietic SCT patients with diffuse alveolar hemorrhage. *Bone Marrow Transplantation, 50,* 420–426. https://doi.org/10.1038/bmt.2014.287

Roncolato, F.T., Chatfield, M., Houghton, B., Toner, G., Stockler, M., Thomson, D., ... Grimison, P. (2016). The effect of pulmonary function testing on bleomycin dosing in germ cell tumours. *Internal Medicine Journal, 46,* 893–898. https://doi.org/10.1111/imj.13158

Russi, E.W., & Negrin, R.S. (2018). Busulfan-induced pulmonary toxicity. In H. Hollingsworth & D.M.F. Savarese (Eds.), *UpToDate.* Retrieved May 4, 2018, from https://www.uptodate.com/contents/busulfan-induced-pulmonary-injury

Ryu, J.H., Moua, T., Daniels, C.E., Hartman, T.E., Yi, E.S., Utz, J.P., & Limper, A.H. (2014). Idiopathic pulmonary fibrosis: Evolving concepts. *Mayo Clinic Proceedings, 89,* 1130–1142. https://doi.org/10.1016/j.mayocp.2014.03.016

Sakai, M., Kubota, T., Takaoka, M., Tsukuda, T., Arakawa, Y., Anabuki, K., … Yokoyama, A. (2015). Successful re-administration of lenalidomide after lenalidomide-induced pulmonary alveolar hemorrhage in a patient with refractory myeloma. *Annals of Hematology, 94,* 891–892. https://doi.org/10.1007/s00277-014-2260-4

Sakamoto, K., Ito, S., Hashimoto, N., & Hasegawa, Y. (2017). Pirfenidone as salvage treatment for refractory bleomycin-induced lung injury: A case report of seminoma. *BMC Cancer, 17,* 526. https://doi.org/10.1186/s12885-017-3521-0

Saleem, S.A., Ammannagari, N., Winans, A.R.M., & Leonardo, J.M. (2015). Diffuse alveolar hemorrhage: A fatal complication of rituximab. *Global Journal of Hematology and Blood Transfusion, 2,* 1–3. https://doi.org/10.15379/2408-9877.2015.02.01.01

Sanofi-Aventis U.S. LLC. (2015a). *Eloxatin® (oxaliplatin)* [Package insert]. Bridgewater, NJ: Author.

Sanofi-Aventis U.S. LLC. (2015b). *Taxotere® (docetaxel)* [Package insert]. Bridgewater, NJ: Author.

Sanz, M.A., & Montesinos, P. (2014). How we prevent and treat differentiation syndrome in patients with acute promyelocytic leukemia. *Blood, 123,* 2777–2782. https://doi.org/10.1182/blood-2013-10-512640

Satoh, H., Tazawa, R., Sakakibara, T., Ohkouchi, S., Ebina, M., Miki, M., … Nukiwa, T. (2012). Bilateral peripheral infiltrates refractory to immunosuppressants were diagnosed as autoimmune pulmonary alveolar proteinosis and improved by inhalation of granulocyte/macrophage-colony stimulating factor. *Internal Medicine, 51,* 1737–1742. https://doi.org/10.2169/internalmedicine.51.6093

Schiffer, C.A., Cortes, J.E., Hochhaus, A., Saglio, G., le Coutre, P., Porkka, K., … Shah, N.P. (2016). Lymphocytosis after treatment with dasatinib in chronic myeloid leukemia: Effects on response and toxicity. *Cancer, 112,* 1398–1407. https://doi.org/10.1002/cncr.29933

Schwaiblmair, M., Behr, W., Haeckel, T., Märkl, B., Foerg, W., & Berghaus, T. (2012). Drug induced interstitial lung disease. *Open Respiratory Medicine Journal, 6,* 63–74. https://doi.org/10.2174/1874306401206010063

Schwarz, M.I. (2017). The diffuse alveolar hemorrhage syndromes. In H. Hollingsworth (Ed.), *UpToDate.* Retrieved May 4, 2018, from https://www.uptodate.com/contents/the-diffuse-alveolar-hemorrhage-syndromes

Seattle Genetics, Inc. (2016). *Adcetris® (brentuximab vedotin)* [Package insert]. Bothell, WA: Author.

Shannon, V.R. (2017). Pneumotoxicity associated with immune checkpoint inhibitor therapies. *Current Opinion in Pulmonary Medicine, 23,* 305–316. https://doi.org/10.1097/MCP.0000000000000382

Shattuck, T.M., & Bean, S.M. (2013). Pulmonary alveolar proteinosis. *Diagnostic Cytopathology, 41,* 620–622. https://doi.org/10.1002/dc.22857

Shelton, B.K. (2012). Drugs affecting the immune response. In D.S. Aschenbrenner & S.J. Venable (Eds.), *Drug therapy in nursing* (4th ed., pp. 644–668). Philadelphia, PA: Lippincott Williams & Wilkins.

Shogbon, A.O., Hap, J., Dretler, R., & Dalvi, A.G. (2013). Cryptogenic organizing pneumonia during adjuvant chemotherapy with oxaliplatin, 5-fluorouracil, and leucovorin (FOLFOX) for colon cancer. *Journal of Pharmacy Practice, 26,* 62–66. https://doi.org/10.1177/0897190012451929

Sigma-Tau Pharmaceuticals, Inc. (2014). *DepoCyt® (cytarabine liposome injection)* [Package insert]. Gaithersburg, MD: Author.

Specks, U. (2017). Cyclophosphamide pulmonary toxicity. In H. Hollingsworth & D.M.F. Savarese (Eds.), *UpToDate.* Retrieved May 4, 2018, from http://www.uptodate.com/contents/cyclophosphamide-pulmonary-toxicity

Spira, D., Wirths, S., Skowronski, F., Pintoffl, J., Kaufmann, S., Brodoefel, H., & Horger, M. (2013). Diffuse alveolar hemorrhage in patients with hematological malignancies: HRCT patterns of pulmonary involvement and disease course. *Clinical Imaging, 37,* 680–686. https://doi.org/10.1016/j.clinimag.2012.11.005

Stark, P. (2017). Evaluation of diffuse lung disease by conventional chest radiography. In G. Finlay & S.I. Lee (Eds.), *UpToDate.* Retrieved May 4, 2018, from http://www.uptodate.com/contents/evaluation-of-diffuse-lung-disease-by-conventional-chest-radiography

Stein, M.E., Zidan, J., Charas, T., Gershuny, A., & Ben-Yosef, R. (2015). Bleomycin-induced pneumonitis in three patients treated with chemotherapy for primary advanced seminoma. *Journal of B.U.ON., 20,* 928–932.

Sugita, Y., Ohwada, C., Nagao, Y., Kawajiri, C., Shimizu, R., Togasaki, E., … Nakaseko, C. (2015). Early-onset severe diffuse alveolar hemorrhage after bortezomib administration suggestive of pulmonary involvement of myeloma cells. *Journal of Clinical and Experimental Hematopathology, 55,* 163–168. https://doi.org/10.3960/jslrt.55.163

Sun Pharmaceutical Industries, Inc. (2017). *Temozolomide* [Package insert]. Cranbury, NJ: Author.

Suzuki, T., & Trapnell, B.C. (2016). Pulmonary alveolar proteinosis syndrome. *Clinics in Chest Medicine, 37,* 431–440. https://doi.org/10.1016/j.ccm.2016.04.006

Sverzellati, N., Lynch, D.A., Hansell, D.M., Johkoh, T., King, T.E., Jr., & Travis, W.D. (2015). American Thoracic Society–European Respiratory Society classification of the idiopathic interstitial pneumonias: Advances in knowledge since 2002. *RadioGraphics, 35,* 1849–1871. https://doi.org/10.1148/rg.2015140334

Syrigou, E., Dannos, I., Kotteas, E., Makrilia, N., Tourkantonis, I., Dilana, K., … Syrigos, K.N. (2011). Hypersensitivity reactions to docetaxel: Retrospective evaluation and development of a desensitization protocol. *International Archives of Allergy and Immunology, 156,* 320–324. https://doi.org/10.1159/000324454

Takeda, A., Kunieda, E., Ohashi, T., Aoki, Y., Oku, Y., Enomoto, T., … Sugiura, M. (2012). Severe COPD is correlated with mild radiation pneumonitis following stereotactic body radiotherapy. *Chest, 141,* 858–866. https://doi.org/10.1378/chest.11-1193

Tamiya, A., Naito, T., Miura, S., Morii, S., Tsuya, A., Nakamura, Y., … Endo, M. (2012). Interstitial lung disease associated with docetaxel in patients with advanced non-small cell lung cancer. *Anticancer Research, 32,* 1103–1106. Retrieved from http://ar.iiarjournals.org/content/32/3/1103.long

Tamura, M., Saraya, T., Fujiwara, M., Hiraoka, S., Yokoyama, T., Yano, K., … Goto, H. (2013). High-resolution computed tomography findings for patients with drug-induced pulmonary toxicity, with special reference to hypersensitivity pneumonitis-like patterns in gemcitabine-induced cases. *Oncologist, 18,* 454–459. https://doi.org/10.1634/theoncologist.2012-0248

Tan, H.E., & Lake, F. (2016). Interstitial pneumonitis secondary to leuprorelin acetate for prostate cancer. *Respirology Case Reports, 4,* e00146. https://doi.org/10.1002/rcr2.146

Tanaka, K.-I., Azuma, A., Miyazaki, Y., Sato, K., & Mizushima, T. (2012). Effects of lecithinized superoxide dismutase and/or pirfenidone against bleomycin-induced pulmonary fibrosis. *Chest, 142,* 1011–1019. https://doi.org/10.1378/chest.11-2879

Tazawa, R., Inoue, Y., Arai, T., Takada, T., Kasahara, Y., Hojo, M., ... Nakata, K. (2014). Duration of benefit in patients with autoimmune pulmonary alveolar proteinosis after inhaled granulocyte-macrophage colony-stimulating factor therapy. *Chest, 145,* 729–737. https://doi.org/10.1378/chest.13-0603

Teuwen, L.-A., Van den Mooter, T., & Dirix, L. (2015). Management of pulmonary toxicity associated with targeted anticancer therapies. *Expert Opinion on Drug Metabolism and Toxicology, 11,* 1695–1707. https://doi.org/10.1517/17425255.2015.1080687

Teva Pharmaceuticals USA, Inc. (2016). *Trisenox® (arsenic trioxide)* [Package insert]. North Wales, PA: Author.

Tewari, P., Wallis, W., & Kebriaei, P. (2017). Manifestations and management of veno-occlusive disease/sinusoid obstruction syndrome in the era of contemporary therapies. *Clinical Advances in Hematology and Oncology, 15,* 130–139. Retrieved from http://www.hematologyandoncology.net/archives/february-2017/manifestations-and-management-of-veno-occlusive-diseasesinusoidal-obstruction-syndrome-in-the-era-of-contemporary-therapies

Tobiume, M., Shinohara, T., Kuno, T., Mukai, S., Naruse, K., Hatakeyama, N., & Ogushi, F. (2014). BCG-induced pneumonitis with lymphocytic pleurisy in the absence of elevated KL-6. *BMC Pulmonary Medicine, 14,* 35. https://doi.org/10.1186/1471-2466-14-35

Toma, A., Rapoport, A.P., Burke, A., & Sachdeva, A. (2017). Lenalidomide-induced eosinophilic pneumonia. *Respirology Case Reports, 5,* e00233. https://doi.org/10.1002/rcr2.233

Tomii, K., Kato, T., Takahashi, M., Noma, S., Kobashi, Y., Enatsu, S., ... Kudoh, S. (2017). Pemetrexed-related interstitial lung disease reported from post marketing surveillance (malignant pleural mesothelioma/non-small cell lung cancer). *Japanese Journal of Clinical Oncology, 47,* 350–356. https://doi.org/10.1093/jjco/hyx010

Torrisi, J.M., Schwartz, L.H., Gollub, M.J., Ginsberg, M.S., Bosl, G.J., & Hricak, H. (2011). CT findings of chemotherapy-induced toxicity: What radiologists need to know about the clinical and radiologic manifestations of chemotherapy toxicity. *Radiology, 258,* 41–56. https://doi.org/10.1148/radiol.10092129

Travis, W.D., Costabel, U., Hansell, D.M., King, T.E., Jr., Lynch, D.A., Nicholson, A.G., ... Valeyre, D. (2013). An official American Thoracic Society/European Respiratory Society statement: Update of the international multidisciplinary classification of the idiopathic interstitial pneumonias. *American Journal of Respiratory and Critical Care Medicine, 188,* 733–748. https://doi.org/10.1164/rccm.201308-1483ST

Ueda, N., Chihara, D., Kohno, A., Tatekawa, S., Ozeki, K., Watamoto, K., & Morishita, Y. (2014). Predictive value of circulating angiopoietin-2 for endothelial damage–related complications in allogeneic hematopoietic stem cell transplantation. *Biology of Blood and Marrow Transplantation, 20,* 1335–1340. https://doi.org/10.1016/j.bbmt.2014.04.030

Urun, Y., Dincol, D., & Kumbasar, O.O. (2012). Rituximab-related organizing pneumonia and late onset neutropenia in a patient with non-Hodgkin lymphoma: A report of two rare complications and review of the literature. *Journal of the B.U.ON., 17,* 602–603.

Vahid, B., & Marik, P.E. (2008). Pulmonary complications of novel antineoplastic agents for solid tumors. *Chest, 133,* 528–538. https://doi.org/10.1378/chest.07-0851

Vande Vusse, L.K., & Madtes, D.K. (2017). Early onset noninfectious pulmonary syndromes after hematopoietic cell transplantation. *Clinics in Chest Medicine, 38,* 233–248. https://doi.org/10.1016/j.ccm.2016.12.007

Versluys, A.B., & Bresters, D. (2016). Pulmonary complications of childhood cancer treatment. *Paediatric Respiratory Reviews, 17,* 63–70. https://doi.org/10.1016/j.prrv.2015.09.004

Villa, G., Zaragoza, J.J., Sharma, A., Chelazzi, C., Ronco, C., & De Gaudio, A.R. (2014). High cutoff membrane to reduce systemic inflammation due to differentiation syndrome: A case report. *Blood Purification, 38,* 234–238. https://doi.org/10.1159/000369379

Villena Garrido, V., Cases Viedma, E., Fernández Villar, A., de Pablo Gafas, A., Pérez Rodríguez, E., Porcel Pérez, J.M., ... Valdés Cuadrado, L. (2014). Recommendations of diagnosis and treatment of pleural effusion. Update. *Archivos de Bronconeumología, 50,* 235–249. https://doi.org/10.1016/j.arbr.2014.04.007

Vion, A.-C., Pautou, P.-E., Durand, F., Boulanger, C.M., & Valla, D.C. (2015). Interplay of inflammation and endothelial dysfunction in bone marrow transplantation: Focus on hepatic veno-occlusive disease. *Seminars in Thrombosis and Hemostasis, 41,* 629–643. https://doi.org/10.1055/s-0035-1556728

Vymazal, T., & Krecmerova, M. (2015). Respiratory strategies and airway management in patients with pulmonary alveolar proteinosis: A review. *BioMed Research International, 2015,* 639543. https://doi.org/10.1155/2015/639543

Watts, J.M., & Tallman, M.S. (2014). Acute promyelocytic leukemia: What is the new standard of care? *Blood Reviews, 28,* 205–212. https://doi.org/10.1016/j.blre.2014.07.001

Weinberger, S.E., & Larson, R.A. (2017). Differentiation (retinoic acid) syndrome. In H. Hollingsworth & A.G. Rosmarin (Eds.), *UpToDate.* Retrieved May 4, 2018, from http://www.uptodate.com/contents/differentiation-retinoic-acid-syndrome

West-Ward Pharmaceuticals Corp. (2017). *Methotrexate* [Package insert]. Eatontown, NJ: Author.

Willemsen, A.E.C.A.B., Grutters, J.C., Gerritsen, W.R., van Erp, N.P., van Herpen, C.M.L., & Tol, J. (2016). mTOR inhibitor-induced interstitial lung disease in cancer patients: Comprehensive review and a practical management algorithm. *International Journal of Cancer, 138,* 2312–2321. https://doi.org/10.1002/ijc.29887

Wirk, B. (2012). Bortezomib-related diffuse alveolar hemorrhage. *Journal of Clinical Oncology, 30,* e379–e381. https://doi.org/10.1200/JCO.2012.43.6519

Wyeth Pharmaceuticals. (2011). *Neumega® (oprelvekin)* [Package insert]. Philadelphia, PA: Author.

Wyeth Pharmaceuticals. (2017). *Torisel® (temsirolimus)* [Package insert]. Philadelphia, PA: Author.

Xu, J.-F., Washko, G.R., Nakahira, K., Hatabu, H., Patel, A.S., Fernandez, I.E., ... Hunninghake, G.M. (2012). Statins and pulmonary fibrosis: The potential role of NLRP3 inflammasome activation. *American Journal of Respiratory and Critical Care Medicine, 185,* 547–556. https://doi.org/10.1164/rccm.201108-1574OC

Yakabe, T., Kitahara, K., Komiya, K., Sueoka-Aragane, N., Kimura, S., Sugioka, T., & Noshira, H. (2013). Severe eosinophilic pneumonia presenting during gemcitabine adjuvant chemotherapy. *World Journal of Surgical Oncology, 11,* 167. https://doi.org/10.1186/1477-7819-11-167

Yi, X., Li, H., Zeng, Y., Fang, X., Wang, L., Lv, H., ... Li, X. (2012). Transmission electron microscopy of sputum deposition in the diagnosis of pulmonary alveolar proteinosis. *Ultrastructural Pathology, 36,* 153–159. https://doi.org/10.3109/01913123.2011.639134

Yoshimura, M., Kojima, K., Tomimasu, R., Fukushima, N., Hayashi, S., Sueoka, E., & Kimura, S. (2014). ABL tyrosine kinase inhibitor-induced pulmonary alveolar proteinosis in chronic myeloid leukemia. *International Journal of Hematology, 100,* 611–614. https://doi.org/10.1007/s12185-014-1666-z

Zhang, H.-T., Wang, C., Wang, C.-Y., Fang, S.-C., Xu, B., & Zhang, Y.-M. (2016). Efficacy of whole-lung lavage in treatment of pulmonary alveolar proteinosis. *American Journal of Therapeutics, 23,* e1671–e1679. https://doi.org/10.1097/MJT.0000000000000239

CHAPTER 18

Hepatic Toxicities

A. Overview

1. More than 900 drugs and toxins, including antineoplastics and herbs, may cause liver dysfunction (Livshits, Rao, & Smith, 2014; Mehta, 2016).
2. Functions of the liver (Lee & Chan, 2016; Perry, 2012)
   a) Filters toxic substances
   b) Works with spleen to eliminate damaged red blood cells
   c) Produces bile, which aids in absorption and digestion of fats, allowing for excretion of waste products
   d) Synthesizes procoagulant proteins, also referred to as clotting factors (e.g., FII, FV, FVII, FIX, FX, FXI), which promote the maintenance of normal homeostasis (Kujovich, 2015)
   e) Processes and stores vitamins, minerals, proteins, fats, and glucose

B. Pathophysiology

1. Drug toxicity mechanisms (Floyd & Kerr, 2017; Lisi, 2016; Mehta, 2016; Njoku, 2014)
   a) Intrinsic: Directly affect liver; liver toxicity induced by drug that is predictable and dose related
   b) Idiosyncratic: Occur less frequently; associated with less consistent dose–toxicity relationship and varied presentation
2. Mechanisms of injury resulting from cancer therapies (Chen, Suzuki, Borlak, Andrade, & Lucena, 2015; Fontana, 2014; Larson, 2017; Mehta, 2016)
   a) Disruption of hepatocytes: Adenosine triphosphate levels decrease because of covalent binding of drugs to intracellular proteins, leading to actin disruption. Disassembling of actin fibrils on hepatocyte surfaces causes blebs and membrane rupture, resulting in hepatic injury, inflammation, fibrosis, and carcinogenesis (Mehta, 2016).
   b) Disruption of transport proteins: Bile flow may be interrupted by drugs affecting transport proteins at the canalicular membrane. Loss of villous processes and transport pump interruption prevent bile excretion, causing cholestasis.
   c) Cytolytic T-cell activation: Immune response is stimulated by the covalent binding of drugs with cytochrome P450 (CYP) enzymes acting as an immunogen, activating T cells and cytokines and resulting in an immune response to infection or tissue damage (Frick et al., 2017; Mehta, 2016).
   d) Apoptosis of hepatocytes: Apoptotic pathways activated by the tumor necrosis factor-alpha receptor Fas may trigger a cascade of intercellular caspases, resulting in programmed cell death.
   e) Disruption of mitochondria: Specific drugs inhibit synthesis of nicotinamide adenine dinucleotide and flavin adenine dinucleotide, resulting in decreased adenosine triphosphate production.
   f) Injury of bile ducts: Toxic metabolites excreted in bile can cause injury to the bile duct epithelium.
   g) Hypersensitivity/immune-mediated reactions: Antigen recognition by helper T cells occurs in relation with key cytokines.
   h) Genetic differences in CYP protein: These differences can result in abnormal metabolic reactions to drugs; for example, increased toxicity can occur in genetically predisposed individuals such as those who are female or obese (Mehta, 2016; Njoku, 2014).
3. Age-specific considerations
   a) Pediatric considerations (Ali, Charoo, & Abdallah, 2014; Barrett, Patel, Dombrowsky, Bajaj, & Skolnik, 2013; Benn, 2014)
      (1) Developmental changes in liver metabolism from birth to adolescence contribute to the increased sensitivity to toxins in the pediatric population, demonstrated by drug half-life that is more than two to three times longer (Benn, 2014).

(2) Plasma protein binding and partitioning are different in the pediatric population and fluctuate constantly during early years, resulting in how the drug is distributed (Ali et al., 2014).
(3) Age-related differences in pharmacokinetics, particularly in infants and neonates, are important to recognize because pH and motility affect gastrointestinal absorption, body composition alters distribution, and clearance systems are not mature (Ali et al., 2014; Benn, 2014).
(4) Drugs known to cause hepatotoxicity in children (Barrett et al., 2013; Chalasani et al., 2014; Chen et al., 2015)
(a) Analgesics
(b) Antibiotics
(c) Anticonvulsants
(d) Antineoplastic drugs
(5) Frequent monitoring of liver enzymes (Barrett et al., 2013)

b) Geriatric considerations
(1) Developmental changes in liver metabolism in older adults (Mehta, 2016)
(a) Increased risk of hepatic injury
(b) Decreased clearance
(c) Drug–drug interactions
(d) Reduced hepatic blood flow
(e) Varied drug binding
(f) Lower hepatic volume
(2) Drugs known to cause hepatotoxicity in older adults (Stine, Sateesh, & Lewis, 2013)
(a) Analgesics, including nonsteroidal anti-inflammatory drugs
(b) Non-narcotic pain medications, including tricyclic antidepressants, muscles relaxants, and benzodiazepines
(c) Antibiotics
(d) Cardiovascular drugs
(e) Herbal therapies
(f) Psychoneurotic drugs
(g) Antituberculosis drugs
(h) Antineoplastic drugs

C. Incidence (see Table 18-1)

D. Risk factors
1. Race: Variable toxicities (Chalasani et al., 2014; Mehta, 2016)
2. Age: Rare in children, increased in older adults (Chalasani et al., 2014; Chen et al., 2015)
3. Sex: Common in females (Mehta, 2016)
4. History of alcohol use (depletes glutathione); smoking; illicit drug use
5. History of liver disease: Cirrhosis, Budd-Chiari syndrome, alpha-1 antitrypsin deficiency, hemochromatosis, Wilson disease (Leise, Poterucha, & Talwalkar, 2014; Mehta, 2016)
6. History of infections: HIV, hepatitis B, hepatitis C (Chalasani et al., 2014; Leise et al., 2014)
7. Genetic factors: Rate of metabolism of CYP enzymes differs among individuals (Chalasani et al., 2014; Chen et al., 2015; Leise et al., 2014; Mehta, 2016).
8. Comorbidities: Obesity, malnutrition, diabetes mellitus (Mehta, 2016)
9. Drug formulations (intrahepatic chemotherapy), drug interactions, and polypharmacy (noncytotoxic hepatotoxic drugs or herbal products) (Chalasani et al., 2014; Chen et al., 2015; Leise et al., 2014; Mehta, 2016)
10. History of transplantation: Liver, kidney, stem cell transplant (Mehta, 2016)
11. Prior radiation therapy (Chen et al., 2015; Mehta, 2016)

E. Clinical manifestations
1. Variable from asymptomatic laboratory abnormalities to acute illness to overt hepatic failure (Floyd & Kerr, 2017; Mehta, 2016)
2. Elevations in aminotransferases (aspartate aminotransferase, alanine aminotransferase) indicative of hepatocellular injury; portal hypertension (Floyd & Kerr, 2017; Mehta, 2016)
3. Elevations in bilirubin and alkaline phosphatase suggestive of cholestasis
4. Signs and symptoms of cancer treatment–related hepatotoxicity (Floyd & Kerr, 2017; Mehta, 2016; Roesser, 2014)
a) Malaise, myalgia, arthralgia, low-grade fever
b) Gastrointestinal symptoms (anorexia, nausea, vomiting, right upper quadrant pain, acholic stools that are pale, clay-like, or putty-colored due to problems in the biliary system)
c) Jaundice, hyperpigmentation, ascites
d) Dark-colored urine
e) Pruritus
f) Hepatomegaly
g) Coagulopathy; bruising or bleeding
h) Hepatic encephalopathy
i) Hypersensitivity reactions (fever, rash, mononucleosis illness; additional evidence of toxicity to other organs)

F. Pathologic manifestations associated with drug toxicity in the liver (Botti et al., 2016; Gordon et al., 2017; Larson, 2017; Mehta, 2016; Tewari, Wallis, & Kebriaei, 2017)

Table 18-1. Hepatotoxicity of Antineoplastic Agents

Classification	Drug	Side Effects	Nursing Considerations
Chemotherapy Agents			
Alkylating agents	Bendamustine (Bendeka®, Treanda®)	Fatal and severe cases of liver injury reported due to confounding factors including combination therapy, disease progression, or HBV reactivation 3 months after treatment	Monitor LFTs prior to and during treatment. No formal studies have been done on the impact of hepatic dysfunction on drug pharmacokinetics. Avoid administration in patients with preexisting moderate to severe hepatic impairment (transaminases > 2.5 × ULN or total bilirubin > 1.5 × ULN (Floyd & Kerr, 2017; U.S. FDA, n.d.)
	Busulfan (IV: Busulfex®; oral: Myleran®)	Increased risk for SOS (area under the curve greater than 1,500 µM × min) with 8% incidence in setting of allogeneic HSCT; overall incidence of 7.7%–12%; jaundice, hepatic necrosis, hepatomegaly; SOS with incidence of 20%–50% after HSCT	Monitor transaminases, ALP, and bilirubin daily until day +28 post-HSCT to detect hepatotoxicity, which may indicate SOS. Busulfan has not been studied in patients with hepatic dysfunction. Consider therapeutic drug monitoring with high doses. (NIDDK & NLM, n.d.; U.S. FDA, n.d.)
	Chlorambucil (Leukeran®)	Jaundice, hepatotoxicity	No formal studies have been conducted in patients with hepatic dysfunction. Monitor closely in patients with hepatic impairment. Dose reduction may be considered, as no specific recommendations exist because of insufficient data. (U.S. FDA, n.d.)
	Cyclophosphamide (Cytoxan®)	SOS (risk factor with cytoreductive regimen for HSCT using cyclophosphamide, whole body irradiation, busulfan, or other agents), jaundice, cholestatic hepatitis, cytolytic hepatitis, hepatitis, cholestasis, hepatotoxicity with hepatic failure, hepatic encephalopathy, ascites, hepatomegaly, elevated LFTs	Dose reduction of 25% is recommended for serum bilirubin of 3.1–5 mg/dl or AST > 3 × ULN. Do not give if bilirubin > 5 mg/dl. Hepatic impairment reduced conversion of the drug to active metabolite, demonstrating possibly decreased efficacy. Patients with severe hepatic dysfunction have 40% decrease in total body clearance and 64% prolongation in elimination half-life. (Floyd & Kerr, 2017; U.S. FDA, n.d.)
	Dacarbazine	Hepatic necrosis, hepatic vein thrombosis (0.01% incidence)	Monitor for signs of liver toxicity. (Hospira, Inc., 2016)
	Ifosfamide (Ifex®)	Hepatic failure, fulminant hepatitis, SOS, portal vein thrombosis, cytolytic hepatitis, cholestasis (1.8% incidence), jaundice, hepatorenal syndrome, elevated ALT/AST, ALP, GGT, LDH, and bilirubin	Dose reduction of 25% is recommended with significant hepatic dysfunction (AST > 300 IU/L or bilirubin > 3 mg/dl). No formal studies have been conducted in patients with hepatic dysfunction; use caution with administration. (Floyd & Kerr, 2017; U.S. FDA, n.d.)
	Melphalan (Alkeran®, Evomela®)	Transient LFT abnormalities with high-dose use in HSCT; SOS (infrequent), jaundice	Monitor LFTs. (Floyd & Kerr, 2017; U.S. FDA, n.d.)
	Temozolomide (Temodar®)	Fatal and severe hepatotoxicity has been reported; elevated transaminases and bilirubin, cholestasis, hepatitis	Monitor LFTs at baseline, midway through the first cycle, prior to each subsequent cycle, and approximately 2–4 weeks after the last dose. (U.S. FDA, n.d.)

(Continued on next page)

Table 18-1. Hepatotoxicity of Antineoplastic Agents *(Continued)*

Classification	Drug	Side Effects	Nursing Considerations
Chemotherapy Agents *(Cont.)*			
Alkylating agents *(cont.)*	Trabectedin (Yondelis®)	Severe hepatotoxicity including liver failure can occur; one trial reported 35% incidence of grade 3–4 elevations in LFTs (AST/ALT, bilirubin, ALP); 1.3% incidence of drug-induced liver injury (ALT/AST > 3 × ULN, ALP < 2 × ULN, and bilirubin > 2 × ULN); and 18% incidence of ALT/AST > 8 × ULN.	Monitor LFTs prior to each treatment and as clinically indicated. Manage LFT elevations based on severity of LFTs by interrupting treatment, reducing the dose, or permanently discontinuing the drug. (U.S. FDA, n.d.)
Antimetabolites	Capecitabine (Xeloda®)	Hyperbilirubinemia, hepatic fibrosis (0.1%), hepatitis (0.1%), cholestatic hepatitis (0.1%)	Hold drug for grade 3–4 elevations in bilirubin until bilirubin recovers to < 3 × ULN, then resume at 75% of starting dose for first occurrence and 50% of starting dose for second occurrence. Discontinue drug at third occurrence. (U.S. FDA, n.d.)
	Clofarabine (Clolar®)	Increased risk for SOS in HSCT recipients who received clofarabine in combination with other chemotherapy agents (etoposide, cyclophosphamide); severe and fatal hepatotoxicity (hepatitis and hepatic failure) has occurred; elevations in AST/ALT and bilirubin usually occur within 10 days (grade 3–4); decreased AST/ALT, bilirubin (grade 2) within 15 days	Monitor liver function and for signs and symptoms of hepatitis and hepatic failure. Discontinue if grade 3 or greater increase in bilirubin; can restart at 25% dose reduction once patient is stable and organ function is at baseline. (U.S. FDA, n.d.)
	Cytarabine	Elevated bilirubin	Monitor LFTs periodically. Dose reduction of 50% is recommended with any aminotransferase elevations. (Floyd & Kerr, 2017; Pfizer Inc., 2011; U.S. FDA, n.d.)
	5-Fluorouracil (5-FU; Adrucil®)	Transient elevations in aminotransferases associated with hepatic steatosis; rare cases of acute liver injury with jaundice	Omit doses with liver failure (bilirubin > 5 mg/dl). No clear data exist on monitoring of LFTs. (Floyd & Kerr, 2017; NIDDK & NLM, n.d.)
	Floxuridine (FUDR®)	Increased AST/ALT, ALP, and bilirubin; biliary sclerosis (1%–26%)	Check LFTs at least weekly during therapy and after drug has been discontinued if hepatic toxicity is evident. (Floyd & Kerr, 2017)
	Gemcitabine (Gemzar®)	Transient elevation in aminotransferases; liver failure and death (rare); increased ALP, hepatic transaminitis (> 20%)	Monitor hepatic function prior to starting and during treatment. Discontinue drug for severe hepatotoxicity. (Floyd & Kerr, 2017; U.S. FDA, n.d.)

(Continued on next page)

Classification	Drug	Side Effects	Nursing Considerations
Chemotherapy Agents *(Cont.)*			
Antimetabolites *(cont.)*	6-Mercaptopurine (6-MP; Purinethol®)	Intrahepatic cholestasis, parenchymal cell necrosis; jaundice (40%, appearing as early as 1 week or as late as 8 years after starting treatment), ascites, hepatic encephalopathy; hepatotoxicity most common when daily dose > 2 mg/kg; cholestatic liver damage and hepatocellular injury (30 days after initiation, moderate elevations in serum aminotransaminases and ALP, bilirubin of 3–7 mg/dl)	Monitor LFTs (transaminases, ALP, bilirubin) prior to starting, then weekly, followed by monthly thereafter. Consider dose reduction in patients with hepatic impairment. Hold drug if signs of jaundice or hepatomegaly. Discontinue drug if LFTs continue to deteriorate and for toxic hepatitis or biliary stasis. (Floyd & Kerr, 2017; U.S. FDA, n.d.)
	Methotrexate	Acute transaminitis (60%–80% in those receiving high-dose therapy, with return to baseline in 1–2 weeks); risk for cirrhosis and fibrosis (in those receiving chronic low-dose therapy usually after > 2 years)	Obtain baseline hepatic enzymes prior to start of therapy, then every 1–2 months. Discontinue drug for moderate fibrosis. (U.S. FDA, n.d.)
	Nelarabine (Arranon®)	Elevated AST (6%); elevated transaminases (12%) and elevated bilirubin (10%) in pediatric patients	Monitor LFTs closely because of risk for adverse reactions with severe hepatic impairment (total bilirubin > 3 × ULN). (U.S. FDA, n.d.)
	Pemetrexed (Alimta®)	Elevated ALT/AST (8%–10%)	Monitor LFTs periodically. Hold for hepatic toxicity for grade > 3, then resume upon recovery of LFTs to baseline or lower with 75% of previous dose for bilirubin > 3 × ULN or transaminases > 5 × ULN. (Floyd & Kerr, 2017; U.S. FDA, n.d.)
	Pentostatin (Nipent™)	Elevations in LFTs and hepatic disorders (2%)	Monitor LFTs. (Hospira, Inc., 2018; NIDDK & NLM, n.d.)
	Pralatrexate (Folotyn®)	Liver abnormalities observed after drug administration	Monitor LFTs prior to start of first and fourth dose of given cycle. Consider dose modification with persistent LFT abnormalities. Do not give if bilirubin > 3–10 × ULN or transaminases > 5–20 × ULN. Discontinue treatment for bilirubin > 10 × ULN or transaminases > 20 × ULN. (Floyd & Kerr, 2017; U.S. FDA, n.d.)
	Thioguanine (Tabloid®)	Jaundice; development of SOS (hyperbilirubinemia, tender hepatomegaly, weight gain due to fluid retention, ascites); portal hypertension; single case of peliosis hepatis; liver toxicity prevalent in men, high proportion in children	Monitor LFTs (transaminases, ALP, bilirubin) weekly upon starting, then monthly. Hold drug if toxic hepatitis or biliary stasis occurs. Discontinue drug with further liver toxicity, including jaundice. (U.S. FDA, n.d.)
Antitumor antibiotics	Bleomycin (Blenoxane®)	Transient ALT elevations associated when drug given in combination with other agents	Effects of hepatic insufficiency on drug pharmacokinetics have not been evaluated. (NIDDK & NLM, n.d.; U.S. FDA, n.d.)

Table 18-1. Hepatotoxicity of Antineoplastic Agents *(Continued)*

(Continued on next page)

Table 18-1. Hepatotoxicity of Antineoplastic Agents *(Continued)*

Classification	Drug	Side Effects	Nursing Considerations
Chemotherapy Agents *(Cont.)*			
Antitumor antibiotics *(cont.)*	Dactinomycin (Cosmegen®)	Transient elevations in aminotransferases; right upper quadrant pain in pediatric patients (with prior radiation therapy); hepatopathy-thrombocytopenia syndrome in 1% in those treated with Wilms tumor; SOS reported, particularly in children < 48 months; ascites, hepatomegaly, hepatitis, hepatic failure with reports of death, SOS associated with clotting disorder and multiorgan failure	Assess LFTs frequently. (Floyd & Kerr, 2017; U.S. FDA, n.d.)
	Mitomycin (Mitosol®)	Transient ALT elevations; rare cases of SOS with high doses	Dose adjustments from case reports include 50% dose reduction with bilirubin 1.5–3 mg/dl, 75% dose reduction with bilirubin > 3.1 mg/dl, and 50% dose reduction with bilirubin > 3 mg/dl or hepatic enzymes > 3 × ULN. (Floyd & Kerr, 2017; NIDDK & NLM, n.d.)
	Mitoxantrone (Novantrone®)	Increased drug concentration with severe hepatic impairment	Monitor LFTs prior to each course of treatment. Standard dose of 14 mg/m² is recommended for moderate dysfunction (bilirubin 1.5–3.5 mg/dl), and reduction of dose to 8 mg/m² or avoidance of administration is recommended with severe hepatic impairment and bilirubin > 3.5 mg/dl. Patients with multiple sclerosis and hepatic impairment should not receive mitoxantrone. (Floyd & Kerr, 2017; U.S. FDA, n.d.)
Antitumor antibiotics: Anthracyclines	Daunorubicin (Cerubidine®)	May impair liver function and increase risk of toxicity	Dose reduction with hepatic impairment: if bilirubin is 1.2–3 mg/dl, reduce to 75% of usual daily dose; if bilirubin > 3 mg/dl, reduce to 50% of usual daily dose (Floyd & Kerr, 2017; U.S. FDA, n.d.)
	Doxorubicin (Adriamycin®)	Increased aminotransferases and hyperbilirubinemia	Monitor LFTs (ALT/AST, ALP, bilirubin). Dose reduction of 50% is recommended for bilirubin of 1.2–3 mg/dl, and 75% dose reduction is recommended for bilirubin of 3.1–5 mg/dl. Do not give if bilirubin > 5 mg/dl. (Floyd & Kerr, 2017; U.S. FDA, n.d.)
	Doxorubicin liposomal injection (Doxil®)	Impaired liver function, hepatitis (< 1%)	Monitor LFTs (ALT/AST, ALP, bilirubin). Dose reduction of 50% is recommended for bilirubin of 1.2–3 mg/dl, and 75% dose reduction is recommended for bilirubin of 3.1–5 mg/dl. Do not give if bilirubin > 5 mg/dl. (Floyd & Kerr, 2017; U.S. FDA, n.d.)
	Epirubicin (Ellence®)	Elevated bilirubin or AST, which may delay drug clearance, increasing risk for toxicity	Monitor bilirubin and AST before and during treatment. Avoid use in patients with hepatic impairment; no evaluations have been conducted. Dose reduction is recommended for elevated bilirubin or aminotransferase levels: if bilirubin is 1.2–3 mg/dl or AST > 2–4 × ULN, reduce dose to 50% of recommended starting dose; if bilirubin > 3 mg/dl or AST > 4 × ULN, reduce dose to 25% of recommended starting dose. (Floyd & Kerr, 2017; U.S. FDA, n.d.)

(Continued on next page)

Table 18-1. Hepatotoxicity of Antineoplastic Agents *(Continued)*

Classification	Drug	Side Effects	Nursing Considerations
Chemotherapy Agents *(Cont.)*			
Antitumor antibiotics: Anthracyclines *(cont.)*	Idarubicin (Idamycin®)	Impaired drug metabolism caused by moderate to severe hepatic dysfunction, which may lead to elevated drug concentrations; severe hepatic changes (< 5%)	Monitor bilirubin prior to and during treatment. Drug pharmacokinetics have not been evaluated in patients with hepatic impairment. Consider dose reduction with elevated bilirubin. (U.S. FDA, n.d.)
Miscellaneous	Arsenic trioxide (Trisenox®)	Elevations in ALT/AST (> 5%)	Monitor LFTs with patients with severe hepatic impairment. (U.S. FDA, n.d.)
	Asparaginase (Elspar®)	Fulminant hepatic failure; moderate reversible elevation of aminotransferases, bilirubin, and ALP	Monitor LFTs at baseline and periodically during treatment. (Floyd & Kerr, 2017; U.S. FDA, n.d.)
	Asparaginase *Erwinia chrysanthemi* (Erwinaze®)	Mild elevations in bilirubin, transaminases (4%)	Monitor LFTs at baseline and periodically during treatment. (U.S. FDA, n.d.)
	Bexarotene (Targretin®)	Elevations of ALT (2%–9%), AST (5%–7%), and bilirubin (0%–6%)	Monitor LFTs at baseline, after weeks 1, 2, and 4, and if stable, then every 8 weeks thereafter. Consider holding or discontinuing drug if ALT/AST or bilirubin > 3 × ULN. No studies have been done in patients with hepatic insufficiency. (U.S. FDA, n.d.)
	Eribulin mesylate (Halaven®)	Grade 2 or elevated ALT (18%); elevated bilirubin; mild to moderate hepatic dysfunction (increase of drug exposure by 1.8–2.5-fold)	Dose reduction is recommended in patients with hepatic dysfunction, with a dose of 1.1 mg/m² in mild (Child-Pugh A) and 0.7 mg/m² in moderate (Child-Pugh B) hepatic impairment. No studies have been done in patients with severe hepatic impairment. (U.S. FDA, n.d.)
	Hydroxyurea (Hydrea®)	Elevated ALT/AST, ALP, and bilirubin	Monitor LFTs closely. No specific guidance is available on dosing adjustment in patients with hepatic dysfunction. (U.S. FDA, n.d.)
	Ixabepilone (Ixempra®)	Elevated ALT/AST and bilirubin	Monitor LFTs periodically. Recommended dosing is 40 mg/m² for bilirubin ≤ 1 × ULN and ALT/AST ≤ 2.5 × ULN, 32 mg/m² for bilirubin ≤ 1.5 × ULN and ALT/AST ≤ 10 × ULN (32 mg/m²), and 20–30 mg/m² for bilirubin > 1.5 to ≤ 3 × ULN and ALT/AST ≤ 10 × ULN. Drug is not recommended if bilirubin > 3 × ULN and ALT/AST > 10 × ULN; do not give with capecitabine if bilirubin > 2.5 × ULN and ALT/AST > ULN. (Floyd & Kerr, 2017; U.S. FDA, n.d.)
	Procarbazine (Matulane®)	Cause of granulomatous hepatitis; hepatic dysfunction, jaundice	Monitor LFTs prior to treatment and then at least weekly. (Floyd & Kerr, 2017; Sigma-Tau Pharmaceuticals, Inc., 2008)
Nitrosoureas	Carmustine (BiCNU®, Gliadel®)	Increased LFTs (transaminases, ALP, bilirubin) (20%–25%, occurring as late as 4 months after treatment)	Monitor LFTs periodically. (Floyd & Kerr, 2017; U.S. FDA, n.d.)

(Continued on next page)

Classification	Drug	Side Effects	Nursing Considerations
Chemotherapy Agents *(Cont.)*			
Nitrosoureas *(cont.)*	Lomustine (Gleostine®)	Elevated transaminases, ALP, and bilirubin	Monitor LFTs. (U.S. FDA, n.d.)
	Streptozocin (Zanosar®)	Hepatocellular injury (15%–67%, occurring within few days to weeks after treatment)	Monitor LFTs during therapy. (Floyd & Kerr, 2017; Teva Parenteral Medicines, Inc., 2012)
Plant alkaloids: Camptothecins	Irinotecan (Camptosar®)	Elevated bilirubin (> 30%)	Dose reduce with increased bilirubin. Do not administer in patients with bilirubin > 2 mg/dl or transaminases > 3 × ULN if no liver metastasis or transaminases > 5 × ULN with liver metastasis. (U.S. FDA, n.d.)
Plant alkaloids: Epipodophyllotoxins	Etoposide	Transient elevated ALT; not usually hepatotoxic at standard dosing	Monitor LFTs. (Floyd & Kerr, 2017; U.S. FDA, n.d.)
Plant alkaloids: Taxanes	Cabazitaxel (Jevtana®)	Elevated ALT/AST and bilirubin	No studies in patients with impaired hepatic function have been published. It is recommended to not give drug with bilirubin > 3 × ULN and to dose reduce with mild to moderate hepatic dysfunction (bilirubin above ULN or AST > 1.5 × ULN). Drug is not recommended in patients with hepatic impairment. (Floyd & Kerr, 2017; U.S. FDA, n.d.)
	Docetaxel (Taxotere®)	Transient elevations in ALP, ALT/AST, and bilirubin (5%–20%); decreased clearance with elevated bilirubin and/or transaminases	Monitor LFTs prior to each cycle of treatment. It is recommended to not give drug if baseline bilirubin is above ULN or AST > 1.5 × ULN with ALP > 2.5 × ULN. Dose reduce by 20%–40% with grade 2–3 elevations in aminotransferases > 2.5 to < 5 × ULN at baseline with elevated ALP. Discontinue drug if ALT/AST > 5 × ULN and/or ALP > 5 × ULN. (Floyd & Kerr, 2017; U.S. FDA, n.d.)
	Paclitaxel (Taxol®)	Transient elevations in ALP, AST, and bilirubin (5%–20%); hepatic necrosis and hepatic encephalopathy have been reported	Monitor LFTs. Dose modifications for preexisting liver disease include total dose of 175 mg/m² for bilirubin ≤ 1.25 × ULN and AST < 10 × ULN; total dose of 135 mg/m² for bilirubin 1.26–2 × ULN and aminotransferases < 10 × ULN; and total dose of 90 mg/m² for bilirubin 2.01–5 × ULN and aminotransferases < 10 × ULN. Drug is not recommended in patients with bilirubin > 5–7.5 × ULN or aminotransferases ≥ 10 × ULN. (Floyd & Kerr, 2017; U.S. FDA, n.d.)
Plant alkaloids: Vinca alkaloids	Vincristine sulfate (Oncovin®) Vincristine sulfate liposome (Marqibo®)	Severe hepatotoxicity when given with irradiation; SOS has been reported, particularly in pediatric patients; elevated AST	Monitor LFTs. Dose reduction of 50% is recommended with bilirubin > 3 mg/dl. (Floyd & Kerr, 2017; U.S. FDA, n.d.)

(Continued on next page)

Table 18-1. Hepatotoxicity of Antineoplastic Agents *(Continued)*

Classification	Drug	Side Effects	Nursing Considerations
Targeted Therapy Agents			
Small molecule inhibitors	Afatinib (Gilotrif®)	Liver abnormalities (10.1%) with fatal hepatic impairment (0.18%)	Monitor LFTs periodically. No dosing adjustment is recommended for mild (Child-Pugh A) or moderate (Child-Pugh B) hepatic dysfunction. No studies have been done in severe (Child-Pugh C) hepatic dysfunction. Hold or discontinue for severe LFT changes. (U.S. FDA, n.d.)
	Alectinib (Alecensa®)	Elevations of ALT > 5 × ULN (5.3%), AST > 5 × ULN (4.6%), and bilirubin > 3 × ULN (3.7%)	Monitor LFTs every 2 weeks for the first 2 months of treatment, then periodically thereafter; increase frequency with noted ALT/AST or bilirubin elevations. No dose adjustment is recommended for mild hepatic dysfunction (bilirubin ≤ ULN and AST > ULN or bilirubin 1–1.5 × ULN with any AST). For ALT/AST > 5 × ULN with bilirubin ≤ 2 × ULN, hold until patient recovers to baseline or ≤ 3 × ULN, and resume at dose reduction of 450 mg BID. For ALT/AST > 3 × ULN with bilirubin > 2 × ULN without cholestasis or hemolysis, discontinue drug. For bilirubin > 3 × ULN, hold drug until patient recovers to baseline or ≤ 1.5 × ULN, and resume at dose reduction of 450 mg BID. Depending on severity of hepatic dysfunction, consider discontinuation of drug. (Genentech, Inc., 2017; U.S. FDA, n.d.)
	Axitinib (Inlyta®)	Elevated ALT/AST more frequent than elevated ALP	Monitor ALT/AST and bilirubin prior to starting treatment, then periodically throughout treatment. No dosing adjustment is recommended in mild hepatic impairment (Child-Pugh A). Initial dose should be reduced in patients with moderate hepatic dysfunction (Child-Pugh B). (Floyd & Kerr, 2017; U.S. FDA, n.d.)
	Belinostat (Beleodaq®)	Fatal hepatotoxicity and liver abnormalities reported	Monitor LFTs. For grade 3–4 hepatotoxicity, reduce dose by 25% (750 mg/m²). For recurrence of grade 3 or 4 hepatotoxicity, after 2 dose reductions, discontinue drug. (U.S. FDA, n.d.)
	Bortezomib (Velcade®)	Cases of acute liver failure reported; hepatitis; elevated ALT/AST and bilirubin	Monitor LFTs during treatment. No dosing adjustment is recommended with mild hepatic impairment (bilirubin < 1–1.5 × ULN or AST > ULN). In patients with moderate or severe hepatic dysfunction (bilirubin > 1.5–3 × ULN or bilirubin > 3 × ULN with any AST), start at lower dose of 0.7 mg/m² for first cycle and escalate to 1 mg/m² or reduce to 0.5 mg/m² based on tolerance. (U.S. FDA, n.d.)

(Continued on next page)

Table 18-1. Hepatotoxicity of Antineoplastic Agents *(Continued)*			
Classification	**Drug**	**Side Effects**	**Nursing Considerations**
Targeted Therapy Agents *(Cont.)*			
Small molecule inhibitors *(cont.)*	Bosutinib (Bosulif®)	Elevated ALT/AST, bilirubin, and ALP	Monitor LFTs at least monthly for 3 months, then as needed. For baseline hepatic dysfunction, reduce dose to 200 mg daily. For elevated transaminases > 5 × ULN, hold drug until patient recovers to < 2.5 × ULN and resume at 400 mg daily. Discontinue drug if recovery takes > 4 weeks. Discontinue drug if transaminases > 3 × ULN with bilirubin > 2 × ULN and ALP < 2 × ULN. (U.S. FDA, n.d.)
	Cabozantinib (Cabometyx®)	Elevations in transaminases and bilirubin	Reduce starting dose to 40 mg daily with mild or moderate (Child-Pugh A or B) hepatic dysfunction. Drug is not recommended in patients with severe hepatic impairment. (U.S. FDA, n.d.)
	Carfilzomib (Kyprolis®)	Hepatic failure (< 1%), elevated transaminases	Monitor LFTs regularly. Consider dose reduction when appropriate. (U.S. FDA, n.d.)
	Ceritinib (Zykadia®)	Elevations of ALT/AST, bilirubin, and ALP	Monitor LFTs monthly and as clinically indicated; increase frequency if elevated transaminases are noted. For ALT/AST > 5 × ULN with bilirubin ≤ 2 × ULN, hold drug until patient recovers to ≤ 3 × ULN, then resume at reduced dose of 150 mg. For ALT/AST > 3 × ULN with bilirubin > 2 × ULN without cholestasis or hemolysis, discontinue drug. (Floyd & Kerr, 2017; U.S. FDA, n.d.)
	Crizotinib (Xalkori®)	Elevated ALT (grade 3–4), elevated bilirubin	Monitor LFTs monthly and as clinically indicated; increase frequency in patients with grade 2–4 LFT elevations. Recommend holding treatment for grade 3 or 4 aminotransferase elevations with bilirubin ≤ 1.5 × ULN until patient recovers to < grade 1 or baseline, then resume at 200 mg BID. Discontinue drug for ≥ grade 2 elevated ALT/AST or bilirubin. (Floyd & Kerr, 2017; U.S. FDA, n.d.)
	Dabrafenib (Tafinlar®)	Elevated ALT/AST, ALP, and bilirubin with drug used in combination with other antineoplastic agents	No formal studies have been done in patients with hepatic dysfunction. No dose adjustment is recommended in mild hepatic impairment. (U.S. FDA, n.d.)
	Dasatinib (Sprycel®)	Elevated transaminases, bilirubin; ascites, cholestasis, cholecystitis, hepatitis	Use caution with hepatic impairment. Consider holding and reducing dose with persistent elevation of ALT/AST > 5 × ULN or bilirubin > 3 × ULN. (NIDDK & NLM, n.d.; U.S. FDA, n.d.).
	Erlotinib (Tarceva®)	Hepatic failure and hepatorenal syndrome reported	Monitor LFTs periodically; increase frequency with noted elevated LFTs. Closely monitor if patient has Child-Pugh A, B, or C cirrhosis. Interrupt or discontinue treatment if bilirubin > 3 × ULN or elevated aminotransferases > 5 × ULN. Discontinue drug with hepatic failure. (Floyd & Kerr, 2017; U.S. FDA, n.d.)

(Continued on next page)

Table 18-1. Hepatotoxicity of Antineoplastic Agents *(Continued)*

Classification	Drug	Side Effects	Nursing Considerations
Targeted Therapy Agents *(Cont.)*			
Small molecule inhibitors *(cont.)*	Everolimus (Afinitor®, Afinitor Disperz® tablets for oral suspension)	Risk for reactivation of viral hepatitis	Dose reduction of 25% is recommended for patients with Child-Pugh A cirrhosis; 50% reduction is recommended for Child-Pugh B cirrhosis. Dose reduction to 5 mg daily is recommended for Child-Pugh B. Avoid use in patients with severe hepatic dysfunction (Child-Pugh C). (Floyd & Kerr, 2017; U.S. FDA, n.d.)
	Gefitinib (Iressa®)	Elevated ALT/AST and bilirubin, fatal hepatotoxicity (0.04%)	Monitor LFTs periodically. Hold drug (up to 14 days) for grade 2 or higher elevated ALT/AST. Discontinue drug for severe hepatic dysfunction. (U.S. FDA, n.d.)
	Idelalisib (Zydelig®)	Elevated ALT/AST (30%), fatal and/or serious hepatotoxicity (14%)	Monitor LFTs prior to and during treatment (every 2 weeks for first 3 months, every 4 weeks for next 3 months, then every 1–3 months thereafter). No dose adjustment is recommended for ALT/AST > 3–5 × ULN and bilirubin > 1.5–3 × ULN. Monitor LFTs weekly until ALT/AST and bilirubin ≤ 1 × ULN. Hold drug if ALT/AST > 5–20 × ULN and bilirubin > 5–10 × ULN. Monitor LFTs weekly until ALT/AST and bilirubin < 1 × ULN, then resume drug at dose reduction of 100 mg BID. Discontinue drug if ALT/AST > 20 × ULN and bilirubin > 10 × ULN or if recurrent hepatotoxicity is present. (U.S. FDA, n.d.)
	Imatinib mesylate (Gleevec®)	Elevated transaminases and bilirubin, severe hepatotoxicity	Monitor LFTs prior to starting treatment, monthly thereafter, and as clinically indicated. No dose adjustment is recommended with mild to moderate hepatic impairment. Dose reduction by 25% is recommended for severe hepatic dysfunction. Hold for elevations of bilirubin > 3 × ULN or transaminases > 5 × ULN, then resume at reduced dosing when bilirubin < 1.5 × ULN or transaminases < 2.5 × ULN. (Floyd & Kerr, 2017; U.S. FDA, n.d.)
	Ixazomib (Ninlaro®)	Drug-induced liver injury, hepatocellular injury, hepatic steatosis, hepatitis cholestasis, and hepatotoxicity reported (< 1%)	Monitor LFTs during treatment. Dose reduction of starting dose to 3 mg is recommended in moderate to severe (total bilirubin > 1.5–3 × ULN) or severe (total bilirubin > 3 × ULN) hepatic impairment. (U.S. FDA, n.d.)
	Lapatinib (Tykerb®)	Elevated ALT/AST and bilirubin (< 1%)	Monitor LFTs prior to starting treatment, every 4–6 weeks during therapy, then as clinically indicated. Discontinue drug for severe changes in LFTs (ALT/AST > 3 × ULN, bilirubin > 2 × ULN). (Floyd & Kerr, 2017; U.S. FDA, n.d.)

(Continued on next page)

Table 18-1. Hepatotoxicity of Antineoplastic Agents *(Continued)*

Classification	Drug	Side Effects	Nursing Considerations
Targeted Therapy Agents *(Cont.)*			
Small molecule inhibitors *(cont.)*	Lenvatinib (Lenvima®)	Elevated ALT/AST	Monitor LFTs prior to starting treatment, every 2 weeks for first 2 months, and at least monthly thereafter during therapy. No dose adjustment is recommended for mild to moderate hepatic dysfunction. Hold drug for grade 3 or higher hepatic impairment. Dose reduction to 14 mg daily is recommended for severe (Child-Pugh C) hepatic dysfunction. Discontinue drug for hepatic failure. (Floyd & Kerr, 2017; U.S. FDA, n.d.)
	Nilotinib (Tasigna®)	Elevated ALT/AST, bilirubin, and ALP	Monitor LFTs periodically. Hold drug for elevated bilirubin and/or transaminases ≥ grade 3 until patient recovers to ≤ grade 1, then resume drug at dose reduction of 400 mg daily. (U.S. FDA, n.d.)
	Panobinostat (Farydak®)	Elevated transaminases and bilirubin	Monitor LFTs prior to and regularly during treatment. Dose reduction is recommended for mild hepatic impairment (starting dose 15 mg) and moderate hepatic impairment (10 mg). Avoid use in severe hepatic dysfunction. (U.S. FDA, n.d.)
	Pazopanib (Votrient®)	Elevated transaminases and bilirubin reported; fatal hepatotoxicity has occurred	Monitor LFTs prior to starting, at least once every 4 weeks for first 4 months or as clinically indicated, and periodically after therapy. No dose adjustment is recommended for isolated ALT > 3–8 × ULN; check weekly LFTs until patient recovers to < grade 1 or baseline. Hold drug for isolated ALT > 8 × ULN until patient recovers to < grade 1 or baseline, then can consider resuming drug at dose reduction to no greater than 400 mg daily. Check LFTs weekly for 8 weeks; discontinue drug if elevated ALT > 3 × ULN recurs or if ALT > 3 × ULN with bilirubin > 2 × ULN occurs. Drug is not recommended for patients with severe hepatic impairment. (U.S. FDA, n.d.)
	Ponatinib (Iclusig®)	Elevated ALT/AST	Monitor LFTs prior to, monthly, and as clinically indicated during therapy. Hold drug with elevation of transaminases > 3 × ULN (≥ grade 2) until patient recovers to < 3 × ULN (grade 1), then resume drug at reduced dose. Discontinue drug with elevations of ALT/AST > 3 × ULN with elevated bilirubin > 2 × ULN and ALP < 2 × ULN. Avoid giving drug in patients with moderate to severe (Child-Pugh B or C) hepatic dysfunction. (U.S. FDA, n.d.)

(Continued on next page)

Table 18-1. Hepatotoxicity of Antineoplastic Agents *(Continued)*

Classification	Drug	Side Effects	Nursing Considerations
Targeted Therapy Agents *(Cont.)*			
Small molecule inhibitors *(cont.)*	Regorafenib (Stivarga®)	Elevated LFTs, hepatocellular necrosis	Obtain baseline LFTs prior to initiation of therapy, at least every 2 weeks during first 2 months of treatment, then monthly. Dose reduction is recommended for grade 2 hepatic impairment. Discontinue drug for ALT/AST > 20 × ULN or ALT/AST > 3 × ULN with bilirubin > 2 × ULN or recurrence of ALT/AST > 5 × ULN despite dose reduction. Drug is not recommended for patients with severe hepatic impairment (Child-Pugh C). (Floyd & Kerr, 2017; U.S. FDA, n.d.)
	Ribociclib (Kisqali®)	Elevated transaminases; elevated ALT/AST (7%–10% grade 3 or 4), bilirubin (1%)	Monitor LFTs at baseline, every 2 weeks for first 2 cycles, at beginning of each subsequent 4 cycles, then as clinically indicated. Dose reduction of 400 mg in patients with moderate to severe hepatic impairment (Child-Pugh B or C). Hold for ALT/AST > 3–20 × ULN until patient recovers to baseline or < grade 2 or 3 toxicity, then consider resuming at same dose or reducing dose depending on toxicity. Discontinue drug for elevated ALT/AST > 3 × ULN with bilirubin > 2 × ULN or if ALT/AST > 20 × ULN. (Floyd & Kerr, 2017; U.S. FDA, n.d.)
	Sorafenib (Nexavar®)	Elevated transaminases, bilirubin	Monitor LFTs regularly. Discontinuation of drug is recommended if transaminases are significantly increased without other etiology. No dosing adjustment is recommended for Child-Pugh A or B hepatic impairment. (Floyd & Kerr, 2017; U.S. FDA, n.d.)
	Sunitinib (Sutent®)	Jaundice, elevated transaminases and/or bilirubin	Monitor LFTs prior to starting treatment, during each cycle, and as clinically indicated. Hold drug for grade 3 or 4 drug-related hepatic adverse events. Discontinue if patient has no resolution, experiences severe changes in LFTs after stopping drug, or has other signs or symptoms of liver failure. Safety with ALT/AST > 2.5 × ULN, or ALT/AST > 5 × ULN if due to liver metastases, has not been established. No dose adjustment is recommended with Child-Pugh A or B hepatic impairment. (U.S. FDA, n.d.)
	Temsirolimus (Torisel®)	Elevated ALT, ALP, and bilirubin	Monitor LFTs. Dose reduction to 15 mg weekly is recommended for mild hepatic impairment (bilirubin > 1–1.5 × ULN or AST > ULN). Do not give drug if bilirubin > 1.5 × ULN. (Floyd & Kerr, 2017; U.S. FDA, n.d.)
	Trametinib (Mekinist®)	Elevated ALT/AST and ALP	Baseline and periodic monitoring of LFTs is recommended. No dosing adjustment is recommended for mild hepatic impairment. (Floyd & Kerr, 2017; U.S. FDA, n.d.)

(Continued on next page)

Table 18-1. Hepatotoxicity of Antineoplastic Agents *(Continued)*			
Classification	**Drug**	**Side Effects**	**Nursing Considerations**
Targeted Therapy Agents ***(Cont.)***			
Small molecule inhibitors *(cont.)*	Vandetanib (Caprelsa®)	Elevated ALT/AST (20%); elevated bilirubin	Dose reduction is recommended for grade 3 or higher toxicity. Drug is not recommended to be given in patients with moderate or severe hepatic impairment. It is recommended to avoid use in severe hepatic impairment (Child-Pugh B or C cirrhosis). (Floyd & Kerr, 2017; U.S. FDA, n.d.)
	Vemurafenib (Zelboraf®)	Elevated ALT/AST, ALP, and bilirubin	Monitor LFTs prior to starting therapy and monthly during therapy or as clinically indicated. Hold drug for grade 2 or 3 toxicities until patient recovers to < grade 1 toxicity or baseline, then resume at recommended dose reductions. Discontinue for grade 4 toxicity. (U.S. FDA, n.d.)
Immunotherapy Agents			
Checkpoint inhibitors: CTLA-4	Ipilimumab (Yervoy®)	Immune-related hepatitis T-cell activation and proliferation, leading to immune-mediated organ failure	Monitor LFTs and assess for signs and symptoms of hepatotoxicity prior to each dose. No dose adjustment is recommended for mild hepatic dysfunction (bilirubin > 1–1.5 × ULN or ALT/AST > ULN). Hold drug for grade 2. Discontinue drug for grade 3 or 4; initiate steroids 1–2 mg/kg/day prednisone or equivalent until LFTs return to baseline or evidence of sustained improvement is seen, then taper steroids over 1 month. Mycophenolate has been given in the setting of persistent severe hepatitis despite high-dose steroids. (U.S. FDA, n.d.)
Checkpoint inhibitors: PD-1	Nivolumab (Opdivo®)	Elevated ALT (16%), AST (28%), ALP (22%), and bilirubin (9%); immune-mediated hepatitis (1.1%)	Monitor LFTs prior to and periodically during treatment. For grade 2 or higher elevations in transaminases and/or bilirubin, start steroids 1–2 mg/kg/day prednisone or equivalent. Discontinue drug for grade 3 or 4 hepatitis. (U.S. FDA, n.d.)
	Pembrolizumab (Keytruda®)	Immune-mediated hepatitis (0.7%; grade 2: 0.1%; grade 3: 0.4%; grade 4: < 0.1%), elevated ALP (26%; grade 3–4: 3.1%), elevated AST (22%; grade 3–4: 2.1%), elevated ALT (21%; grade 3–4: 1.8%)	Monitor for LFT changes. For grade 2 LFT changes, start steroids 0.5–1 mg/kg/day; for grade 3 or higher, start steroids 1–2 mg/kg/day prednisone or equivalent followed by a taper. Depending on severity of LFT changes, may hold or discontinue drug. (U.S. FDA, n.d.)
Checkpoint inhibitors: PD-L1	Atezolizumab (Tecentriq®)	Across clinical trials (N = 1,978): grade 3 or 4 elevations in ALT (2.5%), AST (2.3%), and total bilirubin (1.6%); in patients with urothelial carcinoma (n = 523): immune-mediated hepatitis (1.3%), grade 3 or 4 elevations in ALT (2.5%), AST (2.5%), and total bilirubin (2.1%), with median time to onset of 1.1 months (range: 0.4–7.7 months)	Monitor for LFT changes, including signs and symptoms of hepatitis. Monitor AST, ALT, and bilirubin prior to and periodically during treatment. Administer corticosteroids at dose of 1–2 mg/kg/day prednisone equivalents for grade 2 or greater transaminase elevations, with or without concurrent total bilirubin elevation, followed by corticosteroid taper. Hold drug for moderate hepatic impairment (ALT or ALT > 3–5 × ULN or total bilirubin > 1.5–3 × ULN). Permanently discontinue drug for severe or life-threatening hepatic impairment (AST or ALT > 5 × ULN or total bilirubin > 3 × ULN). (U.S. FDA, n.d.)

(Continued on next page)

Table 18-1. Hepatotoxicity of Antineoplastic Agents *(Continued)*

Classification	Drug	Side Effects	Nursing Considerations
Immunotherapy Agents *(Cont.)*			
Checkpoint inhibitors: PD-L1 *(cont.)*	Durvalumab (Imfinzi®)	Immune-mediated hepatitis (1.1%; grade 3: 0.6%; median time to onset of 51.5 days [range: 15–312 days]); grade 3 or 4 elevations in ALT (3.0%), AST (4.3%), and total bilirubin (2.8%)	Monitor LFTs for changes in each cycle during treatment. For grade 2 or 3 elevations in transaminases with or without concurrent total bilirubin elevation, initiate dose of 1–2 mg/kg/day prednisone or equivalent followed by taper. Hold drug for moderate hepatic impairment (grade 2 ALT/AST > 3–5 × ULN or total bilirubin > 1.5–3 × ULN; grade 3 ALT/AST ≤ 8 × ULN or total bilirubin ≤ 5 × ULN). Permanently discontinue drug for severe or life-threatening hepatic impairment (grade 3 ALT or AST > 8 × ULN or total bilirubin > 5 × ULN; concurrent ALT or AST > 3 × ULN and total bilirubin > 2 × ULN with no other cause). (U.S. FDA, n.d.)
Cytokines: Interferons	Pegylated interferon alfa-2b (Pegasys®)	Significant elevation in aminotransferases (> 10 × ULN)	Monitor LFTs (weeks 1, 2, 4, 6, and 8, then every 4–6 weeks and more frequently if abnormalities). It is recommended to hold dose if aminotransferases > 5 × ULN until resolution to grade 1, then reduce dose by 33%. (Floyd & Kerr, 2017; U.S. FDA, n.d.)
Cytokines: Interleukins	IL-2, aldesleukin (Proleukin®)	Hepatitis, hepatosplenomegaly, cholecystitis	Monitor LFTs prior to starting therapy, then daily during treatment (U.S. FDA, n.d.).
Miscellaneous: Immunomodulators	Lenalidomide (Revlimid®)	Hepatic failure including fatalities (15% with hepatocellular, cholestatic, and mixed characteristic); patients with multiple myeloma (2%) and myelodysplasia (1%) had serious hepatotoxicity events (hyperbilirubinemia, cholecystitis, acute cholecystitis, hepatic failure); risk factors: preexisting viral liver disease, elevated baseline liver enzymes, and concomitant medications	Monitor LFTs periodically; stop drug and evaluate if hepatotoxicity is suspected. Treatment at lower dose may be considered if LFTs return to baseline values. (U.S. FDA, n.d.)
	Pomalidomide (Pomalyst®)	Elevated bilirubin	Avoid in patients with bilirubin > 2 mg/dl or ALT/AST > 3 × ULN. Dose reduction of 25% is recommended for mild or moderate (Child-Pugh A or B) hepatic impairment; 50% dose reduction is recommended for severe (Child-Pugh C) hepatic impairment. (Floyd & Kerr, 2017; U.S. FDA, n.d.)
Monoclonal antibodies: Human	Ado-trastuzumab emtansine (Kadcyla®)	Mixed pattern of elevated ALP, aminotransferases (ALT/AST), and bilirubin	Monitor LFTs prior to starting therapy and before each dose. Clinical trials excluded patients with known active HBV or HCV infection, baseline transaminases > 2.5 × ULN, or bilirubin > 1.5 × ULN (treat at same dose level of 3.6 mg/kg). Hold for grade 3 (> 5–20 × ULN) elevations in ALT/AST or grade 2–3 (> 1.5–10 × ULN) elevations in bilirubin; resume at one lower dose level only if ALT/AST recover to ≤ grade 2 and bilirubin recovers to ≤ grade 1.

(Continued on next page)

Table 18-1. Hepatotoxicity of Antineoplastic Agents *(Continued)*

Classification	Drug	Side Effects	Nursing Considerations
Immunotherapy Agents *(Cont.)*			
Monoclonal antibodies: Human *(cont.)*	Ado-trastuzumab emtansine (Kadcyla®) *(cont.)*		Discontinue if hepatotoxicity recurs when restarting drug or if grade 4 increased transaminases (ALT/AST > 20 × ULN) or hyperbilirubinemia (bilirubin > 10 × ULN) occurs at any time during treatment. Discontinue if ALT/AST > 3 × ULN with bilirubin > 2 × ULN. (Floyd & Kerr, 2017; U.S. FDA, n.d.)
Monoclonal antibodies: Humanized	Alemtuzumab (Campath®, Lemtrada®)	Risk of HBV and HCV reactivation; intrinsic hepatotoxicity and idiosyncratic liver injury rare	Screen for HBV and HCV prior to starting treatment. Provide prophylaxis or treatment of HBV/HCV before or during treatment. (NIDDK & NLM, n.d.; U.S. FDA, n.d.)
	Brentuximab (Adcetris®)	Severe and potentially fatal hepatotoxicity reported, including elevated transaminases and bilirubin	Monitor LFTs. Avoid drug with Child-Pugh B or C hepatic impairment. (Floyd & Kerr, 2017; U.S. FDA, n.d.)
	Elotuzumab (Empliciti™)	ALT/AST > 3 × ULN, bilirubin > 2 × ULN, ALP < 2 × ULN	Monitor LFTs periodically. Recommend periodic monitoring of liver enzymes; temporarily discontinue drug for ≥ grade 3 hepatotoxicity. (Floyd & Kerr, 2017; U.S. FDA, n.d.)
	Inotuzumab ozogamicin (Besponsa®)	Hepatotoxicity including SOS (life-threatening with increased risk in HSCT recipients); SOS signs/symptoms: elevated total bilirubin, hepatomegaly, rapid weight gain, ascites	Monitor LFTs (AST/ALT, bilirubin, ALP) prior to and following each dose. No adjustment to starting dose is required if total bilirubin ≤ 1.5 × ULN and AST/ALT ≤ 2.5 × ULN. Interrupt drug if total bilirubin > 1.5 × ULN and AST/ALT > 2.5 × ULN. Permanently discontinue drug if SOS or severe liver toxicity occurs or if LFTs do not recover to baseline. (U.S. FDA, n.d.)
	Obinutuzumab (Gazyva®)	Reactivation of HBV, with some cases resulting in fulminant hepatitis, hepatic failure, and death	Screen for HBV infection (HBsAg and anti-HBc) prior to starting treatment; if patient is positive for HBV infection, consult expert for monitoring and consideration of antiviral therapy. Monitor patients with current or prior HBV infection for signs of hepatitis or HBV reactivation during therapy and for several months after treatment. Discontinue drug for HBV reactivation while on treatment. Insufficient data exist on safety of resuming drug in patients with HBV reactivation. (U.S. FDA, n.d.)
	Ofatumumab (Arzerra®)	Risk of HBV reactivation, fulminant hepatitis	Screen high-risk patients prior to starting treatment. Monitor carriers of HBV closely for clinical and laboratory signs of active HBV infection during treatment and for 6–12 months following last dose. Discontinue drug in patients who develop viral hepatitis or viral hepatitis reactivation. (U.S. FDA, n.d.)
	Thalidomide (Thalomid®)	Increased ALP and bilirubinemia	No pharmacokinetic studies have been done in patients with hepatic impairment. (U.S. FDA, n.d.)

(Continued on next page)

Table 18-1. Hepatotoxicity of Antineoplastic Agents *(Continued)*

Classification	Drug	Side Effects	Nursing Considerations
Hormone Therapy Agents			
Androgen inhibitor	Abiraterone acetate (Zytiga®)	Elevated ALT/AST and bilirubin	Monitor ALT/AST and bilirubin prior to starting therapy, every week for the first month, every 2 weeks for the following 2 months of treatment, then monthly thereafter. For moderate hepatic impairment, reduce dose to 250 mg daily. Hold drug if ALT/AST > 5 × ULN or bilirubin > 3 × ULN until patient recovers to baseline or ALT/AST ≤ 2.5 × ULN or bilirubin ≤ 1.5 × ULN. Resume at reduced dose of 750 mg daily at first occurrence and 500 mg daily at second occurrence. Discontinue if ALT/AST > 5 × ULN or bilirubin > 3 × ULN with moderate hepatic impairment or if the patient is unable to tolerate 500 mg daily. Avoid drug in patients with severe hepatic impairment (Child-Pugh C). (U.S. FDA, n.d.)

ALP—alkaline phosphatase; ALT—alanine aminotransferase; AST—aspartate aminotransferase; anti-HBc—hepatitis B core antibody; BID—twice a day; CTLA-4—cytotoxic T-lymphocyte antigen 4; 5-FU—5-fluorouracil; GGT—gamma glutamyl transferase; HBsAg—hepatitis B surface antigen; HBV—hepatitis B virus; HCV—hepatitis C virus; HSCT—hematopoietic stem cell transplantation; IL—interleukin; LDH—lactate dehydrogenase; LFTs—liver function tests; NIDDK—National Institute of Diabetes and Digestive and Kidney Diseases; NLM—National Library of Medicine; PD-1—programmed cell death protein 1; PD-L1—programmed cell death-ligand 1; SOS—sinusoidal obstruction syndrome; ULN—upper limit of normal; U.S. FDA—U.S. Food and Drug Administration

1. Acute hepatocellular injury (Larson, 2017; Mehta, 2016)
   a) Incidence: 90% of cases
   b) Pathophysiology
      (1) Can lead to hepatocellular apoptosis, steatosis, or cellular degeneration
      (2) Liver cells appear spotty (minute clusters of hepatocytes) or confluent (larger groups of hepatocytes involving multiple lobules under microscopy) (Krishna, 2017).
      (3) The hepatic acinus is the functional unit in the liver that is divided into different zones. Zone 1 encircles the portal tracts, where oxygenated blood from hepatic arteries enters; zone 3 is located around the central veins, where oxygenation is poor; and zone 2 is located between zones 1 and 3. Zone 3 is most commonly affected (Larson, 2017).
         (a) Zonal necrosis occurs with compounds with predictable, dose-dependent, intrinsic toxicity.
         (b) Nonzonal necrosis (diffuse, irregular, patchy injury involving all parts of the acinus) occurs with compounds with unpredictable idiosyncratic injury (Fisher, Vuppalanchi, & Saxena, 2015).
      (4) Most recover without developing significant fibrosis.
   c) Signs/symptoms: Jaundice, painful hepatomegaly, abdominal distension, nausea and vomiting, malaise, confusion, sleepiness
2. Chronic hepatocellular injury (Larson, 2017; Mehta, 2016)
   a) Incidence: 5%–10% of cases
   b) Pathophysiology
      (1) Pigment accumulation (excessive iron): Lipofuscin (fine yellow-brown pigment granules) is found in hepatic cells as a result of certain drugs. Additionally, excessive iron may accumulate in the liver due to overingestion or parenteral therapy (Mehta, 2016).
      (2) Steatosis, steatohepatitis, and phospholipidosis
      (3) Hepatic fibrosis and cirrhosis
   c) Signs/symptoms: Nausea, diarrhea, poor appetite, weight loss, fatigue, jaundice, easy bruising or bleeding, pruritus, lower extremity swelling
3. Acute cholestasis: Decrease in bile flow due to impaired secretion by hepatocytes or bile flow obstruction through intra- or extrahepatic bile ducts (Larson, 2017; Mehta, 2016; Nazer, 2017)
   a) Incidence: 2%–5% of cases
   b) Pathophysiology

(1) Reduction in bile flow due to decreased secretion or biliary tree obstruction
(2) Pure cholestasis (canalicular, bland, or noninflammatory) characterized by prominent hepatocellular or canalicular cholestasis with minimal hepatocellular injury or inflammation
(3) Cholestatic hepatitis (hepatocanalicular, cholangiolitic, or inflammatory) characterized by inflammation, prominent cholestasis, and hepatocellular injury

c) Signs/symptoms: Pruritus, jaundice, pale stools, dark urine

4. Chronic cholestasis (Larson, 2017; Mehta, 2016)
   a) Incidence
   (1) About 1% of cases
   (2) Rare cases progress to cirrhosis
   b) Pathophysiology
   (1) Bile duct loss or cholate stasis (rim of pale hepatocytes adjacent to portal tracts)
   (2) Prolonged damage leads to bile duct loss and overt ductopenia.
   c) Signs/symptoms: Pruritus, jaundice, pale stools, dark urine
5. Steatosis: Infiltration of liver cells with fat, which is associated with metabolism being disturbed by drug therapy (Larson, 2017; Mehta, 2016; Rabinowich & Shibolet, 2015)
   a) Incidence: 20%–30% of cases
   b) Pathophysiology
   (1) Acute steatosis causes hepatic cells to appear microvesicular (small vesicles of fat droplets), whereas chronic steatosis causes hepatic cells to appear macrovesicular (large vesicles of fat droplets) under microscopy.
   (2) Hepatocytes are filled with excess fatty cells, which are composed of triglycerides.
   (3) Disruption occurs in mitochondrial beta-oxidation of lipids.
   (4) Steatohepatitis includes variable steatosis, lobular inflammation, and hepatocellular injury.
   c) Signs/symptoms: Ascites, jaundice, confusion, tendency to bleed easily
6. Granulomas: Macrophages that have accumulated in the liver because of chronic exposure to drug therapy (Coash, Forouhar, Wu, & Wu, 2012; Larson, 2017; Mehta, 2016)
   a) Incidence: 15% of cases
   b) Pathophysiology
   (1) Inflammatory process
   (2) Seen in periportal and portal areas
   (3) Temporary injury
   c) Signs/symptoms: Fevers, myalgias, fatigue
7. Budd-Chiari syndrome: Hepatic venous outflow obstruction (Larson, 2017; Mehta, 2016)
   a) Incidence: 10% of cases
   b) Pathophysiology
   (1) Drug-induced thrombosis of hepatic veins or inferior vena cava
   (2) Centrizonal congestion, hepatocellular necrosis, and hemorrhage
   (3) Large regenerative nodules and obstructive portal venopathy may be noted.
   c) Signs/symptoms: Painful hepatomegaly, jaundice, ascites
8. Hepatic sinusoidal obstruction syndrome (SOS; formerly known as veno-occlusive disease or VOD): Syndrome comprising weight gain, ascites, painful hepatomegaly, and jaundice that is caused by damage to the sinusoidal endothelial cells leading to obstruction of the hepatic vessels (Botti et al., 2016; Carreras et al., 2011; Larson, 2017; Mehta, 2016; Mohty et al., 2015; Tewari et al., 2017; Valla & Cazals-Hatem, 2016).
   a) Incidence: Approximately 14% of patients following allogeneic hematopoietic stem cell transplantation (HSCT) (range 0%–62%, depending on the series)
   (1) SOS is a complication of HSCT that most often occurs 20–30 days or later after receiving the conditioning regimen (Valla & Cazals-Hatem, 2016).
   (2) The incidence of SOS following allogeneic HSCT has diminished and the outcome improved over the past decade (Carreras et al., 2011).
   b) Pathophysiology
   (1) Injury occurs to the sinusoids, hepatic veins, and hepatic arteries.
   (2) Luminal narrowing of sinusoids leads to increased resistance to blood flow, resulting in hepatic congestion, sinusoidal dilation, and portal hypertension culminating in fibrosis.
   c) Risk factors include the use of myeloablative conditioning and stem cell source other than a matched sibling donor, preexisting liver disease, and poor performance status (Coppell et al., 2010).
   d) Signs/symptoms: Painful hepatomegaly, ascites (Tewari et al., 2017)
   e) Assessment: Two grading systems have historically been used to diagnose and stage SOS: the Baltimore Criteria (Jones et al., 1987)

and the Seattle Criteria (Shulman & Hinterberger, 1992).

(1) The Baltimore criteria are more stringent, with an absolute requirement for hyperbilirubinemia. The severity of SOS can be classified retrospectively using the Seattle Criteria (Carreras et al., 2011).

(2) The European Society for Blood and Marrow Transplantation have proposed revised criteria for diagnosis and grading in adults and children (Corbacioglu et al., 2018; Dignan et al., 2013; Mohty et al., 2015; see Table 18-2).

9. Neoplastic lesions: Focal nodular hyperplasia and hepatocellular adenomas have been seen with hepatotoxic drugs (Mehta, 2016).
   a) Incidence: 6% of cases
   b) Pathophysiology: Focal nodular hyperplasia and hepatocellular adenomas
   c) Signs/symptoms: Abdominal distension, jaundice, weight loss, easy bruising, right upper quadrant pain
10. Immune-related adverse events (Gordon et al., 2017; Larson, 2017; see Table 18-1)
    a) Incidence: 3%–9% of cases
       (1) May occur with checkpoint inhibitors (cytotoxic T-lymphocyte antigen-4–blocking antibodies, programmed cell death protein 1 and programmed cell death-ligand 1 inhibitors), chimeric antigen receptor T-cell therapies, and monoclonal antibodies (Teply & Lipson, 2014)
       (2) May present 8–12 weeks after initiation of therapy
    b) Pathophysiology
       (1) Inflammation of hepatocytes or bile ducts
       (2) Diffuse T-cell infiltrates of the liver
    c) Signs/symptoms: Asymptomatic elevations in liver enzymes (at least three times the upper limit of normal of aspartate aminotransferase [AST] and alanine aminotransferase [ALT] and/or twice the total bilirubin), hepatomegaly, enlarged perihepatic lymph nodes

G. Assessment (Botti et al., 2016; Helissey, Vicier, & Champiat, 2016; Herrine, 2016; Postow, 2015; Skood, Conrad, Luu, & Slabinski, 2017; Teply & Lipson, 2014; Weber, Yang, Atkins, & Disis, 2015)

1. Medical history
   a) Previous medications (prescription, illicit or recreational, herbal)
   b) Alcohol use
   c) Hepatitis
   d) Familial history of liver disease
   e) Risk factor exposure for viral hepatitis (transfusions, travel, sexual contacts, occupation, body piercing or tattoos)
   f) Exposure to hepatic toxins
   g) Organ transplants
   h) Previous complications (bleeding, infection, renal failure)
2. Vital signs (fever, hypotension/hypertension, bradycardia/tachycardia)
3. Laboratory testing should be obtained prior to each treatment and every 6–12 weeks for the first 6 months following completion of cancer therapies. Depending on treatment response or occurrence of toxicities, increased frequency of follow-up workup may be necessary.
   a) Complete blood counts
   b) Thyroid function tests
   c) Liver function tests (bilirubin, ALT, AST, lactate dehydrogenase, alkaline phosphatase)
   d) Complete metabolic panels
   e) Coagulation factors
   f) Hepatitis titers
4. Physical examination should include thorough head-to-toe assessment to identify signs and symptoms of hepatic toxicity.
   a) Neurologic examination: Assess level of consciousness, orientation, and behavioral changes.
   b) Examination of skin and head, eyes, ears, nose, and throat: Assess for jaundice of the skin, sclerae (icteric), and mucous membranes; rash; ecchymosis; and petechiae.
   c) Cardiac and pulmonary examination: Assess for hypotension or hypertension, bradycardia or tachycardia, jugular venous distension, peripheral edema, crackles and rales, and weight gain.
   d) Abdominal examination: Assess for bowel sounds, ascites, hepatosplenomegaly, abdominal pain, and hematemesis.

H. Collaborative management (Lee & Chan, 2016; Roesser, 2014)

1. An interprofessional approach and collaboration among providers, nurses, patients, caregivers, and consultants is essential in the management of patients who may develop hepatotoxicity. Liver abnormalities may increase, fluctuate, or possibly resolve without intervention (Economopoulou & Psyrri, 2016; Fecher, Agarwala, Hodi, & Weber, 2013).
   a) Monitoring of liver function tests should increase to every one to three days until stabilization followed by weekly monitoring (Fecher et al., 2013)

Table 18-2. Diagnosis and Grading of Sinusoidal Obstruction Syndrome

System	Diagnostic Criteria	Grading/Severity
Modified Seattle criteria (Shulman & Hinterberger, 1992)	At least 2 of the following, occurring within 20 days of transplantation: • Serum bilirubin > 34 mcmol/L (> 2 mg/dl) • Hepatomegaly with right upper quadrant pain • > 2% weight gain from baseline due to fluid retention	Mild: • No adverse effects of liver disease, and • No medications required for diuresis or hepatic pain, and • All symptoms, signs, and laboratory features reversible Moderate: • Adverse effects of liver disease present, and • Sodium restriction or diuretics required, or • Medication for hepatic pain required, and • All symptoms, signs, and laboratory features reversible Severe: • Adverse effects of liver disease present, and • Symptoms, signs, or laboratory features not resolved by day +100, or • Death
Baltimore criteria (Jones et al., 1987)	Serum bilirubin > 34 mcmol/L (> 2 mg/dl) within 21 days of transplantation and at least 2 of the following criteria: • Hepatomegaly • > 5% weight gain from baseline • Ascites	–
EBMT diagnostic criteria for diagnosis of SOS in adults (Mohty et al., 2016)	In first 21 days after transplantation: • Bilirubin > 34 mcmol/L (> 2 mg/dl) plus 2 of the following criteria: – Painful hepatomegaly – Weight gain > 5% from baseline – Ascites Greater than 21 days after transplantation: • Classical SOS, or • Histologically proved SOS, or • 2 or more of the following: – Painful hepatomegaly – Weight gain > 5% from baseline – Ascites – And hemodynamic or ultrasound evidence of SOS	–
EBMT diagnostic criteria for diagnosis of SOS in children (Corbacioglu et al., 2018)	No time limitation for onset of SOS Presence of 2 or more of the following criteria: • Steroid-refractory thrombocytopenia (unexplained) • Unexplained weight gain for 3 consecutive days unresponsive to treatment or weight gain > 5% above baseline • Hepatomegaly above baseline value (preferably confirmed with imaging) • Ascites above baseline value (preferably confirmed with imaging) • Elevated bilirubin above baseline for 3 consecutive days or ≥ 2 mg/dl within 72 hours	–

EBMT—European Society for Blood and Marrow Transplantation; SOS—sinusoidal obstruction syndrome

b) Nurses should rule out other causes such as disease progression, infection, effects of other medications, hemochromatosis, or alcohol intake (Tarhini, 2013; Teply & Lipson, 2014).

c) Standardized toxicity grading tools should be used.

(1) The National Cancer Institute Cancer Therapy Evaluation Program's

Common Terminology Criteria for Adverse Events (2017) is a standardized classification to quantify or grade severity of treatment-related adverse effects, including liver enzyme elevations (Floyd & Kerr, 2017; Grigorian & O'Brien, 2014; see Table 18-3).

(2) The Child-Pugh classification is a scoring system used to measure the severity of chronic liver disease, including cirrhosis, and provides clinicians a way to communicate objectively about liver function (Floyd & Kerr, 2017; Grigorian & O'Brien, 2014; Peng, Qi, & Guo, 2016; see Table 18-4). The modified Child-Pugh score classifies liver disease severity according to the degree of ascites, serum concentrations of bilirubin and albumin, prothrombin time, and degree of encephalopathy.

d) Consider autoimmunity workup: Serum antinuclear antibody, smooth muscle antibody, antimitochondrial antibodies, antisoluble liver antigen/liver-pancreas antibodies, anti–liver-kidney microsomal type 1 antibodies, and additional studies as appropriate.

e) Consider viral screening: Epstein-Barr virus, cytomegalovirus, hepatitis B and C, and hepatitis A, D, and E if the patient has a recent history of travel outside of the country (DeSouza & Savva, 2016).

f) Additional laboratory tests to consider include complete metabolic panel, complete blood counts, ammonia level, and coagulation factors.

g) Consider consultation with a gastroenterologist or hepatologist.

h) Consider imaging (DeSouza & Savva, 2016; Gordon et al., 2017).

(1) Ultrasound of the liver: Rule out obstruction of the biliary tree and assess for masses in the liver parenchyma.

(2) Computed tomography scan: May identify hepatomegaly, periportal edema, or periportal lymphadenopathy. Other findings that may be noted include liver abnormalities such as fatty liver, pseudocirrhosis, biliary sclerosis, and SOS (Torrisi et al., 2011).

i) Rarely, liver biopsy may be considered if the diagnosis remains unclear (DeSouza & Savva, 2016; Postow, 2015).

(1) Autoimmune hepatitis and drug-induced liver injury may present similarly, and liver biopsy would provide definitive diagnosis of the causative agent (Kleiner & Berman, 2012). Severe inflammation of the lobules in the liver with thickening of the surrounding hepatic veins, which could lead to necrosis, has been seen.

(2) Primary biliary pattern with mild portal mononuclear infiltration around proliferated bile ductules has been seen.

(a) Consider dose adjustment of drugs if hepatic dysfunction is noted at baseline (Wilkes & Barton-Burke, 2018).

(b) Consider avoidance of hepatotoxic drugs in patients with preexisting liver dysfunction (Floyd & Kerr, 2017).

(c) Consider withdrawal of the offending hepatotoxic drug and monitoring for normalization of liver function tests (Larson, 2017).

2. Management of immune-mediated hepatitis: The primary mode of treatment for hepatotoxicity is withdrawal of the offending drug. Management algorithms have been developed based on the severity of the toxicity (Brahmer et al., 2018; Fay, Moreira, Nunes Filho, Albuquerque, & Barrios, 2016; Friedman, Proverbs-Singh, & Postow, 2016; Mistry, Forbes, & Fowler, 2017; Naidoo et al., 2015; Postow & Wolchok, 2017; Spain, Diem, & Larkin, 2016; Teply & Lipson, 2014; Villadolid & Amin, 2015).

a) Moderate or severe (grade 2) immune-related adverse events necessitate holding the drug and initiating corticosteroids (Economopoulou & Psyrri, 2016).

b) The drug is resumed when toxicity is grade 1 or less.

c) Severe or life-threatening (grade 3 or 4) immune-related adverse events require permanent discontinuation of the drug and initiation of high-dose corticosteroids.

d) Steroids are tapered gradually over at least one month.

e) In the presence of steroid-refractory hepatitis, consider adding mycophenolate or antithymocyte globulin (DeSouza & Savva, 2016; Economopoulou & Psyrri, 2016; Eigentler et al., 2016; Gangadhar & Vonderheide, 2014; Kim et al., 2013; Lampson et al., 2016; Weber, Kähler, & Hauschild, 2012).

I. Patient and family education (Chalasani et al., 2014; Champiat et al., 2016; Economopoulou & Psyrri, 2016; Fecher et al., 2013)

1. Patient and caregiver education about the potential side effects of drugs is essential. Communi-

Table 18-3. Common Terminology Criteria for Adverse Events Grading for Liver Toxicity[a]

Adverse Event	Grade 1	Grade 2	Grade 3	Grade 4	Grade 5
Alanine aminotransferase increased	> ULN–3 × ULN if baseline was normal; 1.5–3 × baseline if baseline was abnormal	> 3–5 × ULN if baseline was normal; > 3–5 × baseline if baseline was abnormal	> 5–20 × ULN if baseline was normal; > 5–20 × baseline if baseline was abnormal	> 20 × ULN if baseline was normal; > 20 × baseline if baseline was abnormal	–
Alkaline phosphatase increased	> ULN–2.5 × ULN if baseline was normal; 2–2.5 × baseline if baseline was abnormal	> 2.5–5 × ULN if baseline was normal; > 2.5–5 × baseline if baseline was abnormal	> 5–20 × ULN if baseline was normal; > 5–20 × baseline if baseline was abnormal	> 20 × ULN if baseline was normal; > 20 × baseline if baseline was abnormal	–
Aspartate aminotransferase increased	> ULN–3 × ULN if baseline was normal; 1.5–3 × baseline if baseline was abnormal	> 3–5 × ULN if baseline was normal; > 3–5 × baseline if baseline was abnormal	> 5–20 × ULN if baseline was normal; > 5–20 × baseline if baseline was abnormal	> 20 × ULN if baseline was normal; > 20 × baseline if baseline was abnormal	–
Gamma-glutamyl transpeptidase increased	> ULN–2.5 × ULN if baseline was normal; 2–2.5 × baseline if baseline was abnormal	> 2.5–5 × ULN if baseline was normal; 2.5–5 × baseline if baseline was abnormal	> 5–20 × ULN if baseline was normal; > 5–20 × baseline if baseline was abnormal	> 20 × ULN if baseline was normal; > 20 × baseline if baseline was abnormal	–
Liver failure (clinical)	–	–	Asterixis; mild encephalopathy; drug-induced liver injury; limiting self-care activities of daily living	Life-threatening consequences; moderate to severe encephalopathy; coma	Death
Portal hypertension	–	Decreased portal vein flow	Reversal/retrograde portal vein flow; associated with varices and/or ascites	Life-threatening consequences; urgent intervention indicated	Death
Total bilirubin increased	> ULN–1.5 × ULN if baseline was normal; > 1–1.5 × baseline if baseline was abnormal	> 1.5–3 × ULN if baseline was normal; > 1.5–3 × baseline if baseline was abnormal	> 3–10 × ULN if baseline was normal; > 3–10 × baseline if baseline was abnormal	> 10 × ULN if baseline was normal; > 10 × baseline if baseline was abnormal	–

[a] Grading criteria for additional hepatobiliary disorders are available in the *Common Terminology Criteria for Adverse Events*.

ULN—upper limit of normal

Note. From *Common Terminology Criteria for Adverse Events* [v.5.0], by National Cancer Institute Cancer Therapy Evaluation Program, 2017. Retrieved from https://ctep.cancer.gov/protocoldevelopment/electronic_applications/docs/CTCAE_v5_Quick_Reference_5x7.pdf.

Table 18-4. Child-Pugh Classification of Severity of Cirrhosis

Clinical and Laboratory Criteria	Points Assigned		
	1	2	3
Albumin	> 3.5 g/dl (35 g/L)	2.8–3.5 g/dl (28–35 g/L)	< 2.8 g/dl (< 28 g/L)
Ascites	None	Mild to moderate (responsive to diuretics)	Severe (refractory to diuretics)
Bilirubin	< 2 mg/dl (< 34.2 mcmol/L)	2–3 mg/dl (34.2–51.3 mcmol/L)	> 3 mg/dl (> 51.3 mcmol/L)
Encephalopathy	Grade 0 (none)	Grade 1–2	Grade 3–4
Prothrombin time (PT; in seconds over normal value)/international normalized ratio (INR)	PT < 4; INR < 1.7	PT 4–6; INR 1.7–2.3	PT > 6; INR > 2.3

Total Score	Grade	Description	1- and 2-Year Survival
5–6	A	Well-compensated disease	100%; 85%
7–9	B	Significant functional compromise	80%; 60%
10–15	C	Decompensated disease	45%; 35%

Note. Based on information from Durand & Valla, 2005; Pugh et al., 1973.

cation is critical, including an emphasis on the importance of prompt identification and reporting of the following signs and symptoms:

a) Change in level of consciousness (increased sedation, confusion)
b) Malaise, fever
c) Jaundice, icteric sclera
d) Abdominal pain, bleeding or persistent bruising, hematemesis, changes in stool or urine (including the presence of blood)
e) Edema of extremities, weight gain

2. Items to include in patient instructions
   a) Avoidance of other hepatotoxins, including herbal supplements and over-the-counter medications
   b) Close follow-up with healthcare providers, including periodic monitoring of liver function studies
   c) Maintenance of a well-balanced diet and hydration
   d) Skin care (e.g., avoidance of scratching; use of lotions; daily showers)
   e) Fall prevention

References

Ali, A.A., Charoo, N.A., & Abdallah, D.B. (2014). Pediatric drug development: Formulation considerations. *Drug Development and Industrial Pharmacy, 40,* 1283–1299. https://doi.org/10.3109/03639045.2013.850713

Barrett, J.S., Patel, D., Dombrowsky, E., Bajaj, G., & Skolnik, J.M. (2013). Risk assessment of drug interaction potential and concomitant dosing pattern on targeted toxicities in pediatric cancer patients. *AAPS Journal, 15,* 775–786. https://doi.org/10.1208/s12248-013-9489-z

Benn, C.E. (2014). Optimising medicines for children: Considerations for clinical pharmacists. *European Journal of Hospital Pharmacy, 21,* 350–354. https://doi.org/10.1136/ejhpharm-2013-000396

Botti, S., Orlando, L., Gargiulo, G., De Cecco, V., Banfi, M., Duranti, L., … Bonifazi, F. (2016). Veno-occlusive disease nurse management: Development of a dynamic monitoring tool by the GITMO nursing group. *Ecancermedicalscience, 10,* 661. https://doi.org/10.3332/ecancer.2016.661

Brahmer, J.R., Lacchetti, C., Schneider, B.J., Atkins, M.B., Brassil, K.J., Caterino, J.M., … National Comprehensive Cancer Network. (2018). Management of immune-related adverse events in patients treated with immune checkpoint inhibitor therapy: American Society of Clinical Oncology clinical practice guideline. *Journal of Clinical Oncology, 36,* 1714–1768. https://doi.org/10.1200/jco.2017.77.6385

Carreras, E., Díaz-Beyá, M., Rosiñol, L., Martínez, C., Fernández-Avilés, F., & Rovira, M. (2011). The incidence of veno-occlusive disease following allogeneic hematopoietic stem cell transplantation has diminished and the outcome improved over the last decade. *Biology of Blood and Marrow Transplantation, 17,* 1713–1720. https://doi.org/10.1016/j.bbmt.2011.06.006

Chalasani, N.P., Hayashi, P.H., Bonkovsky, H.L., Navarro, V.J., Lee, W.M., & Fontana, R.J. (2014). ACG clinical guideline: The diagnosis and management of idiosyncratic drug-induced liver injury. *American Journal of Gastroenterology, 109,* 950–966. https://doi.org/10.1038/ajg.2014.131

Champiat, S., Lambotte, O., Barreau, E., Belkhir, R., Berdelou, A., Carbonnel, F., … Marabelle, A. (2016). Management of immune checkpoint blockade dysimmune toxicities: A collaborative position paper. *Annals of Oncology, 27,* 559–574. https://doi.org/10.1093/annonc/mdv623

Chen, M., Suzuki, A., Borlak, J., Andrade, R.J., & Lucena, M.I. (2015). Drug-induced liver injury: Interactions between drug properties and host factors. *Journal of Hepatology, 63,* 503–514. https://doi.org/10.1016/j.jhep.2015.04.016

Coash, M., Forouhar, F., Wu, C.H., & Wu, G.Y. (2012). Granulomatous liver diseases: A review. *Journal of the Formosan Medical Association, 111,* 3–13. https://doi.org/10.1016/j.jfma.2011.11.023

Coppell, J.A., Richardson, P.G., Soiffer, R., Martin, P.L., Kernan, N.A., Chen, A., ... Niederwieser, D. (2010). Hepatic veno-occlusive disease following stem cell transplantation: Incidence, clinical course, and outcome. *Biology of Blood and Marrow Transplantation, 16,* 157–168. https://doi.org/10.1016/j.bbmt.2009.08.024

Corbacioglu, S., Carreras, E., Ansari, M., Balduzzi, A., Cesaro, S., Dalle, J.-H., ... Bader, P. (2018). Diagnosis and severity criteria for sinusoidal obstruction syndrome/veno-occlusive disease in pediatric patients: A new classification from the European Society for Blood and Marrow Transplantation. *Bone Marrow Transplantation, 53,* 138–145. https://doi.org/10.1038/bmt.2017.161

DeSouza, K., & Savva, C. (2016). Management of immunotherapy related adverse effects. *Journal of Cancer Prevention and Current Research, 6,* 00187. https://doi.org/10.15406/jcpcr.2016.06.00187

Dignan, F.L., Wynn, R.F., Hadzic, N., Karani, J., Quaglia, A., Pagliuca, A., ... Potter, M. (2013). BCSH/BSBMT guideline: Diagnosis and management of veno-occlusive disease (sinusoidal obstruction syndrome) following haematopoietic stem cell transplantation. *British Journal of Haematology, 163,* 444–457. https://doi.org/10.1111/bjh.12558

Durand, F., & Valla, D. (2005). Assessment of the prognosis of cirrhosis: Child–Pugh versus MELD. *Journal of Hepatology, 42,* S100–S107. https://doi.org/10.1016/j.jhep.2004.11.015

Economopoulou, P., & Psyrri, A. (2016). Overview and management of toxicities of immune checkpoint-blocking drugs. *Forum of Clinical Oncology, 7,* 28–37. https://doi.org/10.1515/fco-2016-0004

Eigentler, T.K., Hassel, J.C., Berking, C., Aberle, J., Bachmann, O., Grünwald, V., ... Gutzmer, R. (2016). Diagnosis, monitoring and management of immune-related adverse drug reactions of anti-PD-1 antibody therapy. *Cancer Treatment Reviews, 45,* 7–18. https://doi.org/10.1016/j.ctrv.2016.02.003

Fay, A.P., Moreira, R.B., Nunes Filho, P.R.S., Albuquerque, C., & Barrios, C.H. (2016). The management of immune-related adverse events associated with immune checkpoint blockade. *Expert Review of Quality of Life in Cancer Care, 1,* 89–97. https://doi.org/10.1080/23809000.2016.1142827

Fecher, L.A., Agarwala, S.S., Hodi, F.S., & Weber, J.S. (2013). Ipilimumab and its toxicities: A multidisciplinary approach. *Oncologist, 18,* 733–743. https://doi.org/10.1634/theoncologist.2012-0483

Fisher, K., Vuppalanchi, R., & Saxena, R. (2015). Drug-induced liver injury. *Archives of Pathology and Laboratory Medicine, 139,* 876–887. https://doi.org/10.5858/arpa.2014-0214-RA

Floyd, J., & Kerr, T.A. (2017). Chemotherapy hepatotoxicity and dose modification in patients with liver disease. In D.M.F. Savarese (Ed.), *UpToDate.* Retrieved July 10, 2017, from https://www.uptodate.com/contents/chemotherapy-hepatotoxicity-and-dose-modification-in-patients-with-liver-disease

Fontana, R.J. (2014). Pathogenesis of idiosyncratic drug-induced liver injury and clinical perspectives. *Gastroenterology, 146,* 914–928. https://doi.org/10.1053/j.gastro.2013.12.032

Frick, M., Mouchacca, P., Verdeil, G., Hamon, Y., Billaudeau, C., Buferne, M., ... Boyer, C. (2017). Distinct patterns of cytolytic T-cell activation by different tumour cells revealed by Ca^{2+} signalling and granule mobilization. *Immunology, 150,* 199–212. https://doi.org/10.1111/imm.12679

Friedman, C.F., Proverbs-Singh, T.A., & Postow, M.A. (2016). Treatment of the immune-related adverse effects of immune checkpoint inhibitors: A review. *JAMA Oncology, 2,* 1346–1353. https://doi.org/10.1001/jamaoncol.2016.1051

Gangadhar, T.C., & Vonderheide, R.H. (2014). Mitigating the toxic effects of anticancer immunotherapy. *Nature Reviews Clinical Oncology, 11,* 91–99. https://doi.org/10.1038/nrclinonc.2013.245

Genentech, Inc. (2017). *Alecensa® (alectinib)* [Package insert]. South San Francisco, CA: Author.

Gordon, RA., Kasler, M.K., Stasi, K., Shames, Y., Errante, M., Ciccolini, K., ... Fischer-Cartlidge, E. (2017). Checkpoint inhibitors: Common immune-related adverse events and their management. *Clinical Journal of Oncology Nursing, 21*(Suppl. 2), 45–52. https://doi.org/10.1188/17.CJON.S2.45-52

Grigorian, A., & O'Brien, C.B. (2014). Hepatotoxicity secondary to chemotherapy. *Journal of Clinical and Translational Hepatology,* 2, 95–102. https://doi.org/10.14218/JCTH.2014.00011

Helissey, C., Vicier, C., & Champiat, S. (2016). The development of immunotherapy in older adults: New treatments, new toxicities? *Journal of Geriatric Oncology, 7,* 325–333. https://doi.org/10.1016/j.jgo.2016.05.007

Herrine, S.K. (2016, May). Evaluation of the patient with a liver disorder. In R.S. Porter (Ed.), *Merck manual* (Professional version). Retrieved from http://www.merckmanuals.com/professional/hepatic-and-biliary-disorders/approach-to-the-patient-with-liver-disease/evaluation-of-the-patient-with-a-liver-disorder

Hospira, Inc. (2016). *Dacarbazine* [Package insert]. Lake Forest, IL: Author.

Hospira, Inc. (2018). *Nipent™ (pentostatin)* [Package insert]. Lake Forest, IL: Author.

Jones, R.J., Lee, K.S.K., Beschorner, W.E., Vogel, V.G., Grochow, L.B., Braine, H.G., ... Saral, R. (1987). Venoocclusive disease of the liver following bone marrow transplantation. *Transplantation, 44,* 778–783. https://doi.org/10.1097/00007890-198712000-00011

Kim, K.W., Ramaiya, N.H., Krajewski, K.M., Jagannathan, J.P., Tirumani, S.H., Srivastava, A., & Ibrahim, N. (2013). Ipilimumab associated hepatitis: Imaging and clinicopathologic findings. *Investigational New Drugs, 31,* 1071–1077. https://doi.org/10.1007/s10637-013-9939-6

Kleiner, D.E., & Berman, D. (2012). Pathologic changes in ipilimumab-related hepatitis in patients with metastatic melanoma. *Digestive Diseases and Sciences, 57,* 2233–2240. https://doi.org/10.1007/s10620-012-2140-5

Krishna, M. (2017). Patterns of necrosis in liver disease. *Clinical Liver Disease, 10,* 53–56. https://doi.org/10.1002/cld.653

Kujovich, J.L. (2015). Coagulopathy in liver disease: A balancing act. *Hematology: American Society of Hematology Education Program Book, 2015,* 243–249. https://doi.org/10.1182/asheducation-2015.1.243

Lampson, B.L., Kasar, S.N., Matos, T.R., Morgan, E.A., Rassenti, L., Davids, M.S., ... Brown, J.R. (2016). Idelalisib given front-line for treatment of chronic lymphocytic leukemia causes frequent immune-mediated hepatotoxicity. *Blood, 128,* 195–203. https://doi.org/10.1182/blood-2016-03-707133

Larson, A.M. (2017). Drug-induced liver injury. In K.M. Robson (Ed.), *UpToDate.* Retrieved July 11, 2017, from https://www.uptodate.com/contents/drug-induced-liver-injury

Lee, K.W.-C., & Chan, S.L. (2016). Hepatotoxicity of targeted therapy for cancer. *Expert Opinion on Drug Metabolism and Toxicology, 12,* 789–802. https://doi.org/10.1080/17425255.2016.1190831

Leise, M.D., Poterucha, J.J., & Talwalkar, J.A. (2014). Drug-induced liver injury. *Mayo Clinic Proceedings, 89,* 95–106. https://doi.org/10.1016/j.mayocp.2013.09.016

Lisi, D.M. (2016). Drug-induced liver injury: An overview. *U.S. Pharmacist, 41*(12), 30–34. Retrieved from https://www.uspharmacist.com/article/druginduced-liver-injury-an-overview

Livshits, Z., Rao, R.B., & Smith, S.W. (2014). An approach to chemotherapy-associated toxicity. *Emergency Medicine Clinics of North America, 32,* 167–203. https://doi.org/10.1016/j.emc.2013.09.002

Mehta, N. (2016). Drug-induced hepatotoxicity. Retrieved from http://emedicine.medscape.com/article/169814-overview

Mistry, H.E., Forbes, S.G., & Fowler, N. (2017). Toxicity management: Development of a novel and immune-mediated adverse events algorithm. *Clinical Journal of Oncology Nursing, 21*(Suppl. 2), 53–59. https://doi.org/10.1188/17.CJON.S2.53-59

Mohty, M., Malard, F., Abecassis, M., Aerts, E., Alaskar, A.S., Aljurf, M., … Carreras, E. (2015). Sinusoidal obstruction syndrome/veno-occlusive disease: Current situation and perspectives—a position statement from the European Society for Blood and Marrow Transplantation (ESBMT). *Bone Marrow Transplantation, 50,* 781–789. https://doi.org/10.1038/bmt.2015.52

Naidoo, J., Page, D.B., Li, B.T., Connell, L.C., Schindler, K., Lacouture, M.E., … Wolchok, J.D. (2015). Toxicities of the anti-PD-1 and anti-PD-L1 immune checkpoint antibodies. *Annals of Oncology, 26,* 2375–2391. https://doi.org/10.1093/annonc/mdv383

National Cancer Institute Cancer Therapy Evaluation Program. (2017). *Common terminology criteria for adverse events* [v.5.0]. Retrieved from https://evs.nci.nih.gov/ftp1/CTCAE/CTCAE_4.03_2010-06-14_QuickReference_5x7.pdf

National Institute of Diabetes and Digestive and Kidney Diseases & National Library of Medicine. (n.d.). LiverTox®. Retrieved from https://livertox.nlm.nih.gov/index.html

Nazer, H. (2017). Cholestasis. Retrieved from https://emedicine.medscape.com/article/927624-overview

Njoku, D.B. (2014). Drug-induced hepatotoxicity: Metabolic, genetic and immunological basis. *International Journal of Molecular Sciences, 15,* 6990–7003. https://doi.org/10.3390/ijms15046990

Peng, Y., Qi, X., & Guo, X. (2016). Child–Pugh versus MELD score for the assessment of prognosis in liver cirrhosis: A systematic review and meta-analysis of observational studies. *Medicine, 95,* e2877. https://doi.org/10.1097/MD.0000000000002877

Perry, M.C. (2012). Hepatotoxicity of chemotherapeutic agents. In M.C. Perry (Ed.), *The chemotherapy source book* (5th ed., pp. 234–251). Philadelphia, PA: Wolters Kluwer Health/Lippincott Williams & Wilkins.

Pfizer Inc. (2011). *Cytarabine injection* [Package insert]. New York, NY: Author.

Postow, M.A. (2015). Managing immune checkpoint-blocking antibody side effects. *American Society of Clinical Oncology Educational Book, 35,* 76–83. https://doi.org/10.14694/EdBook_AM.2015.35.76

Postow, M.A., & Wolchok, J. (2017). Toxicities associated with checkpoint inhibitor immunotherapy. In M.E. Ross (Ed.), *UpToDate.* Retrieved June 29, 2017, from https://www.uptodate.com/contents/toxicities-associated-with-checkpoint-inhibitor-immunotherapy

Pugh, R.N.H., Murray-Lyon, I.M., Dawson, J.L., Pietroni, M.C., & Williams, R. (1973). Transection of the oesophagus for bleeding oesophageal varices. *British Journal of Surgery, 60,* 646–649. https://doi.org/10.1002/bjs.1800600817

Rabinowich, L., & Shibolet, O. (2015). Drug induced steatohepatitis: An uncommon culprit of a common disease. *BioMed Research International, 2015,* 1–14. https://doi.org/10.1155/2015/168905

Roesser, K.A. (2014). Hepatotoxicity. In D. Camp-Sorrell & R.A. Hawkins (Eds.), *Clinical manual for the oncology advanced practice nurse* (3rd ed., pp. 663–671). Pittsburgh, PA: Oncology Nursing Society.

Shulman, H.M., & Hinterberger, W. (1992). Hepatic veno-occlusive disease—Liver toxicity syndrome after bone marrow transplantation. *Bone Marrow Transplantation, 10,* 197–214.

Sigma-Tau Pharmaceuticals, Inc. (2008). *Matulane® (procarbazine hydrochloride capsules)* [Package insert]. Gaithersburg, MD: Author.

Skood, G.K., Conrad, S.A., Luu, L., & Slabinski, M.S. (2017). Acute liver failure clinical presentation. Retrieved from http://emedicine.medscape.com/article/177354-clinical

Spain, L., Diem, S., & Larkin, J. (2016). Management of toxicities of immune checkpoint inhibitors. *Cancer Treatment Reviews, 44,* 51–60. https://doi.org/10.1016/j.ctrv.2016.02.001

Stine, J.G., Sateesh, P., & Lewis, J.H. (2013). Drug-induced liver injury in the elderly. *Current Gastroenterology Reports, 15,* 299. https://doi.org/10.1007/s11894-012-0299-8

Tarhini, A. (2013). Immune-mediated adverse events associated with ipilimumab CTLA-4 blockade therapy: The underlying mechanisms and clinical management. *Scientifica, 2013,* 1–19. https://doi.org/10.1155/2013/857519

Teply, B.A., & Lipson, E.J. (2014). Identification and management of toxicities from immune checkpoint-blocking drugs. *Oncology, 28*(11, Suppl. 3), 30–38. Retrieved from http://www.cancernetwork.com/oncology-journal/identification-and-management-toxicities-immune-checkpointblocking-drugs

Teva Parenteral Medicines, Inc. (2012). *Zanosar® (streptozocin sterile powder)* [Package insert]. Irvine, CA: Author.

Tewari, P., Wallis, W., & Kebriaei, P. (2017). Manifestations and management of veno-occlusive disease/sinusoidal obstruction syndrome in the era of contemporary therapies. *Clinical Advances in Hematology and Oncology, 15,* 130–139.

Torrisi, J.M., Schwartz, L.H., Gollub, M.J., Ginsberg, M.S., Bosl, G.J., & Hricak, H. (2011). CT findings of chemotherapy-induced toxicity: What radiologists need to know about the clinical and radiologic manifestations of chemotherapy toxicity. *Radiology, 258,* 41–56. https://doi.org/10.1148/radiol.10092129

U.S. Food and Drug Administration. (n.d.). Drugs@FDA: FDA approved drug products. Retrieved from https://www.accessdata.fda.gov/scripts/cder/daf

Valla, D.-C., & Cazals-Hatem, D. (2016). Sinusoidal obstruction syndrome. *Clinics and Research in Hepatology and Gastroenterology, 40,* 378–385. https://doi.org/10.1016/j.clinre.2016.01.006

Villadolid, J., & Amin, A. (2015). Immune checkpoint inhibitors in clinical practice: Update on management of immune-related toxicities. *Translational Lung Cancer Research, 4,* 560–575. https://doi.org/10.3978/j.issn.2218-6751.2015.06.06

Weber, J.S., Kähler, K.C., & Hauschild, A. (2012). Management of immune-related adverse events and kinetics of response with ipilimumab. *Journal of Clinical Oncology, 30,* 2691–2697. https://doi.org/10.1200/JCO.2012.41.6750

Weber, J.S., Yang, J.C., Atkins, M.B., & Disis, M.L. (2015). Toxicities of immunotherapy for the practitioner. *Journal of Clinical Oncology, 33,* 2092–2099. https://doi.org/10.1200/JCO.2014.60.0379

Wilkes, G.M., & Barton-Burke, M. (2018). *2018 oncology nursing drug handbook.* Burlington, MA: Jones & Bartlett Learning.

CHAPTER 19

Genitourinary Toxicities

A. Overview

1. The kidneys have multiple roles within the human body, with their primary functions including blood filtration, metabolism, excretion of endogenous and exogenous compounds, and endocrine functions (Perlman, Heung, & Ix, 2013).
   a) Anatomically, the kidney comprises roughly one million nephrons, each of which include a glomerulus (the site of blood filtration) and a renal tubule, where water and salts are reclaimed (Perlman et al., 2013).
   b) Many anticancer treatments, including certain chemotherapy and immunotherapy agents, are considered nephrotoxic because they are metabolized via the renal system. Therefore, many therapies necessitate careful monitoring and possible dose modifications to prevent kidney injury, which in some cases can be irreversible (Shahinian, Bahl, Niepel, & Lorusso, 2017).
2. The bladder consists of three layers, the mucosa, submucosa, and muscularis, each of which are sensitive to damage by chemotherapy and radiation therapy, alone or in combination. Chemotherapy- and radiation therapy–induced damage to the bladder, specifically hemorrhagic cystitis, is thought to be induced by damage to the glycosaminoglycan layer of the bladder, resulting in loss of barrier function (Çetinel, 2015).

B. Antineoplastic-associated genitourinary toxicities

1. Acute kidney injury (AKI)
   a) Definition/pathophysiology: AKI is characterized by rapid deterioration in renal function leading to accumulation of blood nitrogenous waste that is typically excreted in urine (Perlman et al., 2013). Initial presentation includes increasing blood urea nitrogen and serum creatinine but can also include oliguria, anuria, edema, hypertension, proteinuria, electrolyte disturbances, and flank pain (Perlman et al., 2013). Kidney function is a crucial consideration when developing treatment plans in patients with cancer because of the propensity of certain antineoplastic agents, as well as certain cancer types, to cause kidney damage. AKI and electrolyte disturbances are the most common renal complications seen in patients with cancer (Lameire, Vanholder, Van Biesen, & Benoit, 2016).
   b) Incidence: Exact incidence is unknown. See Table 19-1 for drug-related incidence.
   c) Risk factors
      (1) Pharmacologic agents
         (a) Chemotherapy: Aldesleukin, azacitidine, carboplatin, carmustine, diaziquone, cisplatin, gallium nitrate, ifosfamide, methotrexate, mitomycin C, nitrosoureas, pentostatin, plicamycin, semustine, streptozocin (Aapro & Launay-Vacher, 2012)
         (b) Targeted therapies: Bevacizumab, cabozantinib, sorafenib, sunitinib (Aapro & Launay-Vacher, 2012; Choueiri et al., 2017)
         (c) Immunotherapy agents: Combination nivolumab and ipilimumab (Cortazar et al., 2016)
         (d) Other drugs: IV bisphosphonates, including ibandronate, pamidronate, and zoledronic acid (Aapro & Launay-Vacher, 2012; Arellano et al., 2015)
      (2) Preexisting conditions
         (a) Syndrome of inappropriate antidiuretic hormone secretion (SIADH)
         (b) Tumor lysis syndrome
         (c) Preexisting renal disease
         (d) Chronic comorbidities: Diabetes, chronic kidney disease, hypertension, cardiac insufficiency, autoimmune disease
         (e) Urinary stones
         (f) Urinary tract infections
         (g) Lower urinary tract obstruction
         (h) Hydronephrosis

Table 19-1. Genitourinary Toxicities With Specific Chemotherapy, Targeted Therapy, and Immunotherapy Agents

Classification	Drug	Side Effects	Nursing Considerations
Chemotherapy Agents			
Alkylating agents	Bendamustine (Bendeka®, Treanda®)	Increased serum creatinine (grade 3–4): 2%	Drug is associated with TLS. Use with caution in patients with mild to moderate renal impairment. Drug is not recommended in patients with CrCl < 40 ml/min.
	Cisplatin (Platinol®, Platinol®-AQ)	Acute renal failure and chronic renal insufficiency: 28%–36%	Monitor CrCl and electrolytes. Dose adjust for CrCl < 50 ml/min. Prehydration with 1–2 L of fluid is recommended. Replete electrolytes as needed
	Cyclophosphamide (Cytoxan®)	SIADH: < 1% Hemorrhagic cystitis	Dose adjust for CrCl < 10 ml/min. Increase fluid intake 1–2 days after dose to avoid bladder toxicity (hemorrhagic cystitis).
	Ifosfamide (Ifex®)	Renal insufficiency: 6% Hemorrhagic cystitis	Drug may cause severe nephrotoxicity resulting in renal failure. Drug is associated with proteinuria and SIADH.
	Melphalan (Alkeran®, Evomela®)	Hypokalemia: 74% Renal failure: 1%–10%	Drug is associated with SIADH. Reduce dose 50% for CrCl < 10 ml/min.
	Oxaliplatin (Eloxatin®)	Increased serum creatinine: 5%–10%	Drug is associated with hypokalemia and dehydration. Dose adjust for CrCl < 30 ml/min.
Antimetabolites	Azacitidine (Vidaza®)	Renal failure: < 5%	Monitor serum creatinine. Drug is associated with TLS.
	Capecitabine (Xeloda®)	Renal insufficiency: < 1% Dehydration: 7%	Drug is contraindicated in patients with CrCl < 30 ml/min. Drug is associated with risk of dehydration resulting in acute renal failure. Exercise caution with concomitant use with nephrotoxic agents.
	Fludarabine	Renal failure: ≤ 1%	Monitor CrCl. Dose adjust for CrCl < 80 ml/min.
	Gemcitabine (Gemzar®)	Increased BUN: 16% Proteinuria: 45% Increased serum creatinine: 8%	Drug is associated with capillary leak syndrome. Monitor serum creatinine and BUN.
	Methotrexate	Not defined	Drug is associated with AKI. Drug can cause crystal nephropathy when given at high doses. Maintain adequate hydration and urinary alkalization.
	Pemetrexed (Alimta®)	Increased serum creatinine: ≤ 5%	Drug is not recommended in patients with CrCl < 45 ml/min. Drug can be retained in pleural effusions and ascites.
	Pentostatin (Nipent™)	Increased serum creatinine: 3%–10% Nephrolithiasis: < 3% Renal failure: < 3%	Severe renal toxicities can result with higher-than-recommended doses. Discontinue if CrCl < 30 ml/min.
Antitumor antibiotics	Bleomycin (Blenoxane®)	Nephrotoxicity: < 1%	Dose adjust if CrCl < 60 ml/min.
	Mitomycin (Mitosol®)	Increased serum creatinine: 2%	Do not administer if serum creatinine > 1.7 mg/dl Associated with hemolytic-uremic syndrome

(Continued on next page)

Table 19-1. Genitourinary Toxicities With Specific Chemotherapy, Targeted Therapy, and Immunotherapy Agents *(Continued)*

Classification	Drug	Side Effects	Nursing Considerations
Chemotherapy Agents *(Cont.)*			
Antitumor antibiotics: Anthracyclines	Idarubicin (Idamycin®)	Not defined	Dose adjust for CrCl < 50 ml/min.
Miscellaneous	Hydroxyurea (Hydrea®)	Not defined	Drug is associated with increased serum creatinine, BUN, uric acid, and renal tubular disease.
Plant alkaloids: Taxanes	Cabazitaxel (Jevtana®)	Renal failure: 4%	Use with caution if CrCl < 30 ml/min.
Plant alkaloids: Vinca alkaloids	Vincristine sulfate, vincristine sulfate liposomal (Oncovin®, Marqibo®)	Not defined	Drug is associated with SIADH.
Targeted Therapy Agents			
Small molecule inhibitors	Cabozantinib (Cabometyx®)	Increased serum creatinine: 58%	Drug is associated with proteinuria and HTN. Monitor serum creatinine.
	Gefitinib (Iressa®)	Increased serum creatinine: 2% Proteinuria: 8%–35%	Monitor serum creatinine and UA.
	Imatinib mesylate (Gleevec®)	Increased serum creatinine: ≤ 44%	Drug is associated with AKI and SIADH. Dose adjust for CrCl < 60 ml/min.
	Sunitinib (Sutent®)	Increased serum creatinine: 70% in patients with renal cell carcinoma	Drug is associated with proteinuria, HTN, and TLS.
Immunotherapy Agents			
Cytokines: Interleukins	Interleukin-2 (IL-2), aldesleukin (Proleukin®)	Hypomagnesemia: 12% Increased serum creatinine: 33% Acute renal failure: 1%	Drug is associated with capillary leak syndrome. Patients must have serum creatinine ≤ 1.5 mg/dl prior to treatment. Monitor vital signs and intake and output frequently.
Miscellaneous: Biologic response modifiers	Lenalidomide (Revlimid®)	Hypomagnesemia: 6%–7% Hypokalemia: 7%–17% Renal failure: 4%–10%	Dose adjust for CrCl < 60 ml/min. Drug is associated with TLS. Use with caution in patients with renal impairment.
Monoclonal antibodies	Bevacizumab (Avastin®)	Increased serum creatinine: 16%	Drug can cause elevated blood pressure. Drug is associated with proteinuria and increased serum creatinine.
Miscellaneous			
Bisphosphonates	Pamidronate (Aredia®)	Increased serum creatinine: ≤ 19%	Drug can cause electrolyte abnormalities. Initial doses have been associated with renal failure and dialysis. Drug is associated with glomerulosclerosis. Do not use in patients with renal impairment.
	Zoledronic acid (Zometa®)	Renal insufficiency: 8%–17%	Risk of AKI is increased with abnormal baseline creatinine.

(Continued on next page)

Table 19-1. Genitourinary Toxicities With Specific Chemotherapy, Targeted Therapy, and Immunotherapy Agents *(Continued)*

Classification	Drug	Side Effects	Nursing Considerations
Miscellaneous *(Cont.)*			
Calcineurin inhibitors	Cyclosporine (Sandimmune®)	Increased serum creatinine: 16% to > 50% Renal insufficiency: 10%–38%	Monitor serum creatinine, electrolytes, UA, and HTN. Drug is associated with interstitial nephritis.
	Tacrolimus (Prograf®)	Nephrotoxicity: > 10%	Nephrotoxicity is associated with higher doses. Drug is associated with AKI, hydronephrosis, increased BUN and creatinine, interstitial nephritis, and renal tubular necrosis.

AKI—acute kidney injury; BUN—blood urea nitrogen; CrCl—creatinine clearance; HTN—hypertension; SIADH—syndrome of inappropriate antidiuretic hormone secretion; TLS—tumor lysis syndrome; UA—urinalysis

Note. Based on information from Wolters Kluwer Health, 2017.

(3) Cancer types: Multiple myeloma and renal involvement of tumor
(4) Patient characteristics
  (*a*) Age older than 65
  (*b*) Family history of chronic kidney disease

d) Clinical manifestations (Perlman et al., 2013)
(1) Hematuria, pyuria
(2) Edema
(3) Hypertension
(4) Oliguria
(5) Weight gain

e) Assessment
(1) Laboratory assessment
  (*a*) Serum creatinine
  (*b*) Creatinine clearance (CrCl) using Cockcroft-Gault formula or 24-hour urine (Cockcroft & Gault, 1976)
  (*c*) Proteinuria (best assessed with 24-hour urine)
  (*d*) Electrolyte abnormalities
  (*e*) Albumin
(2) Imaging: Renal ultrasound
(3) Physical assessment
  (*a*) Intake and output
  (*b*) Vital signs
  (*c*) Daily weights
  (*d*) Edema
  (*e*) Costovertebral angle tenderness

f) Collaborative management
(1) Assess for risk factors prior to initiating nephrotoxic agents.
(2) Optimize hydration status and evaluation prior to starting therapy.
(3) Follow dosing adjustments for patients with impaired renal function.
(4) Minimize coadministration of nonsteroidal anti-inflammatory drugs (NSAIDs) or cyclooxygenase-2 inhibitors (Aapro & Launay-Vacher, 2012).
(5) Optimize treatment of comorbidities such as hypertension and diabetes.
(6) See Drug-Specific Considerations section later in chapter.

g) Patient and family education
(1) Educate patients and families regarding the risk of AKI with cytotoxic agents.
(2) Educate patients and families on the signs and symptoms of AKI.
(3) Instruct patients to notify the healthcare team if the following symptoms occur (Forman, 2017):
  (*a*) No urine output for more than 12 hours
  (*b*) Very small amounts of dark urine
  (*c*) Appearance of urine is dark, concentrated, or cloudy, or blood is present
  (*d*) Occurrence of edema or acute weight gain
(4) Encourage patients to monitor their blood pressure at home.
(5) Educate patients and families about the importance of adequate oral hydration—up to 3 L per day while they are receiving nephrotoxic cytotoxic agents (e.g., cisplatin, methotrexate) (Almanric, Marceau, Cantin, & Bertin, 2017; Howard, McCormick, Pui, Buddington, & Harvey, 2016).

2. SIADH
   a) Definition/pathophysiology: SIADH is a paraneoplastic syndrome characterized by impaired water excretion secondary to excess antidiuretic hormone, which causes the kidneys to reabsorb water. Water retention in turn leads to hyponatremia (Sterns, 2017). Paraneoplastic SIADH is thought to be the result of ectopic secretion of antidiuretic hormone from tumor cells (Gralla et al., 2017). Certain antineoplastic agents can cause hyponatremia; therefore, it is important to determine the cause of SIADH, as SIADH is typically a diagnosis of exclusion (Burst et al., 2017).
   b) Diagnostic criteria (Spasovski et al., 2014)
      (1) Effective serum osmolality less than 275 mOsm/kg
      (2) Urine osmolality greater than 100 mOsm/kg at some level of decreased effective osmolality
      (3) Clinical euvolemia
      (4) Urine sodium concentration greater than 30 mmol/L with normal dietary salt and water intake
      (5) Absence of adrenal, thyroid, pituitary, or renal insufficiency
      (6) No recent diuretic agents
   c) Incidence: SIADH occurs in 1%–2% of all patients with cancer and is more prevalent in patients with non-small cell lung cancer, as well as prostate, breast, adrenal, and small cell lung cancer (Dimitriadis et al., 2017).
   d) Risk factors
      (1) Pharmacologic agents
         (a) Chemotherapy: Cisplatin, ifosfamide, melphalan, methotrexate, vinblastine, vincristine, vinorelbine
         (b) Immunotherapy: Immunotherapy agents can cause hypophysitis, which is inflammation of the pituitary gland. When the pituitary gland is inflamed, the normal body functions it controls, such as regulation of the endocrine system and storage of hormones produced by the hypothalamus, can be significantly altered (Vazquez, 2017).
         (c) Other drugs: Amiodarone, amitriptyline, ciprofloxacin, haloperidol, NSAIDs, selective serotonin reuptake inhibitors, thiazides
      (2) Preexisting conditions: Cerebrovascular accident, infection, mental illness, hypopituitarism, hypothyroidism, HIV (Sterns, 2017)
      (3) Cancer types: Non-small cell lung cancer, prostate cancer, breast cancer, adrenal cancer, head and neck cancer, olfactory neuroblastoma
      (4) Patient characteristics: Older than age 65
   e) Clinical manifestations (dependent on serum sodium concentration)
      (1) Serum sodium less than 125 mEq/L: Altered mental status, seizures, coma, respiratory collapse (Dimitriadis et al., 2017)
      (2) Serum sodium 125–135 mEq/L: Increased thirst, anorexia, nausea, weakness, fatigue, muscle cramps, headache (Dimitriadis et al., 2017)
   f) Assessment
      (1) Laboratory assessment
         (a) Serum sodium
         (b) Serum osmolality
         (c) Urine sodium
         (d) Urine osmolality
         (e) Serum cortisol
         (f) Thyroid-stimulating hormone, free T4
         (g) CrCl
      (2) Imaging: Brain magnetic resonance imaging if concern for SIADH secondary to immune-related hypophysitis
      (3) Physical assessment
         (a) Thorough patient history including current medications and comorbidities
         (b) Neurologic examination
         (c) Assessment for signs and symptoms of fluid volume overload
            i. Hypertension
            ii. Edema
            iii. Weight gain
            iv. Decreased urine output
            v. Altered respiratory status
   g) Collaborative management
      (1) Consulting endocrinology colleagues has been shown to improve patient outcomes (Dimitriadis et al., 2017).
      (2) Treatment (Peri, Grohé, Berardi, & Runkle, 2017)
         (a) Fluid restriction
         (b) Hypertonic saline
         (c) Tolvaptan, an oral V_2 receptor antagonist indicated for clinically significant hypovolemic and euvolemic hyponatremia (Gralla et al., 2017)
         (d) Salt tablets

(e) Loop diuretics
(f) Treatment of the underlying cause (e.g., malignancy); if related to hypophysitis—treat with corticosteroids (Vazquez, 2017).

h) Patient and family education
(1) Educate patients and families on the risk factors for SIADH.
(2) Educate patients and families on the clinical signs and symptoms of SIADH, and stress the importance of notifying the healthcare team if signs or symptoms appear.

3. Tumor lysis syndrome
a) Definition/pathophysiology: Tumor lysis syndrome is an oncologic emergency that results when a large number of tumor cells are killed, or lysed, causing the intracellular components to be dumped into circulation. This can lead to a variety of metabolic abnormalities, including hyperkalemia, hyperphosphatemia, hypocalcemia, and hyperuricemia, which in turn cause AKI (Kaplow & Iyere, 2016; Weeks & Kimple, 2015). The syndrome is most commonly seen in hematologic malignancies treated with cytotoxic therapies/chemotherapy, although it can also occur in solid tumors carrying significant tumor burden with strong chemosensitivity (Weeks & Kimple, 2015). Early identification and treatment is critical to avoid life-threatening consequences (Cairo, Coiffier, Reiter, & Younes, 2010). The most widely accepted definition was described by Cairo and Bishop (2004) with both laboratory and clinical considerations.
b) Diagnostic criteria: The following laboratory results and clinical data must be within three days before or seven days after cytotoxic therapy (Cairo & Bishop, 2004).
(1) Laboratory tumor lysis syndrome: Must contain two or more of the following:
(a) Uric acid 8 mg/dl or higher, or 25% increase from baseline
(b) Potassium 6 mmol/L or higher, or 25% increase from baseline
(c) Phosphorus 4.5 mg/dl or higher, or 25% increase from baseline
(d) Calcium 7 mg/dl or lower, or 25% decrease from baseline
(2) Clinical tumor lysis syndrome: Meets laboratory criteria plus one of the following:
(a) Creatinine at least 1.5 times the upper limit of normal
(b) Cardiac arrhythmias/sudden death
(c) New-onset seizure
c) Incidence: Exact incidence unknown
d) Risk factors: Medications/treatments cause tumor lysis syndrome by causing rapid cell death (Kaplow & Iyere, 2016).
(1) Pharmacologic agents
(a) Chemotherapy: Alemtuzumab, cisplatin, cladribine, cytarabine, doxorubicin, etoposide, fludarabine, gemtuzumab, imatinib mesylate, mitoxantrone, paclitaxel, rituximab, tamoxifen
(b) Radiation: Total body irradiation
(c) Other drugs: Corticosteroids
(2) Cancer types
(a) Hematologic malignancies: Burkitt lymphoma, acute lymphoblastic lymphoma, acute lymphoblastic leukemia, acute myeloid leukemia, chronic leukemia, T-cell lymphoma, metastatic lymphoma, multiple myeloma (Coiffier, Altman, Pui, Younes, & Cairo, 2008; Kaplow & Iyere, 2016)
(b) Solid tumors with high tumor burden: Breast cancer, colorectal cancer, germ cell cancer, lymphosarcoma, metastatic medulloblastoma, neuroblastoma, ovarian cancer, small cell lung cancer, thymoma, vulvar cancer (Kaplow & Iyere, 2016)
(3) Patient characteristics: Acidic urine, dehydration, extensive lymph node involvement, hyperuricemia, increased lactate dehydrogenase, leukocytosis, hyperkalemia, hyperphosphatemia, large tumor burden, nephrotoxic agent exposure, oliguria, renal dysfunction, renal involvement of cancer at diagnosis (Cairo et al., 2010; Kaplow & Iyere, 2016)
e) Clinical manifestations result from metabolic abnormalities (Kaplow & Iyere, 2016).
(1) Weakness
(2) Nausea and/or vomiting
(3) Diarrhea
(4) Electrocardiogram abnormalities
(5) Muscle twitching
(6) Confusion and/or delirium
(7) Seizures
(8) Peripheral edema
(9) Oliguria

(10) Flank pain
(11) Paralysis
(12) Paresthesias
(13) Muscle cramps

f) Assessment

(1) Laboratory assessment: Complete blood count, comprehensive metabolic panel, magnesium, phosphorus, uric acid, lactate dehydrogenase, urinalysis, arterial blood gases, CrCl (using Cockcroft-Gault formula)
(2) Imaging: Electrocardiogram
(3) Physical examination
(a) Vital signs
(b) Chvostek sign: Contraction of the ipsilateral facial muscles elicited by tapping the facial nerve just in front of the ear (Goltzman, 2017)
(c) Trousseau sign: Adduction of the thumb, flexion of wrist and metacarpophalangeal joints, and extension of the interphalangeal joints as induced by a blood pressure cuff inflated above systolic blood pressure on the upper arm for three minutes (Goltzman, 2017)
(d) Weight changes
(e) Daily intake and output
(f) Changes in mental status

g) Collaborative management

(1) Prevention: Close monitoring and assessment of high-risk patients is essential to prevent and treat tumor lysis syndrome (Coiffier et al., 2008).
(2) Treatment and management options
(a) Hydration: Aggressive hydration and diuresis are the cornerstone of management and prevention (Coiffier et al., 2008).
i. Hydration should begin 24–72 hours prior to initiating antineoplastic therapy, with a goal of 2–3 L per day (Kaplow & Iyere, 2016).
ii. Diuretics may be necessary to maintain adequate urine output (Coiffier et al., 2008).
(b) Alkalinization: No longer recommended (Coiffier et al., 2008)
(c) Allopurinol: Prevents the conversion of purine metabolites to uric acid (Coiffier et al., 2008)
i. It is used in combination with vigorous hydration in low-risk patients (Shaikh, Marini, Hough, & Perissinotti, 2018).
ii. The dosing is 300 mg PO daily starting several days prior to chemotherapy administration.
(d) Recombinant urate oxidase (rasburicase)
i. The U.S. Food and Drug Administration (FDA) approved rasburicase in 2002 for the management of tumor lysis syndrome. It works by rapidly reducing uric acid levels, preventing or reversing AKI (Shaikh et al., 2018).
ii. It is for use in high-risk patients and should be avoided in patients with glucose-6-phosphate dehydrogenase deficiency (Coiffier et al., 2008).
iii. FDA dosing for rasburicase is 6 mg flat dose; however, recent evidence has suggested using a flat dose of 3 mg for patients with uric acid levels of 8–15 mg/dl is noninferior (Shaikh et al., 2018).
(3) Nursing considerations
(a) Collaborate with providers to determine if cardiac monitoring is indicated (Kaplow & Iyere, 2016).
(b) Closely monitor laboratory results, specifically paying attention to electrolytes, uric acid, and renal function.
(c) Ensure adequate hydration of at-risk patients.
(d) Closely monitor for changes in cognition or mental status.

h) Patient and family education

(1) Educate patients and families on the risk factors and treatment strategies for tumor lysis syndrome.
(2) Educate patients and families on the clinical signs and symptoms, and stress the importance of notifying the healthcare team if signs or symptoms appear.

4. Chronic kidney disease

a) Pathophysiology: Chronic kidney disease is defined as abnormal kidney function or structure for a period greater than three months (McManus & Wynter-Minott, 2017). Many patients with cancer may have preexisting chronic kidney disease or be at higher risk because of comorbidities or exposure to nephrotoxic cytotoxic agents. The disease is best managed in consultation with nephrology specialists (Shahinian et al., 2017).

b) Incidence: The exact incidence in patients with cancer is unknown, although renal impairment is present in more than half of patients with solid tumors (Aapro & Launay-Vacher, 2012).

c) Risk factors
- (1) Chemotherapy: Cisplatin, ifosfamide, melphalan, methotrexate, vinblastine, vincristine, vinorelbine
- (2) Preexisting conditions: Type 2 diabetes, hypertension, history of kidney transplantation, vitamin D deficiency
- (3) Cancer types: Solid tumor malignances, multiple myeloma, bone metastasis
- (4) Patient characteristics
  - *(a)* Older than age 70
  - *(b)* Male gender
  - *(c)* Cigarette use

d) Clinical manifestations
- (1) Hypertension
- (2) Edema
- (3) Weight gain
- (4) Decreased urine output

e) Assessment
- (1) Laboratory assessment
  - *(a)* Serum creatinine
  - *(b)* Blood urea nitrogen
  - *(c)* CrCl using Cockcroft-Gault formula or 24-hour urine (Cockcroft & Gault, 1976)
  - *(d)* Proteinuria (best assessed with 24-hour urine)
  - *(e)* Electrolyte abnormalities
  - *(f)* Albumin
- (2) Imaging: Renal ultrasound
- (3) Physical assessment
  - *(a)* Intake and output
  - *(b)* Vital signs
  - *(c)* Daily weights
  - *(d)* Edema
  - *(e)* Costovertebral angle tenderness

f) Collaborative management: Patients with preexisting chronic kidney disease should be followed by a nephrologist while undergoing cancer treatment.

g) Patient and family education
- (1) Educate patients and families regarding the risk of chronic kidney disease with cytotoxic agents.
- (2) Educate patients and families on the signs and symptoms of worsening chronic kidney disease.
- (3) Encourage patients to monitor their blood pressure at home.
- (4) Educate patients and families about the importance of adequate oral hydration—up to 3 L per day while receiving nephrotoxic cytotoxic agents (e.g., cisplatin, methotrexate).
- (5) Educate patients and families on the importance of continued follow-up with nephrology while undergoing cancer treatment.

5. Hemorrhagic cystitis

a) Definition/pathophysiology: Hemorrhagic cystitis is defined as diffused inflammatory condition of the urinary bladder due to an infection or noninfectious etiology resulting in bleeding from the bladder mucosa (Manikandan, Kumar, & Dorairanjan, 2010). Treatment-related causes include both chemotherapy and radiation (Haldar, Dru, & Bhowmick, 2014). Although bacteria and fungi pathogens promote inflammation of the urinary tract, they seldom cause hemorrhagic cystitis. Viruses have a high incidence of causing hemorrhagic cystitis in immunocompromised patients. Hemorrhagic cystitis can be acute or chronic, and severity can range from mild discomfort in the lower abdomen to severe life-threatening hemorrhage characterized by frequency, lower abdominal pain, and dysuria (Dosin et al., 2017).

b) Incidence
- (1) May affect up to 70% of immunocompromised population (Ruggeri et al., 2015).
- (2) BK viruria occurs in 25%–100% of hematopoietic stem cell transplantation (HSCT) recipients and can lead to BK polyomavirus–associated hemorrhagic cystitis in up to 40% (Schneidewind et al., 2017).
- (3) The incidence of hemorrhagic cystitis in the adult and pediatric population after HSCT ranges from 10% to 70% in the literature (Au et al., 2017; Ruggeri et al., 2015).
- (4) Early-onset hemorrhagic cystitis, occurring two to three days after HSCT, is usually associated with thrombocytopenia, conditioning regimens with high-dose alkylating chemotherapy agents, and radiation therapy.

Delayed-onset hemorrhagic cystitis occurs two to three weeks after HSCT, is usually caused by viral infections due to depressed immune cell response or graft-versus-host disease (GVHD), and is often fatal (Au et al., 2017).

c) Risk factors

(1) Pharmacologic agents

(a) Chemotherapy agents are known to cause hemorrhagic cystitis as a result of hepatic breakdown of antineoplastic agents to toxic compounds that affect the internal membrane of the bladder or urothelium (Johnston et al., 2015).

i. Cyclophosphamide and ifosfamide are metabolized by the liver and converted into antineoplastic agents phosphoramide mustard and iphosphoramide mustard, respectively, and into a compound called acrolein that is responsible for injury to the urothelium in the bladder (Haldar et al., 2014). Accumulation of acrolein in the bladder induces release of inflammatory mediators including tumor necrosis factor-alpha, interleukin-1-beta, and endogenous nitric oxide, which provokes vascular dilation, mucosal inflammation, and increased capillary fragility, causing hemorrhage of the bladder (Haldar et al., 2014).

ii. Busulfan and thiotepa are alkylating agents known to induce trauma to the urothelium wall of the bladder. These are often used in the conditioning regimen for HSCT (Lam, Storek, Li, Geddes, & Daly, 2017).

(b) Although immunotherapies can be associated with inflammatory response (e.g., cytokine release syndrome), there is no evidence to date of correlation with hemorrhagic cystitis.

(c) Radiation therapy in combination with chemotherapy causes hemorrhagic cystitis in approximately 15%–20% of patients with cancer. The effect of radiation and chemotherapy causes single- and double-stranded DNA to break, leading to activation of DNA damage repair genes and apoptosis in a vicious circle that depletes the energy sources of the cells, resulting in loss of bladder muscle expansion, hyperplasia, and progressively worsening hemorrhagic cystitis (Haldar et al., 2014).

i. External beam radiation causes ischemia to the bladder mucosa as a result of endarteritis progressing to hypovascular, hypocellular, and hypoxic tissue, leading to ulcerative tissue formation and bleeding (Kaplan & Wolf, 2009).

ii. Radiation causes cellular depletion, fibrosis, and obliterative endarteritis of the urothelial wall in the bladder, causing late onset of hemorrhagic cystitis (A. Thompson et al., 2014).

(2) Preexisting conditions

(a) GVHD, a complication after HSCT, is a condition where the matured T lymphocytes from the donor bone marrow attack the host tissues of the transplant recipient.

i. GVHD in the bladder may also cause hemorrhagic cystitis as T lymphocytes induce urothelial damage and hematuria (Lunde et al., 2015).

ii. Immunosuppressive therapies to treat GVHD aid in microorganism infections that exacerbate hemorrhagic cystitis (Lunde et al., 2015; Scadden & Raaijmakers, 2017).

(b) Infection may lead to hemorrhagic cystitis by acquired or reactivation of microorganisms in the presence of an exacerbated immunosuppression state (Schneidewind et al., 2017).

i. BK virus, JC virus, adenovirus type 11, cytomegalovirus, and herpesvirus play a crucial role in inflammatory processes and breakdown of epithelial cells of the bladder mucosa, leading to painful hematuria in patients with cancer (Dosin et al., 2017; Fu et al., 2013).

ii. Fungal organisms, such as *Candida albicans* and *tropicalis*, *Cryptococcus neoformans*, *Aspergillus fumigatus*, and *Torulopsis glabrata*, cause inner bladder inflammation and damage of the urothelium in the bladder (Manikandan et al., 2010; Wang et al., 2015).

iii. Bacterial infections affecting the bladder's mucosa, specifically *Escherichia coli*, *Staphylococcus saprophyticus*, *Proteus mirabilis*, and *Klebsiella*, contribute to loss of cellular urothelial protective function in the bladder (Manikandan et al., 2010).

d) Clinical manifestations

(1) Signs and symptoms of patients presenting with hemorrhagic cystitis should be classified based on the grade of bleeding with the purpose of providing prognosis of survival and treatments. Grading ranges from 1 to 4; higher grade indicates higher mortality risk (Au et al., 2017).

(a) Grade 1: Presenting microscopic hematuria

(b) Grade 2: Macroscopic hematuria

(c) Grade 3: Macroscopic hematuria with small clots

(d) Grade 4: Gross hematuria with clots causing urinary tract obstruction requiring clot evacuation

(2) In addition to the severity of hemorrhage, hemorrhagic cystitis is classified according to time of occurrence after cancer treatments: early stage is within 72 hours, and late stage is after the first 72 hours post-treatment. Patients experiencing hemorrhagic cystitis may present with pain in the lower abdominal area, fever, weakness, palpitations, and frustration due to the prolonged period of discomfort (Au et al., 2017; Dosin et al., 2017).

e) Collaborative management

(1) Assessment

(a) Review past infections that may be reactivated by a neutropenic state, such as BK virus (Graham, 2017; Wilkinson, Treas, Barnett, & Smith, 2015).

(b) Collaborate with medical teams to expedite obtaining urine culture and polymerase chain reaction to identify pathogen infections and viral load (Klein et al., 2015).

(c) Assess renal function by obtaining the following laboratory levels: blood urea nitrogen, creatinine, glomerular filtration rate, and urinalysis. Collaborate in obtaining an interstitial biopsy to verify and monitor bladder and renal infections (Klein et al., 2015).

(d) Identify drinking and voiding patterns to formulate plans of care in the presence of possible hemorrhagic cystitis.

(e) Assess patients' menstrual cycle to prevent misinterpretation with hematuria.

(f) Review treatment plans to correlate potential risk factors for hemorrhagic cystitis, including chemotherapy agents, radiation therapy, pathogen infections, and neutropenia. Identify antineoplastic therapies associated with hemorrhagic cystitis (e.g., cyclophosphamide, ifosfamide, radiation) and monitor for associated clinical manifestations.

(2) Monitoring

(a) Monitor urinalysis to identify possible occurrences of hematuria (D.L. Thompson, 2017).

(b) Monitor urinalysis and sensitivity to screen for potential pathogens associated with hemorrhagic cystitis (D.L. Thompson, 2017).

(c) Monitor complete blood count to anticipate risks of anemia, neutropenia, and thrombocytopenia in the presence of hemorrhagic cystitis (D.L. Thompson, 2017; Wilkinson et al., 2015).

(*d*) Monitor fluid intake and output to maintain fluid balance at all times (D.L. Thompson, 2017).

(3) Treatment: Management of hemorrhagic cystitis varies depending on etiology and symptomatic presentation. Some antineoplastic protocols include initiating continuous bladder irrigation in the presence of conditioning regimens known to cause hemorrhagic cystitis.

(*a*) Bladder irrigation: Continuous bladder irrigation is the treatment of choice for hemorrhagic cystitis. A three-way urethral catheter to continuously irrigate the bladder will decompress any clots formed and often will stop the bleeding. In addition, continuous bladder irrigation decreases concentration of acrolein and its contact time with the bladder urothelium. Some antineoplastic protocols include initiating it prior to cyclophosphamide chemotherapy or in combination with the bladder protectant mesna, hyperhydration with forced diuresis and frequent voiding, antibiotic prophylaxis with fluoroquinolones, and urethral catheterization (Gonella, di Pasquale, & Palese, 2015).

i. Continuous bladder irrigation with 0.9% sodium chloride isotonic solution or manual irrigation of clots reduces bleeding by removing urokinase, an anticoagulant substance secreted into the urine by the kidney (Gonella et al., 2015).

ii. Alum may be added to the bladder irrigation to cause reduced protein precipitation, vasoconstriction, and decreased capillary permeability (Ziegelmann, Boorjian, Joyce, Montgomery, & Linder, 2017).

iii. Silver nitrate bladder instillation causes chemical coagulation and scarring at bleeding site (Ziegelmann et al., 2017).

iv. Formalin bladder instillation stops bleeding by causing chemical corrosion in the bladder mucosa without scar tissue formation (Ziegelmann et al., 2017).

v. Aminocaproic acid (Amicar®) may also be used for the management of hemorrhagic cystitis, but caution should be taken because of the risk for formation of hard clots in the bladder that are difficult to evacuate (A. Thompson et al., 2014).

vi. 2-Mercaptoethane sodium sulfonate (mesna) is the most widely used uroprotective agent that acts to neutralize the corrosive metabolite acrolein, which is responsible for induction of hemorrhagic cystitis. Throughout the years, varying dosages and timings of mesna and hyperhydration have been tested as prophylaxis against hemorrhagic cystitis. In 2002, the American Society of Clinical Oncology established clinical practice guidelines for the use of mesna (Schuchter, Hensley, Meropol, & Winer, 2002).

(*b*) Mesna dosing with ifosfamide therapy

i. With a standard dose of ifosfamide less than 2.5 g/m^2 daily, dosing of mesna should equal 60% of the total daily dose of ifosfamide and be divided between three bolus doses administered 15 minutes before and 4 and 8 hours after the administration of each dose of ifosfamide (Matz & Hsieh, 2017).

ii. For an ifosfamide dosage greater than 2.5 g/m^2 daily, mesna dosing has not been established, although it has been given in divided doses equivalent to 60%–160% of the ifosfamide daily dose. Example regimen:

- Before ifosfamide: Mesna equivalent of 20% of the

total daily ifosfamide dose given as IV bolus

- During ifosfamide: Mesna equivalent of 100%–120% of the total daily ifosfamide dose given as IV infusion over 24 hours (mixed in bags with ifosfamide)
- After ifosfamide: Mesna equivalent of 60% of the total daily ifosfamide dose given as IV infusion over 12 hours
- Alternatively, mesna can be administered intravenously at a dose equivalent of 20% of the ifosfamide dosage, followed by two oral doses, each at the equivalent of 40% of the antineoplastic agent. Mesna oral doses should be administered at two and six hours after each dose of ifosfamide (Schuchter et al., 2002).

iii. For patients receiving cyclophosphamide, mesna should be administered at the milligram equivalent of 60%–160% of the total dose of cyclophosphamide, divided in five doses given 15 minutes before and 3, 6, 9, and 12 hours after each dose of cyclophosphamide.

- Mesna can be given concomitantly with both antineoplastic agents cyclophosphamide and ifosfamide (Zhang et al., 2013).
- Mesna dosing with high-dose cyclophosphamide (greater than 1 g/m^2, e.g., HSCT mobilization with cyclophosphamide 1.5 g/m^2) requires mesna equivalent of 60%–160% total dose of cyclophosphamide daily dosage given intravenously. Mesna must be given by IV administration in three to five divided doses or by continuous infusion. Mesna should be administered each day cyclophosphamide is administered and continued for at least 24 hours after cyclophosphamide is discontinued.
- Alternatively, if cyclophosphamide is given orally, mesna can initially be administered via IV at a dose equivalent of 20% of the antineoplastic agent, followed by two oral doses, each at the equivalent of 40% of the antineoplastic agent. Oral doses of mesna should be administered at two and six hours after each dose of cyclophosphamide (Schuchter et al., 2002).

iv. Mesna administration

- Mesna equivalent of 40% of the total daily cyclophosphamide dose given as IV bolus before cyclophosphamide
- Mesna equivalent of 40% of the total daily cyclophosphamide dose given as IV bolus 3, 6, 9, and 12 hours after the start of the cyclophosphamide infusion
- Mesna can be given by mouth, taking into consideration that its bioavailability and half-life is approximately 50% of those observed after IV infusion (Jeelani et al., 2017).
- Dexamethasone is also used as an adjunct to mesna to effectively prevent hemorrhagic cystitis (Matz & Hsieh, 2017).
- In the setting of patients receiving cyclophosphamide for HSCT, mesna plus saline diuresis is recommended to prevent hemorrhagic cystitis (Matz & Hsieh, 2017).

(c) Hyperbaric oxygen therapy may be used, as it causes vasoconstriction, enhances angiogenesis and granulation tissue formation, and optimizes immune function at the cellular level (Haldar et al., 2014).

(d) Surgical interventions

i. Cystoscopy and fulguration using high-frequency electrocautery; energy channeled using either electrocautery or laser

ii. Intravesical formalin instillation using a large-bore catheter and cystogram under general anesthesia (Ziegelmann et al., 2017)

iii. Cystectomy with urinary diversion (Au et al., 2017)

(4) Care coordination: Coordinate care with social work services, case management, home health, and pharmacy for patients undergoing hemorrhagic cystitis treatment.

f) Patient and family education

(1) Educate patients and caregivers about the importance of actively participating in the prevention and management of hemorrhagic cystitis.

(2) Explain the importance of oral hydration, if not contraindicated, to stimulate frequent voiding while receiving oncologic treatments. Pollakiuria, or frequent voiding, minimizes the time that acrolein and microorganisms are in the bladder.

(3) Teach patients and families neutropenic precautions to avoid new and recurrent infections during the recovery state that may exacerbate hemorrhagic cystitis.

(4) Educate about the importance of assessing the urine and symptoms associated with hemorrhagic cystitis (e.g., pink and dark color, burning sensation while voiding, difficulty voiding, lack of sensation to urinate, frequency, lower abdomen pain).

(5) Explain to patients and caregivers the process of continuous bladder irrigation and symptom management (D.L. Thompson, 2017; Wilkinson et al., 2015).

C. Drug-specific considerations

1. Chemotherapy

a) Cisplatin: Cisplatin is a platinum-based antineoplastic agent used in many different malignancies. Nephrotoxicity is the primary dose-limiting toxicity, and thus treating with cisplatin-based regimens necessitates careful evaluation, prevention, and management of associated nephrotoxicity (Crona et al., 2017). Cisplatin can also cause salt wasting, magnesium wasting, SIADH, and hypokalemia, which can lead to nephrotoxicity (Almanric et al., 2017).

(1) Incidence: See Table 19-1.

(2) Risk factors (Almanric et al., 2017)

(a) Pharmacologic agents

i. Chemotherapy: Previous cisplatin exposure

ii. Other agents: Angiotensin-converting enzyme inhibitors, angiotensin receptor blockers, and hydrochlorothiazide

(b) Preexisting conditions: Hypertension, arteriosclerotic heart disease, myocardial infarction, coronary artery bypass surgery, type 2 diabetes

(c) Patient characteristics: Hypomagnesemia, hypokalemia

(3) Clinical manifestations

(a) Hypertension

(b) Electrolyte disturbances

(c) Edema

(4) Assessment: Assess CrCl using the Cockcroft-Gault formula prior to administration of cisplatin.

(5) Collaborative management

(a) Hydration: Patients should receive 2–4 L of normal saline over two to six hours with cisplatin administration (Crona et al., 2017).

(b) Mannitol: Reduces concentration of cisplatin in the kidneys; some studies suggest it should only be used for high-dose cisplatin (100 mg/m^2) or with preexisting hypertension (Crona et al., 2017).

(c) Monitoring: Electrolytes, specifically magnesium and potassium; add to IV hydration accordingly.

b) Methotrexate: Methotrexate is an antimetabolite chemotherapy drug that disrupts folic acid metabolism and is used for a range of different malignances. AKI is a well-documented toxicity, and methotrexate, like cisplatin, requires close monitoring and prompt intervention to avoid kidney damage (Howard et al., 2016). Nephrotoxicity occurs through crystal nephropathy, which is a result of methotrexate and its metabolites forming precipitate within the renal tubules. Crystal-induced nephropathy initially might cause an elevation in serum creatinine and then progress to tubular necrosis (Howard et al., 2016).

(1) Incidence: See Table 19-1.

(2) Risk factors

(a) Pharmacologic agents

i. Chemotherapy: High-dose methotrexate dosing (i.e., greater than 500 mg/m^2)

ii. Other agents: Concurrent use of drugs that impair methotrexate clearance, such as NSAIDs, penicillin, salicylates, probenecid, gemfibrozil, trimethoprim-sulfamethoxazole, proton pump inhibitors, levetiracetam, amphotericin, aminoglycosides, radiographic contrast dyes

(b) Preexisting conditions: History of nephrotoxicity with previous methotrexate therapy

(c) Cancer types: Lymphomas

(d) Patient characteristics: Volume depletion

(3) Clinical manifestations

(a) Edema

(b) Electrolyte disturbances

(c) Hypertension

(4) Assessment

(a) Laboratory assessment

i. Monitor blood urea nitrogen and creatinine.

ii. Monitor urine pH and maintain above 7.

(b) Physical assessment

i. Assess for signs and symptoms of fluid overload.

ii. Perform strict intake and output monitoring.

(5) Collaborative management (Howard et al., 2016)

(a) Discontinue medications that interfere with methotrexate elimination.

(b) Hydration: Administer prehydration with IV fluids containing bicarbonate at a rate of 150–200 ml/hr for a total of 2 L prior to high-dose methotrexate administration.

(c) Perform strict monitoring of intake and output during and after high-dose methotrexate infusion.

(d) Urine alkalinization: Because methotrexate and its metabolites are poorly soluble in an acidic pH, using sodium bicarbonate for hydration increases urine pH to 7 and thus increases the solubility of methotrexate, minimizing the risk of intratubular crystal formation (Howard et al., 2016).

(e) Monitor plasma methotrexate levels closely and adjust leucovorin dosing accordingly.

(f) Glucarpidase is the antidote for methotrexate, indicated only for toxic methotrexate plasma concentrations greater than 1 mcmol/L in patients with delayed clearance due to renal impairment (Wolters Kluwer Health, 2017).

2. Immunotherapy

a) Immune checkpoint inhibitors, first approved for use in melanoma, have quickly emerged in a number of different neoplasms. They work by enhancing tumor-directed immune response by targeting inhibitory receptors seen on T cells and other tumor cells (Cortazar et al., 2016). The toxicities associated with immunotherapy agents are immune-related events with the most common being dermatitis, colitis, hepatitis, pneumonitis, and hypophysitis, with minimal effects to the kidneys. However, a small number of case reports cite immune-related nephritis, with ipilimumab, a cytotoxic T-lymphocyte antigen 4 inhibitor, as the most common offender (Izzedine et al., 2014). Although no standard of care exists for immune-related nephritis, as with other immune-related toxicities, it is typically managed with steroids (Cortazar et al., 2016; Izzedine et al., 2014; Thajudeen, Madhrira, Bracamonte, & Cranmer, 2015).

b) Management: Once immune-related etiology is confirmed, usually via biopsy, patients are treated with prednisone or equivalent, at a dose of 1 mg/kg (Izzedine et al., 2014). Immune-mediated toxicity may require temporary or permanent discontinuation of the offending agent.

c) Patient and family education
(1) Educate patients and families regarding the risks of nephrotoxicity with the specific antineoplastic/cytotoxic regimens.
(2) Provide patients with a list of warning signs and symptoms that necessitate contacting their provider.
(3) Educate patients and families regarding the need for extra oral hydration while receiving nephrotoxic therapies.
(4) Provide patients with a list of drugs to avoid to decrease the risk of nephrotoxicity.

References

Aapro, M., & Launay-Vacher, V. (2012). Importance of monitoring renal function in patients with cancer. *Cancer Treatment Reviews, 38,* 235–240. https://doi.org/10.1016/j.ctrv.2011.05.001

Almanric, K., Marceau, N., Cantin, A., & Bertin, É. (2017). Risk factors for nephrotoxicity associated with cisplatin. *Canadian Journal of Hospital Pharmacy, 70,* 99–106. https://doi.org/10.4212/cjhp.v70i2.1641

Arellano, J., Hernandez, R.K., Wade, S.W., Chen, K., Pirolli, M., Quach, D., … Shahinian, V.B. (2015). Prevalence of renal impairment and use of nephrotoxic agents among patients with bone metastases from solid tumors in the United States. *Cancer Medicine, 4,* 713–720. https://doi.org/10.1002/cam4.403

Au, J.K., Graziano, C., Elizondo, R.A., Ryan, S., Roth, D.R., Koh, C.J., … Seth, A. (2017). Urologic outcomes of children with hemorrhagic cystitis after bone marrow transplant at a single institution. *Urology, 101,* 126–132. https://doi.org/10.1016/j.urology.2016.10.030

Burst, V., Grundmann, F., Kubacki, T., Greenberg, A., Rudolf, D., Salahudeen, A., … Grohé, C. (2017). Euvolemic hyponatremia in cancer patients. Report of the Hyponatremia Registry: An observational multicenter international study. *Supportive Care in Cancer, 25,* 2275–2283. https://doi.org/10.1007/s00520-017-3638-3

Cairo, M.S., & Bishop, M. (2004). Tumour lysis syndrome: New therapeutic strategies and classification. *British Journal of Haematology, 127,* 3–11. https://doi.org/10.1111/j.1365-2141.2004.05094.x

Cairo, M.S., Coiffier, B., Reiter, A., & Younes, A. (2010). Recommendations for the evaluation of risk and prophylaxis of tumour lysis syndrome (TLS) in adults and children with malignant diseases: An expert TLS panel consensus. *British Journal of Haematology, 149,* 578–586. https://doi.org/10.1111/j.1365-2141.2010.08143.x

Çetinel, B. (2015). Chemotherapy and pelvic radiotherapy-induced bladder injury. *Urologia Journal, 82*(Suppl. 3), S2–S5. https://doi.org/10.5301/uro.5000144

Choueiri, T.K., Halabi, S., Sanford, B.L., Hahn, O., Michaelson, M.D., Walsh, M.K., … Morris, M.J. (2017). Cabozantinib versus sunitinib as initial targeted therapy for patients with metastatic renal cell carcinoma of poor or intermediate risk: The Alliance A031203 CABOSUN Trial. *Journal of Clinical Oncology, 35,* 591–597. https://doi.org/10.1200/JCO.2016.70.7398

Cockcroft, D.W., & Gault, M.H. (1976). Prediction of creatinine clearance from serum creatinine. *Nephron, 16,* 31–41. https://doi.org/10.1159/000180580

Coiffier, B., Altman, A., Pui, C.-H., Younes, A., & Cairo, M.S. (2008). Guidelines for the management of pediatric and adult tumor lysis syndrome: An evidence-based review. *Journal of Clinical Oncology, 26,* 2767–2778. https://doi.org/10.1200/JCO.2007.15.0177

Cortazar, F.B., Marrone, K.A., Troxell, M.L., Ralto, K.M., Hoenig, M.P., Brahmer, J.R., … Leaf, D.E. (2016). Clinicopathological features of acute kidney injury associated with immune checkpoint inhibitors. *Kidney International, 90,* 638–647. https://doi.org/10.1016/j.kint.2016.04.008

Crona, D.J., Faso, A., Nishijima, T.F., McGraw, K.A., Galsky, M.D., & Milowsky, M.I. (2017). A systematic review of strategies to prevent cisplatin-induced nephrotoxicity. *Oncologist, 22,* 609–619. https://doi.org/10.1634/theoncologist.2016-0319

Dimitriadis, G.K., Angelousi, A., Weickert, M.O., Randeva, H.S., Kaltsas, G., & Grossman, A. (2017). Paraneoplastic endocrine syndromes. *Endocrine-Related Cancer, 24,* R173–R190. https://doi.org/10.1530/ERC-17-0036

Dosin, G., Aoun, F., El Rassy, E., Assi, T., Lewalle, P., Blanc, J., … Bron, D. (2017). Viral-induced hemorrhagic cystitis after allogeneic hematopoietic stem cell transplant. *Clinical Lymphoma, Myeloma and Leukemia, 17,* 438–442. https://doi.org/10.1016/j.clml.2017.05.013

Forman, J.P. (2017). Patient education: Acute kidney injury (The basics). In *UpToDate.* Retrieved April 19, 2018, from https://www.uptodate.com

Fu, H., Xu, L., Liu, D., Zhang, X., Liu, K., Chen, H., … Huang, X. (2013). Late-onset hemorrhagic cystitis after haploidentical hematopoietic stem cell transplantation in patients with advanced leukemia: Differences in ATG dosage are key. *International Journal of Hematology, 98,* 89–95. https://doi.org/10.1007/s12185-013-1350-8

Goltzman, D. (2017). Clinical manifestations of hypocalcemia. In J.E. Mulder (Ed.), *UpToDate.* Retrieved April 19, 2018, from https://www.uptodate.com/contents/clinical-manifestations-of-hypocalcemia

Gonella, S., di Pasquale, T., & Palese, A. (2015). Preventive measures for cyclophosphamide-related hemorrhagic cystitis in blood and bone marrow transplantation: An Italian multicenter retrospective study [Online exclusive]. *Clinical Journal of Oncology Nursing, 19,* E8–E14. https://doi.org/10.1188/15.CJON.E8-E14

Graham, L.A. (2017). Infection prevention and control. In P.A. Potter, A.G. Perry, P.A. Stockert, & A.M. Hall (Eds.), *Fundamentals of nursing* (9th ed., pp. 442–485). St. Louis, MO: Elsevier.

Gralla, R.J., Ahmad, F., Blais, J.D., Chiodo, J., III, Zhou, W., Glaser, L.A., & Czerwiec, F.S. (2017). Tolvaptan use in cancer patients with hyponatremia due to the syndrome of inappropriate antidiuretic hormone: A post hoc analysis of the SALT-1 and SALT-2 trials. *Cancer Medicine, 6,* 723–729. https://doi.org/10.1002/cam4.805

Haldar, S., Dru, C., & Bhowmick, N.A. (2014). Mechanisms of hemorrhagic cystitis. *American Journal of Clinical and Experimental Urology, 2,* 199–208.

Howard, S.C., McCormick, J., Pui, C.-H., Buddington, R.K., & Harvey, R.D. (2016). Preventing and managing toxicities of high-dose methotrexate. *Oncologist, 21,* 1471–1482. https://doi.org/10.1634/theoncologist.2015-0164

Izzedine, H., Gueutin, V., Gharbi, C., Mateus, C., Robert, C., Routier, E., … Rouvier, P. (2014). Kidney injuries related to ipilimumab. *Investigational New Drugs, 32,* 769–773. https://doi.org/10.1007/s10637-014-0092-7

Jeelani, R., Jahanbakhsh, S., Kohan-Ghadr, H.-R., Thakur, M., Khan, S., Aldhaheri, S.R., … Abu-Soud, H.M. (2017). Mesna

(2-mercaptoethane sodium sulfonate) functions as a regulator of myeloperoxidase. *Free Radical Biology and Medicine, 110,* 54–62. https://doi.org/10.1016/j.freeradbiomed.2017.05.019

Johnston, D., Schurtz, E., Tourville, E., Jones, T., Boemer, A., & Giel, D. (2015). Risk factors associated with severity and outcomes in pediatric patients with hemorrhagic cystitis. *Journal of Urology, 195,* 1312–1317. https://doi.org/10.1016/j.juro.2015.11.035

Kaplan, J.R., & Wolf, J.S., Jr. (2009). Efficacy and survival associated with cystoscopy and clot evaluation for radiation or cyclophosphamide induced hemorrhagic cystitis. *Journal of Urology, 181,* 641–646. https://doi.org/10.1016/j.juro.2008.10.037

Kaplow, R., & Iyere, K. (2016). Recognizing and preventing tumor lysis syndrome. *Nursing, 46*(11), 26–32. https://doi.org/10.1097/01.NURSE.0000502751.87828.2d

Klein, J., Kuperman, M., Haley, C., Barri, Y., Chandrakantan, A., Fischbach, B., … Rajagopal, B. (2015). Late presentation of adenovirus-induced hemorrhagic cystitis and ureteral obstruction in a kidney-pancreas transplant recipient. *Baylor University Medical Center Proceedings, 28,* 488–491. https://doi.org/10.1080/08998280.2015.11929318

Lam, W., Storek, J., Li, H., Geddes, M., & Daly, A. (2017). Incidence and risk factor of hemorrhagic cystitis after allogeneic transplantation with fludarabine, busulfan, and anti-thymocyte globulin myeloablative conditioning. *Transplant Infectious Disease, 19,* e12677. https://doi.org/10.1111/tid.12677

Lameire, N., Vanholder, R., Van Biesen, W., & Benoit, D. (2016). Acute kidney injury in critically ill cancer patients: An update. *Critical Care, 20,* 209. https://doi.org/10.1186/s13054-016-1382-6

Lunde, L.E., Dasaraju, S., Cao, Q., Cohn, C.S., Reding, M., Bejanyan, N., … Ustun, C. (2015). Hemorrhagic cystitis after allogeneic hematopoietic cell transplantation: Risk factors, graft source, and survival. *Bone Marrow Transplantation, 50,* 1432–1437. http://doi.org/10.1038/bmt.2015.162

Manikandan, R., Kumar, S., & Dorairanjan, L.N. (2010). Hemorrhagic cystitis: A challenge to the urologist. *Indian Journal of Urology, 26,* 159–166. https://doi.org/10.4103/0970-1591.65380

Matz, E.L., & Hsieh, M.H. (2017). Review of advances in uroprotective agents for cyclophosphamide- and ifosfamide-induced hemorrhagic cystitis. *Urology, 100,* 16–19. https://doi.org/10.1016/j.urology.2016.07.030

McManus, M.S., & Wynter-Minott, S. (2017). Guidelines for chronic kidney disease: Defining, staging, and managing in primary care. *Journal for Nurse Practitioners, 13,* 400–410. https://doi.org/10.1016/j.nurpra.2017.04.017

Peri, A., Grohé, C., Berardi, R., & Runkle, I. (2017). SIADH: Differential diagnosis and clinical management. *Endocrine, 55,* 311–319. https://doi.org/10.1007/s12020-016-0936-3

Perlman, R.L., Heung, M., & Ix, J.H. (2013). Renal disease. In G.D. Hammer & S.J. McPhee (Eds.), *Pathophysiology of disease: An introduction to clinical medicine* (7th ed., pp. 455–482). New York, NY: McGraw-Hill Education.

Ruggeri, A., Roth-Guepin, G., Battipaglia, G., Mamez, A.-C., Malard, F., Gomez, A., … Mohty, M. (2015). Incidence and risk factors for hemorrhagic cystitis in unmanipulated haploidentical transplant recipients. *Transplant Infectious Disease, 17,* 822–830. https://doi.org/10.1111/tid.12455

Scadden, D.T., & Raaijmakers, M.H.G.P. (2017). Overview of stem cells. In J.S. Tirnauer (Ed.), *UpToDate.* Retrieved April 24, 2018, from https://www.uptodate.com/contents/overview-of-stem-cells

Schneidewind, L., Neumann, T., Kranz, J., Knoll, F., Pelzer, A.E., Schmidt, C., & Krüger, W. (2017). Nationwide survey of BK polyomavirus associated hemorrhagic cystitis in adult allogeneic stem cell transplantation among haematologists and urologists. *Annals of Hematology, 96,* 797–803. https://doi.org/10.1007/s00277-017-2935-8

Schuchter, L.M., Hensley, M.L., Meropol, N.J., & Winer, E.P. (2002). 2002 update of recommendations for the use of chemotherapy and radiotherapy protectants: Clinical practice guidelines of the American Society of Clinical Oncology. *Journal of Clinical Oncology, 20,* 2895–2903. https://doi.org/10.1200/JCO.2002.04.178

Shahinian, V.B., Bahl, A., Niepel, D., & Lorusso, V. (2017). Considering renal risk while managing cancer. *Cancer Management and Research, 9,* 167–178. https://doi.org/10.2147/CMAR.S125864

Shaikh, S.A., Marini, B.L., Hough, S.M., & Perissinotti, A.J. (2018). Rational use of rasburicase for the treatment and management of tumor lysis syndrome. *Journal of Oncology Pharmacy Practice, 24,* 176–184. https://doi.org/10.1177/1078155216687152

Spasovski, G., Vanholder, R., Allolio, B., Annane, D., Ball, S., Bichet, D., … Nagler, E. (2014). Clinical practice guideline on diagnosis and treatment of hyponatraemia. *Intensive Care Medicine, 40,* 320–331. https://doi.org/10.1007/s00134-014-3210-2

Sterns, R.H. (2017). Pathophysiology and etiology of the syndrome of inappropriate antidiuretic hormone secretion (SIADH). In J.P. Forman (Ed.), *UpToDate.* Retrieved April 19, 2018, from https://www.uptodate.com/contents/pathophysiology-and-etiology-of-the-syndrome-of-inappropriate-antidiuretic-hormone-secretion-siadh

Thajudeen, B., Madhrira, M., Bracamonte, E., & Cranmer, L.D. (2015). Ipilimumab granulomatous interstitial nephritis. *American Journal of Therapeutics, 22,* e84–e87. https://doi.org/10.1097/MJT.0b013e3182a32ddc

Thompson, A., Adamson, A., Bahl, A., Borwell, J., Dodds, D., Heath, C., … Payne, H. (2014). Guidelines for the diagnosis and management of chemical- and radiation-induced cystitis. *Journal of Clinical Urology, 7,* 25–35. https://doi.org/10.1177/2051415813512647

Thompson, D.L. (2017). Urinary elimination. In P.A. Potter, A.G. Perry, P.A. Stockert, & A.M. Hall (Eds.), *Fundamentals of nursing* (9th ed., pp. 1101–1148). St. Louis, MO: Elsevier.

Vazquez, A. (2017). Hypophysitis: Nursing management of immune-related adverse events. *Clinical Journal of Oncology Nursing, 21,* 154–156. https://doi.org/10.1188/17.CJON.154-156

Wang, L., Ji, X., Sun, G.-F., Qin, Y.-C., Gong, M.-Z., Zhang, J.-X., … Na, Y.-Q. (2015). Fungus ball and emphysematous cystitis secondary to Candida tropicalis: A case report. *Canadian Urological Association Journal, 9,* E683–E686. https://doi.org/10.5489/cuaj.3008

Weeks, A.C., & Kimple, M.E. (2015). Spontaneous tumor lysis syndrome: A case report and critical evaluation of current diagnostic criteria and optimal treatment regimens. *Journal of Investigative Medicine—High Impact Case Reports, 3.* https://doi.org/10.1177/2324709615603199

Wilkinson, J.M., Treas, L.S., Barnett, K.L., & Smith, M.H. (2015). *Fundamentals of nursing* (3rd ed.). Philadelphia, PA: F.A. Davis.

Wolters Kluwer Health. (2017). Lexicomp Online. Retrieved from https://online.lexi.com

Zhang, Y., Kawedia, J.D., Myers, A.L., McIntyre, C.M., Anderson, P.M., Kramer, M.A., & Culotta, K.S. (2013). Physical and chemical stability of high-dose ifosfamide and mesna for prolonged 14-day continuous infusion. *Journal of Oncology Pharmacy Practice, 20,* 51–57. https://doi.org/10.1177/1078155213478284

Ziegelmann, M.J., Boorjian, S.A., Joyce, D.D., Montgomery, B.D., & Linder, B.J. (2017). Intravesical formalin for hemorrhagic cystitis: A contemporary cohort. *Canadian Urological Association Journal, 11,* E79–E82. https://doi.org/10.5489/cuaj.4047

CHAPTER 20

Altered Sexual and Reproductive Functioning

A. Alterations in sexual functioning
   1. Overview: Sexuality is both a high priority and an unmet need for cancer survivors. Sexual dysfunction after cancer has consistently been reported and associated with poor quality of life among survivors (Sears, Robinson, & Walker, 2018). Sexuality, and therefore sexual toxicities, are a concern for individuals across the age spectrum, although most notably are reported among individuals younger than age 65 or those who reported being sexually active at the time of cancer diagnosis (Schover et al., 2014). Studies suggest that despite advances in knowledge about how cancer treatment affects both sexuality and fertility, many individuals with cancer are not informed about these changes, resulting in unmet educational needs about potential options to restore sexual function (Schover et al., 2014). Further, interventions are primarily focused on individuals with cancers affecting sexual or reproductive organs (Ussher, Perz, Gilbert, & Australian Cancer and Sexuality Study Team, 2015). Approximately 20% of men with treatment-related problems ever consult with a healthcare provider about them (Schover, 2016), and women tend to be asked about this less than men (Ben Charif et al., 2016).
   2. Pathophysiology: Sexual dysfunction resulting from cancer treatment often is linked to nerve and blood vessel damage, as well as alterations in hormones associated with sexual function (Schover et al., 2014).
      a) Women
         (1) Premature ovarian failure resulting in loss of ovarian androgen and precursor sex hormones (estrogen, progesterone, and testosterone) (Bennett et al., 2016)
         (2) Neurotoxic chemotherapy hypothesized to damage genital sensory neurons (Marchand & Bradford, 2017)
         (3) Estrogen deprivation resulting from hormonal manipulation (Bennett et al., 2016)
      b) Men
         (1) Alterations in testosterone levels
         (2) Chemotherapy that may be neurotoxic to erectile nerves and impact on penile blood supply causing erectile problems (Voznesensky, Annam, & Kreder, 2016)
         (3) Pathophysiologically, erectile dysfunction is classified as vascular, neurogenic, endocrinologic, or psychogenic (Costabile, 2000; Dean & Lue, 2005).
            (a) Vascular: Associated with alterations in penile blood flow or damage to the pudendal or penile arteries
               i. Veno-occlusive dysfunction also may occur, in which there is a failure of passive venous outflow obstructive mechanism, resulting in the inability of sinusoids to trap blood.
               ii. Pelvic irradiation is a major cause, with erectile dysfunction occurring in 90% of patients receiving this treatment, likely due to arterial sclerosis (Costabile, 2000).
            (b) Neurogenic: Associated with any disease or dysfunction involving the brain, spinal cord, or cavernous and pudendal nerves. Causes can include surgical (iatrogenic) damage and tumor impingement.
            (c) Endocrinologic: Of or related to altered androgen (testosterone) levels. Testosterone enhances sexual interest, increases frequency of sexual acts, contributes to the

development of secondary sex characteristics and sperm, and influences secretion of fluid from the prostate gland, seminal vesicles, and Cowper glands (Dean & Lue, 2005).

i. Testosterone production can be influenced by tumor growth or treatment contributing to hypogonadotropic hypogonadism.
ii. Treatment-related hyperprolactinemia may suppress the production of testosterone.
iii. Pure hormonal-driven erectile dysfunction is rare.

(d) Psychogenic

i. May result from anxiety, fatigue, or depression that often manifests as lack of interest in sexual activity or decline in arousability
ii. May be partner, performance, or mood related

3. Incidence: Sexual dysfunction affects at least 50% of individuals (both men and women) treated for pelvic malignancies and more than 25% of individuals with other types of cancer (Schover et al., 2014). As more than 60% of all cancer survivors in the United States have been treated for pelvic or breast tumors, sexual toxicities are a potential concern for a significant population of individuals in cancer survivorship (American Cancer Society, 2016; Miller et al., 2016). Up to 33% of childhood cancer survivors experience sexual problems, with women reporting sexual dysfunction at twice the rate of men (Bober et al., 2013). The probability of sexual dysfunction increases over time for young adults (Acquati et al., 2018).

a) In men with cancer, 30.9% are dissatisfied with sexual functioning (compared to 19.8% of healthy controls), and in women with cancer, 18.2% are dissatisfied, compared to 11.8% of healthy controls (Jackson, Wardle, Steptoe, & Fisher, 2016).

b) Women: Incidence is 30%–100% across female survivors of diverse cancer types (Dizon, Suzin, & McIlvenna, 2014).

(1) Desire: Decrease in desire occurs in 31%–56%, although this may be underreported (Rellini, Farmer, & Golden, 2011).

(2) Dyspareunia: Among women with breast cancer, 56.5% of women being treated with aromatase inhibitors and 31.3% of those being treated with tamoxifen reported dyspareunia (Baumgart, Nilsson, Evers, Kallak, & Poromaa, 2013).

(3) Vaginal stenosis/obstruction: Incidence is 1.2%–88% and is primarily linked to radiation therapy, but it also may result from graft-versus-host disease following hematopoietic stem cell transplantation, with an incidence of 3%–15% (Falk & Dizon, 2013).

(4) Among young adult breast cancer survivors, 52% report sexual dysfunction (Acquati et al., 2018).

c) Men

(1) Erectile dysfunction

(a) Following radical prostatectomy, 81% of men reported erectile dysfunction two years after surgery (Dadhich, Hockenberry, Kirby, & Lipshultz, 2017).

(b) Rates of erectile dysfunction in long-term survivorship (more than 10 years) were 84%–95% (Resnick et al., 2013; Schover et al., 2014; Taylor et al., 2012).

(c) Less than 25% of men retain or recover former erection quality (Ussher et al., 2015).

(2) Genital shrinkage as a result of loss of erections is reported in half of men after radical prostatectomy (Carlsson et al., 2012).

(3) Loss of desire and ejaculation: Among testicular cancer survivors, 11% report loss of desire, and 51% report ejaculation problems (Acquati et al., 2018).

4. Risk factors

a) General (DeSimone et al., 2014)

(1) Individuals with cancer with other chronic illness states, specifically hypertension, endocrine disorders (both hypo- and hyperthyroidism), fatigue, and depression, are at an increased risk for sexual dysfunction.

(a) Diuretics and beta-blockers are associated with decreased libido and orgasm.

(b) Similarly, selective serotonin reuptake inhibitors may inhibit sexual desire, arousal, and orgasm.

(2) Among young adults, those who were female, older, married or in a committed relationship, or treated with che-

motherapy and those who reported comorbid psychological distress and lower social support had a higher probability of reporting sexual dysfunction (Acquati et al., 2018).

(3) Anticancer agents affecting sexual health: All of the following agents are used in various combinations; thus, the side effects may be cumulative.

(a) Alkylating agents (e.g., busulfan, cyclophosphamide, ifosfamide, nitrogen mustard) cause nausea and vomiting, which significantly decrease desire (Pinto, 2013).

(b) Antimetabolites (e.g., cladribine, cytarabine, hydroxyurea, methotrexate) cause general malaise, mucositis, nausea, and vomiting (Pinto, 2013).

(c) Antitumor antibiotics (e.g., daunorubicin, doxorubicin, mitoxantrone) cause nausea, vomiting, and mucositis (Pinto, 2013).

(d) Plant alkaloids (e.g., vincristine) cause peripheral neuropathy, which may affect sensation in the hands and fingers.

(e) Immunotherapy agents: Many of these agents cause fatigue, flu-like symptoms, and changes to body image (Krebs, 2012).

(f) Targeted therapy agents: No evidence exists regarding direct sexual effects, but these agents cause fatigue, diarrhea, and rash with the potential to affect body image (Krebs, 2012).

b) Women

(1) Premature ovarian failure resulting from cancer treatment (Ford et al., 2014)

(a) Risk for sexual dysfunction increases among women with permanent ovarian failure.

(b) Risk for permanent ovarian failure increases with age, particularly in women older than age 35.

(2) Anticancer therapies

(a) Chemotherapy

i. Alkylating agents and higher cumulative doses of chemotherapy contribute to sexual dysfunction.

ii. Chemotherapy can cause hair loss, nausea, and vomiting that decrease sexual desire and frequency (Dizon et al., 2014).

iii. Agents also can cause direct toxicity to the pelvis and vagina (Dizon et al., 2014).

(b) Hormone therapy (see Chapter 7)

i. Aromatase inhibitors: Risk to sexual health is believed to be higher than that of estrogen receptor modulators (Dizon et al., 2014).

ii. Estrogen receptor modulators: Tamoxifen may cause venous congestion and a resulting lack of vaginal lubrication, although a causal relationship has not yet been demonstrated in the literature (DeSimone et al., 2014).

(c) Pelvic or anal irradiation

(d) Bilateral oophorectomy (for cancer treatment or prevention)

(e) Use of gonadotropin agonists or antagonists (however, sexual dysfunction may resolve when hormonal agents are discontinued)

(3) Systemic graft-versus-host disease, which can potentially make vaginal intercourse impossible because of severe tissue damage to the vulva and vagina

(4) Subjectively, women report that tiredness, general pain, body and appearance changes, and feelings of unattractiveness contribute to changes in sexual frequency and activities (DeSimone et al., 2014; Ussher et al., 2015).

c) Men (Schover et al., 2014)

(1) Disease factors

(a) History of prostate cancer, including men on active surveillance

(b) Hypogonadism

(2) Treatment factors

(a) Surgery for bladder or rectal cancer

(b) Chemotherapy plus radiation therapy for anal cancer

(c) Prostatectomy (both radical and nerve sparing)

(d) Damage to pelvic nerves

(e) Pelvic or total body irradiation

(3) Multimodality treatment (chemotherapy with radiation therapy) is more

likely to cause sexual problems (Capogrosso et al., 2016).

(4) Subjectively, men report that erectile dysfunction, surgery, and aging were the primary causes of changes in their sexual functioning (Ussher et al., 2015).

5. Clinical manifestations: Sexual dysfunction often is associated with fatigue, nausea, or incontinence and can result in discontinuation of sexual activity. Sexual dysfunction also may result in psychosocial sequelae, including depression, anxiety, relationship conflict, and loss of self-esteem (Schover et al., 2014).
   a) General: Both men and women report decreases in sexual frequency and satisfaction, as well as changes in sexual behaviors with decreased sexual engagement with partners after cancer (Ussher et al., 2015).
   b) Women (Marchand & Bradford, 2017; Schover et al., 2014)
      (1) Most common manifestations
         (a) Dyspareunia (painful intercourse)
         (b) Vaginal dryness
         (c) Low sexual desire
      (2) Effects may also include difficulty with sexual self-image, arousal, feeling pleasure, or achieving orgasm during sexual activity. Hair loss due to chemotherapy can contribute to negative body image, which in turn affects sexual functioning.
      (3) Chemotherapy-induced menopause: Symptoms of chemically induced menopause are dramatic and may be worse for women who are premenopausal when diagnosed. Symptoms include the following (Farthmann et al., 2016):
         (a) Menstrual cycle changes with eventual cessation
         (b) Hot flashes, insomnia
         (c) Vaginal or vulvar dryness
         (d) Dyspareunia
         (e) Weight gain
   c) Men (Nelson, Scardino, Eastham, & Mulhall, 2013; Ussher et al., 2015)
      (1) Most common manifestations are loss of desire and erectile dysfunction.
      (2) Additional possible manifestations
         (a) Diminished genital size
         (b) Changes in quality of and ability to achieve orgasm, pain associated with orgasm
         (c) Absence of sexual dreams or fantasies
         (d) Feminization as a result of androgen deprivation

6. Collaborative management: Management of treatment-related sexual dysfunction should involve an interprofessional approach, consisting of both medical and psychosocial treatment options (Schover et al., 2014). This is important because sexual dysfunction emerges from physiologic changes related to cancer and its treatment and from the psychological sequelae of cancer, which can include negative body image and depression.
   a) General recommendations (Schover et al., 2014)
      (1) Address sexual needs early in cancer treatment rather than trying to address sexual dysfunction after it has progressed.
      (2) Obtain a prior history of sexual experience, including the cultural and religious attitudes and beliefs that may influence them (DeSimone et al., 2014).
      (3) Focus on communication between patient and partner.
      (4) Emphasize that sexual pleasure and intimacy can be found beyond penetrative intercourse.
      (5) Identify coping mechanisms for the limitations of sex after cancer.
      (6) Educate patients on the need for barrier protection (Kelvin, Steed, & Jarrett, 2014).
         (a) Patients are usually advised to use a barrier (condom or dental dam) for penetrative intercourse and oral sex to protect their partner from exposure to metabolites of chemotherapy.
         (b) Barrier protection should be used on the day of and for a week after chemotherapy administration.
   b) Women (Barbera et al., 2017)
      (1) Assessment: In addition to physical examination, psychosocial assessment should focus on changes in spontaneous versus receptive sexual desire, barriers to sexual activity (e.g., pain), changes in relationship adjustment (if applicable), and assessment of risk factors (Marchand & Bradford, 2017). Validated instruments include the following (Marchand & Bradford, 2017):
         (a) Female Sexual Function Index (Rosen et al., 2000)

(b) Sexual Activity Questionnaire (Thirlaway, Fallowfield, & Cuzick, 1996)

(c) Menopausal Sexual Interest Questionnaire (Rosen, Lobo, Block, Yang, & Zipfel, 2004)

(d) Patient-Reported Outcomes Measurement Information System Sexual Function and Satisfaction Measure (PROMIS SexFS) (Flynn et al., 2013)

(2) Psychosocial counseling is recommended to improve desire, arousal, orgasm, intimacy in relationships, and body image. Couple-based interventions have demonstrated efficacy in improving sexual functioning among individuals with partners.

(3) Sex therapy: Distinct from psychosocial counseling, sex therapy may use a multimodal approach (e.g., education, communication, sensate focus, mindfulness) to enhance sexual desire (Marchand & Bradford, 2017).

(4) Physical interventions

(a) Regular stimulation (e.g., masturbation) can also help to improve sexual response.

(b) Physical exercise and/or pelvic floor exercises can be helpful.

(5) First-line choice for managing menopausal symptoms should be nonhormonal.

(a) Four nonhormonal treatments appear to be beneficial management of vasomotor symptoms (Drewe, Bucher, & Zahner, 2015).

i. Gabapentin/pregabalin

ii. Selective serotonin reuptake inhibitors

- Fluoxetine (Prozac®) and paroxetine (Paxil®) have been shown to increase the risk of recurrence of breast cancer in women taking tamoxifen (Drewe et al., 2015).
- Tamoxifen competes for the same metabolic pathway as paroxetine and fluoxetine; therefore, those agents should not be used in women receiving tamoxifen therapy for breast cancer.

iii. Venlafaxine/desvenlafaxine

iv. Black cohosh: A phytopharmaceutical agent derived from a flowering perennial plant that has been shown to have mixed efficacy on menopausal symptoms, including hot flashes.

- As with all herbal supplements, use of black cohosh should be reviewed with a provider, as it may influence the metabolism and efficacy of various medications.
- Mixed evidence exists that suggests potential for inhibition of the drug-metabolizing enzyme CYP3A4, as well as potentiating effects when used in combination with tamoxifen, 5-fluorouracil, paclitaxel, doxorubicin, and docetaxel in patients with breast cancer (Antoine, Liebens, Carly, Pastijn, & Rozenberg, 2007).

(6) Hormone therapies: The decision to use hormonal treatment in women with hormone-dependent cancer should be made in conjunction with oncologist and detailed discussion with the patient (American Cancer Society, 2016).

(a) Local estrogen therapy for vaginal atrophy

i. The use of vaginal estrogen creams, pessaries, or rings can significantly reduce vulvovaginal dryness (Pfeiler et al., 2011). Estriol is the preferred form of local estrogen (Lammerink, de Bock, Schröder, & Mourits, 2012).

ii. Annual estradiol exposure in women using local estradiol tablets (10 mcg) is 1.14 mg (Simon & Maamari, 2013).

iii. Local estrogen use did not increase risk of recurrence in women with breast cancer on adjuvant tamoxifen (Le Ray, Dell'Aniello, Bonnetain, Azoulay, & Suissa, 2012).

iv. The safety of local estrogen for women on aromatase inhibitors is not yet established (Sulaica et al., 2016).

v. Vaginal testosterone has shown efficacy in reducing vulvovaginal atrophy in women with breast cancer on aromatase inhibitors (Witherby et al., 2011).

(b) Systemic therapy: Three to five years of hormone therapy may be considered in patients with nonhormonal cancers if menopausal symptoms are refractory to other treatments. The woman's quality of life should be considered in the decision (Biglia, Bounous, Sgro, D'Alonzo, & Gallo, 2015).

(7) Other therapeutic agents—available as gels, creams, and suppositories (Barbera et al., 2017; Marchand & Bradford, 2017)

(a) Vaginal moisturizers and lubricants: Moisturizers can be used for daily comfort; lubricants can be used during intercourse.

(b) Topical anesthetics may also be used to reduce pain during intercourse.

(c) Topical steroids can be used to treat graft-versus-host disease.

(d) Additional agents include polycarbophil gel, hyaluronic acid, and olive oil.

(8) Vaginal dilators may be beneficial in the presence of vaginismus or vaginal stenosis, particularly among women who received radiation treatment for cervical cancer.

c) Men

(1) Assessment should be conducted at each visit and include examination of genital appearance, testing of testosterone levels, and prostate examination, if appropriate (Marchand & Bradford, 2017).

(a) The International Index of Erectile Function may be used to quickly assess erectile dysfunction concerns; however, it focuses on penile-vaginal intercourse and may not be appropriate to assess erectile dysfunction in men who have sex with men (Marchand & Bradford, 2017).

(b) The PROMIS SexFS (Flynn et al., 2013)

(2) Care coordination (Schover, 2016; Schover et al., 2014)

(a) Coordinate interprofessional referrals, including urology and sex therapy.

(b) Ensure that female partners receive care for postmenopausal sexual dysfunction.

(c) Psychosocial counseling is recommended to improve desire, arousal, orgasm, intimacy, and relationships (Barbera et al., 2017).

(3) Treatment options for erectile dysfunction

(a) Phosphodiesterase type 5 (PDE5) inhibitors: PDE5 inhibitors, including sildenafil (Viagra®), tadalafil (Cialis®), and vardenafil (Levitra®), are a drug class that has demonstrated efficacy in supporting erectile function following nerve-sparing radical prostatectomy (Limoncin et al., 2017). This drug class increases perfusion to the blood vessels of the corpus cavernosum of the penis by blocking the degradative action of cyclic granulocyte-macrophage inhibitor–specific PDE5 in smooth muscle cells. They are contraindicated with the use of nitrates (Deng et al., 2017).

(b) Vacuum erection devices: Devices consist of a closed-ended clear plastic cylinder and a vacuum pump and can be hand or battery operated; they use negative pressure to increase blood flow to the penis through distension of the corporeal sinusoids (Hoyland, Vasdev, & Adshead, 2013).

i. Advantages: Easy to use, noninvasive, quick response with an average time to erection of two to three minutes, can be incorporated into foreplay (Hoyland et al., 2013)

ii. Disadvantages: Potential for pivoting of penis because of instability at base due to constriction ring, inability to ejaculate due to urethral constriction (12%–30%), petechiae (25%–39%), pain due to suction and constriction (Hoyland et al., 2013)

iii. Contraindicated with coagulation abnormalities and sickle cell disease

iv. May be used in combination with PDE5 inhibitors (Deng et al., 2017)

(c) Prostaglandin injection/suppository: Prostaglandin E1 is a naturally occurring prostaglandin that can be administered by suppository or intracavernosal injection to induce vasodilation and expansion of the corpora spongiosum, causing rapid arterial inflow that supports the achievement of erection (Hakky et al., 2014).

i. Typically used as second-line therapy in patients in whom PDE5 inhibitor therapy was not successful

ii. Intracavernosal injection is most effective when administered within three months of nerve-sparing radical prostatectomy.

iii. May use suppositories alone or in combination with a vacuum erection device or PDE5 inhibitor; have demonstrated increased efficacy when used in combination

(d) Penile prosthetic implants: Implants are surgically implanted devices that may be noninflatable, semirigid, or inflatable, allowing for erection through manual manipulation or pump-facilitated inflation.

i. Advantages: Some studies suggest higher scores on measures of erectile function with implanted inflatable prosthetics compared to medical management (Dadhich et al., 2017).

ii. Disadvantages: Invasive procedure; rare complications including bladder injury, reservoir hernia, and reservoir erosion (Dadhich et al., 2017)

iii. Minimally used, with less than 1% of patients reporting progression to prosthesis placement after cancer treatment (Dadhich et al., 2017)

(e) Other treatment modalities (Barbera et al., 2017)

i. Venlafaxine, medroxyprogesterone acetate, cyproterone acetate, or gabapentin may be used to improve vasomotor symptoms.

ii. Some studies have suggested acupuncture may also be used to treat these symptoms.

d) Assessment tools: A number of models are helpful in communicating with patients about sexuality. The most frequently used model is the PLISSIT model (Annon, 1976). A more recent model specifically designed for the oncology population is the BETTER model (Mick, Hughes, & Cohen, 2004), and the 5 A's model (Bober & Varela, 2012) is increasingly being used in clinical practice.

(1) PLISSIT model (Annon, 1976)

(a) The first level in this model involves giving the patient or client *permission* to talk about sexual issues.

(b) The second level, *limited information*, refers to factual information given to the patient in response to a question or observation.

(c) The third level involves making a *specific suggestion* to the client or patient.

(d) The fourth level refers to *intensive therapy* needed for severe or more long-standing sexual problems or referral to a specialist, such as a urologist or gynecologist.

(2) BETTER model (Mick et al., 2004)

(a) The first level of intervention involves *bringing up* the topic.

(b) The second level involves *explaining* that sexuality is part of quality of life and that patients can talk about this with the nurse.

(c) Care providers should then *tell* patients that appropriate resources will be found to address their concerns.

(d) Care providers should state that while the *timing* may not be appropriate now, patients can ask for information at any time.
(e) Patients should be *educated* about the sexual side effects of their treatment.
(f) Finally, a *record* should be made in the patient's medical record stating that this topic has been discussed.

(3) The 5 A's model (Bober & Varela, 2012)
(a) *Ask* about changes to sexuality or sexual functioning.
(b) *Assess* the severity and frequency of any issues raised in response to the initial question.
(c) *Advise* the patient that help can be found and that sexual changes are common after treatment.
(d) *Assist* the patient by providing resources and referrals as necessary.
(e) *Arrange* for follow-up and ask about resolution of problems.

7. Patient and partner education
a) Education and counseling should begin early to promote effective rehabilitation and to limit sexual inactivity (Schover, 2016).
(1) Encourage affected individuals to communicate openly about sex with their partner.
(2) Internet-based resources are recommended as self-help tools that affected individuals and their partners can use in the privacy of their home.
(3) Encourage patients and their partners to explore ways of expressing affection in the context of sexual dysfunction.
(4) Encourage individuals or couples to view sexual activity as a chance to explore variety and fantasy rather than as a performance that needs to be done correctly.
b) Social support has a protective effect related to sexual dysfunction for young adults (Acquati et al., 2018); therefore, social connectivity should be emphasized to and supported for young adults during and following cancer treatment.

B. Alterations in reproductive functioning

1. Overview: Although they affect a small percentage of all patients with cancer and survivors, reproductive problems are among the most distressing treatment sequelae for individuals of childbearing age (Schover et al., 2014). Despite this, information about fertility preservation may be underreported to patients, and fertility preservation resources underutilized (Schover et al., 2014). Alterations in reproductive functioning may result from specific cancers but are more often attributed to cancer treatments (Schover et al., 2014).
a) Attention to fertility concerns was cited as an unmet need in 93% of adolescent and young adult survivors (Wong et al., 2017).
b) Uncertainty about fertility status is common in young adult cancer survivors (Benedict, Shuk, & Ford, 2016).
c) Lack of fertility counseling is common and is associated with regret (Chan et al., 2017).

2. Pathophysiology
a) Women: Chemotherapy causes effects such as damage to ovarian follicles, decreased ovarian volume, and decreased ovarian reserve.
b) Men: Damage to gonadal tissue results in reduced or absent (azoospermia) sperm production; damage can occur to germinal stem cells in the testes (Tournaye, Dohle, & Barratt, 2014).

3. Incidence
a) Women: Rates of chemotherapy-induced amenorrhea increase with age (Zavos & Valachis, 2016).
(1) Women younger than age 35: 26%
(2) Women aged 35–40 years: 39%
(3) Women older than age 40: 77%
b) Men: Infertility is dependent on the chemotherapy regimen and other therapies such as total body irradiation or orchiectomy in testicular cancer. Azoospermia rates range from 10% with newer, less toxic regimens to 100% with older, more toxic regimens (Kort, Eisenberg, Millheiser, & Westphal, 2014).

4. Risk factors
a) Disease-related risk factors
(1) Women: Individuals with ovarian cancer and hormone-sensitive breast cancer may have increased risk for childlessness; in addition, those with *BRCA1* mutations may have increased risk for early menopause (Schover et al., 2014).
(2) Men: Individuals with testicular cancer may have poorer sperm quality and genetic viability (Bujan et al., 2013).
b) Treatment-related risk factors
(1) Combination therapy: The addition of radiation to the treatment regimen significantly increases the risk of per-

manent infertility (Kort et al., 2014; Vakalopoulos, Dimou, Anagnostou, & Zeginiadou, 2015).

(2) Alkylating agents pose the highest risk for infertility in both men and women related to damage to reproductive cells that increases with higher cumulative doses of these agents (Gracia et al., 2012; Meistrich, 2013).

(a) Women: Procarbazine and the CMF (cyclophosphamide, methotrexate, 5-fluorouracil) regimen are associated with increased risk of infertility (Overbeek et al., 2017).

(b) Men: Alkylating agents and platinum analogs are gonadotoxic, and the risk to spermatogenesis increases with combination therapy (Vakalopoulos et al., 2015).

i. Cyclophosphamide, ifosfamide, and procarbazine are gonadotoxic and are associated with azoospermia (Moss, Keeter, Brannigan, & Kim, 2016).

ii. Studies among pediatric patients receiving cyclophosphamide suggest a dose less than 4,000 mg/m^2 is associated with a lower risk (Green et al., 2014).

iii. Antimetabolites can cause temporary reduction in sperm count (Vakalopoulos et al., 2015).

(3) Age

(a) Older age increases the risk for infertility in both men and women.

(b) Chemotherapy accelerates reproductive aging in childhood cancer survivors (Anderson & Wallace, 2016).

5. Clinical manifestations

a) Women: Psychosocial effects

(1) Women with high levels of concern about fertility are more likely to experience depression (Gorman, Su, Roberts, Dominick, & Malcarne, 2015).

(2) Women are also concerned about the effects of cancer treatment on the health of future offspring (Benedict, Thom, et al., 2016).

(3) Women who receive fertility preservation counseling experience less long-term regret, better physical quality of life, and improved coping (Deshpande, Braun, & Meyer, 2015).

b) Men

(1) Oligozoospermia: Semen with a low concentration of sperm occurs in approximately 50% of men before treatment begins (Giwercman, 2017).

(2) Azoospermia: Absence of sperm in ejaculate occurs in 3%–18% of men at diagnosis (Berookhim & Mulhall, 2014).

(a) Recovery of spermatogenesis is typically observed within two to five years after chemotherapy, after which 8% of men remain azoospermic, with prolonged azoospermia occurring in up to 65% of individuals receiving greater than 600 mg/m^2 of cisplatin (Giwercman, 2017).

(b) Among male survivors of childhood cancer, approximately 20% present with azoospermia, with incidence ranging from 15% in individuals treated with chemotherapy alone versus 33% among those treated with chemotherapy plus radiation (Giwercman, 2017).

6. Collaborative management: Patients interested in exploring fertility preservation options should be referred to a reproductive specialist (Loren et al., 2013). In addition, referral to a psychologist may be appropriate for patients expressing distress related to potential or actual infertility.

a) Women

(1) Oocyte and embryo cryopreservation techniques are established methods.

(2) Cryopreservation requires 8–14 days for ovarian stimulation (Levine, Kelvin, Quinn, & Gracia, 2015).

(3) Limited data are available on the safety of ovarian stimulation in women with cancer (Levine et al., 2015).

(4) Ovarian cortex or immature oocyte cryopreservation is regarded as experimental (De Vos, Smitz, & Woodruff, 2014).

(5) Controversy exists about the use of gonadotropin-releasing hormone analogs to protect the ovaries from damage (Oktay & Bedoschi, 2016).

(6) Ovarian suppression is not likely to be of benefit despite support for this strategy and apparent safety (Demeestere et al., 2016; Hickman, Valentine, & Falcone, 2016; Kim, Turan, & Oktay, 2016).

(7) The return of menstrual periods does not necessarily indicate good ovarian function, and, in turn, lack of menstruation does not mean that ovarian function has ceased.

b) Men

(1) Sperm cryopreservation before treatment is highly effective, as sperm remain viable after freezing and can be used to fertilize ovum.

(2) Ideally, semen samples should be collected 48 hours apart (Tournaye et al., 2014).

(3) Electroejaculation can be used in peripubertal males who are embarrassed or unable to produce a semen sample. This requires general anesthesia but can be done at the time of another surgical procedure, such as bone marrow aspiration (Romao & Lorenzo, 2017).

(4) Cryopreservation of testicular tissue is an experimental procedure that may offer hope to prepubertal boys (Wise, 2016).

7. Patient and family education

a) Decisions about treatments that affect fertility must be made when the patient is trying to cope with the diagnosis of cancer; priorities may change over time. It is important to educate patients honestly and directly, as they may assume that modern reproductive technologies will result in a future pregnancy. A strong desire to be a biological parent motivates some patients to attempt to preserve fertility (Hershberger, Sipsma, Finnegan, & Hirshfeld-Cytron, 2016; Shnorhavorian et al., 2015).

b) Educate patients and caregivers about challenges to fertility preservation, which include the following (Flink, Sheeder, & Kondapalli, 2017):

(1) Urgency to start treatment

(2) Inadequate information

(3) Cost

(4) Sociodemographic factors (e.g., race, relationship status)

c) Parents of a child with cancer may have to make decisions about treatment for their child and may not be capable of discussing sperm banking or ovarian preservation with their child or healthcare providers, as their priority is to save the life of their child (Li, Jayasinghe, Kemertzis, Moore, & Peate, 2017).

d) Discuss access to fertility services.

(1) An interprofessional approach is regarded as optimal to address the complex ethical and psychological issues. Nurses who have longitudinal relationships with patients are vital to ensuring that information is provided to patients (Quinn et al., 2016).

(2) Identify barriers to fertility services.

(a) Disparity in access to fertility services is related to age (older than 35), previous children, ethnicity, and sexual orientation (Letourneau et al., 2012).

(b) Age-appropriate information and services are an unmet need for adolescents and young adults with cancer, as is fertility-related follow-up after the completion of treatment (Bibby, White, Thompson, & Anazodo, 2017).

(c) Referrals for sperm banking remain low—29% of young men reported receiving counseling, and 11% attempted sperm banking (Grover, Deal, Wood, & Mersereau, 2016).

(d) Women are less likely to receive counseling about fertility preservation (Quinn et al., 2015).

(e) Information provided after treatment is over leaves patients living with the consequences and struggling to find out what they can do (Giles, 2017).

e) General education (Loren et al., 2013)

(1) Address the risk of infertility as well as fertility preservation options with patients as part of informed consent before cancer therapy. Sperm and embryo cryopreservation are well established as the standard of care.

(2) Encourage patients to participate in registries and clinical trials related to fertility preservation.

(3) Provide information about the timeline for fertility preservation and how it may affect treatment.

(4) Advise patients of the potential toxicity to reproductive material or the loss of opportunity to preserve reproductive material after the start of chemotherapy.

(5) Engage both patients and their caregivers (if the patient is underage) in discussions of cryopreservation options.

References

Acquati, C., Zebrack, B.J., Faul, A.C., Embry, L., Aguilar, C., Block, R., ... Cole, S. (2018). Sexual functioning among young adult cancer patients: A 2-year longitudinal study. *Cancer, 124,* 398–405. https://doi.org/10.1002/cncr.31030

American Cancer Society. (2016). *Cancer treatment and survivorship facts and figures 2016–2017.* Retrieved from https://www.cancer.org/content/dam/cancer-org/research/cancer-facts-and-statistics/cancer-treatment-and-survivorship-facts-and-figures/cancer-treatment-and-survivorship-facts-and-figures-2016-2017.pdf

Anderson, R.A., & Wallace, W.H.B. (2016). Chemotherapy risks to fertility of childhood cancer survivors. *Lancet Oncology, 17,* 540–541. https://doi.org/10.1016/S1470-2045(16)00116-9

Annon, J.S. (1976). The PLISSIT model: A proposed conceptual scheme for the behavioral treatment of sexual problems. *Journal of Sex Education and Therapy, 2,* 1–15. https://doi.org/10.1080/01614576.1976.11074483

Antoine, C., Liebens, F., Carly, B., Pastijn, A., & Rozenberg, S. (2007). Safety of alternative treatments for menopausal symptoms after breast cancer: A qualitative systematic review. *Climacteric, 10,* 23–26. https://doi.org/10.1080/13697130601176734

Barbera, L., Zwaal, C., Elterman, D., McPherson, K., Wolfman, W., Katz, A., & Matthew, A. (2017). Interventions to address sexual problems in people with cancer. *Current Oncology, 24,* 192–200. https://doi.org/10.3747/co.24.3583

Baumgart, J., Nilsson, K., Evers, A.S., Kallak, T.K., & Poromaa, I.S. (2013). Sexual dysfunction in women on adjuvant endocrine therapy after breast cancer. *Menopause, 20,* 162–168. Retrieved from https://journals.lww.com/menopausejournal/Abstract/2013/02000/Sexual_dysfunction_in_women_on_adjuvant_endocrine.10.aspx

Ben Charif, A., Bouhnik, A.-D., Courbiere, B., Rey, D., Préau, M., Bendiane, M.-K., ... Mancini, J. (2016). Patient discussion about sexual health with health care providers after cancer—A national survey. *Journal of Sexual Medicine, 13,* 1686–1694. https://doi.org/10.1016/j.jsxm.2016.09.005

Benedict, C., Shuk, E., & Ford, J.S. (2016). Fertility issues in adolescent and young adult cancer survivors. *Journal of Adolescent and Young Adult Oncology, 5,* 48–57. https://doi.org/10.1089/jayao.2015.0024

Benedict, C., Thom, B., Friedman, D.N., Diotallevi, D., Pottenger, E.M., Raghunathan, N.J., & Kelvin, J.F. (2016). Young adult female cancer survivors' unmet information needs and reproductive concerns contribute to decisional conflict regarding posttreatment fertility preservation. *Cancer, 122,* 2101–2109. https://doi.org/10.1002/cncr.29917

Bennett, N., Incrocci, L., Baldwin, D., Hackett, G., El-Zawahry, A., Graziottin, A., ... Krychman, M. (2016). Cancer, benign gynecology, and sexual function—Issues and answers. *Journal of Sexual Medicine, 13,* 519–537. https://doi.org/10.1016/j.jsxm.2016.01.018

Berookhim, B.M., & Mulhall, J.P. (2014). Outcomes of operative sperm retrieval strategies for fertility preservation among males scheduled to undergo cancer treatment. *Fertility and Sterility, 101,* 805–811. https://doi.org/10.1016/j.fertnstert.2013.11.122

Bibby, H., White, V., Thompson, K., & Anazodo, A. (2017). What are the unmet needs and care experiences of adolescents and young adults with cancer? A systematic review. *Journal of Adolescent and Young Adult Oncology, 6,* 6–30. https://doi.org/10.1089/jayao.2016.0012

Biglia, N., Bounous, V.E., Sgro, L.G., D'Alonzo, M., & Gallo, M. (2015). Treatment of climacteric symptoms in survivors of gynaecological cancer. *Maturitas, 82,* 296–298. https://doi.org/10.1016/j.maturitas.2015.07.006

Bober, S.L., & Varela, V.S. (2012). Sexuality in adult cancer survivors: Challenges and intervention. *Journal of Clinical Oncology, 30,* 3712–3719. https://doi.org/10.1200/JCO.2012.41.7915

Bober, S.L., Zhou, E.S., Chen, B., Manley, P.E., Kenney, L.B., & Recklitis, C.J. (2013). Sexual function in childhood cancer survivors: A report from Project REACH. *Journal of Sexual Medicine, 10,* 2084–2093. https://doi.org/10.1111/jsm.12193

Bujan, L., Walschaerts, M., Moinard, N., Hennebicq, S., Saias, J., Brugnon, F., ... Rives, N. (2013). Impact of chemotherapy and radiotherapy for testicular germ cell tumors on spermatogenesis and sperm DNA: A multicenter prospective study from the CECOS network. *Fertility and Sterility, 100,* 673–680.e2. https://doi.org/10.1016/j.fertnstert.2013.05.018

Capogrosso, P., Boeri, L., Ferrari, M., Ventimiglia, E., La Croce, G., Capitanio, U., ... Salonia, A. (2016). Long-term recovery of normal sexual function in testicular cancer survivors. *Asian Journal of Andrology, 18,* 85–89. https://doi.org/10.4103/1008-682X.149180

Carlsson, S., Nilsson, A.E., Johansson, E., Nyberg, T., Akre, O., & Steineck, G. (2012). Self-perceived penile shortening after radical prostatectomy. *International Journal of Impotence Research, 24,* 179–184. https://doi.org/10.1038/ijir.2012.13

Chan, J.L., Letourneau, J., Salem, W., Cil, A.P., Chan, S.-W., Chen, L.-M., & Rosen, M.P. (2017). Regret around fertility choices is decreased with pre-treatment counseling in gynecologic cancer patients. *Journal of Cancer Survivorship, 11,* 58–63. https://doi.org/10.1007/s11764-016-0563-2

Costabile, R.A. (2000). Cancer and male sexual dysfunction. *Oncology, 14,* 195–205. Retrieved from http://www.cancernetwork.com/prostate-cancer/cancer-and-male-sexual-dysfunction

Dadhich, P., Hockenberry, M., Kirby, E.W., & Lipshultz, L. (2017). Penile prosthesis in the management of erectile dysfunction following cancer therapy. *Translational Andrology and Urology, 6,* S881–S889. https://doi.org/10.21037/tau.2017.07.05

Dean, R.C., & Lue, T.F. (2005). Physiology of penile erection and pathophysiology of erectile dysfunction. *Urologic Clinics of North America, 32,* 379–395. https://doi.org/10.1016/j.ucl.2005.08.007

Demeestere, I., Brice, P., Peccatori, F.A., Kentos, A., Dupuis, J., Zachee, P., ... Englert, Y. (2016). No evidence for the benefit of gonadotropin-releasing hormone agonist in preserving ovarian function and fertility in lymphoma survivors treated with chemotherapy: Final long-term report of a prospective randomized trial. *Journal of Clinical Oncology, 34,* 2568–2574. https://doi.org/10.1200/JCO.2015.65.8864

Deng, H., Liu, D., Mao, X., Lan, X., Liu, H., & Li, G. (2017). Phosphodiesterase-5 inhibitors and vacuum erection device for penile rehabilitation after laparoscopic nerve-preserving radical proctectomy for rectal cancer: A prospective controlled trial. *American Journal of Men's Health, 11,* 641–646. https://doi.org/10.1177/1557988316665084

Deshpande, N.A., Braun, I.M., & Meyer, F.L. (2015). Impact of fertility preservation counseling and treatment on psychological outcomes among women with cancer: A systematic review. *Cancer, 121,* 3938–3947. https://doi.org/10.1002/cncr.29637

DeSimone, M., Spriggs, E., Gass, J.S., Carson, S.A., Krychman, M.L., & Dizon, D.S. (2014). Sexual dysfunction in female cancer survivors. *American Journal of Clinical Oncology, 37,* 101–106. https://doi.org/10.1097/COC.0b013e318248d89d

De Vos, M., Smitz, J., & Woodruff, T.K. (2014). Fertility preservation in women with cancer. *Lancet, 384,* 1302–1310. https://doi.org/10.1016/S0140-6736(14)60834-5

Dizon, D.S., Suzin, D., & McIlvenna, S. (2014). Sexual health as a survivorship issue for female cancer survivors. *Oncologist, 19,* 202–210. https://doi.org/10.1634/theoncologist.2013-0302

Drewe, J., Bucher, K.A., & Zahner, C. (2015). A systematic review of non-hormonal treatments of vasomotor symptoms in climacteric and cancer patients. *SpringerPlus, 4,* 65. https://doi.org/10.1186/s40064-015-0808-y

Falk, S.J., & Dizon, D.S. (2013). Sexual dysfunction in women with cancer. *Fertility and Sterility, 10,* 916–921. https://doi.org/10.1016/j.fertnstert.2013.08.018

Farthmann, J., Hanjalic-Beck, A., Veit, J., Rautenberg, B., Stickeler, E., Erbes, T., ... Hasenburg, A. (2016). The impact of chemotherapy for breast cancer on sexual function and health-related quality of life. *Supportive Care in Cancer, 24,* 2603–2609. https://doi.org/10.1007/s00520-015-3073-2

Flink, D.M., Sheeder, J., & Kondapalli, L.A. (2017). A review of the oncology patient's challenges for utilizing fertility preservation services. *Journal of Adolescent and Young Adult Oncology, 6,* 31–44. https://doi.org/10.1089/jayao.2015.0065

Flynn, K.E., Lin, L., Cyranowski, J.M., Reeve, B.B., Reese, J.B., Jeffery, D.D., ... Weinfurt, K.P. (2013). Development of the NIH PROMIS® sexual function and satisfaction measures in patients with cancer. *Journal of Sexual Medicine, 10*(Suppl. 1), 43–52. https://doi.org/10.1111/j.1743-6109.2012.02995.x

Ford, J.S., Kawashima, T., Whitton, J., Leisenring, W., Laverdière, C., Stovall, M., ... Sklar, C.A. (2014). Psychosexual functioning among adult female survivors of childhood cancer: A report from the childhood cancer survivor study. *Journal of Clinical Oncology, 32,* 3126–3136. https://doi.org/10.1200/JCO.2013.54.1086

Giles, C. (2017). Young people with cancer lack clear information about preserving fertility. *BMJ, 356,* i6790. https://doi.org/10.1136/bmj.i6790

Giwercman, A. (2017). Effect of cancer treatments on testicular function. In A. Lenzi & E.A. Jannini (Series Eds.), *Endocrinology: Endocrinology of the testis and male reproduction* (pp. 881–898). https://doi.org/10.1007/978-3-319-44441-3_29

Gorman, J.R., Su, H.I., Roberts, S.C., Dominick, S.A., & Malcarne, V.L. (2015). Experiencing reproductive concerns as a female cancer survivor is associated with depression. *Cancer, 121,* 935–942. https://doi.org/10.1002/cncr.29133

Gracia, C.R., Sammel, M.D., Freeman, E., Prewitt, M., Carlson, C., Ray, A., ... Ginsberg, J.P. (2012). Impact of cancer therapies on ovarian reserve. *Fertility and Sterility, 97,* 134–140.e1. https://doi.org/10.1016/j.fertnstert.2011.10.040

Green, D.M., Liu, W., Kutteh, W.H., Ke, R.W., Shelton, K.C., Sklar, C.A., ... Hudson, M.M. (2014). Cumulative alkylating agent exposure and semen parameters in adult survivors of childhood cancer: A report from the St Jude Lifetime Cohort Study. *Lancet Oncology, 15,* 1215–1223. https://doi.org/10.1016/S1470-2045(14)70408-5

Grover, N.S., Deal, A.M., Wood, W.A., & Mersereau, J.E. (2016). Young men with cancer experience low referral rates for fertility counseling and sperm banking. *Journal of Oncology Practice, 12,* 465–471. https://doi.org/10.1200/JOP.2015.010579

Hakky, T.S., Baumgarten, A.S., Parker, J., Zheng, Y., Kongnyuy, M., Martinez, D., & Carrion, R.E. (2014). Penile rehabilitation: The evolutionary concept in the management of erectile dysfunction. *Current Urology Reports, 15,* 393. https://doi.org/10.1007/s11934-014-0393-6

Hershberger, P.E., Sipsma, H., Finnegan, L., & Hirshfeld-Cytron, J. (2016). Reasons why young women accept or decline fertility preservation after cancer diagnosis. *Journal of Obstetric, Gynecologic and Neonatal Nursing, 45,* 123–134. https://doi.org/10.1016/j.jogn.2015.10.003

Hickman, L.C., Valentine, L.N., & Falcone, T. (2016). Preservation of gonadal function in women undergoing chemotherapy: A review of the potential role for gonadotropin-releasing hormone agonists. *American Journal of Obstetrics and Gynecology, 215,* 415–422. https://doi.org/10.1016/j.ajog.2016.06.053

Hoyland, K., Vasdev, N., & Adshead, J. (2013). The use of vacuum erection devices in erectile dysfunction after radical prostatectomy. *Reviews in Urology, 15,* 67–71.

Jackson, S.E., Wardle, J., Steptoe, A., & Fisher, A. (2016). Sexuality after a cancer diagnosis: A population-based study. *Cancer, 122,* 3883–3891. https://doi.org/10.1002/cncr.30263

Kelvin, J.F., Steed, R., & Jarrett, B. (2014). Discussing safe sexual practices during cancer treatment. *Clinical Journal of Oncology Nursing, 18,* 449–453. https://doi.org/10.1188/14.CJON.449-453

Kim, J., Turan, V., & Oktay, K. (2016). Long-term safety of letrozole and gonadotropin stimulation for fertility preservation in women with breast cancer. *Journal of Clinical Endocrinology and Metabolism, 101,* 1364–1371. https://doi.org/10.1210/jc.2015-3878

Kort, J.D., Eisenberg, M.L., Millheiser, L.S., & Westphal, L.M. (2014). Fertility issues in cancer survivorship. *CA: A Cancer Journal for Clinicians, 64,* 118–134. https://doi.org/10.3322/caac.21205

Krebs, L.U. (2012). Sexual health during cancer treatment. In I.R. Cohen, A. Lajtha, J.D. Lambris, R. Paoletti, & N. Rezaei (Series Eds.), *Advances in Experimental Medicine and Biology: Vol. 732. Reproductive health and cancer in adolescents and young adults* (pp. 61–76). https://doi.org/10.1007/978-94-007-2492-1_5

Lammerink, E.A.G., de Bock, G.H., Schröder, C.P., & Mourits, M.J.E. (2012). The management of menopausal symptoms in breast cancer survivors: A case-based approach. *Maturitas, 73,* 265–268. https://doi.org/10.1016/j.maturitas.2012.07.010

Le Ray, I., Dell'Aniello, S., Bonnetain, F., Azoulay, L., & Suissa, S. (2012). Local estrogen therapy and risk of breast cancer recurrence among hormone-treated patients: A nested case–control study. Breast *Cancer Research and Treatment, 135,* 603–609. https://doi.org/10.1007/s10549-012-2198-y

Letourneau, J.M., Smith, J.F., Ebbel, E.E., Craig, A., Katz, P.P., Cedars, M.I., & Rosen, M.P. (2012). Racial, socioeconomic, and demographic disparities in access to fertility preservation in young women diagnosed with cancer. *Cancer, 118,* 4579–4588. https://doi.org/10.1002/cncr.26649

Levine, J.M., Kelvin, J.F., Quinn, G.P., & Gracia, C.R. (2015). Infertility in reproductive-age female cancer survivors. *Cancer, 121,* 1532–1539. https://doi.org/10.1002/cncr.29181

Li, N., Jayasinghe, Y., Kemertzis, M.A., Moore, P., & Peate, M. (2017). Fertility preservation in pediatric and adolescent oncology patients: The decision-making process of parents. *Journal of Adolescent and Young Adult Oncology, 6,* 213–222. https://doi.org/10.1089/jayao.2016.0061

Limoncin, E., Gravina, G.L., Corona, G., Maggi, M., Ciocca, G., Lenzi, A., & Jannini, E.A. (2017). Erectile function recovery in men treated with phosphodiesterase type 5 inhibitor administration after bilateral nerve-sparing radical prostatectomy: A systematic review of placebo-controlled randomized trials with trial sequential analysis. *Andrology, 5,* 863–872. https://doi.org/10.1111/andr.12403

Loren, A.W., Mangu, P.B., Beck, L.N., Brennan, L., Magdalinski, A.J., Partridge, A.H., ... Oktay, K. (2013). Fertility preservation for patients with cancer: American Society of Clinical Oncology clinical practice guideline update. *Journal of Clinical Oncology, 31,* 2500–2510. https://doi.org/10.1200/JCO.2013.49.2678

Marchand, E., & Bradford, A. (2017). Sex and cancer. In W.W. IsHak (Ed.), *The textbook of clinical sexual medicine* (pp. 455–477). https://doi.org/10.1007/978-3-319-52539-6_30

Meistrich, M.L. (2013). Effects of chemotherapy and radiotherapy on spermatogenesis in humans. *Fertility and Sterility, 100,* 1180–1186. https://doi.org/10.1016/j.fertnstert.2013.08.010

Mick, J., Hughes, M., & Cohen, M.Z. (2004). Using the BETTER model to assess sexuality. *Clinical Journal of Oncology Nursing, 8,* 84–86. https://doi.org/10.1188/04.CJON.84-86

Miller, K.D., Siegel, R.L., Lin, C.C., Mariotto, A.B., Kramer, J.L., Rowland, J.H., … Jemal, A. (2016). Cancer treatment and survivorship statistics, 2016. *CA: A Cancer Journal for Clinicians, 66,* 271–289. https://doi.org/10.3322/caac.21349

Moss, J.L., Keeter, M.K.F., Brannigan, R.E., & Kim, E.D. (2016). Erectile dysfunction and infertility in male cancer patients: Addressing unmet needs. *Future Oncology, 12,* 2293–2296. https://doi.org/10.2217/fon-2016-0335

Nelson, C.J., Scardino, P.T., Eastham, J.A., & Mulhall, J.P. (2013). Back to baseline: Erectile function recovery after radical prostatectomy from the patients' perspective. *Journal of Sexual Medicine, 10,* 1636–1643. https://doi.org/10.1111/jsm.12135

Oktay, K., & Bedoschi, G. (2016). Appraising the biological evidence for and against the utility of GnRHa for preservation of fertility in patients with cancer. *Journal of Clinical Oncology, 34,* 2563–2565. https://doi.org/10.1200/JCO.2016.67.1693

Overbeek, A., van den Berg, M.H., van Leeuwen, F.E., Kaspers, G.J.L., Lambalk, C.B., & van Dulmen-den Broeder, E. (2017). Chemotherapy-related late adverse effects on ovarian function in female survivors of childhood and young adult cancer: A systematic review. *Cancer Treatment Reviews, 53,* 10–24. https://doi.org/10.1016/j.ctrv.2016.11.006

Pfeiler, G., Glatz, C., Königsberg, R., Geisendorfer, T., Fink-Retter, A., Kubista, E., … Seifert, M. (2011). Vaginal estriol to overcome side-effects of aromatase inhibitors in breast cancer patients. *Climacteric, 14,* 339–344. https://doi.org/10.3109/13697137.2010.529967

Pinto, A.C. (2013). Sexuality and breast cancer: Prime time for young patients. *Journal of Thoracic Disease, 5*(Suppl. 1), S81–S86. https://doi.org/10.3978/j.issn.2072-1439.2013.05.23

Quinn, G.P., Block, R.G., Clayman, M.L., Kelvin, J., Arvey, S.R., Lee, J.-H., … Hayes-Lattin, B. (2015). If you did not document it, it did not happen: Rates of documentation of discussion of infertility risk in adolescent and young adult oncology patients' medical records. *Journal of Oncology Practice, 11,* 137–144. https://doi.org/10.1200/JOP.2014.000786

Quinn, G.P., Woodruff, T.K., Knapp, C.A., Bowman, M.L., Reinecke, J., & Vadaparampil, S.T. (2016). Expanding the oncofertility workforce: Training allied health professionals to improve health outcomes for adolescents and young adults. *Journal of Adolescent and Young Adult Oncology, 5,* 292–296. https://doi.org/10.1089/jayao.2016.0003

Rellini, A.H., Farmer, M.A., & Golden, G.H. (2011). Hypoactive sexual desire disorder. In E.A. Klein (Series Ed.), *Current Clinical Urology: Cancer and sexual health* (pp. 105–123). https://doi.org/10.1007/978-1-60761-916-1_9

Resnick, M.J., Koyama, T., Fan, K.-H., Albertsen, P.C., Goodman, M., Hamilton, A.S., … Penson, D.F. (2013). Long-term functional outcomes after treatment for localized prostate cancer. *New England Journal of Medicine, 368,* 436–445. https://doi.org/10.1056/NEJMoa1209978

Romao, R.L.P., & Lorenzo, A.J. (2017). Fertility preservation options for children and adolescents with cancer. *Canadian Urological Association Journal, 11*(Suppl. 1), S97–S102. https://doi.org/10.5489/cuaj.4410

Rosen, R.C., Brown, C., Heiman, J., Leiblum, S., Meston, C., Shabsigh, R., … D'Agostino, R., Jr. (2000). The Female Sexual Function Index (FSFI): A multidimensional self-report instrument for the assessment of female sexual function. *Journal of Sex and Marital Therapy, 26,* 191–208. https://doi.org/10.1080/009262300278597

Rosen, R.C., Lobo, R.A., Block, B.A., Yang, H.-M., & Zipfel, L.M. (2004). Menopausal Sexual Interest Questionnaire (MSIQ): A unidimensional scale for the assessment of sexual interest in postmenopausal women. *Journal of Sex and Marital Therapy, 30,* 235–250. https://doi.org/10.1080/00926230490422340

Schover, L.R. (2016). Managing erectile dysfunction after cancer: More than penile rigidity. *Journal of Oncology Practice, 12,* 307–308. https://doi.org/10.1200/JOP.2016.011569

Schover, L.R., van der Kaaij, M., van Dorst, E., Creutzberg, C., Huyghe, E., & Kiserud, C.E. (2014). Sexual dysfunction and infertility as late effects of cancer treatment. *European Journal of Cancer Supplements, 12,* 41–53. Retrieved from https://www.sciencedirect.com/science/article/pii/S1359634914000068

Sears, C.S., Robinson, J.W., & Walker, L.M. (2018). A comprehensive review of sexual health concerns after cancer treatment and the biopsychosocial treatment options available to female patients. *European Journal of Cancer Care, 27,* e12738. https://doi.org/10.1111/ecc.12738

Shnorhavorian, M., Harlan, L.C., Smith, A.W., Keegan, T.H.M., Lynch, C.F., Prasad, P.K., … Schwartz, S.M. (2015). Fertility preservation knowledge, counseling, and actions among adolescent and young adult patients with cancer: A population-based study. *Cancer, 121,* 3499–3506. https://doi.org/10.1002/cncr.29328

Simon, J.A., & Maamari, R. (2013). Ultra-low-dose vaginal estrogen tablets for the treatment of postmenopausal vaginal atrophy. *Climacteric, 16*(Suppl. 1), 37–43. https://doi.org/10.3109/13697137.2013.807606

Sulaica, E., Han, T., Wang, W., Bhat, R., Trivedi, M.V., & Niravath, P. (2016). Vaginal estrogen products in hormone receptor-positive breast cancer patients on aromatase inhibitor therapy. *Breast Cancer Research and Treatment, 157,* 203–210. https://doi.org/10.1007/s10549-016-3827-7

Taylor, K.L., Luta, G., Miller, A.B., Church, T.R., Kelly, S.P., Muenz, L.R., … Riley, T.L. (2012). Long-term disease-specific functioning among prostate cancer survivors and noncancer controls in the prostate, lung, colorectal, and ovarian cancer screening trial. *Journal of Clinical Oncology, 30,* 2768–2775. https://doi.org/10.1200/JCO.2011.41.2767

Thirlaway, K., Fallowfield, L., & Cuzick, J. (1996). The Sexual Activity Questionnaire: A measure of women's sexual functioning. *Quality of Life Research, 5,* 81–90. https://doi.org/10.1007/BF00435972

Tournaye, H., Dohle, G.R., & Barratt, C.L.R. (2014). Fertility preservation in men with cancer. *Lancet, 384,* 1295–1301. https://doi.org/10.1016/S0140-6736(14)60495-5

Ussher, J.M., Perz, J., Gilbert, E., & Australian Cancer and Sexuality Study Team. (2015). Perceived causes and consequences of sexual changes after cancer for women and men: A mixed method study. *BMC Cancer, 15,* 268. https://doi.org/10.1186/s12885-015-1243-8

Vakalopoulos, I., Dimou, P., Anagnostou, I., & Zeginiadou, T. (2015). Impact of cancer and cancer treatment on male fertility. *Hormones, 14,* 579–589. https://doi.org/10.14310/horm.2002.1620

Voznesensky, M., Annam, K., & Kreder, K.J. (2016). Understanding and managing erectile dysfunction in patients treated for cancer. *Journal of Oncology Practice, 12,* 297–304. https://doi.org/10.1200/JOP.2016.010678

Wise, J. (2016). Frozen tissue service offers fertility hope to young people with cancer. *BMJ, 354,* i3955. https://doi.org/10.1136/bmj.i3955

Witherby, S., Johnson, J., Demers, L., Mount, S., Littenberg, B., Maclean, C.D., … Muss, H. (2011). Topical testosterone for breast cancer patients with vaginal atrophy related to aromatase inhibitors: A phase I/II study. *Oncologist, 16,* 424–431. https://doi.org/10.1634/theoncologist.2010-0435

Wong, A.W.K., Chang, T.-T., Christopher, K., Lau, S.C.L., Beaupin, L.K., Love, B., ... Feuerstein, M. (2017). Patterns of unmet needs in adolescent and young adult (AYA) cancer survivors: In their own words. *Journal of Cancer Survivorship, 11,* 751–764. https://doi.org/10.1007/s11764-017-0613-4

Zavos, A., & Valachis, A. (2016). Risk of chemotherapy-induced amenorrhea in patients with breast cancer: A systematic review and meta-analysis. *Acta Oncologica, 55,* 664–670. https://doi.org/10.3109/0284186X.2016.1155738

CHAPTER 21

Cutaneous Toxicities and Alopecia

A. Cutaneous toxicity
1. Overview: For years, the cutaneous side effects from conventional cytotoxic chemotherapy agents have been observed and described in detail. More recently, the emergence of targeted therapy and immunotherapy agents has widened the spectrum of cutaneous adverse effects seen in patients with cancer (Shi, Levy, & Choi, 2016; Sibaud et al., 2016). As the number of agents and uses for targeted therapy and immunotherapy agents increases, so does the need to recognize and treat the dermatologic side effects of these agents (Shi et al., 2016). See Table 21-1 for cutaneous reactions and management of toxicities from chemotherapy, targeted therapy, and immunotherapy agents.
2. Pathophysiology, incidence, risk factors, and clinical manifestations
   a) Chemotherapy
      (1) Numerous cutaneous side effects have been reported from traditional chemotherapy drugs, including cytarabine, anthracyclines (including doxorubicin), 5-fluorouracil (5-FU), capecitabine (5-FU prodrug), taxanes (including docetaxel), and methotrexate.
         (a) Reports include clinical and histologic findings that have significant overlap. Cutaneous adverse events from chemotherapy can affect the skin, hair, nails, and mucosa.
         (b) Cutaneous side effects from chemotherapy occur due to disruptions in the cell cycle phases. The specific phase in which the disruption occurs will cause a specific type of cutaneous reaction (Reyes-Habito & Roh, 2014a).
            i. Alkylating agents, such as cyclophosphamide, cause damage in all phases of the cell cycle and tend to cause hyperpigmentation.
            ii. Antimetabolites, such as gemcitabine, damage cells in the S phase and cause a range of cutaneous effects, such as maculopapular rash, hand-foot syndrome, and hyperpigmentation.
            iii. Antitumor antibiotic agents, such as doxorubicin, cause damage in all phases of the cell cycle and lead to reactions such as hand-foot syndrome and follicular rash.
            iv. Mitotic inhibitors, which include the taxanes and vinca alkaloids, cause damage in the M phase of the cell cycle. Cutaneous reactions that occur from these agents include hand-foot syndrome, nail changes, and erythema multiforme.
            v. Topoisomerase inhibitors, such as topotecan and etoposide, affect the cell cycle during the S or G_2 phase. Cutaneous reactions seen with these agents include hand-foot syndrome and paronychia (Reyes-Habito & Roh, 2014a).
      (2) The clinically descriptive term *toxic erythema of chemotherapy* (TEC) has been introduced as an easily understood clinical name for numerous entities (Shi et al., 2016).
         (a) Clinical findings of TEC include areas of erythema that may be accompanied by edema, most often involving the hands, feet, and intertriginous zones, such as the axillae and inguinal folds. Less

Table 21-1. Cutaneous Reactions to Antineoplastic Agents

Cutaneous Reaction	General Comments	Chemotherapy	Targeted Therapy	Immunotherapy
Hair changes: Alopecia, hirsutism, hypertrichosis	A number of chemotherapy drugs can cause hair changes and hair loss. Dose, route of administration, combination of drugs, and other individual characteristics will influence occurrence as well as degree of hair loss. Hair changes may occur 2–3 months after initiation of EGFRI therapy, with hair thinning and developing a dry, brittle, or curly texture. Hirsutism is characterized by excess hair growth in women in anatomic sites where growth is typically a male characteristic (beard, mustache, hair on chest and abdomen). Hypertrichosis is characterized by hair density or length beyond the accepted limits of normal in a particular body region or a particular age or race.	Hair changes: Bexarotene, carboplatin, cisplatin, cyclophosphamide, dactinomycin, doxorubicin, etoposide, hexamethylmelamine, ifosfamide, paclitaxel, vincristine Alopecia: Bleomycin, carboplatin, cisplatin, cyclophosphamide, cytarabine, dacarbazine, dactinomycin, daunorubicin, docetaxel, doxorubicin, epirubicin, eribulin, etoposide, 5-FU, hydroxyurea, ifosfamide, ixabepilone, methotrexate, paclitaxel	Alopecia: Axitinib, dabrafenib, dasatinib, eribulin, erlotinib, gefitinib, lapatinib, nilotinib, pazopanib, pegylated IFN alfa-2b, sorafenib, vemurafenib Alopecia, hirsutism, and hypertrichosis: Everolimus Hair color changes and alopecia: Cabozantinib, pazopanib, sunitinib Hair color changes: Imatinib	Cetuximab, panitumumab
Trichomegaly	Increased hair growth of the eyelashes and eyebrows is rare but can occur. Trichomegaly is associated with patient discomfort and can lead to corneal abrasions and further ocular complications. Ocular changes may occur within 1–2 weeks of treatment. Trichomegaly can be treated with lash clipping every 2–4 weeks. Referral to an ophthalmologist is indicated for patients with irritation or persistent discomfort. Topical eflornithine cream has been well tolerated.	Gemcitabine	Erlotinib, gefitinib, IFN alfa-2b	Cetuximab, panitumumab
Paronychia	Paronychia is characterized by tender, edematous, often purulent inflammation of the nail fold. Fingernails and toenails may be affected, with the first digits the most commonly affected. It often is delayed, developing 4–8 weeks after the start of therapy and occurring in 10%–15% of patients. Encourage preventive measures, such as keeping hands dry and out of water if possible, wearing gloves while cleaning (e.g., household, dishes), avoiding friction and pressure on the nail fold or manipulation of the nail, and wearing comfortable shoes. Treatment includes topical steroids with antiseptic soaks to prevent infections.	Bleomycin, cyclophosphamide, docetaxel, doxorubicin, hydroxyurea, methotrexate	Afatinib, erlotinib, gefitinib, lapatinib	Cetuximab, necitumumab, panitumumab

(Continued on next page)

Table 21-1. Cutaneous Reactions to Antineoplastic Agents *(Continued)*

Cutaneous Reaction	General Comments	Chemotherapy	Targeted Therapy	Immunotherapy
Nail changes	–	Cyclophosphamide, daunorubicin, docetaxel, doxorubicin, ifosfamide	Gefitinib, osimertinib, sorafenib, sunitinib, temsirolimus	Cetuximab, panitumumab
Nail shedding (onycholysis)	Loss of all or a portion of the nail	Bleomycin, capecitabine, cisplatin, cyclophosphamide, docetaxel, doxorubicin, etoposide, hydroxyurea, ixabepilone, melphalan, mitoxantrone, topical 5-FU, vinblastine, vincristine, weekly paclitaxel administration	Everolimus	–
Dystrophy	Dystrophy is a transverse midline linear groove in the nail plate.	Bleomycin, hydroxyurea	Dystrophy and nail changes are common with EGFRIs.	–
Beau lines	Beau lines are transverse ridges across the nail plate. These findings are benign, dose related, and resolve with cessation of chemotherapy.	Bleomycin, cisplatin, docetaxel (taxanes), doxorubicin, melphalan, vincristine; capecitabine, hydroxyurea	Beau lines and nail changes are common with EGFRIs.	–
Hyperpigmentation	Hyperpigmentation is the darkening of an area of skin or nails caused by increased melanin. Cutaneous hyperpigmentation associated with chemotherapy can present in localized or generalized patterns affecting the skin, teeth, or nails. Patients should avoid sun exposure or use effective sun barrier preparations to minimize the risk of hyperpigmentation. Sun exposure aggravates hyperpigmentation. It occurs most commonly in people of Mediterranean descent. Darkening may occur within 2–3 weeks of chemotherapy or immunotherapy and persist for months following the completion of therapy. Postinflammatory hyperpigmentation is seen following acneform eruption or other causes of skin inflammation such as eczema or an inflamed sebaceous cyst. No treatment or prevention methods exist, but these changes will usually resolve within months after cessation of therapy.	Bleomycin, busulfan, capecitabine, carboplatin, cisplatin, cyclophosphamide, dacarbazine, dactinomycin, daunorubicin, docetaxel, doxorubicin, etoposide, 5-FU, hydroxyurea, idarubicin, ifosfamide, melphalan, methotrexate, mitomycin C, mitoxantrone, nitrogen mustard, nitrosoureas, oxaliplatin, paclitaxel, prednisolone, 6-mercaptopurine, thiotepa, vincristine Flagellate streaks of hyperpigmentation caused by nails scratching the skin have been reported with parenteral and intrapleural administration of bleomycin.	Imatinib, sunitinib	–

(Continued on next page)

Table 21-1. Cutaneous Reactions to Antineoplastic Agents *(Continued)*

Cutaneous Reaction	General Comments	Chemotherapy	Targeted Therapy	Immunotherapy
Rash	Manifestation of monoclonal antibody–induced skin rash: Rash appears to be dose related and generally evolves within 2–3 weeks of the start of treatment. Tyrosine kinase inhibitors can cause a dose-dependent maculopapular rash that usually affects the trunk and forearms.	Asparaginase, bendamustine HCl, carboplatin, cladribine, cyclophosphamide, cytarabine, dacarbazine, docetaxel, 5-FU, fludarabine, gemcitabine, hydroxyurea, ifosfamide, lomustine, methotrexate, paclitaxel, pemetrexed, pralatrexate, vinblastine, vincristine Cytarabine can cause skin peeling.	Afatinib, axitinib, bortezomib, crizotinib, dabrafenib, dasatinib, eltrombopag, erlotinib, everolimus, gefitinib, imatinib, lapatinib, nilotinib, pazopanib, romidepsin, sorafenib, sunitinib, trametinib, vandetanib, vemurafenib	Atezolizumab, cetuximab, denosumab, ipilimumab, lenalidomide, necitumumab, nivolumab, ofatumumab, panitumumab, pegylated IFN alfa-2b, pembrolizumab, pertuzumab, ramucirumab, trastuzumab
Acneform eruptions or papulopustular rash	EGFRI-mediated rashes generally follow a well-characterized clinical course. Within the first week of treatment, patients experience sensory disturbance with erythema and edema; from weeks 1–3, the papulopustular eruption manifests, followed by crusting at week 4. Despite successful treatment, erythema and dry skin may persist in the areas previously affected by skin rash through weeks 4–6. It generally presents as a diffuse erythema over the face and body, progressing to follicular papules and pustules resembling acne. Causative chemotherapy agents should be discontinued. Causative EGFRIs may not need to be discontinued. The disorder is characterized by an eruption consisting of papules (a small, raised pimple) and pustules (a small pus-filled blister), typically appearing on the face, scalp, and upper chest and back. Unlike acne, this rash does not present with whiteheads or blackheads and can be symptomatic, with itchy or tender lesions. See text for grading and management of papulopustular rash.	–	Dabrafenib, erlotinib, everolimus, gefitinib, lapatinib, temsirolimus, trametinib, vandetanib	Cetuximab, panitumumab

(Continued on next page)

Table 21-1. Cutaneous Reactions to Antineoplastic Agents *(Continued)*

Cutaneous Reaction	General Comments	Chemotherapy	Targeted Therapy	Immunotherapy
Erythema multiforme	Condition generally presents as a maculopapular erythematous lesion that may progress to vesicles and also can progress to Stevens-Johnson syndrome and toxic epidermal necrolysis. Record description, presentation, and severity (use a grading scale). Consult with physician regarding possible etiology. Consider discontinuing offending chemotherapy agent. Causative EGFRIs may not need to be discontinued. Examine areas of tissue breakdown, and attend to comfort measures with skin care and pain management strategies (see guidelines in text).	Infrequently associated with chemotherapy. High-dose combination chemotherapy produces highest risk. Characterized by lesions over the extremities and often involving mucous membranes. Bleomycin, busulfan, cytarabine, etoposide, hydroxyurea, methotrexate, and procarbazine are associated with these lesions, which sometimes progress to generalized blistering. Amifostine, cladribine, cyclophosphamide, daunorubicin, doxorubicin, docetaxel, 5-FU, ifosfamide, mechlorethamine, mitomycin C, mitotane, paclitaxel, vinblastine Hormone therapy: Tamoxifen	Gefitinib, vemurafenib	Bexarotene
Skin blistering	–	5-FU, vinblastine	–	IL-2
Xerosis	Xerosis is abnormal dryness of the skin, mucous membranes, or conjunctiva. Treatment of mild or moderate xerosis consists of thick moisturizing creams without fragrances or potential irritants. Moisturizers should be occlusive, emollient creams that are generally packaged in a jar or tub rather than a lotion that can be pumped or poured. Specific creams can include urea, colloidal oatmeal, and petroleum-based creams. For scaly areas of xerosis, ammonium lactate or lactic acid creams can be used. Greasy creams may be used on the limbs for better control of xerosis but should be used with caution on the face, chest, and extremely hairy sites because of the risk for folliculitis secondary to occlusion. For more severe xerosis causing inflammation with or without eczema, topical steroid creams may be necessary. Topical retinoids and benzoyl peroxide gels are not recommended because of their drying effect.	–	Afatinib, axitinib, cabozantinib, dasatinib, erlotinib, everolimus, gefitinib, imatinib, lapatinib, nilotinib, osimertinib, pazopanib, pegylated IFN alfa-2b, regorafenib, sorafenib, sunitinib, temsirolimus, trametinib, trametinib, vandetanib, vemurafenib, vorinostat	Alemtuzumab, bexarotene, cetuximab, necitumumab, panitumumab

(Continued on next page)

Table 21-1. Cutaneous Reactions to Antineoplastic Agents *(Continued)*

Cutaneous Reaction	General Comments	Chemotherapy	Targeted Therapy	Immunotherapy
Painful fissures	Skin fissures and deep cracks in the skin can form as a result of significant xerosis and often occur in the fingertips, palms or knuckles, and the soles. Fissures are a late side effect of EGFRI therapy, occurring around 30–60 days into therapy. They can be very painful and create risk for infection. Cyanoacrylate glue (liquid bandage formulations) may be helpful in protecting the fissures. Treat topically with propylene glycol 50% in water for 30 minutes under plastic occlusion every night, followed by application of hydrocolloid dressing, antiseptic baths, or topical application of silver nitrate. For painful fissures on toes, use protective footwear and a topical corticosteroid, thick moisturizer, or barrier cream (e.g., petroleum jelly, zinc oxide).	–	EGFRI therapy can lead to painful fissures.	Panitumumab
Telangiectasia	Disorder is characterized by local dilation of small vessels resulting in red discoloration of the skin or mucous membranes. Early during the development of acneform eruption or with subsequent flares of the rash, scattered telangiectasia may appear on the face, on and behind the ears, and on the chest, back, and limbs, usually in the vicinity of a follicular pustule. Unlike other telangiectasia, the lesions tend to fade over months, usually leaving some hyperpigmentation. Telangiectasia caused by treatment with EGFRIs, unlike spontaneous telangiectasia, will gradually disappear over months. In select cases, electrocoagulation or pulsed dye laser therapy can be applied to accelerate disappearance. Radiation may cause telangiectasia, which is thought to be related to the destruction of the capillary bed. It generally is considered a permanent change in the vessel.	Topical carmustine and mechlorethamine (nitrogen mustard) cause vessel fragility and destruction.	Scattered telangiectasia can be seen with the development of any acneform eruption caused by EGFRIs.	–

(Continued on next page)

Table 21-1. Cutaneous Reactions to Antineoplastic Agents *(Continued)*

Cutaneous Reaction	General Comments	Chemotherapy	Targeted Therapy	Immunotherapy
Stevens-Johnson syndrome	Stevens-Johnson syndrome (also known as erythema multiforme major) is a rare, serious disorder in which the skin and mucous membranes react severely to a medication or infection. It often begins with flu-like symptoms, followed by a painful red or purplish rash that spreads and blisters, eventually causing the top layer of the skin to die and shed. Stevens-Johnson syndrome presents a medical emergency that usually requires hospitalization. Treatment focuses on eliminating the underlying cause, controlling symptoms, and minimizing complications.	Cases of Stevens-Johnson syndrome and toxic epidermal necrolysis, some fatal, have been reported when bendamustine HCl (Treanda®) was administered concomitantly with allopurinol and other medications known to cause these syndromes. The relationship to Treanda cannot be determined. Stevens-Johnson syndrome has been reported with amifostine, asparaginase, bleomycin, capecitabine, chlorambucil, cladribine, cyclophosphamide, cytarabine, docetaxel, doxorubicin, etoposide, 5-FU, imatinib, methotrexate, paclitaxel, and procarbazine. Hormone therapy: Letrozole	Bortezomib, cetuximab, gefitinib Sunitinib: If signs or symptoms are present, discontinue treatment and do not restart. Vemurafenib: Stevens-Johnson syndrome has been observed. Discontinue drug permanently.	Cetuximab, ipilimumab, lenalidomide, levamisole, rituximab, thalidomide
Toxic epidermal necrolysis	Toxic epidermal necrolysis is most commonly drug induced. However, the disorder has other potential etiologies, including infection, malignancy, and vaccinations. Toxic epidermal necrolysis is idiosyncratic, and its occurrence is not easily predicted. Some authors believe that Stevens-Johnson syndrome is a manifestation of the same process involved in toxic epidermal necrolysis, with the latter involving more extensive necrotic epidermal detachment. Toxic epidermal necrolysis involves > 30% of the body surface, whereas Stevens-Johnson syndrome involves < 10%. It may be hard to distinguish from grade 4 acute GVHD of the skin.	Bendamustine HCl: In combination with rituximab, one case of toxic epidermal necrolysis occurred. Toxic epidermal necrolysis has been reported with rituximab. Report and withhold bendamustine and/or rituximab. Toxic epidermal necrolysis has been reported with asparaginase, chlorambucil, cladribine, cytarabine, docetaxel, doxorubicin, gemcitabine, methotrexate, mithramycin, pemetrexed, procarbazine, and 6-mercaptopurine.	Gefitinib Vemurafenib: Toxic epidermal necrolysis has been observed. Discontinue drug permanently.	Aldesleukin (IL-2), cetuximab, denileukin, ipilimumab

(Continued on next page)

Table 21-1. Cutaneous Reactions to Antineoplastic Agents *(Continued)*

Cutaneous Reaction	General Comments	Chemotherapy	Targeted Therapy	Immunotherapy
Acral erythema	Acral erythema consists of erythema, swelling, and pain of the digits. It usually occurs 1–14 days after treatment starts and lasts for 1–2 weeks. It generally presents as dysesthesia (altered sensation of the skin) with tingling in the hands and feet progressing to pain. After 4 or 5 days of intense edematous erythema and even fissures of the palms, soles, and digital joints, progression to desquamation and reepithelialization occurs. It resolves 5–7 days after therapy is discontinued. The etiology is not clear but may be related to drug concentration in eccrine glands of the palms and soles. Applying cold compresses and elevating the hands and feet during drug administration may minimize the incidence and degree of toxicity. Skin care and comfort measures are instituted as soon as symptoms are evident. Supportive care may include wound dressings, analgesia (pain relief), and cold compresses.	Amsacrine, bleomycin, capecitabine, cyclophosphamide, cytarabine, etoposide, docetaxel, doxorubicin, 5-FU, floxuridine, gemcitabine, hydroxyurea, liposomal doxorubicin, mercaptopurine, methotrexate, mitotane, paclitaxel, teniposide, vinblastine	Axitinib, dasatinib, everolimus, sorafenib, sunitinib	–
Palmar-plantar erythrodysesthesia (hand-foot syndrome)	It first appears as mild redness on the palms and soles with tingling sensations in the hands, usually at the fingertips; symptoms progress to a more intense burning pain and tenderness. Palms and soles appear edematous, and patients may have difficulty walking or grasping objects. Ulceration may occur if therapy is not stopped. Incidence and severity of symptoms are related to protracted exposure of cells to the drug. Symptoms usually develop 2–12 days after administration of chemotherapy. Early recognition and cessation of drug administration are critical to symptom management. Symptoms may include flaking, swelling, small blisters, or small sores. Prevention and treatment include reducing exposure of hands and feet to friction and heat by having patients avoid hot water (washing dishes, long showers, hot baths), impact on their feet (jogging, aerobics, walking, jumping), use of tools that require them to squeeze their hand on a hard surface (garden tools, household tools, kitchen knives), and rubbing (applying lotion, massaging). Dose reduction may minimize the risk of recurrence.	Bleomycin, capecitabine, cisplatin, cyclophosphamide, cytarabine, daunorubicin, docetaxel, doxorubicin, etoposide, 5-FU (given in prolonged infusion), floxuridine, fludarabine, gemcitabine, hydroxyurea, idarubicin, ixabepilone, liposomal encapsulated doxorubicin, methotrexate, mitotane, thiotepa, vinorelbine Incidence of 50% (although reports vary) in patients receiving liposomal encapsulated doxorubicin. Incidence correlates with higher doses and increased number of cycles. Combination therapy: • Docetaxel + capecitabine—56%–63% • Doxorubicin + continuous 5-FU—89%	Hand-foot skin reaction is common with multikinase inhibitors and develops within the first 1–4 weeks of treatment. Axitinib, everolimus, lapatinib, pazopanib, sorafenib, sunitinib	–

(Continued on next page)

Table 21-1. Cutaneous Reactions to Antineoplastic Agents *(Continued)*

Cutaneous Reaction	General Comments	Chemotherapy	Targeted Therapy	Immunotherapy
Photosensitivity	Photosensitivity presents as sunburn occurring after minimal sun exposure. It is an erythematous response to UV radiation; skin appears red with erythema, edema, and possibly vesicles. Patients are instructed to wear protective clothing and a hat when in the sun; avoid direct sunlight when possible, especially during peak hours between 10 am and 3 pm; and avoid tanning beds. They should wear a sunscreen with an SPF higher than 15. In addition to measures taken to avoid sun exposure, patients treated with EGFRIs are advised to wear sunscreen with an SPF of 30 or higher.	Dacarbazine, 5-FU, high-dose methotrexate, vinblastine	Patients treated with EGFRIs may develop photosensitivity characterized by erythema from UV-induced damage. Erythema may be painful and associated with desquamation. In severe cases, photosensitivity and erythema may be disabling or life threatening. Dabrafenib, dasatinib, imatinib, nilotinib, vandetanib, vemurafenib	Cetuximab, panitumumab, tretinoin
Transient erythema or urticaria	Urticaria is characterized as multiple swollen, raised areas on the skin that are intensely itchy and appear primarily on the chest, back, extremities, face, and scalp. It usually occurs within hours of chemotherapy and disappears within a few hours. It may be generalized or local at the site of chemotherapy or along the vein.	Arsenic trioxide, asparaginase, carboplatin, cytarabine, daunorubicin, and prednisolone can cause urticaria. Asparaginase can cause urticaria, fever, chills, and hypotension (skin testing is advised). Bleomycin can cause erythema over pressure points and hyperpigmentation. Chlorambucil, melphalan, methotrexate, and thiotepa can cause urticaria and angioedema. Cytarabine can cause transient erythema. Doxorubicin can cause an erythematous flare with pruritus at the IV site and along the vein. Oxaliplatin can cause delayed urticaria.	The offending agent may need to be discontinued if the reaction is severe or associated with systemic reactions such as a generalized rash. IFN alfa-2a and IFN alfa-2b can cause dry, scaling, itchy skin or a pruritic maculopapular reaction. Dasatinib, sunitinib, vemurafenib	Aldesleukin can cause erythema and pruritus that may progress into a pruritic papular rash. Ofatumumab, panitumumab
Skin depigmentation and vitiligo	Pigment changes occur due to inhibition of c-KIT, which is the protein that regulates melanocytes. Changes may be localized, patchy, or diffuse. They occur more often in darker skin. Effects can be reversed with dose reduction or discontinuation.	–	Dasatinib, imatinib, nilotinib, pazopanib	–

(Continued on next page)

Table 21-1. Cutaneous Reactions to Antineoplastic Agents *(Continued)*

Cutaneous Reaction	General Comments	Chemotherapy	Targeted Therapy	Immunotherapy
Pruritus or itching	Pruritus may be localized or generalized; symptoms may worsen with dehydration. Encourage patients to drink 8–10 glasses of fluid per day and minimize salt and alcohol intake. Recommended skin care includes the use of medicated baths, anesthetic creams, and emollient creams. Mild soap designed for sensitive skin should be used, and perfumes, deodorants, cosmetics, and starch-based powders should be avoided. Massage, pressure, or rubbing with a soft cloth should be suggested instead of scratching. Wearing loose-fitting clothing and clothing made of cotton or other soft fabrics can alleviate pruritus. Use antibiotics if pruritus is secondary to infection. Use oral antihistamines, with increased doses at bedtime. Sedatives, tranquilizers, and antidepressants may be useful treatments. Aspirin seems to reduce itching in some patients but increases it for others. Aspirin combined with cimetidine may be effective for patients with Hodgkin lymphoma or polycythemia vera. Use of distraction, relaxation, positive imagery, or cutaneous stimulation is encouraged. A cool, humid environment may prevent skin from itching. Skin moisturizer and urea- or polidocanol-containing lotions are suitable to soothe pruritus. Systemic treatment with oral H_1-antihistamines such as cetirizine, fexofenadine, or loratadine, as well as clemastine, may provide relief of itching for patients with grade 2–3 pruritus.	Alkylating agents, antimetabolites, antibiotics, plant alkaloids, and nitrosoureas can cause pruritus. Agents most associated with hypersensitivities include cisplatin, cytarabine, daunorubicin, doxorubicin, L-asparaginase, and paclitaxel. Asparaginase, carboplatin, cisplatin, cytarabine, daunorubicin, doxorubicin, etoposide, IFN alfa-2a and IFN alfa-2b, melphalan, and teniposide can all cause a rash. Actinic keratoses: Topical 5-FU, cisplatin, cytarabine, dacarbazine, dactinomycin, docetaxel, doxorubicin, pentostatin, 6-thioguanine, vincristine Bendamustine HCl, pralatrexate	Afatinib, axitinib, dasatinib, erlotinib, gefitinib, imatinib, lapatinib, nilotinib, osimertinib, sorafenib, sunitinib, temsirolimus, trametinib, vandetanib, vemurafenib	Atezolizumab, cetuximab, ipilimumab, necitumumab, nivolumab, panitumumab, pegylated IFN alfa-2b, pembrolizumab

EGFRI—epidermal growth factor receptor inhibitor; 5-FU—5-fluorouracil; GVHD—graft-versus-host disease; HCl—hydrochloride; IFN—interferon; IL—interleukin; IV—intravenous; SPF—sun protection factor; UV—ultraviolet

Note. Based on information from Amgen Inc., 2017; Anforth et al., 2015; AstraZeneca Pharmaceuticals LP, 2015, 2016, 2017; Bayer HealthCare Pharmaceuticals Inc., 2015; Bouché et al., 2005; Boucher et al., 2011; Bristol-Myers Squibb Co., 2015; Caccavale & Ruocco, 2017; Camp-Sorrell, 2018; Cephalon, Inc., 2016; Chon et al., 2012; Degen et al., 2010; Fabbrocini et al., 2015; Genentech, Inc., 2016, 2017; Genentech, Inc., & Astellas Pharma US, Inc., 2016; Gill & Dominguez, 2016; GlaxoSmithKline, 2017; Hoffmann-La Roche Inc., 2008; Huang & Anadkat, 2011; ImClone LLC, 2016; Kamil et al., 2010; Kaur & Mahajan, 2015; Kheir et al., 2014; Lacouture et al., 2010, 2011; Ligand Pharmaceuticals Inc., 2015, Lupu et al., 2016; Merck and Co., Inc., 2015; Morse, 2014; National Cancer Institute, 2016; Novartis Pharmaceuticals Corp., 2016, 2017a, 2017b; Pfizer Inc., 2017; Potthoff et al., 2011; Prometheus Laboratories Inc., 2015; Reyes-Habito & Roh, 2014b; Rosen et al., 2014; Sanofi-Aventis U.S. LLC, 2015; Segaert & Van Cutsem, 2005; Shi et al., 2016; Sibaud et al., 2016; Thebeau et al., 2017; Tischer et al., 2017; Tummino et al., 2007; Valentine et al., 2015; Villée et al., 2010; White & Cox, 2006; Wolters Kluwer Health, 2017; Wu et al., 2011; Wyeth Pharmaceuticals Inc., 2017.

frequently, the elbows, knees, and ears are involved (Shi et al., 2016).

(b) Patches or plaques typically develop within two days to three weeks following drug administration. Associated symptoms of pain, burning, paresthesia, and pruritus are frequently present. Areas of intense erythema can be accompanied by development of a dusky discoloration, petechiae, or sterile bullae, which can be followed by erosions. Typically, spontaneous resolution and desquamation occur without specific therapy, and if the chemotherapy agent is given again at the same or higher dose, recurrences are possible and may be more intense with higher doses. In certain cases, a delayed onset of 2–10 months can be seen, particularly in patients receiving lower-dose, continuous IV infusions (Shi et al., 2016).

(c) Treatment options for TEC have been of variable success and include bland emollients, analgesics, cool compresses, topical corticosteroids, and topical antibiotics for erosions. It is important for nurses, oncologists, and dermatologists to recognize TEC, understanding that the reaction is not allergic or infectious in nature and thus avoiding unnecessary labeling of drug allergies or use of antimicrobials (Shi et al., 2016).

b) Epidermal growth factor receptor (EGFR) inhibitors (EGFRIs), which can include both targeted agents (e.g., gefitinib, erlotinib, lapatinib, afatinib) and monoclonal antibodies (e.g., cetuximab, panitumumab)

(1) EGFRIs are associated with many cutaneous reactions due to the prevention of epidermal keratinocytes from controlling the intercellular signal transduction pathways, which control cell proliferation, apoptosis, angiogenesis, adhesion, and motility (Wallner, Köck-Hódi, Booze, White, & Mayer, 2016). More than 80% of patients will have a cutaneous reaction from treatment with EGFRIs (Wallner et al., 2016).

(2) Skin toxicities from EGFRIs include acneform eruption; xerosis; paronychia; abnormal scalp, facial hair, and eyelash growth; maculopapular rash; and postinflammatory hyperpigmentation (see Figure 21-1). EGFRI cutaneous reactions are labeled as PRIDE syndrome (papulopustules and/or paronychia, regulatory abnormalities of hair growth, itching, and dryness due to an EGFRI) (Lupu et al., 2016).

(3) Acneform eruption is the most common reaction associated with EGFRIs. The presentation can be divided into four stages, beginning with sensory disturbance accompanied by edema and erythema. The characteristic rash of papules and pustules, which is predominantly but not exclusively folliculocentric in distribution, appears subsequently. This is followed by a postinflammatory phase of erythema and telangiectasias. For patients with darker skin tone, a fourth phase of postinflammatory hyperpigmentation may be present and can be long lasting. Most patients will have complete or significant resolution despite continuing treatment with EGFRIs, and the rash will completely disappear one month after the end of treatment (Lupu et al., 2016).

(4) Refer to Figure 21-2 for treatment options.

(5) Patients who are also being treated with radiation therapy have an increased risk of developing severe radiation dermatitis (Wolters Kluwer Health, 2017). Prophylactic antibiotics have been shown to prevent the rash from occurring (Lacouture, 2015).

c) Multikinase inhibitors

(1) The multikinase inhibitors sorafenib and sunitinib cause cutaneous reactions in 74% and 81% of patients, respectively. The pathophysiology is unknown but thought to be related to vessel damage or extravasation of the drug (Reyes-Habito & Roh, 2014b).

(2) Skin toxicities from multikinase inhibitors include hand-foot skin reaction, rash, pruritus, subungual splinter hemorrhage, yellow skin discoloration, hair depigmentation, pigment dilution, scrotal erythema, and nail splinter hemorrhage (Shi et al., 2016).

Figure 21-1. Pustular/Papular Rash Presentations

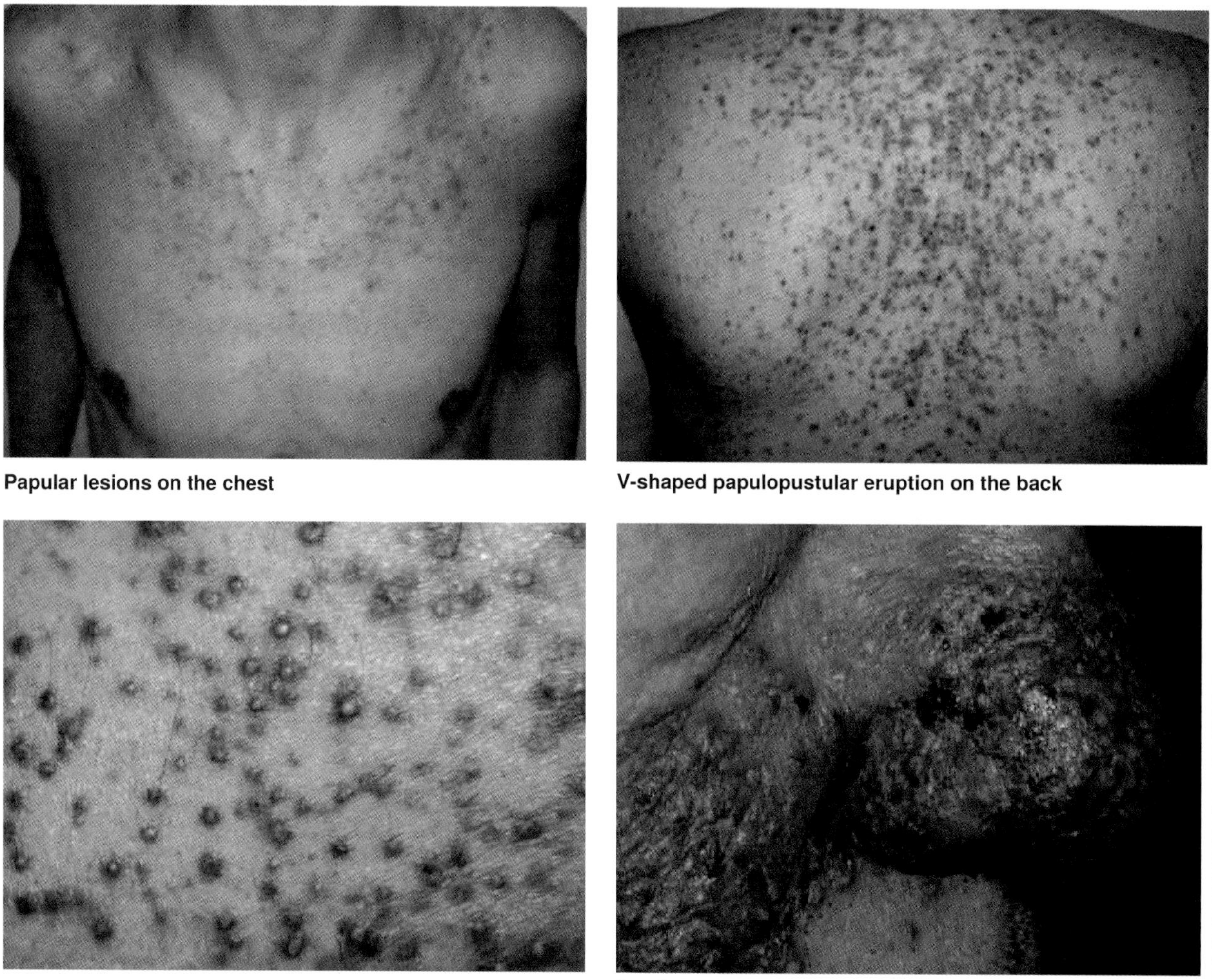

Papular lesions on the chest

V-shaped papulopustular eruption on the back

Follicular pustules

Confluent pustules on the nose

Note. From "Clinical Signs, Pathophysiology and Management of Skin Toxicity During Therapy With Epidermal Growth Factor Receptor Inhibitors," by S. Segaert and E. Van Cutsem, 2005, *Annals of Oncology, 16,* p. 1427. Copyright 2005 by European Society for Medical Oncology. Reprinted with permission.

(3) Hand-foot skin reaction, which differs from the classical hand-foot syndrome seen with nontargeted chemotherapy, presents in the first two to four weeks of treatment with the development of localized painful, symmetric erythematous plaques on palms and soles (Shi et al., 2016). Symptoms of hand-foot skin reaction can include paresthesia, tingling, burning, and painful sensation in the palms and soles. Prior to treatment, prophylactic measures can be taken, including pretreatment pedicure, orthotic evaluation, reduced exposure of hands and feet to heat, and avoidance of excessive friction. One randomized study showed that prophylactic celecoxib 200 mg/day reduced the incidence of grade 2 or greater hand-foot skin reaction in patients receiving capecitabine by more than 50% (Lacouture, 2015).

(4) Treatment of hand-foot skin reaction includes keratolytics such as urea 20%–40% cream, topical corticosteroids, topical retinoids, and topical analgesics, which can reduce symptoms (Shi et al., 2016).

d) BRAF inhibitors (e.g., dabrafenib, vemurafenib) and MEK inhibitors (e.g., selumetinib, trametinib)

(1) Dermatologic side effects are the most common adverse events seen with

Figure 21-2. Recommendations for Prevention and Management of Epidermal Growth Factor Receptor Inhibitor–Induced Rash

Multinational Association of Supportive Care in Cancer

Preventive/Prophylactic
- Systemic: Minocycline 100 mg daily[a] or doxycycline 100 mg BID[b]
- Topical: Hydrocortisone 1% cream with moisturizer and sunscreen BID

Treatment
- Topical
  - Alclometasone 0.05% cream
  - Fluocinonide 0.05% cream BID
  - Clindamycin 1%
- Systemic
  - Doxycycline 100 mg BID
  - Minocycline 100 mg daily
  - Isotretinoin at low doses of 20–30 mg/day

National Comprehensive Cancer Network

Preventive/Prophylactic
- Systemic
  - Oral semisynthetic tetracycline agents (doxycycline or minocycline)
  - Doxycycline 100 mg BID in combination with the following topical agents
- Topical: Hydrocortisone 1%, skin moisturizer, and sunscreen

Treatment
- Topical: Topical steroids and antibiotics, such as clindamycin and erythromycin, may be useful.
- Systemic
  - Oral antibiotics include doxycycline or minocycline.
  - Systemic steroids are not typically used, but published case reports have suggested their use in specific settings.
  - Administer isotretinoin reactively (based on anecdotal or nonrandomized studies).

Not Recommended

Acitretin, oil-in-water topical trolamine emulsion, pimecrolimus 1% cream, sunscreen as a single agent, tazarotene 0.05% cream, tetracycline 500 mg BID, vitamin K_1 cream

[a] Minocycline is less photosensitizing.

[b] Doxycycline should be used in patients with renal impairment.

BID—twice daily

Note. Based on information from Burtness et al., 2009; Eaby-Sandy et al., 2012; Lacouture et al., 2011.

BRAF inhibitors. Pathophysiology is thought to be hypersensitivity reaction (Shi et al., 2016).

(2) The most common dermatologic side effect is rash, which can be maculopapular, papulopustular, or folliculocentric and appears most often on the face, upper torso, and arms. Other cutaneous reactions include photosensitivity, which usually occurs within 24 hours of sun exposure and can include painful blistering. It is important to provide patient education related to good sun protection. Squamoproliferative lesions are also common and can present as skin papillomas, verrucous keratosis, and seborrheic keratosis. Vemurafenib or dabrafenib have been associated with keratoacanthomas or squamous cell carcinomas, as well as melanocytic changes with all BRAF inhibitors, so regular dermatologic follow-up is recommended for these patients. Other dermatologic effects include hand-foot skin reaction and altered hair growth. MEK inhibitors have similar cutaneous effects as seen with EGFRIs, including papulopustular eruption, most commonly on the scalp, face, chest, and back; xerosis; and pruritus (Shi et al., 2016).

(3) Treatment for rash includes topical antibiotics, oral antibiotics, and topical corticosteroids. Treatments for squamoproliferative lesions include shave removal and cryotherapy (Shi et al., 2016).

e) Immunotherapies

(1) Cytotoxic T-lymphocyte antigen 4 (known as CTLA-4) inhibitors such as ipilimumab are commonly associated with rash, usually occurring in the first three to four weeks. The rash is typically erythematous macules and papules that coalesce into thick plaques on the extremities and trunk. Vitiligo also can occur (Shi et al., 2016).

(2) The cutaneous adverse effects of programmed cell death protein 1 (PD-1) inhibitors, such as nivolumab and pembrolizumab, and programmed cell death-ligand 1 (PD-L1) inhibitors, such as atezolizumab, have yet to be fully described but are known to include vitiligo, rash, and pruritus. Cutaneous complications most often

are mild and easily managed with supportive care (Sibaud et al., 2016). The rash is a lichenoid rash and presents with erythematous papules and plaques on the chest, back, abdomen, and extremities. The most common rash occurring from PD-1 inhibitor therapy is a nonspecific maculopapular rash occurring most often on the trunk and extremities (see Figures 21-3 through 21-5). PD-L1 inhibitors may have a slightly lower incidence of rash than PD-1 inhibitors (Sibaud et al., 2016).

(3) Treatment includes topical corticosteroids for low-grade eruptions and systemic corticosteroids for high-grade eruptions (Shi et al., 2016).

f) Combination radiation and targeted therapy

(1) Significant in-field toxicity can occur when radiation therapy and targeted agents are given concomitantly (Lacouture, 2015).

(2) The best prevention for radiation dermatitis is to wash with soap and water. This can prevent the risk of radiation dermatitis by half (Lacouture, 2015).

(3) Topical nonsteroidal agents and moisturizer can significantly reduce discomfort, redness, and itching (Lacouture, 2015).

g) Chemotherapy agents associated with radiation enhancement and radiation recall

(1) Radiation enhancement: Bleomycin, capecitabine, chlorambucil, dacti-

Figure 21-3. Immunotherapy-Mediated Rash: Metastatic Melanoma

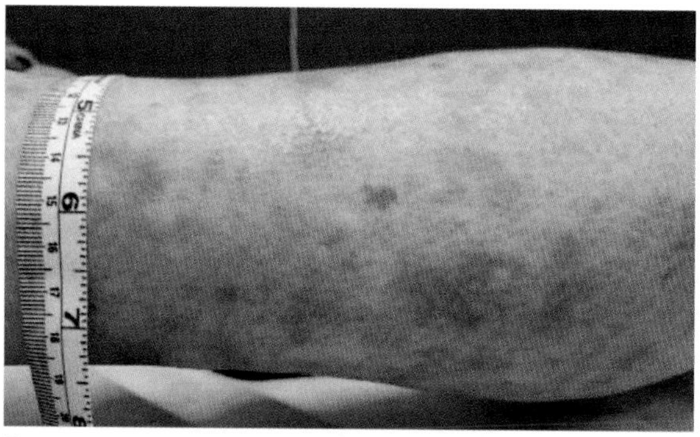

Patient is a 67-year-old woman with metastatic melanoma status post 3 doses of pembrolizumab with diffuse rash to bilateral legs.

Note. Image courtesy of Johns Hopkins Hospital. Used with permission.

Figure 21-4. Immunotherapy-Mediated Rash: Merkel Cell Carcinoma

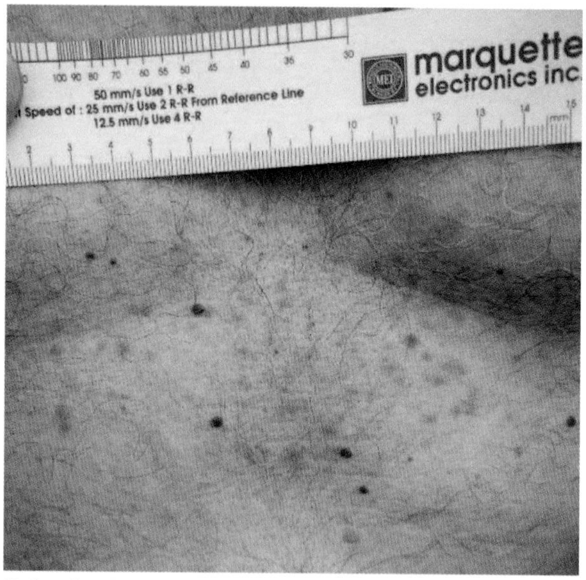

Patient is a 71-year-old man with Merkel cell carcinoma status post 22 doses of every-3-week pembrolizumab.

Note. Image courtesy of Johns Hopkins Hospital. Used with permission.

Figure 21-5. Immunotherapy-Mediated Rash: Full-Body Rash

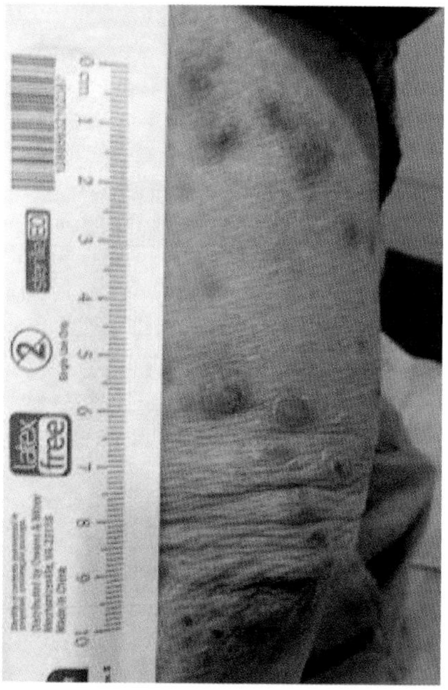

Patient is a 59-year-old man with prostate cancer with biopsy-proven immune-mediated full-body rash after 4 doses of a PD-1 inhibitor, with oral mucositis requiring steroids and discontinuation of immunotherapy.

Note. Image courtesy of Johns Hopkins Hospital. Used with permission.

nomycin, doxorubicin, 5-FU with and without cisplatin, gemcitabine, hydroxyurea, methotrexate, paclitaxel, and 6-mercaptopurine (Wolters Kluwer Health, 2017)

(2) Radiation recall: Arsenic trioxide, bleomycin, capecitabine, cyclophosphamide, cytarabine, dactinomycin, daunorubicin, docetaxel, doxorubicin (free and liposomal), etoposide, 5-FU, gemcitabine, hydroxyurea, idarubicin, lomustine, melphalan, methotrexate, paclitaxel, pemetrexed, tamoxifen, and vinblastine (Wolters Kluwer Health, 2017)

(3) See Figures 21-6 through 21-9 for examples of specific cutaneous manifestations of EGFRI- and chemotherapy-induced toxicities.

3. Assessment

a) Accurate grading of dermatologic adverse events is necessary for drug toxicity determination, integrant comparisons, and supportive grading scale. The Common Terminology Criteria for Adverse Events (CTCAE) (National Cancer Institute Cancer Therapy Evaluation Program, 2017; see Table 21-2) is widely accepted throughout the oncology community as the standard classification and severity grading scale for adverse events in cancer therapy clinical trials and other oncology settings. However, it was not designed specifically for the newer agents and may result in underreporting and poor grading of distinctive adverse events (Wallner et al., 2016).

b) The Multinational Association of Supportive Care in Cancer Study Group has proposed a new grading scale for EGFRI-induced dermatologic adverse events. The group believes that a class-specific grading scale is needed to help standardize assessment and improve reporting of these dermatologic adverse events (Lacouture, 2015).

Figure 21-6. Trichomegaly

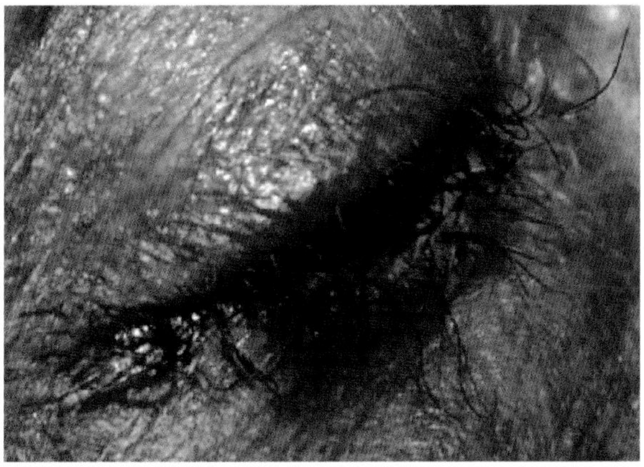

Note. From "Clinical Signs, Pathophysiology and Management of Skin Toxicity During Therapy With Epidermal Growth Factor Receptor Inhibitors," by S. Segaert and E. Van Cutsem, 2005, *Annals of Oncology, 16,* p. 1428. Copyright 2005 by European Society for Medical Oncology. Reprinted with permission.

Figure 21-7. Paronychia of the Nail

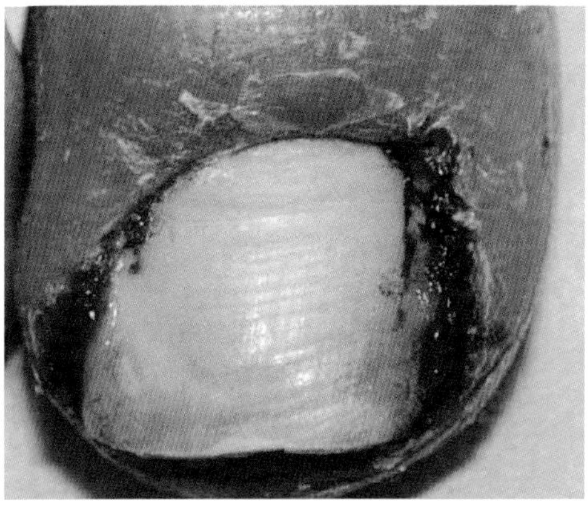

Note. From "Clinical Signs, Pathophysiology and Management of Skin Toxicity During Therapy With Epidermal Growth Factor Receptor Inhibitors," by S. Segaert and E. Van Cutsem, 2005, *Annals of Oncology, 16,* p. 1428. Copyright 2005 by European Society for Medical Oncology. Reprinted with permission.

Figure 21-8. Hyperpigmentation

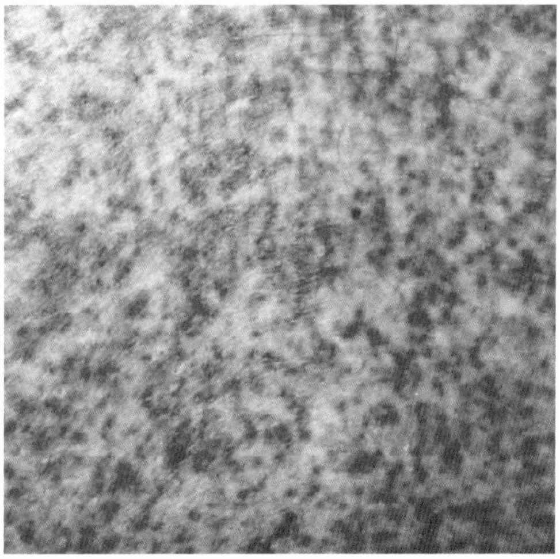

Note. From "Clinical Signs, Pathophysiology and Management of Skin Toxicity During Therapy With Epidermal Growth Factor Receptor Inhibitors," by S. Segaert and E. Van Cutsem, 2005, *Annals of Oncology, 16,* p. 1429. Copyright 2005 by European Society for Medical Oncology. Reprinted with permission.

Figure 21-9. Fissure

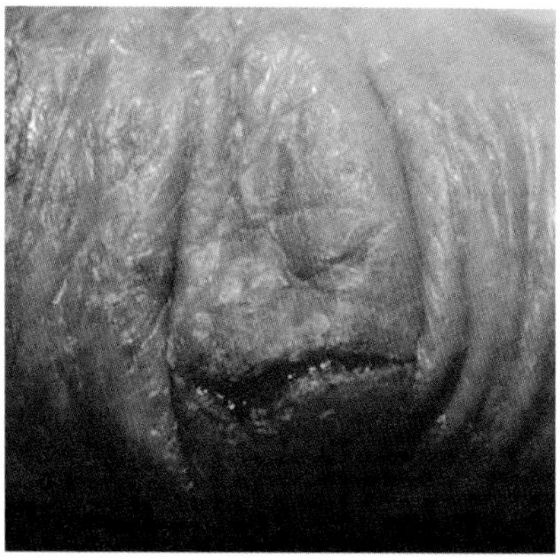

Note. From "Clinical Signs, Pathophysiology and Management of Skin Toxicity During Therapy With Epidermal Growth Factor Receptor Inhibitors," by S. Segaert and E. Van Cutsem, 2005, *Annals of Oncology, 16,* p. 1428. Copyright 2005 by European Society for Medical Oncology. Reprinted with permission

4. Collaborative management
   a) General management
      (1) Prior to initiation of therapy, a full medical history should be taken, including a history of prior or active skin diseases. Partner with an interprofessional team and refer patients to a dermatologist if necessary. Provide patient education regarding reporting of any adverse events (Thebeau et al., 2017).
      (2) Skin reactions are associated with significant morbidity and can lead to dose reductions or premature discontinuation of chemotherapy. The adverse effect of cutaneous reactions on patients' quality of life is only beginning to be understood. The use of patient-reported outcome questionnaires should be included in routine clinical care to improve the accuracy of reported adverse events (Tischer, Huber, Kraemer, & Lacouture, 2017).
      (3) Treatment of rash is largely dependent on symptoms. Intervention should be recommended based on the severity of the symptoms, with the goal of alleviation or minimization (Thebeau et al., 2017).
      (4) Instruct patients to avoid sun exposure. They should apply sunscreen daily to exposed skin areas regardless of the season. Sunscreens with the following characteristics are recommended: hypoallergenic, high sun protection factor (at least 30), PABA free, UVA and UVB protection (broad spectrum), and containing zinc oxide or titanium dioxide. Recommend that patients wear a hat and protective clothing for sun protection (Fabbrocini, Panariello, Caro, & Monfrecola, 2015).
   b) Secondary infection: Secondary bacterial, viral, or fungal infection occurs in 40% of patients taking EGFRIs. Providers should have a low threshold for sending cultures of any lesions that have signs of infection, such as discharge. Although secondary infections can occur in any patient with cutaneous toxicity, they are most common with EGFRI rashes (Lacouture, 2015).
   c) Rash and response/survival
      (1) Incidence and severity of papulopustular rashes are associated with a better prognosis and therefore are considered to predict response of a tumor to the EGFRI. Studies addressing EGFRI-induced rash suggest that its severity is a surrogate marker for efficacy of the therapy (Tischer et al., 2017).
      (2) Data suggest a correlation of rash incidence and severity with clinical response and increased survival time, leading investigators to implement "dose-to-rash" strategies, in which a patient's EGFRI dose is progressively escalated until rash of a specified grade appears. A consistent relationship between rash and response has not been observed with all EGFRIs studied in clinical trials to date (Tischer et al., 2017).
   d) Psychosocial issues
      (1) Skin toxicities from antineoplastic therapy can have a significant impact on patients' physical, emotional, and social function. Patients are at risk for low self-esteem, altered self-image, depression, anxiety, and vulnerability. These side effects may interfere with treatment adherence, but patients may accept them as part of their experience with cancer or as a sign of response to therapy (Charalambous & Charalambous, 2016).
      (2) Cutaneous toxicity effects on quality of life (Charalambous & Charalambous, 2016)

Table 21-2. Common Terminology Criteria for Adverse Events Grading Relevant to Targeted Therapy–Associated Dermatologic Toxicity

	Grade				
Adverse Event	1	2	3	4	5
Alopecia	Hair loss of < 50% of normal for that individual that is not obvious from a distance but only on close inspection; a different hairstyle may be required to cover the hair loss but it does not require a wig or hairpiece to camouflage	Hair loss of ≥ 50% of normal for that individual that is readily apparent to others; a wig or hairpiece is necessary if the patient desires to completely camouflage the hair loss; associated with psychosocial impact	–	–	–
Dry skin	Covering < 10% BSA and no associated erythema or pruritus	Covering 10%–30% BSA and associated with erythema or pruritus; limiting instrumental ADL	Covering > 30% BSA and associated with pruritus; limiting self-care ADL	–	–
Paronychia	Nail fold edema or erythema; disruption of the cuticle	Localized intervention indicated; oral intervention indicated (e.g., antibiotic, antifungal, antiviral); nail fold edema or erythema with pain; associated with discharge or nail plate separation; limiting instrumental ADL	Operative intervention indicated; IV antibiotics indicated; limiting self-care ADL	–	–
Pruritus	Mild or localized; topical intervention indicated	Widespread and intermittent; skin changes from scratching (e.g., edema, papulation, excoriations, lichenification, oozing/crusts); oral intervention indicated; limiting instrumental ADL	Widespread and constant; limiting self-care ADL or sleep; systemic corticosteroid or immunosuppressive therapy indicated	–	–
Rash acneform	Papules and/or pustules covering < 10% BSA, which may or may not be associated with symptoms of pruritus or tenderness	Papules and/or pustules covering 10%–30% BSA, which may or may not be associated with symptoms of pruritus or tenderness; associated with psychosocial impact; limiting instrumental ADL; papules and/or pustules covering > 30% BSA with or without mild symptoms	Papules and/or pustules covering > 30% BSA with moderate or severe symptoms; limiting self-care ADL; associated with local superinfection with oral antibiotics indicated	Life-threatening consequences; papules and/or pustules covering any % BSA, which may or may not be associated with symptoms of pruritus or tenderness and are associated with extensive superinfection with IV antibiotics indicated	Death
Rash maculopapular	Macules/papules covering < 10% BSA with or without symptoms (e.g., pruritus, burning, tightness)	Macules/papules covering 10%–30% BSA with or without symptoms (e.g., pruritus, burning, tightness); limiting instrumental ADL; rash covering > 30% BSA with or without mild symptoms	Macules/papules covering > 30% BSA with moderate or severe symptoms; limiting self-care ADL	–	–

ADL—activities of daily living; BSA—body surface area; IV—intravenous

Note. From *Common Terminology Criteria for Adverse Events* [v.5.0], by National Cancer Institute Cancer Therapy Evaluation Program, 2017. Retrieved from https://ctep.cancer.gov/protocoldevelopment/electronic_applications/docs/CTCAE_v5_Quick_Reference_5x7.pdf.

(a) Loss of dignity
(b) Hopelessness
(c) Living in fear
(d) Isolation
(e) Feeling insecure
(f) Loss of independence

5. Patient and family education
   a) Instruct patients about the potential treatment-related symptoms of dermatologic toxicities as part of supportive measures (Thebeau et al., 2017; Wallner et al., 2016).
   b) Include information about the potential toxicities associated with the agent being used.
   c) Provide information on preventive and management measures.
   d) Ensure that family and other support systems (friends, clergy, visiting nurses, homecare personnel) can provide encouragement to patients to help rebuild their self-esteem and self-belief. Discuss the potential for anxiety or depression.
   e) Perform follow-up phone calls to promote communication with patients regarding their treatment experience. It is an opportunity for nurses to educate and give supportive care.

B. Alopecia

1. Overview: Alopecia is one of the most common and distressing side effects of chemotherapy. Hair loss has been identified as the most traumatic aspect of chemotherapy by 77% of patients (Ron, Kalmus, Kalmus, Inbar, & Chaitchik, 1997). A portion of these patients may choose not to receive chemotherapy because of an intense fear of this side effect (Ross & Fischer-Cartlidge, 2017). In young adults aged 18–38 years, men and women reported equally negative experiences related to chemotherapy-induced alopecia (Chon, Champion, Geddes, & Rashid, 2012). Chemotherapy-induced alopecia most commonly occurs on the scalp; however, it can occur anywhere on the body, including facial (beards, eyebrows, eyelashes), axillary, and pubic hair. Chemotherapy-induced alopecia negatively affects an individual's perceptions of body image, sexuality, and self-esteem.
2. Pathophysiology
   a) The pathobiology of the response of human hair follicles to chemotherapy remains largely unknown. Cells responsible for hair growth have high mitotic and metabolic rates. Certain cytotoxic agents disrupt the proliferative phase of hair growth. Approximately 90% of hair follicles on the scalp are in the anagen (growth) phase of the hair cycle at any given time (Fabbrocini et al., 2015).
   b) Two major types of chemotherapy-induced alopecia exist: telogen effluvium and anagen effluvium.
      (1) Telogen effluvium involves less than 50% of the scalp and results in hair thinning. Hair enters the telogen, or resting, phase and results in shedding three to four months after drug administration. Antineoplastic drugs that can cause this type of alopecia are methotrexate, 5-FU, and retinoids (Paus, Haslam, Sharov, & Botchkarev, 2013).
      (2) Anagen effluvium is the most common form of chemotherapy-induced alopecia. Because most hair follicles are in the anagen (growth) phase, chemotherapy damages these rapidly growing cells, leading to damage of the inner root sheath cells or the hair shaft integrity. The hair shaft is no longer anchored and falls out easily or breaks off at the scalp. Hair falls out spontaneously or during washing or combing. Chemotherapy agents such as cyclophosphamide, daunorubicin, doxorubicin, etoposide, ifosfamide, and paclitaxel are associated with this type of damage. The hairs remain in the telogen phase after damage occurs until the chemotherapy is completed, at which time they can enter the anagen phase again, and hair regrowth resumes (Paus et al., 2013).
3. Incidence
   a) As many as 65% of patients receiving chemotherapy will experience alopecia to some degree (Chon et al., 2012). The overall risk is lower in patients receiving targeted therapies, with the incidence at 14.7% (Belum et al., 2015).
   b) The extent of alopecia depends on the mechanism of action of the drug, administration route, drug dose, serum half-life, duration (e.g., bolus vs. continuous infusion), the response of the patient, the use of combination chemotherapy, and the condition of the hair prior to treatment (Chon et al., 2012).
4. Risk factors
   a) Type of antineoplastic drugs administered
      (1) The drugs that present the highest risk of alopecia are camptothecins, cyclophosphamide, daunorubicin, docetaxel, doxorubicin, epirubicin,

etoposide, ifosfamide, paclitaxel, and vinorelbine (Fabbrocini et al., 2015; see Table 21-3).

(2) Combination chemotherapy is associated with a higher incidence of alopecia than single-agent therapy (Fabbrocini et al., 2015).

(3) Molecularly targeted agents, such as monoclonal antibodies, which target EGFR, and small molecule inhibitors of EGFR, have been associated with diffuse alopecia that is generally reversible (Lacouture, 2015).

(4) Multitargeted tyrosine kinase inhibitors (e.g., sorafenib, sunitinib) have been associated with alopecia, although incidence is lower than with chemotherapy (Lacouture, 2015).

b) Certain noncytotoxic medications (e.g., propranolol hydrochloride, heparin sodium, lithium carbonate, prednisone, vitamin A, androgen preparations)

c) Certain medical conditions (e.g., hypothyroidism, aging)

d) Poor hair condition before cytotoxic treatment

e) Concomitant or previous radiation therapy to the head (local effect)

5. Clinical manifestations

a) Scalp dryness, soreness, pruritus, and rash can occur before, during, or after hair loss.

b) Expected time frame and pattern (Fabbrocini et al., 2015)

(1) Hair shedding begins approximately one to three weeks after administration of the drug and may last one to two months after initiation of therapy.

(2) Pattern: Hair loss tends to occur first on the crown and sides of head above the ears.

(3) Chemotherapy-induced alopecia generally is reversible.

(4) Hair regrowth begins one to three months after discontinuation of chemotherapy.

(5) Regrown hair may demonstrate changes in color, structure, or texture, and in some patients, hair density may continue to be reduced after treatment (Paus et al., 2013).

(6) Permanent alopecia following chemotherapy, although rare, can occur with high-dose busulfan and cyclophosphamide following hematopoietic stem cell transplantation, long-term use of EGFRIs, and treatment with taxanes (Fabbrocini et al., 2015; Fonia et al., 2017).

6. Assessment: See Table 21-2 for CTCAE grading for alopecia.

7. Collaborative management: Alopecia is a constant reminder of disease and greatly affects patients' sense of self. Patients may experience privacy issues because alopecia often is associated with having cancer.

Table 21-3. Risk of Chemotherapy-Induced Alopecia for Antineoplastic Agents

Classification	High Risk	Moderate Risk	Mild Risk
Chemotherapy agents	Cyclophosphamide Daunorubicin Docetaxel Doxorubicin Epirubicin Eribulin Etoposide Ifosfamide Irinotecan Ixabepilone Paclitaxel Topotecan Vinorelbine	Amsacrine Busulfan Carboplatin (AUC 5–6) Cytarabine Gemcitabine Mechlorethamine Methotrexate Oxaliplatin	Bleomycin Capecitabine Carboplatin (weekly) Cisplatin Cyclophosphamide (oral) 5-Fluorouracil Fludarabine Hydroxyurea Mitoxantrone Thiotepa Vinblastine Vincristine
Immunotherapy agents	–	Cetuximab	–
Targeted therapy agents	–	Dabrafenib Vemurafenib	Dasatinib Pazopanib

AUC—area under the plasma concentration versus time curve

Note. Based on information from Rugo et al., 2017; Wolters Kluwer Health, 2017.

a) Currently, no approved pharmacologic treatment is available for prevention of alopecia caused by cytotoxic therapy. Multiple pharmacologic and biologic therapies are being studied, such as epidermal growth factor, keratinocyte growth factor, cytokines, antioxidants, and apoptosis inhibitors (Paus et al., 2013).

b) Scalp cooling is a strategy created to prevent or limit chemotherapy-induced alopecia. It is routinely used in the United Kingdom, France, Netherlands, and Canada and has been around for more than 40 years.

(1) The process works by inducing vasoconstriction and decreased follicle metabolism. The decreased blood flow to the hair follicles limits the uptake of the chemotherapy agents, and decreased metabolism makes the follicles less susceptible to damage from the chemotherapy agent.

(2) Scalp cooling has been shown to be effective in reducing chemotherapy-induced alopecia (Ross & Fischer-Cartlidge, 2017). Previously, scalp cooling was not recommended, because of concerns of scalp metastasis and secondary seeding to other organs from cancer cells that remained in the scalp. However, a literature review found a lack of data showing any concern for scalp metastases or secondary seeding.

(3) The majority of patients who have been studied at this time are patients with breast cancer (Ross & Fischer-Cartlidge, 2017). A recent prospective cohort study conducted at five U.S. medical centers in women with breast cancer found that the use of scalp cooling was associated with less hair loss four weeks after the last dose of chemotherapy (Rugo et al., 2017). The study also found that quality-of-life measures were better in the group that received scalp cooling (Rugo et al., 2017).

(4) Contraindications exist for scalp cooling and include patients with known hematologic malignancies because of reports of scalp metastasis and lack of safety data, as well as patients with cold sensitivity, cold agglutinin disease, cryoglobulinemia, and cryofibrinogenemia. Patients may experience headaches, excessive coldness, or feelings of claustrophobia (Rugo et al., 2017).

(5) Four systematic reviews looking at percentage of successful hair preservation showed success rates of 10%–100%, with the majority around 50% (Ross & Fischer-Cartlidge, 2017). Another systematic review found that the use of scalp cooling decreased relative risk of alopecia by 43% (Rugo & Voigt, 2018).

(6) The U.S. Food and Drug Administration approved the DigniCap® Scalp Cooling System and the Paxman Scalp Cooler to be used in patients with solid tumors (U.S. Food and Drug Administration, 2017).

(a) The DigniCap system gradually decreases from room temperature to the target temperature of 37°F–41°F (2.8°C–5°C), with a safety mechanism in place to ensure the temperature always stays above freezing at 32°F (Dignitana, Inc., n.d.). Contraindications to the use of DigniCap include pediatric patients, cold sensitivities, central nervous system malignancies, squamous cell carcinoma of the lung, small cell carcinoma of the lung, cancers of the head and neck, skin cancers, hematologic malignancies, solid tumor malignancies with a high likelihood of metastases in transit, current use of myeloablative chemotherapy, and current or previous skull irradiation (Dignitana, Inc., n.d.).

(b) The Paxman cooling system works by using inline temperature sensors to ensure the cooling cap maintains a constant temperature (Paxman, n.d.). Contraindications to the use of the Paxman system include hematologic malignancies, cold allergy, cold agglutinins, scalp metastases, and current use of myeloablative chemotherapy or skull irradiation (Paxman, n.d.).

c) Topical minoxidil had been associated with decreased severity and duration of alopecia, but this has not held up in further studies (Gill & Dominguez, 2016).

8. Patient and family education

a) Ask patients to verbalize feelings related to hair loss. Increasing patients' knowledge may give them a sense of control as their appearance changes (Ishida, Ishida, & Kiyoko, 2014).

b) Advise patients and caregivers about the following (Can, Yildiz, & Özdemir, 2017):

(1) The cause of alopecia and the time frame of hair loss and regrowth

(2) Strategies to manage hair loss and regrowth

(a) Be aware that most strategies are literature based and have not been tested in randomized controlled clinical trials.

(b) Use baby shampoo with a neutral pH balance.

(c) Avoid using permanent waves, bleach, and coloring agents on hair, as well as vigorous brushing, hot rollers, and excessive heat with hair dryer use.

(d) Avoid excessive brushing or combing. Use a soft brush or a wide-tooth comb.

(e) Consider cutting hair in a short style or shaving the head (Fabbrocini et al., 2015).

(f) Protect the scalp from the cold and sun with hats, scarves, wigs, and sunscreen. Consider cotton head coverings.

(g) Instruct patients that new hair that grows after completion of therapy may differ from the original hair in color or texture.

(3) Local resources for support (e.g., wig salons, scarf and turban catalogs, support groups)

(a) Look Good Feel Better is a program offered by the Look Good Feel Better Foundation through community organizations such as the American Cancer Society to provide guidance and support regarding wigs and other head coverings, makeup, and skin care (Look Good Feel Better Foundation, n.d.).

(b) Computerized imaging programs to simulate baldness and the look of various types and colors of wigs may be useful and can decrease distress related to hair loss (Chon et al., 2012).

(4) A wig may be covered by the patient's insurance, which will help to defray costs. A prescription written for "hair prosthesis" may be required.

(a) Wigs can be synthetic or made of human hair, with the latter being more expensive. Representatives at salons or stores that specialize in wigs can discuss the pros and cons of each type of wig with the patient. Synthetic wigs may be damaged by excessive heat during styling. Manufacturers' care guidelines should be followed.

(b) Wig specialists may have an easier time matching a wig to the patient's usual style if the patient consults the stylist before hair loss begins or provides pictures. It may be helpful to preserve a portion of normal hair prior to complete hair loss to allow for color and texture matching.

(c) If a wig is purchased prior to hair loss, it should be adjustable so that the size can be decreased as the hair loss occurs (Look Good Feel Better Foundation, n.d.).

(d) A variety of scarves and turbans are available and assist with protection of the scalp and prevention of heat loss.

References

Amgen Inc. (2017). *Vectibix® (panitumumab)* [Package insert]. Thousand Oaks, CA: Author.

Anforth, R., Carlos, G., Clements, A., Kefford, R., & Fernandez-Peñas, P. (2015). Cutaneous adverse events in patients treated with BRAF inhibitor-based therapies for metastatic melanoma for longer than 52 weeks. *British Journal of Dermatology, 172,* 239–243. https://doi.org/10.1111/bjd.13200

AstraZeneca Pharmaceuticals LP. (2015). *Iressa® (gefitinib)* [Package insert]. Wilmington, DE: Author.

AstraZeneca Pharmaceuticals LP. (2016). *Caprelsa® (vandetanib)* [Package insert]. Wilmington, DE: Author.

AstraZeneca Pharmaceuticals LP. (2017). *Tagrisso® (osimertinib)* [Package insert]. Wilmington, DE: Author.

Bayer HealthCare Pharmaceuticals Inc. (2015). *Nexavar® (sorafenib)* [Package insert]. Whippany, NJ: Author.

Belum, V.R., Marulanda, K., Ensslin, C., Gorcey, L., Parikh, T., Wu, S., … Lacouture, M.E. (2015). Alopecia in patients treated with molecularly targeted anticancer therapies. *Annals of Oncology, 26,* 2495–2502. https://doi.org/10.1093/annonc/mdv390

Bouché, O., Brixi-Benmansour, H., Bertin, A., Perceau, G., & Lagarde, S. (2005). Trichomegaly of the eyelashes following treatment with cetuximab. *Annals of Oncology, 16,* 1711–1712. https://doi.org/10.1093/annonc/mdi300

Boucher, J., Olson, L., & Piperdi, B. (2011). Preemptive management of dermatologic toxicities associated with epidermal growth factor receptor inhibitors. *Clinical Journal of Oncology*

Nursing, 15, 501–508. https://doi.org/10.1188/11.CJON.501-508

Bristol-Myers Squibb Co. (2015). *Taxol® (paclitaxel)* [Package insert]. Princeton, NJ: Author.

Burtness, B., Anadkat, M., Basti, S., Hughes, M., Lacouture, M.E., McClure, J.S., … Spencer, S. (2009). NCCN Task Force report: Management of dermatologic and other toxicities associated with EGFR inhibition in patients with cancer. *Journal of the National Comprehensive Cancer Network, 7*(Suppl. 1), S5–S21. Retrieved from http://www.jnccn.org/content/7/Suppl_1/S-5.full.pdf+html

Caccavale, S., & Ruocco, E. (2017). Acral manifestations of systemic diseases: Drug-induced and infectious diseases. *Clinics in Dermatology, 35,* 55–63. https://doi.org/10.1016/j.clindermatol.2016.09.008

Camp-Sorrell, D. (2018). Chemotherapy toxicities and management. In C.H. Yarbro, D. Wujcik, & B.H. Gobel (Eds.), *Cancer nursing: Principles and practice* (8th ed., pp. 497–554). Burlington, MA: Jones & Bartlett Learning.

Can, G., Yildiz, M., & Özdemir, E.E. (2017). Supportive care for chemotherapy induced alopecia: Challenges and solutions. *Clinical Research in Infectious Diseases, 4,* 1048. Retrieved from https://www.jscimedcentral.com/InfectiousDiseases/infectiousdiseases-4-1048.pdf

Cephalon, Inc. (2016). *Treanda® (bendamustine hydrochloride)* [Package insert]. Frazer, PA: Author.

Charalambous, A., & Charalambous, M. (2016). "I lost my image, the image others know me by": Findings from a hermeneutic phenomenological study of patients living with treatment-induced cutaneous toxicities. *Research in Nursing and Health, 39,* 187–196. https://doi.org/10.1002/nur.21722

Chon, S.Y., Champion, R.W., Geddes, E.R., & Rashid, R.M. (2012). Chemotherapy-induced alopecia. *Journal of the American Academy of Dermatology, 67,* e37–e47. https://doi.org/10.1016/j.jaad.2011.02.026

Degen, A., Alter, M., Schenck, F., Satzger, I., Völker, B., Kapp, A., & Gutzmer, R. (2010). The hand-foot-syndrome associated with medical tumor therapy—Classification and management. *Journal of the German Society of Dermatology, 8,* 652–661. https://doi.org/10.1111/j.1610-0387.2010.07449.x

Dignitana, Inc. (n.d.). DigniCap®. Retrieved from https://dignicap.com

Eaby-Sandy, B., Grande, C., & Viale, P.H. (2012). Dermatologic toxicities in epidermal growth factor receptor and multikinase inhibitors. *Journal of the Advanced Practitioner in Oncology, 3,* 138–150.

Fabbrocini, G., Panariello, L., Caro, G., & Monfrecola, G. (2015). Chemotherapy and cutaneous drug reactions. In J.C. Hall & B.J. Hall (Eds.), *Cutaneous drug eruptions: Diagnosis, histopathology and therapy* (pp. 309–321). https://doi.org/10.1007/978-1-4471-6729-7_29

Fonia, A., Cota, C., Setterfield, J.F., Goldberg, L.J., Fenton, D.A., & Stefanato, C.M. (2017). Permanent alopecia in patients with breast cancer after taxane chemotherapy and adjuvant hormonal therapy: Clinicopathologic findings in a cohort of 10 patients. *Journal of the American Academy of Dermatology, 76,* 948–957. https://doi.org/10.1016/j.jaad.2016.12.027

Genentech, Inc. (2016). *Zelboraf® (vemurafenib)* [Package insert]. South San Francisco, CA: Author.

Genentech, Inc. (2017). *Herceptin® (trastuzumab)* [Package insert]. South San Francisco, CA: Author.

Genentech, Inc., & Astellas Pharma US, Inc. (2016). *Tarceva® (erlotinib)* [Package insert]. South San Francisco, CA, and Northbrook, IL: Authors.

Gill, J., & Dominguez, A.R. (2016). Cutaneous manifestations of chemotherapeutic drugs. *Current Dermatology Reports, 5,* 58–69. https://doi.org/10.1007/s13671-016-0130-0

GlaxoSmithKline. (2017). *Tykerb® (lapatinib)* [Package insert]. Research Triangle Park, NC: Author.

Hoffmann-La Roche Inc. (2008). *Roferon-A® (interferon alfa-2a, recombinant)* [Package insert]. Nutley, NJ: Author.

Huang, V., & Anadkat, M. (2011). Dermatologic manifestations of cytotoxic therapy. *Dermatologic Therapy, 24,* 401–410. https://doi.org/10.1111/j.1529-8019.2011.01432.x

ImClone LLC. (2016). *Erbitux® (cetuximab)* [Package insert]. Branchburg, NJ: Author.

Ishida, K., Ishida, J., & Kiyoko, K. (2014). Psychosocial reaction patterns to alopecia in female patients with gynecological cancer undergoing chemotherapy. *Asian Pacific Journal of Cancer Prevention, 16,* 1225–1233. https://doi.org/10.7314/APJCP.2015.16.3.1225

Kamil, N., Kamil, S., Ahmed, S.P., Ashraf, R., Khurram, M., & Ali, M.O. (2010). Toxic effects of multiple anticancer drugs on skin. *Pakistan Journal of Pharmaceutical Sciences, 23,* 7–14.

Kaur, S., & Mahajan, B.B. (2015). Eyelash trichomegaly. *Indian Journal of Dermatology, 60,* 378–380. https://doi.org/10.4103/0019-5154.160484

Kheir, W.J., Sniegowski, M.C., El-Sawy, T., Li, A., & Esmaeli, B. (2014). Ophthalmic complications of targeted cancer therapy and recently recognized ophthalmic complications of traditional chemotherapy. *Survey of Ophthalmology, 59,* 493–502. https://doi.org/10.1016/j.survophthal.2014.02.004

Lacouture, M.E. (2015). Management of dermatologic toxicities. *Journal of the National Comprehensive Cancer Network, 13*(Suppl. 5), 686–689. https://doi.org/10.6004/jnccn.2015.0204

Lacouture, M.E., Anadkat, M.J., Bensadoun, R.-J., Bryce, J., Chan, A., Epstein, J.B., … Murphy, B.A. (2011). Clinical practice guidelines for the prevention and treatment of EGFR inhibitor-associated dermatologic toxicities. *Supportive Care in Cancer, 19,* 1079–1095. https://doi.org/10.1007/s00520-011-1197-6

Lacouture, M.E., Maitland, M.L., Segaert, S., Setser, A., Baran, R., Fox, L.P., … Trotti, A. (2010). A proposed EGFR inhibitor dermatologic adverse event-specific grading scale from the MASCC skin toxicity study group. *Supportive Care in Cancer, 18,* 509–522. https://doi.org/10.1007/s00520-009-0744-x

Ligand Pharmaceuticals Inc. (2015). *Targretin® (bexarotene)* [Package insert]. San Diego, CA: Author.

Look Good Feel Better Foundation. (n.d.). Look Good Feel Better. Retrieved from http://lookgoodfeelbetter.org

Lupu, I., Voiculescu, N., Bacalbasa, N., Cojocaru, I., Vrancian, V., & Giurcaneanu, C. (2016). Cutaneous complications of molecular targeted therapy used in oncology. *Journal of Medicine and Life, 9,* 19–25.

Merck and Co., Inc. (2015). *Intron® A (interferon alfa-2b, recombinant)* [Package insert]. Whitehouse Station, NJ: Author.

Morse, L. (2014). Skin and nail bed changes. In C.H. Yarbro, D. Wujcik, & B.H. Gobel (Eds.), *Cancer symptom management* (4th ed., pp. 587–616). Burlington, MA: Jones & Bartlett Learning.

National Cancer Institute. (2016). Pruritus (PDQ®) [Health professional version]. Retrieved from http://www.cancer.gov/cancertopics/pdq/supportivecare/pruritus/HealthProfessional

National Cancer Institute Cancer Therapy Evaluation Program. (2017). *Common terminology criteria for adverse events* [v.5.0]. Retrieved from https://ctep.cancer.gov/protocoldevelopment/electronic_applications/docs/CTCAE_v5_Quick_Reference_5x7.pdf

Novartis Pharmaceuticals Corp. (2016). *Afinitor® (everolimus)* [Package insert]. East Hanover, NJ: Author.

Novartis Pharmaceuticals Corp. (2017a). *Mekinist® (trametinib)* [Package insert]. East Hanover, NJ: Author.

Novartis Pharmaceuticals Corp. (2017b). *Tasigna® (nilotinib)* [Package insert]. East Hanover, NJ: Author.

Paus, R., Haslam, I.S., Sharov, A.A., & Botchkarev, V.A. (2013). Pathobiology of chemotherapy-induced hair loss. *Lancet Oncology, 14,* e50–e59. https://doi.org/10.1016/S1470-2045(12)70553-3

Paxman. (n.d.). Scalp cooling. Retrieved from https://paxmanscalpcooling.com/scalp-cooling

Pfizer Inc. (2017). *Sutent® (sunitinib malate)* [Package insert]. New York, NY: Author.

Potthoff, K., Hofheinz, R., Hassel, J.C., Volkenandt, M., Lordick, F., Hartmann, J.T., ... Wollenberg, A. (2011). Interdisciplinary management of EGFR-inhibitor-induced skin reactions: A German expert opinion. *Annals of Oncology, 22,* 524–535. https://doi.org/10.1093/annonc/mdq387

Prometheus Laboratories Inc. (2015). *Proleukin® (aldesleukin)* [Package insert]. San Diego, CA: Author.

Reyes-Habito, C.M., & Roh, E.K. (2014a). Cutaneous reactions to chemotherapeutic drugs and targeted therapy for cancer: Part I. Conventional chemotherapeutic drugs. *Journal of the American Academy of Dermatology, 71,* 203.e1–203.e12. https://doi.org/10.1016/j.jaad.2014.04.014

Reyes-Habito, C.M., & Roh, E.K. (2014b). Cutaneous reactions to chemotherapeutic drugs and targeted therapy for cancer: Part II. Targeted therapy. *Journal of the American Academy of Dermatology, 71,* 217.e1–217.e11. https://doi.org/10.1016/j.jaad.2014.04.013

Ron, I.G., Kalmus, Y., Kalmus, Z., Inbar, M., & Chaitchik, S. (1997). Scalp cooling system in prevention of alopecia in patients receiving depilating chemotherapy. *Supportive Care in Cancer, 5,* 136–138. https://doi.org/10.1007/BF01262571

Rosen, A.C., Balagula, Y., Raisch, D.W., Garg, V., Nardone, B., Larsen, N., ... Lacouture, M.E. (2014). Life-threatening dermatologic adverse events in oncology. *Anti-Cancer Drugs, 25,* 225–234. https://doi.org/10.1097/CAD.0000000000000032

Ross, M., & Fischer-Cartlidge, E. (2017). Scalp cooling: A literature review of efficacy, safety, and tolerability for chemotherapy-induced alopecia. *Clinical Journal of Oncology Nursing, 21,* 226–233. https://doi.org/10.1188/17.CJON.226-233

Rugo, H.S., Klein, P., Melin, S.A., Hurvitz, S.A., Melisko, M.E., Moore, A., ... Cigler, T. (2017). Association between use of a scalp cooling device and alopecia after chemotherapy for breast cancer. *JAMA, 317,* 606–614. https://doi.org/10.1001/jama.2016.21038

Rugo, H.S., & Voigt, J. (2018). Scalp hypothermia for preventing alopecia during chemotherapy. A systematic review and meta-analysis of randomized controlled trials. *Clinical Breast Cancer, 18,* 19–28. https://doi.org/10.1016/j.clbc.2017.07.012

Sanofi-Aventis U.S. LLC. (2015) *Taxotere® (docetaxel)* [Package insert]. Bridgewater, NJ: Author.

Segaert, S., & Van Cutsem, E. (2005). Clinical signs, pathophysiology and management of skin toxicity during therapy with epidermal growth factor receptor inhibitors. *Annals of Oncology, 16,* 1425–1433. https://doi.org/10.1093/annonc/mdi279

Shi, V.J., Levy, L.L., & Choi, J.N. (2016). Cutaneous manifestations of nontargeted and targeted chemotherapies. *Seminars in Oncology, 43,* 419–425. https://doi.org/10.1053/j.seminoncol.2016.02.018

Sibaud, V., Meyer, N., Lamant, L., Vigarios, E., Mazieres, J., & Delord, J.P. (2016). Dermatologic complications of anti-PD-1/PD-L1 immune checkpoint antibodies. *Current Opinion in Oncology, 28,* 254–263. https://doi.org/10.1097/CCO.0000000000000290

Thebeau, M., Rubin, K., Hofmann, M., Grimm, J., Weinstein, A., & Choi, J.N. (2017). Management of skin adverse events associated with immune checkpoint inhibitors in patients with melanoma: A nursing perspective. *Journal of the American Association of Nurse Practitioners, 29,* 294–303. https://doi.org/10.1002/2327-6924.12458

Tischer, B., Huber, R., Kraemer, M., & Lacouture, M.E. (2017). Dermatologic events from EGFR inhibitors: The issue of the missing patient voice. *Supportive Care in Cancer, 25,* 651–660. https://doi.org/10.1007/s00520-016-3419-4

Tummino, C., Barlesi, F., Tchouhadjian, C., Tasei, A.M., Gaudy-Marqueste, C., Richard, M.A., & Astoul, P. (2007). [Severe cutaneous toxicity after pemetrexed as second line treatment for a refractory non small cell lung cancer]. *Revue des Maladies Respiratoires, 24,* 635–638.

U.S. Food and Drug Administration. (2017, July 3). FDA clears expanded use of cooling cap to reduce hair loss during chemotherapy. Retrieved from https://www.fda.gov/NewsEvents/Newsroom/PressAnnouncements/ucm565599.htm

Valentine, J., Belum, V.R., Duran, J., Ciccolini, K., Schindler, K., Wu, S., & Lacouture, M.E. (2015). Incidence and risk of xerosis with targeted anticancer therapies. *Journal of the American Academy of Dermatology, 72,* 656–667. https://doi.org/10.1016/j.jaad.2014.12.010

Villée, C., Tennstedt, D., Marot, L., Goossens, A., & Baeck, M. (2010). Delayed urticaria with oxaliplatin. *Contact Dermatitis, 63,* 50–53. https://doi.org/10.1111/j.1600-0536.2010.01738.x

Wallner, M., Köck-Hódi, S., Booze, S., White, K.J., & Mayer, H. (2016). Nursing management of cutaneous toxicities from epidermal growth factor receptor inhibitors. *Clinical Journal of Oncology Nursing, 20,* 529–536. https://doi.org/10.1188/16.CJON.529-536

White, G.M., & Cox, N.H. (2006). *Diseases of the skin* (2nd ed.). St. Louis, MO: Elsevier Mosby.

Wolters Kluwer Health. (2017). Lexicomp® and UpToDate® drug information. Retrieved from http://www.wolterskluwerhealth.com

Wu, P.A., Balagula, Y., Lacouture, M.E., & Anadkat, M.J. (2011). Prophylaxis and treatment of dermatologic adverse events from epidermal growth factor inhibitors. *Current Opinion in Oncology, 23,* 343–351. https://doi.org/10.1097/CCO.0b013e3283474063

Wyeth Pharmaceuticals Inc. (2017). *Torisel® (temsirolimus)* [Package insert]. Philadelphia, PA: Author.

CHAPTER 22

Endocrine Toxicities

A. Overview
1. Aside from steroids administered as part of the chemotherapy, which are known to cause hyperglycemia, several other chemotherapy agents are reported to cause endocrine disorders.
2. Endocrinopathies are one of the adverse side effects of cancer treatment and are primarily associated with immunotherapy.
   a) Adrenal, thyroid, and pituitary glands are the endocrine organs that are most commonly affected by immune checkpoint inhibitors (Sznol et al., 2017).
   b) Adverse effects include hyperthyroidism, hypothyroidism, hypophysitis, hyperglycemia (diabetes), myxedema, and adrenal insufficiency.
   c) Most of these are associated with repeated administration of immunotherapy agents.
3. These side effects may often go unnoticed and therefore underreported, underdiagnosed, and undertreated. It is important that prior to initiation of treatment, as well as during and after completion of treatment, every patient be evaluated for the presence of these endocrine disorders.
4. Although endocrinopathies may not be considered the most common adverse side effects of antineoplastics, they have been associated with the following:
   a) Mammalian target of rapamycin (mTOR) inhibitors
   b) Recombinant human interferon (IFN) alfa
   c) Cytokine interleukin (IL)-2
   d) Checkpoint inhibitors
      (1) Cytotoxic T-lymphocyte antigen 4 (CTLA-4)
      (2) Programmed cell death protein 1 (PD-1)
      (3) Programmed cell death-ligand 1 (PD-L1)
   e) These therapies upregulate the immune system, thereby combating tumor cells (Gonzalez-Rodriguez & Rodriguez-Abreu, 2016). See Table 22-1 for a list of these drugs, side effects, and nursing considerations.

B. Drug-specific endocrinopathies
1. Hyperglycemia with mTOR inhibitors (Dy & Adjei, 2013; Hwangbo & Lee, 2017)
   a) Pathophysiology
      (1) Decrease in glucose-stimulated insulin secretion from beta cells
      (2) Increase in apoptosis
      (3) Increase in peripheral insulin resistance
      (4) Promotion of gluconeogenesis in the liver
   b) Incidence: Hyperglycemia has been found to occur in 12% of patients treated with everolimus and in 11% of those treated with temsirolimus.
   c) Risk factors: May be similar to the risk factors for cancer
      (1) Obesity
      (2) Decreased physical activity
      (3) Older age
   d) Manifestations: Hyperglycemia usually occurs with the first six weeks of treatment and resolves between doses.
   e) Assessment: Patients should have fasting blood glucose levels checked prior to initiating and during treatment.
   f) Prevention and treatment: Lifestyle modification should be initiated (diet and exercise), and antidiabetic medication should be started if indicated.
      (1) For patients with a history of hyperglycemia or diabetes—optimize blood glucose control prior to treatment.
      (2) For blood glucose levels of 250–500 mg/dl, hold the drug temporarily, and restart at a decreased dose.
      (3) For blood glucose greater than 500 mg/dl, discontinue the drug.
   g) Patient and family education: Educate patients and families on the signs and symp-

Table 22-1. Endocrine Toxicities of Antineoplastics

Classification	Drug	Side Effects	Nursing Considerations
Chemotherapy Agents			
Antimetabolites	Decitabine (Dacogen®)	Hyperglycemia observed in clinical trials: 6%–33%	Monitor blood glucose, and educate patients and families on the signs and symptoms of hyperglycemia.
Antitumor antibiotics	Valrubicin (Valstar®)	Hyperglycemia observed in clinical trials: 1%	Monitor blood glucose, and educate patients and families on the signs and symptoms of hyperglycemia.
Miscellaneous	Asparaginase *Erwinia chrysanthemi* (Erwinaze®)	Hyperglycemia secondary to inhibition of insulin or insulin receptor synthesis: 2%–17% Malabsorption of glucose: 5% Potentially irreversible glucose intolerance Diabetic ketoacidosis Transient diabetes mellitus was observed in pediatric patients undergoing treatment with L-asparaginase and prednisone. Death	Monitor blood glucose, and educate patients and families on the signs and symptoms of hyperglycemia. In the presence of increased serum insulin, discontinue the drug; IV fluids and insulin may be used to reverse hyperglycemia.
	Mitotane (Lysodren®)	Acute adrenal injury (adrenal crisis can occur with shock or severe trauma) Adrenal insufficiency	In the presence of acute adrenal injury, hold drug and administer hydrocortisone; monitor for worsening signs of shock. In the presence of adrenal insufficiency, steroid replacement may be used, and free cortisol and corticotropin should be monitored until steroid replacement normalizes levels.
	Omacetaxine (Synribo®)	Hyperglycemia (grade 3–4: 11%) and hyperosmolar hyperglycemic state have been observed.	Avoid use in patients with poorly controlled diabetes mellitus unless good glycemic control is achieved. Monitor blood glucose, and educate patients and families on the signs and symptoms of hyperglycemia.
	Pegaspargase (Oncaspar®)	Irreversible glucose intolerance may occur. Hyperglycemia: 5%	Monitor blood glucose, and educate patients and families on the signs and symptoms of hyperglycemia.
	Vorinostat (Zolinza®)	Hyperglycemia: 8.1% Increased serum glucose	Monitor blood glucose, and educate patients and families on the signs and symptoms of hyperglycemia. Monitor serum glucose every 2 weeks during the first 2 months of treatment and monthly thereafter.
Nitrosoureas	Streptozocin (Zanosar®)	Impaired glucose tolerance Hyperglycemia secondary to islet cell inflammation and destruction	Monitor blood glucose, and educate patients and families on the signs and symptoms of hyperglycemia.

(Continued on next page)

Table 22-1. Endocrine Toxicities of Antineoplastics *(Continued)*			
Classification	**Drug**	**Side Effects**	**Nursing Considerations**
Targeted Therapy Agents			
Small molecule inhibitors	Axitinib (Inlyta®)	Hyperthyroidism: 1% Hypothyroidism: 19%	Monitor TSH levels.
	Brigatinib (Alunbrig®)	Hyperglycemia	Monitor blood glucose, and educate patients and families on the signs and symptoms of hyperglycemia. In the presence of grade 3 or greater hyperglycemia (> 250 mg/dl or 13.9 mmol/L), hold brigatinib until adequate hyperglycemic control is achieved. Once hyperglycemic control is achieved, consider reduction to next lower dose or permanently discontinue.
	Ceritinib (Zykadia®)	Hyperglycemia	Monitor blood glucose, and educate patients and families on the signs and symptoms of hyperglycemia. Withhold ceritinib if the patient develops treatment-resistant hyperglycemia > 250 mg/dl. If hyperglycemia is controlled, resume with a 150 mg dose reduction. Discontinue if unable to tolerate 300 mg once daily or if hyperglycemia remains uncontrolled with medical intervention.
	Dabrafenib (Tafinlar®)	Hyperglycemia: 50%–60%	Monitor blood glucose, and educate patients and families on the signs and symptoms of hyperglycemia. Dabrafenib, alone or in combination with trametinib, may require more intensive hypoglycemic therapy.
	Everolimus (Afinitor®, Afinitor Disperz® tablets for oral suspension)	Diabetes mellitus (both new onset and exacerbation): 1%–10% Hyperglycemia: 13%–75% (grade 3–4: 5%–17%) Hypoglycemia: 1 instance of death related to hypoglycemia and cardiac arrest reported in a clinical trial	Monitor blood glucose, and educate patients and families on the signs and symptoms of hyperglycemia. Drug may need to be interrupted, dose adjusted, or discontinued based on resolution of hyperglycemia. Monitor fasting serum glucose prior to therapy and periodically during therapy.
	Imatinib mesylate (Gleevec®)	Hypothyroidism Decreased glucose level (mean decrease of 4.7% alone, 23.9% with dasatinib, 12.2% with sunitinib, and 12.8% with sorafenib)	Monitor blood glucose, and for patients on hypoglycemic agents, instruct on the signs and symptoms of hypoglycemia.
	Midostaurin (Rydapt®)	Hyperglycemia: 20%	Monitor blood glucose, and educate patients and families on the signs and symptoms of hyperglycemia.
	Pazopanib (Votrient®)	Decreased glucose level: 17% (grade 3: 0%; grade 4: < 1%) Increased glucose levels: 41% in patients with RCC; 45% in patients with soft tissue sarcoma Hypothyroidism: 4%–7%	Monitor blood glucose, and educate patients and families on the signs and symptoms of hypo- and hyperglycemia.

(Continued on next page)

Table 22-1. Endocrine Toxicities of Antineoplastics *(Continued)*

Classification	Drug	Side Effects	Nursing Considerations
Targeted Therapy Agents *(Cont.)*			
Small molecule inhibitors *(cont.)*	Sunitinib (Sutent®)	Hyperthyroidism Hypoglycemia: 2% in patients with GIST and RCC; 10% in patients with pNET Hypothyroidism: 4%–36% in patients with GIST; 16% in patients with RCC; 7% in patients with pNET	Monitor blood glucose, and educate patients and families on the signs and symptoms of hypoglycemia. Monitor TSH levels. Oral levothyroxine and IV methylprednisolone may be initiated for management of severe hypothyroidism.
	Temsirolimus (Torisel®)	Hyperglycemia: 89%	Monitor blood glucose, and educate patients and families on the signs and symptoms of hyperglycemia. Test glucose prior to and during treatment. Patients may require insulin or oral hypoglycemic agents for management.
	Trametinib (Mekinist®)	Hyperglycemia has been observed in combination with dabrafenib.	Monitor blood glucose, and educate patients and families on the signs and symptoms of hyperglycemia.
	Vandetanib (Caprelsa®)	Decreased glucose level: 24% Hypothyroidism: 6%	Monitor blood glucose, and educate patients and families on the signs and symptoms of hypoglycemia. Consider monitoring TSH levels.
	Vorinostat (Zolinza®)	Hyperglycemia: 8.1%	Monitor serum glucose every 2 weeks during the first 2 months of treatment and monthly thereafter. Educate patients and families on the signs and symptoms of hyperglycemia.
Immunotherapy Agents			
Checkpoint inhibitors: PD-1	Pembrolizumab (Keytruda®)	Hyperglycemia: 40%–48% Hyperthyroidism: 3.4% Hypophysitis: 0.6% Hypothyroidism: 8.5%–14% Thyroiditis: 0.6% Type 1 diabetes mellitus: 0.2%	Type 1 diabetes mellitus: Administer insulin. For severe hyperglycemia, withhold pembrolizumab, and administer antihyperglycemics. May resume once toxicity recovers to grade 0 or 1. Administer thioamides and beta-blockers as appropriate. Withhold or discontinue for severe (grade 3) or life-threatening (grade 4) hyperthyroidism. May resume once toxicity recovers to grade 0 or 1. Administer corticosteroids and hormone replacement as clinically indicated. For moderate (grade 2) hypophysitis, withhold pembrolizumab. Withhold or discontinue for severe (grade 3) or life-threatening (grade 4) hypophysitis. May resume once toxicity recovers to grade 0 or 1.
Checkpoint inhibitors: PD-L1	Avelumab (Bavencio®)	Adrenal insufficiency: 0.5% Thyroid gland disorder: 6% Hyperthyroidism: 0.4% Hypothyroidism: 5% Thyroiditis: 0.2% Type 1 diabetes mellitus: 0.1%	For grade 3 or 4 endocrinopathies, withhold avelumab, and initiate appropriate medical management of toxicity. May resume avelumab after resolution of grade 0–1 and corticosteroid taper. For persistent grade 2–3 immune-mediated toxicity (lasting 12 weeks or longer), permanently discontinue avelumab. For patients who require 10 mg/day or greater prednisone or equivalent for > 12 weeks, permanently discontinue avelumab.

(Continued on next page)

Table 22-1. Endocrine Toxicities of Antineoplastics *(Continued)*

Classification	Drug	Side Effects	Nursing Considerations
Immunotherapy Agents *(Cont.)*			
Cytokines	Interferon alfa-2b (Intron-A®)	Diabetes mellitus: < 5% Thyroid gland disorder: < 5%	Patients whose glucose levels cannot be maintained with medication should not begin interferon alfa-2b therapy. In patients who develop this condition during therapy, which cannot be controlled with medication, discontinue interferon treatment. Discontinuation of interferon therapy has not always reversed dysfunction occurring during treatment. TSH should be evaluated prior to starting interferon alfa-2b, and therapy should be discontinued if patients develop thyroid abnormalities during treatment.
Cytokines: Hematopoietic growth factors	Epoetin alfa (Procrit®)	Hyperglycemia: 6%	Monitor blood glucose, and educate patients and families on the signs and symptoms of hyperglycemia.
Miscellaneous: Immunomodulators	Lenalidomide (Revlimid®)	Hyperglycemia: 11.7% Hypothyroidism has been observed in patients with myelodysplastic syndrome.	Monitor blood glucose, and educate patients and families on the signs and symptoms of hyperglycemia. Clinical monitoring of thyroid function is recommended.
Monoclonal antibodies: Human	Bevacizumab (anti-VEGF antibody; Avastin®)	Hyperglycemia: 26%–31%	Monitor blood glucose, and educate patients and families on the signs and symptoms of hyperglycemia.
	Elotuzumab (anti-SLAMF7 antibody; Empliciti™)	Hyperglycemia: 89.3%	Monitor blood glucose, and educate patients and families on the signs and symptoms of hyperglycemia.
Miscellaneous Therapies			
Calcineurin inhibitors	Tacrolimus (Prograf®)	Hyperglycemia secondary to inhibition of insulin secretion and peripheral insulin resistance: 16%–70% New-onset diabetes mellitus: 10%–37% (increased risk in African American and Hispanic transplant recipients)	Monitor blood glucose, and educate patients and families on the signs and symptoms of hyperglycemia.
Hormones	Octreotide (Sandostatin®)	Hyperglycemia secondary to inhibition of insulin secretion: 16%–27% Hypoglycemia: 3%–4% Hypothyroidism: 2%–12%	Monitor blood glucose, and educate patients and families on the signs and symptoms of hyper- and hypoglycemia. Baseline and periodic assessments of thyroid function tests are recommended during chronic therapy. Thyroid replacement therapy may be needed in the presence of hypothyroidism.
	Leuprolide (Lupron®)	Diabetes mellitus has been observed in men with locoregional prostate cancer receiving leuprolide.	Monitor blood glucose, and educate patients and families on the signs and symptoms of diabetes mellitus.
Steroids	Glucocorticoids	Hyperglycemia secondary to increased hepatic glucose Decreased insulin effectiveness Decreased insulin secretion	Monitor blood glucose, and educate patients and families on the signs and symptoms of hyperglycemia.

GIST—gastrointestinal stromal tumor; IV—intravenous; PD-1—programmed cell death protein 1; PD-L1—programmed cell death-ligand 1; pNET—pancreatic neuroendocrine tumor; RCC—renal cell carcinoma; TSH—thyroid-stimulating hormone; VEGF—vascular endothelial growth factor

Note. Based on information from Otsuka America Pharmaceutical, Inc., 2014; Truven Health Analytics, 2017.

toms of hyperglycemia (e.g., increased thirst, increased urination), with instructions to report them if they develop.

2. Hyperthyroidism/hypothyroidism and biphasic thyroiditis with recombinant human IFN alfa used in the treatment of hairy cell leukemia and resected high-risk melanoma (Hauschild et al., 2008; Weber, Yang, Atkins, & Disis, 2015)
   a) Pathophysiology: Stimulation of autoreactive lymphocytes resulting in autoimmune thyroiditis (Corsello et al., 2013)
   b) Incidence: Occurs in 5%–31% of patients receiving treatment
   c) Risk factors
      (1) Presence of thyroid antibodies
      (2) Preexisting thyroid disease leads to increased severity of hypothyroidism
   d) Manifestations
      (1) Symptoms of hyperthyroidism
         (a) Palpitations
         (b) Weight loss
         (c) Diarrhea
         (d) Cold intolerance
      (2) Symptoms of hypothyroidism
         (a) Constipation
         (b) Heat intolerance
         (c) Weight gain, which usually occurs 3–12 weeks after initiation of therapy
   e) Assessment: Assess thyroid function at induction/maintenance and every three months.
      (1) Thyroid-stimulating hormone (TSH)
      (2) Free T4
      (3) Thyroid peroxidase antibodies and thyroglobulin
   f) Prevention and treatment
      (1) Levothyroxine (1.6 mcg/kg) is used for the treatment of hypothyroidism.
      (2) Beta-blockers or corticosteroids may also be used.
      (3) Symptoms may resolve when therapy is stopped.
      (4) If thyroid functions do not normalize, therapy should be stopped.
   g) Patient and family education
      (1) Instruct patients and families to report symptoms of hypo- or hyperthyroidism as listed previously.
      (2) If thyroid hormone replacement has been initiated, instruct patients to take medications in the morning on an empty stomach.

3. Thyroiditis with cytokine IL-2 used for the treatment of advanced renal cell carcinoma and melanoma (Schwartz, Stover, & Dutcher, 2002; Weber et al., 2015)
   a) Pathophysiology: Thyroiditis is believed to occur due to the release of nitric oxide, IL-1, IFN gamma, and tumor necrosis factor-alpha and increased infiltration of lymphocytes into the thyroid gland. Pathophysiology remains to be fully elucidated.
   b) Incidence: Thirty-five percent of patients may experience hypothyroidism, and 7% may experience hyperthyroidism.
   c) Risk factors: Hypothyroidism is related to duration of therapy.
   d) Manifestations
      (1) Hyperthyroidism
         (a) Palpitations
         (b) Weight loss
         (c) Diarrhea
         (d) Cold intolerance
      (2) Hypothyroidism
         (a) Weight gain
         (b) Constipation
         (c) Heat intolerance
   e) Assessment: Routine testing of thyroid hormones (TSH and free T4) should be performed.
   f) Prevention and treatment
      (1) If hypothyroidism is detected before initiation of treatment, hormone replacement therapy should be started and treatment delayed for at least two weeks.
      (2) Hormone replacement therapy should be continued for one year or until levels return to normal. Symptoms resolve upon withholding of the drug and usually are completely resolved in 6–10 months.
   g) Patient and family education
      (1) Instruct patients and families to report symptoms of hypo- or hyperthyroidism as previously listed.
      (2) If thyroid hormone replacement has been initiated, instruct patients to take medication in the morning on an empty stomach.

4. Glucocorticoids
   a) Background: Glucocorticoids are known to cause the following (Oyer, Shah, & Bettenhausen, 2006; Simmons, Molyneaux, Yue, & Chua, 2012; Trence, 2003; Vigneri, Frasca, Sciacca, Pandini, & Vigneri, 2009):
      (1) Decreased beta cell mass
      (2) Increased glucose intolerance
      (3) Decreased insulin effectiveness

(4) Increased hepatic glucose output
(5) Hyperinsulinemia
(6) Decreased beta cell effectiveness (van Raalte, Ouwens, & Diamant, 2009)

b) Pathophysiology
(1) Glucocorticoids inhibit glucose transport/phosphorylation, thereby decreasing available intracellular energy.
(2) They impede cell mitotic division.
(3) They inhibit protein synthesis, resulting in apoptotic cell death (Coleman, 1992; Laane et al., 2009).

c) Risk factors (Handy, Olsen, & Zitella, 2013)
(1) Preexisting diabetes mellitus (prolonged or undiagnosed)
(2) Family history of diabetes mellitus
(3) Down syndrome
(4) Increased age
(5) Increased body mass index
(6) Central nervous system disease
(7) Concurrent administration of tacrolimus, cyclosporine, or asparaginase

d) Manifestations: (Handy et al., 2013)
(1) Hyperglycemia (blood glucose > 180 mg/dl)
(2) Tachycardia
(3) Elevated systolic blood pressure
(4) Anxiety
(5) Irritability
(6) Drowsiness
(7) Blurred vision
(8) Confusion
(9) Dry mouth
(10) Dehydration
(11) Nausea and vomiting
(12) Shortness of breath
(13) Tremor
(14) Hunger
(15) Dry, itchy skin
(16) Polydipsia
(17) Polyuria
(18) Seizures
(19) Coma

e) Assessment (Handy et al., 2013)
(1) Monitor blood glucose, both fasting and two hours postprandial.
(2) Assess for diabetic ketoacidosis.
(3) Monitor for glucocorticoid-induced osteonecrosis, which includes joint pain, weakness, and gait changes.

f) Prevention and treatment: See Figure 22-1.

g) Patient and family education: The degree of hyperglycemia often is related to the potency and duration of action of the steroid administered.
(1) For example, hydrocortisone has a short duration of action (2–10 hours) compared to dexamethasone, which has a duration of action of about 72 hours.
(2) Repeated exposure to steroids can result in sustained hyperglycemia requiring long-term use of antidiabetic medications.

C. Checkpoint inhibitor–related endocrinopathies (Spain, Diem, & Larkin, 2016; Villadolid & Amin, 2015)

1. CTLA-4 is an inhibitory checkpoint protein expressed on the surface of activated T cells that bind to B7 molecules and inhibit the T cell. This category includes ipilimumab and is used to treat melanoma.
2. PD-1 is an immune inhibitory checkpoint expressed on the surface of activated T cells.
   a) This category of drugs includes pembrolizumab and nivolumab.
   b) They have been used in the treatment of melanoma, Hodgkin lymphoma, renal cell, lung, and mesothelioma.
3. PD-L1 is expressed on T cells and interacts with B7 molecules, resulting in T cells switching off.
4. The adverse side effects from CTLA-4, PD-1, and PD-L1 inhibitors are similar and usually dose related.
   a) Hypothyroidism (Dy & Adjei, 2013; González-Rodríguez & Rodríguez-Abreu, 2016; Khan, Rizvi, Sano, Chiu, & Hadid, 2017; Spain et al., 2016; Villadolid & Amin, 2015)
   (1) Pathophysiology: Has not been fully elucidated
   (2) Incidence: Hypothyroidism occurs in 4%–10% of patients treated with PD-1 inhibitors and 2%–4% of patients treated with CTLA-4 inhibitors.
   (3) Risk factors: More common in women
   (4) Manifestations: The time to manifestations (increased TSH and decreased free T4) is usually two to three months for CTLA-4 inhibitors and 0.7 weeks to 19 months with PD-1 inhibitors.
   (5) Assessment: TSH and free T4 should be measured prior to treatment, at the time of each treatment, and every 6–12 weeks for the first six months after treatment.
   (6) Prevention and treatment: Levothyroxine replacement at dose of 1.6 mcg/kg/day

(7) Patient and family education
(*a*) Instruct patients and families to report symptoms of hypothyroidism as listed previously.
(*b*) If thyroid hormone replacement has been initiated, instruct patients to take medication in the morning on an empty stomach.

b) Hyperthyroidism (Spain et al., 2016)
(1) Pathophysiology: Currently no histopathologic findings
(2) Incidence: Hyperthyroidism occurs in 1%–8% of patients treated with checkpoint inhibitors.
(3) Risk factors
(*a*) Transient thyroiditis proceeding hypothyroidism
(*b*) TSH receptor antibody development
(*c*) Graves disease
(4) Manifestations: Symptoms usually occur 24 days to 11.7 months after

Figure 22-1. Glucocorticoid-Induced Hyperglycemia

Glucocorticoid-Induced Hyperglycemia	Treatments
Mechanism: • Impairs glucose uptake in peripheral tissues • Increases hepatic glucose production • Stimulates protein catabolism, which increases concentrations of circulating amino acids, providing precursors for gluconeogenesis **Risk Factors:** • Total steroid dose and duration of therapy • Preexisting diabetes mellitus (prolonged or undiagnosed) • Family history of diabetes mellitus • Down syndrome • Increased age • Increased BMI • CNS disease • Concurrent administration of tacrolimus, cyclosporine, or asparaginase **Characteristics:** • Associated with normal fasting glucose (once a day steroids), which may lead to underdiagnosis if labs are only checked in AM • Blood glucose rises after lunch and throughout evening. – Monitor blood glucose for patients on glucocorticoids 2 hours postprandial. • Postprandial hyperglycemia is often the first indication. • Most common during ALL induction therapy • Spontaneously resolves in most patients who were not previously diabetic • Can be associated with diabetic ketoacidosis **Consequences of Glucocorticoid-Induced Hyperglycemia:** • Increased risk of infection (impairs phagocytic and microbicidal activities of WBCs and may inhibit endogenous production of interleukins) • Decreased survival in adults with ALL **Glucocorticosteroids:** • Prednisone peak effect 4–8 hours with duration of 12–16 hours – NPH beneficial • Dexamethasone peak effect 20 hours – Glargine beneficial	**Insulin** ***Benefits:*** • Few contraindications • Few drug interactions • Frequent adjustments can be made as steroids are tapered. • Type and peak duration can be matched to steroid duration and dosage. • May be administered SC or IV as a continuous infusion • Long-acting and quick-acting formulations can be combined to provide basal, correctional, and nutritional coverage. – Nutritional insulin will comprise 70%–80% of total daily insulin needs because of the effect of glucocorticoids, and basal insulin will comprise 20%–30% of daily insulin needs. ***Challenges:*** • Patient's ability to learn, self-monitor, and administer insulin • Insulin dosing must be carefully managed and individualized depending on severity of hyperglycemia, glucocorticoid dosing, and schedule. • Lack of insurance coverage • Lack of availability of trained and knowledgeable providers for diabetic teaching • Complexity of multiple injections of insulin per day may deter providers and patients from choosing SC insulin. • For patients with anasarca: SC injections are not recommended; convert patient to an IV insulin drip. **Oral Antidiabetic Agents** ***Benefits:*** • Easy for patients to take ***Challenges:*** • Difficult to adjust because of long half-life • Increased drug interactions • May be contraindicated in patients with renal dysfunction, edema, or cardiac disease • Discontinuation of oral antidiabetic medications is recommended in glucocorticoid-induced hyperglycemia. ***Diet:*** • Carbohydrate-controlled diet • Nutritional insulin if postprandial glucose > 180 mg/dl based on a carbohydrate/insulin ratio

ALL—acute lymphoblastic leukemia/lymphoma; BMI—body mass index; CNS—central nervous system; IV—intravenous; NPH—neutral protamine Hagedorn; SC—subcutaneous; WBC—white blood cell

Note. Based on information from Clore & Thurby-Hay, 2009; Umpierrez et al., 2012.

From "Precursor Lymphoid Neoplasms" (p. 193), by C.M. Handy, M. Olsen, and L.J. Zitella in M. Olsen and L.J. Zitella (Eds.), *Hematologic Malignancies in Adults,* 2013, Pittsburgh, PA: Oncology Nursing Society. Copyright 2013 by Oncology Nursing Society. Reprinted with permission.

treatment and consist of tachycardia and tremors.

(5) Assessment
  (a) Thyroid function test
  (b) Thyroid autoantibodies
  (c) Nuclear medicine scan

(6) Prevention and treatment
  (a) Beta-blockers
  (b) Carbimazole
  (c) For thyroiditis, the treatment is steroids.
  (d) If hypothyroidism results following prolonged hyperthyroidism, the treatment is levothyroxine 1.6 mcg/kg.

(7) Patient and family education
  (a) Instruct patients and families to report symptoms, such as the following:
    i. Palpitations
    ii. Diarrhea
    iii. Tremors
  (b) If thyroid replacement hormone has been initiated, instruct patients to take medication taken in the morning on an empty stomach.

c) Hypophysitis (González-Rodríguez & Rodríguez-Abreu, 2016; Sznol et al., 2017; Vazquez, 2017; Villadolid & Amin, 2015; Weber et al., 2015)

(1) Pathophysiology: Hypophysitis may be due to T-cell–mediated pituitary destruction due to CTLA-4 blockade.

(2) Incidence: The prevalence of hypophysitis is reported as 3.3%–17%.

(3) Risk factors: Male predominance (65% of cases)

(4) Manifestations: The most frequent complaints associated with hypophysitis are fatigue and headache, with magnetic resonance imaging (MRI) showing swelling of the pituitary. Patient may also have visual field defects. Other manifestations include arthralgias, behavioral changes, and loss of libido. The usual time to manifestation of symptoms is 4–24 weeks, and they are likely permanent.

(5) Assessment: Prior to treatment, a detailed history and physical examination should be completed. Each patient should have laboratory work done consisting of the following:
  (a) TSH
  (b) Free T4
  (c) Pituitary function tests (luteinizing hormone, follicle-stimulating hormone, growth hormone)
  (d) Prolactin
  (e) Adrenocorticotropic hormone
  (f) Cortisol
  (g) Testosterone (in men)
  (h) Estradiol (in women)

(6) Prevention and treatment
  (a) Corticosteroids
  (b) For grade 3–4: Withhold treatment.
  (c) Asymptomatic: MRI, hormone replacement, cortisol replacement one week prior to initiation of levothyroxine
  (d) Symptomatic: Prednisolone (1–2 mg/kg), MRI, IV fluids for hypotension, taper steroids over two to four weeks followed by hormone replacement

(7) Patient and family education: Instruct patients and families to report any changes.

d) Hyperglycemia (Hwangbo & Lee, 2017)

(1) Pathophysiology: PD-1, which is expressed on beta cells of islets (in pancreas), is inhibited.

(2) Incidence: Hyperglycemia was found to occur in 45%–49% of patients, with 3%–6% being grade 3–4. The incidence of type 1 diabetes was 0.1%.

(3) Risk factors
  (a) Underlying positive glutamic acid decarboxylase
  (b) Human leukocyte antigen antibodies
  (c) Low C-peptide

(4) Manifestations: Elevated blood glucose, which manifests in 1 week to 12 months

(5) Assessment
  (a) Check fasting blood glucose and A1c prior to initiation of treatment.
  (b) Closely monitor blood glucose during treatment.

(6) Prevention and treatment
  (a) Blood glucose should be adequately controlled with use of antidiabetic medications (oral agents or insulin) as well as adequate hydration.
  (b) In the case of a sudden onset of severely elevated blood glucose,

admission to the intensive care unit and administration of an insulin drip may be required.
(7) Patient and family education
(a) Depending on the severity of the blood glucose elevations, the patient may need to learn how to perform self-monitoring of blood glucose as well as insulin injections.
(b) It may also be beneficial for patients and their families to attend a diabetes self-management education class.
(c) All patients should be educated on the signs and symptoms of hyperglycemia and instructed to report any symptoms related to diabetic ketoacidosis.

e) Diabetes (Alhusseini & Samantray, 2017; Godwin et al., 2017)

(1) Pathophysiology: Destruction of pancreatic beta cells by autoreactive T cells

(2) Incidence: Data are limited to two case studies (Alhusseini & Samantray, 2017; Godwin et al., 2017).

(3) Risk factors

(a) Previous history of diabetes

(b) Positive antibodies (glutamic acid decarboxylase, insulin autoantibodies, insulin antibodies)

(4) Manifestations

(a) Elevated blood glucose

(b) Worsening of hyperglycemia in patients with history of type 2 diabetes

(c) These glucose elevations are commonly seen two weeks after initiation of therapy.

(5) Assessment: Blood glucose levels should be monitored closely during therapy.

(6) Prevention and treatment

(a) Blood glucose should be adequately controlled with use of antidiabetic medications (oral agents or insulin) as well as adequate hydration.

(b) In the case of a sudden onset of severely elevated blood glucose, admission to the intensive care unit and administration of an insulin drip may be required.

(7) Patient and family education

(a) Depending on the severity of the blood glucose elevations, the patient may need to learn how to perform self-monitoring of blood glucose as well as insulin injections.

(b) It may also be beneficial for patients and their families to attend a diabetes self-management education class.

(c) All patients should be educated on the signs and symptoms of hyperglycemia and instructed to report any symptoms related to diabetic ketoacidosis.

f) Adrenal insufficiency (Dy & Adjei, 2013; Postow & Wolchok, 2018; Villadolid & Amin, 2015; Weber et al., 2015)

(1) Pathophysiology: Not fully elucidated

(2) Incidence: Occurs more commonly with PD-1 and PD-L1 inhibitors, but less than 2%

(3) Risk factors: Adrenal insufficiency was associated with higher doses (3–10 mg/kg).

(4) Manifestations

(a) Dehydration

(b) Hypotension

(c) Electrolyte imbalances: Hyperkalemia, hyponatremia

(5) Assessment

(a) Check thyroid hormones, electrolytes, adrenocorticotropic hormone, and cortisol levels in one to three weeks.

(b) Perform imaging of pituitary gland (MRI) within one month.

(c) Obtain an endocrinology consult.

(6) Prevention and treatment

(a) Hormone replacement therapy should be given if needed.

(b) Withhold treatment.

(c) If symptoms of adrenal insufficiency are detected, the patient should be hospitalized immediately and IV steroids initiated.

(7) Patient and family education: Instruct patients and families to report signs and symptoms of the following:

(a) Dehydration

(b) Hypotension

(c) Hyperkalemia

(d) Hyponatremia

References

Alhusseini, M., & Samantray, J. (2017). Autoimmune diabetes superimposed on type 2 diabetes in a patient initiated on immunotherapy for lung cancer. *Diabetes and Metabolism, 43,* 86–88. https://doi.org/10.1016/j.diabet.2016.05.007

Clore, J.N., & Thurby-Hay, L. (2009). Glucocorticoid-induced hyperglycemia. *Endocrine Practice, 15,* 469–474. https://doi.org/10.4158/ep08331.rar

Coleman, R.E. (1992). Glucocorticoids in cancer therapy. *Biotherapy, 4,* 37–44. https://doi.org/10.1007/BF02171708

Corsello, S.M., Barnabei, A., Marchetti, P., De Vecchis, L., Salvatori, R., & Torino, F. (2013). Endocrine side effects induced by immune checkpoint inhibitors. *Journal of Clinical Endocrinology and Metabolism, 98,* 1361–1375. https://doi.org/10.1210/jc.2012-4075

Dy, G.K., & Adjei, A.A. (2013). Understanding, recognizing, and managing toxicities of targeted anticancer therapies. *CA: A Cancer Journal for Clinicians, 63,* 249–279. https://doi.org/10.3322/caac.21184

Godwin, J.L., Jaggi, S., Sirisena, I., Sharda, P., Rao, A.D., Mehra, R., & Veloski, C. (2017). Nivolumab-induced autoimmune diabetes mellitus presenting as diabetic ketoacidosis in a patient with metastatic lung cancer. *Journal for ImmunoTherapy of Cancer, 5,* 40. https://doi.org/10.1186/s40425-017-0245-2

González-Rodríguez, E., & Rodríguez-Abreu, D. (2016). Immune checkpoint inhibitors: Review and management of endocrine adverse events. *Oncologist, 21,* 804–816. https://doi.org/10.1634/theoncologist.2015-0509

Handy, C.M., Olsen, M., & Zitella, L. (2013). Precursor lymphoid neoplasms. In M. Olsen & L.J. Zitella (Eds.), *Hematologic malignancies in adults* (pp. 157–200). Pittsburgh, PA: Oncology Nursing Society.

Hauschild, A., Gogas, H., Tarhini, A., Middleton, M.R., Testori, A., Dréno, B., & Kirkwood, J.M. (2008). Practical guidelines for the management of interferon-α-2b side effects in patients receiving adjuvant treatment for melanoma. *Cancer, 112,* 982–994. https://doi.org/10.1002/cncr.23251

Hwangbo, Y., & Lee, E.K. (2017). Acute hyperglycemia associated with anti-cancer medication. *Endocrinology and Metabolism, 32,* 23–29, https://doi.org/10.3803/EnM.2017.32.1.23

Khan, U., Rizvi, H., Sano, D., Chiu, J., & Hadid, T. (2017). Nivolumab induced myxedema crisis. *Journal for ImmunoTherapy of Cancer, 5,* 13. https://doi.org/10.1186/s40425-017-0213-x

Laane, E., Tamm, K.P., Buentke, E., Ito, K., Kharaziha, P., Oscarsson, J., ... Grandér, D. (2009). Cell death induced by dexamethasone in lymphoid leukemia is mediated through initiation of autophagy. *Cell Death and Differentiation, 16,* 1018–1029. https://doi.org/10.1038/cdd.2009.46

Otsuka America Pharmaceutical, Inc. (2014). *Dacogen® (decitabine)* [Package insert]. Rockville, MD: Author.

Oyer, D.S., Shah, A., & Bettenhausen, S. (2006). How to manage steroid diabetes in the patient with cancer. *Journal of Supportive Oncology, 4,* 479–483.

Postow, M., & Wolchok, J. (2018). Toxicities associated with checkpoint inhibitor immunotherapy. In M.E. Ross (Ed.), *UpToDate.* Retrieved April 29, 2018, from http://www.uptodate.com/contents/toxicities-associated-with-checkpoint-inhibitor-immunotherapy

Schwartz, R.N., Stover, L., & Dutcher, J.P. (2002). Managing toxicities of high-dose interleukin-2. *Oncology, 16*(11, Suppl. 13), 11–20. Retrieved from http://www.cancernetwork.com/renal-cell-carcinoma/managing-toxicities-high-dose-interleukin-2

Simmons, L.R., Molyneaux, L., Yue, D.K., & Chua, E.L. (2012). Steroid-induced diabetes: Is it just unmasking of type 2 diabetes? *ISRN Endocrinology, 2012,* 910905. https://doi.org/10.5402/2012/910905

Spain, L., Diem, S., & Larkin, J. (2016). Management of toxicities of immune checkpoint inhibitors. *Cancer Treatment Reviews, 44,* 51–60. https://doi.org/10.1016/j.ctrv.2016.02.001

Sznol, M., Postow, M.A., Davies, M.J., Pavlick, A.C., Plimack, E.R., Shaheen, M., ... Robert, C. (2017). Endocrine-related adverse events associated with immune checkpoint blockade and expert insights on their management. *Cancer Treatment Reviews, 58,* 70–78. https://doi.org/10.1016/j.ctrv.2017.06.002

Trence, D.L. (2003). Management of patients on chronic glucocorticoid therapy: An endocrine perspective. *Primary Care: Clinics in Office Practice, 30,* 593–605. https://doi.org/10.1016/S0095-4543(03)00038-1

Truven Health Analytics. (2017). Micromedex® Solutions [Web application]. Retrieved from http://www.micromedexsolutions.com/micromedex2/librarian

Umpierrez, G.E., Hellman, R., Korytkowski, M.T., Kosiborod, M., Maynard, G.A., Montori, V.M., ... Van den Berghe, G. (2012). Management of hyperglycemia in hospitalized patients in non-critical care setting: An Endocrine Society clinical practice guideline. *Journal of Clinical Endocrinology and Metabolism, 97,* 16–38. https://doi.org/10.1210/jc.2011-2098

van Raalte, D.H., Ouwens, D.M., & Diamant, M. (2009). Novel insights into glucocorticoid-mediated diabetogenic effects: Towards expansion of therapeutic options? *European Journal of Clinical Investigation, 39,* 81–93. https://doi.org/10.1111/j.1365-2362.2008.02067.x

Vazquez, A. (2017). Hypophysitis: Nursing management of immune-related adverse events. *Clinical Journal of Oncology Nursing, 21,* 154–156. https://doi.org/10.1188/17.CJON.154-156

Vigneri, P., Frasca, F., Sciacca, L., Pandini, G., & Vigneri, R. (2009). Diabetes and cancer. *Endocrine-Related Cancer, 16,* 1103–1123. https://doi.org/10.1677/ERC-09-0087

Villadolid, J., & Amin, A. (2015). Immune checkpoint inhibitors in clinical practice: Update on management of immune-related toxicities. *Translational Lung Cancer Research, 4,* 560–575. https://doi.org/10.3978/j.issn.2218-6751.2015.06.06

Weber, J.S., Yang, J.C., Atkins, M.B., & Disis, M.L. (2015). Toxicities of immunotherapy for the practitioner. *Journal of Clinical Oncology, 33,* 2092–2099. https://doi.org/10.1200/JCO.2014.60.0379

CHAPTER 23

Fatigue

A. Overview
   1. Cancer-related fatigue (CRF) is a "distressing, persistent, subjective sense of physical, emotional, and/or cognitive tiredness or exhaustion related to cancer or cancer treatment that is not proportional to recent activity and interferes with usual functioning" (National Comprehensive Cancer Network® [NCCN®], 2018, p. FT-1).
   2. Multiple factors contribute to this complex syndrome in patients with cancer, making it difficult to identify a clear underlying cause (Bower, 2014; Gerber, 2017).
   3. CRF is underreported, underdiagnosed, and undertreated, and healthcare professionals may not fully appreciate the degree of distress and functional loss that fatigue produces (Borthwick, Knowles, McNamara, O'Dea, & Stroner, 2003; Hockenberry-Eaton & Hinds, 2000; Vogelzang et al., 1997). Fatigue is among the most common, distressing, and disabling side effects of cancer treatment; it is experienced by patients receiving cancer treatment, cancer survivors, and those at the end of life (Goedendorp, Gielissen, Verhagen, & Bleijenberg, 2013; Ness et al., 2013; Nishimori, Maeda, & Tanimoto, 2013).
   4. It can produce profound decrements in physical, social, cognitive, and vocational functioning (Curt & Johnston, 2003; de Jong, Candel, Schouten, Abu-Saad, & Courtens, 2006; Escalante & Manzullo, 2009); sleep disturbances (Lindqvist, Widmark, & Rasmussen, 2004); adverse mood changes (Dimeo et al., 2004); and emotional and spiritual distress for both patients and families (Borneman et al., 2012; Brown & Kroenke, 2009; Fitzgerald et al., 2013).
   5. NCCN (2018) guidelines recommend that all patients with cancer be screened for fatigue at their initial visit and at regular intervals across the cancer continuum and that fatigue in both adults and children should be treated promptly.

B. Pathophysiology: Exact mechanisms are unknown. Clinical studies have focused on understanding the factors that contribute to CRF. Factors include the tumor itself, treatments, and comorbid conditions (Davis & Goforth, 2014; H.-J. Kim, Barsevick, Beck, & Dudley, 2012; H.T. Kim & Armand, 2013; Kiserud et al., 2015; Peters, Goedendorp, Verhagen, van der Graaf, & Bleijenberg, 2014; Trudel-Fitzgerald, Savard, & Ivers, 2013a, 2013b).
   1. Underlying mechanisms of CRF (see Figure 23-1) are believed to involve several physiologic and biochemical systems (Bower, 2014; Saligan & Kim, 2012; Saligan et al., 2015). Accumulating evidence suggests that gene polymorphisms, hypothalamic-pituitary-adrenal axis disruption, altered circadian rhythmicity, diminished heart rate variability, immune dysfunction, serotonin dysregulation, mitochondrial dysfunction, 5-hydroxytryptophan dysregulation, and proinflammatory cytokine activity are among the mechanisms that directly or indirectly contribute to CRF (Barsevick, Frost, Zwinderman, Hall, & Halyard, 2010; Bower & Lamkin, 2013; Dantzer, Heijnen, Kavelaars, Laye, & Capuron, 2014; de Jong, Courtens, Abu-Saad, & Schouten, 2002; Filler et al., 2014; Goldberg & Giralt, 2013; Hsiao, Wang, Kaushal, Chen, & Saligan, 2014; Kamath, 2012; E.-J. Kim, Kim, & Cho, 2013; Kisiel-Sajewicz et al., 2012; Lacourt & Heijnen, 2017; Liu et al., 2012; Saligan & Kim, 2012; Wood & Weymann, 2013). Studies also suggest that fatigue may be related to impairments in neuromuscular metabolism and function, distressing symptoms such as pain and dyspnea, psychological and coping responses, and imbalanced neuroendocrine-immune stress responses (Bower, 2014; Karshikoff, Sundelin, & Lasselin, 2017). Screening for treatable contributors to CRF is discussed in D.4.
   2. Treatment-related causes: Direct effects of chemotherapy, hormone therapy, radiation therapy, molecularly targeted agents, immunotherapy, and combined-modality therapies have all been implicated as contributors to the intensity of fatigue in patients with cancer (Abdel-Rahman et al., 2016; Li & Gu, 2017; Santoni et al., 2015;

Figure 23-1. Etiology of Cancer-Related Fatigue

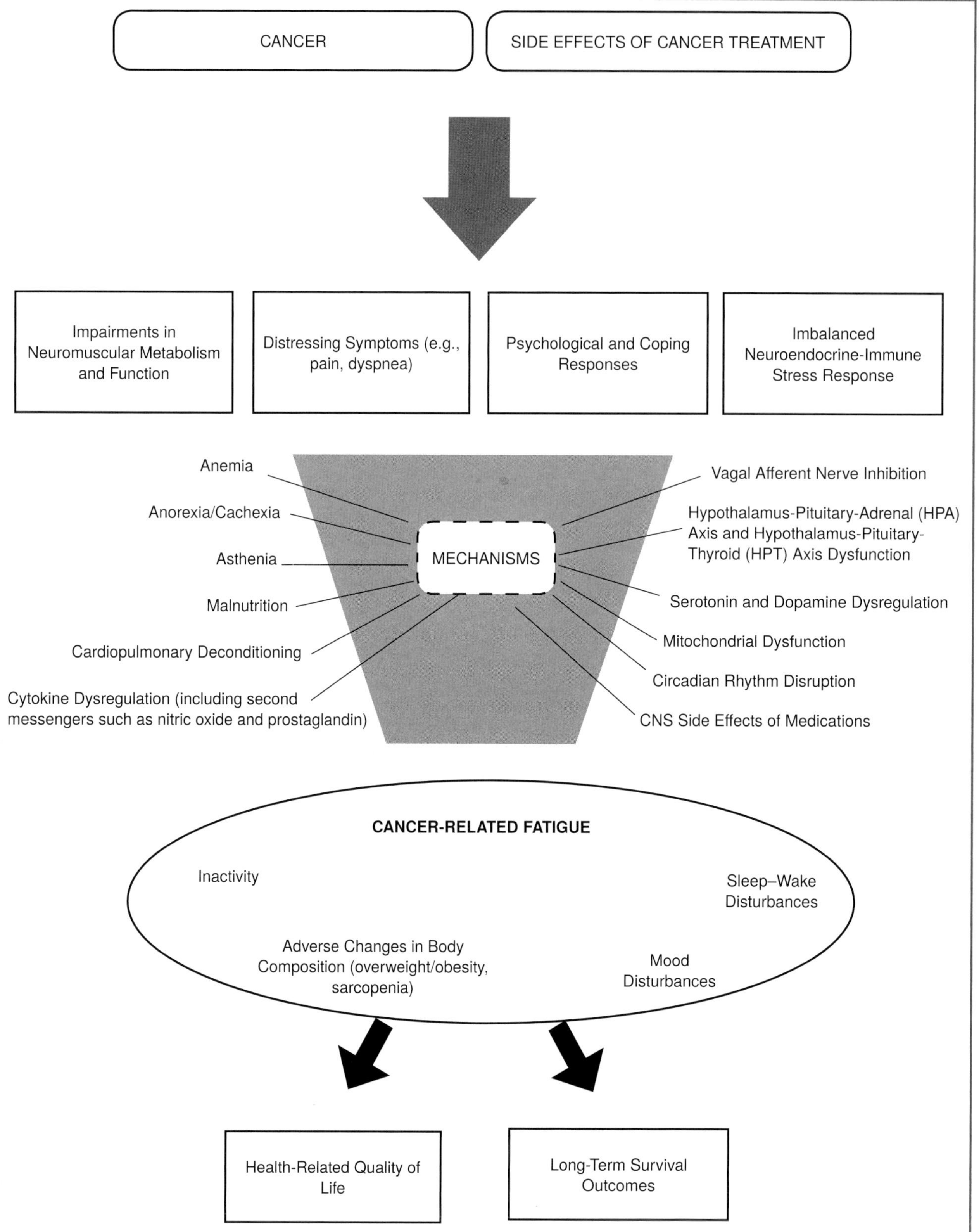

CNS—central nervous system

Note. Image copyright 2010 by Sandra A. Mitchell and Ann M. Berger. Used with permission.

Wagland et al., 2016). The burden of traveling to and from a clinic for treatments and office visits, along with the requirements for self-management during treatment, can amplify a patient's level of fatigue.

3. Disease process and comorbid conditions, including metabolic disorders
   a) Endocrine dysfunction, including hypothyroidism, adrenal insufficiency, and, in males, testicular hypogonadism or androgen deficiency (low testosterone levels)
   b) Cardiopulmonary dysfunction (cardiomyopathy, bronchiolitis, pneumonitis)
   c) Dehydration and electrolyte imbalances
   d) Infection
   e) Insulin sensitivity: Insulin resistance causes abnormal uptake of glucose by muscle and increases body fat, contributing to CRF (Berger, Gerber, & Mayer, 2012).
   f) Uncontrolled concurrent symptoms, such as pain, nausea and vomiting, dyspnea, and anxiety
   g) Side effects of medications that act on the central nervous system (e.g., narcotics, anxiolytics, antiemetics)
   h) Sleep disturbances (NCCN, 2018)
      (1) Obstructive sleep apnea
      (2) Restless legs syndrome/periodic limb movements
      (3) Narcolepsy
      (4) Insomnia (difficulty falling or staying asleep, early morning awakening)
      (5) Hypersomnia
   i) Disease recurrence
   j) Anemia: A relationship clearly exists between low hemoglobin and fatigue. A decrease in red blood cells increases hypoxia-related compromise in organ function, which contributes to fatigue (Balducci, 2010).
   k) Nutritional deficiencies: Reduced caloric intake and imbalances in serum levels of sodium, potassium, calcium, iron, and magnesium may contribute to fatigue and affect quality of life (NCCN, 2018).
   l) Sarcopenia, physical deconditioning, and inactivity: Direct effects of the tumor or side effects of the treatment regimen often contribute to fatigue through sarcopenia (loss of muscle mass), reduced physical activity, cardiopulmonary deconditioning, and reduced muscle strength (Powers, Lynch, Murphy, Reid, & Zijdewind, 2016).
   m) Psychological distress
   n) Depression: Depression may occur concurrently or independently of fatigue and has a different pattern of expression over time (Bower, 2014).
   o) Phenotypes/genotypes: Single nucleotide polymorphisms, especially in the regulatory regions of relevant genes, are thought to contribute to the development of CRF (T. Wang, Yin, Miller, & Xiao, 2017).

C. Incidence: Fatigue is one of the most commonly reported symptoms experienced by patients receiving treatment for cancer, and it often persists beyond the conclusion of active treatment. Across the cancer care continuum, depending on how fatigue is defined and measured, estimates of prevalence vary from 25% to 99% (Campos, Hassan, Riechelmann, & Del Giglio, 2011; Dhruva et al., 2013; Humpel & Iverson, 2010; Langston, Armes, Levy, Tidey, & Ream, 2013; Neefjes, van der Vorst, Blauwhoff-Buskermolen, & Verheul, 2013; Peters et al., 2014; Weis, 2011).

D. Assessment: Oncology nurses are responsible for ensuring that screening for CRF occurs and is documented at regular intervals across the cancer control continuum (Howell et al., 2013). When CRF is present, a detailed evaluation of the characteristics, consequences, and potential contributing factors should be performed, and fatigue should be managed with evidence-based interventions (NCCN, 2018).

1. Brief measures to screen for fatigue are rapid and sensitive and can be applied efficiently in the clinic to identify individuals who would benefit from more systematic evaluation (Danjoux, Gardner, & Fitch, 2007; Goedendorp, Jacobsen, & Andrykowski, 2016; Kirsh, Passik, Holtsclaw, Donaghy, & Theobald, 2001; Temel, Pirl, Recklitis, Cashavelly, & Lynch, 2006).
2. Increased availability of item banks, computerized adaptive testing, electronic collection of patient-reported outcomes, and integration of patient-reported outcomes into the electronic health record may advance the precision, efficiency, interpretation, and actionability of screening measures for CRF (Lai et al., 2005, 2011, 2013; Wagner et al., 2015).
3. Multiple measures for CRF screening and evaluation are available (Seyidova-Khoshknabi, Davis, & Walsh, 2011; Tomlinson et al., 2013).
   a) Single-item, single-dimension measures are easy to administer. These include a 0–10 scale, a visual analog scale, or Likert scales.
      (1) On a 0–10 scale (0 = no fatigue, and 10 = worst fatigue imaginable), mild fatigue is reflected by a score of 1–3; moderate fatigue, a score of 4–6; and severe fatigue, a score of 7–10 (NCCN, 2018).

(2) Fatigue measurement in children is simplified. Young children (younger than six years old) may just be asked if they are "tired" or "not tired." Valid and reliable instruments are available to measure fatigue in children and adolescents (NCCN, 2018).

(3) If fatigue is absent or mild (score 0–3), patients and family members should receive anticipatory guidance about fatigue and available strategies for prevention and management (e.g., exercise, relaxation, stress management).

(4) When fatigue is rated as moderate to severe (4–10), a focused history and physical examination should be conducted as part of the primary evaluation phase.

b) More than 20 self-report measures (including single-item measures, multi-item unidimensional scales, and multidimensional inventories) have been developed to measure fatigue in adults and children with cancer (Seyidova-Khoshknabi et al., 2011; Tomlinson et al., 2013). Consideration of the measurement properties and strengths and limitations of these instruments, including psychometric properties, sensitivity to change, and the availability of normative values to aid interpretation, together with practical issues such as respondent burden and availability of the measure in multiple languages, should guide decisions about the feasibility and utility of a measure for specific clinical or research purposes (Barsevick, Cleeland, et al., 2010).

4. NCCN (2018) guidelines recommend that CRF be assessed using a two-tiered approach. Every patient should be screened for the presence of fatigue, and if present, fatigue should be assessed quantitatively on a 0–10 scale (0 = no fatigue, and 10 = worst fatigue imaginable). Patients with a severity of 4 or greater should be further evaluated by history and physical examination.

a) A detailed history includes the presence, intensity, and pervasiveness of fatigue; its course over time; exacerbating or relieving factors; the effectiveness of the self-management interventions the patient has tried for fatigue; and the impact of fatigue on functioning and level of distress.

b) A complete review of systems should be performed.

c) Etiologic or potentiating factors that may contribute to CRF and that may be treatable should be evaluated. These factors include hypothyroidism, hypogonadism, adrenal insufficiency, cardiomyopathy, pulmonary dysfunction, anemia, neutropenia, cachexia, sleep disturbance, fluid and electrolyte imbalances, emotional distress, and uncontrolled concurrent symptoms (Alesi & del Fabbro, 2014; Berger, Yennu, & Million, 2013; Horneber, Fischer, Dimeo, Rüffer, & Weis, 2012; Koornstra, Peters, Donofrio, van den Borne, & de Jong, 2014; Neefjes et al., 2013; X.S. Wang & Woodruff, 2015; Weis, 2011).

d) Evaluation should also include whether disease progression or recurrence could be among the causes of fatigue.

e) The medication profile should be reviewed to identify specific classes of medications (including over-the-counter medications) that have fatigue as a potential side effect. Polypharmacy is common in patients with cancer. Many drugs alone (e.g., antihistamines, beta-blockers) or in combination may significantly compound fatigue (Savard, Ivers, Savard, & Morin, 2015; X.S. Wang et al., 2014; Zlott & Byrne, 2010). See Table 23-1.

f) Other components of a comprehensive fatigue evaluation

(1) Nutritional and metabolic evaluation: Improving dietary intake, with appropriate caloric intake, often can improve fatigue symptoms. Fluids and electrolytes should be assessed. Specifically, imbalances in sodium, potassium, calcium, iron, and magnesium can be reversed with appropriate supplementation, which may improve fatigue (NCCN, 2018).

(2) Evaluation for symptoms such as nausea and vomiting, taste changes, and bowel changes (e.g., obstruction, constipation, diarrhea), which may interfere with nutritional intake and affect fatigue level

(3) Physical activity level

E. Collaborative management

1. Screen for treatable causes of fatigue and manage as indicated, including concurrent distressing symptoms, physical deconditioning, endocrinopathies, emotional distress, and sedation secondary to specific medication classes.
2. Exercise (physical activity): Across tumor types and at different places on the cancer continuum, the accumulated evidence strongly supports exercise as an intervention to manage CRF

Table 23-1. Drug Classifications and Pharmacologic Agents Associated With Fatigue

Drug Classification	Examples	Potential Adverse Effects
Anticholinergics	Oxybutynin, tolterodine, trospium chloride	Fatigue, sedation
Anticonvulsants	Carbamazepine, gabapentin, pregabalin	Sedation, daytime sleepiness
Antidepressants	Paroxetine, sertraline	Sedation, daytime sleepiness
Antiemetics	Haloperidol, metoclopramide, prochlorperazine, scopolamine	Sedation, daytime sleepiness
Antihistamines	Diphenhydramine, hydroxyzine	Sedation, daytime sleepiness
Anxiolytics, sedatives, hypnotics	Alprazolam, chloral hydrate, chlordiazepoxide, clonazepam, diazepam, doxepin, lorazepam, zolpidem	Sedation, daytime sleepiness
Barbiturates	Phenobarbital, secobarbital	Sedation, daytime sleepiness
Beta-blockers	Atenolol, carvedilol, metoprolol	Bradycardia
Cannabinoids	Dronabinol, nabilone	Sedation, daytime sleepiness
Corticosteroids	Dexamethasone, prednisone	Sleep disturbances, proximal muscle weakness
Hormonal anticancer treatments	Androgen deprivation therapy, aromatase inhibitors, selective estrogen receptor modulators	Sarcopenia, fatigue, muscle weakness
Opioid analgesics	Codeine, fentanyl, hydrocodone, hydromorphone, methadone, morphine, oxycodone	Sedation, daytime sleepiness
Skeletal muscle relaxants	Baclofen	Sedation, daytime sleepiness, muscle weakness

Note. Based on information from Savard et al., 2015; X.S. Wang et al., 2014; Zlott & Byrne, 2010.

(Hilfiker et al., 2017; Mitchell et al., 2014; NCCN, 2018; Schmitz et al., 2010). All patients with cancer should be encouraged to maintain an optimum level of physical activity during and following cancer treatment. Exercise improves aerobic capacity, prevents muscle loss and deconditioning, and may favorably affect sleep quality, psychological stress, mood, and quality of life (Gerritsen & Vincent, 2016).

a) Exercise intensity, frequency, and type of activity need further study to determine the most beneficial program for each individual and stage of disease. Referral for structured rehabilitation may be helpful and has been shown to be an effective intervention for CRF (Mitchell et al., 2014; NCCN, 2018).

b) National guidelines recommend that patients aim for at least 150 minutes of moderate-intensity physical activity (brisk walking, bicycling, swimming, deep water walking/running) each week. Strength training (all major muscle groups, 10 repetitions, 1–3 sets per exercise) should be performed two times weekly.

c) Other types of physical activity, including yoga, Pilates, tai chi, or organized sports, can also be incorporated.

d) Provide referrals to community-based exercise programs, comprehensive rehabilitation programs, or an exercise professional (e.g., physical therapist, exercise trainer, physiatrist).

e) Exercise programs must be undertaken with caution and only after medical clearance for patients with bone metastasis, immunosuppression or neutropenia, fever, thrombocytopenia, anemia, peripheral neuropathy, risk for falls, or treatment complications.

f) Medical clearance should be obtained prior to initiating an exercise program for patients with osteoporosis, bone metastases, neuropathy, neurologic disorders, weakness, cardiopulmonary dysfunction, arrhythmia, chest pain, shortness of breath, peripheral edema, or history of coronary artery disease. Patients with compromised immunity require clearance before using public gyms or pools. Patients with a tunneled or peripherally inserted central venous catheter must avoid swimming.

g) Programs should be initiated slowly so the patient's tolerance can be assessed. Activity can be modified or advanced as the patient's condition changes (NCCN, 2018). Walking, cycling, swimming, resistance training, and a combination of these have been evaluated and are reasonable modalities for patients to choose. Programs that are too vigorous during treatment may increase fatigue.

h) Mobile health tools such as activity monitors, smartphone apps, and social media may help to strengthen motivation and adherence.

i) Relative contraindications to exercise include nonhealed surgical wounds, extreme fatigue, severe anemia, ataxia, and acute arm or shoulder problems, including lymphedema (avoid upper body exercises).

j) Instruct patients to stop exercise and contact a member of their healthcare team if they experience dizziness, blurred vision, fainting, sudden onset of nausea or vomiting, unusual or sudden shortness of breath, irregular heartbeat, palpitations, chest pain, leg or calf pain, bone or joint pain, muscle cramping, or sudden onset of muscle weakness. During treatment and immediately following its completion, patients should be encouraged to exercise with a partner, caregiver, or exercise professional for safety reasons.

3. Yoga: Evidence from controlled trials shows that yoga is effective in reducing fatigue, particularly in breast cancer survivors (Bower et al., 2012; Kiecolt-Glaser et al., 2014; Vardar Yağlı et al., 2015). However, five systematic reviews (Buffart et al., 2012; Felbel, Meerpohl, Monsef, Engert, & Skoetz, 2014; Harder, Parlour, & Jenkins, 2012; Sadja & Mills, 2013; Zhang, Yang, Tian, & Wang, 2012) all concluded that due to a high risk of bias in the studies, the effectiveness of yoga on fatigue outcomes has not been sufficiently established as effective in reducing fatigue across a wide range of patient populations or at all points in the cancer continuum.

4. Tai chi and qigong have shown beneficial effects on fatigue outcomes in randomized clinical trials; however, study results should be interpreted cautiously because of heterogeneous study quality and high risk of bias (Xiang, Lu, Chen, & Wen, 2017; Zeng, Luo, Xie, Huang, & Cheng, 2014).

5. Structured rehabilitation improves fatigue outcomes, particularly in cancer survivors (Egan et al., 2013; Mitchell et al., 2014; Scott et al., 2013). The rehabilitation interventions tested were generally multicomponent interventions that included a combination of exercise, psychoeducational support, mind–body therapies, and physical modalities such as manual lymph drainage.

6. Psychoeducational interventions: Consistent evidence shows that psychoeducational interventions including anticipatory guidance, energy conservation, coaching to enhance self-efficacy, goal setting, and emotional support improve fatigue outcomes, although effect sizes may be small (Bennett et al., 2016; Duijts, Faber, Oldenburg, van Beurden, & Aaronson, 2011; Fors et al., 2011; Goedendorp, Gielissen, Verhagen, & Bleijenberg, 2009; Howell, Harth, Brown, Bennett, & Boyko, 2017; Kangas, Bovbjerg, & Montgomery, 2008; Larkin, Lopez, & Aromataris, 2014; Pachman, Price, & Carey, 2014).

a) Psychoeducational interventions that have been shown to be effective include anticipatory guidance about patterns of fatigue, counseling and supportive psychotherapy, cognitive behavioral therapy (CBT), care coordination, and recommendations for energy conservation and self-management (e.g., exercise, lifestyle changes to improve sleep quality), together with coaching, praise, and encouragement to augment feelings of control and promote self-efficacy. Principles of patient and family education are detailed later in this chapter.

b) CBT approaches (with or without hypnosis) for fatigue, depression, or pain are generally promising for the relief of CRF in a variety of patient populations during and following cancer treatment (Carlson et al., 2017; Cramer et al., 2015; Duijts et al., 2011; Kwekkeboom, Cherwin, Lee, & Wanta, 2010).

c) Energy conservation: NCCN (2018) guidelines describe the goal of energy conservation as maintaining balance between rest and activity so that valued activities can be maintained during periods of high fatigue. This is a learned process for each patient and is dictated by the patient's disease experience.

(1) Instruct patients to delegate activities, pace themselves, take extra rest periods, plan high-energy activities at times of peak energy, and conserve energy for valued activities (NCCN, 2018).

(2) Recommend energy-saving devices (e.g., raised toilet seats, grabber tools, seated walkers, wheelchairs).

7. Control concurrent symptoms (e.g., pain, depression, shortness of breath): Interven-

tions for management of concurrent symptoms that have demonstrated an impact on fatigue outcomes include an advanced practice nursing intervention that incorporated systematic symptom monitoring (de Raaf et al., 2013) and symptom-focused palliative care interventions (Kao, Hu, Chiu, & Chen, 2014; Yennurajalingam et al., 2011).

8. Improve sleep quality: CBT for insomnia (CBT-I) to optimize sleep quality has been shown to decrease CRF (Johnson et al., 2016; Mitchell et al., 2014; NCCN, 2018).
   a) These interventions to improve sleep quality can be effectively delivered individually, in a group setting, or via the web.
   b) CBT-I may take several weeks of steady practice to become fully effective and usually requires four to eight 30-minute sessions with a behavioral sleep therapist, such as a nurse, psychologist, or other professional.
   c) Components of CBT-I
      (1) Stimulus control: Go to bed only when sleepy, use the bed/bedroom for sleep and sexual activities only, and maintain a consistent presleep routine and a consistent time to lie down and get up.
      (2) Sleep consolidation: Limit the amount of time in bed, including naps.
      (3) Sleep hygiene: Avoid caffeine late in the day, and provide a comfortable sleep environment to promote a good night's sleep.
      (4) Intervention components also include relaxation training and strategies to reduce cognitive-emotional arousal (e.g., keep at least an hour to relax before going to bed, establish a presleep routine to be used every night).
9. Meditation, mindfulness-based stress reduction, and cognitive behavioral stress management have been shown in several randomized controlled trials to improve both fatigue severity and fatigue-related daytime interference in women receiving treatment for breast cancer and in survivors who have completed treatment for breast or colorectal cancer (Haller et al., 2017; Mitchell et al., 2014; NCCN, 2018). These interventions also favorably affect fatigue-related biomarkers (Carlson et al., 2017).
10. Progressive muscle relaxation with or without imagery, relaxation breathing, coping skills training, or distraction delivered in a series of sessions has demonstrated effectiveness in improving fatigue outcomes (Carlson et al., 2017; Hilfiker et al., 2017).
11. Bright-light therapy has been shown in controlled trials to prevent deterioration in patients with CRF during chemotherapy for breast cancer (Ancoli-Israel et al., 2012; Redd et al., 2014) and in cancer survivors post-treatment (Johnson et al., 2018), potentially by protecting recipients from circadian rhythm desynchronization (Neikrug et al., 2012). Trials of this promising therapy are ongoing in other patient populations.
12. Evidence for the effectiveness of acupuncture, acupressure, self-acupuncture, and electroacupuncture in reducing CRF has been summarized in nearly a dozen meta-analyses or systematic reviews (Chien, Liu, & Hsu, 2013; Finnegan-John, Molassiotis, Richardson, & Ream, 2013; Garcia et al., 2013; He, Wang, & Li, 2013; Johnston et al., 2011; Kilian-Kita, Puskulluoglu, Konopka, & Krzemieniecki, 2016; Lau et al., 2016; Molassiotis et al., 2012, 2013; O'Regan & Filshie, 2010; Posadzki et al., 2013; Smith, Carmady, Thornton, Perz, & Ussher, 2013; Tao et al., 2016; Towler, Molassiotis, & Brearley, 2013; Zeng et al., 2014). While a majority of these reviews concluded that acupuncture and acupressure interventions are beneficial, acceptable, and well tolerated, the authors drew somewhat conflicting conclusions about whether these interventions were ready for translation into practice (Azad & John, 2013; Ernst & Posadzki, 2013; Molassiotis, 2013a, 2013b; Molassiotis & Richardson, 2013), and all have urged for additional study using rigorous trial designs.
13. Complementary and integrative therapies: Evidence is emerging from small trials that complementary therapies including polarity therapy, moxibustion, healing touch, Reiki, and massage may improve CRF (Carlson et al., 2017; Hilfiker et al., 2017; Mao et al., 2016; Mitchell et al., 2014; Viscuse et al., 2017). Continued study of these potentially promising interventions with longer follow-up and active control conditions is warranted. Complementary and integrative medicine strategies such as these are well tolerated and may be particularly useful when strategies such as exercise are contraindicated or infeasible. They can be considered to augment other treatment approaches for fatigue such as yoga, relaxation, or CBT.
14. Pharmacologic interventions: Because the exact pathophysiology of CRF is obscure, pharmacotherapy is empiric or geared toward reversing possible contributing factors such as anemia, poor nutrition, or depression (Bower, 2014; Minton, Richardson, Sharpe, Hotopf, & Stone, 2008).

a) Erythropoiesis-stimulating agents (ESAs): Data from several systematic reviews suggest that patients receiving recombinant human erythropoietin to correct anemia less than 10 g/dl may experience increased vigor and diminished fatigue (Bohlius, Tonia, & Schwarzer, 2011; Eton & Cella, 2011; Tonia & Bohlius, 2011), but only limited evidence supports that ESAs improve fatigue when anemia is less severe (Bohlius et al., 2014; Grant et al., 2013). A target hemoglobin level of 11–12 g/dl will produce the greatest gains in fatigue and other quality-of-life outcomes (Eton & Cella, 2011). Although ESAs are generally well tolerated, because of safety issues, the use of these agents specifically for the management of fatigue is not recommended (Bormanis et al., 2013; Gao, Ma, & Lu, 2013; Wauters & Vansteenkiste, 2012). National clinical practice guidelines (Lichtin, 2011; NCCN, 2018; Rizzo et al., 2010) and the guidance of the U.S. Food and Drug Administration (2016) should be used to weigh risks and benefits and to guide the management of patients receiving ESAs.

b) Antidepressants have been recommended as treatment for fatigue when depression is suggested as a causal factor. In particular, paroxetine, bupropion, and venlafaxine have been studied. Although these drugs may be helpful in alleviating depression, studies have not demonstrated a benefit compared to placebo in nondepressed patients with fatigue, and they are not recommended specifically to lessen fatigue (Mitchell et al., 2014; Mücke et al., 2016; NCCN, 2018). Small trials have also shown a trend toward a possible benefit for antidepressant agents in treating fatigue in two distinct subpopulations: women experiencing hot flashes (Carpenter et al., 2007; Weitzner, Moncello, Jacobsen, & Minton, 2002) and patients receiving interferon alfa (Capuron et al., 2002).

c) Several systematic reviews have concluded that preliminary evidence supports the use of psychostimulants (methylphenidate, dexmethylphenidate, modafinil) to treat CRF (Breitbart & Alici, 2010; Gong et al., 2014; Minton, Richardson, Sharpe, Hotopf, & Stone, 2011; Portela, Rubiales, & Centeno, 2011; Qu et al., 2016; Yennurajalingam & Bruera, 2014a). However, given the mixed evidence for efficacy (Moraska et al., 2010; Spathis et al., 2014) and a concern about the potential for side effects (headache, insomnia, agitation, anorexia, nausea, vomiting, and dry mouth), the use of these agents outside of clinical trials has been discouraged (Barton, 2014; Ruddy, Barton, & Loprinzi, 2014).

d) Corticosteroids (prednisone and dexamethasone) have short-term efficacy in ameliorating CRF. Given the potential detrimental side effects of muscle wasting and infection with long-term use, it is difficult to draw definitive conclusions about the risk–benefit profile (Franco, William, Poon, & Azad, 2014; Yennurajalingam & Bruera, 2014a, 2014b; Yennurajalingam et al., 2013).

e) Megestrol acetate is widely used for appetite improvement, and its safety and efficacy have been confirmed in treating cancer cachexia. However, a meta-analysis of the four trials that compared progestational steroids with placebo found no difference in the two arms for reducing CRF (NCCN, 2018; Payne, Wiffen, & Martin, 2012).

f) Androgen replacement therapy: Although male hypogonadism is thought to be a contributor to fatigue (Vigano et al., 2010), a blinded, placebo-controlled trial of testosterone replacement in a small sample of men with advanced cancer did not improve fatigue endpoints (Del Fabbro et al., 2013).

g) Thyrotropin-releasing hormone improved fatigue outcomes in a small, pilot, randomized, placebo-controlled crossover study in eight patients with cancer who also had significant fatigue (Kamath, Feinn, & Winokur, 2012).

h) Targeted anticytokine therapy may have favorable effects on CRF (Monk et al., 2006; Tookman, Jones, DeWitte, & Lodge, 2008); however, small sample sizes and the nonrandomized uncontrolled study design limit the strength of the conclusions that can be drawn.

i) Ginseng: Wisconsin ginseng, Asian ginseng, and fermented red ginseng extract were effective in improving fatigue outcomes in patients during and following cancer treatment (Barton et al., 2013; Jiang et al., 2017; H.S. Kim et al., 2017; Yennurajalingam et al., 2015).

j) Several nutritional and herbal supplements (e.g., guarana, essiac, valerian, vitamin supplements, zinc, levocarnitine, coenzyme Q10, mistletoe extract) and combined modality interventions that incorporate several complementary therapies (e.g., megestrol acetate and omega-3 fatty acid supplementation) have also been evaluated with mixed evidence for efficacy (Mitchell et al., 2014; NCCN, 2018).

Interpretation of the study outcomes in these trials is limited by small sample sizes and the predominantly single-arm, open-label study designs (Mitchell et al., 2014).

F. Patient and family education
1. Management of fatigue originates with the primary oncology team with assessment of fatigue as a symptom related to treatment and disease status. This begins with an initial screening and then expands to a more focused evaluation for moderate to higher levels of fatigue (NCCN, 2018).
2. Inform patients and family members that fatigue is a major symptom related to the disease and treatment process and that patterns are variable and not necessarily an indication of treatment failure or disease progression. Explain the multifactorial causes of fatigue, including psychosocial stressors, concurrent symptoms, sleep disturbances, muscle weakness and deconditioning, sedating side effects of medications, and proinflammatory cytokine release.
3. Daily self-monitoring of fatigue levels in a log or diary can be helpful (NCCN, 2018). Encourage patients to differentiate facets of the fatigue experience (fatigue, tiredness, weakness, cognitive slowing) and to document the use and effectiveness of self-management interventions (exercise, sleep, progressive muscle relaxation, meditation).
4. Offer anticipatory guidance about possible patterns of fatigue occurrence (e.g., at nadir; with conclusion of radiation therapy; in association with boredom, excess activity, and impaired sleep quality or stress).
5. Develop and tailor an individualized plan for fatigue management.
6. Inform patients and families that interventions such as energy conservation, exercise, relaxation and stress management, psychosocial support, and measures to optimize sleep quality and reduce concurrent symptoms have been shown to be effective in limiting the severity of fatigue during treatment.
7. Teach energy conservation strategies and other self-management techniques and provide coaching to enhance self-efficacy and to integrate these techniques into daily life.
8. Provide information concerning the importance of a balanced diet with adequate intake of fluid, calories, protein, carbohydrates, fat, vitamins, and minerals (NCCN, 2018).
9. Instruct patients in implementing a balanced exercise program (e.g., walking, stretching, and strength training). Encourage patients to continue normal activities and to remain as active as possible during treatment. Following treatment, the exercise program should be advanced as tolerated, gradually building up the length and intensity of physical activity to meet national guidelines of at least 150 minutes of moderate-intensity physical activity each week. Offer referrals to exercise professionals and community-based exercise programs.
10. Offer information and referrals to counseling or a support group (in person or online). Supportive expressive therapies, counseling, and journal writing may serve as an emotional outlet, as well as an avenue for support and encouragement (NCCN, 2018). Oncology nurses frequently provide this one-on-one education and support for patients.
11. Care planning
    a) Causes of CRF often are overlapping and may evolve across the cancer continuum from diagnosis to treatment to survivorship or end of life. Intervention approaches for each patient are therefore symptom oriented and individualized.
    b) The care plan should be regularly revised based on goals, preferences, response, and tolerance.
    c) A multimodal approach that includes exercise, psychoeducational interventions, management of concurrent symptoms, and efforts to improve sleep quality, together with judicious use of complementary therapies such as relaxation, massage, acupuncture or bright-light therapy, offers the greatest likelihood of success and is consistent with evidence-based guidelines from NCCN (2018) and the Oncology Nursing Society (Mitchell et al., 2014).
    d) Consideration may be given to a trial of antidepressants, psychostimulants, wakefulness-promoting agents, corticosteroids, or ginseng in specific clinical circumstances.

References

Abdel-Rahman, O., Helbling, D., Schmidt, J., Petrausch, U., Giryes, A., Mehrabi, A., ... Oweira, H. (2016). Treatment-associated fatigue in cancer patients treated with immune checkpoint inhibitors: A systematic review and meta-analysis. *Clinical Oncology, 28,* e127–e138. https://doi.org/10.1016/j.clon.2016.06.008

Alesi, E.R., & del Fabbro, E. (2014). Opportunities for targeting the fatigue-anorexia-cachexia symptom cluster. *Cancer Journal, 20,* 325–329. https://doi.org/10.1097/PPO.0000000000000065

Ancoli-Israel, S., Rissling, M., Neikrug, A., Trofimenko, V., Natarajan, L., Parker, B.A., … Liu, L. (2012). Light treatment prevents fatigue in women undergoing chemotherapy for breast cancer. *Supportive Care in Cancer, 20,* 1211–1219. https://doi.org/10.1007/s00520-011-1203-z

Azad, A., & John, T. (2013). Do randomized acupuncture studies in patients with cancer need a sham acupuncture control arm? *Journal of Clinical Oncology, 31,* 2057–2058. https://doi.org/10.1200/JCO.2012.47.8750

Balducci, L. (2010). Anemia, fatigue and aging. *Transfusion Clinique et Biologique, 17,* 375–381. https://doi.org/10.1016/j.tracli.2010.09.169

Barsevick, A.M., Cleeland, C.S., Manning, D.C., O'Mara, A.M., Reeve, B.B., Scott, J.A., & Sloan, J.A. (2010). ASCPRO recommendations for the assessment of fatigue as an outcome in clinical trials. *Journal of Pain and Symptom Management, 39,* 1086–1099. https://doi.org/10.1016/j.jpainsymman.2010.02.006

Barsevick, A., Frost, M., Zwinderman, A., Hall, P., & Halyard, M. (2010). I'm so tired: Biological and genetic mechanisms of cancer-related fatigue. *Quality of Life Research, 19,* 1419–1427. https://doi.org/10.1007/s11136-010-9757-7

Barton, D. (2014). Journey to Oz in search of a remedy for fatigue. *Cancer Journal, 20,* 15–17. https://doi.org/10.1097/PPO.0000000000000019

Barton, D.L., Liu, H., Dakhil, S.R., Linquist, B., Sloan, J.A., Nichols, C.R., … Loprinzi, C.L. (2013). Wisconsin ginseng (*Panax quinquefolius*) to improve cancer-related fatigue: A randomized, double-blind trial, N07C2. *Journal of the National Cancer Institute, 105,* 1230–1238. https://doi.org/10.1093/jnci/djt181

Bennett, S., Pigott, A., Beller, E.M., Haines, T., Meredith, P., & Delaney, C. (2016). Educational interventions for the management of cancer-related fatigue in adults. *Cochrane Database of Systematic Reviews, 2016*(11). https://doi.org/10.1002/14651858.CD008144.pub2

Berger, A.M., Gerber, L.H., & Mayer, D.K. (2012). Cancer-related fatigue: Implications for breast cancer survivors. *Cancer, 118*(Suppl. 8), 2261–2269. https://doi.org/10.1002/cncr.27475

Berger, A.M., Yennu, S., & Million, R. (2013). Update on interventions focused on symptom clusters: What has been tried and what have we learned? *Current Opinion in Supportive and Palliative Care, 7,* 60–66. https://doi.org/10.1097/SPC.0b013e32835c7d88

Bohlius, J., Tonia, T., Nüesch, E., Jüni, P., Fey, M.F., Egger, M., & Bernhard, J. (2014). Effects of erythropoiesis-stimulating agents on fatigue- and anaemia-related symptoms in cancer patients: Systematic review and meta-analyses of published and unpublished data. *British Journal of Cancer, 111,* 33–45. https://doi.org/10.1038/bjc.2014.171

Bohlius, J., Tonia, T., & Schwarzer, G. (2011). Twist and shout: One decade of meta-analyses of erythropoiesis-stimulating agents in cancer patients. *Acta Haematologica, 125,* 55–67. https://doi.org/10.1159/000318897

Bormanis, J., Quirt, I., Chang, J., Kouroukis, C.T., MacDonald, D., Melosky, B., … Couture, F. (2013). Erythropoiesis-stimulating agents (ESAs): Do they still have a role in chemotherapy-induced anemia (CIA)? *Critical Reviews in Oncology/Hematology, 87,* 132–139. https://doi.org/10.1016/j.critrevonc.2012.12.010

Borneman, T., Piper, B.F., Koczywas, M., Munevar, C.M., Sun, V., Uman, G.C., & Ferrell, B.R. (2012). A qualitative analysis of cancer-related fatigue in ambulatory oncology [Online exclusive]. *Clinical Journal of Oncology Nursing, 16,* E26–E32. https://doi.org/10.1188/12.CJON.E26-E32

Borthwick, D., Knowles, G., McNamara, S., O'Dea, R., & Stroner, P. (2003). Assessing fatigue and self-care strategies in patients receiving radiotherapy for non-small cell lung cancer. *European Journal of Oncology Nursing, 7,* 231–241. https://doi.org/10.1016/S1462-3889(03)00046-2

Bower, J.E. (2014). Cancer-related fatigue—Mechanisms, risk factors, and treatments. *Nature Reviews Clinical Oncology, 11,* 597–609. https://doi.org/10.1038/nrclinonc.2014.127

Bower, J.E., Garet, D., Sternlieb, B., Ganz, P.A., Irwin, M.R., Olmstead, R., & Greendale, G. (2012). Yoga for persistent fatigue in breast cancer survivors: A randomized controlled trial. *Cancer, 118,* 3766–3775. https://doi.org/10.1002/cncr.26702

Bower, J.E., & Lamkin, D.M. (2013). Inflammation and cancer-related fatigue: Mechanisms, contributing factors, and treatment implications. *Brain, Behavior, and Immunity, 30*(Suppl.), S48–S57. https://doi.org/10.1016/j.bbi.2012.06.011

Breitbart, W., & Alici, Y. (2010). Psychostimulants for cancer-related fatigue. *Journal of the National Comprehensive Cancer Network, 8,* 933–942. https://doi.org/10.6004/jnccn.2010.0068

Brown, L.F., & Kroenke, K. (2009). Cancer-related fatigue and its associations with depression and anxiety: A systematic review. *Psychosomatics, 50,* 440–447. https://doi.org/10.1016/S0033-3182(09)70835-7

Buffart, L.M., van Uffelen, J.G.Z., Riphagen, I.I., Brug, J., van Mechelen, W., Brown, W.J., & Chinapaw, M.J.M. (2012). Physical and psychosocial benefits of yoga in cancer patients and survivors, a systematic review and meta-analysis of randomized controlled trials. *BMC Cancer, 12,* 559. https://doi.org/10.1186/1471-2407-12-559

Campos, M.P.O., Hassan, B.J., Riechelmann, R., & Del Giglio, A. (2011). Cancer-related fatigue: A practical review. *Annals of Oncology, 22,* 1273–1279. https://doi.org/10.1093/annonc/mdq458

Capuron, L., Gumnick, J.F., Musselman, D.L., Lawson, D.H., Reemsnyder, A., Nemeroff, C.B., & Miller, A.H. (2002). Neurobehavioral effects of interferon-α in cancer patients: Phenomenology and paroxetine responsiveness of symptom dimensions. *Neuropsychopharmacology, 26,* 643–652. https://doi.org/10.1016/S0893-133X(01)00407-9

Carlson, L.E., Zelinski, E., Toivonen, K., Flynn, M., Qureshi, M., Piedalue, K.-A., & Grant, R. (2017). Mind-body therapies in cancer: What is the latest evidence? *Current Oncology Reports, 19,* 67. https://doi.org/10.1007/s11912-017-0626-1

Carpenter, J.S., Storniolo, A.M., Johns, S., Monahan, P.O., Azzouz, F., Elam, J.L., … Shelton, R.C. (2007). Randomized, double-blind, placebo-controlled crossover trials of venlafaxine for hot flashes after breast cancer. *Oncologist, 12,* 124–135. https://doi.org/10.1634/theoncologist.12-1-124

Chien, T.-J., Liu, C.-Y., & Hsu, C.-H. (2013). Integrating acupuncture into cancer care. *Journal of Traditional and Complementary Medicine, 3,* 234–239. https://doi.org/10.4103/2225-4110.119733

Cramer, H., Lauche, R., Paul, A., Langhorst, J., Kümmel, S., & Dobos, G.J. (2015). Hypnosis in breast cancer care: A systematic review of randomized controlled trials. *Integrative Cancer Therapies, 14,* 5–15. https://doi.org/10.1177/1534735414550035

Curt, G., & Johnston, P.G. (2003). Cancer fatigue: The way forward. *Oncologist, 8*(Suppl. 1), 27–30. https://doi.org/10.1634/theoncologist.8-suppl_1-27

Danjoux, C., Gardner, S., & Fitch, M. (2007). Prospective evaluation of fatigue during a course of curative radiotherapy for localised prostate cancer. *Supportive Care in Cancer, 15,* 1169–1176. https://doi.org/10.1007/s00520-007-0229-8

Dantzer, R., Heijnen, C.J., Kavelaars, A., Laye, S., & Capuron, L. (2014). The neuroimmune basis of fatigue. *Trends in Neurosciences, 37,* 39–46. https://doi.org/10.1016/j.tins.2013.10.003

Davis, M.P., & Goforth, H. (2014). Fighting insomnia and battling lethargy: The yin and yang of palliative care. *Current Oncology Reports, 16,* 377. https://doi.org/10.1007/s11912-014-0377-1

de Jong, N., Candel, M.J.J.M., Schouten, H.C., Abu-Saad, H.H., & Courtens, A.M. (2006). Course of the fatigue dimension "activity level" and the interference of fatigue with daily living activities for patients with breast cancer receiving adjuvant chemotherapy. *Cancer Nursing, 29,* E1–E13. https://doi.org/10.1097/00002820-200609000-00013

de Jong, N., Courtens, A.M., Abu-Saad, H.H., & Schouten, H.C. (2002). Fatigue in patients with breast cancer receiving adjuvant chemotherapy: A review of the literature. *Cancer Nursing, 25,* 283–297. https://doi.org/10.1097/00002820-200208000-00004

Del Fabbro, E., Garcia, J.M., Dev, R., Hui, D., Williams, J., Engineer, D., ... Bruera, E. (2013). Testosterone replacement for fatigue in hypogonadal ambulatory males with advanced cancer: A preliminary double-blind placebo-controlled trial. *Supportive Care in Cancer, 21,* 2599–2607. https://doi.org/10.1007/s00520-013-1832-5

de Raaf, P.J., de Klerk, C., Timman, R., Busschbach, J.J.V., Oldenmenger, W.H., & van der Rijt, C.C.D. (2013). Systematic monitoring and treatment of physical symptoms to alleviate fatigue in patients with advanced cancer: A randomized controlled trial. *Journal of Clinical Oncology, 31,* 716–723. https://doi.org/10.1200/JCO.2012.44.4216

Dhruva, A., Aouizerat, B.E., Cooper, B., Paul, S.M., Dodd, M., West, C., ... Miaskowski, C. (2013). Differences in morning and evening fatigue in oncology patients and their family caregivers. *European Journal of Oncology Nursing, 17,* 841–848. https://doi.org/10.1016/j.ejon.2013.06.002

Dimeo, F., Schmittel, A., Fietz, T., Schwartz, S., Köhler, P., Böning, D., & Thiel, E. (2004). Physical performance, depression, immune status and fatigue in patients with hematological malignancies after treatment. *Annals of Oncology, 15,* 1237–1242. https://doi.org/10.1093/annonc/mdh314

Duijts, S.F., Faber, M.M., Oldenburg, H.S.A., van Beurden, M., & Aaronson, N.K. (2011). Effectiveness of behavioral techniques and physical exercise on psychosocial functioning and health-related quality of life in breast cancer patients and survivors—A meta-analysis. *Psycho-Oncology, 20,* 115–126. https://doi.org/10.1002/pon.1728

Egan, M.Y., McEwen, S., Sikora, L., Chasen, M., Fitch, M., & Eldred, S. (2013). Rehabilitation following cancer treatment. *Disability and Rehabilitation, 35,* 2245–2258. https://doi.org/10.3109/09638288.2013.774441

Ernst, E., & Posadzki, P. (2013). Reply to Molassiotis. *Supportive Care in Cancer, 21,* 3257. https://doi.org/10.1007/s00520-013-1990-5

Escalante, C.P., & Manzullo, E.F. (2009). Cancer-related fatigue: The approach and treatment. *Journal of General Internal Medicine, 24*(Suppl. 2), 412–416. https://doi.org/10.1007/s11606-009-1056-z

Eton, D.T., & Cella, D. (2011). Do erythropoietic-stimulating agents relieve fatigue? A review of reviews. In G.H. Lyman & D.C. Dale (Eds.), *Cancer Treatment Research: Vol. 157. Hematopoietic growth factors in oncology* (pp. 181–194). https://doi.org/10.1007/978-1-4419-7073-2_11

Felbel, S., Meerpohl, J.J., Monsef, I., Engert, A., & Skoetz, N. (2014). Yoga in addition to standard care for patients with haematological malignancies. *Cochrane Database of Systematic Reviews, 2014*(6). https://doi.org/10.1002/14651858.CD010146.pub2

Filler, K., Lyon, D., Bennett, J., McCain, N., Elswick, R., Lukkahatai, N., & Saligan, L.N. (2014). Association of mitochondrial dysfunction and fatigue: A review of the literature. *BBA Clinical, 1,* 12–23. https://doi.org/10.1016/j.bbacli.2014.04.001

Finnegan-John, J., Molassiotis, A., Richardson, A., & Ream, E. (2013). A systematic review of complementary and alternative medicine interventions for the management of cancer-related fatigue. *Integrative Cancer Therapies, 12,* 276–290. https://doi.org/10.1177/1534735413485816

Fitzgerald, P., Lo, C., Li, M., Gagliese, L., Zimmermann, C., & Rodin, G. (2013). The relationship between depression and physical symptom burden in advanced cancer. *BMJ Supportive and Palliative Care, 5,* 381–388. https://doi.org/10.1136/bmjspcare-2012-000380

Fors, E.A., Bertheussen, G.F., Thune, I., Juvet, L.K., Elvsaas, I.-K.Ø., Oldervoll, L., ... Leivseth, G. (2011). Psychosocial interventions as part of breast cancer rehabilitation programs? Results from a systematic review. *Psycho-Oncology, 20,* 909–918. https://doi.org/10.1002/pon.1844

Franco, M., William, L., Poon, P., & Azad, A. (2014). Dexamethasone for cancer-related fatigue. *Journal of Clinical Oncology, 32,* 608–609. https://doi.org/10.1200/JCO.2013.53.7878

Gao, S., Ma, J.-J., & Lu, C. (2013). Venous thromboembolism risk and erythropoiesis-stimulating agents for the treatment of cancer-associated anemia: A meta-analysis. *Tumor Biology, 35,* 603–613. https://doi.org/10.1007/s13277-013-1084-5

Garcia, M.K., McQuade, J., Haddad, R., Patel, S., Lee, R., Yang, P., ... Cohen, L. (2013). Systematic review of acupuncture in cancer care: A synthesis of the evidence. *Journal of Clinical Oncology, 31,* 952–960. https://doi.org/10.1200/JCO.2012.43.5818

Gerber, L.H. (2017). Cancer-related fatigue: Persistent, pervasive, and problematic. *Physical Medicine and Rehabilitation Clinics of North America, 28,* 65–88. https://doi.org/10.1016/j.pmr.2016.08.004

Gerritsen, J.K.W., & Vincent, A.J.P.E. (2016). Exercise improves quality of life in patients with cancer: A systematic review and meta-analysis of randomised controlled trials. *British Journal of Sports Medicine, 50,* 796–803. https://doi.org/10.1136/bjsports-2015-094787

Goedendorp, M.M., Gielissen, M.F.M., Verhagen, C.A.H.H.V.M., & Bleijenberg, G. (2009). Psychosocial interventions for reducing fatigue during cancer treatment in adults. *Cochrane Database of Systematic Reviews, 2009*(1). https://doi.org/10.1002/14651858.CD006953.pub2

Goedendorp, M.M., Gielissen, M.F., Verhagen, C.A.H.H.V.M., & Bleijenberg, G. (2013). Development of fatigue in cancer survivors: A prospective follow-up study from diagnosis into the year after treatment. *Journal of Pain and Symptom Management, 45,* 213–222. https://doi.org/10.1016/j.jpainsymman.2012.02.009

Goedendorp, M.M., Jacobsen, P.B., & Andrykowski, M.A. (2016). Fatigue screening in breast cancer patients: Identifying likely cases of cancer-related fatigue. *Psycho-Oncology, 25,* 275–281. https://doi.org/10.1002/pon.3907

Goldberg, J.D., & Giralt, S. (2013). Assessing response of therapy for acute and chronic graft-versus-host disease. *Expert Review of Hematology, 6,* 103–107. https://doi.org/10.1586/ehm.12.65

Gong, S., Sheng, P., Jin, H., He, H., Qi, E., Chen, W., ... Hou, L. (2014). Effect of methylphenidate in patients with cancer-related fatigue: A systematic review and meta-analysis. *PLOS ONE, 9,* e84391. https://doi.org/10.1371/journal.pone.0084391

Grant, M.D., Piper, M., Bohlius, J., Tonia, T., Robert, N., Vats, V., ... Aronson, N. (2013). *Epoetin and darbepoetin for managing anemia in patients undergoing cancer treatment: Comparative effectiveness update* (AHRQ Publication No. 13-EHC077-EF). Rockville, MD: Agency for Healthcare Research and Quality.

Haller, H., Winkler, M.M., Klose, P., Dobos, G., Kümmel, S., & Cramer, H. (2017). Mindfulness-based interventions for women with breast cancer: An updated systematic review and meta-analysis. *Acta Oncologica, 56,* 1665–1676. https://doi.org/10.1080/0284186X.2017.1342862

Harder, H., Parlour, L., & Jenkins, V. (2012). Randomised controlled trials of yoga interventions for women with breast cancer: A systematic literature review. *Supportive Care in Cancer, 20,* 3055–3064. https://doi.org/10.1007/s00520-012-1611-8

He, X.-R., Wang, Q., & Li, P.-P. (2013). Acupuncture and moxibustion for cancer-related fatigue: A systematic review and meta-analysis. *Asian Pacific Journal of Cancer Prevention, 14,* 3067–3074. https://doi.org/10.7314/APJCP.2013.14.5.3067

Hilfiker, R., Meichtry, A., Eicher, M., Nilsson, B.L., Knols, R.H., Verra, M.L., & Taeymans, J. (2017). Exercise and other non-pharmaceutical interventions for cancer-related fatigue in patients during or after cancer treatment: A systematic review incorporating an indirect-comparisons meta-analysis. *British Journal of Sports Medicine, 53,* 651–658. https://doi.org/10.1136/bjsports-2016-096422

Hockenberry-Eaton, M., & Hinds, P.S. (2000). Fatigue in children and adolescents with cancer: Evolution of a program of study. *Seminars in Oncology Nursing, 16,* 261–272. https://doi.org/10.1053/sonu.2000.16577

Horneber, M., Fischer, I., Dimeo, F., Rüffer, J.U., & Weis, J. (2012). Cancer-related fatigue: Epidemiology, pathogenesis, diagnosis, and treatment. *Deutsches Ärzteblatt International, 109,* 161–172. https://doi.org/10.3238/arztebl.2012.0161

Howell, D., Harth, T., Brown, J., Bennett, C., & Boyko, S. (2017). Self-management education interventions for patients with cancer: A systematic review. *Supportive Care in Cancer, 25,* 1323–1355. https://doi.org/10.1007/s00520-016-3500-z

Howell, D., Keller-Olaman, S., Oliver, T.K., Hack, T.F., Broadfield, L., Biggs, K., … Olson, K. (2013). A pan-Canadian practice guideline and algorithm: Screening, assessment, and supportive care of adults with cancer-related fatigue. *Current Oncology, 20,* e233–e246. https://doi.org/10.3747/co.20.1302

Hsiao, C.-P., Wang, D., Kaushal, A., Chen, M.-K., & Saligan, L. (2014). Differential expression of genes related to mitochondrial biogenesis and bioenergetics in fatigued prostate cancer men receiving external beam radiation therapy. *Journal of Pain and Symptom Management, 48,* 1080–1090. https://doi.org/10.1016/j.jpainsymman.2014.03.010

Humpel, N., & Iverson, D.C. (2010). Sleep quality, fatigue and physical activity following a cancer diagnosis. *European Journal of Cancer Care, 19,* 761–768. https://doi.org/10.1111/j.1365-2354.2009.01126.x

Jiang, S.-L., Liu, H.-J., Liu, Z.-C., Liu, N., Liu, R., Kang, Y.-R., … Kang, S.-J. (2017). Adjuvant effects of fermented red ginseng extract on advanced non-small cell lung cancer patients treated with chemotherapy. *Chinese Journal of Integrative Medicine, 23,* 331–337. https://doi.org/10.1007/s11655-015-2146-x

Johnson, J.A., Garland, S.N., Carlson, L.E., Savard, J., Simpson, J.S.A., Ancoli-Israel, S., & Campbell, T.S. (2018). Bright light therapy improves cancer-related fatigue in cancer survivors: A randomized controlled trial. *Journal of Cancer Survivorship, 12,* 206–215. https://doi.org/10.1007/s11764-017-0659-3

Johnson, J.A., Rash, J.A., Campbell, T.S., Savard, J., Gehrman, P.R., Perlis, M., … Garland, S.N. (2016). A systematic review and meta-analysis of randomized controlled trials of cognitive behavior therapy for insomnia (CBT-I) in cancer survivors. *Sleep Medicine Reviews, 27,* 20–28. https://doi.org/10.1016/j.smrv.2015.07.001

Johnston, M.F., Hays, R.D., Subramanian, S.K., Elashoff, R.M., Axe, E.K., Li, J.-J., … Hui, K.-K. (2011). Patient education integrated with acupuncture for relief of cancer-related fatigue randomized controlled feasibility study. *BMC Complementary and Alternative Medicine, 11,* 49. https://doi.org/10.1186/1472-6882-11-49

Kamath, J. (2012). Cancer-related fatigue, inflammation and thyrotropin-releasing hormone. *Current Aging Science, 5,* 195–202. https://doi.org/10.2174/1874609811205030005

Kamath, J., Feinn, R., & Winokur, A. (2012). Thyrotropin-releasing hormone as a treatment for cancer-related fatigue: A randomized controlled study. *Supportive Care in Cancer, 20,* 1745–1753. https://doi.org/10.1007/s00520-011-1268-8

Kangas, M., Bovbjerg, D.H., & Montgomery, G.H. (2008). Cancer-related fatigue: A systematic and meta-analytic review of non-pharmacological therapies for cancer patients. *Psychology Bulletin, 134,* 700–741. https://doi.org/10.1037/a0012825

Kao, C.-Y., Hu, W.-Y., Chiu, T.-Y., & Chen, C.-Y. (2014). Effects of the hospital-based palliative care team on the care for cancer patients: An evaluation study. *International Journal of Nursing Studies, 51,* 226–235. https://doi.org/10.1016/j.ijnurstu.2013.05.008

Karshikoff, B., Sundelin, T., & Lasselin, J. (2017). Role of inflammation in human fatigue: Relevance of multidimensional assessments and potential neuronal mechanisms. *Frontiers in Immunology, 8,* 21. https://doi.org/10.3389/fimmu.2017.00021

Kiecolt-Glaser, J.K., Bennett, J.M., Andridge, R., Peng, J., Shapiro, C.L., Malarkey, W.B., … Glaser, R. (2014). Yoga's impact on inflammation, mood, and fatigue in breast cancer survivors: A randomized controlled trial. *Journal of Clinical Oncology, 32,* 1040–1049. https://doi.org/10.1200/JCO.2013.51.8860

Kilian-Kita, A., Puskulluoglu, M., Konopka, K., & Krzemieniecki, K. (2016). Acupuncture: Could it become everyday practice in oncology? *Contemporary Oncology, 20,* 119–123. https://doi.org/10.5114/wo.2016.60065

Kim, E.-J., Kim, N., & Cho, S.-G. (2013). The potential use of mesenchymal stem cells in hematopoietic stem cell transplantation. *Experimental and Molecular Medicine, 45,* e2. https://doi.org/10.1038/emm.2013.2

Kim, H.-J., Barsevick, A.M., Beck, S.L., & Dudley, W. (2012). Clinical subgroups of a psychoneurologic symptom cluster in women receiving treatment for breast cancer: A secondary analysis [Online exclusive]. *Oncology Nursing Forum, 39,* E20–E30. https://doi.org/10.1188/12.ONF.E20-E30

Kim, H.S., Kim, M.-K., Lee, M., Kwon, B.-S., Suh, D.H., & Song, Y.S. (2017). Effect of red ginseng on genotoxicity and health-related quality of life after adjuvant chemotherapy in patients with epithelial ovarian cancer: A randomized, double blind, placebo-controlled trial. *Nutrients, 9,* 772. https://doi.org/10.3390/nu9070772

Kim, H.T., & Armand, P. (2013). Clinical endpoints in allogeneic hematopoietic stem cell transplantation studies: The cost of freedom. *Biology of Blood and Marrow Transplantation, 19,* 860–866. https://doi.org/10.1016/j.bbmt.2013.01.003

Kirsh, K.L., Passik, S., Holtsclaw, E., Donaghy, K., & Theobald, D. (2001). I get tired for no reason: A single item screening for cancer-related fatigue. *Journal of Pain and Symptom Management, 22,* 931–937. https://doi.org/10.1016/S0885-3924(01)00350-5

Kiserud, C.E., Seland, M., Holte, H., Fosså, A., Fosså, S.D., Bollerslev, J., … Loge, J.H. (2015). Fatigue in male lymphoma survivors differs between diagnostic groups and is associated with latent hypothyroidism. *Acta Oncologica, 54,* 49–59. https://doi.org/10.3109/0284186X.2014.948057

Kisiel-Sajewicz, K., Davis, M.P., Siemionow, V., Seyidova-Khoshknabi, D., Wyant, A., Walsh, D., … Yue, G.H. (2012). Lack of muscle contractile property changes at the time of perceived physical exhaustion suggests central mechanisms contributing to early motor task failure in patients with cancer-related fatigue. *Journal of Pain and Symptom Management, 44,* 351–361. https://doi.org/10.1016/j.jpainsymman.2011.08.007

Koornstra, R.H.T., Peters, M., Donofrio, S., van den Borne, B., & de Jong, F.A. (2014). Management of fatigue in patients with cancer—A practical overview. *Cancer Treatment Reviews, 40,* 791–799. https://doi.org/10.1016/j.ctrv.2014.01.004

Kwekkeboom, K.L., Cherwin, C.H., Lee, J.W., & Wanta, B. (2010). Mind-body treatments for the pain-fatigue-sleep disturbance symptom cluster in persons with cancer. *Journal of Pain and Symptom Management, 39,* 126–138. https://doi.org/10.1016/j.jpainsymman.2009.05.022

Lacourt, T.E., & Heijnen, C.J. (2017). Mechanisms of neurotoxic symptoms as a result of breast cancer and its treatment: Considerations on the contribution of stress, inflammation, and cellular bioenergetics. *Current Breast Cancer Reports, 9,* 70–81. https://doi.org/10.1007/s12609-017-0245-8

Lai, J.-S., Cella, D., Choi, S., Junghaenel, D.U., Christodoulou, C., Gershon, R., & Stone, A. (2011). How item banks and their application can influence measurement practice in rehabilitation medicine: A PROMIS fatigue item bank example. *Archives of Physical and Medical Rehabilitation, 92*(Suppl. 10), S20–S27. https://doi.org/10.1016/j.apmr.2010.08.033

Lai, J.-S., Cella, D., Dineen, K., Bode, R., Von Roenn, J., Gershon, R.C., & Shevrin, D. (2005). An item bank was created to improve the measurement of cancer-related fatigue. *Journal of Clinical Epidemiology, 58,* 190–197. https://doi.org/10.1016/j.jclinepi.2003.07.016

Lai, J.-S., Stucky, B.D., Thissen, D., Varni, J.W., Dewitt, E.M., Irwin, D.F., … DeWalt, D.A. (2013). Development and psychometric properties of the PROMIS® pediatric fatigue item banks. *Quality of Life Research, 22,* 2417–2427. https://doi.org/10.1007/s11136-013-0357-1

Langston, B., Armes, J., Levy, A., Tidey, E., & Ream, E. (2013). The prevalence and severity of fatigue in men with prostate cancer: A systematic review of the literature. *Supportive Care in Cancer, 21,* 1761–1771. https://doi.org/10.1007/s00520-013-1751-5

Larkin, D., Lopez, V., & Aromataris, E. (2014). Managing cancer-related fatigue in men with prostate cancer: A systematic review of non-pharmacological interventions. *International Journal of Nursing Practice, 20,* 549–560. https://doi.org/10.1111/ijn.12211

Lau, C.H.Y., Wu, X., Chung, V.C., Liu, X., Hui, E.P., Cramer, H., … Wu, J.C.Y. (2016). Acupuncture and related therapies for symptom management in palliative cancer care: Systematic review and meta-analysis. *Medicine, 95,* e2901. https://doi.org/10.1097/MD.0000000000002901

Li, J., & Gu, J. (2017). Fatigue associated with newly approved vascular endothelial growth factor receptor tyrosine kinase inhibitors in cancer patients: An up-to-date meta-analysis. *International Journal of Clinical Oncology, 22,* 807–816. https://doi.org/10.1007/s10147-017-1167-1

Lichtin, A.E. (2011). Clinical practice guidelines for the use of erythroid-stimulating agents: ASCO, EORTC, NCCN. In G.H. Lyman & D.C. Dale (Eds.), *Cancer Treatment and Research: Vol. 157. Hematopoietic growth factors in oncology* (pp. 239–248). https://doi.org/10.1007/978-1-4419-7073-2_14

Lindqvist, O., Widmark, A., & Rasmussen, B.H. (2004). Meanings of the phenomenon of fatigue as narrated by 4 patients with cancer in palliative care. *Cancer Nursing, 27,* 237–243. https://doi.org/10.1097/00002820-200405000-00010

Liu, L., Mills, P.J., Rissling, M., Fiorentino, L., Natarajan, L., Dimsdale, J.E., … Ancoli-Israel, S. (2012). Fatigue and sleep quality are associated with changes in inflammatory markers in breast cancer patients undergoing chemotherapy. *Brain, Behavior, and Immunity, 26,* 706–713. https://doi.org/10.1016/j.bbi.2012.02.001

Mao, H., Mao, J.J., Guo, M., Cheng, K., Wei, J., Shen, X., & Shen, X. (2016). Effects of infrared laser moxibustion on cancer-related fatigue: A randomized, double-blind, placebo-controlled trial. *Cancer, 122,* 3667–3672. https://doi.org/10.1002/cncr.30189

Minton, O., Richardson, A., Sharpe, M., Hotopf, M., & Stone, P. (2008). A systematic review and meta-analysis of the pharmacological treatment of cancer-related fatigue. *Journal of the National Cancer Institute, 100,* 1155–1166. https://doi.org/10.1093/jnci/djn250

Minton, O., Richardson, A., Sharpe, M., Hotopf, M., & Stone, P.C. (2011). Psychostimulants for the management of cancer-related fatigue: A systematic review and meta-analysis. *Journal of Pain and Symptom Management, 41,* 761–767. https://doi.org/10.1016/j.jpainsymman.2010.06.020

Mitchell, S.A., Hoffman, A.J., Clark, J.C., DeGennaro, R.M., Poirier, P., Robinson, C.B., & Weisbrod, B.L. (2014). Putting evidence into practice: An update of evidence-based interventions for cancer-related fatigue during and following treatment. *Clinical Journal of Oncology Nursing, 18*(Suppl. 6), 38–58. https://doi.org/10.1188/14.CJON.S3.38-58

Molassiotis, A. (2013a). Evidence is in the eye of the beholder. *Supportive Care in Cancer, 21,* 3259–3260. https://doi.org/10.1007/s00520-013-1929-x

Molassiotis, A. (2013b). Managing cancer-related fatigue with acupuncture: Is it all good news for patients? *Acupuncture in Medicine, 31,* 3–4. https://doi.org/10.1136/acupmed-2012-010292

Molassiotis, A., Bardy, J., Finnegan-John, J., Mackereth, P., Ryder, D.W., Filshie, J., … Richardson, A. (2012). Acupuncture for cancer-related fatigue in patients with breast cancer: A pragmatic randomized controlled trial. *Journal of Clinical Oncology, 30,* 4470–4476. https://doi.org/10.1200/JCO.2012.41.6222

Molassiotis, A., Bardy, J., Finnegan-John, J., Mackereth, P., Ryder, W.D., Filshie, J., … Richardson, A. (2013). A randomized, controlled trial of acupuncture self-needling as maintenance therapy for cancer-related fatigue after therapist-delivered acupuncture. *Annals of Oncology, 24,* 1645–1652. https://doi.org/10.1093/annonc/mdt034

Molassiotis, A., & Richardson, A. (2013). Reply to A. Azad et al. *Journal of Clinical Oncology, 31,* 2058–2059. https://doi.org/10.1200/JCO.2013.49.2470

Monk, J.P., Phillips, G., Waite, R., Kuhn, J., Schaaf, L.J., Otterson, G.A., … Villalona-Calero, M.A. (2006). Assessment of tumor necrosis factor alpha blockade as an intervention to improve tolerability of dose-intensive chemotherapy in cancer patients. *Journal of Clinical Oncology, 24,* 1852–1859. https://doi.org/10.1200/JCO.2005.04.2838

Moraska, A.R., Sood, A., Dakhil, S.R., Sloan, J.A., Barton, D., Atherton, P.J., … Loprinzi, C.L. (2010). Phase III, randomized, double-blind, placebo-controlled study of long-acting methylphenidate for cancer-related fatigue: North Central Cancer Treatment Group NCCTG-N05C7 trial. *Journal of Clinical Oncology, 28,* 3673–3679. https://doi.org/10.1200/JCO.2010.28.1444

Mücke, M., Mochamat, Cuhls, H., Peuckmann-Post, V., Minton, O., Stone, P., & Radbruch, L. (2016). Pharmacological treatments for fatigue associated with palliative care: Executive summary of a Cochrane Collaboration systematic review. *Journal of Cachexia, Sarcopenia and Muscle, 7,* 23–27. https://doi.org/10.1002/jcsm.12101

National Comprehensive Cancer Network. (2018). *NCCN Clinical Practice Guidelines in Oncology (NCCN Guidelines®): Cancer-related fatigue* [v.2.2018]. Retrieved from https://www.nccn.org/professionals/physician_gls/PDF/fatigue.pdf

Neefjes, E.C.W., van der Vorst, M.J.D.L., Blauwhoff-Buskermolen, S., & Verheul, H.M.W. (2013). Aiming for a better understanding and management of cancer-related fatigue. *Oncologist, 18,* 1135–1143. https://doi.org/10.1634/theoncologist.2013-0076

Neikrug, A.B., Rissling, M., Trofimenko, V., Liu, L., Natarajan, L., Lawton, S., … Ancoli-Israel, S. (2012). Bright light therapy protects women from circadian rhythm desynchronization during chemotherapy for breast cancer. *Behavioral Sleep Medicine, 10,* 202–216. https://doi.org/10.1080/15402002.2011.634940

Ness, S., Kokal, J., Fee-Schroeder, K., Novotny, P., Satele, D., & Barton, D. (2013). Concerns across the survivorship trajectory: Results from a survey of cancer survivors. *Oncology Nursing Forum, 40,* 35–42. https://doi.org/10.1188/13.ONF.35-42

Nishimori, H., Maeda, Y., & Tanimoto, M. (2013). Chronic graft-versus-host disease: Disease biology and novel therapeutic strategies. *Acta Medica Okayama, 67,* 1–8. Retrieved from http://www.lib.okayama-u.ac.jp/www/acta/pdf/67_1_1.pdf

O'Regan, D., & Filshie, J. (2010). Acupuncture and cancer. *Autonomic Neuroscience, 157,* 96–100. https://doi.org/10.1016/j.autneu.2010.05.001

Pachman, D.R., Price, K.A., & Carey, E.C. (2014). Nonpharmacologic approach to fatigue in patients with cancer. *Cancer Journal, 20,* 313–318. https://doi.org/10.1097/PPO.0000000000000064

Payne, C., Wiffen, P.J., & Martin, S. (2012). Interventions for fatigue and weight loss in adults with advanced progressive illness. *Cochrane Database of Systematic Reviews, 2012*(1). https://doi.org/10.1002/14651858.CD008427.pub2

Peters, M.E., Goedendorp, M.M., Verhagen, C.A., van der Graaf, W.T., & Bleijenberg, G. (2014). Severe fatigue during the palliative treatment phase of cancer: An exploratory study. *Cancer Nursing, 37,* 139–145. https://doi.org/10.1097/NCC.0b013e318291bd2d

Portela, M.A., Rubiales, A.S., & Centeno, C. (2011). The use of psychostimulants in cancer patients. *Current Opinion in Supportive and Palliative Care, 5,* 164–168. https://doi.org/10.1097/SPC.0b013e3283462ff3

Posadzki, P., Moon, T.-W., Choi, T.-Y., Park, T.-Y., Lee, M.S., & Ernst, E. (2013). Acupuncture for cancer-related fatigue: A systematic review of randomized clinical trials. *Supportive Care in Cancer, 21,* 2067–2073. https://doi.org/10.1007/s00520-013-1765-z

Powers, S.K., Lynch, G.S., Murphy, K.T., Reid, M.B., & Zijdewind, I. (2016). Disease-induced skeletal muscle atrophy and fatigue. *Medicine and Science in Sports and Exercise, 48,* 2307–2319. https://doi.org/10.1249/MSS.0000000000000975

Qu, D., Zhang, Z., Yu, X., Zhao, J., Qiu, F., & Huang, J. (2016). Psychotropic drugs for the management of cancer-related fatigue: A systematic review and meta-analysis. *European Journal of Cancer Care, 25,* 970–979. https://doi.org/10.1111/ecc.12397

Redd, W.H., Valdimarsdottir, H., Wu, L.M., Winkel, G., Byrne, E.E., Beltre, M.A., ... Ancoli-Israel, S. (2014). Systematic light exposure in the treatment of cancer-related fatigue: A preliminary study. *Psycho-Oncology, 23,* 1431–1434. https://doi.org/10.1002/pon.3553

Rizzo, J.D., Brouwers, M., Hurley, P., Seidenfeld, J., Arcasoy, M.O., Spivak, J.L., ... Somerfield, M.R. (2010). American Society of Clinical Oncology/American Society of Hematology clinical practice guideline update on the use of epoetin and darbepoetin in adult patients with cancer. *Journal of Clinical Oncology, 28,* 4996–5010. https://doi.org/10.1200/JCO.2010.29.2201

Ruddy, K.J., Barton, D., & Loprinzi, C.L. (2014). Laying to rest psychostimulants for cancer-related fatigue? *Journal of Clinical Oncology, 32,* 1865–1867. https://doi.org/10.1200/JCO.2014.55.8353

Sadja, J., & Mills, P.J. (2013). Effects of yoga interventions on fatigue in cancer patients and survivors: A systematic review of randomized controlled trials. *Explore, 9,* 232–243. https://doi.org/10.1016/j.explore.2013.04.005

Saligan, L.N., & Kim, H.S. (2012). A systematic review of the association between immunogenomic markers and cancer-related fatigue. *Brain, Behavior, and Immunity, 26,* 830–848. https://doi.org/10.1016/j.bbi.2012.05.004

Saligan, L.N., Olson, K., Filler, K., Larkin, D., Cramp, F., Yennurajalingam, S., ... Mustian, K. (2015). The biology of cancer-related fatigue: A review of the literature. *Supportive Care in Cancer, 23,* 2461–2478. https://doi.org/10.1007/s00520-015-2763-0

Santoni, M., Conti, A., Massari, F., Arnaldi, G., Iacovelli, R., Rizzo, M., ... Cascinu, S. (2015). Treatment-related fatigue with sorafenib, sunitinib and pazopanib in patients with advanced solid tumors: An up-to-date review and meta-analysis of clinical trials. *International Journal of Cancer, 136,* 1–10. https://doi.org/10.1002/ijc.28715

Savard, J., Ivers, H., Savard, M.-H., & Morin, C.M. (2015). Cancer treatments and their side effects are associated with aggravation of insomnia: Results of a longitudinal study. *Cancer, 121,* 1703–1711. https://doi.org/10.1002/cncr.29244

Schmitz, K.H., Courneya, K.S., Matthews, C., Demark-Wahnefried, W., Galvao, D.A., Pinto, B.M., ... Schwartz, A.L. (2010). American College of Sports Medicine roundtable on exercise guidelines for cancer survivors. *Medicine and Science in Sports and Exercise, 42,* 1409–1426. https://doi.org/10.1249/MSS.0b013e3181e0c112

Scott, D.A., Mills, M., Black, A., Cantwell, M., Campbell, A., Cardwell, C.R., ... Donnelly, M. (2013). Multidimensional rehabilitation programmes for adult cancer survivors. *Cochrane Database of Systematic Reviews, 2013*(3). https://doi.org/10.1002/14651858.CD007730.pub2

Seyidova-Khoshknabi, D., Davis, M.P., & Walsh, D. (2011). Review article: A systematic review of cancer-related fatigue measurement questionnaires. *American Journal of Hospice and Palliative Care, 28,* 119–129. https://doi.org/10.1177/1049909110381590

Smith, C., Carmady, B., Thornton, C., Perz, J., & Ussher, J.M. (2013). The effect of acupuncture on post-cancer fatigue and well-being for women recovering from breast cancer: A pilot randomised controlled trial. *Acupuncture in Medicine, 31,* 9–15. https://doi.org/10.1136/acupmed-2012-010228

Spathis, A., Fife, K., Blackhall, F., Dutton, S., Bahadori, R., Wharton, R., ... Wee, B. (2014). Modafinil for the treatment of fatigue in lung cancer: Results of a placebo-controlled, double-blind, randomized trial. *Journal of Clinical Oncology, 32,* 1882–1888. https://doi.org/10.1200/JCO.2013.54.4346

Tao, W.-W., Jiang, H., Tao, X.-M., Jiang, P., Sha, L.-Y., & Sun, X.-C. (2016). Effects of acupuncture, tuina, tai chi, qigong, and traditional Chinese medicine five-element music therapy on symptom management and quality of life for cancer patients: A meta-analysis. *Journal of Pain and Symptom Management, 51,* 728–747. https://doi.org/10.1016/j.jpainsymman.2015.11.027

Temel, J.S., Pirl, W.F., Recklitis, C.J., Cashavelly, B., & Lynch, T.J. (2006). Feasibility and validity of a one-item fatigue screen in a thoracic oncology clinic. *Journal of Thoracic Oncology, 1,* 454–459. https://doi.org/10.1016/S1556-0864(15)31611-7

Tomlinson, D., Hinds, P.S., Ethier, M.C., Ness, K.K., Zupanec, S., & Sung, L. (2013). Psychometric properties of instruments used to measure fatigue in children and adolescents with cancer: A systematic review. *Journal of Pain and Symptom Management, 45,* 83–91. https://doi.org/10.1016/j.jpainsymman.2012.02.010

Tonia, T., & Bohlius, J. (2011). Ten years of meta-analyses on erythropoiesis-stimulating agents in cancer patients. In G.H. Lyman & D.C. Dale (Eds.), *Cancer Treatment and Research: Vol. 157. Hematopoietic growth factors in oncology* (pp. 217–238). https://doi.org/10.1007/978-1-4419-7073-2_13

Tookman, A.J., Jones, C.L., DeWitte, M., & Lodge, P.J. (2008). Fatigue in patients with advanced cancer: A pilot study of an intervention with infliximab. *Supportive Care in Cancer, 16,* 1131–1140. https://doi.org/10.1007/s00520-008-0429-x

Towler, P., Molassiotis, A., & Brearley, S.G. (2013). What is the evidence for the use of acupuncture as an intervention for symptom management in cancer supportive and palliative care: An integrative overview of reviews. *Supportive Care in Cancer, 21,* 2913–2923. https://doi.org/10.1007/s00520-013-1882-8

Trudel-Fitzgerald, C., Savard, J., & Ivers, H. (2013a). Evolution of cancer-related symptoms over an 18-month period. *Journal of*

Pain and Symptom Management, 45, 1007–1018. https://doi.org/10.1016/j.jpainsymman.2012.06.009

Trudel-Fitzgerald, C., Savard, J., & Ivers, H. (2013b). Which symptoms come first? Exploration of temporal relationships between cancer-related symptoms over an 18-month period. *Annals of Behavioral Medicine, 45,* 329–337. https://doi.org/10.1007/s12160-012-9459-1

U.S. Food and Drug Administration. (2016). FDA drug safety communication: Erythropoiesis-stimulating agents (ESAs): Procrit, Epogen and Aranesp. Retrieved from https://www.fda.gov/Drugs/DrugSafety/PostmarketDrugSafetyInformationforPatientsandProviders/ucm200297.htm

Vardar Yağlı, N., Şener, G., Arıkan, H., Sağlam, M., İnal İnce, D., Savcı, S., … Özışık, Y. (2015). Do yoga and aerobic exercise training have impact on functional capacity, fatigue, peripheral muscle strength, and quality of life in breast cancer survivors? *Integrative Cancer Therapies, 14,* 125–132. https://doi.org/10.1177/1534735414565699

Vigano, A., Piccioni, M., Trutschnigg, B., Hornby, L., Chaudhury, P., & Kilgour, R. (2010). Male hypogonadism associated with advanced cancer: A systematic review. *Lancet Oncology, 11,* 679–684. https://doi.org/10.1016/S1470-2045(10)70021-8

Viscuse, P.V., Price, K., Millstine, D., Bhagra, A., Bauer, B., & Ruddy, K.J. (2017). Integrative medicine in cancer survivors. *Current Opinion in Oncology, 29,* 235–242. https://doi.org/10.1097/CCO.0000000000000376

Vogelzang, N.J., Breitbart, W., Cella, D., Curt, G.A., Groopman, J.E., Horning, S.J., … Portenoy, R.K. (1997). Patient, caregiver, and oncologist perceptions of cancer-related fatigue: Results of a tripart assessment survey. *Seminars in Hematology, 34*(Suppl. 3), 4–12.

Wagland, R., Richardson, A., Ewings, S., Armes, J., Lennan, E., Hankins, M., & Griffiths, P. (2016). Prevalence of cancer chemotherapy-related problems, their relation to health-related quality of life and associated supportive care: A cross-sectional survey. *Supportive Care in Cancer, 24,* 4901–4911. https://doi.org/10.1007/s00520-016-3346-4

Wagner, L.I., Schink, J., Bass, M., Patel, S., Diaz, M.V., Rothrock, N., … Cella, D. (2015). Bringing PROMIS to practice: Brief and precise symptom screening in ambulatory cancer care. *Cancer, 121,* 917–934. https://doi.org/10.1002/cncr.29104

Wang, T., Yin, J., Miller, A.H., & Xiao, C. (2017). A systematic review of the association between fatigue and genetic polymorphisms. *Brain, Behavior, and Immunity, 62,* 230–244. https://doi.org/10.1016/j.bbi.2017.01.007

Wang, X.S., & Woodruff, J.F. (2015). Cancer-related and treatment-related fatigue. *Gynecologic Oncology, 136,* 446–452. https://doi.org/10.1016/j.ygyno.2014.10.013

Wang, X.S., Zhao, F., Fisch, M.J., O'Mara, A.M., Cella, D., Mendoza, T.R., & Cleeland, C.S. (2014). Prevalence and characteristics of moderate to severe fatigue: A multicenter study in cancer patients and survivors. *Cancer, 120,* 425–432. https://doi.org/10.1002/cncr.28434

Wauters, I., & Vansteenkiste, J. (2012). Darbepoetin alfa in the treatment of anemia in cancer patients undergoing chemotherapy. *Expert Review of Anticancer Therapy, 12,* 1383–1390. https://doi.org/10.1586/era.12.117

Weis, J. (2011). Cancer-related fatigue: Prevalence, assessment and treatment strategies. *Expert Review of Pharmacoeconomics and Outcomes Research, 11,* 441–446. https://doi.org/10.1586/erp.11.44

Weitzner, M.A., Moncello, J., Jacobsen, P.B., & Minton, S. (2002). A pilot trial of paroxetine for the treatment of hot flashes and associated symptoms in women with breast cancer. *Journal of Pain and Symptom Management, 23,* 337–345. https://doi.org/10.1016/S0885-3924(02)00379-2

Wood, L.J., & Weymann, K. (2013). Inflammation and neural signaling: Etiologic mechanisms of the cancer treatment-related symptom cluster. *Current Opinion in Supportive and Palliative Care, 7,* 54–59. https://doi.org/10.1097/SPC.0b013e32835dabe3

Xiang, Y., Lu, L., Chen, X., & Wen, Z. (2017). Does tai chi relieve fatigue? A systematic review and meta-analysis of randomized controlled trials. *PLOS ONE, 12,* e0174872. https://doi.org/10.1371/journal.pone.0174872

Yennurajalingam, S., & Bruera, E. (2014a). Review of clinical trials of pharmacologic interventions for cancer-related fatigue: Focus on psychostimulants and steroids. *Cancer Journal, 20,* 319–324. https://doi.org/10.1097/PPO.0000000000000069

Yennurajalingam, S., & Bruera, E. (2014b). Role of corticosteroids for fatigue in advanced incurable cancer: Is it a "wonder drug" or "deal with the devil." *Current Opinion in Supportive and Palliative Care, 8,* 346–351. https://doi.org/10.1097/SPC.0000000000000093

Yennurajalingam, S., Frisbee-Hume, S., Palmer, J.L., Delgado-Guay, M.O., Bull, J., Phan, A.T., … Bruera, E. (2013). Reduction of cancer-related fatigue with dexamethasone: A double-blind, randomized, placebo-controlled trial in patients with advanced cancer. *Journal of Clinical Oncology, 31,* 3076–3082. https://doi.org/10.1200/JCO.2012.44.4661

Yennurajalingam, S., Reddy, A., Tannir, N.M., Chisholm, G.B., Lee, R.T., Lopez, G., … Bruera, E. (2015). High-dose Asian ginseng (Panax ginseng) for cancer-related fatigue: A preliminary report. *Integrative Cancer Therapies, 14,* 419–427. https://doi.org/10.1177/1534735415580676

Yennurajalingam, S., Urbauer, D.L., Casper, K.L.B., Reyes-Gibby, C.C., Chacko, R., Poulter, V., & Bruera, E. (2011). Impact of a palliative care consultation team on cancer-related symptoms in advanced cancer patients referred to an outpatient supportive care clinic. *Journal of Pain and Symptom Management, 41,* 49–56. https://doi.org/10.1016/j.jpainsymman.2010.03.017

Zeng, Y., Luo, T., Xie, H., Huang, M., & Cheng, A.S. (2014). Health benefits of qigong or tai chi for cancer patients: A systematic review and meta-analyses. *Complementary Therapies in Medicine, 22,* 173–186. https://doi.org/10.1016/j.ctim.2013.11.010

Zhang, J., Yang, K.-H., Tian, J.-H., & Wang, C.-M. (2012). Effects of yoga on psychologic function and quality of life in women with breast cancer: A meta-analysis of randomized controlled trials. *Journal of Alternative and Complementary Medicine, 18,* 994–1002. https://doi.org/10.1089/acm.2011.0514

Zlott, D.A., & Byrne, M. (2010). Mechanisms by which pharmacologic agents may contribute to fatigue. *PM&R, 2,* 451–455. https://doi.org/10.1016/j.pmrj.2010.04.018

CHAPTER 24

Neurologic Toxicities

A. Overview

1. *Neurotoxicity* refers to injury to the brain and spinal cord (central nervous system [CNS]) or the peripheral nervous system (nervous system outside of the brain and spinal cord) caused by exposure to natural or manufactured toxic substances.
2. Cancer therapies can induce a range of toxic side effects (see Table 24-1) on nervous tissue, resulting in significant morbidity and mortality, many of which persist beyond the treatment period.
3. Neurologic toxicity from cancer therapies is a common problem for patients and second only to myelosuppression as a root cause of dose modification or discontinuation (Magge & DeAngelis, 2015).
4. Besides this potential to limit the overall therapeutic efficacy of the cancer treatment itself, neurologic sequelae have become some of the most important challenges in patient survivorship (Wick, Hertenstein, & Platten, 2016).
5. Neurotoxicity presents most frequently as fatigue and peripheral neuropathies (see Table 24-2), although a wide range of clinical symptoms have been reported.
6. Acute toxicities such as seizure, encephalopathy, and cerebrovascular events such as thromboembolic stroke or hemorrhage require immediate intervention.
7. It therefore is critical that oncology nurses regularly assess for and recognize early neurotoxicity to allow for rapid diagnosis, treatment, and dose adjustment to mitigate the risk of irreversible neurologic impairment.

B. Radiation-induced CNS toxicity

1. Neurotoxicity is often the result of synergistic effects of concurrent chemotherapy and radiation.
2. General neurotoxicities: Direct or ancillary exposure of nervous tissue to radiation therapy carries risk of neurologic injury. General neurotoxicities result from permeating injury to brain tissue with accompanying nonspecific symptoms, such as headache, fatigue, and nausea.
   a) Pathophysiology: Radiation delivered to the entire brain (whole brain radiation therapy), partial brain radiation therapy, or targeted radiation therapy (stereotactic radiosurgery, Gamma Knife®) causes irreversible injury to brain tissue that frequently results in the death of healthy brain tissue as well as tumor tissue. Swelling of the brain and meninges following radiation can further potentiate injury, and this edema often is the root cause of acute neurotoxicity. Delayed neurotoxicities are frequently attributed to demyelination or vasculopathy (E.L. Lee & Westcarth, 2012).
   b) Incidence: Radiation therapy is often synergistic with chemotherapy but carries an independent risk of neurotoxicity. Incidence and severity vary according to multiple factors, including radiation dose and type, sites treated, and body mass index. Generally, the most frequently reported toxicities include fatigue and headache, whereas the least common are radiation-induced secondary tumors.
   c) Clinical manifestations: Neurologic sequelae often are described temporally to the administration of radiation therapy as acute (during or immediately after treatment), early-delayed (weeks to months following treatment), and late-delayed (months to years following treatment).
      (1) Acute through early-delayed symptoms are generally reversible and include headache, fatigue, nausea, irritability, somnolence, and encephalopathy and may be associated with fever, vomiting, drowsiness, and exacerbation of focal deficits (Arrillaga-Romany & Dietrich, 2012).
      (2) Delayed neurotoxicity from radiation therapy includes leukoencephalopathy, necrosis, cystic degeneration, hydrocephalus, cerebrovascular events such as infarct or hemor-

Table 24-1. Central Neurotoxicity in Chemotherapy, Immunotherapy, and Targeted Therapies

Adverse Effect	Signs and Symptoms	Reported Agents	Potential Treatment
Cerebellar syndrome	Ataxia Altered mental status Dysarthria Dysmetria Dysphagia Gait imbalance Nystagmus Somnolence	Altretamine Bortezomib Capecitabine Cytarabine 5-Fluorouracil Nelarabine Oxaliplatin Procarbazine Rituximab Thalidomide Trastuzumab Vincristine	Discontinue drug.
Acute encephalopathy	Agitation Cerebellar ataxia Cognitive dysfunction Confusion Disorientation Lethargy Loss of consciousness Seizure	Altretamine Azacitidine Blinatumomab Bortezomib CAR T cells Carmustine Cisplatin Cytarabine Etoposide Fludarabine Ifosfamide Interferon alfa Interleukin-2 L-Asparaginase Methotrexate Mitomycin C Nelarabine Nitrosoureas Procarbazine Tamoxifen Thalidomide Thiotepa Vincristine	Implement drug interruption with steroid course, or discontinue drug.
Posterior reversible encephalopathy syndrome	Altered mental status Confusion Headache Hypertension Lethargy Seizure Visual disturbances Vomiting	Bevacizumab Carboplatin Cisplatin Doxorubicin 5-Fluorouracil Gemcitabine Ifosfamide Imatinib Ipilimumab Methotrexate Nelarabine Rituximab Sirolimus Sorafenib Sunitinib Tacrolimus Vincristine	Discontinue drug. Stabilize blood pressure. Consider antiepileptic therapy/prophylaxis.
Myelopathy	Back pain Incontinence Numbness Weakness	Cytarabine Methotrexate Thiotepa	Initiate steroids.

(Continued on next page)

Table 24-1. Central Neurotoxicity in Chemotherapy, Immunotherapy, and Targeted Therapies *(Continued)*

Adverse Effect	Signs and Symptoms	Reported Agents	Potential Treatment
Cerebrovascular events (thromboembolism, hemorrhage, ischemia)	Decreased alertness Difficulty speaking Headache Loss of consciousness Nausea/vomiting Neurologic deficit Seizure Weakness	Bevacizumab Cisplatin L-Asparaginase Methotrexate Sorafenib Sunitinib Vandetanib VEGF Trap	Replace electrolytes. Pause or discontinue drug.
Aseptic meningitis	Fever Headache Nausea/vomiting Photophobia Protein, white blood cells in cerebrospinal fluid Stiff neck	Cetuximab Cytarabine Ipilimumab IV immunoglobulin Methotrexate Rituximab	Discontinue drug. Reverse immune deficiency. Initiate steroids.
Seizures	Altered mental status Involuntary jerking Loss of consciousness Staring spells Temporary confusion Violent movements of arms/legs	Amsacrine Busulfan CAR T cells Carmustine Chlorambucil Cisplatin Cytarabine Dacarbazine Etoposide 5-Fluorouracil Fludarabine Gemcitabine Ifosfamide L-Asparaginase Methotrexate Nelarabine Paclitaxel Teniposide Thalidomide Vincristine	Replace electrolytes. Pause or discontinue drug.
Progressive multifocal leukoencephalopathy	Ataxia Confusion Loss of vision Personality change Speech disturbance	Alemtuzumab Brentuximab Carmustine Cytarabine Fludarabine Ibrutinib Ifosfamide Infliximab Methotrexate Rituximab Thalidomide Vincristine	Discontinue drug. Reverse immune deficiency. Initiate steroids.
Hypophysitis	Fatigue Headache Visual disturbances	Atezolizumab Ipilimumab Nivolumab Pembrolizumab	Discontinue drug. Initiate steroids. Consider hormone replacement.

(Continued on next page)

Table 24-1. Central Neurotoxicity in Chemotherapy, Immunotherapy, and Targeted Therapies *(Continued)*

Adverse Effect	Signs and Symptoms	Reported Agents	Potential Treatment
Headache	Pain Pressure	Altretamine Bevacizumab CAR T cells Cetuximab Dabrafenib Dasatinib Etoposide Fludarabine Imatinib Ipilimumab Ixabepilone L-Asparaginase Mechlorethamine Methotrexate Nelarabine Retinoic acid Rituximab Tamoxifen Temozolomide Trastuzumab Vemurafenib	Discontinue drug. Initiate steroids. Consider hormone replacement.
Ototoxicity	Hearing loss Tinnitus	Carboplatin Cisplatin Oxaliplatin	Discontinue drug.

CAR—chimeric antigen receptor; VEGF—vascular endothelial growth factor receptor

Note. Based on information from Arrillaga-Romany & Dietrich, 2012; Stone & DeAngelis, 2016; Wick et al., 2016.

rhage, radiation-induced tumors, parenchymal calcifications, brain atrophy, and cognitive impairment (Arrillaga-Romany & Dietrich, 2012).

d) Assessment: Diagnosis is typically by patient self-report of symptoms. Careful neurologic assessment may reveal focal deficits or altered mental status and encephalopathy. Leukoencephalopathy, cystic degeneration, hydrocephalus, cerebrovascular events, secondary tumors, and parenchymal calcifications usually are seen radiographically; however, surgical biopsy may be required to achieve the final diagnosis.

e) Collaborative management: Acute toxicities are managed with careful treatment planning and directed pharmacologic intervention—for example, steroids for swelling or antiemetics for nausea and vomiting. Delayed toxicities such as hydrocephalus, cerebrovascular events, and the development of radiation-induced tumors often require surgical intervention. For other types (e.g., brain atrophy, cognitive impairment, parenchymal calcifications), no treatment options may be available.

3. SMART syndrome: *SMART* stands for **s**troke-like **m**igraine **a**ttacks after **r**adiation **t**herapy. It is a delayed neurotoxic effect occurring 1–30 years following radiation treatment to the brain (Stone & DeAngelis, 2016).

a) Pathophysiology: The etiology is uncertain, but symptoms likely stem from neuronal dysfunction rather than cerebral vascular pathology (Stone & DeAngelis, 2016).

b) Incidence: SMART syndrome is rare, but the condition is likely underreported.

c) Clinical manifestations: Symptoms can include headache, focal neurologic deficits, drowsiness, altered mental status, and seizures (Lim, Brooke, Dineen, & O'Donoghue, 2016; Stone & DeAngelis, 2016).

d) Assessment: Radiographic imaging may help rule out other differential diagnoses (e.g., secondary mass, radiation necrosis), but findings are otherwise nonspecific and nondiagnostic. Diagnosis is achieved by patient report of symptoms, treatment history, careful neurologic examination, and the elimination of organic causes (Lim et al., 2016; Stone & DeAngelis, 2016).

e) Collaborative management: Antimigraine therapies (e.g., valproic acid) have been used with some success to prevent the onset

Table 24-2. Chemotherapy-Induced Peripheral Neuropathy[a]

Classification	Agents	Type of Neuropathy	Symptoms
Alkylating Agents			
Hydrazines and triazines	Altretamine Procarbazine	Sensory	Myalgia Paresthesias
Metal salts	Carboplatin Cisplatin Oxaliplatin	Sensory	Coasting phenomenon[b] Hearing loss Jaw spasm Lhermitte syndrome Muscle cramps Numbness Paresthesias Reduced deep tendon reflexes (DTR) Sense vibration Tingling Tinnitus
Plant Alkaloids			
Antimetabolites	Azacitidine Capecitabine Cladribine Cytarabine Fludarabine Gemcitabine Nelarabine	Sensory	Brachial plexopathy Paresthesias
Taxanes	Cabazitaxel Docetaxel Nab-paclitaxel Paclitaxel	Autonomic Motor Sensory	Arrhythmia Impaired/lost sensation Neuropathic pain Orthostatic hypotension Paresthesias Reduced/lost DTR Weakness
Vinca alkaloids	Vinblastine Vincristine Vinorelbine	Autonomic Cranial nerves Sensorimotor	Constipation Foot drop Lower limb weakness Muscle cramps Neuropathic pain Orthostatic hypotension Paralytic ileus Reduced/lost DTR Sensory impairment
Targeted Therapy Agents			
Monoclonal antibodies	Alemtuzumab Bevacizumab Brentuximab Ibritumomab Ipilimumab Pertuzumab Rituximab	Sensorimotor Sensory	Muscle cramps Myalgias Radicular neuropathy Weakness

(Continued on next page)

Table 24-2. Chemotherapy-Induced Peripheral Neuropathy[a] *(Continued)*

Classification	Agents	Type of Neuropathy	Symptoms
Targeted Therapy Agents *(Cont.)*			
Small molecules	Bortezomib Carfilzomib Imatinib Regorafenib Selumetinib Sorafenib Sunitinib Vemurafenib	Painful sensory	Muscle wasting Muscle weakness Paresthesias Reduced/lost DTR Severe neuropathic pain Tingling/burning sensation
Miscellaneous Antineoplastics			
Chemotherapy	Arsenic trioxide Eribulin Ixabepilone Sagopilone	Sensorimotor Sensory	Dysesthesias Impaired/lost sensation Neuralgia Neuropathic pain Reduced/lost DTR
Immunomodulatory agents	Lenalidomide Pomalidomide Thalidomide	Autonomic Sensory	Bradycardia Constipation Impotence Neuropathic pain Paresthesias

[a] To date, peripheral neuropathy has not been reported with antitumor antibiotics or immunotherapy such as chimeric antigen receptor T cells.

[b] *Coasting* refers to worsening of neuropathy signs or symptoms after drug withdrawal.

Note. Based on information from Stone & DeAngelis, 2016; Taillibert et al., 2016; Wick et al., 2016.

of SMART syndrome (Stone & DeAngelis, 2016).

4. Leukoencephalopathy: Toxicity of treatment caused by injury to white matter, specifically, when the myelin sheaths that cover nerve fibers degenerate (Arrillaga-Romany & Dietrich, 2012). It is a late effect characterized by white matter changes on magnetic resonance imaging (MRI) with or without variable neurocognitive changes.
   a) Pathophysiology: The exact pathophysiology of leukoencephalopathy is unknown but globally attributed to injury of the brain parenchyma, as well as small blood vessel damage (Arrillaga-Romany & Dietrich, 2012).
   b) Incidence: The incidence of leukoencephalopathy varies widely according to radiation dose and type and when imaging was obtained, as well as how the diagnosis was achieved, with reports citing incidences of 5.4%–92% (Cummings et al., 2016). It is possible that subclinical cases (e.g., mild or no symptoms) are not recognized and are unreported.
   c) Clinical manifestations: Patients may report no symptoms or a range of minor symptoms (mild cognitive impairment) to a progressive cognitive decline including dementia, altered consciousness, ataxia, focal deficits, and seizure (Taillibert, Le Rhun, & Chamberlain, 2016). Gait abnormalities and urinary incontinence are noteworthy to correlate with higher severity (Arrillaga-Romany & Dietrich, 2012). Although acute white matter injury in the immediate aftermath of treatment can lead to headache, fever, vomiting, drowsiness, and encephalopathy, symptoms are more commonly experienced more than one month to a year following radiation.
   d) Assessment: Diagnosis is achieved radiographically with MRI, which typically shows deep and periventricular white matter abnormalities characterized by T2 flair hyperintensities in the absence of focal lesions (Arrillaga-Romany & Dietrich, 2012; Cummings et al., 2016). Additional findings may include cortical atrophy and dilated ventricles, as well as necrosis and demyelination, if tissue is obtained for biopsy (Arrillaga-Romany & Dietrich, 2012).
   e) Collaborative management: No specific treatment exists for leukoencephalopathy.

The focus is on palliative support for clinical manifestations.

5. Radiation necrosis: In the setting of cancers requiring radiation therapy to the head, radiation necrosis is a form of delayed cell injury and death of healthy brain tissue that results in the formation of a necrotic mass (Arrillaga-Romany & Dietrich, 2012).
   a) Pathophysiology: Radiation exposure provokes damage to the vascular endothelium in the noncancerous neural tissue surrounding the original tumor or surgical bed, eventually resulting in small artery thrombosis, arterial occlusion, and tissue death (Arrillaga-Romany & Dietrich, 2012).
   b) Incidence: Incidence varies widely according to how radiation necrosis is defined and ultimately diagnosed, as well as the type of radiation and presence of concurrent systemic agents, with estimates ranging from 2.5% to 24% (Chao et al., 2013). Importantly, emerging evidence concludes that the incidence of radiation necrosis has increased in the setting of concomitant immunotherapy (e.g., ipilimumab) or select targeted agents (e.g., BRAF inhibitors) compared with rates in the chemotherapy/radiation-only era (Colaco, Martin, Kluger, Yu, & Chiang, 2016; Kim et al., 2017; K.R. Patel et al., 2016).
   c) Clinical manifestations: Patients typically present months to years after radiation treatment with new neurologic symptoms stemming from a mass effect of the necrotic tissue plug, including headache, focal neurologic deficits, seizures, and cognitive impairment.
   d) Assessment: MRI often shows an enhancing mass that is radiographically indistinguishable from tumor recurrence or progression. Biopsy or surgical resection often is required to definitively determine whether the mass represents true tumor progression/recurrence or radiation necrosis (Chao et al., 2013).
   e) Collaborative management: No approved treatment exists, although numerous off-label treatment modalities for radiation necrosis have been reported in the literature, including anticoagulation with heparin or warfarin, hyperbaric oxygen, focused interstitial laser therapy, and bevacizumab (Chao et al., 2013). Of these, bevacizumab is the most supported in the literature. Therapies for the secondary effects of brain swelling include systemic steroids. Left untreated, radiation necrosis typically self-resolves.

6. Pseudoprogression: Pseudoprogression occurs when a CNS-based tumor increases in size radiographically during or immediately (first few weeks to six months) following active treatment with radiation therapy alone or with combination radiation/chemotherapy. Although the appearance of pseudoprogression on MRI can be similar to radiation necrosis, time is the primary distinction; pseudoprogression occurs in the immediate aftermath of treatment, whereas radiation necrosis presents months to years following treatment.
   a) Pathophysiology: The mechanism by which pseudoprogression occurs is poorly understood but is thought to be a secondary effect of blood–brain barrier breakdown, which causes edema and increased uptake of contrast material (Magge & DeAngelis, 2015).
   b) Incidence: The reported incidences of pseudoprogression vary widely, according to how it is defined and which diagnostics are used (e.g., Response Assessment in Neuro-Oncology, Macdonald, Response Evaluation Criteria in Solid Tumors), with reports specifying the overall incidence across all categories of solid tumors ranging from less than 10% (Chiou & Burotto, 2015) to as high as 36% in patients with high-grade gliomas (Abbasi et al., 2017). More recently, pseudoprogression has also been reported with the use of targeted therapies, especially checkpoint inhibitors, such as nivolumab and pembrolizumab (Chae, Wang, Nimeiri, Kalyan, & Giles, 2017; Cohen et al., 2016).
   c) Clinical manifestations: Typically, pseudoprogression is a treatment-related effect only seen radiographically, and patients often do not report symptoms.
   d) Assessment: The enhancing lesion is seen on MRI and often followed serially until resolution.
   e) Collaborative management: No approved treatment exists for pseudoprogression, and in the absence of symptoms, patients typically only require surveillance with serial imaging until the condition self-resolves. For symptomatic patients, supportive therapies mirror those for radiation necrosis, as discussed previously (Miyatake et al., 2013).

C. Radiation-induced peripheral nervous system toxicity: Radiation fibrosis syndrome
   1. Overview: Radiation fibrosis syndrome describes a specific and late toxicity of radiation therapy causing progressive fibrotic sclerosis to the mus-

culoskeletal, soft, neural, and cardiopulmonary tissues within the irradiation field (Straub et al., 2015). Specific forms of radiation fibrosis are lumbosacral plexopathy and brachial plexopathy.

a) Lumbosacral plexopathy is a rare but serious form of radiation fibrosis affecting the lumbar or sacral plexuses following radiation therapy of pelvic-area cancers (e.g., cervical).

b) Brachial plexopathy can occur in patients who have had radiation therapy directed at the chest, axillary region, thorax, or neck (e.g., radiation therapy for breast cancer), injuring the network of nerves (brachial plexus) that innervate the sensorimotor function of the shoulder, arm, and hand.

2. Pathophysiology: The pathologic mechanism is not fully delineated but involves capillary network/vascular disruption, vascular endothelial damage, and microvascular injury with subsequent tissue sclerosis, fibrosis, and atrophy (Straub et al., 2015).
3. Incidence: Radiation fibrosis syndrome is a late (4–12 months following radiation therapy) and rare effect, with the incidence varying according to type of cancer, specific radiation therapy, and radiation dose (Straub et al., 2015). However, its occurrence is probably underestimated because it is not commonly evaluated by radiation oncologists, and symptoms often are overlooked or attributed to other causes.
4. Clinical manifestations: Skin changes may be seen in the radiation field. Symptoms vary according to site. For example, in head and neck cancers, radiation fibrosis can cause inability to fully open the mouth, swallowing difficulties, and associated speech pathologies (Stubblefield, 2017). In lung cancer, postradiation pulmonary fibrosis manifests as difficulty breathing, dry cough, fatigue, and inspirational pain. Symptoms of lumbosacral plexopathy typically include lower leg pain; reduced sensation; different degrees of weakness, paresis, or paralysis; and, in severe cases, urinary or fecal incontinence. Numbness, weakness, pain, or abnormal sensations (tingling, burning) are often reported along the wrist, hand, arm, or shoulder in brachial plexopathy (Straub et al., 2015; Stubblefield, 2017).
5. Assessment: Diagnosis is based on report of symptoms in the context of time, location, and dose of radiation therapy. Histopathologic evaluation of fibrotic masses, if present, can provide definitive diagnosis.
6. Collaborative management: Radiation fibrosis is a permanent effect of radiation therapy; no cure exists. Treatment consists of education, physical therapy, occupational therapy, orthotics, and medication to increase function, decrease sensory abnormalities, and protect from further injury (Stubblefield, 2017).

D. Chemotherapy-induced CNS toxicity

1. Fatigue

a) Overview: Fatigue, the feeling of extreme tiredness, is the most common CNS complication of cancer therapies and is not agent specific (Wick et al., 2016). It is an adverse effect of traditional chemotherapy agents, as well as radiation therapy, targeted agents, including all epidermal growth factor receptor inhibitors, and immunotherapies, including chimeric antigen receptor (CAR) T cells (Wick et al., 2016; Zhu et al., 2016). For additional information, see Chapter 23.

b) Pathophysiology: Fatigue occurs as either a direct effect of the cancer therapy itself (e.g., anemia, hormonal changes) or indirectly, through reactions with the immune system. Recent literature further suggests interdependent relationships and shared mechanisms with the greater disease process, as well as a patient's innate stress and coping responses (e.g., depression, anxiety) (Lacourt & Heijnen, 2017; Wick et al., 2016).

c) Incidence: The incidence of fatigue varies widely according to disease phase, treatment modality, and cancer diagnosis, with general estimates across all diagnostic categories, treatment phases, and cancer stages as high as 75%–99% (Barsevick et al., 2013).

d) Clinical manifestations: Patients with fatigue commonly describe themselves as weak, tired, exhausted, slow, having no energy, or worn out.

e) Assessment: Fatigue is a self-perceived symptom and is identified by the patient. It may be assessed clinically using one of many validated patient-reported outcome measures.

f) Collaborative management: Acute fatigue management focuses on identifying associated target factors, such as anemia, alterations in mood, or sleep disturbances. The only intervention currently described at level 1 evidence for chronic fatigue is exercise (Barsevick et al., 2013).

2. Acute or chronic encephalopathy

a) Overview: *Encephalopathy* is a general term referring to a syndrome of overall brain dysfunction that commonly manifests as confusion and altered mental status. Encephalopathy may be acute or chronic. Toxic leukoencephalopathy is an encephalopathy specifically of white matter resulting from exposure to antineoplastic therapies or other toxic agents (see previous discussion in Radiation-Induced CNS Toxicity section). In addition to treatment temporality (acute vs. chronic), specific types of toxic leukoencephalopathy are further distinguished by stability (i.e., reversible vs. permanent).

(1) Acute encephalopathy emerges within a few hours or days after chemotherapy, often resolves spontaneously, and rarely confers long-term sequelae. It is highly associated with specific agents—namely, methotrexate, ifosfamide, and cytarabine (Taillibert et al., 2016). For example, somnolence, confusion, seizures, and headaches are signs and symptoms of acute encephalopathy occurring in the setting of high-dose methotrexate (greater than 500 mg/m^2).

(a) Posterior reversible encephalopathy syndrome (PRES) is an acute leukoencephalopathy that occurs with multiple anticancer agents, particularly certain tyrosine kinase inhibitors (imatinib), as well as immunosuppressants (cyclosporine, tacrolimus, sirolimus) used for patients undergoing stem cell transplant. It also can occur in patients who have received CAR T cells. It occurs with higher frequency when these agents are given in combination with radiation therapy (Magge & DeAngelis, 2015).

(b) Other classes of chemotherapy agents have been associated with PRES, including platinum analogs (cisplatin and carboplatin), folate antagonists (methotrexate), antimetabolites (gemcitabine and 5-fluorouracil), anthracyclines (doxorubicin), vinca alkaloids (vincristine), and targeted agents (bevacizumab and rituximab) (Arrillaga-Romany & Dietrich, 2012).

(c) Radiographically, PRES is characterized by vasogenic edema throughout the brain. Symptoms include headache, seizure, altered mental status, vomiting, alterations in vision (from visual field cuts to cortical blindness), lethargy, and confusion (Arrillaga-Romany & Dietrich, 2012; Magge & DeAngelis, 2015). Hypertension is often a preceding or accompanying clinical sign (Magge & DeAngelis, 2015).

(d) Treatment is primarily supportive to reduce the severity of symptoms (e.g., analgesic for headache) and stabilize blood pressure (Magge & DeAngelis, 2015). Discontinuation of drug is necessary to reduce the risk of progression to irreversible cytotoxic edema. Generally, symptoms of PRES improve or dissipate entirely with drug discontinuation and supportive therapy.

(e) Concomitant hemorrhage or ischemia indicates poorer prognosis (Arrillaga-Romany & Dietrich, 2012).

(2) Chronic encephalopathy is typically observed more than six months post-treatment and even several years beyond treatment (Taillibert et al., 2016). It is generally irreversible and occasionally even progressive. Patients typically report mild to moderate neurocognitive deficits, such as memory impairment or inability to focus, whereas more severe symptoms, such as ataxia, urinary incontinence, and spasticity, correlate with greater neurotoxicity. Some patients report no symptoms.

(a) Progressive multifocal leukoencephalopathy (PML): PML is a neuroinfectious disease causing demyelinating injury to the CNS that can manifest during treatment or months to years following treatment with immunomodulatory therapy.

(b) PML is caused by reactivation of latent John Cunningham virus, a type of human polyomavirus that is normally innocuous and present in a majority of healthy adults. Treatment-related immunosuppression with brentuximab, rituximab, alemtuzumab, and ofatumumab therapy leads to lytic infection of CNS white matter, with resultant demyelination (Bohra, Sokol,

& Dalia, 2017; Magge & DeAngelis, 2015). Symptoms can include hemiparesis, visual impairment, altered mental status, ataxia, dysmetria, dysarthria, headache, vertigo, seizures, sensory deficits, parkinsonism, aphasia, and neglect (Bohra et al., 2017).

(c) PML is untreatable, progressive, and nearly always fatal (case fatality rate of 90%) (Bohra et al., 2017; Magge & DeAngelis, 2015).

b) Pathophysiology: Exact pathologic mechanisms vary according to agent and subtype of encephalopathy. PML, for example, results from opportunistic infection in the setting of an immunocompromised host.

c) Incidence: Incidence varies, with chronic encephalopathy being more common and occurring in 16%–75% of adult survivors of solid tumors (Yust-Katz & Gilbert, 2014). Although rare (incidence of 0.07% in the setting of hematologic malignancies), PML in the setting of cancer may be underreported given the challenges of achieving diagnosis (Bohra et al., 2017). However, with increasing use of immunomodulatory therapies in the oncology setting, clinicians should be familiar with PML as a differential diagnosis in the setting of neurologic symptoms.

d) Clinical manifestation: The permeating symptom of all forms of encephalopathy is varying levels of altered mental status. Acute encephalopathy can develop as a constellation of symptoms including focal neurologic deficits, neurobehavioral problems, seizure, or alterations in consciousness. Chronic encephalopathy is frequently described in terms of "chemobrain" or "chemo fog" and typically includes global impairment in attention, memory, and executive function (Magge & DeAngelis, 2015).

e) Assessment: Diagnosis can be difficult, as the list of differential diagnoses is extensive (e.g., brain metastases, aseptic meningitis), but is typically achieved based on report of symptoms, neurologic examination, and treatment context and timing. Because of the structural changes within white matter, PRES and PML can often be identified radiographically, but brain biopsy is required for definitive diagnosis of PML.

f) Collaborative management: Acute encephalopathy typically self-resolves with discontinuation of the agent. No cure exists for chronic encephalopathy. Supportive therapies for toxic leukoencephalopathy is as described previously in the Radiation-induced CNS Toxicity section.

3. Focal deficits: Focal neurologic deficits are limited failures of neurologic function that affect a specific part of the body. Vision, speech, and hearing impairments during or immediately following treatment for cancer are considered focal neurologic toxicities, as are isolated sensory and motor losses, among others.

a) Pathophysiology: All focal nerve deficits originate from injury to the nerve, either as a direct result of chemotherapy or as a secondary effect (e.g., swelling). The exact pathogenesis of cranial nerve involvement is uncertain. It is important to note that focal deficits may be a direct consequence of malignancy as well.

b) Incidence: Transient focal deficits are relatively common over the trajectory of cancer and are sometimes difficult to attribute exclusively to the cancer or its treatment.

c) Clinical manifestations: Each cranial nerve operates a distinct neurologic function and can be useful to help localize neurotoxic injury (see Table 24-3). For example, double vision has been reported with capecitabine use and correlated with neurotoxic palsy of cranial nerve VI (Dasgupta, Adilieje, Bhattacharya, Smith, & Sheikh, 2010).

d) Assessment: Diagnosis is achieved with careful neurologic examination.

e) Collaborative management: Treatment typically involves supportive therapy or, in severe cases, discontinuation of the agent.

4. Cerebellar syndrome: Neurotoxic injury to the cerebellum may result in cerebellar syndrome, characterized by ataxia, dysmetria, dizziness, nystagmus, and gait imbalance.

a) Pathophysiology: Cerebellar syndrome has been reported as an acute event with traditional chemotherapy agents, including capecitabine, cytarabine, 5-fluorouracil, hexamethylmelamine, nelarabine, oxaliplatin, procarbazine, and vincristine (Stone & DeAngelis, 2016), as well as targeted agents, including bortezomib, rituximab, thalidomide, and trastuzumab (Wick et al., 2016). It generally is dose related and self-limiting, but some patients may experience permanent dysfunction secondary to loss of Purkinje cells in the cerebellum (Stone & DeAngelis, 2016). Exact pathologic mechanisms

Table 24-3. Focal Deficits Involving the Cranial Nerves

Signs and Symptoms	Cranial Nerve	Name	Origination	Function
Loss of smell (anosmia)	I	Olfactory	Olfactory bulb	Special sensory: smell
Visual disturbances; vision loss	II	Optic	Thalamus	Special sensory: vision
Loss of pupillary light reflex: papilledema; ptosis; double vision (diplopia); blurry vision	III	Oculomotor	Midbrain	Motor: eyeball movement; controls eyelid Parasympathetic: pupil constrictor
Diplopia; nystagmus	IV	Trochlear	Midbrain	Motor: eyeball movement
Loss of sensations (see function column); difficulty chewing, abnormal jaw-jerk reflex	V	Trigeminal	Pons	Motor: chewing muscles Sensory: touch, pain, temperature, vibration for face, mouth, anterior two-thirds of tongue
Strabismus; nystagmus; diplopia	VI	Abducens	Pons	Motor: eyeball movement
Facial paresis or plegia; loss of taste	VII	Facial	Pons	Motor: face muscles Sensory: sense near ears Special sensory: taste in anterior two-thirds of tongue
Hearing loss; balance issues	VIII	Auditory	Pons/medulla	Special sensory: hearing and balance
Absent gag; impaired or absent swallow; loss of taste; loss of pharyngeal movement	IX	Glossopharyngeal	Pons/medulla	Motor: pharyngeal movement Sensory: middle ear; pharynx, posterior one-third of tongue Parasympathetic: parotid gland
Absent gag; impaired or absent swallow; loss of velar movement; loss of voice or hoarseness, dyspnea, dysarthria	X	Vagus	Medulla	Motor: pharyngeal and laryngeal muscles Sensory: pharynx and blood pressure Special sensory: taste from epiglottis/pharynx Parasympathetic: heart, lungs, digestive tract
Droopy shoulder, movement of neck	XI	Spinal accessory	Medulla	Motor: neck and shoulder muscles
Loss of tongue movement; tongue fasciculation, tongue atrophy	XII	Hypoglossal	Medulla	Motor: tongue muscles

Note. From *Neuroanatomy for Speech Language Pathology and Audiology* (pp. 84–85), by M.H. Rouse, 2016, Burlington, MA: Jones & Bartlett Learning. Copyright 2016 by Jones & Bartlett Learning, www.jblearning.com. Adapted with permission.

vary according to the agent, but symptoms arise from loss or delay of nerve conduction through the cerebellum, which is responsible for coordinating muscle activity and movement.

b) Incidence: Overall, the incidence of cerebellar syndrome is low, with variation by agent. Cerebellar syndrome manifests most commonly in 10%–20% of patients with acute myeloid leukemia and lymphoma treated with high-dose cytarabine 1 g/m^2 or greater given as a bolus infusion (Arrillaga-Romany & Dietrich, 2012).

c) Risk factors: Several risk factors have been associated with the development of cerebellar syndrome in the setting of cytarabine, including a cumulative dose of 36 g/m^2 or greater, older age, renal dysfunction, previous history of neurologic dysfunction, or elevated alkaline phosphatase (Magge & DeAngelis, 2015). The incidence of cerebellar syndrome with 5-fluorouracil, a pyrimidine analog, is much lower at 2%–4% (Arrillaga-Romany & Dietrich, 2012).

d) Clinical manifestations: Early signs include nystagmus, speech difficulties (dysarthria), uncoordinated movements, abnormal gait, and trouble writing (dysmetria). Rarely, somnolence or lethargy, altered mental status, and encephalopathy can co-occur (Magge & DeAngelis, 2015). Symptoms typically resolve with drug discontinuation, but up to 30% of patients suffer permanent cerebellar injury (Magge & DeAngelis, 2015). Cerebellar atrophy is a late effect, particularly with the use of cytarabine (Arrillaga-Romany & Dietrich, 2012).

e) Assessment: Diagnosis is achieved from report of symptoms with careful neurologic examination before each cytarabine infusion. This includes assessment of the patient's coordination (e.g., finger-to-nose and finger-to-finger test, rapid alternating hand movements, ability to write), speech pattern, gait and balance, and presence of abnormal eye movements (nystagmus). When signs and symptoms are present, the causative medication should be held, and the prescriber should be notified immediately.

f) Collaborative management: Symptoms typically resolve over time or with discontinuation of therapy immediately when symptoms occur. Depending on the extent of injury, some sequelae may be permanent.

5. Adverse cerebrovascular events

a) Overview: Cerebrovascular events are a constellation of clinical syndromes that disrupt blood supply to the brain with resultant neurologic symptom or symptom complex. Cerebrovascular events are classified according to etiology, location, and duration of symptoms. Common cerebrovascular events manifesting in the setting of chemotherapy include thromboembolism, intracranial hemorrhage, and ischemic stroke.

(1) Cerebral thromboembolism is a blood clot that occludes the small and large cerebral arteries.

(2) Intracranial hemorrhage is bleeding inside the cranial vault, resulting in accumulation of blood and, frequently, increased intracranial pressure.

(3) Ischemic stroke is the sudden loss of blood circulation to an area of the brain, resulting in a corresponding loss of neurologic function. It occurs in the setting of thrombotic or embolic occlusion of a cerebral artery.

b) Pathophysiology: Cancer stimulates the coagulation system, predisposing patients to a baseline hypercoagulable or prothrombotic state. Many cancer therapies further potentiate this risk of thrombosis through procoagulant release, endothelial damage, or stimulation of tissue factors. Ischemic stroke, a direct effect of arterial occlusion by thromboembolism, is associated with antiangiogenic agents such as bevacizumab, sorafenib, sunitinib, and vandetanib, and to a lesser extent with traditional chemotherapy agents such as cisplatin, L-asparaginase, and intrathecal methotrexate (Arrillaga-Romany & Dietrich, 2012). In contrast, intracranial hemorrhage, including intratumoral hemorrhage, in patients with cancer is typically a secondary effect of disseminated intravascular coagulation, thrombocytopenia due to bone marrow suppression, or vitamin K deficiency. An increased risk exists in the setting of bevacizumab (Arrillaga-Romany & Dietrich, 2012).

c) Incidence: Incidence varies according to the type of event and agent. For example, the risk of thromboembolism can be as high as 35% with L-asparaginase, which is approved for use in acute lymphocytic leukemia (Arrillaga-Romany & Dietrich, 2012). Patients frequently continue the full regimen of L-asparaginase if therapeutically anticoagulated. The risk of hemorrhage or ischemic stroke is reported to be higher with newer agents, particularly bevacizumab. The overall intracranial hemorrhage rate among patients with cancer treated with bevacizumab is 0.3%–0.9% and increases to 0.9%–1.5% in those with known primary or metastatic brain tumors (Schiff et al., 2015). The rate of stroke approached 2% in patients with glioblastoma treated with bevacizumab (Schiff et al., 2015).

d) Clinical manifestations: The cardinal clinical feature of many cerebrovascular events is pain (headache). Additional symptoms include nausea, vomiting, altered mental status, seizure, or focal neurologic symptoms. Depending on when the patient is seen and the underlying cause, the deficit may be stable, progressive, or completely resolved.

e) Assessment: Diagnosis is made radiographically.

f) Collaborative management: Patients with thromboembolism and ischemic stroke typically are given multimodality therapy such as anticoagulation, thrombolysis, and platelet inhibition. Hemorrhage may require neurosurgical intervention to decompress the brain, initiate invasive pressure monitoring, or evacuate a clot. Supportive treatment includes pain medication, steroids, and antiseizure medication.

6. Aseptic meningitis: Aseptic meningitis is irritation and inflammation of the meninges in the absence of infection. It is the most commonly reported toxicity of intrathecal chemotherapy, especially methotrexate and cytarabine (Magge & DeAngelis, 2015; Taillibert et al., 2016). Other agents reported to induce aseptic meningitis include cetuximab, ipilimumab, IV immunoglobulin, and rituximab (Magge & DeAngelis, 2015; Maritaz, Metz, Baba-Hamed, Jardin-Szucs, & Deplanque, 2016; Wick et al., 2016).
   a) Pathophysiology: The pathologic mechanism of aseptic meningitis is indeterminate and likely varies by agent. For example, aseptic meningitis following cetuximab administration is thought to stem from an allergic hypersensitivity reaction or serum immunoglobulin crossing the blood–brain barrier, causing meningeal inflammation (Maritaz et al., 2016).
   b) Incidence: Incidence of aseptic meningitis varies widely according to agent and dose. For example, meningitis following intrathecal methotrexate administration is reported to occur in 9.8%–90% of patients with overt CNS disease and is dose dependent (Jacob et al., 2015). However, the incidence of meningitis following cetuximab administration is much lower, with fewer than a dozen reports in the literature (Maritaz et al., 2016).
   c) Clinical manifestations: Symptoms include fever, headache, stiff neck, nausea, vomiting, photophobia, and increased cell presence (white blood cells, protein) in the cerebrospinal fluid (Taillibert et al., 2016).
   d) Assessment: The diagnosis is usually presumptive based on symptoms and temporality and route of chemotherapy. A lumbar puncture showing cerebrospinal fluid pleocytosis may or may not help to improve diagnostic certainty (Taillibert et al., 2016).
   e) Collaborative management: Prophylactic dosing with dexamethasone prior to intrathecal chemotherapy may help reduce the risk of aseptic meningitis (Magge & DeAngelis, 2015). Symptoms can be managed with supportive therapy, which includes analgesics, antiemetics, steroids if not already given prophylactically, and IV fluids. Otherwise, spontaneous recovery is seen without any neurologic sequelae when the agent is discontinued.

7. Myelopathy: Myelopathy is a rare complication (approximately 3%) of swelling and spinal cord compression during or following administration of intrathecal chemotherapy such as methotrexate and cytarabine (Cachia et al., 2015; Magge & DeAngelis, 2015).
   a) Pathophysiology: The etiology of myelopathy following intrathecal chemotherapy remains unclear (Cachia et al., 2015; Magge & DeAngelis, 2015), but symptoms result from swelling and cord compression.
   b) Incidence: Myelopathy as a complication of intrathecal chemotherapy is rare in adults, with most of the cases described in the literature occurring in the pediatric population (Cachia et al., 2015).
   c) Clinical manifestations: Symptoms include low back pain, sensory or motor deficits in the lower extremities, and bowel or bladder incontinence (Magge & DeAngelis, 2015). Lhermitte sign, an electric shock–like sensation, may be elicited when the neck is extended (Arrillaga-Romany & Dietrich, 2012).
   d) Assessment: MRI is the most sensitive radiologic technique in the diagnosis of myelopathy, but MRI abnormalities are nonspecific and include cord swelling, T2 hyperintensity, and contrast enhancement (Cachia et al., 2015).
   e) Collaborative management: No approved treatment exists for chemotherapy-induced myelopathy. Symptoms and swelling typically resolve with discontinuation of drug.

8. Seizures: A seizure is the manifestation of an abnormal, hypersynchronous electrical discharge of a population of cortical neurons. This discharge may produce symptoms or objective signs (clinical seizure) or may be subclinical, materializing only on electroencephalogram.
   a) Pathophysiology: The underlying etiology of seizures in patients with cancer can be complex, involving anatomic and metabolic disruptions caused by brain tumors themselves, tumor- or medication-related stroke or opportunistic infection, chemotherapy, or neuroradiotherapy. Seizures may be caused directly by agents themselves (e.g., busulfan, used commonly during stem cell transplant) or may result from hyponatremia as a secondary effect of hormonal or electrolyte imbalances (Taillibert et al., 2016). For example, syndrome of inappropriate antidiuretic hormone secretion is a known effect of vinca alkaloids and cisplatin that can result in hyponatremia, leading to severe confusion,

coma, and seizures (Bénit & Vecht, 2016). Cisplatin-induced renal injury can result in salt wasting, hyponatremia, and seizures (Bénit & Vecht, 2016). Targeted therapies that inhibit epidermal growth factor receptor pathways, such as the monoclonal antibodies cetuximab and panitumumab and the tyrosine kinase inhibitors gefitinib and erlotinib, also cause secondary electrolyte depletion, which increases the risk of seizure (Wick et al., 2016).

b) Incidence: Incidence varies according to cancer type, location, and agent. Busulfan, an agent used during conditioning for stem cell transplant, carries a 10% risk of seizures (Taillibert et al., 2016). For patients with primary brain tumor, greater than 65% of patients with gliomas and 33% of patients with meningiomas will have epilepsy (Bénit & Vecht, 2016). For patients with systemic cancer, the overall incidence of seizure is higher: 60% of patients with brain metastases will also develop epilepsy (Bénit & Vecht, 2016).

c) Clinical manifestations: Signs and symptoms of seizure can include temporary confusion, staring spells, involuntary jerking or violent movements of the arms and legs, and altered mental status, including loss of consciousness.

d) Assessment: A thorough neurologic examination is first done to explore differential diagnoses. Diagnosis is typically achieved via electroencephalogram (EEG), although a witnessed tonic-clonic seizure can be enough to initiate treatment.

e) Collaborative management: Seizures are treated with antiepileptics. In the case of high-dose busulfan (greater than 9 mg/kg oral or IV equivalent), prophylaxis with antiepileptics prior to therapy is recommended, as the risk of seizure is significantly high (Magge & DeAngelis, 2015; Stone & DeAngelis, 2016; Taillibert et al., 2016).

9. Headache: Headache is pain with or without pressure in the head.

a) Pathophysiology

(1) Headache can be caused directly by mass effect of intracranial malignancy, malignant infiltration of the meninges or pituitary gland, or as a direct effect of anticancer therapies such as radiation, chemotherapy (e.g., 5-fluorouracil, procarbazine), targeted therapies (e.g., ipilimumab, imatinib, rituximab), and immunotherapies (e.g., CAR T cells) (Stone & DeAngelis, 2016). As a result, attributing a single causative agent is challenging, but temporality of headache emergence to treatment can be instructive. Mechanisms of action are varied based on the agent. For example, headache during rituximab infusion likely results from the release of inflammatory cytokines (Wick et al., 2016), whereas bevacizumab-induced hypertension can lead to headache (Magge & DeAngelis, 2015).

(2) Headache can also be a secondary effect of treatment—for example, post-procedural complications of cancer diagnostics such as lumbar puncture or brain biopsy; stress, fatigue, anxiety, or sleep disturbances resulting from the cancer or its treatment; cancer- or treatment-associated anemia; and hypercalcemia and dehydration from vomiting and diarrhea.

b) Incidence: Incidence varies widely according to the causative agent.

c) Clinical manifestation: Patients may report pain, tightness, or pressure in the head or upper neck.

d) Assessment: Diagnosis is based on patient self-report.

e) Collaborative management: Treatment typically involves administration of analgesics and, if warranted, intervention to correct the proximate cause, such as a blood patch for post–lumbar puncture headache, correction of anemia or hypercalcemia, or treatment of hypertension following bevacizumab infusion.

E. Chemotherapy-induced peripheral neuropathy (CIPN): General neurotoxicities

1. Overview: CIPN is damage to nerve cells, nerve fibers (axons), and nerve coverings (myelin) due to exposure to a neurotoxic chemotherapy agent that results in inhibition or deceleration of nerve signals. The three major categories of CIPN are sensory, motor, and autonomic.

a) Sensory neuropathy is damage to sensory nerves causing problems with sensation—for example, a patient's ability to feel pain or light touch.

b) Motor neuropathy is injury to motor nerves, affecting movement.

c) Autonomic neuropathy is impairment of the nonsensory, involuntary nervous system that controls and regulates smooth muscles, cardiac muscles, and glands (e.g., the nerves innervating the heart, the bladder, salivary glands).

2. Pathophysiology: Antineoplastics differentially impair specific structures within the neuron according to their mechanism of action. In general, the predominant pathophysiologic mechanism of CIPN across all chemotherapy agents is induction of mitochondrial abnormalities and inhibition of mitochondrial function (Brewer, Morrison, Dolan, & Fleming, 2016). CIPN can be broadly attributed to the resultant demyelination and axonal degeneration.
3. Incidence: Incidence and severity of CIPN vary by the specific type (sensory, motor, autonomic), agent, agent combinations, and dosages and is likely underreported. In aggregate, CIPN occurs in 30%–40% of patients receiving neurotoxic chemotherapy, most notably platinum agents, vinca alkaloids, and taxanes (Staff, Grisold, Grisold, & Windebank, 2017).
4. Clinical manifestations
   a) Sensory: Sensory neuropathies may be subtle and not consistently present during physical examination. Symptoms may be "positive," in which sensations are present in the absence of external stimuli and perceived as tingling, burning, pins and needles, or pain that is typically described as stabbing or shooting. Sensory disturbances can also manifest as "negative" phenomena (e.g., numbness, loss of sensation, impaired proprioception), in which sensation is completely absent with external stimulation; for example, the patient reports inability to feel a pinprick.
   b) Motor: Motor neuropathies may manifest as weakness, muscle fatigue, or atrophy. Patients also may report abnormally frequent and painful muscle cramps or fasciculation causing problems with ambulation and manual dexterity. Motor neuropathy may co-occur with sensory neuropathy (sensorimotor neuropathy).
   c) Autonomic: Autonomic neuropathy is seen most commonly with vinca alkaloids and can be associated with orthostatic hypotension, erectile dysfunction, and bowel and bladder dysfunction, including paralytic ileus, constipation, and urinary retention.
5. Assessment: Results from the physical examination may be normal or show sensory loss. Loss of the Achilles tendon reflex is usually the first clinical sign of CIPN (Tzatha & DeAngelis, 2016). Nerve conduction studies and an electromyogram can assist with diagnostic evaluation (Tzatha & DeAngelis, 2016).
6. Collaborative management: CIPN is managed by empirical dose modifications or discontinuation of treatment at the discretion of the treating physician. An autonomic neuropathy consisting of abdominal colic and constipation often requires concomitant bowel prophylaxis to prevent paralytic ileus (Magge & DeAngelis, 2015). Treatment of urinary retention may include intermittent catheterization until recovery of function.

F. Common antineoplastics conferring increased neurotoxicity
1. Chemotherapy
   a) Vinca alkaloids: Vinca alkaloids (e.g., vinblastine, vincristine, vinorelbine) inhibit cell proliferation and promote cytotoxicity by direct binding to tubulin, a critical component of microtubules. Microtubules perform the essential function of aligning chromosomes during metaphase (the third phase of mitosis). The binding of vinca to the microtubules ultimately results in inhibition of mitotic spindle function and arrests cancer cells in metaphase, rendering them unable to divide. However, throughout the nervous system, microtubules also help direct axonal transport of neuronal signals. Peripheral neuropathies of vinca alkaloids that target microtubules result from interruption of the axonal transport and nerve degeneration, most commonly resulting in axonal sensorimotor neuropathy characterized by paresthesias and weakness, such as wrist or foot drop (Magge & DeAngelis, 2015). Muscle cramps in the upper and lower extremities often are the first sign of neurotoxicity (Magge & DeAngelis, 2015). Rarely, vincristine also may cause focal neuropathies of the cranial nerves, resulting in hoarseness, diplopia, jaw pain, and facial palsies. Autonomic neuropathies rarely occur but can include urinary retention, orthostatic hypotension, and hypertension. Additional but infrequent neurotoxicities have been reported, including confusion and seizures from hyponatremia following syndrome of inappropriate antidiuretic hormone secretion, cortical blindness, ataxia, and Parkinson disease–like symptoms (Magge & DeAngelis, 2015).
   b) Platinum-based agents: Cisplatin and oxaliplatin are two widely used neurotoxic agents.
      (1) Peripheral neurotoxicity seen with cisplatin is dose dependent and usually manifests at cumulative doses of 400 mg/m^2 (Magge & DeAngelis, 2015).

Symptoms include numbness, tingling, and pain in the extremities. Additional neurotoxicity may present as Lhermitte sign, ototoxicity (e.g., tinnitus, hearing loss), and, more relevant to IV administration, encephalopathy typified by seizures and focal neurologic deficits (Magge & DeAngelis, 2015).

(2) Oxaliplatin induces a peripheral neurotoxicity as two clinically distinct syndromes.

(a) Acute transient paresthesia in the distal extremities usually occurs within the early phase of drug administration, during or just following infusion. Symptoms can be cold-triggered and include paresthesias, dysesthesias, and jaw tightening, which typically improve within a day following administration (Magge & DeAngelis, 2015).

(b) Chronic cumulative sensory neuropathy causes more persistent clinical impairments, including eye and jaw pain, ptosis, visual impairment, voice changes, sensory ataxia, and muscle cramps that may persist for several months (Magge & DeAngelis, 2015).

(c) Ocular toxicity is a rarer but overlooked effect of oxaliplatin, occurring acutely during infusion or as a late effect. Symptoms include tearing, dry eyes, conjunctivitis, blurred vision, photosensitivity, altered color vision, and eye pain triggered by cold (Cidon & Alonso, 2016).

c) Taxanes: Cabazitaxel, docetaxel, nab-paclitaxel, and paclitaxel are associated with sensory neuropathies involving the feet and occasionally the hands, with painful paresthesias, mild weakness, and myalgias (Magge & DeAngelis, 2015). Symptoms usually improve after treatment discontinuation but may persist. Symptoms associated with changes in autonomic function are rarer but must be carefully evaluated in patients receiving taxanes; cardiac and vascular dysfunction reported as arrhythmias and orthostatic hypotension has been reported in patients receiving paclitaxel (Velasco & Bruna, 2015).

d) Antitumor antibiotics: Of note, antitumor antibiotics (e.g., bleomycin, doxorubicin) produce highly selective neurotoxic effects (to dorsal root ganglia) and peripheral neurologic toxicity. CNS toxicity is mostly described in terms of cognitive impairment (Kesler & Blayney, 2016).

2. Immunotherapy

a) Thalidomide and its synthetic analogs: Neurotoxic effects from thalidomide are dose dependent. The most common toxicity seen with thalidomide is somnolence (thalidomide was first marketed as a sedative). At typical doses, 50% of patients taking thalidomide develop peripheral neuropathy (10% with severe symptoms), including distal paresthesias or dysesthesias with or without sensory loss (Stone & DeAngelis, 2016). Autonomic neuropathies include constipation and, rarely, impotence and bradycardia (Stone & DeAngelis, 2016). Lhermitte sign is sometimes seen (Magge & DeAngelis, 2015).

b) CAR T cells: CAR T cells are manufactured for each individual patient using T cells drawn from the patient's blood. The T cells are then genetically coded to express a CAR specific to an antigen expressed by the patient's cancer cells. The binding of CAR T cells to cancer antigens in the body results in T-cell proliferation and expansion, as well as further immune activation, including elevations in cytokines (Magge & DeAngelis, 2015), ultimately resulting in cancer cell death. Neurotoxicity from CAR T cells is largely a secondary result of cytokine-associated toxicity, also known as cytokine release syndrome (CRS). CRS is characterized by fever, hypotension, capillary leak, and neurotoxicity and can result in death. Encephalopathic-type symptoms consisting of headache, mental status changes, confusion, delirium, focal deficits, word-finding difficulty or aphasia, hallucinations, tremor, dysmetria, altered gait, and seizures have been reported in the context of CRS (D.W. Lee et al., 2014; Wick et al., 2016) but may represent a separate, parallel process from CRS (Turtle et al., 2016). Ischemic events have also been observed (Wick et al., 2016). Steroids are typically not used to palliate symptoms, because they would also blunt the intended immune activation.

3. Targeted therapy

a) Bortezomib: Bortezomib, a proteasome inhibitor, is a primary treatment consideration in relapsed or resistant multiple myeloma but can induce painful sensory neuropathy characterized by paresthesias in limbs and neuropathic pain in a stocking-and-glove distribution in approximately 22% of patients (Meregalli, 2015).

b) Milder neuropathy is reported to occur in 50%–75% of patients (Stone & DeAngelis, 2016; Wick et al., 2016). The mechanisms underlying the pathogenesis of bortezomib-induced peripheral neuropathy are unknown. No approved treatment exists, but symptoms typically resolve with dose modification or discontinuation.

c) Subcutaneous administration is recommended for individuals with preexisting or at high risk for peripheral neuropathy (Truven Health Analytics, 2017) because incidence of peripheral neuropathy is lower with the subcutaneous formulation than the IV formulation (38% vs. 53%, respectively) (Mateos & San Miguel, 2012).

G. Risk factors and prophylaxis

1. Risk factors: The clinical sequelae of neurotoxicity from antineoplastic therapies are complex functions of dose, mode of administration, exposure time, and the unique genetic susceptibilities of the patient. Risk factors for the development of CIPN include preexisting neuropathies due to diabetes, alcohol abuse, folate/vitamin B_{12} deficiency, hereditary sensorimotor neuropathy (e.g., Charcot-Marie-Tooth disease), or neuropathies caused by the malignancy itself (Magge & DeAngelis, 2015).

2. Prophylaxis: Only a few prophylactic agents have been supported in the literature to reduce specific neurotoxic effects. Most (e.g., amifostine, glutathione, infusions of calcium and magnesium, venlafaxine, xaliproden) have ultimately had inconsistent and generally negative results (Albers, Chaudhry, Cavaletti, & Donehower, 2014; Taillibert et al., 2016). Some strategies, such as vitamin E supplementation, have been shown to be ineffective as a neuroprotective agent (Albers et al., 2014). For specific neurotoxic effects, the following have demonstrated efficacy.

a) Aseptic meningitis: Prophylactic dosing with dexamethasone prior to intrathecal chemotherapy may help reduce the risk of aseptic meningitis (Magge & DeAngelis, 2015).

b) Seizures: For agents with known seizure risk (e.g., busulfan), prophylaxis with antiepileptics is highly effective at reducing the development of seizures (Taillibert et al., 2016).

c) Autonomic neuropathy affecting gastrointestinal motility: Prevention of functional bowel disorders such as paralytic ileus often requires concomitant bowel prophylaxis with high fiber intake, fluid balance, and the use of opioid-sparing analgesia, stool softeners, and laxatives (Taillibert et al., 2016).

d) General CIPN: Increased physical activity and exercise has been shown to consistently mitigate the general effects of CIPN during treatment with antineoplastics (Taillibert et al., 2016).

H. Cognitive impairment

1. Cognitive function is a multidimensional concept that encompasses several domains (e.g., attention and concentration, executive function, information processing speed, language, motor function, visuospatial skill, learning, memory) regulated by the brain (Jansen, 2017; see Figure 24-1). Cognitive impairment is a decline in function in either one or multiple domains of cognitive function and may represent a single, highly specific deficit or a cluster of related deficits (Lezak, Howieson, Bigler, & Tranel, 2012; Von Ah, Jansen, & Allen, 2014).

2. Pathophysiology: Although cancer therapies, including surgery, radiation therapy, chemotherapy, hormone therapy, and immunotherapy, have been associated with cognitive changes, the use of multimodal therapy makes it difficult to determine the underlying mechanism for cognitive impairment. The presence of cancer and tumor burden also may contribute to cognitive impairment prior to the initiation of treatment (Wefel, Kesler, Noll, & Schagen, 2015).

a) The mechanisms of cancer treatment–related cognitive changes are thought to be multifactorial. Although animal studies have elucidated many hypotheses, the actual mechanisms for individual and multimodal treatments are still not fully understood (Jansen, 2017).

b) Suggested pathophysiologic mechanisms

(1) Structural and functional damage of the brain due to direct tumor involvement or surgical removal of CNS tumors: Effects are specific to the area of the tumor location (Bohan, 2013; Jansen, 2017). In contrast, patients with non-CNS cancers who receive chemotherapy may demonstrate declines in gray matter volume most often in the prefrontal lobe, whereas decreases in white matter integrity and brain activity are more widespread (Holohan, Von Ah, McDonald, & Saykin, 2013; Janelsins, Kesler, Ahles, & Morrow, 2014).

Figure 24-1. Anatomic Correlates of Cognitive Function

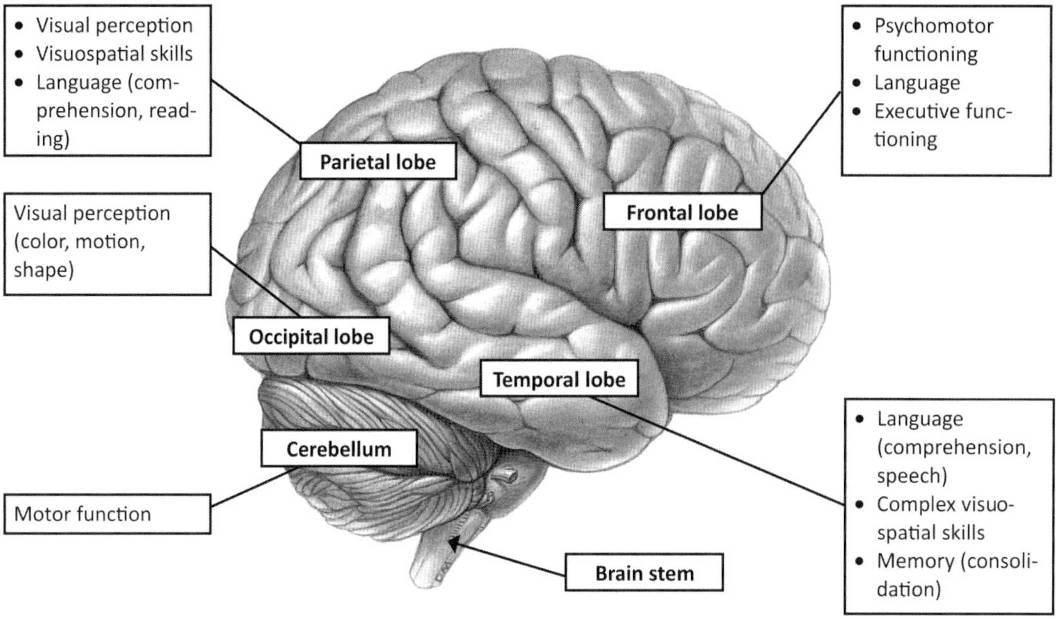

Note. Based on information from Filley, 2012; Gazzaniga et al., 2014; Lisberger & Thach, 2013; Olson & Colby, 2013; Pearl & Emsellem, 2014.

(2) Direct injury to neurons or other brain structures (including oligodendrocytes, glial cells, and white matter tracts) from chemotherapy or radiation therapy (de Ruiter & Schagen, 2013; Edelstein, Richard, & Bernstein, 2017; Greene-Schloesser, Moore, & Robbins, 2013; Jansen, 2017; Kaiser, Bledowski, & Dietrich, 2014; Koppelmans et al., 2014; McDonald & Saykin, 2013; Parihar & Limoli, 2013; Scherling & Smith, 2013; Seigers, Schagen, Van Tellingen, & Dietrich, 2013; Simó et al., 2015): Neurotoxic effects result in disruption of neural stem and progenitor cells within the CNS, which appear to be more sensitive than cancer cells to various chemotherapy agents (Dietrich, 2010; Kaiser et al., 2014; Wefel et al., 2015). Specific chemotherapy and hormonal drugs shown to target neural progenitor cells in experimental studies include carmustine, cisplatin, cyclophosphamide, cytarabine, docetaxel, doxorubicin, 5-fluorouracil, ifosfamide, methotrexate, oxaliplatin, paclitaxel, tamoxifen, temozolomide, and thiotepa (Dietrich, Prust, & Kaiser, 2015; Kaiser et al., 2014).

(3) Disruption of the blood–brain barrier: Chemotherapy drugs unable to cross the blood–brain barrier cause damage to blood vessels, thereby adversely affecting the brain (Merriman, Von Ah, Miaskowski, & Aouizerat, 2013; Wardill et al., 2016; Wefel et al., 2015).

(4) DNA damage due to chemotherapy or ionizing irradiation (Conroy, McDonald, Smith, et al., 2013; Edelstein et al., 2017; Hoeffner, 2016; Jansen, 2017; Joly et al., 2015; Mandelblatt, Jacobsen, & Ahles, 2014; Merriman et al., 2013)

(5) Cytokine dysregulation: Cytokines are proteins that have a role in neural function and repair and the metabolism of neurotransmitters. Increased levels of cytokines may activate a stress cascade that can cause inflammation and affect cognition (Castel et al., 2017; Merriman et al., 2013). Although many che-

motherapy agents are not able to cross the blood–brain barrier, they can stimulate a release of proinflammatory cytokines in response to cell injury. This release leads to an elevation in circulating tumor necrosis factor-alpha that can cross the blood–brain barrier and cause excessive levels of CNS cytokines, resulting in cognitive impairment. Evidence for increases in cytokine levels exists for all treatment modalities (Bender & Thelen, 2013; Cheung et al., 2015; Conroy, McDonald, Smith, et al., 2013; Ganz et al., 2013; Kesler, 2014; Kesler et al., 2013; Lacourt & Heijnen, 2017; Pomykala, Ganz, et al., 2013; Shibayama et al., 2014; Smith et al., 2014; Wang et al., 2015). Increased cytokine levels may also exist prior to the initiation of treatment (S.K. Patel et al., 2015). Studies have found higher levels of inflammatory markers (e.g., interleukin-1β, interleukin-6) associated with lower self-perceived memory (Ganz et al., 2013; Henneghan, 2016) and global cognitive functioning (Cheung et al., 2015, Pomykala, Ganz, et al., 2013). One study found significant associations between interleukin-6 and tumor necrosis factor-alpha levels and logical memory ($p = 0.006$; Kesler et al., 2013).

(6) Oxidative damage: Various chemotherapy drugs (e.g., carmustine, cyclophosphamide, doxorubicin, methotrexate) may initiate oxidative stress that can trigger cell membrane damage and produce large amounts of free radicals (Dietrich et al., 2015; Seigers et al., 2103; Wardill et al., 2016). Evidence of oxidative stress was associated with lower gray matter density ($p = 0.011$) in one study of breast cancer survivors (Conroy, McDonald, Smith, et al., 2013). Oxidative damage, or inflammatory responses, can occur with radiation therapy, are dose dependent, and may last from weeks to months (Edelstein et al., 2017; Greene-Schloesser et al., 2013).

(7) Anemia: Insufficient brain oxygenation is associated with cognitive problems in multiple domains, such as attention and concentration, executive functioning, motor function, and memory (Lezak et al., 2012). Patients with cancer may experience anemia as a result of primary or metastatic cancer involvement of the bone marrow or bones or because of cancer treatments such as chemotherapy and radiation therapy (Jansen, 2017).

(8) Hormone-mediated effects: Estrogen and androgen are neuroprotective, and receptors for these hormones are widely distributed throughout the brain (Boss, Kang, Marcus, & Bergstrom, 2014; Hogervorst, 2013; Lobo, 2014; Wu & Amidi, 2017). Although hormonal agents work by different mechanisms—selective estrogen receptor modulators (e.g., tamoxifen, raloxifene) act as estrogen agonists or estrogen antagonists and block estrogen receptors; aromatase inhibitors (e.g., anastrozole, exemestane, letrozole) decrease estrogen synthesis in the peripheral tissues; and androgen deprivation therapy reduces testosterone levels—their use can affect cognitive functioning (Bakoyiannis, Tsigka, Perrea, & Pergialiotis, 2016; Boss et al., 2014; Gonzalez et al., 2015; P.E. Lee, Tierney, Wu, Pritchard, & Rochon, 2016; McGinty et al., 2014; Merriman et al., 2013; Wefel et al., 2015; Wu & Amidi, 2017; Zwart, Terra, Linn, & Schagen, 2015). Chemotherapy often induces menopause with a more accelerated decline in estrogen levels, but the significance of this to cognitive functioning is still unclear (Conroy, McDonald, Ahles, West, & Saykin, 2013; Jansen, 2017; Lobo, 2014).

(9) Leukoencephalopathy: Structural alterations in cerebral white matter can occur with cranial irradiation (Hoeffner, 2016). White matter changes have also been reported with various chemotherapy and targeted agents, such as bevacizumab, brentuximab, busulfan, carmustine, cisplatin, cytarabine, 5-fluorouracil, fludarabine, ifosfamide, infliximab, interleukin-2, lenalidomide, levamisole, methotrexate, natalizumab, procarbazine, rituximab, sorafenib, sunitinib, temozolomide, and thiotepa (Fernandez-Robles, Greenberg, & Pirl, 2016; Magge & DeAngelis, 2015; Mann, Dail, & Bai-

ley, 2016; Westin, Sood, & Coleman, 2018; Wick et al., 2016).

3. Incidence: The incidence of treatment-related cognitive changes is difficult to determine because many factors influence cognition. Many studies are limited by their cross-sectional study design (lacking baseline neuropsychological testing) or small sample sizes. There is a growing evidence base for cancer and cancer treatment–related cognitive changes that incorporates objective and subjective measures, as well as genetic and radiologic tests. It is important to include predisposing factors and to evaluate for impairment prior to treatment, as well as to include combination therapies and differences in sample characteristics, to attempt to differentiate what cognitive changes are truly treatment related.
   a) Chemotherapy-related cognitive changes have been predominantly studied in patients with breast cancer. Evidence to support whether chemotherapy-induced cognitive changes exist or are due solely to chemotherapy is inconclusive. However, it is estimated that up to 75% of patients with cancer experience cognitive impairment during or after cancer treatment (Allen, Myers, Jansen, Merriman, & Von Ah, 2018; Janelsins et al., 2014).
   b) Evidence of cognitive impairment in 20%–30% of patients prior to treatment has been reported, with incidences up to 40% reported in older adult patients (Joly et al., 2015; Lange et al., 2014; Wefel et al., 2015).
   c) Cognitive problems are estimated to persist for months or up to 20 years following the completion of treatment in up to 35% of survivors (Janelsins et al., 2014).
   d) Cognitive problems, especially difficulties with concentration, memory, and the ability to multitask, are a major concern to cancer survivors, especially when reentering the workplace (Von Ah et al., 2016). Studies have confirmed that cognitive issues continue to have a negative impact on survivors in the workplace for at least one if not many years after treatment (Duijts, van der Beek, Boelhouwer, & Schagen, 2017; Kanaskie & Loeb, 2015; Von Ah et al., 2016).
4. Risk factors: Predisposing factors that influence cognitive function are not consistent, but the following have been suggested.
   a) Individual risk factors
      (1) Gender: Women excel in language, information processing speed, and motor function, whereas men perform better in visuospatial skills and mathematics (Lezak et al., 2012).
      (2) Age: Cognitive decline occurs with aging, which is associated with several proposed mechanisms for cognitive impairment, including but not limited to increased cell senescence, DNA damage, oxidative stress, inflammation, mitochondrial dysfunction, and decreased telomere length (Vega, Dumas, & Newhouse, 2017). Although younger patients report worse cognitive problems, older patients perform worse on objective tests (Merriman et al., 2013). Of note, normative data for neuropsychological tests are based on age.
      (3) Comorbidities: Patients with greater comorbidity levels, especially illnesses such as diabetes and cardiovascular disease, have been reported to have cognitive impairment prior to initiating cancer treatments (Allen et al., 2018; Mandelblatt, Stern, et al., 2014).
      (4) Genetics: As is true with other side effects, not all patients are equally affected by the same regimen. Consequently, several genetic polymorphisms are being evaluated to determine those that might influence an individual's risk of cognitive changes during cancer and cancer treatments (Mandelblatt, Jacobsen, & Ahles, 2014). Genetic mutations may influence the impact of cancer and cancer treatments on brain activity and cognitive function (Wefel, Noll, & Scheurer, 2016). For example, the presence of the apolipoprotein E (*APOE*) gene ε4 variant has been associated with decreased cognitive functioning (e.g., executive function, memory), and several other candidate genes are being studied for their potential role in chemotherapy-induced cognitive changes (Correa et al., 2014; Wefel et al., 2016). In one study of patients with breast cancer receiving chemotherapy, those with the brain-derived neurotrophic factor (*BDNF*) Val/Met heterozygous genotype had lower odds of impairment in executive function ($p = 0.030$), whereas the *BDNF* Met/Met homozygous genotype was found to be protective of language ($p = 0.043$), executive function ($p = 0.030$), and subjective cognitive functioning ($p = 0.036$)

compared to those with *BDNF* Val/Val genotypes (Ng et al., 2016).

(5) Psychological factors such as stress, anxiety, and depression can affect performance on neuropsychological testing (Lezak et al., 2012). However, these psychological factors are generally not correlated with objective measures in studies of patients with cancer. It has been suggested that patients' perceptions of cognitive impairments may indicate emotional distress, as anxiety and depression often are correlated with subjective measures of cognitive functioning (Kaiser et al., 2014). Stress related to cognitive impairment has also been characterized as post-traumatic stress disorder (Hermelink et al., 2017).

(a) Increased anxiety at baseline was found to correlate with lower performance on objective cognitive measures in one study (Lyon et al., 2016). Although anxiety has not been consistently related to objective measures, higher levels have been found to be predictive of poorer perceived cognitive functioning over time (Janelsins et al., 2017; Merriman et al., 2017).

(b) Higher levels of depressive symptoms prior to treatment have been found to be predictive of worse perceived cognitive functioning over time (Lyon et al., 2016; Merriman et al., 2017).

(c) Fatigue can negatively affect cognitive function and also is related to subjective measures of cognitive functioning (Oh, 2017). In one longitudinal study of patients with breast cancer, a strong inverse relationship was found between fatigue and multiple cognitive domains over time (Lyon et al., 2016).

(d) Sleep disturbance has been found to be associated with perceived cognitive impairment ($p < 0.001$; Myers, Wick, & Klemp, 2015). In one study, more hours of sleep was associated with better performance on objective measures of verbal function ($p = 0.007$; Hartman, Marinac, Natarajan, & Patterson, 2015).

b) Risk factors related to cancer treatments

(1) Regimens: Because most patients receive multimodal therapy, it is difficult to determine if specific drugs or regimens promote higher incidences of cognitive changes.

(2) Dose intensity and cumulative effects: Cognitive changes in patients who receive cranial irradiation are related to the total dose received (Bohan, 2013). Exposure to higher doses of chemotherapy (or higher concentrations due to impaired clearance), as well as the additive or synergistic effects of multiagent regimens, also may increase risk (Wefel & Schagen, 2012). In addition, cumulative chemotherapy cycles have been reported as a predictor of cognitive decline (Oh, 2017).

(3) Concomitant medications such as analgesics, antidepressants, antiepileptics, anxiolytics, antipsychotics, immunosuppressants, and steroids also may contribute to cognitive deficits (Jansen, 2017).

5. Clinical manifestations: Although cognitive changes may be subtle, patients report difficulties with their ability to concentrate, think clearly, retain or learn new information, be efficient, organize and prioritize, manage responsibility, interact socially, and cope with problems (Kanaskie & Loeb, 2015; Myers, 2013).

6. Assessment: Patients who report cognitive problems should be screened for potentially reversible factors that may contribute to cognitive impairment (Allen et al., 2018; Jansen, 2013; National Comprehensive Cancer Network® [NCCN®], 2018; Roebuck-Spencer et al., 2017). Many neuropsychological tests are available to measure cognitive function but are generally used only in studies and require a referral to a neuropsychologist. Imaging (e.g., MRI, positron-emission tomography, EEG) has been used to study structural and electrophysiologic outcomes related to cognitive impairment, but these are generally not considered feasible for routine cognitive evaluation (Pomykala, de Ruiter, Deprez, McDonald, & Silverman, 2013). NCCN (2018) guidelines recommend using imaging only for ruling out structural abnormalities in high-risk patients or individuals with focal neurologic deficits.

a) Assess the patient for cognitive complaints (e.g., inability to focus on tasks or follow instructions; difficulties with concentration, memory, and word finding), including duration and intensity.

b) Assess for any focal neurologic deficits, and refer to physician for further workup (neuroimaging) as indicated.

c) Assess the patient's social history (e.g., living situation, lifestyle factors including alcohol or drug use, work history) and any potential influencing factors, such as anxiety, depression, emotional distress, pain, sleep disturbances, or fatigue. Manage any symptoms that may be contributing.

d) Review cancer and treatment history (e.g., tumor type, staging, treatments received, disease trajectory).

e) Review coexisting medical conditions (e.g., cardiovascular disease, diabetes, neurologic conditions, psychiatric illness) and menopausal status.

f) Review current medications (e.g., analgesics, antidepressants, antiemetics, antiepileptics, antipsychotics, immunosuppressants, steroids) and evaluate for new medications, supplements, or potential medication interactions, and adjust regimens as needed.

g) Monitor laboratory results to determine if the patient has anemia, metabolic abnormalities, or liver or renal dysfunction, and take appropriate action as indicated.

h) Consider referral for neuropsychological testing if indicated (Block, Johnson-Greene, Pliskin, & Boake, 2017).

7. Collaborative management: Currently, the only evidence-based recommendation for the prevention or treatment of cognitive impairment is cognitive training (Von Ah, 2015; Von Ah et al., 2014). Although the mechanisms of cancer treatment–related cognitive changes are still unclear, several pharmacologic and nonpharmacologic interventions have been studied. Many of these focus on preventing cognitive impairment by targeting the potential mechanisms discussed earlier. Further research is needed to determine potential interventions for patients experiencing cognitive impairments.

a) Nonpharmacologic interventions that have been studied

(1) Cognitive training that involves interventions aimed at improving, maintaining, or restoring attention, concentration, and memory through repeated and structured practice of tasks. This intervention is the most promising to improve cognitive functioning.

(2) Cognitive behavioral interventions that are focused on adaptive strategies to compensate for cognitive impairment require further research to determine their effectiveness.

(3) Exercise (e.g., aerobic, resistance training, mindfulness based) as an intervention for cognitive impairment has not been established to be effective.

(4) EEG/neurofeedback, which consists of real-time display of brain electrical activity, may have benefit for several symptoms but requires additional research to determine its effectiveness.

(5) Natural restorative environment intervention that involves the participant spending time in a natural environment has not been established to be effective.

(6) Vitamin E, a fat-soluble vitamin, has not shown effectiveness for treating cognitive impairment, but results are limited by small studies.

b) Pharmacologic interventions

(1) Psychostimulants (e.g., methylphenidate/dexmethylphenidate, modafinil): The role of psychostimulants as an intervention for cognitive impairment is an area of investigation with equivocal results and therefore lacks sufficient evidence (Von Ah, 2015; Von Ah et al., 2014). A trial use of psychostimulants may be considered (NCCN, 2018).

(2) Cholinesterase inhibitors (e.g., donepezil), antioxidants (e.g., ginkgo biloba, melatonin), memantine, and erythropoiesis-stimulating agents (e.g., erythropoietin) have also been studied, and effectiveness has not been established. Of note, current evidence suggests that ginkgo biloba is unlikely to be effective, and erythropoiesis-stimulating agents are not recommended for practice because of U.S. Food and Drug Administration warnings regarding risks associated with its use (Von Ah et al., 2014).

I. Patient and family education

1. Teach patients and caregivers the general signs and symptoms of neurotoxicity and provide written information describing both immediate and delayed effects for specific treatment agents. Provide information on how, when, and to whom signs and symptoms should be reported.

2. Teach patients and caregivers to recognize signs and symptoms that may indicate life-threatening toxicities (e.g., cerebrovascular events) and instruct them to immediately seek medical attention.
3. When neurotoxic effects manifest, orient patients and caregivers to the relevant safety issues and precautions.
   a) Seizures: Patients with a known seizure event or who are prophylactically treated for seizures should be instructed not to drive, operate heavy machinery, swim, take baths (showers only), or use heated appliances while alone (e.g., stoves, curling irons, barbecue grills). A medical alert bracelet or similar disclosure tool should be worn or carried at all times.
   b) Sensory neuropathy: Patients with loss of sensation in their extremities are at risk for thermal or ischemic injuries. Teach patients and caregivers to pay particular attention to hands and feet, including regular inspection of the feet, and emphasize the importance of wearing properly fitted shoes. Notably, patients without laboratory evidence of vitamin deficiencies should be instructed to avoid nutritional supplements because they may worsen the neuropathy (Tzatha & DeAngelis, 2016). Additionally, cold pain is a frequent symptom in neuropathic pain, manifesting as a pain response to a normally innocuous cold stimulus (cold allodynia) or heightened sensitivity to a painful cold stimulus (cold hyperalgesia). When these symptoms are present, patients should be taught to avoid exposure to cold environments and objects.
   c) Motor neuropathy: Patient counseling should focus on strategies to avoid falls and injury, especially when navigating changing surfaces, such as bare floor to carpet. Patients should consider walking shoes, which provide good traction and support, and should generally opt for shoes that tie versus those that slip on (e.g., flip-flops, sandals, slippers). Removing throw rugs, clearing walkways of clutter, and using skid strips on slippery surfaces (e.g., shower and tub floors) can help reduce the risk of falls. When possible, patients should be offered physical or occupational therapy to preserve function and limit further injury.
   d) Autonomic neuropathy: Teach strategies to manage symptoms of autonomic dysfunction (postural hypotension, constipation, and urinary retention), such as dangling the legs prior to standing, increasing oral intake, and adding dietary fiber or a formalized bowel regimen.
4. Cognitive impairment: Inform patients that cognitive changes are a possible side effect of treatment and that studies elucidating this phenomenon, its mechanisms, and subsequent interventions are ongoing.
   a) Acknowledge, validate, and record patient reports of cognitive changes.
   b) Encourage patients and family members to report cognitive problems.
   c) Acknowledge that although studies have been done for various interventions, there is limited evidence to make treatment recommendations.
   d) Encourage routine physical activity.
   e) Recommend optimizing management of anxiety, depression, fatigue, sleep disturbances, and other contributing symptoms (NCCN, 2018).
   f) Strategies reported by patients as helpful (Kanaskie & Loeb, 2015; Myers, 2013; Von Ah, 2015; Von Ah, Storey, Jansen, & Allen, 2013)
      (1) Healthy lifestyle practices
         (a) Ensure adequate sleep and rest.
         (b) Eat a well-balanced diet.
         (c) Engage in physical exercise.
      (2) Intellectual activities (e.g., reading, learning new skills, solving puzzles, working out math problems)
      (3) Social activities (e.g., support groups)
      (4) Practical management
         (a) Use technology (e.g., smartphones, voice recorders).
         (b) Keep a daily planner or calendar.
         (c) Keep things in the same place.
         (d) Write reminders and use notes.
         (e) Focus on one task at a time.
         (f) Develop a routine schedule.
      (5) Focus on the future.

References

Abbasi, A.W., Westerlaan, H.E., Holtman, G.A., Aden, K.M., van Laar, P.J., & van der Hoorn, A. (2017). Incidence of tumour progression and pseudoprogression in high-grade gliomas: A systematic review and meta-analysis. *Clinical Neuroradiology.* https://doi.org/10.1007/s00062-017-0584-x

Albers, J.W., Chaudhry, V., Cavaletti, G., & Donehower, R.C. (2014). Interventions for preventing neuropathy caused by cisplatin and related compounds. *Cochrane Database of Systematic Reviews, 2014*(3). https://doi.org/10.1002/14651858.CD005228.pub4

Allen, D.H., Myers, J.A., Jansen, C.E., Merriman, J.D., & Von Ah, D. (2018). Assessment and management of cancer- and cancer treatment-related cognitive impairment. *Journal for Nurse Practitioners, 14,* 217–224. https://doi.org/10-116

Arrillaga-Romany, I.C., & Dietrich, J. (2012). Imaging findings in cancer therapy-associated neurotoxicity. *Seminars in Neurology, 32,* 476–486. https://doi.org/10.1055/s-0032-1331817

Bakoyiannis, I., Tsigka, E.A., Perrea, D., & Pergialiotis, V. (2016). The impact of endocrine therapy on cognitive functions of breast cancer patients: A systematic review. *Clinical Drug Investigation, 36,* 109–118. https://doi.org/10.1007/s40261-015-0364-9

Barsevick, A.M., Irwin, M.R., Hinds, P., Miller, A., Berger, A., Jacobsen, P., ... Cella, D. (2013). Recommendations for high-priority research on cancer-related fatigue in children and adults. *Journal of the National Cancer Institute, 105,* 1432–1440. https://doi.org/10.1093/jnci/djt242

Bender, C.M., & Thelen, B.D. (2013). Cancer and cognitive changes: The complexity of the problem. *Seminars in Oncology Nursing, 29,* 232–237. https://doi.org/10.1016/j.soncn.2013.08.003

Bénit, C.P., & Vecht, C.J. (2016). Seizures and cancer: Drug interactions of anticonvulsants with chemotherapeutic agents, tyrosine kinase inhibitors and glucocorticoids. *Neuro-Oncology Practice, 3,* 245–260. https://doi.org/10.1093/nop/npv038

Block, C.K., Johnson-Greene, D., Pliskin, N., & Boake, C. (2017). Discriminating cognitive screening and cognitive testing from neuropsychological assessment: Implications for professional practice. *Clinical Neuropsychologist, 31,* 487–500. https://doi.org/10.1080/13854046.2016.1267803

Bohan, E.M. (2013). Cognitive changes associated with central nervous system malignancies and treatment. *Seminars in Oncology Nursing, 29,* 238–247. https://doi.org/10.1016/j.soncn.2013.08.004

Bohra, C., Sokol, L., & Dalia, S. (2017). Progressive multifocal leukoencephalopathy and monoclonal antibodies: A review. *Cancer Control, 24,* 1–9. https://doi.org/10.1177/1073274817729901

Boss, L., Kang, D.-H., Marcus, M., & Bergstrom, N. (2014). Endogenous sex hormones and cognitive function in older adults: A systematic review. *Western Journal of Nursing Research, 36,* 388–426. https://doi.org/10.1177/0193945913500566

Brewer, J.R., Morrison, G., Dolan, M.E., & Fleming, G.F. (2016). Chemotherapy-induced peripheral neuropathy: Current status and progress. *Gynecologic Oncology, 140,* 176–183. https://doi.org/10.1016/j.ygyno.2015.11.011

Cachia, D., Kamiya-Matsuoka, C., Pinnix, C.C., Chi, L., Kantarjian, H.M., Cortes, J.E., ... Woodman, K. (2015). Myelopathy following intrathecal chemotherapy in adults: A single institution experience. *Journal of Neuro-Oncology, 122,* 391–398. https://doi.org/10.1007/s11060-015-1727-z

Castel, H., Denouel, A., Lange, M., Tonon, M.-C., Dubois, M., & Joly, F. (2017). Biomarkers associated with cognitive impairment in treated cancer patients: Potential predisposition and risk factors. *Frontiers in Pharmacology, 8,* 138. https://doi.org/10.3389/fphar.2017.00138

Chae, Y.K., Wang, S., Nimeiri, H., Kalyan, A., & Giles, F.J. (2017). Pseudoprogression in microsatellite instability-high colorectal cancer during treatment with combination T cell mediated immunotherapy: A case report and literature review. *Oncotarget, 8,* 57889–57897. https://doi.org/10.18632/oncotarget.18361

Chao, S.T., Ahluwalia, M.S., Barnett, G.H., Stevens, G.H.J., Murphy, E.S., Stockham, A.L., ... Suh, J.H. (2013). Challenges with the diagnosis and treatment of cerebral radiation necrosis. *International Journal of Radiation Oncology, Biology, Physics, 87,* 449–457. https://doi.org/10.1016/j.ijrobp.2013.05.015

Cheung, Y.T., Ng, T., Shwe, M., Ho, H.K., Foo, K.M., Cham, M.T., ... Chan, A. (2015). Association of proinflammatory cytokines and chemotherapy-associated cognitive impairment in breast cancer patients: A multi-centered, prospective, cohort study. *Annals of Oncology, 26,* 1446–1451. https://doi.org/10.1093/annonc/mdv206

Chiou, V.L., & Burotto, M. (2015). Pseudoprogression and immune-related response in solid tumors. *Journal of Clinical Oncology, 33,* 3541–3543. https://doi.org/10.1200/JCO.2015.61.6870

Cidon, E.U., & Alonso, P. (2016). Oxaliplatin-induced ocular toxicities remain overlooked [Poster P-195]. *Annals of Oncology, 27*(Suppl. 2), ii57. https://doi.org/10.1093/annonc/mdw199.187

Cohen, J.V., Alomari, A.K., Vortmeyer, A.O., Jilaveanu, L.B., Goldberg, S.B., Mahajan, A., ... Kluger, H.M. (2016). Melanoma brain metastasis pseudoprogression after pembrolizumab treatment. *Cancer Immunology Research, 4,* 179–182. https://doi.org/10.1158/2326-6066.CIR-15-0160

Colaco, R.J., Martin, P., Kluger, H.M., Yu, J.B., & Chiang, V.L. (2016). Does immunotherapy increase the rate of radiation necrosis after radiosurgical treatment of brain metastases? *Journal of Neurosurgery, 125,* 17–23. https://doi.org/10.3171/2015.6.JNS142763

Conroy, S.K., McDonald, B.C., Ahles, T.A., West, J.D., & Saykin, A.J. (2013). Chemotherapy-induced amenorrhea: A prospective study of brain activation changes and neurocognitive correlates. *Brain Imaging and Behavior, 7,* 491–500. https://doi.org/10.1007/s11682-013-9240-5

Conroy, S.K., McDonald, B.C., Smith, D.J., Moser, L.R., West, J.D., Kamendulis, L.M., ... Saykin, A.J. (2013). Alterations in brain structure and function in breast cancer survivors: Effect of post-chemotherapy interval and relation to oxidative DNA damage. *Breast Cancer Research and Treatment, 137,* 493–502. https://doi.org/10.1007/s10549-012-2385-x

Correa, D.D., Satagopan, J., Baser, R.E., Cheung, K., Richards, E., Lin, M., ... Orlow, I. (2014). *APOE* polymorphisms and cognitive functions in patients with brain tumors. *Neurology, 83,* 320–327. https://doi.org/10.1212/WNL.0000000000000617

Cummings, M., Dougherty, D.W., Mohile, N.A., Walter, K.A., Usuki, K.Y., & Milano, M.T. (2016). Severe radiation-induced leukoencephalopathy: Case report and literature review. *Advances in Radiation Oncology, 1,* 17. https://doi.org/10.1016/j.adro.2016.01.002

Dasgupta, S., Adilieje, C., Bhattacharya, A., Smith, B., & Sheikh, M. (2010). Capecitabine and sixth cranial nerve palsy. *Journal of Cancer Research and Therapeutics, 6,* 80–81. https://doi.org/10.4103/0973-1482.63555

de Ruiter, M.B., & Schagen, S.B. (2013). Functional MRI studies in non-CNS cancers. *Brain Imaging and Behavior, 7,* 388–408. https://doi.org/10.1007/s11682-013-9249-9

Dietrich, J. (2010). Chemotherapy associated central nervous system damage. In R.B. Raffa & R.J. Tallarida (Eds.), *Chemo fog: Cancer chemotherapy-related cognitive impairment* (pp. 77–85). https://doi.org/10.1007/978-1-4419-6306-2_11

Dietrich, J., Prust, M., & Kaiser, J. (2015). Chemotherapy, cognitive impairment and hippocampal toxicity. *Neuroscience, 309,* 224–232. https://doi.org/10.1016/j.neuroscience.2015.06.016

Duijts, S.F.A., van der Beek, A.J., Boelhouwer, I.G., & Schagen, S.B. (2017). Cancer-related cognitive impairment and patients' ability to work: A current perspective. *Current Opinion in Supportive and Palliative Care, 11,* 19–23. https://doi.org/10.1097/SPC.0000000000000248

Edelstein, K., Richard, N.M., & Bernstein, L.J. (2017). Neurocognitive impact of cranial radiation in adults with cancer: An update of recent findings. *Current Opinion in Supportive and Palliative Care, 11,* 32–37. https://doi.org/10.1097/SPC.0000000000000255

Fernandez-Robles, C., Greenberg, D.B., & Pirl, W.F. (2016). Psycho-oncology: Psychiatric co-morbidities and complications of cancer and cancer treatment. In T.A. Stern, M. Fava, T.E.

Wilens, & J.F. Rosenbaum (Eds.), *Massachusetts General Hospital comprehensive clinical psychiatry* (2nd ed., pp. 618–626). New York, NY: Elsevier.

Filley, C.M. (2012). *The behavioral neurology of white matter* (2nd ed.). New York, NY: Oxford University Press.

Ganz, P.A., Bower, J.E., Kwan, L., Castellon, S.A., Silverman, D.H.S., Geist, C., … Cole, S.W. (2013). Does tumor necrosis factor-alpha (TNF-α) play a role in post-chemotherapy cerebral dysfunction? *Brain, Behavior, and Immunity, 30*(Suppl.), S99–S108. https://doi.org/10.1016/j.bbi.2012.07.015

Gazzaniga, M.S., Ivry, R.B., & Mangun, G.R. (2014). *Cognitive neuroscience: The biology of the mind* (4th ed.). New York, NY: Norton.

Gonzalez, B.D., Jim, H.S.L., Booth-Jones, M., Small, B.J., Sutton, S.K., Lin, H.Y., … Jacobsen, P.B. (2015). Course and predictors of cognitive function in patients with prostate cancer receiving androgen-deprivation therapy: A controlled comparison. *Journal of Clinical Oncology, 33,* 2021–2027. https://doi.org/10.1200/JCO.2014.60.1963

Greene-Schloesser, D., Moore, E., & Robbins, M.E. (2013). Molecular pathways: Radiation-induced cognitive impairment. *Clinical Cancer Research, 19,* 2294–2300. https://doi.org/10.1158/1078-0432.CCR-11-2903

Hartman, S.J., Marinac, C.R., Natarajan, L., & Patterson, R.E. (2015). Lifestyle factors associated with cognition functioning in breast cancer survivors. *Psycho-Oncology, 24,* 669–675. https://doi.org/10.1002/pon.3626

Henneghan, A. (2016). Modifiable factors and cognition dysfunction in breast cancer survivors: A mixed-method systematic review. *Supportive Care in Cancer, 24,* 481–497. https://doi.org/10.1007/s00520-015-2927-y

Hermelink, K., Bühner, M., Sckopke, P., Neufeld, F., Kaste, J., Voigt, V., … Harbeck, N. (2017). Chemotherapy and post-traumatic stress in the causation of cognitive dysfunction in breast cancer patients. *Journal of the National Cancer Institute, 109,* djx0457. https://doi.org/10.1093/jnci/djx057

Hoeffner, E.G. (2016). Central nervous system complications of oncologic therapy. *Hematology/Oncology Clinics of North America, 30,* 899–920. https://doi.org/10.1016/j.hoc.2016.03.010

Hogervorst, E. (2013). Effects of gonadal hormones on cognitive behaviour in elderly men and women. *Journal of Neuroendocrinology, 25,* 1182–1195. https://doi.org/10.1111/jne.12080

Holohan, K.N., Von Ah, D., McDonald, B.C., & Saykin, A.J. (2013). Neuroimaging, cancer, and cognition: State of the knowledge. *Seminars in Oncology Nursing, 29,* 280–287. https://doi.org/10.1016/j.soncn.2013.08.008

Jacob, L.A., Sreevatsa, A., Chinnagiriyappa, L.K., Dasappa, L., Suresh, T.M., & Babu, G. (2015). Methotrexate-induced chemical meningitis in patients with acute lymphoblastic leukemia/lymphoma. *Annals of Indian Academy of Neurology, 18,* 206–209. https://doi.org/10.4103/0972-2327.150586

Janelsins, M.C., Heckler, C.E., Peppone, L.J., Kamen, C., Mustian, K.M., Mohile, S.G., … Morrow, G.R. (2017). Cognitive complaints in survivors of breast cancer after chemotherapy compared with age-matched controls: An analysis from a nationwide, multicenter, prospective longitudinal study. *Journal of Clinical Oncology, 35,* 506–514. https://doi.org/10.1200/JCO.2016.68.5826

Janelsins, M.C., Kesler, S.R., Ahles, T.A., & Morrow, G.R. (2014). Prevalence, mechanisms, and management of cancer-related cognitive impairment. *International Review of Psychiatry, 26,* 102–113. https://doi.org/10.3109/09540261.2013.864260

Jansen, C.E. (2013). Cognitive changes associated with cancer and cancer therapy: Patient assessment and education. *Seminars in Oncology Nursing, 29,* 270–279. https://doi.org/10.1016/j.soncn.2013.08.007

Jansen, C. (2017). Cognitive changes. In J. Eggert (Ed.), *Cancer basics* (2nd ed., pp. 381–395). Pittsburgh, PA: Oncology Nursing Society.

Joly, F., Giffard, B., Rigal, O., De Ruiter, M.B., Small, B.J., Dubois, M., … Castel, H. (2015). Impact of cancer and its treatments on cognitive function: Advances in research from the Paris International Cognition and Cancer Task Force symposium and update since 2012. *Journal of Pain and Symptom Management,50,* 830–841. https://doi.org/10.1016/j.jpainsymman.2015.06.019

Kaiser, J., Bledowski, C., & Dietrich, J. (2014). Neural correlates of chemotherapy-related cognitive impairment. *Cortex, 54,* 33–50. https://doi.org/10.1016/j.cortex.2014.01.010

Kanaskie, M.L., & Loeb, S.J. (2015). The experience of cognitive change in women with breast cancer following chemotherapy. *Journal of Cancer Survivorship, 9,* 375–387. https://doi.org/10.1007/s11764-014-0387-x

Kesler, S.R. (2014). Default mode network as a potential biomarker of chemotherapy-related brain injury. *Neurobiology of Aging, 35*(Suppl. 2), S11–S19. https://doi.org/10.1016/j.neurobiolaging.2014.03.036

Kesler, S.R., & Blayney, D.W. (2016). Neurotoxic effects of anthracycline- vs nonanthracycline-based chemotherapy on cognition in breast cancer survivors. *JAMA Oncology, 2,* 185–192. https://doi.org/10.1001/jamaoncol.2015.4333

Kesler, S.R., Janselsins, M., Koovakkattu, D., Palesh, O., Mustian, K., Morrow, G., & Dhabhar, F.S. (2013). Reduced hippocampal volume and verbal memory performance associated with interleukein-6 and tumor necrosis factor-alpha levels in chemotherapy-treated breast cancer survivors. *Brain, Behavior, and Immunity, 30*(Suppl.), S109–S116. https://doi.org/10.1016/j.bbi.2012.05.017

Kim, J.M., Miller, J.A., Kotecha, R., Xiao, R., Juloori, A., Ward, M.C., … Chao, S.T. (2017). The risk of radiation necrosis following stereotactic radiosurgery with concurrent systemic therapies. *Journal of Neuro-Oncology, 133,* 357–368. https://doi.org/10.1007/s11060-017-2442-8

Koppelmans, V., de Groot, M., de Ruiter, M.B., Boogerd, W., Seynaeve, C., Vernooij, M.W., … Breteler, M.M. (2014). Global and focal white matter integrity in breast cancer survivors 20 years after adjuvant chemotherapy. *Human Brain Mapping, 35,* 889–899. https://doi.org/10.1002/hbm.22221

Lacourt, T.E., & Heijnen, C.J. (2017). Mechanisms of neurotoxic symptoms as a result of breast cancer and its treatment: Considerations on the contribution of stress, inflammation, and cellular bioenergetics. *Current Breast Cancer Reports, 9,* 70–81. https://doi.org/10.1007/s12609-017-0245-8

Lange, M., Giffard, B., Noal, S., Rigal, O., Kurtz, J.-E., Heutte, N., … Joly, F. (2014). Baseline cognitive functions among elderly patients with localised breast cancer. *European Journal of Cancer, 50,* 2181–2189. https://doi.org/10.1016/j.ejca.2014.05.026

Lee, D.W., Gardner, R., Porter, D.L., Louis, C.U., Ahmed, N., Jensen, M., … Mackall, C.L. (2014). Current concepts in the diagnosis and management of cytokine release syndrome. *Blood, 124,* 188–195. https://doi.org/10.1182/blood-2014-05-552729

Lee, E.L., & Westcarth, L. (2012). Neurotoxicity associated with cancer therapy. *Journal of the Advanced Practitioner in Oncology, 3,* 11–21.

Lee, P.E., Tierney, M.C., Wu, W., Pritchard, K.I., & Rochon, P.A. (2016). Endocrine treatment-associated cognitive impairment in breast cancer survivors: Evidence from published studies. *Breast Cancer Research and Treatment, 158,* 407–420. https://doi.org/10.1007/s10549-016-3906-9

Lezak, M.D., Howieson, D.B., Bigler, E.D., & Tranel, D. (2012). *Neuropsychological assessment* (5th ed.). New York, NY: Oxford University Press.

Lim, S.Y., Brooke, J., Dineen, R., & O'Donoghue, M. (2016). Stroke-like migraine attack after cranial radiation therapy: The SMART syndrome. *Practical Neurology, 16,* 406–408. https://doi.org/10.1136/practneurol-2016-001385

Lisberger, S.G., & Thach, W.T. (2013). The cerebellum. In E.R. Kandel, J.H. Schwartz, T.M. Jessell, S.A. Siegelbaum, & A.J. Hudspeth (Eds.), *Principles of neural science* (5th ed., pp. 960–981). New York, NY: McGraw-Hill Companies.

Lobo, R.A. (2014). Menopause and aging. In J.F. Strauss III & R.L. Barbieri (Eds.), *Yen and Jaffe's reproductive endocrinology* (7th ed., pp. 308–339.e8). https://doi.org/10.1016/B978-1-4557-2758-2.00015-9

Lyon, D.E., Cohen, R., Chen, H., Kelly, D.L., Starkweather, A., Ahn, H.-C., & Jackson-Cook, C.K. (2016). The relationship of cognitive performance to concurrent symptoms, cancer- and cancer-treatment-related variables in women with early-stage breast cancer: A 2-year longitudinal study. *Journal of Cancer Research and Clinical Oncology, 142,* 1461–1474. https://doi.org/10.1007/s00432-016-2163-y

Magge, R.S., & DeAngelis, L.M. (2015). The double-edged sword: Neurotoxicity of chemotherapy. *Blood Reviews, 29,* 93–100. https://doi.org/10.1016/j.blre.2014.09.012

Mandelblatt, J.S., Jacobsen, P.B., & Ahles, T. (2014). Cognitive effects of cancer systemic therapy: Implications for the care of older patients and survivors. *Journal of Clinical Oncology, 32,* 2617–2626. https://doi.org/10.1200/JCO.2014.55.1259

Mandelblatt, J.S., Stern, R.A., Luta, G., McGuckin, M., Clapp, J.D., Hurria, A., ... Ahles, T. (2014). Cognitive impairment in older patients with breast cancer before systemic therapy: Is there an interaction between cancer and comorbidity? *Journal of Clinical Oncology, 32,* 1909–1918. https://doi.org/10.1200/JCO.2013.54.2050

Mann, T.K., Dail, R.B., & Bailey, D.E., Jr. (2016). Cognitive and affective symptoms experienced by cancer patients receiving high-dose intravenous interleukin 2 therapy: An integrative literature review. *Cancer Nursing, 39,* 349–357. https://doi.org/10.1097/NCC.0000000000000317

Maritaz, C., Metz, C., Baba-Hamed, N., Jardin-Szucs, M., & Deplanque, G. (2016). Cetuximab-induced aseptic meningitis: Case report and review of a rare adverse event. *BMC Cancer, 16,* 384. https://doi.org/10.1186/s12885-016-2434-7

Mateos, M.-V., & San Miguel, J.F. (2012). Safety and efficacy of subcutaneous formulation of bortezomib versus the conventional intravenous formulation in multiple myeloma. *Therapeutic Advances in Hematology, 3,* 117–124. https://doi.org/10.1177/2040620711432020

McDonald, B.C., & Saykin, A.J. (2013). Alterations in brain structure related to breast cancer and its treatment: Chemotherapy and other considerations. *Brain Imaging and Behavior, 7,* 374–387. https://doi.org/10.1007/s11682-013-9256-x

McGinty, H.L., Phillips, K.M., Jim, H.S.L., Cessna, J.M., Asvat, Y., Cases, M.G., ... Jacobsen, P.B. (2014). Cognitive functioning in men receiving androgen deprivation therapy for prostate cancer: A systematic review and meta-analysis. *Supportive Care in Cancer, 22,* 2271–2280. https://doi.org/10.1007/s00520-014-2285-1

Meregalli, C. (2015). An overview of bortezomib-induced neurotoxicity. *Toxics, 3,* 294–303. https://doi.org/10.3390/toxics3030294

Merriman, J.D., Sereika, S.M., Brufsky, A.M., McAuliffe, P.F., McGuire, K.P., Myers, J.S., ... Bender, C.M. (2017). Trajectories of self-reported cognitive function in postmenopausal women during adjuvant systemic therapy for breast cancer. *Psycho-Oncology, 26,* 44–52. https://doi.org/10.1002/pon.4009

Merriman, J.D., Von Ah, D., Miaskowski, C., & Aouizerat, B.E. (2013). Proposed mechanisms for cancer- and treatment-related cognitive changes. *Seminars in Oncology Nursing, 29,* 260–269. https://doi.org/10.1016/j.soncn.2013.08.006

Miyatake, S.-I., Furuse, M., Kawabata, S., Maruyama, T., Kumabe, T., Kuroiwa, T., & Ono, K. (2013). Bevacizumab treatment of symptomatic pseudoprogression after boron neutron capture therapy for recurrent malignant gliomas. Report of 2 cases. *Neuro-Oncology, 15,* 650–655. https://doi.org/10.1093/neuonc/not020

Myers, J.S. (2013). Cancer- and chemotherapy-related cognitive changes: The patient experience. *Seminars in Oncology Nursing, 29,* 300–307. https://doi.org/10.1016/j.soncn.2013.08.010

Myers, J.S., Wick, J.A., & Klemp, J. (2015). Potential factors associated with perceived cognitive impairment in breast cancer survivors. *Supportive Care in Cancer, 23,* 3219–3228. https://doi.org/10.1007/s00520-015-2708-7

National Comprehensive Cancer Network. (2018). *NCCN Clinical Practice Guidelines in Oncology (NCCN Guidelines®): Survivorship* [v.3.2017]. Retrieved from https://www.nccn.org/professionals/physician_gls/pdf/survivorship.pdf

Ng, T., Teo, S.M., Yeo, H.L., Shwe, M., Gan, Y.X., Cheung, Y.T., ... Chan, A. (2016). Brain-derived neurotrophic factor genetic polymorphism (rs6265) is protective against chemotherapy-associated cognitive impairment in patients with early-stage breast cancer. *Neuro-Oncology, 18,* 244–251. https://doi.org/10.1093/neuonc/nov162

Oh, P.-J. (2017). Predictors of cognitive decline in people with cancer undergoing chemotherapy. *European Journal of Oncology Nursing, 27,* 53–59. https://doi.org/10.1016/j.ejon.2016.12.007

Olson, C.R., & Colby, C.L. (2013). The organization of cognition. In E.R. Kandel, J.H. Schwartz, T.M. Jessell, S.A. Siegelbaum, & A.J. Hudspeth (Eds.), *Principles of neural science* (5th ed., pp. 392–411). New York, NY: McGraw-Hill Companies.

Parihar, V.K., & Limoli, C.L. (2013). Cranial irradiation compromises neuronal architecture in the hippocampus. *Proceedings of the National Academy of Sciences of the United States of America, 110,* 12822–12827. https://doi.org/10.1073/pnas.1307301110

Patel, K.R., Chowdhary, M., Switchenko, J.M., Kudchadkar, R., Lawson, D.H., Cassidy, R.J., ... Khan, M.K. (2016). BRAF inhibitor and stereotactic radiosurgery is associated with an increased risk of radiation necrosis. *Melanoma Research, 26,* 387–394. https://doi.org/10.1097/CMR.0000000000000268

Patel, S.K., Wong, A.L., Wong, F.L., Breen, E.C., Hurria, A., Smith, M., ... Bhatia, S. (2015). Inflammatory biomarkers, comorbidity, and neurocognition in women with newly diagnosed breast cancer. *Journal of the National Cancer Institute, 107,* djv131. https://doi.org/10.1093/jnci/djv131

Pearl, P.L., & Emsellem, H.A. (2014). *Neuro-logic: A primer on localization.* New York, NY: Demos Medical Publishing.

Pomykala, K.L., de Ruiter, M.B., Deprez, S., McDonald, B.C., & Silverman, D.H.S. (2013). Integrating imaging findings in evaluating the post-chemotherapy brain. *Brain Imaging and Behavior, 7,* 436–452. https://doi.org/10.1007/s11682-013-9239-y

Pomykala, K.L., Ganz, P.A., Bower, J.E., Kwan, L., Castellon, S.A., Mallam, S., ... Silverman, D.H.S. (2013). The association between pro-inflammatory cytokines, regional cerebral metabolism, and cognitive complaints following adjuvant chemotherapy for breast cancer. *Brain Imaging and Behavior, 7,* 511–523. https://doi.org/10.1007/s11682-013-9243-2

Roebuck-Spencer, T.M., Glen, T., Puente, A.E., Denney, R.L., Ruff, R.M., Hostetter, G., & Bianchini, K.J. (2017). Cognitive screening tests versus comprehensive neuropsychological test batteries: A National Academy of Neuropsychology education paper. *Archives of Clinical Neuropsychology, 32,* 491–498. https://doi.org/10.1093/arclin/acx021

Rouse, M.H. (2016). *Neuroanatomy for speech language pathology and audiology*. Burlington, MA: Jones & Bartlett Learning.

Scherling, C.S., & Smith, A. (2013). Opening up the window into "chemobrain": A neuroimaging review. *Sensors, 13,* 3169–3203. https://doi.org/10.3390/s130303169

Schiff, D., Lee, E.Q., Nayak, L., Norden, A.D., Reardon, D.A., & Wen, P.Y. (2015). Medical management of brain tumors and the sequelae of treatment. *Neuro-Oncology, 17,* 488–504. https://doi.org/10.1093/neuonc/nou304

Seigers, R., Schagen, S.B., Van Tellingen, O., & Dietrich, J. (2013). Chemotherapy-related cognitive dysfunction: Current animal studies and future directions. *Brain Imaging and Behavior, 7,* 453–459. https://doi.org/10.1007/s11682-013-9250-3

Shibayama, O., Yoshiuchi, K., Inagaki, M., Matsuoka, Y., Yoshikawa, E., Sugawara, Y., … Uchitomi, Y. (2014). Association between adjuvant regional radiotherapy and cognitive function in breast cancer patients treated with conservation therapy. *Cancer Medicine, 3,* 702–709. https://doi.org/10.1002/cam4.174

Simó, M., Root, J.C., Vaquero, L., Ripollés, P., Jové, J., Ahles, T., … Rodríguez-Fornells, A. (2015). Cognitive and brain structural changes in a lung cancer population. *Journal of Thoracic Oncology, 10,* 38–45. https://doi.org/10.1097/JTO.0000000000000345

Smith, A.K., Conneely, K.N., Pace, T.W.W., Mister, D., Felger, J.C., Kilaru, V., … Torres, M.A. (2014). Epigenetic changes associated with inflammation in breast cancer patients treated with chemotherapy. *Brain, Behavior, and Immunity, 38,* 227–236. https://doi.org/10.1016/j.bbi.2014.02.010

Staff, N.P., Grisold, A., Grisold, W., & Windebank, A.J. (2017). Chemotherapy-induced peripheral neuropathy: A current review. *Annals of Neurology, 81,* 772–781. https://doi.org/10.1002/ana.24951

Stone, J.B., & DeAngelis, L.M. (2016). Cancer-treatment-induced neurotoxicity—Focus on newer treatments. *Nature Reviews Clinical Oncology, 13,* 92–105. https://doi.org/10.1038/nrclinonc.2015.152

Straub, J.M., New, J., Hamilton, C.D., Lominska, C., Shnayder, Y., & Thomas, S.M. (2015). Radiation-induced fibrosis: Mechanisms and implications for therapy. *Journal of Cancer Research and Clinical Oncology, 141,* 1985–1994. https://doi.org/10.1007/s00432-015-1974-6

Stubblefield, M.D. (2017). Clinical evaluation and management of radiation fibrosis syndrome. *Physical Medicine and Rehabilitation Clinics of North America, 28,* 89–100. https://doi.org/10.1016/j.pmr.2016.08.003

Taillibert, S., Le Rhun, E., & Chamberlain, M.C. (2016). Chemotherapy-related neurotoxicity. *Current Neurology and Neuroscience Reports, 16,* 81. https://doi.org/10.1007/s11910-016-0686-x

Truven Health Analytics. (2017). Bortezomib. In *Micromedex Solutions.* Retrieved from http://www.micromedexsolutions.com/micromedex2/librarian

Turtle, C.J., Hanafi, L.-A., Berger, C., Gooley, T.A., Cherian, S., Hudecek, M., … Maloney, D.G. (2016). CD19 CAR-T cells of defined $CD4^+$:$CD8^+$ composition in adult B cell ALL patients. *Journal of Clinical Investigation, 126,* 2123–2138. https://doi.org/10.1172/JCI85309

Tzatha, E., & DeAngelis, L.M. (2016). Chemotherapy-induced peripheral neuropathy. *Oncology, 30,* 240–244.

Vega, J.N., Dumas, J., & Newhouse, P.A. (2017). Cognitive effects of chemotherapy and cancer-related treatments in older adults. *American Journal of Geriatric Psychiatry, 25,* 1415–1426. https://doi.org/10.1016/j.jagp.2017.04.001

Velasco, R., & Bruna, J. (2015). Taxane-induced peripheral neurotoxicity. *Toxics, 3,* 152–169. https://doi.org/10.3390/toxics3020152

Von Ah, D. (2015). Cognitive changes associated with cancer and cancer treatment: State of the science. *Clinical Journal of Oncology Nursing, 19,* 47–56. https://doi.org/10.1188/15.CJON.19-01AP

Von Ah, D., Jansen, C.E., & Allen, D.H. (2014). Evidence-based interventions for cancer- and treatment-related cognitive impairment. *Clinical Journal of Oncology Nursing, 18*(Suppl. 6), 17–25. https://doi.org/10.1188/14.CJON.S3.17-25

Von Ah, D., Storey, S., Jansen, C.E., & Allen, D.H. (2013). Coping strategies and interventions for cognitive changes in patients with cancer. *Seminars in Oncology Nursing, 29,* 288–299. https://doi.org/10.1016/j.soncn.2013.08.009

Von Ah, D., Storey, S., Tallman, E., Nielsen, A., Johns, S.A., & Pressler, S.J. (2016). Cancer, cognitive impairment, and work-related outcomes: An integrative review. *Oncology Nursing Forum, 43,* 602–616. https://doi.org/10.1188/16.ONF.602-616

Wang, X.-M., Walitt, B., Saligan, L., Tiwari, A.F.Y., Cheung, C.W., & Zhang, Z.-J. (2015). Chemobrain: A critical review and causal hypothesis of link between cytokines and epigenetic reprogramming associated with chemotherapy. *Cytokine, 72,* 86–96. https://doi.org/10.1016/j.cyto.2014.12.006

Wardill, H.R., Mander, K.A., Van Sebille, Y.Z.A., Gibson, R.J., Logan, R.M., Bowen, J.M., & Sonis, S.T. (2016). Cytokine-mediated blood brain barrier disruption as a conduit for cancer/chemotherapy-associated neurotoxicity and cognitive dysfunction. *International Journal of Cancer, 139,* 2635–2645. https://doi.org/10.1002/ijc.30252

Wefel, J.S., Kesler, S.R., Noll, K.R., & Schagen, S.B. (2015). Clinical characteristics, pathophysiology, and management of non-central nervous system cancer-related cognitive impairment in adults. *CA: A Cancer Journal for Clinicians, 65,* 123–138. https://doi.org/10.3322/caac.21258

Wefel, J.S., Noll, K.R., & Scheurer, M.E. (2016). Neurocognitive functioning and genetic variation in patients with primary brain tumors. *Lancet Oncology, 17,* e97–e108. https://doi.org/10.1016/S1470-2045(15)00380-0

Wefel, J.S., & Schagen, S.B. (2012). Chemotherapy-related cognitive dysfunction. *Current Neurology and Neuroscience Reports, 12,* 267–275. https://doi.org/10.1007/s11910-012-0264-9

Westin, S.N., Sood, A.K., & Coleman, R.L. (2018). Targeted therapy and molecular genetics. In P.J. DiSaia, W.T. Creasman, R.S. Mannell, S. McMeekin, & D.G. Mutch (Eds.), *Clinical gynecologic oncology* (9th ed., pp. 470–492.e10). https://doi.org/10.1016/B978-0-323-40067-1.00018-8

Wick, W., Hertenstein, A., & Platten, M. (2016). Neurological sequelae of cancer immunotherapies and targeted therapies. *Lancet Oncology, 17,* e529–e541. https://doi.org/10.1016/S1470-2045(16)30571-X

Wu, L.M., & Amidi, A. (2017). Cognitive impairment following hormone therapy: Current opinion of research in breast and prostate cancer patients. *Current Opinion in Supportive and Palliative Care, 11,* 38–45. https://doi.org/10.1097/SPC.0000000000000251

Yust-Katz, S., & Gilbert, M.R. (2014). Neurologic complications. In J.E. Niederhuber, J.O. Armitage, J.H. Doroshow, M.B. Kastan, & J.E. Tepper (Eds.), *Abeloff's clinical oncology* (5th ed., pp. 822–844). Philadelphia, PA: Elsevier Saunders.

Zhu, Y., Tan, Y., Ou, R., Zhong, Q., Zheng, L., Du, Y., … Huang, J. (2016). Anti-CD19 chimeric antigen receptor-modified T cells for B-cell malignancies: A systematic review of efficacy and safety in clinical trials. *European Journal of Haematology, 96,* 389–396. https://doi.org/10.1111/ejh.12602

Zwart, W., Terra, H., Linn, S.C., & Schagen, S.B. (2015). Cognitive effects of endocrine therapy for breast cancer: Keep calm and carry on? *Nature Reviews Clinical Oncology, 12,* 597–606. https://doi.org/10.1038/nrclinonc.2015.124

CHAPTER 25

Ocular Toxicities

A. Overview: Patients may develop ocular toxicities as a result of cancer treatments, with the onset, presentation, and incidence varying by drug and dose. Nurses should be familiar with the signs and symptoms, assessment, and management of these potential complications, as well as with patient and family education.

B. Pathophysiology
   1. The causes of ocular toxicity are not fully understood and may include the following (see Table 25-1):
      a) Damage to the eye or eye structures related directly to treatment (e.g., distribution of cytotoxic drugs in tears, direct vascular injury during intracarotid administration, direct nerve injury from chemotherapy or radiation therapy, solubility characteristics of the drug and its ability to gain access through barriers such as the blood–ocular barrier) (DeAngelis, 2017; Palmer et al., 2008)
      b) A secondary process related to treatment (e.g., eye irritation caused from loss of eyelashes in the presence of neutropenia)
      c) A secondary process related to concurrent disease, such as diabetes or Graves disease leading to diplopia or ptosis (DeAngelis, 2017)
      d) Metastases to the eyes or central nervous system resulting in increased intracranial pressure
      e) Factors unrelated to cytotoxic therapy, such as head trauma or drug toxicity from narcotics or anticonvulsants leading to diplopia (DeAngelis, 2017)
      f) Checkpoint inhibitors: Checkpoint inhibitors are new immunologic agents that block inhibitory receptors of immune system elements, such as cytotoxic T-lymphocyte antigen-4, programmed cell death protein 1, and its ligand, leading to the activation of specific antitumor T-cell responses.
         (1) The mechanisms of immune-related adverse events (irAEs) have been hypothesized to involve a breakdown of peripheral tolerance and induction of organ-specific inflammatory processes.
         (2) Ophthalmic irAEs have been reported in less than 1% of patients (Antoun et al., 2016).
         (3) Examples of ophthalmic irAEs include iritis, uveitis, conjunctivitis, dry eyes, and blurred vision. These irAEs can be treated with topical nonsteroidal or steroidal therapy (Antoun et al., 2016; Zimmer et al., 2016).
      g) Epidermal growth factor receptor inhibitors (EGFRIs): Epidermal growth factor receptor (EGFR) is a normal part of epidermal cells. It is widely distributed on the eye surface in the conjunctival and corneal epithelium, as well as in the eyelid skin, lash follicles, tear glands, and sebaceous and sweat glands (Burtness et al., 2009; Hager & Seitz, 2014). Inhibiting EGFR can lead to damage to the epidermal cells found in the ocular region, which includes the eye and surrounding skin (Garibaldi & Adler, 2007).
         (1) Examples of EGFRI-induced effects are tear film dysfunction and unusual hyper- or hypopigmentation (Zhang, Basti, & Jampol, 2007). EGFRIs have led to dry eyes, inflammation of the lid margin (blepharitis), dysfunction of the sebaceous glands of the eyelid (meibomitis), corneal erosion, and inversion or eversion of the eyelid margin (Burtness et al., 2009).
         (2) EGFR also has a crucial role in the regulation of the hair growth cycle.
            (a) An EGFRI can hinder this cycle, leading to loss of eyelashes and eyebrows (Robert et al., 2005; Zhang et al., 2007) or an accelerated growth and curling of the eyelashes, leading to tortuous eyelashes or eyelash

Table 25-1. Ocular Toxicities and Their Treatments		
Toxicity	**Definition/Symptoms**	**Treatment**
Blepharitis	Inflammation of the eyelids, mainly at the margin; main signs are redness and flaking of the skin on the eyelids and crusting that is worse on waking.	Use warm compress, eyelid hygiene, and corticosteroids or anti-inflammatory medications.
Blurred vision	Decreased clarity or sharpness in vision	Refer to ophthalmologist; discontinue agent.
Central serous retinopathy	Localized serous retinal detachment observable only on fundoscopy; manifests as slightly blurry vision and the perception of objects smaller than they really are (micropsia)	–
Conjunctivitis	Inflammation and redness of the conjunctiva	Hold agent; use corticosteroids or anti-inflammatory medications and artificial tears.
Corneal edema	Swelling of the cornea	Refer to ophthalmologist.
Corneal epithelial defect	Significant eye pain, sensitivity to light	Refer to ophthalmologist.
Cystoid macular edema	Chronic inflammation of the macular area only observable on fundoscopy and confirmed by fluorescein angiography	Refer to ophthalmologist; hold agent.
Diplopia	Double vision	Refer to ophthalmologist and neurologist.
Dysfunctional tear syndrome (tear film changes)	Fluctuating or mild decrease in vision, transient eye pain, burning or foreign body sensation in the eye, eye fatigue	Mild symptoms: Apply supplemental tears 4–6 times a day. Severe symptoms or no relief: Refer to ophthalmologist (treatment may consist of punctal plugs and/or anti-inflammatory medications).
Epiphora	Excessive tear production, usually caused by eye irritation	Refer to ophthalmologist; use topical lubricants.
Hemianopia	Visual field defect that respects the vertical midline in both eyes; can be homonymous or bitemporal	–
Iridocyclitis	Sensitivity to light, sustained eye pain, decrease in vision	Refer to ophthalmologist. Treatment involves use of anti-inflammatory medications.
Keratitis	Inflammation of the cornea, usually referring to the corneal surface (epithelium); manifests as pain, photophobia, and increased lacrimation; more evident in slit-lamp examination with the aid of a dye	Refer to ophthalmologist; use topical lubricants.
Lacrimal duct stenosis	Narrowing of the tear duct	Refer to ophthalmologist; hold agent.
Maculopathy	Disease or damage to the central part of the retina or macula	Refer to ophthalmologist; discontinue agent.
Meibomitis (meibomian gland dysfunction)	Fluctuations in vision (varying degrees), burning sensation in the eye, some mucous discharge, eye redness (may occur only on awakening)	Clean eyelid and apply warm compresses to the eyelid for at least 4 minutes twice daily. Use artificial lubricants. If lid scrubs and warm compresses are ineffective, consider topical or oral antibiotics.
Optic neuritis	Inflammation of the optic nerve	Refer to ophthalmologist and neurologist; discontinue agent.

(Continued on next page)

Table 25-1. Ocular Toxicities and Their Treatments *(Continued)*

Toxicity	Definition/Symptoms	Treatment
Papilledema	Optic disc swelling caused by increased intracranial pressure	Use corticosteroids or anti-inflammatory medications; discontinue agent.
Periorbital edema	Inflammation and increased fluid accumulation of the interstitial tissues from the eyelid into the orbital septum; manifests as a hard swelling of the eyelid	Apply warm compress; refer to ophthalmologist; discontinue agent.
Periorbital rash	Discoloration of the tissue around the eye	Use corticosteroids or anti-inflammatory medications, warm compress, and eyelid hygiene.
Photopsia/photophobia	Ocular pain and sensitivity to light	Use topical lubricants; avoid light exposure.
Ptosis	Drooping or falling of the upper eyelid over the eye; also known as "drooping eyes"	Refer to ophthalmologist and neurologist.
Retinal vein occlusion	Blockage of the small veins that carry blood away from the retina	Refer to ophthalmologist; discontinue agent.
Retinopathy	Damage to the retina caused by abnormal blood flow	Refer to ophthalmologist and neurologist; discontinue agent.
Squamous blepharitis (i.e., eyelid skin changes)	Hyperemia, papulopustular rash, crusting; eyelids become sore and irritated, with discomfort described as severe. Eyelid margins may have mild redness to significant edema and soreness of the eyelid margin. Small pustules at the base of the eyelashes may be seen.	Acute reactions: Apply warm compresses with a moist washcloth; ensure regular cleaning of the eyelid; use artificial lubricant. Apply fluorometholone (0.1%) ointment to eyelid (both skin and lid margin) for 1 week. Do not use for > 2 weeks. An ophthalmologist must examine patient within 4 weeks. Chronic reactions: Apply tacrolimus 0.03% ointment or pimecrolimus cream twice daily to skin of eyelid only. If treatment is minimally effective or not effective at all, try tacrolimus 0.1%. This treatment should not be used for > 6 months.
Trichomegaly	Pathologically long eyelashes that can get misdirected and cause ocular surface abrasions	Refer to ophthalmologist; trim long or misdirected eyelashes.
Uveitis	Inflammation of the uveal tract; can be anterior (involving the anterior chamber and iris) or posterior (involving the vitreous and choroid)	Refer to ophthalmologist.

Note. Based on information from Agustoni et al., 2014; Basti, 2007; Burtness et al., 2009; International Workshop on Meibomian Gland Dysfunction, 2011; Ouwerkerk & Boers-Doets, 2010.

trichomegaly (Hager & Seitz, 2014; Robert et al., 2005).

(b) Most ocular side effects are not vision threatening but should be followed by an ophthalmologist to quickly treat the discomfort and prevent ocular injury (Burtness et al., 2009).

2. A broad spectrum of disorders have been documented, including the inflammatory conditions uveitis, conjunctivitis, keratitis, blepharitis, iritis, and the development of retinal opacities, cataract formation, lid and lacrimation disorders, optic neuritis, and other neurologic injuries (F.T. Fraunfelder, Fraunfelder, & Chambers, 2008). For site-specific disorders, see Table 25-2.
3. With frequent use of combination therapy, it may be difficult to determine which specific drug is causing complications (F.T. Fraunfelder et al., 2008).
4. Patients may experience toxicity-related visual impairment during chemotherapy and up to two weeks after chemotherapy (Kende, Sirkin, Thomas, & Freeman, 1979). Neurologic damage to the eye has occurred up to 43 days following chemotherapy (Warrell & Berman, 1986).
5. The toxic effect of certain drugs may be cumulative and dose dependent (Palmer et al., 2008).

Table 25-2. Specific Ocular Toxicities by Anatomic Site

Site	Ocular Toxicity
Orbit	Arteriovenous shunts, cavernous sinus syndrome, edema, exophthalmos, pallor, pain
Lids	Cicatricial ectropion, ankyloblepharon, increased lid necrosis after cryotherapy, hyperpigmentation
Lacrimal drainage	Tear duct fibrosis and punctal occlusion
Lacrimal gland	Keratoconjunctivitis sicca
Conjunctiva	Conjunctivitis
Sclera	Discoloration
Cornea	Keratopathy, keratitis
Pupil	Pinpoint pupils, internal ophthalmoplegia
Uvea	Uveitis
Trabecular meshwork and/or ciliary body	Increased intraocular pressure
Lens	Cataract
Retina	Toxic retinopathy
Vitreous	Opacification
Optic nerve	Disc edema, optic neuritis, optic atrophy
Cranial nerves III, IV, V, VI	Ptosis, paresis with or without diplopia, corneal hypesthesia
Extraocular muscles	Fibrosis
Central nervous system	Cortical blindness, internuclear ophthalmoplegia, blepharospasm

Note. Based on information from Palmer et al., 2008.

6. Ocular changes may go unnoticed until damage is irreversible.
7. Ocular signs and symptoms may precede the development of peripheral neuropathies and thus may be an important marker of neurologic status (Bobba & Klein, 2012).
8. The presence of ocular signs or symptoms may predict the development of graft-versus-host disease in patients who have received an allogeneic hematopoietic stem cell transplant (Kim et al., 2002).
9. Ocular changes may be incorrectly attributed to the aging process.

C. Incidence
   1. Incidence varies according to drug classification, dose, and route of administration (see Table 25-3).
   2. Ophthalmologic effects of chemotherapy occur less frequently and tend to be less severe than other chemotherapy-related side effects. Most ocular side effects tend to improve or even resolve completely upon discontinuation of the drug. Early detection often minimizes sequelae (Teitelbaum, 2011).

D. Risk factors: Causal relationships between agents and ocular toxicities are difficult to establish. Risk factors are equally difficult to establish.

E. Clinical manifestations: See Table 25-3.

F. Assessment: Ask patients about a history of any eye disturbance. In addition, assess the following (Bickley, 2017):
   1. Visual acuity: Use a Snellen eye chart if possible. Position the patient 20 feet from the chart. Have the patient wear glasses or contacts for the examination if the corrective lenses are normally used other than for reading. Ask the patient to cover one eye with a card and to read the smallest line possible. Have the patient repeat with the other eye. Acuity can be assessed using a near-vision card held at arm's length; patients who wear glasses or contact lenses should remove them. Record any visual disturbances.
   2. Visual fields: Sit or stand in front of the patient and have the patient look with both eyes into your eyes. While the patient gazes into your eyes, place your hands two feet apart, lateral to the patient's ears. Instruct the patient to point to your fingers as soon as they are seen. Slowly move your fingers along an imaginary bowl and toward the line of gaze until the patient identifies them. Repeat this pattern in upper and lower temporal quadrants.
   3. Position of eyes, eyebrows, and eyelids: While standing or sitting in front of the patient, observe the eyes for position and alignment with each other. Inspect the eyebrows, noting their quantity and distribution and any flaking of the underlying skin. Survey the eyelids, observing and palpating for signs of erythema and edema. Assess for signs of exudates, crusting, and presence of ptosis. Observe condition of lashes.
   4. Lacrimation: Note dryness, foreign body sensation, excessive tearing, or swelling of the lacrimal sac.

Table 25-3. Ocular Toxicities of Antineoplastic Agents			
Classification	**Drug**	**Side Effects**	**Nursing Considerations**
Chemotherapy Agents			
Alkylating agents	Busulfan (intravenous [IV]: Busulfex®; oral: Myleran®)	Long-standing reports of cataract formation and blurred vision ; rare cases of keratoconjunctivitis sicca (Bobba & Klein, 2012; Palmer et al., 2008; Singh & Singh, 2012)	Toxic effects are believed to act on proliferating lens epithelial cells. (Bobba & Klein, 2012)
	Carboplatin	IV: Rare cases of blurred vision, eye pain; reports of maculopathy and optic neuropathy with transient cortical blindness when given to patients with renal dysfunction Intracarotid: Reports of severe ocular and orbital toxicity in ipsilateral eye following intracarotid injection (Al-Tweigeri et al., 1996; Singh & Singh, 2012; W. Watanabe et al., 2002)	–
	Chlorambucil (Leukeran®)	Keratitis, diplopia, bilateral papilledema, retinal hemorrhages; oculomotor disturbance, disc edema, retinopathy (Bobba & Klein, 2012; Palmer et al., 2008)	Ocular toxicity is rare. (Bobba & Klein, 2012)
	Cisplatin	IV: Blurred vision, altered color perception, papilledema, decreased visual acuity, retrobulbar neuritis, transient cortical blindness, disc edema, retinopathy, electroretinogram abnormalities, cavernous sinus syndrome, color blindness Intracarotid: Ipsilateral visual loss (15%–60%) from retinal or optic nerve ischemia, possibly prevented by infusion distal to ophthalmic artery; optic neuropathy, unilateral vision loss; retinal pigment disturbances, altered color perception, cotton wool spots, intraretinal hemorrhages (Bobba & Klein, 2012; Kwan et al., 2006; Palmer et al., 2008)	Ocular toxicity has generally been reported after the use of regimens with higher doses or greater dose frequency than those recommended by the manufacturer. Improvement or total recovery usually occurs after discontinuation of cisplatin. (Agustoni et al., 2014)
	Cyclophosphamide	Blurred vision (reversible), keratoconjunctivitis sicca, pinpoint pupils (Palmer et al., 2008; Singh & Singh, 2012)	–
	Ifosfamide (Ifex®)	IV: Blurred vision (reversible), conjunctivitis (Bobba & Klein, 2012; Singh & Singh, 2012)	–
	Mechlorethamine (nitrogen mustard; Mustargen®, Valchlor®)	Intracarotid: Rare reports of ipsilateral necrotizing uveitis and necrotizing vasculitis of choroids (Bobba & Klein, 2012)	No reports exist of ocular toxicity with IV administration. (Bobba & Klein, 2012)
	Oxaliplatin (Eloxatin®)	Mild changes: Dry eyes, excessive tearing, severe ocular irritation, conjunctivitis, abnormal lacrimation Severe changes: Retinal damages, visual field cuts (Mesquida et al., 2010; Oncology.TV, 2011; Singh & Singh, 2012)	Look for patients complaining of blurred vision, visual loss, tunnel vision, or altered color vision. Most changes are transient and reversible once treatment is stopped. (Mesquida et al., 2010)
Antimetabolites	Capecitabine (Xeloda®)	Ocular irritation, decreased vision, corneal deposits (Singh & Singh, 2012; Walkhom et al., 2000)	–

(Continued on next page)

Table 25-3. Ocular Toxicities of Antineoplastic Agents *(Continued)*			
Classification	**Drug**	**Side Effects**	**Nursing Considerations**
Chemotherapy Agents *(Cont.)*			
Antimetabolites *(cont.)*	Cytarabine	IV: Keratitis and conjunctivitis most common; blurred vision with evidence of bilateral conjunctival hyperemia, ocular pain, photophobia, and foreign body sensation at high doses; case reports of corneal toxicity with low dose of cytarabine Intrathecal: Optic neuropathy leading to severe visual loss (may be potentiated by cranial radiation therapy) (Bobba & Klein, 2012; Haddadin & Perry, 2012; Hopen et al., 1981; Lochhead et al., 2003)	Hydrocortisone or dexamethasone eye drops may prevent keratitis. It is recommended to start eye drops the evening before therapy begins. (Cleri & Haywood, 2002)
	5-Fluorouracil (5-FU; Adrucil®)	Conjunctivitis, excessive lacrimation; tear duct fibrosis; blepharitis. Other ocular toxicities include keratoconjunctivitis, cicatricial ectropion, ankyloblepharon, blepharospasm, punctal occlusion, oculomotor disturbances, blurred vision, photophobia, nystagmus, increased lid necrosis after cryotherapy, ocular pain, circumorbital edemas, dry eyes, and excessive tearing (F.T. Fraunfelder et al., 2008; Haidak et al., 1978; Jansman et al., 2001; Oncology.TV, 2011; Palmer et al., 2008; Singh & Singh, 2012)	Loprinzi et al. (1994) studied the use of ice packs to decrease ocular irritation; effectiveness was also reinforced in a North Central Cancer Treatment Group clinical trial (ice applied for 30 minutes, starting 5 minutes before infusion). The use of dexamethasone eye drops decreased ocular toxicities. (Jansman et al., 2001)
	Fludarabine	Decreased visual acuity (most common presenting sign before development of progressive encephalopathy); rare cases of diplopia, photophobia, and optic neuritis (Palmer et al., 2008; Singh & Singh, 2012)	Effects are dose dependent. (Bobba & Klein, 2012)
	Gemcitabine (Gemzar®)	Retinopathy (Agustoni et al., 2014)	–
	Methotrexate	IV: Blepharitis, conjunctival hyperemia, increased lacrimation, periorbital edema, photophobia, optic pain Intrathecal: With concurrent radiation, case reports of bilateral ophthalmoplegia with exotropia; optic nerve atrophy Intra-arterial: Retinal changes in ipsilateral eye (Bobba & Klein, 2012; F.T. Fraunfelder et al., 2008; Palmer et al., 2008; Singh & Singh, 2012)	Up to 25% of patients may develop ocular toxicity. Toxicity is more common with higher doses. Drug is found in tears. (Bobba & Klein, 2012; F.T. Fraunfelder et al., 2008; Palmer et al., 2008; Singh & Singh, 2012)
	Pemetrexed (Alimta®)	Conjunctivitis—generally associated with hyperemia, irritation, and serous secretions (Agustoni et al., 2014)	Treatment usually involves use of artificial tears, withdrawal of the agent, and short course of topical steroids. Treatment is usually curative. (Agustoni et al., 2014)
	Pentostatin (Nipent™)	Conjunctivitis, photophobia, diplopia; abnormal vision, amblyopia, conjunctivitis, dry eye, problems with lacrimation, photophobia, retinopathy, watery eyes (Haddadin & Perry, 2012; Singh & Singh, 2012)	–
Antitumor antibiotics	Doxorubicin (Adriamycin®)	Conjunctivitis, increased lacrimation; increased lacrimation in up to 25% of patients receiving doxorubicin (Bobba & Klein, 2012; Singh & Singh, 2012)	Serious ocular side effects are rare. (Bobba & Klein, 2012)

(Continued on next page)

Table 25-3. Ocular Toxicities of Antineoplastic Agents *(Continued)*

Classification	Drug	Side Effects	Nursing Considerations
Chemotherapy Agents *(Cont.)*			
Antitumor antibiotics *(cont.)*	Mitomycin (Mutamycin®)	IV: Blurred vision Topical: Keratoconjunctivitis (Bobba & Klein, 2012; Palmer et al., 2008; Singh & Singh, 2012)	Other than blurred vision, keratoconjunctivitis was reported after topical use in ophthalmologic surgeries. (Bobba & Klein, 2012; Singh & Singh, 2012)
	Mitoxantrone	Conjunctivitis, discoloration of sclera (Karch, 2014)	Drug is secreted in tears.
Epipodophyllotoxins	Etoposide (Toposar™); Etoposide phosphate (Etopophos®)	Intracarotid: Optic neuritis, transient cortical blindness (Lauer et al., 1999)	Effects occur when etoposide is given in combination with carboplatin. (Lauer et al., 1999)
Nitrosoureas	Carmustine (BiCNU®); Lomustine (Gleostine®)	Optic neuritis and atrophy, hyperemia, orbital pain, retinopathy, corneal opacities and edema, orbital IV shunts, secondary glaucoma, internal ophthalmoplegia, blurred vision, vitreous opacification, extraocular muscle fibrosis, diplopia IV: Rare reports of delayed blurred vision and loss of depth perception Intracarotid: Severe, ipsilateral occurrences including arterial narrowing, disc edema, and intraretinal hemorrhages (Bobba & Klein, 2012; Palmer et al., 2008; Singh & Singh, 2012)	–
Miscellaneous	Mitotane (Lysodren®)	Visual blurring, diplopia, lens opacity, toxic retinopathy (Bristol-Myers Squibb Co., 2017; Palmer et al., 2008)	Ocular side effects are infrequent. (Bristol-Myers Squibb Co., 2017)
	Procarbazine (Matulane®)	Retinal hemorrhage, papilledema, photophobia, diplopia, inability to focus (Sigma-Tau Pharmaceuticals, Inc., 2008)	Ophthalmic side effects are rare. (Cleri & Haywood, 2002)
Taxanes	Docetaxel (Taxotere®)	Epiphora, canalicular stenosis, nasolacrimal duct obstruction; conjunctivitis, punctal stenosis; optic neuropathy (Agustoni et al., 2014; Esmaeli, Valero, et al., 2001; Moloney et al., 2014; Singh & Singh, 2012)	Drug is secreted in tears. Successful treatment is achieved with bicanalicular silicone intubation. Optic neuropathy is treated with steroids. (Ahmadi & Esmaeli, 2001; Esmaeli et al., 2002; Moloney et al., 2014)
	Paclitaxel (Taxol®)	Scintillating scotomas or "shooting lights" in 20% of cases, which resolved spontaneously; transient scintillating scotoma, visual impairment, photopsia, possible ischemic optic neuropathy; bilateral cystoid macular edema, retinal capillary leakage, intracellular fluid accumulation, glaucoma; dry eye, keratitis (Agustoni et al., 2014; Bobba & Klein, 2012; Rao & Choudhry, 2016; Singh & Singh, 2012)	Scotomas usually occur toward the end of the 3-hour infusion. Photopsia usually appears during the last 30 minutes of the infusion and resolves within 3 hours. Toxicities are treated by stopping the agent and using topical carbonic anhydrase agents and injection of anti–vascular endothelial growth factor antibodies. (Agustoni et al., 2014; Bobba & Klein, 2012; Rao & Choudhry, 2016)

(Continued on next page)

Table 25-3. Ocular Toxicities of Antineoplastic Agents *(Continued)*			
Classification	**Drug**	**Side Effects**	**Nursing Considerations**
Chemotherapy Agents *(Cont.)*			
Vinca alkaloids	Vinblastine (Velban®)	Extraocular muscle palsies; cranial nerve palsies, optic neuropathy, optic atrophy, cortical blindness, night blindness (F.W. Fraunfelder & Fraunfelder, 2004; Singh & Singh, 2012)	–
	Vincristine (Marqibo®)	Cranial nerve palsies, optic neuropathy, optic atrophy, case reports of transient cortical blindness, night blindness (Bobba & Klein, 2012; Palmer et al., 2008; Singh & Singh, 2012)	Effects usually are reversible after discontinuation of vincristine. (Bobba & Klein, 2012)
Hormone Therapy Agents			
Aromatase inhibitors	Anastrozole (Arimidex®); exemestane (Aromasin®); letrozole (Femara®)	Visual disturbances, retinal hemorrhages, hemiretinal artery occlusion, vitreoretinal traction, corneal epithelial cysts, dry eye, impact on retinal and optic nerve function (Chatziralli et al., 2016)	–
	Tamoxifen (Nolvadex®)	Cataracts and decreased color vision; increased risk with doses > 20 mg/day; retinal toxicity (small refractile or crystalline dot-like yellowish deposits in the area surrounding the macula, in the nerve, and in plexiform layers); corneal opacities, retinopathy (Bommireddy & Carrim, 2016; Gianni et al., 2006; Palmer et al., 2008; Singh & Singh, 2012; Tsai et al., 2003)	A baseline ophthalmic examination is recommended within the first year. Visual acuity along with macular edema may improve with tamoxifen withdrawal, but retinal deposits often do not. Small doses of tamoxifen (20–40 mg/day) can cause ocular side effects. The incidence rises with increasing total cumulative dose and duration of treatment. (Bommireddy & Carrim, 2016 Gianni et al., 2006; Gorin et al., 1998)
Immunotherapy Agents			
Checkpoint inhibitors: CTLA-4	Ipilimumab (Yervoy®)	Uveitis, iritis, papillitis; rare (< 1%) conjunctivitis, scleritis, episcleritis, blepharitis, and temporal arteritis; tearing, diplopia, orbital inflammation, keratitis, dry eyes, blurred vision (Huillard et al., 2014; Papavasileiou et al., 2016; Renouf et al., 2012; Zimmer et al., 2016)	Uveitis, iritis, and papillitis were successfully treated with topical corticosteroid drops. Treatment consisted of stopping the agent and initiating adjunctive systemic and/or topical corticosteroids. (Cunningham et al., 2016; Renouf et al., 2012; Zimmer et al., 2016)
Cytokines: Interferons	Interferon (IFN) alfa, IFN beta, and IFN gamma	Retinopathy, primarily retinal hemorrhages; cotton wool spots; disc edema Vision changes, nonspecific conjunctivitis, and ocular pain are the most frequently reported ocular side effects. (Esmaeli, Koller, et al., 2001; Palmer et al., 2008; Teitelbaum, 2011; Willson, 2004)	Risk is increased in patients with hypertension or diabetes and those receiving higher doses. Effects may occur as soon as 15 minutes after initial exposure or take many months to be apparent. Less than 1% of patients receiving IFN develop ocular toxicities. (Teitelbaum, 2011)

(Continued on next page)

Table 25-3. Ocular Toxicities of Antineoplastic Agents *(Continued)*

Classification	Drug	Side Effects	Nursing Considerations
Immunotherapy Agents *(Cont.)*			
Cytokines: Interleukins	Interleukin-2	Neuro-ophthalmic effects including scotoma, diplopia, transient blindness, and visual hallucinations (Teitelbaum, 2011)	–
Miscellaneous	Retinoid	Blepharoconjunctivitis, corneal opacities, papilledema, pseudotumor cerebri, night blindness (Al-Tweigeri et al., 1996)	Avoid concurrent use of tetracyclines and drugs causing intracranial hypertension. (F.T. Fraunfelder et al., 2008)
Monoclonal antibodies: Chimeric	Cetuximab (Erbitux®)	Blurred vision, eye pain, visual field cuts; blepharitis; eyelid dermatitis, conjunctivitis, poliosis (whitening of the eyelashes), corneal erosions, punctate keratitis Relatively common: Loss of eyelashes/eyebrows (madarosis) and/or cicatricial ectropion, loss of color of the skin around the eye with weekly infusions; trichomegaly Very rare: Bilateral ocular discomfort with itchiness around both eyelids, foreign body sensation, tearing associated with exfoliated skin, oil secretions, crusty scaling (Basti, 2007; Garibaldi & Adler, 2007; Huillard et al., 2014; Liu & Kurzrock, 2015; Oncology.TV, 2011; Ramírez-Soria et al., 2008; Renouf et al., 2012; Robert et al., 2005; Tonini et al., 2005)	Ocular side effects occurred in < 20% of patients and resolved after treatment was discontinued. Blepharitis was treated with oxytetracycline cream three times a day for 20 days. Madarosis and cicatricial ectropion resolved after discontinuation of cetuximab. Ocular discomfort cleared up with topical antibiotics and holding therapy. Many researchers recommend an ophthalmologist referral for patients experiencing trichomegaly if eye irritations occur and eyelashes may be carefully and safely trimmed. However, Basti (2007) advises patients to not cut their lashes or have them cut. Waxing or electrolysis may be recommended. (Basti, 2007; Braiteh et al., 2008; Eaby et al., 2008; Esper et al., 2007; Garibaldi & Adler, 2007; Oncology.TV, 2011; Ramírez-Soria et al., 2008; Segaert & Van Cutsem, 2005; Tonini et al., 2005)
	Rituximab (Rituxan®)	Conjunctivitis, transient ocular edema, burning sensation, transient visual changes or permanent and severe loss of visual acuity (Singh & Singh, 2012)	–
Monoclonal antibodies: Human	Panitumumab (Vectibix®)	Keratitis and ulcerative keratitis, conjunctivitis, ocular hyperemia, increased lacrimation, eye/eyelid irritation, growth of eyelashes (Amgen Inc., 2017; Cunningham et al., 2016; Huillard et al., 2014; Liu & Kurzrock, 2015; Oncology.TV, 2011; Singh & Singh, 2012)	Onset of ocular symptoms is 14–15 days after first dose of panitumumab. Symptoms resolve after panitumumab is stopped. Median time of resolution is 84 days. (Amgen Inc., 2017)
Monoclonal antibodies: Humanized	Bevacizumab (Avastin®)	Lacrimation disorder, eye disorder, blurred vision; glaucoma (Eadie et al., 2017; Huillard et al., 2014)	The risk of glaucoma and having glaucoma surgery was greatly increased when patients received 7 or more injections. (Eadie et al., 2017)

(Continued on next page)

Table 25-3. Ocular Toxicities of Antineoplastic Agents *(Continued)*

Classification	Drug	Side Effects	Nursing Considerations
Immunotherapy Agents *(Cont.)*			
Monoclonal antibodies: Humanized *(cont.)*	Pertuzumab (Perjeta®)	Increased lacrimation (Huillard et al., 2014)	–
	Trastuzumab (Herceptin®)	Conjunctivitis, papilledema, retinal hemorrhage, dry eye, increased lacrimation (Huillard et al., 2014)	–
Miscellaneous Agents			
Miscellaneous	Bisphosphonates	Conjunctivitis, uveitis, scleritis; episcleritis, eyelid edema, optic neuritis, periorbital edema; orbital inflammation (Cunningham et al., 2016; F.T. Fraunfelder et al., 2008; Renouf et al., 2012)	Bisphosphonates must be discontinued for symptoms to resolve. Oral corticosteroids are used for severe inflammation or other symptoms. Most reports describe the onset of symptoms within 48 hours of the initial infusion, along with flu-like symptoms, fever, or myalgia. (Cunningham et al., 2016; F.T. Fraunfelder et al., 2008; Renouf et al., 2012)
	Corticosteroids	Posterior subcapsular cataracts, glaucoma, retinal hemorrhage; opportunistic eye infections, visual field defects, blurred vision, diplopia, exophthalmos, scleral discoloration Increased intraocular pressure and subsequent glaucoma have been noted with long-term use. (Loredo et al., 1972; Palmer et al., 2008; Teitelbaum, 2011)	–
	Cyclosporine A	Optic neuropathy; blurred vision, retinopathy, case reports of cortical blindness (Mejico et al., 2000; Palmer et al., 2008)	Combination of cyclosporine A and total body irradiation may increase susceptibility to develop radiation-induced optic neuropathy; patients' symptoms improved to some extent when cyclosporine was discontinued. (Mejico et al., 2000)
	Deferoxamine mesylate/ desferrioxamine (Deseferal®)	Night blindness, visual field constriction, cataracts, pigmentary retinopathy, optic neuropathy; blurring vision, decreased visual acuity, vision loss, visual defects, scotoma, optic neuritis, corneal opacities, and impaired peripheral, color, and night vision (Arora et al., 2004; Novartis Pharmaceuticals Corp., 2015)	Ocular side effects occurred related to prolonged use and high doses or in patients with low ferritin levels; ocular disturbances were reversible upon cessation of treatment. (Arora et al., 2004; Novartis Pharmaceuticals Corp., 2015)

(Continued on next page)

Table 25-3. Ocular Toxicities of Antineoplastic Agents *(Continued)*

Classification	Drug	Side Effects	Nursing Considerations
Miscellaneous Agents *(Cont.)*			
Miscellaneous *(cont.)*	Ethambutol hydrochloride	Decreased visual acuity, color blindness, visual defect, possible irreversible blindness, optic neuritis (STI Pharma, LLC, 2017)	Ocular toxicity can happen at any dose but is increased at doses > 50 mg/kg; change in visual acuity can be unilateral or bilateral. Testing for visual acuity should be performed before treatment begins and periodically during treatment, unless dose is > 15 mg/kg/day, in which monthly testing is needed. (Donald et al., 2006; STI Pharma, LLC, 2017)
	Mannitol (Osmitrol®)	Blurred vision (Baxter Healthcare Corp., 2011)	Because of fluid and electrolyte shift, side effects can be prevented with close monitoring and test dose to evaluate degree of renal failure when indicated. (Baxter Healthcare Corp., 2011)
	Tacrolimus (Prograf®)	Optic neuropathy (Mejico et al., 2000)	–
Radiation therapy	–	Xerophthalmia, keratoconjunctivitis (dry eye syndrome), pain, sensation of a foreign body in the eye, corneal ulceration (Brigden & McKenzie, 2000)	Xerophthalmia is caused by the radiation effect on the lacrimal and other adnexal glands that contribute to tear production. Lubricants and an ophthalmologic consultation are helpful. (Brigden & McKenzie, 2000)
Targeted Therapy Agents			
Small molecule inhibitors	Afatinib (Gilotrif®)	Conjunctivitis, keratitis; blepharitis, corneal thinning and erosion, dry eye syndrome, trichomegaly, uveitis (Agustoni et al., 2014; Davis, 2016; Huillard et al., 2014)	Ocular toxicity occurred in 13%–20% of patients; none were greater than a grade 3. (Agustoni et al., 2014)
	Axitinib (Inlyta®)	Retinal artery occlusion, retinal vein occlusion/thrombosis (Huillard et al., 2014)	–
	Binimetinib (Mektovi®)	Retinopathy (van Dijk et al., 2016; Watanabe et al., 2016)	Stopping the agent would resolve the retinopathy partially to completely. Retinal adverse events were resolved in a majority of patients with stopping the agent or dose reduction. (van Dijk et al., 2016; Watanabe et al., 2016)

(Continued on next page)

References

Agustoni, F., Platania, M., Vitali, M., Zilembo, N., Haspinger, E., Sinno, V., … Garassino, M.C. (2014). Emerging toxicities in the treatment of non-small cell lung cancer: Ocular disorders. *Cancer Treatment Reviews, 40,* 197–203. https://doi.org/10.1016/j.ctrv.2013.05.005

Ahmadi, M.A., & Esmaeli, B. (2001). Surgical treatment of canalicular stenosis in patients receiving docetaxel weekly. *Archives of Ophthalmology, 119,* 1802–1804. https://doi.org/10.1001/archopht.119.12.1802

Al-Tweigeri, T., Nabholtz, J.-M., & Mackey, J.R. (1996). Ocular toxicity and cancer chemotherapy: A review. *Cancer, 78,* 1359–1373. https://doi.org/10.1002/(SICI)1097-0142(19961001)78:7<1359:AID-CNCR1>3.0.CO;2-G

Amgen Inc. (2017). *Vectibix® (panitumumab)* [Package insert]. Thousand Oaks, CA: Author.

Antoun, J., Titah, C., & Cochereau, I. (2016). Ocular and orbital side effects of checkpoint inhibitors: A review article. *Current Opinion in Oncology, 28,* 288–294. https://doi.org/10.1097/CCO.0000000000000296

Arora, A., Wren, S., & Evans, K.G. (2004). Desferrioxamine related maculopathy: A case study. *American Journal of Hematology, 76,* 386–388. https://https://doi.org/10.1002/ajh.20090

Basti, S. (2007). Ocular toxicities of epidermal growth factor receptor inhibitors and their management. *Cancer Nursing, 30*(Suppl. 4), S10–S16. https://doi.org/10.1097/01.NCC.0000281759.23823.82

Baxter Healthcare Corp. (2011). *Osmitrol® (mannitol) injection* [Package insert]. Deerfield, IL: Author.

Bickley, L.S. (2017). *Bates' guide to physical examination and history taking* (12th ed.). Philadelphia, PA: Wolters Kluwer.

Bobba, R.K., & Klein, M. (2012). Ocular side effects of cancer therapeutics. In M.C. Perry (Ed.), *Perry's the chemotherapy source book* (5th ed., pp. 186–193). Philadelphia, PA: Wolters Kluwer Health/Lippincott Williams & Wilkins.

Bommireddy, T., & Carrim, Z.I. (2016). To stop or not? Tamoxifen therapy for secondary prevention of breast cancer in a patient with ocular toxicity. *BMJ Case Reports, 10,* 1136. https://doi.org/10.1136/bcr-2015-213431

Braiteh, F., Kurzrock, R., & Johnson, F.M. (2008). Trichomegaly of the eyelashes after lung cancer treatment with the epidermal growth factor receptor erlotinib. *Journal of Clinical Oncology, 26,* 3460–3462. https://doi.org/10.1200/JCO.2008.16.9391

Brigden, M., & McKenzie, M. (2000). Treating cancer patients: Practical monitoring and management of therapy-related complications. *Canadian Family Physician, 46,* 2258–2268. Retrieved from http://www.cfp.ca/content/46/11/2258.long

Bristol-Myers Squibb Co. (2017). *Lysodren® (mitotane)* [Package insert]. Princeton, NJ: Author.

Burtness, B., Anadkat, M., Basti, S., Hughes, M., Lacouture, M., McClure, J.S., … Spencer, S. (2009). NCCN Task Force report: Management of dermatologic and other toxicities associated with EGFR inhibition in patients with cancer. *Journal of the National Comprehensive Cancer Network, 7*(Suppl. 1), S1–S25 https://doi.org/10.6004/jnccn.2009.0074

Chatziralli, I., Sergentanis, T., Zagouri, F., Chrysikos, D., Ladas, I., Zografos, G.C., & Moschos, M. (2016). Ocular surface disease in breast cancer patients using aromatase inhibitors. *Breast Journal, 22,* 561–563. https://doi.org/10.1111/tbj.12633

Cleri, L.B., & Haywood, R. (2002). *Oncology pocket guide to chemotherapy* (5th ed.). Philadelphia, PA: Mosby.

Cunningham, E.T., London, N.J.S., Moorthy, R., Garg, S.J., & Zierhut, M. (2016). Drugs, inflammation, and the eye. *Ocular Immunology and Inflammation, 24,* 125–127. https://doi.org/10.3109/09273948.2016.1160683

Davis, M.E. (2016). Ocular toxicity of tyrosine kinase inhibitors. *Oncology Nursing Forum, 43,* 235–243. https://doi.org/10.1188/16.ONF.235-243

DeAngelis, L.M. (2017). Neurologic complications of cancer. In R.C. Bast Jr., C.M. Croce, W.N. Hait, W.K. Hong, D.W. Kufe, R.E. Pollock, … J.F. Holland (Eds.), *Holland-Frei cancer medicine* (9th ed., pp. 1701–1716). Hoboken, NJ: Wiley.

Donald, P.R., Maher, D., Maritz, J.S., & Qazi, S. (2006). Ethambutol dosage for the treatment of children: Literature review and recommendations. *International Journal of Tuberculosis and Lung Disease, 10,* 1318–1330.

Eaby, B., Culkin, A., & Lacouture, M.E. (2008). An interdisciplinary consensus on managing skin reactions associated with human epidermal growth factor receptor inhibitors. *Clinical Journal of Oncology Nursing, 12,* 283–290. https://doi.org/10.1188/08.CJON.283-290

Eadie, B.D., Etminan, M., Carelton, B.C., Maberley, D.A., & Mikelberg, F.S. (2017). Association of repeated intravitreous bevacizumab injections with risk of glaucoma surgery. *JAMA Ophthalmology, 135,* 363–368. https://doi.org/10.1001/jamaophthalmol.2017.0059

Esmaeli, B., Ahmadi, M.A., Kim, S., Onan, H., Korbling, M., & Anderlini, P. (2002). Marginal keratitis associated with administration of filgrastim and sargramostim in a healthy peripheral blood progenitor cell donor. *Cornea, 21,* 621–622. https://doi.org/10.1097/00003226-200208000-00021

Esmaeli, B., Koller, C., Papadopoulos, N., & Romaguera, J. (2001). Interferon-induced retinopathy in asymptomatic cancer patients. *Ophthalmology, 108,* 858–860. https://doi.org/10.1016/S0161-6420(01)00546-2

Esmaeli, B., Valero, V., Ahmadi, M.A., & Booser, D. (2001). Canalicular stenosis secondary to docetaxel: A newly recognized side effect. *Ophthalmology, 108,* 994–995. https://doi.org/10.1016/S0161-6420(00)00640-0

Esper, P., Gale, D., & Muehlbauer, P. (2007). What kind of rash is it? Deciphering the dermatologic toxicities of biologic and targeted therapies. *Clinical Journal of Oncology Nursing, 11,* 659–666. https://doi.org/10.1188/07.CJON.659-666

Fraunfelder, F.T., Fraunfelder, F.W., & Chambers, W.A. (2008). *Clinical ocular toxicology.* Philadelphia, PA: Elsevier Saunders.

Fraunfelder, F.W., & Fraunfelder, F.T. (2004). Adverse ocular drug reactions recently identified by the National Registry of Drug-Induced Ocular Side Effects. *Ophthalmology, 111,* 1275–1279. https://doi.org/10.1016/j.ophtha.2003.12.052

Fraunfelder, F.W., & Yang, H.K. (2016). Association between bortezomib therapy and eyelid chalazia. *JAMA Ophthalmology, 134,* 88–90. https://doi.org/10.1001/jamaophthalmol.2015.3963

Garibaldi, D.C., & Adler, R.A. (2007). Cicatricial ectropion associated with treatment of metastatic colorectal cancer in cetuximab. *Ophthalmic Plastic and Reconstructive Surgery, 23,* 62–63. https://doi.org/10.1097/IOP.0b013e31802d9025

Gianni, L., Panzini, I., Li, S., Gelber, R.D., Collins, J., Holmberg, S.B., … Ravaioli, A. (2006). Ocular toxicity during adjuvant chemoendocrine therapy for early breast cancer. *Cancer, 106,* 505–513. https://doi.org/10.1002/cncr.21651

Gorin, M.B., Day, R., Costantino, J.P., Fisher, B., Redmond, C.K., Wickerham, L., … Wolmark, N. (1998). Long-term tamoxifen citrate use and potential ocular toxicity. *American Journal of Ophthalmology, 125,* 493–501. https://doi.org/10.1016/S0002-9394(99)80190-1

Haddadin, S., & Perry, M.C. (2012). Appendix I: Chemotherapeutic agents. In M.C. Perry (Ed.), *The chemotherapy source book* (5th ed., pp. 659–739). Philadelphia, PA: Lippincott Williams & Wilkins.

Hager, T., & Seitz, B. (2014). Ocular side effects of biological agents in oncology: What should the clinician be aware of? *OncoTargets and Therapy, 7,* 69–77. https://doi.org/10.2147/OTT.S54606

Haidak, D.J., Hurwitz, B., & Yeung, K.Y. (1978). Tear-duct fibrosis (dacryostenosis) due to 5-fluorouracil. *Annals of Internal Medicine, 88,* 657. https://doi.org/10.7326/0003-4819-88-5-657_1

Hopen, G., Mondino, B.J., Johnson, B.L., & Chervenick, P.A. (1981). Corneal toxicity with systemic cytarabine. *American Journal of Ophthalmology, 91,* 500–504. https://doi.org/10.1016/0002-9394(81)90240-3

Huillard, O., Bakalian, S., Levy, C., Desjardins, L., Lumbroso-Le Rouic, L., Pop, S., ... Le Tourneau, C. (2014). Ocular adverse events of molecularly targeted agents approved in solid tumours: A systematic review. *European Journal of Cancer, 50,* 638–648. https://doi.org/10.1016/j.ejca.2013.10.016

International Workshop on Meibomian Gland Dysfunction. (2011). *Investigative Ophthalmology and Visual Science, 52,* 1917–2085.

Jansman, F.G.A., Sleijfer, D.T., de Graaf, J.C., Coenen, J.L.L.M., & Brouwers, J.R.B.J. (2001). Management of chemotherapy-induced adverse effects in the treatment of colorectal cancer. *Drug Safety, 24,* 353–367. https://doi.org/10.2165/00002018-200124050-00002

Karch, A.M. (2014). *2014 Lippincott's nursing drug guide.* Philadelphia, PA: Lippincott Williams & Wilkins.

Kende, G., Sirkin, S.R., Thomas, P.R.M., & Freeman, A.I. (1979). Blurring of vision: A previously undescribed complication of cyclophosphamide therapy. *Cancer, 44,* 69–71. https://doi.org/10.1002/1097-0142(197907)44:1<69::AID-CNCR2820440113>3.0.CO;2-O

Kim, R.Y., Anderlini, P., Naderi, A.A., Rivera, P., Ahmadi, M.A., & Esmaeli, B. (2002). Scleritis as the initial clinical manifestation of graft-versus-host disease after allogeneic bone marrow transplantation. *American Journal of Ophthalmology, 133,* 843–845. https://doi.org/10.1016/S0002-9394(02)01425-3

Kosker, M., & Celik, T. (2015). Ocular side effects and trichomegaly of eyelashes induced by erlotinib: A case report and review of the literature. *Contact Lens and Anterior Eye, 38,* 59–60. https://doi.org/10.1016/j.clae.2014.08.005

Kwan, A.S.L., Sahu, A., & Palexes, G. (2006). Retinal ischemia with neovascularization in cisplatin related retinal toxicity. *American Journal of Ophthalmology, 141,* 196–197. https://doi.org/10.1016/j.ajo.2005.07.046

Lauer, A.K., Wobig, J.L., Shults, W.T., Neuwelt, E.A., & Wilson, M.W. (1999). Severe ocular and orbital toxicity after intracarotid etoposide phosphate and carboplatin therapy. *American Journal of Ophthalmology, 127,* 230–233. https://doi.org/10.1016/S0002-9394(98)00346-8

Liu, S., & Kurzrock, R. (2015). Understanding toxicities of targeted agents: Implications for anti-tumor activity and management. *Seminars in Oncology, 42,* 863–875. https://doi.org/10.1053/j.seminoncol.2015.09.032

Lochhead, J., Salmon, J.F., & Bron, A.J. (2003). Cytarabine-induced corneal toxicity [Letter]. *Eye, 17,* 677–678. https://doi.org/10.1038/sj.eye.6700451

Loprinzi, C.L., Wender, D.B., Veeder, M.H., O'Fallon, J.R., Vaught, N.L., Dose, A.M., ... Leitch, J.M. (1994). Inhibition of 5-fluorouracil-induced ocular irritation by ocular ice packs. *Cancer, 74,* 945–948. https://doi.org/10.1002/1097-0142(19940801)74:3<945::AID-CNCR2820740324>3.0.CO;2-C

Loredo, A., Rodriguez, R.S., & Murillo, L. (1972). Cataracts after short-term corticosteroid treatment. *New England Journal of Medicine, 286,* 160. https://doi.org/10.1056/NEJM197201202860317

Mejico, L.J., Bergloeff, J., & Miller, N.R. (2000). New therapies with potential neuro-ophthalmologic toxicity. *Current Opinion in Ophthalmology, 11,* 389–394. https://doi.org/10.1097/00055735-200012000-00002

Mesquida, M., Sanchez-Dalmau, B., Ortiz-Perez, S., Pelegrín, L., Molina-Fernandez, J.M., Figueras-Roca, F., ... Adán, A. (2010). Oxaliplatin-related ocular toxicity. *Case Reports in Oncology, 3,* 423–427. https://doi.org/10.1159/000322675

Methvin, A.B., & Gausas, R.E. (2007). Newly recognized ocular side effects of erlotinib. *Ophthalmic Plastic and Reconstructive Surgery, 23,* 63–65. https://doi.org/10.1097/IOP.0b013e31802d97f0

Moloney, T.P., Xu, W., Rallah-Baker, K., Oliveira, N., Woodward, N., & Farrah, J.J. (2014). Toxic optic neuropathy in the setting of docetaxel chemotherapy: A case report. *BMC Ophthalmology, 14,* 18. https://doi.org/10.1186/1471-2415-14-18

Novartis Pharmaceuticals Corp. (2015). *Desferal® (deferoxamine mesylate for injection USP)* [Package insert]. East Hanover, NJ: Author.

Oncology.TV. (2011). Ocular changes secondary to chemotherapy. Retrieved from http://www.oncology.tv/SymptomManagement/OcularChangesSecondary.aspx

Ouwerkerk, J., & Boers-Doets, C. (2010). Best practices in the management of toxicities related to anti-EGFR agents for metastatic colorectal cancer. *European Journal of Oncology Nursing, 14,* 337–349. https://doi.org/10.1016/j.ejon.2010.03.004

Palmer, M.L., Hyndiuk, R.A., Hughes, M.S., Baker, A.S., Erickson, K., Schroeder, A., ... Mattox, C. (2008). Toxicology of ophthalmic agents by class. In D.M. Albert, J.W. Miller, D.T. Azar, & B.A. Blodi (Eds.), *Albert and Jakobiec's principles and practice of ophthalmology* (3rd ed., pp. 345–377). Philadelphia, PA: Elsevier Saunders.

Papavasileiou, E., Prasad, S., Freitag, S.K., Sobrin, L., & Lobo, A. (2016). Ipilimumab-induced ocular and orbital inflammation—A case series and review of the literature. *Ocular Immunology and Inflammation, 24,* 140–146. https://doi.org/10.3109/09273948.2014.1001858

Purbrick, R.M.J., Osunkunle, O.A., Talbot, D.C., & Downes, S.M. (2017). Ocular toxicity of mitogen-activated protein kinase inhibitors. *JAMA Oncology, 3,* 275–277. https://doi.org/10.1001/jamaoncol.2016.4213

Ramírez-Soria, M.P., España-Gregori, E., Aviñó-Martínez, J., & Pastor-Pascual, F. (2008). Blepharitis related to cetuximab treatment in an advanced colorectal cancer patient. *Archivos de la Sociedad Espanola de Oftalmologia, 83,* 665–668. Retrieved from http://www.oftalmo.com/seo/archivos/maquetas/4/7AD11994-2BDD-E208-7BED-00006F41D9D4/articulo.pdf

Rao, R.C., & Choudhry, N. (2016). Cystoid macular edema associated with chemotherapy. *Canadian Medical Association Journal, 188,* 216. https://doi.org/10.1503/cmaj.131080

Renouf, D.J., Velazquez-Martin, J.P., Simpson, R., Siu, L.L., & Bedard, P.L. (2012). Ocular toxicity of targeted therapies. *Journal of Clinical Oncology, 30,* 3277–3286. https://doi.org/10.1200/JCO.2011.41.5851

Robert, C., Soria, J.-C., Spatz, A., Le Cesne, A., Malka, D., Pautier, P., ... Le Chevalier, T. (2005). Cutaneous side-effects of kinase inhibitors and blocking antibodies. *Lancet Oncology, 6,* 491–500. https://doi.org/10.1016/S1470-2045(05)70243-6

Segaert, S., & Van Cutsem, E. (2005). Clinical signs, pathophysiology and management of skin toxicity during therapy with epidermal growth factor receptor inhibitors. *Annals of Oncology, 16,* 1425–1433. https://doi.org/10.1093/annonc/mdi279

Sigma-Tau Pharmaceuticals, Inc. (2008, March). *Matulane® (procarbazine hydrochloride capsules)* [Package insert]. Gaithersburg, MD: Author.

Singh, P., & Singh, A. (2012). Ocular adverse effects of anti-cancer chemotherapy. *Journal of Cancer Therapeutics and Research, 1,* 5. https://doi.org/10.7243/2049-7962-1-5

STI Pharma, LLC. (2017, May). *Ethambutol HCl USP* [Package insert]. Langhorne, PA: Author.

Teitelbaum, A. (2011). Eye symptoms and toxicities of systemic chemotherapy. In I.N. Olver (Ed.), *The MASCC textbook of cancer supportive care and survivorship* (pp. 333–350). New York, NY: Springer.

Tonini, G., Vincenzi, B., Santini, D., Olzi, D., Lambiase, A., & Bonini, S. (2005). Ocular toxicity related to cetuximab monotherapy in an advanced colorectal cancer patient. *Journal of the National Cancer Institute, 97,* 606–607. https://doi.org/10.1093/jnci/dji104

Tsai, D.-C., Chen, S.-J., Chiou, S.-H., Lee, A.-F., Lee, F.-L., & Hsu, W.-M. (2003). Should we discontinue tamoxifen in a patient with vision-threatening ocular toxicity related to low-dose tamoxifen therapy? [Letter]. *Eye, 17,* 276–278. https://doi.org/10.1038/sj.eye.6700317

van Dijk, E.H.C., Duits, D.E.M., Versluis, M., Luyten, G.P.M., Bergen, A.A.B., Kapiteijn, E.W., ... van der Velden, P.A. (2016). Loss of MAPK pathway activation in post-mitotic retinal cells as mechanism in MEK inhibition-related retinopathy in cancer patients. *Medicine, 95,* e3457. https://doi.org/10.1097/MD.0000000000003457

Walkhom, B., Fraunfelder, F.T., & Henner, W.D. (2000). Severe ocular irritation and corneal deposits associated with capecitabine use [Letter]. *New England Journal of Medicine, 343,* 740–741. https://doi.org/10.1056/NEJM200009073431015

Warrell, R.P., Jr., & Berman, E. (1986). Phase I and II study of fludarabine phosphate in leukemia: Therapeutic efficacy with delayed central nervous system toxicity. *Journal of Clinical Oncology, 4,* 74–79. https://doi.org/10.1200/JCO.1986.4.1.74

Watanabe, K., Otsu, S., Hirashima, Y., Morinaga, R., Nishikawa, K., Hisamatsu, Y., ... Ando, Y. (2016) A phase I study of binimetinib (MEK162) in Japanese patients with advanced solid tumors. *Cancer Chemotherapy and Pharmacology, 77,* 1157–1164. https://doi.org/10.1007/s00280-016-3019-5

Watanabe, W., Kuwabara, R., Nakahara, T., Hamasaki, O., Sakamoto, I., Okada, K., ... Mishima, H.K. (2002). Severe ocular and orbital toxicity after intracarotid injection of carboplatin for recurrent glioblastomas. *Graefe's Archive for Clinical and Experimental Ophthalmology, 240,* 1033–1035. https://doi.org/10.1007/s00417-002-0573-9

Willson, R.A. (2004). Visual side effects of pegylated interferon during therapy for chronic hepatitis C infection. *Journal of Clinical Gastroenterology, 38,* 717–722. https://doi.org/10.1097/01.mcg.0000135897.30038.16

Zhang, G., Basti, S., & Jampol, L.M. (2007). Acquired trichomegaly and symptomatic external ocular changes in patients receiving epidermal growth factor receptor inhibitors: Case reports and a review of literature. *Cornea, 26,* 858–860. https://doi.org/10.1097/ICO.0b013e318064584a

Zimmer, L., Goldinger, S.M., Hofmann, L., Loquai, C., Ugurel, S., Thomas, I., ... Heinzerling, L.M. (2016). Neurological, respiratory, musculoskeletal, cardiac and ocular side-effects of anti-PD-1 therapy. *European Journal of Cancer, 60,* 210–225. https://doi.org/10.1016/j.ejca.2016.02.024

SECTION VI

Post-Treatment

CHAPTER 26

Post-Treatment and Survivorship Care

A. Overview: In 1985, Fitzhugh Mullan famously wrote about his experience with cancer and acknowledged that survivorship "begins at the point of diagnosis" (p. 270). Subsequently, major federal, public, and private cancer organizations have defined survivorship as beginning with diagnosis and continuing for the rest of life. Over the past 30 years, the number of cancer survivors in the United States has increased from 3 million to more than 15.5 million (American Cancer Society, 2016). The number is expected to increase to 20.3 million (a 31% increase) by 2026 (Bluethmann, Mariotto, & Rowland, 2016). Early diagnosis and advances in cancer treatment have led to improved five-year relative survival rates for all cancers from 49% in the 1970s to 69% for those diagnosed between 2008 and 2014 (Noone et al., 2018). The exponential growth in the number of older survivors has been called the "silver tsunami" and has led to the prediction that by 2040, 73% of cancer survivors will be aged 65 years and older (Bluethmann et al., 2016).

1. Childhood cancer survivors: Childhood cancers are now often cured; approximately 84% of children and adolescents survive a cancer diagnosis (Siegel, Miller, & Jemal, 2018). However, long-term survivors of childhood cancer are at risk for long-term effects from their disease and treatment.
   a) Research suggests that approximately 70% of survivors of childhood cancers have one or more treatment- or disease-related long-term effects (Phillips et al., 2015).
   b) The Children's Oncology Group (2013) published long-term follow-up guidelines for screening and management of late effects for survivors of childhood cancer (available at http://survivorshipguidelines.org).
2. Adult cancer survivors: Currently, 62% of cancer survivors are aged 65 years or older and almost half (47%) are aged 70 or older (Siegel et al., 2018). Meanwhile, U.S. survival statistics have improved more slowly for older survivors compared to younger survivors of cancer in the past two decades (Zeng et al., 2015). This trend likely reflects decreased use or efficacy of new therapies in older adults with cancer (Siegel et al., 2018).
3. In addition to the physical long-term and late effects of cancer and its treatment, child, adolescent, adult, and older adult cancer survivors may face a spectrum of psychological, financial, emotional, spiritual, and social challenges. The number and types of continuing, long-term, and late effects experienced by an individual survivor are influenced by the type and dose of treatments received.
4. Nurses have multiple roles in the continuing care of cancer survivors. These roles include monitoring, assessing, and treating survivors for the effects of treatment that emerge after completion of therapy. Nurses have a vital role in teaching survivors about the advantages of a healthy lifestyle and other interventions to minimize the potential effects of a cancer diagnosis and cancer treatment.

B. Survivorship care

1. Follow-up care for cancer survivors is recommended for life. All follow-up care is site and treatment specific. The National Comprehensive Cancer Network® (NCCN®, www.nccn.org) provides evidence-based guidelines for site-specific follow-up care.
2. Early follow-up care occurs frequently and emphasizes management of continuing physical psychological, financial, emotional, spiritual, and social effects of disease and treatment, as well as surveillance for and detection of disease recurrence.
3. Long-term follow-up care focuses on anticipating and identifying late effects of the disease or treatment, as well as continued surveillance for disease recurrence.

4. Essential elements of comprehensive survivorship care
   a) Components include a survivorship care plan (SCP), psychosocial care plan, and treatment summary; screening for new cancers and surveillance for recurrence; care coordination; health promotion education; and symptom management and palliative care (Rechis, Beckjord, Arvey, Reynolds, & McGoldrick, 2011).
   b) Additional recommended elements of survivorship care include education regarding late effects, survivorship, available programs, and self-advocacy; comprehensive medical and psychosocial assessments; rehabilitation and lifestyle services; family and caregiver support; transition visits; and patient navigation (Rechis et al., 2011).
   c) Care coordination may be the most important component of survivorship care (Salz & Baxi, 2016). The interprofessional cancer care team, primary care providers, and other specialist providers participate in post-treatment care.
   d) Nursing assessment and care: RNs and advanced practice nurses have been identified as appropriate members of the cancer care team who are prepared to coordinate care and deliver the SCP to survivors at the completion of their treatment (American College of Surgeons Commission on Cancer [ACoS CoC], 2015).
      (1) Holistic needs assessment: Facilitate person-centered care by gathering information on the patient's physical, emotional, spiritual, mental, social, and environmental well-being (Young, Cund, Renshaw, Quigley, & Snowden, 2015).
      (2) Sleep quality: Sleep quality issues are a challenge for many cancer survivors after treatment and should be part of the patient assessment (Mustian et al., 2013; Phipps et al., 2016).
5. SCPs were recommended in the seminal publication *From Cancer Patient to Cancer Survivor: Lost in Transition* (Hewitt, Greenfield, & Stovall, 2006) and in *The Essential Elements of Survivorship Care* (Rechis et al., 2011). In 2016, ACoS CoC incorporated the provision of a survivorship plan of care as a standard for cancer center accreditation. Despite the promise of SCPs and current requirements from ACoS CoC, research trials have not yet demonstrated efficacy (Salz & Baxi, 2016).
   a) All patients completing primary treatment should be provided with an SCP. It should be communicated and written by the principal care provider(s) who coordinated oncology treatment. The plan should summarize critical information needed for the survivor's long-term care (Mayer et al., 2014). Discussion of the SCP with the patient is required to meet the ACoS CoC standard.
   b) The SCP includes a treatment summary and addresses post-treatment needs and follow-up care to improve health and quality of life. Many organizations have developed templates for SCPs, including the American Society of Clinical Oncology (n.d.) and the Journey Forward initiative, a collaboration of multiple organizations including the Oncology Nursing Society, the National Coalition for Cancer Survivorship, and other academic, community, and industry partners (www.journeyforward.org/about-journey-forward).
   c) The SCP minimally includes general patient information, provider contact information, comprehensive treatment summary, genetic risk assessment, follow-up plan of care including surveillance and screening schedule, potential long-term and late effects specific to the cancer type and the treatment received, and required patient education (ACoS CoC, 2015).
6. Models of survivorship care: Although different models for delivering survivorship care have been implemented, superiority of one model has not yet been demonstrated, and models vary widely by institution. Models may include specialist-led care, nurse-led care, community-based family physician–led care, and interprofessional or shared care (Halpern et al., 2015).

C. Late effects of cancer treatment: Second malignant neoplasms (SMNs) and cardiovascular disease (CVD) are among the most serious and life-threatening late adverse effects of cancer treatment.
   1. Incidence
      a) Cancer survivors have an increased risk of developing another malignancy, given the longer duration of cancer survivorship, with the lifetime risk reaching as high as 33% and a greater risk for mortality (Donin et al., 2016). More than 8% of patients diagnosed with 1 of the 10 most prevalent cancers were found to have an SMN, the most common of which is lung cancer (Donin et al., 2016).
      b) The 30-year cumulative incidence of SMNs among survivors of childhood malignancies is 20.5% when including nonmelanoma skin

cancer and 7.9%, when excluding nonmelanoma skin cancer (Friedman et al., 2010).

2. Therapy-related risk factors
   a) Chemotherapy
      (1) Chemotherapy is associated with a risk of SMN, primarily treatment-related leukemia and, to a lesser extent, solid tumors (Cowell & Austin, 2012; Ng & Travis, 2008; Travis et al., 2010).
      (2) Type of chemotherapy: Alkylating agents are associated with the greatest incidence of late effects (Turcotte et al., 2017).
      (3) Dose: Higher cumulative dose increases the risk of treatment-related leukemia (Leone, Fianchi, & Voso, 2011; Travis et al., 2010). Higher cumulative doses of alkylating agents are associated with an increased risk of multiple health conditions (Oeffinger et al., 2006).
      (4) Agents with known carcinogenic potential are noted in Chapter 12.
   b) Radiation therapy
      (1) Radiation-associated solid tumors are the most common type of SMN (Ng, Kenney, Gilbert, & Travis, 2010).
      (2) Radiation is associated with a risk of solid tumors that develop within or near the radiation fields and have a latency period of 5–10 years (Ng & Travis, 2008; Travis et al., 2012).
      (3) The risk of an SMN from radiation increases with the dose of radiation and the extent of the radiation field (Braunstein & Nakamura, 2013; Travis et al., 2012).
         (a) Advances in three-dimensional imaging of tumors have allowed for reduction of the radiation field (Travis et al., 2014).
         (b) Advances in radiation technology allow for more precise delivery of radiation to the tumor so that increased doses can be delivered to the tumor while sparing healthy tissue (Travis et al., 2014).
         (c) Treatment with 35 gray (Gy) involved-field radiation therapy (IFRT): Compared to 35 Gy mantle radiation therapy, 35 Gy IFRT is estimated to reduce the risk for female breast and lung cancer by approximately 65% and the risk for male lung cancer by approximately 35%. Reducing the dose of IFRT from 35 Gy to 20 Gy is estimated to reduce the risk approximately 40% more (Koh et al., 2007).
   c) Combination chemotherapy and radiation
      (1) Few high-quality studies have reported the association of the combination of radiation and alkylating agents with increased risk of SMNs (Morton et al., 2013; Oeffinger et al., 2006).
      (2) Exposure to one of five specific combinations is associated with a risk of having a severe health condition that is at least 10 times the expected risk (Oeffinger et al., 2006).
         i. Chest irradiation plus bleomycin
         ii. Chest irradiation plus an anthracycline
         iii. Chest irradiation plus abdominal or pelvic irradiation
         iv. An anthracycline plus an alkylating agent
         v. Abdominal or pelvic irradiation plus an alkylating agent
   d) Immunotherapy
      (1) Data on late effects of immunotherapy are emerging as agents are approved and individuals receive standard-of-care treatment with long-term follow-up.
      (2) Most late effects are reported in the context of case studies and in relation to the checkpoint inhibitors and include pneumonitis, pericarditis, and enterocolitis (Blevins Primeau, 2018).
      (3) A unique attribute of immunotherapy treatment is the potential for long-term immunogenicity, surveillance that can protect against future recurrence but may also have adverse sequelae for healthy cells. One example involves the potential for prolonged B-cell aplasia in patients who have undergone CAR T-cell therapy (Kalos et al., 2013).
3. Patient-related risk factors
   a) Age
      (1) Younger age at cancer diagnosis increases the risk of developing an SMN (Friedman et al., 2010). The risk of developing a subsequent cancer in childhood cancer survivors is estimated at three- to sixfold (Reulen et al., 2011).
      (2) Developing organs in younger patients may be especially vulnerable to the effects of medication and radiation

(Ng, Kenney, et al., 2010). Older patients who experience adverse effects from their disease or its treatment may be unable to compensate for lost function.

(3) The cumulative incidence of a chronic health condition in childhood cancer survivors is more than 70% within 30 years of the cancer diagnosis, and more than 40% of these conditions will be severe, disabling, or fatal (Oeffinger et al., 2006). Hospitalization rates of childhood cancer survivors are 1.6 times the rate in the general U.S. population, indicating that while cure may be attainable for many children with cancer, the long-term health effects and costs associated with treatment-related long-term toxicities are notable (Kurt et al., 2012).

b) Sex

(1) Female childhood cancer survivors are more likely than male survivors to have one or more chronic health conditions (Oeffinger et al., 2006).

(2) Overall, women have a slightly higher risk of SMNs than men (Friedman et al., 2010; Miller et al., 2016).

c) Exposures

(1) Tobacco and alcohol exposure increase the risk of developing an SMN in all cancer survivors (Wood et al., 2012).

(2) Infections such as human papillomavirus (HPV) may increase the risk of SMNs in survivors of cervical and head and neck cancers, and HPV and hepatitis B and C increase the risk in hematopoietic stem cell transplant (HSCT) recipients (Diaz et al., 2016; Inamoto et al., 2015; Ng & Travis, 2008).

(3) Sun exposure (Ng & Travis, 2008)

d) Diet and exercise: Caloric excess, a diet low in fruits and vegetables, obesity, and physical inactivity contribute to the risk of SMNs involving the upper aerodigestive tract, colon cancer, breast cancer, and cancers of the female reproductive organs (Rock et al., 2012; Wood et al., 2012).

e) Immunodeficiency increases the risk of SMNs. Immune dysregulation may be associated with primary cancers such as leukemia and lymphoma or with immunosuppressive treatment (Brewer, Habermann, & Shanafelt, 2014; Inamoto et al., 2015; Ng, 2014; Visentin et al., 2017).

f) Genetic predisposition: Patients with genetic phenotypes that contributed to the development of their original cancer are at increased risk for a secondary cancer. Common syndromes identified with increased risk are hereditary breast and ovarian cancer and hereditary nonpolyposis colorectal cancer, or Lynch syndrome (Wood et al., 2012).

4. Types of late effects

a) Nonmalignant physical effects (Treanor & Donnelly, 2014; see Table 26-1)

(1) Cardiovascular: Cardiomyopathy, subclinical left ventricular dysfunction, coronary artery disease, valvular heart disease, pericardial disease, and arrhythmias

(a) The risk of developing anthracycline-associated cardiotoxicity increases with the total lifetime cumulative dose of doxorubicin at 400–550 mg/m^2, with many patients receiving lower doses (Chen, Colan, Diller, & Force, 2011; McGowan et al., 2017). All patients treated with an anthracycline should be considered at risk for cardiac dysfunction.

(b) More than 50% of children treated for childhood cancers are at an increased risk for CVD 5–10 years following chemotherapy (Henning & Harbison, 2017).

(c) Cardiotoxicity from commonly used anticancer drugs (e.g., anthracyclines, monoclonal antibodies, tyrosine inhibitors) may not occur or become clinically evident until 10–20 years after chemotherapy treatment (Henning & Harbison, 2017).

(d) Cisplatin is associated with an increased risk of cardiovascular risk factors, such as obesity, lipid abnormalities (decreased HDL and elevated LDL), and hypertension, and can be detected in the blood up to 20 years after treatment (Carver et al., 2007; Okwuosa, Anzevino, & Rao, 2017).

(2) Pulmonary: Pulmonary fibrosis, dyspnea, radiation pneumonitis, idiopathic pneumonia syndrome, bronchiolitis obliterans, generally impaired pulmonary function (Treanor & Donnelly, 2014)

Table 26-1. Potential Late Medical Effects by Body Function or System and Associated Treatments

Function or System	Associated Treatments	Potential Late Effect(s)
Auditory	Platinum agents, head radiation therapy	Hearing loss, tinnitus
Bladder	Cyclophosphamide, pelvic and lumbar–sacral radiation, spinal surgery, cystectomy, prostatectomy	Bladder fibrosis, incontinence, neurogenic bladder
Cardiovascular	Anthracyclines, cyclophosphamide, cisplatin, fluorouracil, taxanes, trastuzumab, radiation therapy	Cardiomyopathy, ischemia, pericardial disease, arrhythmias, CHF, CAD, valvular heart disease
Cognitive	IT or high-dose methotrexate; high-dose cytarabine; adjuvant chemotherapy for breast cancer; systemic chemotherapy treatment for lung cancer, ovarian cancer, and lymphoma; cranial radiation; neurosurgery	Alterations in attention, concentration, memory, and mental processing speed; visual and auditory impairment; dementia
Endocrine	Corticosteroids, hormone therapy, head/neck radiation therapy, HSCT	Hypothyroidism, hypopituitarism, hyperparathyroidism, adrenal dysfunction
Gastrointestinal	Head/neck, abdominal, and pelvic radiation therapy; head/neck, colorectal, and pelvic/spinal surgery; HSCT with chronic GVHD	Diarrhea, incontinence, constipation, GI tract strictures/fibrosis/vasculitis, obstruction, impaired swallowing, impaired absorption of nutrients, fistulas
Hepatic	Antimetabolites, abdominal radiation therapy, HSCT	Hepatitis B and C, hepatic dysfunction, cirrhosis, cholelithiasis
Lymphatic	Radiation therapy, melanoma excision, pelvic lymph node dissection, axillary lymph node dissection	Lymphedema
Neurologic—central	High-dose IV and IT methotrexate; high-dose cytarabine; head, brain, and neck radiation therapy; neurosurgery	Motor and sensory deficits, leukoencephalopathy, stroke, seizures
Neurologic—peripheral	Brachial or lumbosacral plexus radiation therapy, spinal surgery, vincristine, vinblastine, platinum agents, taxanes, bortezomib, thalidomide	Brachial plexopathy, peripheral neuropathy
Ocular	Corticosteroids, busulfan, tamoxifen, head and TBI radiation therapy, neurosurgery, HSCT with GVHD	Cataracts, glaucoma, retinopathy, ocular nerve palsy, xerophthalmia
Psychosocial	Any cancer treatment	Depression, anxiety, PTSD, financial and health insurance coverage challenges, altered body image
Renal	Cisplatin, methotrexate, nitrosoureas, nephrectomy, abdominal and TBI radiation therapy	Renal dysfunction, HTN, chronic kidney disease
Respiratory	Alkylating agents, bleomycin, busulfan, and nitrosoureas; head/neck, chest, and TBI radiation therapy; head/neck surgery and pulmonary lobectomy; HSCT with GVHD	Dyspnea, pulmonary fibrosis, pneumonitis, idiopathic pneumonia syndrome, bronchiolitis obliterans
Skeletal	Alkylating agents, anthracyclines, taxanes, corticosteroids, hormone therapies, aromatase inhibitors, pelvic radiation therapy, orchiectomy, androgen ablation	Osteopenia, osteoporosis
Sexual/reproductive	Alkylating agents, abdominal/pelvic radiation and surgery, androgen-suppressing treatments	Infertility; higher risk of miscarriage, preterm labor, and low birth-weight infants; erectile dysfunction; painful sex, diminished libido

CAD—coronary artery disease; CHF—congestive heart failure; GI—gastrointestinal; GVHD—graft-versus-host disease; HSCT—hematopoietic stem cell transplantation; HTN—hypertension; IT—intrathecal; IV—intravenous; PTSD—post-traumatic stress disorder; TBI—total body irradiation

Note. Based on information from Andersen et al., 2014; Bower et al., 2014; Hershman et al., 2014; Koelwyn et al., 2012; Lenihan & Cardinale, 2012; Marchese et al., 2011; Travis et al., 2012; Treanor & Donnelly, 2014; Valdivieso et al., 2012.

From "Late Effects of Cancer Treatment" (p. 2031), by K.M. Slusser in C.H. Yarbro, D. Wujcik, and B.H. Gobel (Eds.), *Cancer Nursing: Principles and Practice* (8th ed.), 2018, Burlington, MA: Jones & Bartlett Learning. Copyright 2018 by Jones & Bartlett Learning, www.jblearning.com. Reprinted with permission.

(3) Renal and hepatic: Nephropathy, chronic kidney disease, hepatitis B and C (Treanor & Donnelly, 2014)
(4) Musculoskeletal: Osteopenia, osteoporosis, osteonecrosis (Treanor & Donnelly, 2014)
(5) Endocrine: Hypothyroidism, growth hormone deficiency, gonadal failure, panhypopituitarism, adrenal insufficiency or dysfunction, diabetes mellitus, hypopituitarism, hyperparathyroidism (Treanor & Donnelly, 2014)
(6) Central nervous system: Cognitive impairment, peripheral neuropathy, leukoencephalopathy, cataracts, visual and auditory impairment, brain atrophy, brain necrosis, dementia, brachial plexopathy, peripheral sensory neuropathy, tinnitus (Treanor & Donnelly, 2014; see Chapter 24).
(7) Gastrointestinal: Diarrhea; incontinence; constipation; gastrointestinal tract strictures, fibrosis, or vasculitis; obstruction; impaired swallowing; impaired absorption of nutrients; fistulas (Slusser, 2018)
(8) Lymphatic: Cancer-related lymphedema (Shaitelman et al., 2015)
(9) Sexual/reproductive: Gonadal failure; treatment-induced menopause; infertility; higher risk of miscarriage, preterm labor, and low birth-weight infants; sexual dysfunction, including loss of libido, erectile dysfunction, and pain (Treanor & Donnelly, 2014; see Chapter 20)

b) Malignant effects (SMNs; see Table 26-2)

(1) Definition: A *second malignant neoplasm* is a new cancer that is distinct from the original malignancy and does not rep-

Table 26-2. Second Malignant Neoplasms

Primary Malignancy	Second Malignant Neoplasm[a]	Risk Factors
ALL	• CNS malignancy – Risk is 17-fold after 5 years.	Cranial irradiation at doses of 18–24 Gy
	• Melanoma – Cumulative incidence: 0.43%	Age > 10 years (p < 0.001) Family history of cancer (p = 0.01)
	• Thyroid cancer	RT
Breast cancer	• Any SMN – Elevated risk for women diagnosed at younger than age 40 (SIR: 1.81) but not for women diagnosed after age 40 – Increased risk of salivary gland, esophageal, stomach, colon, breast, uterine corpus, ovarian, thyroid, and soft tissue cancers, melanoma, and acute nonlymphocytic leukemia	Age < 40 years at diagnosis Risk of leukemia associated with alkylating agents Risk of solid tumors associated with radiation therapy
	• Leukemia – Cumulative incidence: < 0.5% at 8–10 years after anthracycline-cyclophosphamide chemotherapy	
	• Endometrial – Associated with 35% increased risk	Tamoxifen
	• Sarcoma – SIR: 3–6 – Latency: 5–10 years	RT
Cervical cancer	• Urogenital cancer – 10 to > 40 years after treatment	RT
CLL/SLL	• HL – SIR: 15.11	Age < 70 years at time of CLL/SLL diagnosis Chemotherapy Risk higher in CLL than SLL
	• Lung cancer – SIR: 1.44	Patients diagnosed before age 55 had higher SIR: 2.32.
	• Melanoma – SIR: 1.92	

(Continued on next page)

Table 26-2. Second Malignant Neoplasms *(Continued)*

Primary Malignancy	Second Malignant Neoplasm[a]	Risk Factors
CML	• Breast cancer (in CML Ph+) – SIR: 0.24 • Colorectal cancer – SIR: 1.12 • Endocrine cancer (in CML Ph+) – SIR: 3.0 • Gastrointestinal cancer (in CML Ph+) – SIR: 0.38 • Head and neck cancer – Buccal cavity, SIR: 1.27 • Lymphoid leukemia – SIR: 5.53 • Myeloid leukemia – SIR: 12.32 • Melanoma – SIR: 1.4 – SIR: 3.0 (CML Ph+) • NHL – SIR: 2.17 • Prostate cancer – SIR: 1.38 • Renal cancer – SIR: 1.5 (CML Ph+) • Stomach cancer – SIR: 2.76 • Skin (nonmelanoma) – SIR: 5.36 • Urogenital cancer – SIR: 1.61	–
DLBCL	• AML – SIR: 4.96	Age < 55 Chemotherapy Female
	• HL – SIR: 9.02	
Follicular lymphoma	• AML – SIR: 5.96 • HL – SIR: 6.78	Age < 55 Chemotherapy
	• Lung cancer – SIR: 1.28	Patients diagnosed before age 55 had higher SIR: 2.01.
	• Melanoma – SIR: 1.6	
HL	• Breast – 20-year cumulative risk after mantle RT: 23% (median dose 40 Gy) – RR: 6.1 for patients diagnosed at age 30 and survived to ≥ 40	Occurs 10–15 years after chest irradiation Highest risk occurs in women treated with chest irradiation at age 35 or younger; risk increases with younger age. Risk increases with dose of radiation. Risk increases with TBI use pretransplantation. RT-related premature menopause is associated with decreased risk.
	• Colorectal cancer	Risk increases with dose of radiation.

(Continued on next page)

Table 26-2. Second Malignant Neoplasms *(Continued)*

Primary Malignancy	Second Malignant Neoplasm[a]	Risk Factors
HL *(cont.)*	• Lung cancer – RR: 7.0 – Chemotherapy-associated lung cancer occurs 1–4 years after therapy up to 15 years. – Radiation-associated lung cancer risk is elevated for 5–9 years after therapy and can last for more than 20 years. • Pleura – RR: 19.5	Thoracic irradiation Risk increases with dose of radiation. Alkylating agents Radiation dose and therapy with alkylating agents has a combined additive risk. RT and smoking significantly increase risk ($p < 0.001$).
	• Melanoma – 1–4 years after treatment – RR: 5.5	May be related to immunosuppression associated with HL
	• NHL – Within 5 years of treatment, then risk remains constant or increases over lifetime – 25-year cumulative risk: 3.5% – RR: 21.5	Immunosuppression associated with the HL or with combined chemoradiation treatment
	• Thyroid cancer – RR: 15.2	RT
	• Mesothelioma – RR is 20-fold for patients diagnosed at age 30 and survived to ≥ age 40.	
NHL	• Bladder cancer – Cyclophosphamide: * 20–49 g, RR: 6.0 * > 50 g, RR: 14.5	Cyclophosphamide > 20 g Risk increases with RT use.
	• Leukemia – Overall RR: 8.8 – Occurs within 15 years – Male, RR: 5.65 – Female, RR: 19.89	ACVBP Carmustine Chlorambucil > 1,300 mg (RR: 6.5) CHOP (RR: 14.2) Mechlorethamine (RR: 13.0) Procarbazine Risk of acute leukemia increases with RT use, especially TBI pre-transplantation.
	• Lung cancer – SIR: 1.6–2.45	Alkylating agents Male gender Smoking is dose-related with higher risk in those who smoked at diagnosis and continue to smoke after therapy.
	• Melanoma – Cumulative incidence: 0.55%	> 10 years old ($p < 0.001$) Family history of cancer ($p = 0.01$)
	• Mesothelioma	Risk increases with RT use.
Multiple myeloma	• 17% at 50 months	Alkylating agents
Lung cancer	• Leukemia – Non-small cell, SIR: 1.47 – Small cell, SIR: 6.57	Increased risk due to use of alkylating agents
Mycosis fungoides/ Sézary syndrome	• Bladder cancer – SIR: 1.71 • HL – SIR: 1.71 • Lung cancer – SIR: 1.42 • Melanoma – SIR: 2.60 • NHL – SIR: 5.08 • Renal cancer – SIR: 1.71	–

(Continued on next page)

Table 26-2. Second Malignant Neoplasms *(Continued)*

Primary Malignancy	Second Malignant Neoplasm[a]	Risk Factors
Ovarian cancer	• Leukemia – Occurs up to 10 years after therapy	Alkylating agents, including cyclophosphamide and melphalan Platinum-containing regimens
Polycythemia vera	• CML – SIR: 1.6 • Lung cancer – SIR: 1.8 • Myeloid leukemia – SIR: 8.5 at 1–2 years – SIR: 14.6 at 2–4 years – SIR: 18.6 at 5 years • NHL – SIR: 1.8	–
Testicular cancer	• Leukemia – SIR: 1.6–6.7 – Median time to occurrence: 4.5 years	Etoposide (Risk appears to be increasing since PEB chemotherapy became standard in the 1990s.)
	• Gastrointestinal cancer – SIR: 1.27–2.1	RT
	• Bladder cancer – SIR: 3.9 – Median time to occurrence: 20 years	RT including the iliac lymph nodes (This risk will likely decrease because from the mid-1980s, RT has been directed to the para-aortic lymph nodes only.) No study noted increased risk of bladder cancer after chemotherapy alone; however, because PEB is carcinogenic to humans, and platinum is excreted in urine up to 20 years after treatment with PEB chemotherapy, prolonged platinum exposure may play a role in bladder cancer development.
Waldenström macroglobulinemia	• AML – SIR: 5.3 • Colorectal cancer – SIR: 2.2 • Lung cancer – SIR: 1.6 • Melanoma – SIR: 1.6 • Multiple myeloma – SIR: 4.4 • NHL – SIR: 4.9 • Prostate cancer – SIR: 1.2 • Renal cancer – SIR: 1.4 • Uterine cancer – SIR: 2.2	–

[a] SIR: Standardized incidence ratio or relative risk (observed cases/expected cases) compares actual cases observed with the number of expected cases in the general population to determine increased (> 1.0) or decreased (< 1.0) risk (Curtis et al., 2006; Ojha & Thertulien, 2012; Verma et al., 2011).

ACVBP—doxorubicin, cyclophosphamide, vindesine, bleomycin, prednisone; ALL—acute lymphocytic leukemia; AML—acute myeloid leukemia; CHOP—cyclophosphamide, doxorubicin, vincristine, prednisone; CLL—chronic lymphocytic leukemia; CML—chronic myeloid leukemia; CNS—central nervous system; DLBCL—diffuse large B-cell lymphoma; Gy—gray; HL—Hodgkin lymphoma; NHL—non-Hodgkin lymphoma; PEB—cisplatin, etoposide, bleomycin; Ph+—Philadelphia chromosome positive; RR—relative risk; RT—radiation therapy; SIR—standardized incidence ratio; SLL—small lymphocytic lymphoma; SMN—second malignant neoplasm; TBI—total body irradiation

Note. Based on information from André et al., 2004; Curtis et al., 2006; Forman & Nakamura, 2015; Frederiksen et al., 2011; Hodgson, 2011; Hodgson et al., 2007; Huang et al., 2007; International Agency for Research on Cancer, 2012a, 2012b; Morton et al., 2010; Ng et al., 2011; Ojha & Thertulien, 2012; Rebora et al., 2010; Travis et al., 2012; Tward et al., 2007; van den Belt-Dusebout et al., 2007; van Leeuwen et al., 2000; van Leeuwen & Travis, 2001; Verma et al., 2011.

From "Management of the Complications of Hematologic Malignancy and Treatment," by C.H. Erb and W.H. Vogel in M. Olsen and L.J. Zitella (Eds.), *Hematologic Malignancies in Adults* (pp. 629–633), 2013, Pittsburgh: PA: Oncology Nursing Society. Copyright 2013 by Oncology Nursing Society. Adapted with permission.

resent metastatic disease from the primary tumor (Wood et al., 2012).

(2) Pathophysiology

(a) Chemotherapy and radiation therapy cause DNA damage, which is the mechanism that leads to cell death. However, if nonlethal DNA damage occurs, DNA repair is critical to prevent the development of a secondary cancer (Cowell & Austin, 2012).

(b) Alkylating agents transfer an alkyl group to DNA, causing DNA mismatch and inhibition of DNA replication and transcription. A DNA mismatch repair mechanism is responsible for repairing this cell damage; otherwise, apoptosis occurs. If cells survive with a dysfunctional DNA mismatch repair or genomic instability, this may lead to malignancy (Allan & Travis, 2005; Cowell & Austin, 2012; Tward, Glenn, Pulsipher, Barnette, & Gaffney, 2007).

(c) Topoisomerase II inhibitors cause double-stranded DNA breaks, which lead to apoptosis. If the cell survives, these DNA breaks may cause chromosomal translocations of the *MLL* gene or other crucial transforming genes that can lead to leukemia (Allan & Travis, 2005; Cowell & Austin, 2012; Tward et al., 2007).

(d) Radiation therapy deposits energy in or near DNA, which results in genetic or epigenetic changes that cause cell death. If radiation induces mutations in the DNA and the cells do not die, the mutations are passed on to cellular progeny and over time may lead to malignant transformation (Travis et al., 2012).

(e) Chemotherapy and radiation therapy interact with other factors such as tobacco exposure, genetic makeup, hormonal status, and immune function, which may contribute to the risk of developing a secondary cancer (Allan & Travis, 2005; Travis et al., 2012).

(3) Types of SMNs: The two major types of SMNs are acute myeloid neoplasms and solid neoplasms. The relative risk of treatment-related leukemia is generally greatest during the first five years after therapy (Wood et al., 2012). Solid tumors occur at least 5–10 years after treatment, with the risk differing across the age spectrum by type of malignancy, latency period, associated risk factors, and modifying influences (Ng, Kenney, et al., 2010).

(a) Treatment-related acute myeloid leukemia (AML)/myelodysplastic syndrome (MDS) generally presents within five years of chemotherapy and is most commonly associated with the use of alkylating agents or topoisomerase inhibitors.

(b) Two types of treatment-related leukemia (Churpek & Larson, 2013)

i. Alkylating agent–induced AML (Churpek & Larson, 2013)
- Risk is associated with alkylating agents such as cyclophosphamide, melphalan, chlorambucil, and nitrosoureas.
- Disease usually occurs 3–10 years after treatment.
- Development is associated with deletion or loss of chromosome 5 or 7 or both.

ii. Topoisomerase II inhibitor–induced acute leukemia (Churpek & Larson, 2013)
- Risk is associated with topoisomerase II inhibitors such as etoposide, teniposide, mitoxantrone, and anthracyclines.
- Risk begins shortly after completion of therapy, and disease usually occurs within a few months to three years after treatment.
- Occurrence is often not associated with preceding MDS.
- Development is associated with chromosomal translocations 11q23 or 21q22, and sometimes t15;17.

(4) Radiation-induced solid tumors, such as Hodgkin lymphoma (HL), sarco-

mas, leukemia, and breast, lung, cervical, prostate, skin, stomach, esophageal, and thyroid tumors, are observed at least 5–10 years after treatment, and the risk persists for decades (Travis et al., 2012; Wood et al., 2012). Radiation-induced SMNs tend to occur within or at the margins of the radiation field, and the risk increases with the extent of tissue irradiated and the dose of radiation (Wood et al., 2012).

c) Psychosocial effects (McFarland & Holland, 2016)
   (1) Psychosocial issues: Social withdrawal, relationship issues, body image changes, sexuality issues
   (2) Mental health disorders: Adjustment, delirium, depression, anxiety, post-traumatic stress
   (3) Political and vocational issues: Employment, access to health care, insurance, and educational assistance

5. Risk of late effects for patients with select primary cancers
   a) HL
      (1) The leading causes of death in HL survivors are SMNs and CVD (Matasar et al., 2015; Ng & van Leeuwen, 2016).
         (a) Patients treated with radiation therapy are at greater risk of SMNs and CVD than those treated with chemotherapy alone (Ng, LaCasce, & Travis, 2011). Compared to chemotherapy, radiation therapy for HL was associated with higher risk for both second and third malignancies during the first five years of follow-up (van Eggermond et al., 2014).
         (b) SMNs: HL survivors are at risk for leukemia and solid tumors, particularly lung and breast cancer (Ng & van Leeuwen, 2016).
            i. Solid tumors account for 75%–80% of all SMNs following treatment for HL, and the risk is greatly increased with radiation (Ng, Kenney, et al., 2010).
               • Cumulative risk of SMN following treatment with 40–45 Gy of extended-field or mantle radiation therapy is approximately 30% at 30 years (Hodgson, 2011).
               • Modern radiation therapy for HL uses IFRT, which treats only the lymph node regions that are initially involved. Prescribed radiation doses are 20–30 Gy. This reduces the volume of healthy tissue exposed to radiation and significantly decreases the risk of SMNs (Hodgson, 2011).
            ii. Breast cancer: Risk of breast cancer in HL survivors is significantly increased, particularly for women who were treated with chest irradiation before age 30 (Oeffinger, Baxi, Friedman, & Moskowitz, 2013). The latency period is 8–10 years following treatment (Oeffinger et al., 2013). The risk of breast cancer appears to be decreased in patients who reduce lifetime exposure to endogenous estrogen, such as those who experience ovarian failure or premature menopause (Oeffinger et al., 2013).
            iii. Lung cancer: The risk of lung cancer is associated with radiation therapy, alkylating agents, and smoking (Oeffinger et al., 2013).
         (c) CVD: HL survivors have a three- to fivefold increased risk of CVD, which generally manifests 10 years after therapy and persists more than 25 years after therapy (Ng et al., 2011).
            i. Coronary artery disease is the most common cardiovascular toxicity among HL survivors and accounts for approximately 40%–50% of adverse cardiac events (Hodgson, 2011).
            ii. Valvular disease is less common. It typically has a late onset (more than 10 years after radiation therapy) and is related to higher

doses (greater than 30 Gy) or young age at treatment (Hodgson, 2011).

iii. Acute pericarditis is uncommon but may occur following radiation therapy that includes a large cardiac volume (Hodgson, 2011).

iv. HL survivors treated with mantle radiation therapy at doses of 35–45 Gy are estimated to have a two- to fourfold increased risk of cardiac morbidity. The cumulative risks of significant heart disease among survivors of adult HL are approximately 5%–10% at 15 years, 16% at 20 years, and 34% at 30 years (Hodgson, 2011).

(2) HL survivors have a risk of treatment-related pulmonary toxicity, including radiation pneumonitis and bleomycin toxicity (Ng et al., 2011).

b) Non-Hodgkin lymphoma (NHL)

(1) Relative risk of a secondary cancer in NHL survivors is 1.8 greater than the risk of the general population (Pirani et al., 2011).

(2) Patients are at increased risk for AML, sarcomas, bladder cancer, head and neck cancer, melanoma, lung cancer, gastrointestinal cancer, kidney cancer, HL, and thyroid cancer (Tward et al., 2007).

(a) Chemotherapy increases the risk of AML, lung cancer, and bladder cancer (Tward et al., 2007).

(b) Radiation therapy increases the risk of sarcomas, breast cancer, and mesothelioma (Tward et al., 2007).

(3) Survivors of NHL have an overall significantly decreased risk of breast cancer, prostate cancer, and myeloma (Tward et al., 2007).

c) Breast cancer: Breast cancer survivors are at risk for SMNs, cardiotoxicity from anthracyclines or trastuzumab, chemotherapy-induced premature menopause, osteoporosis, chemotherapy-induced cognitive impairment, sexual dysfunction, and taxane-related neuropathy (Azim, de Azambuja, Colozza, Bines, & Piccart, 2011; Ganz & Hahn, 2008).

(1) SMNs: Breast cancer survivors are at increased risk for sarcoma, melanoma, AML, and cancers of the salivary gland, esophagus, stomach, colon, breast, uterine corpus, ovary, and thyroid (Curtis et al., 2006; VanderWalde & Hurria, 2011). Increased risk for SMNs may also be attributed to age, treatment modality, and reproductive, environmental, or genetic factors (Molina-Montes et al., 2015).

(2) Risk of SMN is greater in breast cancer survivors who carry a genetic predisposition (e.g., *BRCA2*, *TP53*), were treated with radiation therapy (e.g., risk for secondary lung and esophageal cancer), or were treated with hormone therapy (e.g., risk for uterine cancer secondary to tamoxifen) (Azim et al., 2011).

(3) Radiation to the breast increases the risk of lung cancer, esophageal cancer, and sarcoma in all patients, as well as the risk of contralateral breast cancer in patients younger than 40–45 years of age (Ng, Kenney, et al., 2010; Travis et al., 2012).

d) Prostate cancer: Prostate cancer survivors are at increased risk for subsequent melanoma, small intestine, soft tissue, bladder, thyroid, and thymus cancer (Curtis et al., 2006; Ng, Kenney, et al., 2010).

e) Testicular cancer

(1) Testicular cancer survivors are at risk for SMNs, CVD, neurotoxicity, nephrotoxicity, pulmonary toxicity, hypogonadism, decreased fertility, psychosocial disorders, and cognitive impairment (Travis et al., 2010).

(2) SMNs

(a) Among 10-year testicular cancer survivors, there are statistically significant increased risks of malignant melanoma and cancers of the lung (relative risk [RR] = 1.5, 95% confidence interval [CI] [1.2, 1.7]); thyroid, esophagus, pleura, and stomach (RR = 4.0, 95% CI [3.2, 4.8]); and pancreas, colon, rectum, kidney, bladder, and connective tissue (RR = 4.0, 95% CI [2.3, 6.3]) (Travis et al., 2005, 2012).

(b) Chemotherapy increases the risk of radiation-associated SMNs (van den Belt-Dusebout et al., 2007).

(c) The risk of SMN increases with younger age at time of treatment (van den Belt-Dusebout et al., 2007).
(d) The median time to occurrence of SMN is 20 years (van den Belt-Dusebout et al., 2007).
(e) Etoposide and cisplatin chemotherapy increase the risk of treatment-related leukemia in a dose-related fashion (Travis et al., 2010).

(3) Cardiotoxicity: Increased risk of cardiotoxicity, including myocardial infarction, coronary artery disease, hyperlipidemia, and metabolic syndrome (Carver et al., 2007; Ng et al., 2011; Travis et al., 2010)
(4) Neurotoxicity: Increased risk of sensory peripheral neuropathy and cisplatin-induced ototoxicity (Travis et al., 2010)
(5) Nephrotoxicity: Increased risk of cisplatin-induced chronic renal dysfunction (Travis et al., 2010)
(6) Pulmonary toxicity: Increased risk of bleomycin-induced pneumonitis and increased risk of mortality related to respiratory disease (Travis et al., 2010)

f) Cervical cancer (Chaturvedi et al., 2007)
(1) Cervical cancer survivors have an increased risk for HPV-related cancers (i.e., cancers of the pharynx, genital sites, and rectum/anus) and smoking-related cancers (i.e., cancers of the pharynx, trachea, bronchus, lung, pancreas, and urinary bladder).
(2) Patients with cervical cancer treated with radiation were at increased risk for all SMNs at heavily irradiated sites (colon, rectum/anus, urinary bladder, ovary, and genital sites) beyond 40 years of follow-up compared with women in the general population (Curtis et al., 2006; Travis et al., 2012).
(3) The 40-year cumulative risk of any secondary cancer was 22% among women diagnosed with cervical cancer before age 50 and 16% for those diagnosed after age 50 (Chaturvedi et al., 2007).

g) Pediatric malignancies
(1) The cumulative incidence of SMNs in survivors of childhood cancer treated from 1970 to 1986 at 30 years after diagnosis was 20.5% (95% CI [19.1%, 21.8%]) and was higher for patients who had received radiation therapy than for those who had not (approximately 25% vs. 10%) (Friedman et al., 2010).
(2) The most frequent SMNs were nonmelanoma skin cancer and breast cancer, with 30-year cumulative incidences of 9.1% and 5%, respectively (Friedman et al., 2010). SMNs with a 30-year cumulative incidence less than 1% included bone cancer, soft tissue sarcoma, leukemia, lymphoma, central nervous system tumors, head and neck cancer, gastrointestinal cancer, lung cancer, and thyroid cancer (Friedman et al., 2010).
(3) The risk of SMNs among childhood cancer survivors is associated with radiation therapy, chemotherapy, and genetic predisposition (Henderson et al., 2012; Travis et al., 2012).
(4) The median latency period for development of an SMN was 17.8 years (range 5–35.2 years) (Friedman et al., 2010).

h) HSCT recipients: HSCT recipients are at risk for secondary solid tumors, treatment-related leukemia/MDS, and post-transplant lymphoproliferative disorders.
(1) In patients who underwent autologous HSCT for lymphoma, the cumulative incidence of secondary myelodysplasia/acute leukemia was 3.09% at 5 years and 4.52% at 10 years. The cumulative incidence of solid tumors was 2.54% at 5 years and 6.79% at 10 years. The risk of solid tumors was associated with advanced age and radiation therapy (Tarella et al., 2011).
(2) Allogeneic HSCT recipients were twice as likely to develop a solid tumor when compared to the general population. Risk was related to younger age at the time of transplantation (younger than 30 years) and exposure to radiation therapy (Bhatia, 2014).
(3) The risk of a post-transplant malignancy increases with younger age at time of transplant, especially for those younger than 17 years (Serrano et al., 2017).
(4) Relative risk of thyroid carcinoma in HSCT recipients is 3.26 overall, with

a significantly increased risk associated with age younger than 10 years, radiation therapy, female gender, and chronic graft-versus-host disease (Cohen et al., 2007).

6. Preventive screening recommendations and follow-up care (NCCN, 2018)
   a) Survivors should follow adult cancer screening recommendations. This is especially important for childhood cancer survivors who have additional risk for premature development of adult cancers.
   b) Irradiated skin and soft tissues should be thoroughly evaluated and reassessed for the life of the patient.
   c) Women who have been treated with mantle radiation therapy should perform breast self-examination monthly beginning at puberty, and clinical breast examination should be performed annually. Annual mammograms should begin eight years after irradiation (Memorial Sloan Kettering Cancer Center, n.d.; Ng, Constine, et al., 2010).
   d) Healthcare providers should discuss weight management and exercise regimens with all cancer survivors. Physical activity and a healthy diet reduce the risk of cancer recurrence and decrease overall mortality in multiple cancer survivor groups, including breast, colorectal, prostate, and ovarian cancer (Rutledge & Demark-Wahnefried, 2016).
      (1) Eating a diet high in fruits, vegetables, and whole grains and low in red and processed meats appears to protect against cancer progression, risk of recurrence, and overall mortality for a variety of cancers.
      (2) Regular exercise appears to be associated with a lower risk for recurrence and improved survival following treatment for breast, prostate, ovarian, and colorectal cancers.
      (3) Cancer survivors who are overweight or obese may benefit from intentional weight loss following treatment.
      (4) Cancer survivors should obtain the nutrients they need from foods instead of supplements or vitamins because preliminary evidence has shown that supplements may do more harm than good (Rock et al., 2012).
      (5) Cancer survivors should be advised that food consumption away from home, such as fast food and full-service restaurant food consumption, lead to reduced diet quality (i.e., decrease in daily intake of vitamins A and K, increased sodium and total energy intake) (An & Liu, 2013).
   e) Patients should be counseled regarding smoking cessation (Travis, Wahnefried, Allan, Wood, & Ng, 2013).
   f) Bone density studies are indicated for breast cancer survivors aged 65 years or older or aged 60–64 years with risk factors (e.g., family history, prior nontraumatic fracture), postmenopausal patients on an aromatase inhibitor, and patients with chemotherapy-induced early menopause (Ganz & Hahn, 2008). Osteoporosis is also a concern in prostate cancer survivors, multiple myeloma survivors, gastric cancer survivors, and HSCT recipients (Drake, 2013). Adherence to long-term therapy (e.g., breast and prostate cancer) is important to reduce morbidity and mortality associated with osteoporosis and fractures (Warriner & Curtis, 2009). A better understanding of causes for poor adherence and methods to improve adherence (e.g., patient education, provider–patient communication) is critical (see Chapter 4).
7. Patient and family education
   a) Provide information about the treatment and potential late effects related to the patient's disease and treatment received (see Table 26-3).
   b) Explain the risks of SMNs, the typical time to onset, cancer screening recommendations, and the importance of follow-up visits.
   c) Promote healthy lifestyle practices.
      (1) Diet (Denlinger et al., 2014)
         (a) A diet high in fruits, vegetables, and whole grains is associated with a lower risk of death than one that contains a high intake of processed and red meats, refined grains, sugar, and high-fat dairy products.
         (b) Avoid vitamin supplements, and obtain nutrients from food.
      (2) Regular physical activity
      (3) Smoking cessation
      (4) Sun safety practices
8. Professional education
   a) Educate primary care professionals who may be working with survivors after they are no

Table 26-3. Key Resources for Cancer Survivorship Information

Organization and Website	Description
American Cancer Society www.cancer.org/treatment/survivorship-during-and-after-treatment/survivorship-care-plans.html	Information on survivorship care plans, including the following: • What's Next? Life After Cancer Treatment • Journey Forward • American Society of Clinical Oncology (ASCO) Cancer Treatment Summaries • OncoLife Survivorship Care Plan
American Society of Clinical Oncology Survivorship Care Planning Tools www.asco.org/practice-guidelines/cancer-care-initiatives/prevention-survivorship/survivorship-compendium	Treatment plan and summary resources Survivorship care plan templates for the following cancers: • Breast • Colorectal • Non-small cell lung • Small cell lung • Prostate • Diffuse large B-cell lymphoma
Cancer.Net www.cancer.net/survivorship/survivorship-resources	Comprehensive cancer survivorship information including general resources for cancer survivors of all ages and information for young adults, teens, and kids General resources include Internet links to the following: • American Institute for Cancer Research • Cancer and Careers • Cancer*Care* • Cancer Financial Assistance Coalition • Cancer Support Community • Job Accommodation Network • Journey Forward • Livestrong • Livestrong Survivorship Centers of Excellence • MyOncofertility.org • National Cancer Institute: Office of Cancer Survivorship • National Cancer Survivors Day Foundation • National Coalition for Cancer Survivorship • OncoLink: OncoLife Survivorship Care Plan • Patient Advocate Foundation Age-specific resources: • Childhood Cancer • Teens • Young Adults
Centers for Disease Control and Prevention: Cancer Survivorship www.cdc.gov/cancer/survivorship/resources/index.htm	Comprehensive cancer survivorship information for survivors, caregivers, healthcare professionals, and researchers
Memorial Sloan Kettering Cancer Center www.mskcc.org/referring-physicians/survivorship/survivorship-care-plan	Survivorship care plan resources for healthcare professionals
National Comprehensive Cancer Network www.nccn.org/professionals/physician_gls/f_guidelines.asp#survivorship	Clinical practice guidelines on survivorship, including the following: • General survivorship principles • Late effects/long-term psychosocial and physical problems • Preventive health

longer being followed by an oncologist. An SCP that includes potential long-term effects of treatment and recommended follow-up is helpful for primary providers, patients, and caregivers who may be unfamiliar with cancer and its treatments. A discussion of the SCP with primary care providers may be required (Iyer, Mitchell, Zheng, Ross, & Kadan-Lottick, 2017).

b) Stay informed of current recommendations related to screening for SMNs in order to advise cancer survivors (see Table 26-3).

References

Allan, J.M., & Travis, L.B. (2005). Mechanisms of therapy-related carcinogenesis. *Nature Reviews Cancer, 5,* 943–955. https://doi.org/10.1038/nrc1749

American Cancer Society. (2016). *Cancer treatment and survivorship facts and figures 2016–2017.* Atlanta, GA: Author.

American College of Surgeons Commission on Cancer. (2015). *Cancer program standards: Ensuring patient-centered care* (2016 ed.). Chicago, IL: Author.

American Society of Clinical Oncology. (n.d.). Survivorship care planning tools. Retrieved from https://www.asco.org/practice-guidelines/cancer-care-initiatives/prevention-survivorship/survivorship-compendium

An, R., & Liu, J. (2013). Fast-food and full-service restaurant consumption in relation to daily energy and nutrient intakes among US adult cancer survivors, 2003–2012. *Nutrition and Health, 22,* 181–195. https://doi.org/10.1177/0260106015594098

Andersen, B.L., DeRubeis, R.J., Berman, B.S., Gruman, J., Champion, V.L., Massie, M.J., ... Rowland, J.H. (2014). Screening, assessment, and care of anxiety and depressive symptoms in adults with cancer: An American Society of Clinical Oncology guideline adaptation. *Journal of Clinical Oncology, 32,* 1605–1619. https://doi.org/10.1200/JCO.2013.52.4611

André, M., Mounier, N., Leleu, X., Sonet, A., Brice, P., Henry-Amar, M., ... Gisselbrecht, C. (2004). Second cancers and late toxicities after treatment of aggressive non-Hodgkin lymphoma with the ACVBP regimen: A GELA cohort study on 2837 patients. *Blood, 103,* 1222–1228. https://doi.org/10.1182/blood-2003-04-1124

Azim, H.A., Jr., de Azambuja, E., Colozza, M., Bines, J., & Piccart, M.J. (2011). Long-term toxic effects of adjuvant chemotherapy in breast cancer. *Annals of Oncology, 22,* 1939–1947. https://doi.org/10.1093/annonc/mdq683

Bhatia, S. (2014). Caring for the long-term survivor after allogeneic stem cell transplantation. *Hematology: American Society of Hematology Education Program Book, 2014,* 495–503. https://doi.org/10.1182/asheducation-2014.1.495

Blevins Primeau, A.S. (2018). Late-onset toxicity possible with immunotherapy. Retrieved from https://www.cancertherapyadvisor.com/side-effect-management/immunotherapy-melanoma-late-onset-toxicity-risk/article/759006/

Bluethmann, S.M., Mariotto, A.B., & Rowland, J.H. (2016). Anticipating the "silver tsunami": Prevalence trajectories and comorbidity burden among older cancer survivors in the United States. *Cancer Epidemiology, Biomarkers and Prevention, 25,* 1029–1036. https://doi.org/10.1158/1055-9965.EPI-16-0133

Bower, J.E., Bak, K., Berger, A., Breitbart, W., Escalante, C.P., Ganz, P.A., ... Lyman, G.H. (2014). Screening, assessment, and management of fatigue in adult survivors of cancer: An American Society of Clinical Oncology clinical practice guideline adaptation. *Journal of Clinical Oncology, 32,* 1840–1850. https://doi.org/10.1200/JCO.2013.53.4495

Braunstein, S., & Nakamura, J.L. (2013). Radiotherapy-induced malignancies: Review of clinical features, pathobiology, and evolving approaches for mitigating risk. *Frontiers in Oncology, 3,* 73. https://doi.org/10.3389/fonc.2013.00073

Brewer, J.D., Habermann, T.M., & Shanafelt, T.D. (2014). Lymphoma-associated skin cancer: Incidence, natural history, and clinical management. *International Journal of Dermatology, 53,* 267–274. https://doi.org/10.1111/ijd.12208

Carver, J.R., Shapiro, C.L., Ng, A., Jacobs, L., Schwartz, C., Virgo, K.S., ... Vaughn, D.J. (2007). American Society of Clinical Oncology clinical evidence review on the ongoing care of adult cancer survivors: Cardiac and pulmonary late effects. *Journal of Clinical Oncology, 25,* 3991–4008. https://doi.org/10.1200/JCO.2007.10.9777

Chaturvedi, A.K., Engels, E.A., Gilbert, E.S., Chen, B.E., Storm, H., Lynch, C.F., ... Travis, L.B. (2007). Second cancers among 104,760 survivors of cervical cancer: Evaluation of long-term risk. *Journal of the National Cancer Institute, 99,* 1634–1643. https://doi.org/10.1093/jnci/djm201

Chen, M.H., Colan, S.D., Diller, L., & Force, T. (2011). Cardiovascular disease: Cause of morbidity and mortality in adult survivors of childhood cancers. *Circulation Research, 108,* 619–628. https://doi.org/10.1161/CIRCRESAHA.110.224519

Children's Oncology Group. (2013). *Long-term follow-up guidelines for survivors of childhood, adolescent, and young adult cancers* (Version 4.0). Retrieved from http://survivorshipguidelines.org

Churpek, J.E., & Larson, R.A. (2013). The evolving challenge of therapy-related myeloid neoplasms. *Best Practice and Research Clinical Haematology, 26,* 309–317. https://doi.org/10.1016/j.beha.2013.09.001

Cohen, A., Rovelli, A., Merlo, D.F., van Lint, M.T., Lanino, E., Bresters, D., ... Socié, G. (2007). Risk for secondary thyroid carcinoma after hematopoietic stem-cell transplantation: An EBMT Late Effects Working Party study. *Journal of Clinical Oncology, 25,* 2449–2454. https://doi.org/10.3390/ijerph9062075

Cowell, I.G., & Austin, C.A. (2012). Mechanism of generation of therapy related leukemia in response to anti-topoisomerase II agents. *International Journal of Environmental Research and Public Health, 9,* 2075–2091. https://doi.org/10.3390/ijerph9062075

Curtis, R.E., Freedman, D.M., Ron, E., Ries, L.A.G., Hacker, D.G., Edwards, B.K., ... Fraumeni, J.F., Jr. (Eds.). (2006). *New malignancies among cancer survivors: SEER cancer registries, 1973–2000* (NIH Publ. No. 05-5302). Bethesda, MD: National Cancer Institute.

Denlinger, C.S., Ligibel, J.A., Are, M., Baker, K.S., Demark-Wahnefried, W., Dizon, D., ... Ku, G.H. (2014). Survivorship: Healthy lifestyles, version 2.2014. *Journal of the National Comprehensive Cancer Network, 12,* 1222–1237. https://doi.org/10.6004/jnccn.2014.0121

Diaz, D.A., Reis, I.M., Weed, D.T., Elsayyad, N., Samuels, M., & Abramowitz, M.C. (2016). Head and neck second primary cancer rates in the human papillomavirus era: A population-based analysis. *Head and Neck, 38*(Suppl. 1), E873–E883. https://doi.org/10.1002/hed.24119

Donin, N., Filson, C., Drakaki, A., Tan, H.J., Castillo, A., Kwan, L., ... Chamie, K. (2016). Risk of second primary malignancies among cancer survivors in the United States, 1992 through 2008. *Cancer, 122,* 3075–3086. https://doi.org/10.1002/cncr.30164

Drake, M.T. (2013). Osteoporosis and cancer. *Current Osteoporosis Reports, 11,* 163–170. http://doi.org/10.1007/s11914-013-0154-3

Forman, S.J., & Nakamura, R. (2015). Hematopoietic cell transplantation. Retrieved from http://www.cancernetwork.com/cancer-management/hematopoietic-cell-transplantation

Frederiksen, H., Farkas, D.K., Christiansen, C.F., Hasselbalch, H.C., & Sørensen, H.T. (2011). Chronic myeloproliferative neoplasms and subsequent cancer risk: A Danish population-based cohort study. *Blood, 118,* 6515–6520. https://doi.org/10.1182/blood-2011-04-348755

Friedman, D.L., Whitton, J., Leisenring, W., Mertens, A.C., Hammond, S., Stovall, M., ... Neglia, J.P. (2010). Subsequent neoplasms in 5-year survivors of childhood cancer: The Childhood Cancer Survivor Study. *Journal of the National Cancer Institute, 102,* 1083–1095. https://doi.org/10.1093/jnci/djq238

Ganz, P.A., & Hahn, E.E. (2008). Implementing a survivorship care plan for patients with breast cancer. *Journal of Clinical Oncology, 26,* 759–767. https://doi.org/10.1200/JCO.2007.14.2851

Halpern, M.T., Viswanathan, M., Evans, T.S., Birken, S.A., Basch, E., & Mayer, D.K. (2015). Models of cancer survivorship care: Overview and summary of current evidence. *Journal of Oncology Practice, 11,* e19–e27. https://doi.org/10.1200/JOP.2014.001403

Henderson, T.O., Rajaraman, P., Stovall, M., Constine, L.S., Olive, A., Smith, S.A., … Whitton, J. (2012). Risk factors associated with secondary sarcomas in childhood cancer survivors: A report from the Childhood Cancer Survivor Study. *International Journal of Radiation Oncology, Biology, Physics, 84,* 224–230. https://doi.org/10.1016/j.ijrobp.2011.11.022

Henning, R.J., & Harbison, R.D. (2017). Cardio-oncology: Cardiovascular complications of cancer therapy. *Future Cardiology, 13,* 379–396. https://doi.org/10.2217/fca-2016-0081

Hershman, D.L., Lacchetti, C., Dworkin, R.H., Smith, E.M.L., Bleeker, J., Cavaletti, G., … Loprinzi, C.L. (2014). Prevention and management of chemotherapy-induced peripheral neuropathy in survivors of adult cancers: American Society of Clinical Oncology clinical practice guideline. *Journal of Clinical Oncology, 32,* 1941–1967. https://doi.org/10.1200/JCO.2013.54.0914

Hewitt, M., Greenfield, S., & Stovall, E. (Eds.). (2006). *From cancer patient to cancer survivor: Lost in transition.* Retrieved from https://www.nap.edu/catalog/11468/from-cancer-patient-to-cancer-survivor-lost-in-transition

Hodgson, D.C. (2011). Late effects in the era of modern therapy for Hodgkin lymphoma. *Hematology: American Society of Hematology Education Program Book, 2011,* 323–329. https://doi.org/10.1182/asheducation-2011.1.323

Hodgson, D.C., Gilbert, E.S., Dores, G.M., Schonfeld, S.J., Lynch, C.F., Storm, H., … Travis, L.B. (2007). Long-term solid cancer risk among 5-year survivors of Hodgkin's lymphoma. *Journal of Clinical Oncology, 25,* 1489–1497. https://doi.org/10.1200/JCO.2006.09.0936

Huang, K.P., Weinstock, M.A., Clarke, C.A., McMillan, A., Hoppe, R.T., & Kim, Y.H. (2007). Second lymphomas and other malignant neoplasms in patients with mycosis fungoides and Sézary syndrome: Evidence from population-based and clinical cohorts. *Archives of Dermatology, 143,* 45–50. https://doi.org/10.1001/archderm.143.1.45

Inamoto, Y., Shah, N.N., Savani, B.N., Shaw, B.E., Abraham, A.A., Ahmed, I.A., … Bitan, M. (2015). Secondary solid cancer screening following hematopoietic cell transplantation. *Bone Marrow Transplantation, 50,* 1013–1023. https://doi.org/10.1038/bmt.2015.63

International Agency for Research on Cancer. (2012a). Agents classified by the *IARC Monographs,* volumes 1–103: Classification groups. Retrieved from http://monographs.iarc.fr/ENG/Classification/index.php

International Agency for Research on Cancer. (2012b). Agents classified by the *IARC Monographs,* volumes 1–103: Complete list. Retrieved from http://monographs.iarc.fr/ENG/Classification/ClassificationsGroupOrder.pdf

Iyer, N.S., Mitchell, H., Zheng, D.J., Ross, W.L., & Kadan-Lottick, N.S. (2017). Experiences with the survivorship care plan in primary care providers of childhood cancer survivors: A mixed methods approach. *Supportive Care in Cancer, 25,* 1547–1555. https://doi.org/10.1007/s00520-016-3544-0

Kalos, M., Nazimuddin, F., Finkelstein, J., Gupta, M., Kulikovskaya, I., Ambrose, D.E., … June, C.H. (2013). Long-term functional persistence, B cell aplasia, and anti-leukemic efficacy in refractory B cell malignancies following T cell immunotherapy using CAR-redirected T cells targeting CD19. *Blood, 122,* 163.

Koelwyn, G.J., Khouri, M., Mackey, J.R., Douglas, P.S., & Jones, L.W. (2012). Running on empty: Cardiovascular reserve capacity and late effects of therapy in cancer survivorship. *Journal of Clinical Oncology, 30,* 4458–4461. https://doi.org/10.1200/JCO.2012.44.0891

Koh, E.-S., Tran, T.H., Heydarian, M., Sachs, R.K., Tsang, R.W., Brenner, D.J., … Hodgson, D. (2007). A comparison of mantle versus involved-field radiotherapy for Hodgkin's lymphoma: Reduction in normal tissue dose and second cancer risk. *Radiation Oncology, 2,* 13. https://doi.org/10.1186/1748-717X-2-13

Kurt, B.A., Nolan, V.G., Ness, K.K., Neglia, J.P., Tersak, J.M., Hudson, M.M., … Arora, M. (2012). Hospitalization rates among survivors of childhood cancer in the Childhood Cancer Survivor Study cohort. *Pediatric Blood and Cancer, 59,* 126–132. https://doi.org/10.1002/pbc.24017

Lenihan, D.J., & Cardinale, D.M. (2012). Late cardiac effects of cancer treatment. *Journal of Clinical Oncology, 30,* 3657–3664. https://doi.org/10.1200/JCO.2012.45.2938

Leone, G., Fianchi, L., & Voso, M.T. (2011). Therapy-related myeloid neoplasms. *Current Opinion in Oncology, 23,* 672–680. https://doi.org/10.1097/CCO.0b013e32834bcc2a

Marchese, V.G., Morris, G.S., Gilchrist, L., Ness, K.K., Wampler, M., VanHoose, L., & Galantino, M.L. (2011). Screening for chemotherapy adverse late effects. *Topics in Geriatric Rehabilitation, 27,* 234–243. https://doi.org/10.1097/TGR.0b013e318219912a

Matasar, M.J., Ford, J.S., Riedel, E.R., Salz, T., Oeffinger, K.C., & Straus, D.J. (2015). Late morbidity and mortality in patients with Hodgkin's lymphoma treated during adulthood. *Journal of the National Cancer Institute, 107,* djv018. https://doi.org/10.1093/jnci/djv018

Mayer, D.K., Nekhlyudov, L., Snyder, C.F., Merrill, J.K., Wollins, D.S., & Shulman, L.N. (2014). American Society of Clinical Oncology clinical expert statement on cancer survivorship care planning. *Journal of Oncology Practice, 10,* 345–351. https://doi.org/10.1200/JOP.2014.001321

McFarland, D.C., & Holland, J.C. (2016). The management of psychological issues in oncology. *Clinical Advances in Hematology and Oncology, 14,* 999–1009. Retrieved from http://www.hematologyandoncology.net/archives/december-2016/the-management-of-psychological-issues-in-oncology

McGowan, J.V., Chung, R., Maulik, A., Piotrowska, I., Walker, J.M., & Yellon, D.M. (2017). Anthracycline chemotherapy and cardiotoxicity. *Cardiovascular Drugs and Therapy, 31,* 63–75. https://doi.org/10.1007/s10557-016-6711-0

Memorial Sloan Kettering Cancer Center. (n.d.). Survivorship resources: Survivorship care plan. Retrieved from https://www.mskcc.org/referring-physicians/survivorship/survivorship-care-plan

Miller, K.D., Siegel, R.L., Lin, C.C., Mariotto, A.B., Kramer, J.L., Rowland, J.H., … Jemal, A. (2016). Cancer treatment and survivorship statistics, 2016. *CA: A Cancer Journal for Clinicians, 66,* 271–289. https://doi.org/10.3322/caac.21349

Molina-Montes, E., Requena, M., Sánchez-Cantalejo, E., Fernández, M.F., Arroyo-Morales, M., Espín, J., … Sánchez, M. (2015). Risk of second cancers cancer after a first primary breast cancer: A systematic review and meta-analysis. *Gynecologic Oncology, 136,* 158–171. https://doi.org/10.1016/j.ygyno.2014.10.029

Morton, L.M., Curtis, R.E., Linet, M.S., Bluhm, E.C., Tucker, M.A., Caporaso, N., … Fraumeni, J.F., Jr. (2010). Second malignancy risks after non-Hodgkin lymphoma and chronic lymphocytic leukemia: Differences by lymphoma subtype. *Journal of Clinical Oncology, 28,* 4935–4944. https://doi.org/10.1200/JCO.2010.29.1112

Morton, L.M., Dores, G.M., Curtis, R.E., Lynch, C.F., Stovall, M., Hall, P., … Leeuwen, F.E. (2013). Stomach cancer risk after treatment for Hodgkin lymphoma. *Journal of Clinical Oncology, 31,* 3369–3377. https://doi.org/10.1200/JCO.2013.50.6832

Mullan, F. (1985). Seasons of survival: Reflections of a physician with cancer. *New England Journal of Medicine, 313,* 270–273. https://doi.org/10.1056/NEJM198507253130421

Mustian, K.M., Sprod, L.K., Janelsins, M., Peppone, L.J., Palesh, O.G., & Chandwani, K. (2013). Multicenter, randomized controlled trial of yoga for sleep quality among cancer survivors. *Journal of Clinical Oncology, 31,* 3233–3240. https://doi.org/10.1200/JCO.2012.43.7707

National Comprehensive Cancer Network. (2018). *NCCN Clinical Practice Guidelines in Oncology (NCCN Guidelines®): Survivorship* [v.3.2017]. Retrieved from https://www.nccn.org/professionals/physician_gls/pdf/survivorship.pdf

Ng, A.K. (2014). Current survivorship recommendations for patients with Hodgkin lymphoma: Focus on late effects. *Blood, 124,* 3373–3379. https://doi.org/10.1182/blood-2014-05-579193

Ng, A.K., Constine, L.S., Advani, R., Das, P., Flowers, C., Friedberg, J., … Yunes, M.J. (2010). ACR Appropriateness Criteria®: Follow-up of Hodgkin's lymphoma. Current Problems in Cancer, 34, 211–227. https://doi.org/10.1016/j.currproblcancer.2010.04.007

Ng, A.K., Kenney, L.B., Gilbert, E.S., & Travis, L.B. (2010). Secondary malignancies across the age spectrum. *Seminars in Radiation Oncology, 20,* 67–78. https://doi.org/10.1016/j.semradonc.2009.09.002

Ng, A.K., LaCasce, A., & Travis, L.B. (2011). Long-term complications of lymphoma and its treatment. *Journal of Clinical Oncology, 29,* 1885–1892. https://doi.org/10.1200/JCO.2010.32.8427

Ng, A.K., & Travis, L.B. (2008). Subsequent malignant neoplasms in cancer survivors. *Cancer Journal, 14,* 429–434. https://doi.org/10.1097/PPO.0b013e31818d8779

Ng, A.K., & van Leeuwen, F.E. (2016). Hodgkin lymphoma: Late effects of treatment and guidelines for surveillance. *Seminars in Hematology, 53,* 209–215. https://doi.org/10.1053/j.seminhematol.2016.05.008

Noone, A.M., Howlader, N., Krapcho, M., Miller, D., Brest, A., Yu, M., … Cronin, K.A. (Eds.). (2018, April). *SEER cancer statistics review, 1975–2015.* Retrieved from https://seer.cancer.gov/csr/1975_2015

Oeffinger, K.C., Baxi, S.S., Friedman, D.N., & Moskowitz, C.S. (2013). Solid tumor second primary neoplasms: Who is at risk, what can we do? *Seminars in Oncology, 40,* 676–689. https://doi.org/10.1053/j.seminoncol.2013.09.012

Oeffinger, K.C., Mertens, A.C., Sklar, C.A., Kawashima, T., Hudson, M.M., Meadows, A.T., … Robison, L.L. (2006). Chronic health conditions in adult survivors of childhood cancer. *New England Journal of Medicine, 355,* 1572–1582. https://doi.org/10.1056/NEJMsa060185

Ojha, R.P., & Thertulien, R. (2012). Second malignancies among Waldenstrom macroglobulinemia patients: Small samples and sparse data. *Annals of Oncology, 23,* 542–543. https://doi.org/10.1093/annonc/mdr537

Okwuosa, T.M., Anzevino, S., & Rao, R. (2017). Cardiovascular disease in cancer survivors. *Postgraduate Medicine Journal, 93,* 82–90. https://doi.org/10.1136/postgradmedj-2016-134417

Phillips, S.M., Padgett, L.S., Leisenring, W.M., Stratton, K.K., Bishop, K., Krull, K.R., … Mariotto, A.B. (2015). Survivors of childhood cancer in the United States: Prevalence and burden of morbidity. *Cancer Epidemiology, Biomarkers and Prevention, 24,* 653–663. https://doi.org/10.1158/1055-9965.EPI-14-1418

Phipps, A.I., Bhatti, P., Neuhouser, M.L., Chen, C., Crane, T.E., Kroenke, C.H., … Watson, N.F. (2016). Pre-diagnostic sleep duration and sleep quality in relation to subsequent cancer survival. *Journal of Clinical Sleep Medicine, 12,* 495–503. https://doi.org/10.5664/jcsm.5674

Pirani, M., Marcheselli, R., Marcheselli, L., Bari, A., Federico, M., & Sacchi, S. (2011). Risk for second malignancies in non-Hodgkin's lymphoma survivors: A meta-analysis. *Annals of Oncology, 22,* 1845–1858. https://doi.org/10.1093/annonc/mdq697

Rebora, P., Czene, K., Antolini, L., Passerini, C.G., Reilly, M., & Valsecchi, M.G. (2010). Are chronic myeloid leukemia patients more at risk for second malignancies? A population-based study. *American Journal of Epidemiology, 172,* 1028–1033. https://doi.org/10.1093/aje/kwq262

Rechis, R., Beckjord, E.B., Arvey, S.R., Reynolds, K.A., & McGoldrick, D. (2011). *The essential elements of survivorship care: A Livestrong brief.* Retrieved from https://www.livestrong.org/sites/default/files/what-we-do/reports/EssentialElementsBrief.pdf

Reulen, R.C., Frobisher, C., Winter, D.L., Kelly, J., Lancashire, E.R., Stiller, C.A., … Hawkins, M.M. (2011). Long-term risks of subsequent primary neoplasms among survivors of childhood cancer. *JAMA, 305,* 2311–2319. https://doi.org/10.1001/jama.2011.747

Rock, C.L., Doyle, C., Demark-Wahnefried, W., Meyerhardt, J.H., Courneya, K.S., Schwartz, A.L., … Gansler, T. (2012). Nutrition and physical activity guidelines for cancer survivors. *CA: A Cancer Journal for Clinicians, 62,* 242–274. https://doi.org/10.3322/caac.21142

Rutledge, L., & Demark-Wahnefried, W. (2016). Weight management and exercise for the cancer survivor. *Clinical Journal of Oncology Nursing, 20,* 129–132. https://doi.org/10.1188/16.CJON.129-132

Salz, T., & Baxi, S. (2016). Moving survivorship care plans forward: Focus on care coordination. *Cancer Medicine, 5,* 1717–1722. https://doi.org/10.1002/cam4.733

Serrano, O.K., Bangdiwala, A.S., Vock, D.M., Chinnakotla, S., Dunn, T.B., Finger, E.B., … Chavers, B.M. (2017). Post-transplant malignancy after pediatric kidney transplantation: Retrospective analysis of incidence and risk factors in 884 patients receiving transplants between 1963 and 2015 at the University of Minnesota. *Journal of the American College of Surgeons, 225,* 181–193. https://doi.org/10.1016/j.jamcollsurg.2017.04.012

Shaitelman, S.F., Cromwell, K.D., Rasmussen, J.C., Stout, N.L., Armer, J.M., Lasinski, B.B., & Cormier, J.N. (2015). Recent progress in the treatment and prevention of cancer-related lymphedema. *CA: A Cancer Journal for Clinicians, 65,* 55–81. https://doi.org/10.3322/caac.21253

Siegel, R.L., Miller, K.D., & Jemal, A. (2018). Cancer statistics, 2018. *CA: A Cancer Journal for Clinicians, 68,* 7–30. https://doi.org/10.3322/caac.21442

Slusser, K.M. (2018). Late effects of cancer treatment. In C.H. Yarbro, D. Wujcik, & B.H. Gobel (Eds.), *Cancer nursing: Principles and practice* (8th ed., pp. 2029–2044). Burlington, MA: Jones & Bartlett Learning.

Tarella, C., Passera, R., Magni, M., Benedetti, F., Rossi, A., Gueli, A., … Rambaldi, A. (2011). Risk factors for the development of secondary malignancy after high-dose chemotherapy and autograft, with or without rituximab: A 20-year retrospective follow-up study in patients with lymphoma. *Journal of Clinical Oncology, 29,* 814–824. https://doi.org/10.1200/JCO.2010.28.9777

Travis, L.B., Beard, C., Allan, J.M., Dahl, A.A., Feldman, D.R., Oldenburg, J., … Fossa, S.D. (2010). Testicular cancer survivorship: Research strategies and recommendations. *Journal of the National Cancer Institute, 102,* 1114–1130. https://doi.org/10.1093/jnci/djq216

Travis, L.B., Hill, D., Dores, G.M., Gospodarowicz, M., van Leeuwen, F.E., Holowaty, E., … Gail, M.H. (2005). Cumulative absolute breast cancer risk for young women treated for Hodgkin lymphoma. *Journal of the National Cancer Institute, 97,* 1428–1437. https://doi.org/10.1093/jnci/dji290

Travis, L.B., Ng, A.K., Allan, J.M., Pui, C.-H., Kennedy, A.R., Xu, X.G., … Constine, L.S. (2012). Second malignant neoplasms and cardiovascular disease following radiotherapy. *Journal of the National Cancer Institute, 104,* 357–370. https://doi.org/10.1093/jnci/djr533

Travis, L.B., Ng, A.K., Allan, J.M., Pui, C.-H., Kennedy, A.R., Xu, X.G., … Constine, L.S. (2014). Second malignant neoplasms and cardiovascular disease following radiotherapy. *Health Physics, 106,* 229–246. https://doi.org/10.1097/HP.0000000000000013

Travis, L.B., Wahnefried, W.D., Allan, J.M., Wood, M.E., & Ng, A.K. (2013). Aetiology, genetics and prevention of secondary neoplasms in adult cancer survivors. *Nature Reviews Clinical Oncology, 10,* 289–301. https://doi.org/10.1038/nrclinonc.2013.41

Treanor, C., & Donnelly, M. (2014). The late effects of cancer and cancer treatment: A rapid review. *Journal of Community and Supportive Oncology, 12,* 137–148. https://doi.org/10.12788/jcso.0035

Turcotte, L.M., Liu, Q., Yasui, Y., Arnold, M.A., Hammond, S., Howell, R.M., … Neglia, J.P. (2017). Temporal trends in treatment and subsequent neoplasm risk among 5-year survivors of childhood cancer, 1970-2015. *JAMA, 317,* 814–824. https://doi.org/10.1001/jama.2017.0693

Tward, J., Glenn, M., Pulsipher, M., Barnette, P., & Gaffney, D. (2007). Incidence, risk factors, and pathogenesis of second malignancies in patients with non-Hodgkin lymphoma. *Leukemia and Lymphoma, 48,* 1482–1495. https://doi.org/10.1080/10428190701447346

Valdivieso, M., Kujawa, A.M., Jones, T., & Baker, L.H. (2012). Cancer survivors in the United States: A review of the literature and a call to action. *International Journal of Medical Sciences, 9,* 163–173. https://doi.org/10.7150/ijms.3827

van den Belt-Dusebout, A.W., de Wit, R., Gietema, J.A., Horenblas, S., Louwman, M.W.J., Ribot, J.G., … van Leeuwen, F.E. (2007). Treatment-specific risks of second malignancies and cardiovascular disease in 5-year survivors of testicular cancer. *Journal of Clinical Oncology, 25,* 4370–4378. https://doi.org/10.1200/JCO.2006.10.5296

VanderWalde, A.M., & Hurria, A. (2011). Second malignancies among elderly survivors of cancer. *Oncologist, 16,* 1572–1581. https://doi.org/10.1634/theoncologist.2011-0214

van Eggermond, A.M., Schaapveld, M., Lugtenburg, P.J., Krol, A.D., de Boer, J.P., Zijlstra, J.M., … van Leeuwen, F.E. (2014). Risk of multiple primary malignancies following treatment of Hodgkin lymphoma. *Blood, 124,* 319–327. https://doi.org/10.1182/blood-2013-10-532184

van Leeuwen, F.E., Klokman, W.J., van't Veer, M.B., Hagenbeek, A., Krol, A.D.G., Vetter, U.A.O., … Aleman, B.M.P. (2000). Long-term risk of second malignancy in survivors of Hodgkin's disease treated during adolescence or young adulthood. *Journal of Clinical Oncology, 18,* 487–497. https://doi.org/10.1200/JCO.2000.18.3.487

van Leeuwen, F.E., & Travis, L.B. (2001). Second cancers. In V.T. DeVita Jr., S. Hellman, & S.A. Rosenberg (Eds.), *Cancer: Principles and practice of oncology* (6th ed., vol. 2, pp. 2939–2964). Philadelphia, PA: Lippincott Williams & Wilkins.

Verma, D., Kantarjian, H., Strom, S.S., Rios, M.B., Jabbour, E., Quintas-Cardama, A., … Cortes, J. (2011). Malignancies occurring during therapy with tyrosine kinase inhibitors (TKIs) for chronic myeloid leukemia (CML) and other hematologic malignancies. *Blood, 118,* 4353–4358. https://doi.org/10.1182/blood-2011-06-362889

Visentin, A., Imbergamo, S., Gurrieri, C., Frezzato, F., Trimarco, V., Martini, V., … Piazza, F. (2017). Major infections, secondary cancers and autoimmune diseases occur in different clinical subsets of chronic lymphocytic leukaemia patients. *European Journal of Cancer, 72,* 103–111. https://doi.org/10.1016/j.ejca.2016.11.020

Warriner, A.H., & Curtis, J.R. (2009). Adherence to osteoporosis treatments: Room for improvement. *Current Opinion in Rheumatology, 21,* 356–362. https://doi.org/10.1097/BOR.0b013e32832c6aa4

Wood, M.E., Vogel, V., Ng, A., Foxhall, L., Goodwin, P., & Travis, L.B. (2012). Second malignant neoplasms: Assessment and strategies for risk reduction. *Journal of Clinical Oncology, 30,* 3734–3745. https://doi.org/10.1200/JCO.2012.41.8681

Young, J., Cund, A., Renshaw, M., Quigley, A., & Snowden, A. (2015). Improving the care of cancer patients: Holistic needs assessment. *British Journal of Nursing, 24*(Suppl. 4), S17–S20. https://doi.org/10.12968/bjon.2015.24.Sup4.S17

Zeng, C., Wen, W., Morgans, A.K., Pao, W., Shu, X.-O., & Zheng, W. (2015). Disparities by race, age, and sex in the improvement of survival for major cancers: Results from the National Cancer Institute Surveillance, Epidemiology, and End Results (SEER) Program in the United States, 1990 to 2010. *JAMA Oncology, 1,* 88–96. https://doi.org/10.1001/jamaoncol.2014.161

Appendices

Appendix A. Clinical Practicum Evaluation: Part I

Antineoplastic Therapy Administration Competency

Employee Name ______________________________

The RN evaluator who verifies competence in antineoplastic therapy administration must observe practice and validate that the nurse meets all of the following criteria.

RN Evaluators	Date	Drugs Administered

PRIOR TO ADMINISTRATION	Initials		
Reviews treatment plan with the RN evaluator, verifying regimen, protocol, treatment cycle, and day of cycle			
Coordinates time of administration with pharmacy and others as needed			
Verifies documentation of consent for treatment (if applicable)			
Verifies that criteria to treat (e.g., laboratory data) are within acceptable parameters and reports results to provider as needed			
Performs independent double check of original orders with a second RN for accuracy of the following • Date of treatment • Agents • Dose calculation methodology (e.g., body surface area, area under the curve, mg/kg) • Drug dose • Schedule/sequence • Route			
Verifies patient understanding of treatment goals, administration procedures, potential side effects, and when and how to contact the healthcare team			
Verifies that premedication, prehydration, and other preparations are completed and documented			
Verifies drug appearance and expiration date and/or time			
ADMINISTRATION			
Applies personal protective equipment, closed-system drug-transfer device (when the dosage form allows), and uses safe handling precautions			
Compares original order to dispensed drug label at the bedside or chairside with a second RN			
Verifies two patient identifiers (cannot use a room or chair number)			
Verifies the presence of venous access appropriate to the treatment plan (location, type)			
Assesses patency of venous access device and ensures blood return is present			
Demonstrates safe administration: • For IV push or IV minibag of vesicant medications: Administers through side arm hub closest to patient, through a free-flowing IV; checks patency every 2–5 ml (every 2–3 ml for pediatric patients). • For infusions: Verifies appropriate rate of administration and infusion pump settings with a second RN. Verifies blood return/patency per institutional policy			
Demonstrates appropriate monitoring/observation for specific acute drug effects			
Verbalizes appropriate action in the event of infiltration or extravasation			
Verbalizes appropriate action in the event of hypersensitivity reaction			
Verbalizes appropriate action in the event of a hazardous drug spill			
AFTER ADMINISTRATION			
Flushes line with compatible fluid to clear IV tubing of drug			
Removes peripheral IV device or flushes/maintains venous access device as appropriate to patient needs			
Disposes of hazardous drug waste according to policy			
Documents medications, dose verification, and patient response			
Communicates post-treatment considerations to the patient, caregivers, and appropriate personnel			

Appendix B. Clinical Practicum Evaluation: Part II			
Note the appropriate column to indicate that the nurse has satisfactorily performed the listed activities. Under Comments, provide examples of how the nurse met each objective or performed each activity. Include plans for remediation as applicable.			
Objective/Activity	**Date/Initials**		
Participates in interprofessional care planning with physicians, nurses, and other healthcare professionals (e.g., homecare or dietary workers), providing interventions specific to individual patient needs Comments:			
Provides individualized patient and family education and verifies understanding of the treatment, short- and long-term side effects, symptom management, and monitoring to occur with treatment Comments:			
Documents pretreatment system review, including assessment of symptoms and response to previous therapy Comments:			
Describes anticipated complications and side effects of antineoplastic therapy on body systems • Hematologic and lymphatic • Immunologic • Gastrointestinal and nutritional • Cardiovascular • Pulmonary • Genitourinary and renal • Reproductive and sexual • Dermatologic • Endocrine • Neurologic and musculoskeletal • Head, ears, eyes, nose, and throat • Psychosocial Comments:			
Identifies evidence-based interventions for complications and side effects of therapy Comments:			
Documents patient response and care according to institutional policy and procedures Comments:			
Identifies and takes nursing action to prevent or manage potential or actual infusion reactions Comments:			
Uses appropriate safe handling precautions in the preparation, handling, and disposal of hazardous drugs Comments:			
Demonstrates knowledge and skill in the assessment, management, and follow-up care of infiltrations and extravasations Comments:			
Assesses patients for the most appropriate type of venous access device (peripheral or central) based on type and duration of intended therapy Comments:			
Demonstrates safe and appropriate use of equipment (e.g., IV pumps) used in antineoplastic therapy administration. Comments:			
Supports clinical research, as applicable to setting, by ensuring patient understanding of clinical trials, administering research drugs, documenting patient response to treatment, and contacting the research team as indicated Comments:			

Appendix C. Sample Chemotherapy Order Template

Breast Cancer
AC (DOXOrubicin/Cyclophosphamide) Every 21 Days followed by DOCEtaxel Every 21 Days + Trastuzumab
AC (DOXOrubicin/Cyclophosphamide) Every 21 Days Course

INDICATION:	**REFERENCES:**	**NCCN SUPPORTIVE CARE:**
HER2 positive: Neoadjuvant or Adjuvant	1. NCCN Guidelines® for Breast Cancer V.1.2017. 2. Slamon D, et al. *N Engl J Med.* 2011;365(14):1273-83. 3. Joensuu H, et al. *N Engl J Med.* 2006;354(8):809-20.	1. *Emetic risk:* Day 1 High 2. *Febrile Neutropenia Risk:* Intermediate

CHEMOTHERAPY REGIMEN
21-day cycle for 4 cycles
- **DOXOrubicin** 60 mg/m^2 IV push on Day 1
  - See *Safety Parameters and Special Instructions* for information on slow IV Push administration.
- **Cyclophosphamide** 600 mg/m^2 IV over 30 minutes on Day 1
  - Oral hydration is strongly encouraged with cyclophosphamide; poorly hydrated patients may need supplemental IV hydration. Patients should attain combined oral and IV hydration of 2000 – 3000 mL/day on day of chemotherapy. See *Other Supportive Therapy* for example of IV hydration.

This course is 4 cycles of AC (DOXOrubicin and cyclophosphamide) Every 21 Days. DOCEtaxel Every 21 Days and Trastuzumab course is initiated following completion of this course. Please see Order Template BRS27b for DOCEtaxel Every 21 Days and Trastuzumab course.

SUPPORTIVE CARE

Antiemetic Therapy

Scheduled prophylactic antiemetic therapy should be given for prevention of acute and delayed nausea and vomiting based on the emetic risk of the chemotherapy regimen. This may include antiemetic therapy given on the days following chemotherapy. For more information on emetic prophylaxis, refer to the NCCN Guidelines for Antiemesis and Appendix D to the NCCN Chemotherapy Order Templates.

PRN for breakthrough: All patients should be provided with at least one medication for breakthrough emesis. Please consult the NCCN Guidelines for Antiemesis for appropriate antiemetic therapy.

Myeloid Growth Factor Therapy
- CSFs may be considered for primary prophylaxis based on the febrile neutropenia (FN) risk of the chemotherapy regimen. For more information on prophylaxis of FN, refer to NCCN Guidelines for Myeloid Growth Factors and Appendix C to the NCCN Templates.

Other Supportive Therapy
- For cyclophosphamide: *Example of recommended hydration*: Sodium chloride 0.9% infused IV at a rate of 1.5 – 3 mL/kg/hour for a total of 500 mL on day of chemotherapy.

MONITORING AND HOLD PARAMETERS
- CBC with differential should be monitored as clinically indicated for potential dose modification.
- For DOXOrubicin:
  - Ejection fraction should be monitored prior to initiation of treatment and as clinically indicated.
  - This agent is an anthracycline. Cumulative anthracycline dosage should be monitored.
  - Liver function should be monitored as clinically indicated for potential dose modification or discontinuation.
- For cyclophosphamide: Renal function should be monitored as clinically indicated for potential dose modification or discontinuation.

SAFETY PARAMETERS AND SPECIAL INSTRUCTIONS
- For DOXOrubicin:
  - **This agent is a vesicant.**
  - This agent is administered IV push. The preferred IV push method for a vesicant is administration through the side port of a freely flowing IV; alternatively, the drug can be administered via direct IV push.
  - Secondary malignancies have been associated with this drug. Review drug package insert for additional information.
  - Central venous access is recommended for administration of this agent.
- For cyclophosphamide: Secondary malignancies have been associated with this drug. Review drug package insert for additional information.

Appendix D. Antineoplastic Treatment Safety Checklist	
√	**Criteria**
	Patient, parent and/or caregiver have received written and verbal education.
	Patient reports understanding of treatment plan and elects to proceed.
	Confirm presence of informed consent documentation (as applicable to practice setting).
Pretreatment Assessment	
	Obtain vital signs.
	Ensure measured height and weight are current and documented in metric units.
	Review allergies.
	Review response to previous treatments, including reactions and treatment toxicities.
	Update medication list and reconcile as needed.
	Perform and record physical assessment and pain assessment.
	Perform psychosocial assessment; initiate referral resources if necessary.
	Review laboratory values relevant to treatment.
	Prepare for potential complications, including infusion reaction, infiltration, and extravasation.
Treatment plan is noted in medical record.	
	Document the diagnosis, indication for treatment, antineoplastic agents to be used, doses (with calculation methodology), schedule, and dose modification and rationale for modification (if applicable).
Antineoplastic orders include the following elements:	
	Orders signed and activated per institutional policy
	Doses consistent with standard regimens or research protocols approved by the practice or institution. Rationale for exception orders is documented.
	Patient name and second identifier
	Cycle number and day of cycle or arm, phase per research protocol
	Date order was written and date of drug administration
	All medications identified by generic name, following abbreviation standards
	Cumulative dose calculated for drugs that have an upper lifetime dose limit
	Multiday continuous infusions include total daily dose and total multiday hours of infusion.
	Supportive care treatments are ordered (e.g., hydration, antiemetics, growth factors).
	Sequence of drug administration

(Continued on next page)

Appendix D. Antineoplastic Treatment Safety Checklist *(Continued)*	
Two people approved by the healthcare setting to prepare or administer chemotherapy independently perform each of the following three safety checks:	
	1. Before preparation
	Verify two patient identifiers, drug name, dose, route, rate, calculations for dosing, treatment cycle, and day of cycle.
	2. Upon preparation of parenteral antineoplastic therapy
	Verify drug vial, drug concentration, drug volume or weight, diluent type and volume, drug stability, need for refrigeration, administration fluid, volume and tubing, and filter if needed.
	3. Before administration, verify:
	Drug name
	Drug dose
	Volume
	Route of administration
	Sequence of drug administration
	Expiration date and/or time
	Appearance and physical integrity of drug
	Rate of administration
	Patient identification using two patient identifiers in the presence of the patient
	Rate of infusion (infusion pump settings)

Note. Based on information from Neuss, M.N., Gilmore, T.R., Belderson, K.M., Billett, A.L., Conti-Kalchik, T., Harvey, B.E., ... Polovich, M. (2016). 2016 updated American Society of Clinical Oncology/Oncology Nursing Society chemotherapy administration safety standards, including standards for pediatric oncology. *Journal of Oncology Practice, 12,* 1262–1271. https://doi.org/10.1200/JOP.2016.017905.

Appendix E. Consent for Antineoplastic Drug Treatment

Patient Name: ____ **Date:** __________

Diagnosis: ____

Treatment Medications: ____

Possible side effects may include any of the following or a combination of the following:

- Allergic and allergic-like reactions
- Anemia
- Fatigue
- Constipation
- Diarrhea
- Loss of appetite
- Mouth sores
- Nausea or vomiting
- Weight gain or loss
- Liver damage
- Hair loss
- Skin and nail darkening
- Skin ulceration at injection site
- Skin rash
- Light and temperature sensitivity
- Numbness or tingling
- Hearing loss
- Heart damage
- Lung damage
- Kidney damage
- Thyroid changes
- Low platelet count causing bleeding
- Low white blood cell count
- Risk of infection
- Menopausal symptoms
- Menstrual irregularities
- Sterility
- Dizziness
- Forgetfulness
- Cognitive impairments
- Secondary cancer
- Muscle aching or weakness

Unexpected side effects may occur in addition to those noted above. Cancer treatments can cause long-term toxicities. In rare instances, cancer treatment can cause life-threatening complications and death.

Many anticancer drugs can be harmful to an unborn child. I understand that it is important to tell the doctor if I think I may be pregnant. It is important for both men and women who are being treated with these drugs and who are sexually active and fertile and who have a fertile partner to use a reliable form of birth control (birth control pills, a reliable barrier method, or a hormonal implant as recommended by a physician). I have discussed possible ways of preserving my fertility with my doctor, if applicable.

_________ (Patient Initials) A healthcare professional has provided and reviewed with me written information on the drugs I will receive. I HAVE HAD THE CHANCE TO ASK ANY QUESTIONS ABOUT THE DRUGS I WILL RECEIVE AND AM SATISFIED WITH THE INFORMATION PROVIDED.

My healthcare team has explained my treatment plan in detail. My doctor has discussed with me other methods of treating this disease and the risks and benefits of treatment. There is no guarantee that this treatment will give me the same results that other patients have received. If I change my mind and decide to stop treatment at any time, my doctor will continue to provide for my care in the future.

I have read the above information. I understand the possible risks and benefits of the recommended treatment plan. I agree to accept the treatment and authorize Dr. ______________________ and his/her healthcare team to carry out the treatment plan.

Patient Signature: ____ **Date:** ______________________

I have explained the expected response, side effects, and possibility of risks of the listed drugs to the above named patient.

Physician Signature: ____ **Date:** ________________

Appendix F. Distress Thermometer

NCCN DISTRESS THERMOMETER

Instructions: Please circle the number (0–10) that best describes how much distress you have been experiencing in the past week including today.

Extreme distress

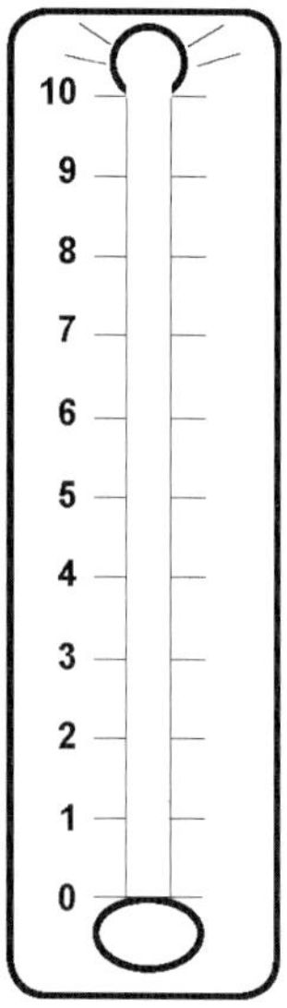

No distress

PROBLEM LIST
Please indicate if any of the following has been a problem for you in the past week including today.
Be sure to check YES or NO for each.

YES	NO	Practical Problems
❑	❑	Child care
❑	❑	Housing
❑	❑	Insurance/financial
❑	❑	Transportation
❑	❑	Work/school
❑	❑	Treatment decisions

YES	NO	Family Problems
❑	❑	Dealing with children
❑	❑	Dealing with partner
❑	❑	Ability to have children
❑	❑	Family health issues

YES	NO	Emotional Problems
❑	❑	Depression
❑	❑	Fears
❑	❑	Nervousness
❑	❑	Sadness
❑	❑	Worry
❑	❑	Loss of interest in usual activities

YES	NO	
❑	❑	Spiritual/religious concerns

YES	NO	Physical Problems
❑	❑	Appearance
❑	❑	Bathing/dressing
❑	❑	Breathing
❑	❑	Changes in urination
❑	❑	Constipation
❑	❑	Diarrhea
❑	❑	Eating
❑	❑	Fatigue
❑	❑	Feeling swollen
❑	❑	Fevers
❑	❑	Getting around
❑	❑	Indigestion
❑	❑	Memory/concentration
❑	❑	Mouth sores
❑	❑	Nausea
❑	❑	Nose dry/congested
❑	❑	Pain
❑	❑	Sexual
❑	❑	Skin dry/itchy
❑	❑	Sleep
❑	❑	Substance abuse
❑	❑	Tingling in hands/feet

Other Problems: ______________________________

____

Note. From *NCCN Distress Thermometer and Problem List for Patients* [v.2.2016], by National Comprehensive Cancer Network. Retrieved from https://www.nccn.org/patients/resources/life_with_cancer/pdf/nccn_distress_thermometer.pdf.

Appendix G. Hazardous Drug Administration Safe Handling Checklist			
Name: ______________ Date of Review and Exam: ______________			
PRIOR TO ADMINISTRATION	**Yes**	**No**	**Initials**
1. Gather equipment required for drug administration.			
2. Select appropriate gloves for hazardous drug administration.			
3. Select appropriate gown for hazardous drug administration.			
4. Identify situations when mask and face protection are required.			
5. Locate hazardous drug spill kit.			
6. Obtain hazardous waste container.			
7. Receive drug(s) from pharmacy in sealed bag.			
ADMINISTRATION			
1. Wash hands and don personal protective equipment before opening drug delivery bag.			
2. Visually inspect the contents of the delivery bag for leaks.			
3. Gather IV administration supplies including closed-system drug-transfer devices.			
4. For IV infusions • Ensure tubing is primed with a nondrug solution. • Utilize plastic backed absorbent pad under work area. Remove cap from IV tubing and connect to patient's IV device. • Utilize closed-system drug-transfer device when compatible. • Tighten locking connections. • When complete, don personal protective equipment and discontinue IV bag with tubing intact (do not unspike bag). • Utilize gauze pads when disconnecting from patient's IV device when a closed-system drug-transfer device cannot be used.			
5. For IV push medications • Utilize closed-system drug-transfer device when possible. • Tighten locking connection. • When complete, do not recap needle. • Discard syringe-needle unit in puncture-proof container.			
6. For intramuscular/subcutaneous injections • Utilize closed-system drug-transfer device when possible. • Attach needle to syringe. • Tighten locking connection. • When complete, do not recap needle. • Discard syringe-needle unit in puncture-proof container.			
7. For oral drugs (tablets/capsules) • If using bar code technology, scan medication prior to removing medication from packaging. • Don gloves. • Open unit-dose package and place into medicine cup (avoid touching drug or inside of package). • Avoid touching tablets/capsules.			
8. For oral drugs in liquid form • Obtain drug in final form in appropriate oral syringe. • Don double gloves, gown, and mask with face protection. • Use plastic-backed absorbent pad during administration. • Discard syringe in hazardous waste container after administration.			
POSTADMINISTRATION			
1. Don personal protective equipment.			
2. Seal hazardous drug–contaminated supplies in sealable plastic bag for transport to hazardous waste container.			

(Continued on next page)

Appendix G. Hazardous Drug Administration Safe Handling Checklist *(Continued)*			
POSTADMINISTRATION *(cont.)*	**Yes**	**No**	**Initials**
3. Place sealed plastic bag in hazardous waste container.			
4. Remove outer gloves.			
5. Close lid on waste container.			
6. Decontaminate equipment in the area appropriately.			
7. Remove and discard inner gloves.			
8. Wash hands thoroughly with soap and water.			

Note. From *Safe Handling of Hazardous Drugs* (3rd ed., pp. 96–97), by M. Polovich and M.M. Olsen (Eds.), 2018, Pittsburgh, PA: Oncology Nursing Society.

Appendix H. Extravasation

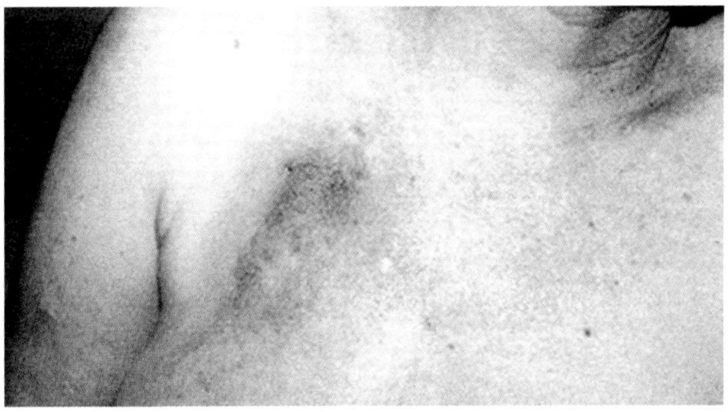

Photo 1. Erythema of site of port extravasation of doxorubicin (February 14)

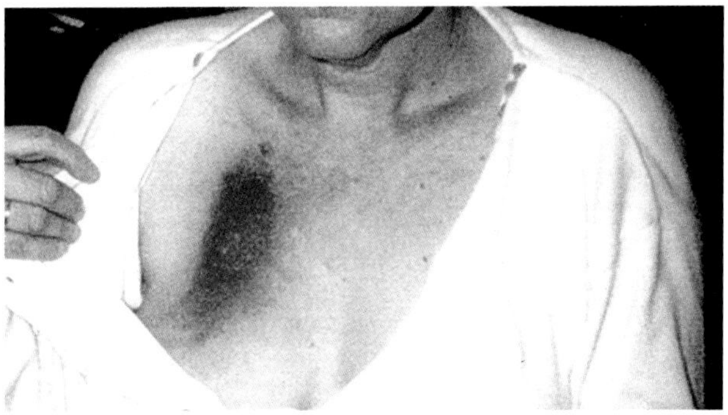

Photo 2. Beginning of skin necrosis (February 28)

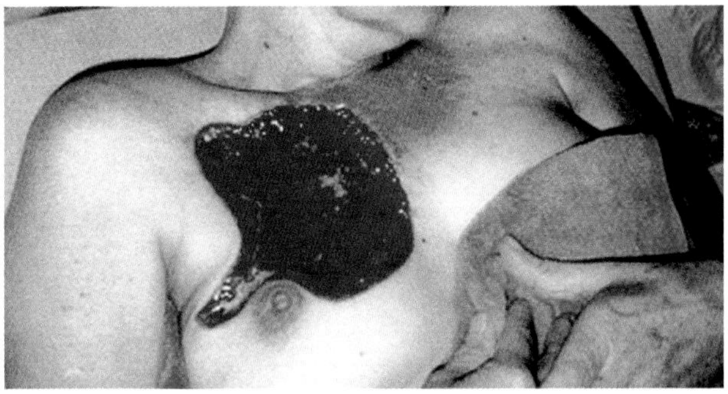

Photo 3. Area of extravasation following debridement (March 18)

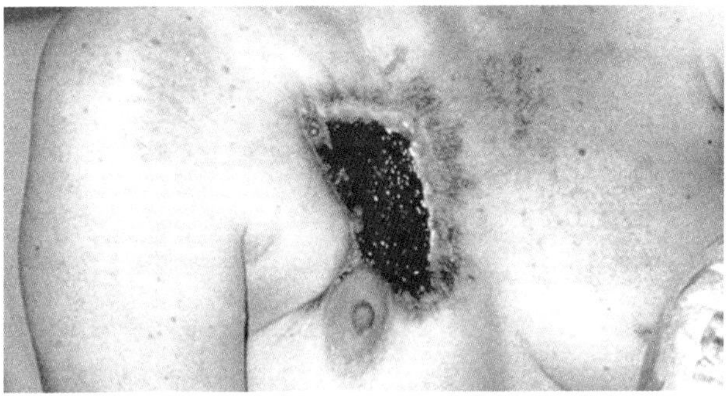

Photo 4. Granulation of outer areas of debrided area (June 5)

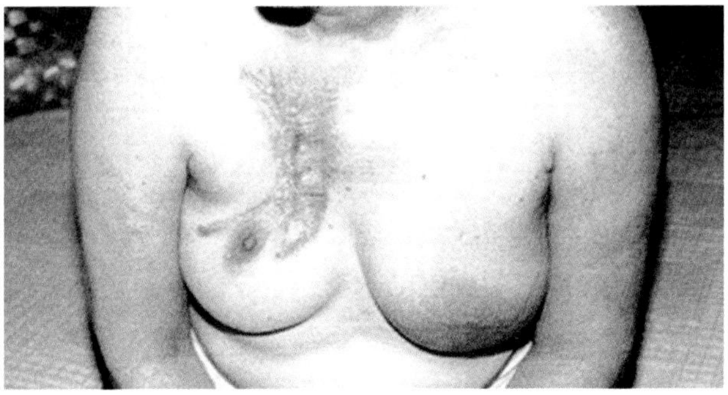

Photo 5. Ten months following extravasation, healing of area and formation of scars (December 10)

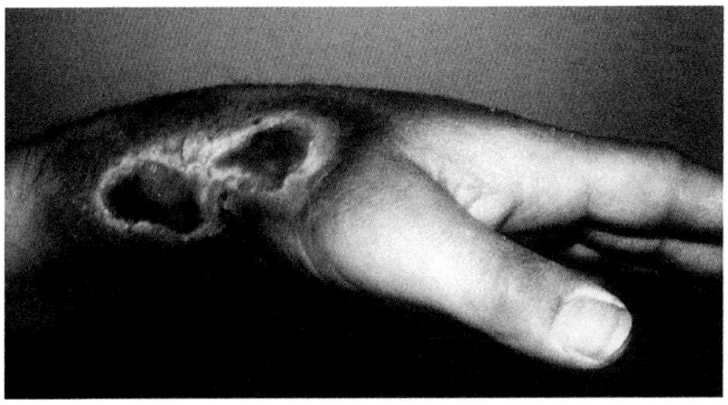

Photo 6. Severe tissue necrosis secondary to vesicant extravasation

Note. Photos 1–5 from "Chemotherapy Extravasation From Implanted Ports," by L. Schulmeister and D. Camp-Sorrell, 2000, *Oncology Nursing Forum, 27,* p. 534. Copyright 2000 by Oncology Nursing Society. Reprinted with permission. Photo 6 courtesy of Rita Wickham, RN, PhD, AOCN®. Used with permission.

Appendix I. Vesicant Drug Extravasation Record

Patient: ______________________ Date of infiltration: __________ Time: ______________

Today's date: ______________

Drug: ______________________ Dilution (mg/ml): ______________

Estimated amount infiltrated: ______________________

Vascular Access	Infusion Method	Pretreatment Assessment
☐ Peripheral IV Location: __________ ☐ Peripherally inserted central catheter ☐ Implanted port Needle size and length: _______ ☐ Tunneled catheter ☐ Other	☐ IV push via side-arm of free-flowing IV ☐ Direct IV push ☐ Minibag infusion ☐ Continuous infusion Infusion pump used? ☐ Yes ☐ No	Location: __________ Type and size of needle/catheter: __________ Description and quality of blood return: __________ Comments: __________ **Consider timed and dated photograph of site to add to medical record.**

Description:
Include topical cooling/heating applied, treatments, antidotes used, measurements of site, edema, and/or redness.
Assess extremity for range of motion and discomfort with movement.

Situation: ______________________

Background: ______________________

Assessment (include photos): ______________________

Recommendations: ______________________

Authorized prescriber notified: ______________________

Patient/Caregiver instructions: ______________________

Comments: ______________________

Consultations:

☐ Plastic surgery Date: ______________

☐ Physical therapy Date: ______________

☐ Other: ______________________

Follow-up:

Include return appointments, patient instructions on skin assessment, temperature monitoring, and reporting of pain.

____

Notes: ______________________

Signature: ______________________ Date: ______________

Index

The letter f *after a page number indicates that relevant information appears in a figure; the letter* t, *in a table.*

B

C

D

E

F

G

H

J

K

L

O

P

T

U

V

W

X

Z

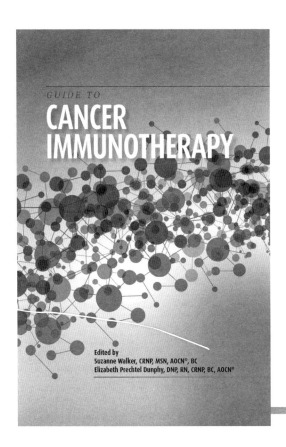

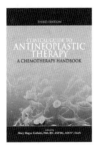